CLINICAL
NUTRITION
Volume **2**

Parenteral Nutrition

JOHN L. ROMBEAU, M.D.

Assistant Professor of Surgery,
University of Pennsylvania School of Medicine
Director, Nutritional Support Service and
   Surgical Metabolic Unit
Veterans Administration Medical Center
Philadelphia, Pennsylvania

MICHAEL D. CALDWELL, M.D., Ph.D.

Associate Professor, Section of Surgery
Brown University
Director, Nutritional Support Service and
   Surgical Metabolism Laboratory
Rhode Island Hospital
Providence, Rhode Island

Illustrations by David Low, M.D.

1986
W.B. SAUNDERS COMPANY

Philadelphia • London • Toronto • Mexico City
Rio de Janeiro • Sydney • Tokyo • Hong Kong

W. B. Saunders Company: West Washington Square
                          Philadelphia, PA   19105

Library of Congress Cataloging in Publication Data

Main entry under title:

Parenteral nutrition.

(Clinical nutrition; v. 2)

1. Parenteral feeding.   I. Rombeau, John L.   II. Caldwell,
   Michael D.   III. Series: Clinical nutrition (Philadelphia,
   Pa.); v. 2. [DNLM: 1. Nutrition.   2. Parenteral Feeding.
   WB 410 P295]
[RM216.C5775 1984 vol. 2]   615.8'54s   85–2501
[RM224]   [615.8'55]

ISBN 0–7216–7645–6

Editor: John Dyson
Designer: Terri Siegel
Production Manager: Bill Preston
Illustration Coordinator: Peg Shaw
Indexer: Betty Gittens

PARENTERAL NUTRITION
Volume 2 of Clinical Nutrition   ISBN   0–7216–7645–6

Last digit is the print number: 9   8   7   6   5   4   3   2   1

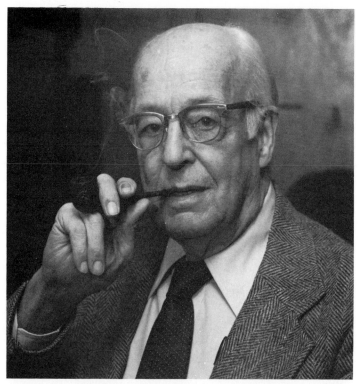

Harry M. Vars, Ph.D., 1903–1983

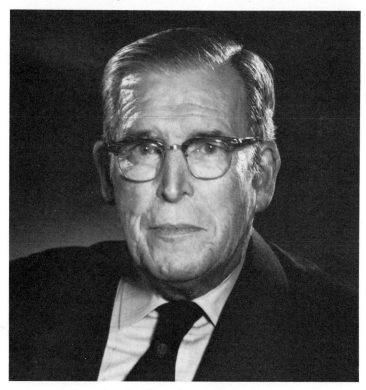

Jonathan E. Rhoads, M.D., D.Sc., 1907–

This text is dedicated to Harry M. Vars, Ph.D., and Jonathan E. Rhoads, M.D., D.Sc., who transformed parenteral nutrition from a clinical dream into the amelioration of human suffering.

Contributors

NAJI N. ABUMRAD, M.D.
Paul W. Sanger Professor of Surgery and Medicine, Vanderbilt University, Nashville, Tennessee; Attending Surgeon, Vanderbilt University Medical Center and Director, S. R. Light Surgical Research Laboratory, Nashville, Tennessee
Hormone-Substrate Interrelationships: The Cellular Reactions

RONALD M. ABEL, M.D.
Associate Professor of Surgery, University of Medicine and Dentistry of New Jersey, Newark, New Jersey; Attending Surgeon and Director, Nutritional Support Service, Newark Beth Israel Medical Center, Newark, New Jersey
Nutritional Support and the Cardiac Patient

BRUCE A. ADYE, M.D.
Associate Surgeon, The Mason Clinic, Seattle, Washington; Staff Surgeon, Virginia Mason Hospital, Seattle, Washington
Enteric Fistulas

JORGE E. ALBINA, M.D.
Assistant Professor of Surgery, Brown University, Providence, Rhode Island; Director, Nutritional Support Service, Miriam Hospital and Assistant Director, Nutritional Support Service, Rhode Island Hospital, Providence, Rhode Island
Fluids, Electrolytes, and Body Composition; Perioperative TPN

MARVIN E. AMENT, M.D.
Professor of Pediatrics, UCLA School of Medicine, Los Angeles, California; Chief, Pediatric Gastroenterology and Chief, Hospital Parenteral and Enteral Nutrition Support, UCLA Medical Center, Los Angeles, California
Home Parenteral Nutrition in Infants and Children

SAMUEL D. ANG, M.D.
Memorial Sloan-Kettering Cancer Center Fellow, New York, New York
Potential Complications and Monitoring of Patients Receiving Total Parenteral Nutrition

THOMAS T. AOKI, M.D.
Professor of Medicine, University of California School of Medicine, Davis, California; Chief, Endocrinology Division, University of California Medical Center, Davis, California
The Metabolic Response to Fasting

KEITH N. APELGREN, M.D.
Assistant Professor, West Virginia University School of Medicine, Morgantown, West Virginia; Attending Surgeon, West Virginia University Hospital, Morgantown, West Virginia
Animal Models in Parenteral Nutrition

PALMER Q. BESSEY, M.D.
Assistant Professor of Surgery, School of Medicine, University of Alabama at Birmingham, Birmingham, Alabama; Chief, Section of Trauma and Burns and Director of UAB Trauma Center, University of Alabama Hospitals, Birmingham, Alabama
Animal Models in Parenteral Nutrition; Parenteral Nutrition and Trauma

BRUCE R. BISTRIAN, M.D., Ph.D.
Associate Professor of Medicine, Harvard Medical School, Boston, Massachusetts; Attending Physician, New England Deaconess Hospital, Boston, Massachusetts
Theoretic and Practical Issues in the Treatment of Obesity

ROBERT H. BOWER, M.D., F.A.C.S.
Associate Professor of Surgery, University of Cincinnati College of Medicine, Cincinnati, Ohio; Director, Nutritional Support, University of Cincinnati Medical Center, Cincinnati, Ohio; Active Staff, University of Cincinnati Medical Center, University Hospital and Holmes Division, Cincinnati, Ohio; Attending Staff, Cincinnati Veterans Administration Medical Center and Children's Hospital Medical Center, Cincinnati, Ohio
Hepatic Indications for Parenteral Nutrition

MURRAY F. BRENNAN, M.D.
Professor of Surgery, Cornell Medical College, New York, New York; Attending Surgeon, New York Hos-

pital-Cornell Medical Center, New York, New York; Chief, Gastric and Mixed Tumor Service, Memorial Sloan-Kettering Cancer Center, New York, New York
Intravenous Feeding of the Cancer Patient

MICHAEL D. CALDWELL M.D., Ph.D.
Associate Professor of Surgery, Brown University, Providence, Rhode Island; Director, Nutritional Support Service and Surgical Metabolism Laboratory, Department of Surgery, Rhode Island Hospital, Providence, Rhode Island
Hormone-Substrate Interrelationships: The Cellular Reactions; Developmental Considerations in Neonatal TPN

CHRISTINE KENNEDY-CALDWELL, R.N.C., M.S.M.
Pediatric Clinical Nurse Specialist, Maternal-Child Health Faculty, School of Nursing, Salve Regina College, Newport, Rhode Island
Developmental Considerations in Neonatal TPN

EMMA L. CATALDI-BETCHER, R.D., M.S.
University of Medicine and Dentistry of New Jersey, Rutgers Medical School, Newark, New Jersey
Parenteral Nutrition Equipment

RONNI CHERNOFF, Ph.D.
Associate Director, Geriatric Research, Education and Clinical Center, John L. McClellan Memorial Veterans Hospital, Little Rock, Arkansas
Total Parenteral Nutrition: Considerations in the Elderly

TERRY P. CLEMMER, M.D.
Associate Professor of Medicine, University of Utah College of Medicine, Salt Lake City, Utah; Director of Critical Care Medicine and Nutritional Support Services, LDS Hospital, Salt Lake City, Utah
Computer Applications in Clinical Nutrition

JOHN M. DALY, M.D.
Associate Professor of Surgery, Cornell University Medical School, New York, New York; Associate Attending Surgeon, Memorial Sloan-Kettering Cancer Center, New York, New York
Potential Complications and Monitoring of Patients Receiving Total Parenteral Nutrition

DANIEL DEMPSEY, M.D.
Instructor in Surgery, University of Pennsylvania School of Medicine, Philadelphia, Pennsylvania; Chief Resident in Surgery, Hospital of the University of Pennsylvania, Philadelphia, Pennsylvania
Parenteral Vitamin Therapy in Hospital Patients

STANLEY J. DUDRICK, M.D., F.A.C.S.
Clinical Professor of Surgery, The University of Texas Medical School at Houston, Houston, Texas; Director,

Nutritional Support Services, St. Luke's Episcopal Hospital, Texas Children's Hospital, Houston, Texas
History of Intravenous Nutrition

EBEN I. FEINSTEIN, M.D.
Associate Professor of Clinical Medicine, University of Southern California Medical School, Los Angeles, California; Attending Physician, Los Angeles County/University of Southern California Medical Center, Los Angeles, California
Nutrition in Acute Renal Failure

IRENE D. FEURER, M.S.Ed.
Coordinator, Metabolic Testing Services, Nutrition Support Service, Hospital of the University of Pennsylvania, Philadelphia, Pennsylvania
Measurement of Energy Expenditure

RICHARD FINLEY, M.D.
Associate Professor of Surgery, University of Western Ontario, London, Ontario, Canada; Chief of Surgery, Victoria Hospital, London, Ontario, Canada
The Metabolic Response to Fasting

JOSEF E. FISCHER, M.D., F.A.C.S.
Christian R. Holmes Professor of Surgery, University of Cincinnati College of Medicine, Cincinnati, Ohio; Professor and Chairman, Department of Surgery, University of Cincinnati Medical Center and Holmes Hospital Divisions, Cincinnati, Ohio
Hepatic Indications for Parenteral Nutrition

LORETTA FORLAW, R.N., M.S.N.
Lieutenant Colonel A.N.C. (Army Nursing Core) and Clinical Nurse Specialist, Nutrition Support Service, Walter Reed Army Medical Center, Washington D.C.
Central Venous Catheter Care

JAMESON FORSTER, M.D.
Assistant Instructor in Surgery, Brown University Rhode Island Hospital, Providence, Rhode Island; Fellow in Surgical Metabolism, Rhode Island Hospital, Providence, Rhode Island
The Use of Total Parenteral Nutrition in the Treatment of Anorexia Nervosa

HERBERT R. FREUND, M.D.
Professor of Surgery, Hebrew University-Hadassah Medical School, Jerusalem, Israel; Chief Physician, Department of Surgery, and Director, Nutritional Support Unit, Hadassah University Medical Center, Jerusalem, Israel
Parenteral Nutrition in the Septic Patient

ROBERT FRIED, M.D.
Assistant Instructor in Surgery, American Cancer Society Fellow, Clinical Nutrition Fellow, Department of Sur

gery, Hospital of the University of Pennsylvania, Philadelphia, Pennsylvania
Malnutrition and Inflammatory Bowel Disease: Indications for and Complications of Parenteral Nutritional Support

MARK S. GLASSMAN, M.D.

Assistant Professor of Pediatrics, Cornell University Medical College, New York, New York; Assistant Attending Physician, New York Hospital-Cornell Medical Center, New York, New York
Parenteral Nutrition in the Neonate

DAVID J. GOLDBERGER, B.S, R.Ph.

Pharmacist, Home Health Care of America, Irvine, California

Parenteral Nutrition Equipment

CLEON W. GOODWIN, M.D, M.P.H.

Associate Professor of Surgery, Cornell University Medical College, New York, New York; Associate Attending Surgeon and Director, Burn Center, New York Hospital, New York, New York
Parenteral Nutrition in Thermal Injuries

JOHN P. GRANT, M.D.

Associate Professor of Surgery, Duke University Medical Center, Durham, North Carolina; Durham VA Medical Center, Durham, North Carolina
Catheter Access

A. DALE GULLEDGE, M.D.

Head Liaison, Psychiatry, Department of Psychiatry, Cleveland Clinic Foundation, Cleveland, Ohio
Home Parenteral Nutrition

ELIE HAMAOUI, M.D.

Assistant Professor of Clinical Medicine, State University of New York, Downstate Medical Center, Brooklyn, New York; Chief, Nutrition Section and Nutrition Support Team, Veterans Administration Medical Center, Brooklyn, New York
The Nutrition Support Team

MICHELENA I. HELBLEY, R.Ph., B.S.

Pharmacology Lecturer, Rupert J. Turnbull School of Enterostomal Therapy, Cleveland Clinic Foundation, Cleveland, Ohio; Staff Pharmacist, Cleveland Clinic Foundation, Cleveland, Ohio
Home Parenteral Nutrition

ROBERT E. HODGES, M.D.

Professor, Department of Family Medicine and Department of Internal Medicine, University of California, Irvine, California
Parenteral Vitamin Therapy in Hospital Patients

L. JOHN HOFFER, M.D.

Assistant Professor, Faculty of Medicine, McGill University, Montreal, Quebec, Canada; Attending Physician, Royal Victoria Hospital, Montreal, Quebec, Canada
Theoretic and Practical Issues in the Treatment of Obesity

DANNY O. JACOBS, M.D.

Fellow in Nutrition and Metabolism, Harrison Department of Surgical Research, Department of Surgery, University of Pennsylvania, Philadelphia, Pennsylvania
Malnutrition and Inflammatory Bowel Disease: Indications for and Complications of Parenteral Nutritional Support

K. N. JEEJEEBHOY, M.B., B.S., Ph.D, F.R.C.P. (Edin., C, Lond.)

Professor and Director of the Division of Gastroenterology, Department of Medicine, University of Toronto, Toronto, Ontario, Canada; Director, Division of Gastroenterology, Toronto General Hospital, Toronto, Ontario, Canada
Malabsorption and the Short-Gut Syndrome

KENNETH W. JONES, M.D.

Attending in Surgery, St. Vincent's Medical Center, Methodist Hospital, and University Hospital of Jacksonville, Jacksonville, Florida
Parenteral Nutrition Equipment

MARK J. KORUDA, M.D.

Assistant Instructor in Surgery, University of Pennsylvania School of Medicine, Philadelphia, Pennsylvania; Nutrition and Metabolic Research Fellow, Veterans Administration Medical Center and University of Pennsylvania School of Medicine, Philadelphia, Pennsylvania
Perioperative Total Parenteral Nutrition

KEITH G. LARSEN, R.Ph.

Adjunct Instructor, University of Utah College of Pharmacy, Salt Lake City, Utah; Director, Clinical Computer Services, LDS Hospital, Salt Lake City, Utah
Computer Applications in Clinical Nutrition

DAVID A. LIPSCHITZ, M.D., Ph.D.

Professor of Medicine, University of Arkansas for Medical Sciences, Little Rock, Arkansas; Director, Geriatric Research, Education and Clinical Center and Chief, Hematology/Oncology, Division of Medicine, Veterans Administration Medical Center and University of Arkansas for Medical Sciences, Little Rock, Arkansas
Total Parenteral Nutrition: Considerations in the Elderly

NANCY LOUIE, M.S., R.Ph.

Assistant Professor of Pharmacy Practice, College of Pharmacy, University of Arizona, Tucson, Arizona; Clinical Pharmacy Coordinator, Tucson Medical Center, Tucson, Arizona
Parenteral Nutrition Solutions

STEPHEN F. LOWRY, M.D.

Assistant Professor of Surgery, Cornell Medical College, New York, New York; Assistant Attending Surgeon and Director, Hyperalimentation Unit, New York Hospital-Cornell Medical Center, New York, New York; Assistant Attending Surgeon, Gastric and Mixed Tumor Service, Memorial Sloan-Kettering Cancer Center, New York, New York
Intravenous Feeding of the Cancer Patient

MAUREEN MacBURNEY, R.D., M.S.

Assistant Director, Nutrition Support Service, Brigham and Women's Hospital, Boston, Massachusetts
Parenteral Nutrition in Pregnancy

CATHLEEN C. MAREIN, R.N., B.S.N.

Nutrition Support Nurse, Department of General Surgery, Cleveland Clinic Foundation, Cleveland, Ohio
Home Parenteral Nutrition

GEORGE MELNIK

Nutritional Support Pharmacist, Pharmacy Service, Veterans Administration Medical Center, Philadelphia, Pennsylvania
Fluids, Electrolytes, and Body Composition

PATRICE M. MISNY, R.N., B.S.N.

Nutrition Support Nurse, Department of General Surgery, Cleveland, Ohio
Home Parenteral Nutrition

JAMES L. MULLEN, M.D.

Associate Professor of Surgery and Director, Nutrition Support Service Hospital of the University of Pennsylvania, Philadelphia, Pennsylvania
Measurement of Energy Expenditure

DENISE M. NEY, M.S., R.D.

Ph.D. Candidate, Nutrition Department, University of California, Davis, California
Lipid Metabolism in Parenteral Nutrition

PAUL W. NIEMIEC, B.S., Ph.D.

Clinical Pharmacy Coordinator, Surgery-Critical Care Division, Johns Hopkins Hospital, Baltimore, Maryland
Parenteral Nutrition Solutions

JAMES F. ORME, Jr., M.D.

Clinical Associate Professor of Medicine, University of Utah College of Medicine, Salt Lake City, Utah; Co-Director, Shock/Trauma ICU and Director, Medical/Surgical ICU, LDS Hospital, Salt Lake City, Utah
Computer Applications in Clinical Nutrition

JOHN PALOMBO, M.D.

Research Associate and Laboratory Supervisor, New England Deaconess Hospital, Boston, Massachusetts
Theoretic and Practical Issues in the Treatment of Obesity

STEVEN C. PATCHING, M.D.

Chief Resident, Department of Surgery, University of California, Davis, California
Cost Effectiveness of Nutritional Support

GILBERTO R. PEREIRA, M.D.

Associate Professor of Pediatrics, University of Pennsylvania School of Medicine, Philadelphia, Pennsylvania; Neonatologist, Children's Hospital of Philadelphia, Philadelphia, Pennsylvania
Parenteral Nutrition in the Neonate

JONATHAN E. RHOADS, M.D.

Professor of Surgery, University of Pennsylvania, Philadelphia, Pennsylvania; Staff Surgeon, Hospital of the University of Pennsylvania and Consultant, Pennsylvania Hospital, Germantown Hospital, and Children's Hospital of Philadelphia, Philadelphia, Pennsylvania
History of Intravenous Nutrition

ROLANDO ROLANDELLI, M.D.

Research Associate, Harrison Department of Surgical Research, University of Pennsylvania School of Medicine, Philadelphia, Pennsylvania
Malnutrition and Inflammatory Bowel Disease: Indications for and Complications of Parenteral Nutritional Support

JOHN L. ROMBEAU, M.D.

Assistant Professor of Surgery, University of Pennsylvania School of Medicine, Philadelphia, Pennsylvania; Hospital of the University of Pennsylvania and Director, Nutrition Support Service, Veterans Administration Medical Center, Philadelphia, Pennsylvania
The Nutrition Support Team; Perioperative Total Parenteral Nutrition; Malnutrition and Inflammatory Bowel Disease: Indications for and Complications of Parenteral Nutritional Support

BRIAN J. ROWLANDS, M.D., F.R.C.S., F.A.C.S.

Associate Professor of Surgery, University of Texas Health Science Center at Houston, Houston, Texas; Attending Surgeon and Director of Nutritional Support Services, Hermann Hospital/The University Hospital, Houston, Texas
Intravenous Nutrition for Acute and Chronic Pancreatitis

JOHN A. RYAN, JR., M.D.

Surgeon and Head, Section of General, Vascular, and Thoracic Surgery, The Mason Clinic, Seattle, Washington; Chairman, Therapeutic Nutrition Committee, Virginia Mason Hospital, Seattle, Washington
Enteric Fistulas

MARTIN H. SAVITZ, M.D., F.A.C.S., F.I.C.S.

Assistant Clinical Professor of Neurosurgery, Mount Sinai School of Medicine, New York, New York; Associate Attending Neurosurgeon, Mount Sinai Hospital, New York, New York, and Chief of Neurosurgery, Nyack and Good Samaritan Hospitals, Rockland County, New York
The Neurologic or Neurosurgical Patient

MURRAY H. SELTZER, M.D.

Chairman, Nutrition Support Committee, Department of Surgery, University of Medicine and Dentistry, Newark, New Jersey; Attending Surgeon, St. Barnabas Medical Center, Livingston, New Jersey
Parenteral Nutrition Equipment

JOHN SHARP, A.C.S.W.

Social Worker, Cleveland Clinic Hospital, Cleveland, Ohio
Home Parenteral Nutrition

HARRY M. SHIZGAL, M.D.

Professor of Surgery, McGill University, Montreal, Quebec, Canada; Senior Surgeon, Royal Victoria Hospital, Montreal, Quebec, Canada
Energy and Nitrogen Interactions

JOHN H. SIEGEL, M.D.

Professor of Surgery, University of Maryland School of Medicine, Baltimore, Maryland, and Professor of Surgery, Johns Hopkins University School of Medicine, Baltimore, Maryland; Director, Clinical Center, Maryland Institute for Emergency Medical Services Systems, University of Maryland Medical System, Baltimore, Maryland
Physiologic and Nutritional Implications of Abnormal Hormone-Substrate Relations and Altered Protein Metabolism in Human Sepsis

BERNADETTE A. SLOCUM, R.N., M.A.

Nutrition Support Service Nurse, St. Barnabas Medical Center Livingston, New Jersey
Parenteral Nutrition Equipment

NOEL W. SOLOMONS, M.D.

Affiliated Investigator, Division of Nutrition and Health, Institute of Nutrition of Central America and Panama, Guatemala City, Guatemala
Trace Minerals

FAITH SRP, R.N.

Nutrition Support Nurse, Department of General Surgery, Cleveland Clinic Foundation, Cleveland, Ohio
Home Parenteral Nutrition

EZRA STEIGER, M.D.

Head, Section of Surgical Nutrition, Department of General Surgery, Cleveland Clinic Foundation, Cleveland, Ohio; Staff Surgeon, Cleveland Clinic Foundation, Cleveland, Ohio
Home Parenteral Nutrition

T. P. STEIN, Ph.D.

Professor of Surgery (Research), University of Medicine and Dentistry of New Jersey, Newark, New Jersey; School of Osteopathic Medicine and Adjunct Professor of Surgery, University of Pennsylvania, Philadelphia, Pennsylvania
Protein Metabolism and Parenteral Nutrition

ROBERT M. SUSKIND, M.D.

Professor of Pediatrics, Louisiana State University School of Medicine, New Orleans, Louisiana; Charity Hospital of New Orleans, Childrens Hospital, New Orleans, Louisiana
Parenteral Nutrition in the Pediatric Patient

RIYAD Y. TARAZI, M.D.

Resident, Department of Thoracic and Cardiovascular Surgery, Cleveland Clinic Foundation, Cleveland, Ohio
Home Parenteral Nutrition

MICHAEL H. TOROSIAN, M.D.

Clinical Instructor of Surgery, Department of Surgery, University of Pennsylvania, Philadelphia, Pennsylvania
Central Venous Catheter Care

PATRICK L. TWOMEY, M.D.

Associate Professor of Surgery, University of California, Davis, California; Chief, Gastrointestinal Surgery, Martinez VA Medical Center, Martinez, California
Cost Effectiveness of Nutritional Support

J. VAN EYS, M.D. Ph.D.

Professor of Pediatrics, The University of Texas System Cancer Center and The University of Texas School of Medicine at Houston, Houston, Texas; Chairman, Department of Pediatrics, Chairman, Department of Experimental Pediatrics, and Head, Division of Pediatrics, The University of Texas System Cancer Center, M. D. Anderson Hospital and Tumor Institute, Houston, Texas
Nonglucose Carbohydrates in Parenteral Nutrition

RAJ N. VARMA, Ph.D.

Assistant Professor of Nutrition, Youngstown State University, Youngstown, Ohio
Parenteral Nutrition in the Pediatric Patient

HARRY M. VARS, Ph.D.

Late Professor Emeritus, Harrison Department of Surgical Research, Department of Surgery, School of Medicine, University of Pennsylvania, Philadelphia, Pennsylvania
History of Intravenous Nutrition

ALEX J. WEINSTEIN, M.D.
Resident in Surgery, Virginia Mason Hospital, Seattle, Washington
Enteric Fistulas

DOUGLAS W. WILMORE, M.D.
Professor of Surgery, Harvard Medical School, Boston, Massachusetts; Senior Staff Surgeon, Brigham and Women's Hospital, Boston, Massachusetts
Animal Models in Parenteral Nutrition; Parenteral Nutrition in Pregnancy

BRUCE M. WOLFE, M.D.
Associate Professor of Surgery, University of California, Davis, California
Lipid Metabolism in Parenteral Nutrition

ROBERT WOLFE, Ph.D.
Associate Professor of Surgery, Anesthesia, and Biochemistry, University of Texas Medical Branch, Galveston, Texas; Chief of Metabolism, Shriners Burns Institute, Galveston, Texas
Carbohydrate Metabolism and Requirements

BYRON YOUNG, M.D.
Professor and Chairman, Division of Neurosurgery, Department of Surgery, Albert B. Chandler Medical Center, University of Kentucky, Lexington, Kentucky
The Neurologic or Neurosurgical Patient

Foreword

Dr. Michael D. Caldwell and Dr. John L. Rombeau edited a very useful volume on Enteral Nutrition and Tube Feeding that was published in 1984. They have followed this, as expected, with this volume on Parenteral Nutrition.

While nearly 100 per cent of the human race take their nourishment orally, and even in hospital populations, over 95 per cent are nourished orally or enterally, parenteral nutrition has a special field of usefulness. Because of the relative abundance of nourishment in the United States and in most Western countries, protein-calorie malnutrition is seldom seen except in patients who have an intrinsic nutritional disability, such as a stricture of the alimentary tract, a fistula, or a very abnormal rate of nutrient loss caused either by a fistula from the alimentary tract or by a protein-losing lesion such as an extensive burn, or in some cases of Ménétrier's syndrome in which albumin escapes through the stomach. Thus, one finds that the very people who need nutritional support most urgently tend to be the same people for whom it cannot be provided by the enteral route. Because so many of these patients have lesions of the alimentary tract, they tend to gravitate toward surgical services, where gastrointestinal surgeons undertake to re-establish functioning alimentary tracts by operative correction of the defects. Unfortunately, patients with severe nutritional deficits are relatively poor surgical risks, a theme that will be expanded in the body of this text. Therefore, methods of restoring the patient's nutritional deficits prior to operation become of crucial importance. It was, indeed, this motive that led to many of the developments in parenteral nutrition, particularly so-called *intravenous hyperalimentation* (IVH), by which we refer to regimens providing substantially more caloric and nitrogen intake than is required even to meet the postoperative hypermetabolic state. Indeed, it was not until the goal of nitrogen equilibrium had been superseded by 30 to 50 per cent that Dudrick, Vars, and Rhoads began to see the dramatic changes that can often be brought about by appropriate intravenous feeding.

Both Dr. Caldwell and Dr. Rombeau have been pioneers in the clinical nutrition field. Dr. Caldwell had the special advantage of being the original editor of the *Journal of Parenteral and Enteral Nutrition*, the official organ of the American Society for Parenteral and Enteral Nutrition (known as ASPEN). He saw most of the reports in this field for a number of years and proved himself to be a superb editor. He is now on the faculty of Brown University School of Medicine, Director of the Nutritional Support Service at the Rhode Island Hospital, and Director of the Surgical Metabolism Laboratory at the same hospital. Dr. Rombeau is on the faculty at the School of Medicine of the University of Pennsylvania and is Director of the Nutrition Support Service at the Philadelphia VA Medical Center. In editing this volume, they have called on many, indeed most, of the people who brought this field from its early laboratory stages at the University of Pennsylvania to the very wide use it serves today. This has been done by careful study and refinement of the details of the parenteral nutrition procedure, resulting in a diminished risk, improved products, advances in the techniques of administration, and far better organization of nutritional support teams.

This volume begins with a chapter on the history of the development of intravenous feeding, going far back in medical history to the many roots of physiologic chemistry and nutritional science, and proceeds in an orderly way to chapters on the basic biochemistry of the nutritional process, the experimental pathology attending nutritional deficits in animals and humans, the assessment of nutritional deficits in patients, and the many phases of the problem, both theoretical and practical. It should serve not only as a book of reference but also as a practical guide to the management of a wide variety of nutritional problems seen in clinical medicine, pediatrics, and surgery.

JONATHAN E. RHOADS, M.D., D.Sc.

Preface

The science of parenteral nutrition has undergone many changes since the report that documented its efficacy in 1967. Similar to what occurred with other medical advances, a period of underutilization was followed by a time of overutilization. More recently, attempts have been made via controlled clinical trials to identify the appropriate utilization of parenteral nutrition and to confirm its metabolic and clinical benefits. Certainly, no one can deny that parenteral nutrition has been life-saving for many individuals, such as those afflicted with short-gut syndromes. It is less clear, however, whether its use is justified in illnesses such as severe hepatic failure or extensive cancer. What can be concluded is that, in most instances, parenteral nutrition functions as a therapy adjuvant to primary treatments such as surgery, antibiotics, and other medical therapies.

The most important need in the field of parenteral nutrition is for the documentation of its effect on clinical outcome. Unfortunately, this may be an impossible task because of the multiple factors that influence clinical outcome. Furthermore, this issue is compounded by the moral and ethical dilemmas that arise when one realizes that the only alternative to parenteral nutrition, in some instances, is starvation.

There are many available texts on parenteral nutrition, and therefore it is important to question the rationale for another book. In our opinion the justification for this text results from the need to communicate the clinical and metabolic advances in parenteral feeding that have occurred so rapidly over the past few years. Furthermore, there has been a recent transition from the general applications of parenteral nutrition to more specific approaches based on nutrient requirements of individual disease states. In other words, parenteral feeding has evolved into an era of prescription nutrition. A major objective of this text has been to reflect these changes and to incorporate them into a reference source for parenteral nutrition. To meet this objective, contributors have been chosen with both clinical and research expertise, and they have been encouraged to document their chapters as extensively as possible.

This is the second volume of a two-volume set. Because of this format, certain general topics that are covered in Volume I, such as nutritional assessment, have not been repeated in Volume II. Other topics covered in Volume I have been included in Volume II when sufficient information specifically relevant to parenteral nutrition is available. It is acknowledged that many readers will be interested only in one volume; therefore, some topics are included in Volume II with the realization that a degree of overlap with Volume I is unavoidable.

Several important new areas are included in this volume. An improved understanding of disease-specific substrate requirements has led to contemporary chapters on this topic. Important advances have occurred in trace element requirements for parenteral nutrition, and this topic is covered extensively. Furthermore, there is now sufficient new information to include specific chapters on the role of parenteral nutrition in the treatment of anorexia nervosa, geriatric illnesses, sepsis, and in ameliorating the gastrointestinal complications associated with pregnancy. Finally, and of major importance, is an objective discussion of the costs and risks and benefits of parenteral nutrition.

It is acknowledged that a major improvement in the delivery of parenteral nutrition has resulted from the formation of multidisciplinary support teams. There is a need to provide updated scientific information to assist these teams in the provision of optimal nutritional care. Therefore, this text includes chapters of interest to such hospital nutrition team members as pharmacists, nurses, and dietitians; however, it is emphasized that its contents are directed primarily to the physician.

We wish to acknowledge the outstanding secretarial support of Jo Ann Graham and Betty Hoaque. A special thanks is extended to Linda Belfus, John Dyson, Evelyn Weiman, and Janet Macnamara-Barnett at the W. B. Saunders Company for their outstanding editorial assistance. Our gratitude is also extended to the many faculty, fellows, and residents who have directly and indirectly made important suggestions in the development of this book. Finally, our deepest gratitude is expressed to our wives and families for their inordinate understanding and forbearance.

JOHN L. ROMBEAU, M.D.
MICHAEL D. CALDWELL, M.D., PH.D.

Contents

History of Intravenous Nutrition

JONATHAN E. RHOADS, M.D., D.Sc.
STANLEY J. DUDRICK, M.D.
HARRY M. VARS, Ph.D.*

In tracing the history of any scientific subject, some judgment is perhaps required as to how far back one should go. Parenteral feeding rests on a knowledge of the physiology of the circulation, a knowledge of chemistry, a knowledge of microbiology, some knowledge of pharmacology and experimental pathology, as well as much clinical investigation.

It appears fair, then, to say that the first basic step was that of William Harvey in demonstrating the circulation of the blood. Once this was demonstrated, it became reasonable to believe first that what was put into the blood would circulate throughout the body and second that the nutritive properties of the food that one ate somehow were carried through the bloodstream to the various tissues of the body. The date of William Harvey's paper was 1628. It was about a generation later when Sir Christopher Wren, known in history as the architect of St. Paul's Cathedral in London, entered the field. He is credited with infusing wine into the veins of dogs in 1656. His apparatus was a goose quill attached to a pig's bladder. He also infused opium, which sedated the dog but did not kill it. This was probably the first instance of the administration of a drug by vein. Fracassato in Pisa carried out a similar procedure by 1658. In 1662, Richard Lower presented a paper before the Royal Society on intravenous feeding and blood transfusion in the dog. In 1666, Lower reported the successful transfusion of blood from an animal into a patient. What is meant by *successful* is not fully defined, but presumably the patient survived the experience.

The equipment used is evidenced in a little volume published in Amsterdam in 1670 entitled *Clysmatic Nova*. Bits of animal veins apparently were used as flexible tubing, and metal cannula tips were evidently available. It is said that some authors used the shafts of feathers with the ends cut off. Veins were entered by cutdown and, of course, without anesthesia.

In 1818, James Blundell transfused blood from man to man in London, and in 1831 Thomas Latta used intravenous saline solutions in the treatment of cholera in Leith, Scotland. Latta chose a patient who "apparently had reached the last moments of her earthly existence and now nothing could injure her. Indeed, so entirely was she reduced that I fear that I shall be unable to get my apparatus ready, ere she expire." He injected many ounces of a solution of water and salt at the elbow, and the patient quickly recovered and survived the attack of cholera. This demonstration of the effectiveness of saline solutions in the cholera epidemic in 1831 led to rather extensive use of intravenous injections despite a certain amount of opposition. Thomas Weatheril injected 15 liters of solution into a 29-year-old blacksmith over 13 hours and the patient subsequently recovered. O'Shaughnessy attributed death from cholera to thickening of the blood and its subsequent inability to circulate.

Claude Bernard, the very productive French physiologist, infused sugar solutions into animals in 1843, and over the next two decades, he infused egg whites, milk, and

*Dr. Harry M. Vars died before this chapter was completed. His work played an important part in many of the developments described, and he made valuable contributions to the preparation of the history. However, responsibility for errors and omissions must rest entirely with the surviving authors.

other nutrients into animals with some degree of success. He observed that cane sugar injected intravenously soon appeared in the urine, but that if it had previously been acted upon by gastric juice, it disappeared and apparently was utilized in the body.

In the middle of the last century, there was a major effort to provide food by subcutaneous injection. One of the first papers was by Menzel and Perco in Vienna, who injected fat, milk, and camphor. In 1875, Krug injected oil and protein extract in a patient who apparently had anorexia nervosa, and in this country, Whitaker described what he considered successful attempts to feed a 20-year-old woman with epigastric pain exacerbated by food by injecting milk, beef extract, and cod liver oil subcutaneously. Abscess formation occurred occasionally during this era. In Canada, Hodder used fresh milk strained through gauze and administered by syringe in an effort to correct fluid and nutrient losses in cholera. He felt the results were generally good; however, he was forced to resign from the hospital staff and was struck off the register and barred from the practice of medicine, so his colleagues apparently did not agree with him.

It seems obvious in retrospect that the field could not progress successfully before much more was known in the basic sciences.

Chemistry could scarcely be called a science before the work of Lavoisier and Priestley, and microbiology could not begin until the discovery of the microscope by Leuwenhoek and the work of Pasteur in the middle of the last century. The applications of Pasteur's work to the problems of surgery were, of course, initiated by Joseph Lister, who published his studies on the use of antisepsis in surgery in 1868 and subsequently. This work was followed by the development of aseptic techniques in Germany. The development of antibiotics is a complicated subject. The first substantial progress against microorganisms may have been the use of quinine against malaria. This practice was wholly empirical. It is said to have been learned from the Central and South American Indians, and it was popularized in western civilization largely by Lady Montague, a lay person. Probably the first scientific approach that succeeded was that of the German chemist Paul Ehrlich. It was known that mercury was sometimes beneficial in certain stages of syphilis, and he made a succession of chemical compounds in the hope of finding one that could circulate in the body and kill the spirochete, *Treponema pallidum*, the causative agent of syphilis. He numbered the compounds, and #606, generally known as salvarsan, was successful. Ehrlich continued his research, and when the combinations reached the 700's, he came up with another effective agent that could be tolerated by most patients, #725, which was called neosalvarsan.

Following these developments, there was an enormous effort to find chemicals that could circulate in the body without doing too much harm to normal tissues and would kill bacteria. The quest was strewn with failures, and most people had given it up. However, Domagh, working for the dye industry in Germany, conceived the idea that one of the supravital dyes might be attached to bacteria circulating in the body via a mordant. The resulting product, called Prontosil, was shown to be highly effective against certain coccal infections in small rodents. Fortunately, just before this was announced, a brother and sister working in a maternity hospital in London, Leonard and Dora Colebrook, had done a rather sophisticated epidemiologic study of puerperal sepsis occurring in the Queen Charlotte Hospital. They were impressed with the announcement of the new drug and applied it to their universe of patients. It was dramatically beneficial. Subsequently, other workers showed that it was not the dye but the mordant, sulfanilamide, that was the effective agent. Sulfanilamide had been discovered as a chemical in 1909, but its antibacterial properties had never been recognized. It revolutionized the treatment not only of puerperal sepsis, which was commonly of streptococcal origin, but also of some staphylococcal infections and some mixed infections. Thus, it was employed in patients with acute appendicitis and for the prophylaxis of infection after large bowel surgery, with conspicuously beneficial results. Patients with so-called blood poisoning, which was generally a coccal infection, erysipelas, and many infections of the upper respiratory tract, including otitis media and mastoiditis, were benefited. This agent was soon followed by modifications, such as sulfathiazine and sulfapyridine, which were effective against most pneumococci. These drugs were concentrated in the urine and were particularly useful against infections of the urinary tract and bladder.

Observations of clearing of culture plates by mold apparently go back at least as far as Tyndale, but their application stems from the experiments of Fleming, who noted the phenomenon in 1927. He did not, however, make application of it clinically at that time; this remained for H. W. Florey and associates to make in 1939. Since then, a galaxy of antibiotic drugs has been developed that gives the clinician the ability to combat a wide range of microbial infections. In the meantime, physiologists defined the fragility of the red cell in terms of concentrations of the solution, and chemists made available glucose in quite pure form as well as fructose and ethyl alcohol.

Much of the methodology used in nutritional studies was developed by Otto Folin, one of the earliest physiologic chemists in the United States. Although trained as an organic chemist at the University of Chicago, he later went to Europe, where physiologic chemistry was really being developed in Germany and Sweden, for what might be called a postdoctoral experience. He returned briefly to teach at the University of West Virginia and then spent seven very productive years at the MacLean Psychiatric Hospital in Waverly, Massachusetts. During these years, he developed analytical methods for measuring urea, uric acid, ammonia, rest nitrogen, and a number of other solutes in urine. He then was called to the Chair of Physiologic Chemistry at Harvard, which he occupied until his death in 1934. During the year 1911, he published only a single paper, but the next year, he wrote 20 papers. What had transpired was, in large part, the development of methods for analyzing nitrogen fractions in blood. He and Willie Denis, who was co-author of more than half of these papers, then published studies on the absorption of various nitrogen-containing products from large bowel loops as well as from the intact small intestine. It was Denis and Folin who introduced and recognized the difference between exogenous and endogenous metabolism, introducing the term *exogenous* in a paper in 1912 and using the term *endogenous metabolism* a few years later. He recognized this distinction as a result of studies on the urinary output of creatinine, which was constant and represented endogenous metabolism, as compared with urea, which fluctuated as a reflection of the nitrogen intake and represented exogenous metabolism. In this series of studies, he showed the prompt disappearance of amino acids from the bloodstream as they were metabolized, and suspected correctly that their metabolism

occurred to a large extent in the liver. By providing the analytical tools, he did much to permit studies of nitrogen and carbohydrate metabolism to proceed.

Another person who contributed greatly to the field was Dr. George Whipple[1] of Rochester, New York. Professor of Pathology and Dean at the then new medical school in New York, he took his early medical education at Johns Hopkins. Whipple showed the effect of infection and nonbacterial injury on nitrogen catabolism. He distinguished between the labile protein reserve, which broke down easily in response to injury and appeared as urea in the nitrogen, and the fixed protein reserves, which did not break down so readily. He and his co-workers showed that if the labile protein reserve was broken down by injury or used up by a protein-deficient diet, the animal lost its ability to respond to injury with a rapid protein catabolism. Beyond this, he and his co-workers demonstrated that various proteins had differing effects on rebuilding plasma proteins in dogs. Thus, it took ten grams of hemoglobin added to a diet in order to produce one gram of plasma protein in the depleted dog, whereas three grams of plasma protein by mouth would accomplish the same thing. These ratios were designated as the biologic value of the food protein. This group also showed that a dog could be kept in nitrogen equilibrium with intravenous plasma alone if given protein-sparing doses of carbohydrate and fat by mouth. This experiment was later repeated by Dr. J. Garrott Allen, who showed that such animals could grow with no protein source except intravenous plasma. Whipple's group, through an ingenious experiment, also obtained evidence that the plasma protein molecules did not have to be broken down all the way to amino acids in order to meet the protein requirements of the animals. They did this by giving the animals a drug that caused the breakdown of amino acids and excretion of the resulting products through the kidneys. The drug was phlorhizin. This drug made the animal temporarily glycosuric, and with the lowering of the blood sugar, many of the amino acids were broken down to yield glucose.

An additional set of data of great importance in nutrition was gleaned from the studies on basal metabolism conducted by F. G. Benedict at the Harvard School of Public Health. These defined a baseline for the caloric requirements of normal human beings and related these to the size of the individual, which is best reflected in the square meters of body surface. The methods of estimating this figure from height and weight were also developed. Thus, the roles of protein, carbohydrate, and fat in nutrition were pretty well defined as biochemistry developed, and W. C. Rose performed his famous and important studies of the essentiality of the various amino acids.

The serious problem of pyrogenic reactions to intravenous infusions had been solved in 1925 by Dr. Florence Seibert,[2] who, working at the Phipps Institute in Philadelphia, showed that the products of bacterial growth, even though the solution was sterile, could cause fever even in very small amounts. It is of interest that the concept of hydrolyzing proteins had been exploited somewhat for rectal infusions both in the experiments of Folin and Denis in 1912 and in the study of the nourishment of a boy by rectal administrations carried out by Abderhalden and Schittenhelm in 1909. Also, in 1913, Henriques and Anderson reported a rather remarkable study of total parenteral nutrition in a goat. Subsequent developments could scarcely have taken place without the information obtained by the individuals listed previously. Yet the reality of total parenteral nutrition or intravenous hyperalimentation was still a good many years away.

Perhaps the second chapter in this development can be conceived of as a demonstration of the dangers of protein-caloric malnutrition. Although undoubtedly these dangers were known in part to doctors and, indeed, to mothers from the time of antiquity, a number of them became well defined and delineated in relation to various disease entities through the 1930s. Although peripheral edema in prisoners was a well-known phenomenon when such individuals were inadequately nourished, as seems frequently to have been the case before 1900, visceral edema due to hypoproteinemia was recognized in patients with gastrointestinal disease by C. M. Jones and F. B. Eaton[3] in Boston and by I. S. Ravdin in Philadelphia. In the belief that such edema might account for the failure of gastroenterostomies to function, Mecray, Ravdin, and Barden[4] created nutritional edema in the dog using the technique of Dr. George Whipple and his associates, which consisted of a one per cent protein diet and plasmapheresis five days a week. With this preparation, it was shown, not only

did animals with fresh gastroenterostomies manifest very slow gastric emptying, but animals with well-healed gastroenterostomies did likewise; indeed, the edema affected the whole process of transit not only out of the stomach but also through the small bowel. In the course of these experiments, the abdominal wounds of some of the hypoproteinemic animals disrupted. On investigation of this phenomenon, Thompson, Ravdin, and Frank[5] found that hypoproteinemia resulted in marked interference with fibroplasia. Retardation in the callus formation after experimental fracture by hypoproteinemia was demonstrated next by J. E. Rhoads and W. Kasinskas,[6] and then poor resistance to hemorrhage by I. S. Ravdin, H. G. McNamee, and associates.[7] Although all of these studies were done in dogs, the human counterparts of these findings were evident clinically, with the possible exception of the fracture findings. The association between increased infectious complications and wounds in patients with hypoproteinemia was demonstrated by Brunschwig and later by Rhoads and Alexander.[8] A more precise animal study of the types of immunologic response affected by hypoproteinemia had been carried out on rats by Cannon, Wissler, and associates[9] at the University of Chicago.[8] Thus, by the end of the 1930s, there was a substantial amount of evidence, some of it from well-controlled studies, to show at least six or seven dangers of hypoproteinemia.

Toward the end of the 1930s the search for a means of compensating for these deficits was intensified. In 1936, Dr. Robert Elman reported the successful administration of an enzymatic hydrolysate of casein to patients. This material was made in the laboratories of Mead Johnson Co. and was so much less expensive than plasma that it made nitrogen equilibrium by this intravenous route a practical possibility. Mixtures of fibrin or casein hydrolysate with glucose, levulose, invert sugar, ossein gelatin, and ethyl alcohol were made available. These mixtures were given intravenously in the support of patients undergoing both small and large operations, with generally helpful results. However, nitrogen balance studies seldom showed that equilibrium was achieved, and a search was on to find out how equilibrium could be attained with regularity.

Equilibrium was harder to obtain because of the phenomenon, measured by D. P. Cuthbertson,[11] known as the catabolic response to injury. This study had been fore-shadowed by work in Whipple's laboratory on dogs in which inflammatory response was caused by the subcutaneous injection of turpentine. Whipple had been particularly interested in the rapid breakdown of what he termed the labile protein reserve. Cuthbertson studied particularly patients with fractures of the femur and showed not only that there was a sudden and fairly protracted breakdown of protein, as measured by nitrogen in the urine, but also that efforts to replace the protein were unsuccessful and generally resulted in the increased excretion of the added protein nitrogen, mainly as urea. In a series of studies done in several hospitals in the early 1940s, it was shown that a 70-kg man with a basal rate of perhaps 1400 calories had an increase in this rate after operations as short as herniorrhaphy. There was a larger increase after cholecystectomy, and after a gastrectomy or colon resection, the increase was about 50 per cent, to around 2100 calories with a liberal intake of nitrogen.

A number of limiting factors had been established for the safe administration of intravenous solutions. One was the volume, which was generally limited to three liters per day for lengthy administration. Often, patients could tolerate 3500 ml for a short period. With larger amounts, there was a tendency to encounter pulmonary edema. The second limitation was the concentration of the solution, which was conventionally administered in peripheral veins, usually those on the flexor side of the elbow or on the adjacent forearm. Glucose, which is isotonic at about five per cent, was usually tolerated at a ten per cent concentration, but when it was increased to 15 per cent, a great deal of thrombosis was encountered, often resulting in closure of the vein and cessation of the infusion. Finally, there were the apparently immutable caloric values of the various solutes, which in round figures are 4 kcal/gm for carbohydrate and protein, 7 kcal/gm for alcohol, and 9 kcal/gm for neutral fat.

A number of authors suggested that the catabolic response to injury must have a teleologic function, possibly that of making protein moieties available for repair of the injured site. The thought was expressed that it probably was unnecessary and perhaps disadvantageous to try to overcome the response by increasing intake. It was believed that a more natural approach might be to let this reaction run its course with a negative balance and then to see if it could not be compensated for later by a good intake during the later phases of convalescence. Although all of this reasoning made a certain amount of sense, experiments on the regeneration of resected rat livers by Vars and Gurd[12] had shown that regeneration was more rapid with a high-protein intake, even though it would occur to some extent at the expense of other body tissues in animals who were not given any protein. Although this experience did not answer the question of whether it was advantageous to overcome the negative nitrogen balance in patients during the catabolic phase of their response to operation, it did seem to us to suggest that there was no harm in doing so. Certainly, for liver regeneration in the rat, doing so was helpful. In any case, it seemed desirable to press for an early intravenous feeding technique in patients who had been seriously depleted of protein and in whom it was known that operation would carry an increased risk of various complications, both infectious and noninfectious. Clearly, the patients affected were those who could not or would not eat, generally those with alimentary tract obstructions or fistulas that resulted in loss of what food they ingested. A number of other groups of patients were likewise affected. Furthermore, it gradually occurred to some of us that one could not build up a reserve in one's bank account simply by depositing the amount that was withdrawn each week. It was desirable, therefore, in nourishing a depleted individual who could not take things by mouth and who was about to undergo an operation, to cover the basal requirements, say 1400 calories, as well as the extra requirement attendant upon surgery, which might be another 700 calories, and then add a clear margin beyond this of perhaps a third, which would make another 700 calories, or 2800 calories in all.

How could this amount be administered? The first thought was to utilize fat with its 9 kcal/gm and its relatively low thrombogenic effect on veins. Although fat emulsions for intravenous use had been prepared as early as the 1930s, the fat particles tended to form globules that might interfere with flow through small vessels and capillaries, so-called fat embolism. In reviewing the history of intravenous fat, one must credit Murlin and Riche, who infused a fat emulsion into animals in Ithaca, New York, in

1915, and also Yamakawa, who infused fat emulsions into humans as early as 1920. The first cotton seed oil fat emulsions were administered by Emmett Holt in Baltimore in 1935. However, these preparations were not developed to the point of clinical usefulness until the papers of Geyer and Stare, who stabilized the droplets with lecithin and tweens, and even then the preparations made in the United States caused a number of febrile reactions and other symptoms. Eventually, Swedish workers led by Wretlind (1961) developed quite satisfactory fat emulsions, but our success with the American products was extremely limited, and we finally abandoned them after more than a decade of clinical trial.

The next approach was to break through the volume limitation with the use of diuretics; this development was reported in 1962 at the meetings of the Federated American Societies for Experimental Biology.[13] The early diuretics had been used sparingly, because many of them contained mercury and there was fear of cumulative renal damage. However, by the 1950s, relatively safe diuretics had become available and were being used long-term in internal medicine for the control of hypertension in certain patients. Thus, we found that one could usually give 5 L/day if the amount was attended with 500 mg of Diuril. Unfortunately, the diuretic response was not fully predictable; unless someone watched the course of the infusion and the resulting diuresis very carefully, the infusion could get ahead of the diuresis, giving rise to pulmonary edema.

This was the first method by which we were able to achieve strongly positive nitrogen balance reliably by the intravenous route. While it was superceded by the delivery of more concentrated solutions into central veins, its success was the stimulus for a fresh attack on the problem, which led to the development of intravenous hyperalimentation at the University of Pennsylvania.

The problem was taken to the laboratory, where Dr. Harry Vars and Dr. C. Martin Rhode[14] had in 1949 developed a method for continuous infusion of dogs. This apparatus was reassembled by Dr. Vars, and a series of experiments was run under his guidance by Jonathan Rhoads, Jr., then a medical student at Harvard. The purpose of these studies was to determine the effects of various diuretics on sodium and potassium loss. After the summer was over, it was concluded that the

problem should be studied to see whether weight gain could be induced in growing puppies. The induction of weight gain in the adult would at best be moderate and would lead to arguments as to whether the weight gain was a real laying down of tissue or simply storage of extra water in the body. Methods were available for measuring total body water, but they were somewhat complicated, so that those who used them could be criticized by those of more experience. If puppies were used, however, the weight gain could be so dramatic as to avoid the possible criticism that the gain in weight was entirely a matter of water retention. A series of experiments was carried out by Spagna and Vars but was not reported because many of the animals did not survive. It was concluded that it would be better to start with animals that had been weaned and were about 12 weeks of age, rather than to battle the problems that had been encountered in younger puppies. This new series of experiments was carried out by Dr. Stanley Dudrick with the active assistance of Dr. Vars, who devised the vitamin and mineral supplement on the basis of his extensive knowledge of the nutritional literature. The animals were pure-bred beagles, and two litters of four were received during the year. From each litter of four, the animals were paired so that the controls would be as comparable as possible with those subjects receiving their nourishment intravenously. The controls received an isocaloric diet by mouth, and the experimental animals received only water by mouth and all of their nourishment through the superior vena cava using the technique of Rhode and Vars, which consisted of a cutdown on the jugular vein with passage of a polyethylene catheter into the superior vena cava. The other end of the catheter was threaded subcutaneously to the back near the posterior edge of the shoulder blades, where it was protected by a harness or a plaster cast, and then led out through a steel speedometer cable casing through the top of the cage. The animal had complete mobility within the cage and could lie down or stand up or turn around at will.

The history of central venous administration deserves some comment. Drs. Rhode and Vars used the method in dogs and reported on it in 1949. Dr. Vars measured the concentration of glucose downstream in the superior vena cava after 50 per cent glucose was injected through another catheter upstream in the superior vena cava. The dilution was so complete that it was difficult to determine any significant elevation of the glucose in the blood aspirated from the downstream cannula when the concentrated glucose solution was injected through the upstream cannula. Various persons employed the method at different times. In 1944 and 1945, Denis in Minneapolis reported that patients could be sustained without oral intake for extended periods when 20 per cent dextrose covered with insulin was added to the bottle and infused peripherally. Human plasma was added as a protein source. Denis also used the central route of administration quite extensively. We had explored the method of inserting the fine sterile catheters from the elbow into the superior vena cava in patients with advanced carcinoma. Autopsies were obtained after the disease had run its course, and it was found that there was a good deal of clot formation about the catheters. We then gave up the method for fear that it would induce a pulmonary embolus. This complication did not seem to occur in dogs, and Dr. Dudrick devised a compromise that was widely adopted. He utilized the subclavian puncture, described by Aubaniac[15] from Viet Nam in 1952 and subsequently used for measurements of central venous pressure by Drs. Mogil, DeLaurentis, and Rosemond[16] in 1967. By this arrangement, it was generally not necessary to perform a cutdown on a vessel, and yet only a relatively short length of catheter lay in a quite large vein. With this technique, it was possible to infuse highly concentrated solutions of glucose and amino acids ranging from 20 to 70 per cent. Thrombosis is occasionally seen, and careful studies have shown that there is almost always an agglutination of thrombocytes and fibrin over the exposed catheter; however, the agglutination has been of little if any clinical significance when the catheter is well placed and its position determined by x-ray. Dr. Dudrick continued to use the jugular vein in children, often with a cutdown, and it is often possible to pass a needle percutaneously into the jugular vein in the adult.

This procedure was carried out in a series of hospitalized patients who had fistulas and other abnormalities of the gastrointestinal tract and who could not be well nourished by mouth. The results were quite astonishing. The patients "perked up," as judged by their reaction to interviews on rounds; granulation tissue that was often gray, edematous, and unhealthy-looking became pink and firm, and epithelium began to grow in to cover it; and the patients were demonstrated to be in strongly positive nitrogen balance and to be gaining weight.

It is one thing to believe that one has learned something and another to convince others of its truth. The case of a small child admitted to the Children's Hospital of Philadelphia with atresia of most of the jejuno-ileum and the distal portion of the colon did more to convince others of the value of the method than anything else. The child was treated and reported by Drs. Wilmore and Dudrick.[17] The patient, whose weight had gone down from a birth weight of seven pounds to a little over four pounds during the period when she had an anastomosis of the proximal jejunum to the distal ileum and a colostomy above the atresia of the colon, was nourished entirely by vein for over six weeks. During this period she not only gained weight in a normal manner but grew, as measured by chest circumference, head circumference, and length, and looked like a wholly different infant within this time span.

There have been many further developments in the field, made in many different laboratories and hospitals. Of these, only a few will be noted here. The use of a modification of this method in patients with urinary shutdown has been helpful in lower nephron necrosis due either to mismatched blood or to a period of shock or muscle crush. In the course of these studies, evidence was obtained to support W. C. Rose's thesis that urea can be recycled.

It was found that many fistulas from the gastrointestinal tract to the body surface would close if patients were nourished solely by vein. The discharge from the fistula decreased in amount and became thin and watery, the granulation tissues about the cutaneous opening of the fistula became pink and healthy-looking, and within a few weeks all drainage often stopped. In a series of 78 patients treated at the Hospital of the University of Pennsylvania by Dr. Dudrick and his colleagues in the early 1970s, 70 per cent of the fistulas closed spontaneously. Others among these patients were in far better condition for surgical closure than they otherwise would have been, and most of those that failed to respond had malignancies. In the course of this study, it was found that some of the patients had inflammatory disease of the bowel, and although the closure rate of fistulas in this disease is not as high as in those following leaking anastomoses, for example, it nevertheless is appreciable, and the method was found useful in inducing remissions in inflammatory disease of the bowel. In some circumstances, these remissions have continued, so that intravenous hyperalimentation can be thought of as a treatment for some cases of Crohn's disease. For others, it is of great adjuvant value in getting the patient in satisfactory condition for surgical intervention.

In 1973, Law, Dudrick, and Abdou[18] tested the effect of protein calorie malnutrition on the mechanism of cellular immunity and showed that deficient patients were frequently anergic and, furthermore, that a substantial proportion of the anergic, nutritionally deprived patients would once again show evidence of improved cellular imunity on intravenous feeding.

A host of further studies in this field have demonstrated the practical usefulness of pure amino acids as opposed to protein hydrolysates. Other studies have been addressed to methods of evaluating patients for nutritional deficits and, surprisingly enough, a number of patients who do not appear ill nourished have been shown to have poor protein nutrition. Another vast body of work has been done on vitamin requirements and mineral requirements. There have been many advances in the methodology of intravenous feeding, such as the use of indwelling Hickman catheters. A vast experience has been gained in the risks as well as the advantages of intravenous feeding, and there have been extensive studies on the branched-chain amino acids in a group of patients with impaired liver function. All of these subjects and many additional problems are developed and elucidated in the ensuing chapters. The purpose of this chapter is merely to give a rapid synopsis of the historical development. It is in no sense a thorough review, and we offer our apologies to the hundreds of productive workers in the field whose accomplishments we have not cited.

REFERENCES

1. Whipple, G. H.: Protein production exchange in the body including hemoglobin, plasma protein and cell protein. Am. J. Med. Sci. 196:609, 1938.
2. Seibert, F. B.: Fever producing substances found in some distilled water. Am. J. Physiol., 67:90, 1923–24.
3. Jones, C. M., and Eaton, F. B.: Postoperative nutritional edema. Arch. Surg., 27:159, 1933.
4. McCray, P. M., Barden, R. P., and Ravdin, I. S.: Nutritional edema, its effect on gastric emptying time before and after gastric operations. Surgery, 1:53, 1937.
5. Thompson, W. B., Ravdin, I. S., and Frank, I. L.: Effect of hypoproteinemia on wound disruption. Arch. Surg., 35:500, 1938.
6. Rhoads, J. E., and Kasinskas, W.: The influence of hypoproteinemia on the formation of callus in experimental fracture. Surgery, 11:38, 1942.
7. Ravdin, I. S., McNamee, H. G., Kamholz, J. H., and Rhoads, J. E.: Effect of hypoproteinemia on susceptibility to shock resulting from hemorrhage. Arch. Surg. 48:491, 1944.
8. Rhoads, J. E., and Alexander, C. E.: Nutritional problems of surgical patients. Ann. N.Y. Acad. Sci., 63:268, 1955.
9. Cannon, P. R., Wissler, R. W., Woolridge, R. L., and Benditt, E. P.: Relationship of protein deficiency to surgical infection. Ann. Surg., 120:514, 1944.
10. Elman, R.: Amino acid content of blood following intravenous injection of hydrolyzed casein. Proc. Soc. Exp. Biol. Med., 37:437, 1937.
11. Cuthbertson, D. P.: Further observations on the disturbance of metabolism caused by injury, with particular reference to the dietary requirements of fracture cases. Br. J. Surg., 23:505, 1936.
12. Vars, H. M., and Gurd, F. N.: Effect of dietary protein upon the regeneration of liver protein in the rat. Am. J. Physiol., 151:399, 1947.
13. Rhoads, J. E.: Diuretics as an adjuvant in disposing of extra water as a vehicle in parenteral hyperalimentation (Abstract). Fed. Proc. 21:389, 1962.
14. Rhode, C. M., Parkins, W., Tourtelotte, D., and Vars, H. M.: Method for continuous intravenous administration of nutritive solutions suitable for prolonged metabolic studies in dogs. Am. J. Physiol., 159:409, 1949.
15. Aubaniac, R.: L'injection intraveineuse sous-claviculaire: Avantages et technique. Presse Med., 60:1456, 1952.
16. Mogil, R. A., DeLaurentis, D. A., and Rosemond, G. P.: The infraclavicular venipuncture. Arch. Surg., 95:320, 1967.
17. Wilmore, D. W., and Dudrick, S. J.: Growth and development of an infant receiving all nutrients exclusively by vein. J.A.M.A., 203:860, 1968.
18. Law, D. K., Dudrick, S. J., and Abdou, N. I.: Immunocompetence of patients with protein-caloric malnutrition. Ann. Intern. Med., 79(4):545, 1973.

CHAPTER 1

The Metabolic Response to Fasting

THOMAS T. AOKI
RICHARD J. FINLEY

For centuries, individuals have voluntarily undergone extended fasts with the hope that certain intellectual or spiritual benefits would be forthcoming. Whether the relative metabolic serenity that accompanies fasting facilitates this objective remains to be determined. It is clear, however, that the ability of primitive humans to go without food for sustained periods with minimal impairment of mobility enabled them to survive very hostile circumstances.

Although our knowledge of normal human metabolism has increased exponentially over the past 50 years, our understanding of the complex metabolic processes associated with trauma has not. The metabolic chaos manifested by the severely injured patient poses a number of questions to the clinician, one of which concerns the mechanism(s) regulating nitrogen metabolism in general and muscle breakdown in particular in such a compromised organism. However, such questions may be best initially addressed using models other than the injured patient. In this respect, studies of diabetic and starving subjects have been especially helpful.

DIABETES MELLITUS

Clinicians have been perplexed by their relative ineffectiveness in treating type I or insulin-dependent diabetic patients. However, certain concepts have emerged recently in this field that appear to be of major importance to the nutritional support of the traumatized patient, in whom insulin and tissue responses to insulin are major factors affecting outcome. These concepts are briefly presented here.

Because the metabolic conditions seen in juvenile-onset or type I diabetes mellitus are primarily attributable to a relative or absolute deficiency of insulin, it would seem reasonable to expect that insulin injections would eliminate the disease. However, although the administration of insulin has significantly prolonged the lives of insulin-dependent diabetic subjects, it has also permitted the development of the complications of chronic diabetes mellitus, e.g., retinopathy, neuropathy, nephropathy, and peripheral vascular disease. It has also become clear that despite our knowledge that a single hormone is lacking in this disease state, administration of the hormone to diabetic patients has not eliminated the disease nor resulted in the reestablishment of euglycemia.

Recent investigations conducted at the Joslin Research Laboratory, however, suggest that the failure of diabetologists over the past 50 years to achieve better metabolic control of the insulin-dependent diabetic subject is due primarily to a lack of appreciation of the pathophysiology of this disease state.[1-3] In brief, the central role of the splanchnic bed and, in particular, the liver in the processing of dietary foodstuffs has been extensively described in normal and diabetic patients[4-8] and then ignored from a therapeutic standpoint with respect to the diabetic patient. Studies of fasting individuals by the authors and their colleagues suggest that it should be possible to gradually reactivate the splanchnic bed and restore it to its dominant role in conventionally treated (one or two injections of insulin per day) diabetic subjects by the administration of insulin in a manner mimicking insulin release

9

in normal humans. This feat has recently been accomplished using the artificial β-cell unit.[1] When the splanchnic bed, particularly the liver, of an insulin-dependent diabetic patient is functioning normally with respect to the processing of dietary carbohydrate, that patient's blood glucose levels remain within the euglycemic range in both the fasting and postprandial states. In addition, once the capacity of the patient to process (oxidize and store) dietary carbohydrate, which is presumably dependent on an enzyme or enzymes (e.g., glucokinase), is restored, it should become to a limited extent insulin-independent. Thus, the capacity of the splanchnic bed to process dietary carbohydrate may be present even in the immediate absence of circulating insulin. Because the liver appears to be central to the metabolic disorder characteristic of the injured patient, and certainly is an important factor in the nutritional support of such a patient, these observations of type I diabetic subjects are of more than passing interest.

THE METABOLISM OF THE FASTING HUMAN

The aforementioned hypothesis regarding the central role (or non-role) played by the splanchnic bed, particularly the liver, of conventionally treated insulin-dependent diabetic subjects was derived largely from ongoing studies of prolonged starved humans by the Metabolism Unit of the Joslin Research Laboratories, which has long been concerned with the characterization of the complex interrelationships that exist among various hormones, substrates, and tissues of normal, diabetic, fasting, and traumatized persons. In particular, we have been interested in the identification of those mechanisms by which fasting individuals are able to conserve body protein. In the remainder of this discussion, both hormonal and nonhormonal mechanisms by which the fasting human accomplishes this extraordinarily important metabolic feat are discussed.

Changes in Circulating Hormone and Substrate Concentrations in Postabsorptive, Briefly Fasted, and Prolonged-Fasted Individuals

The changes in blood, urine, and respiratory gas exchange described in this section are almost wholly derived from studies of overweight but otherwise normal subjects undergoing a prolonged therapeutic fast conducted on the Clinical Research Center at the Brigham and Women's Hospital. In our experience, with certain exceptions that will be noted, similar changes are observed when normal-weight persons fast.

Selection of Subjects. Participants in the fasting program conducted by the Metabolism Unit at the Joslin Research Laboratory are restricted to persons of either sex who are under the age of 40 and have no major illness other than being overweight. They are selected from a list, maintained at the laboratory, of self-referred individuals desiring to undergo a prolonged therapeutic fast for weight reduction and to participate in medical research. They are interviewed, examined, and biochemically screened to ensure their suitability for participation in the program. The biochemical screening procedure includes an intravenous glucose tolerance test, an SMA-18, CBC, and determinations of T_3, T_4, and TSH levels.

Participants are then admitted to the Clinical Research Center at the Brigham and Women's Hospital, where they are put on a balanced 2500-calorie, 3-methylhistidine–free diet for a four- to seven-day equilibration period. They are then started on a complete fast, during which they are urged to drink at least 2 liters of water each day and to ingest tablets containing 17 mEq of sodium chloride and 17 mEq of potassium chloride as well as a multivitamin capsule. Physical activity is encouraged, and participants undergo 30 minutes of physical therapy each day. Because the subjects are entering a highly structured environment significantly different from that at their homes, every attempt is made to encourage their interaction with staff and fellow subjects at the Clinical Research Center. This approach also emphasizes self-care and the performance, if possible, of constructive activities previously performed at home or at work.

Hormonal Changes in the Fasting State. In the transition from the postabsorptive to the prolonged-fasted state, the levels of a number of hormones change in a highly reproducible and consistent manner (Fig. 1–1). Circulating insulin concentrations, which are usually elevated in overweight (compared with normal-weight) subjects, decrease, reaching a nadir at about three days and remaining low for the duration of the fast. This decline presumably reflects the lack

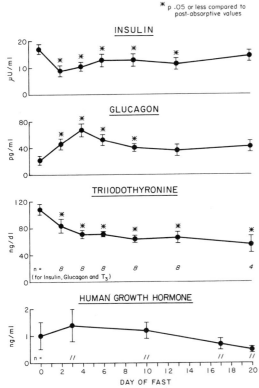

Figure 1–1. Hormonal response to fasting. Note the decline in circulating insulin and triiodothyronine concentrations and the increase in glucagon concentrations. Human growth hormone concentrations do not change significantly during the fast.

In sharp contrast to insulin and triiodothyronine levels, circulating plasma glucagon concentrations gradually increase, peaking at day 3 to 5 of the fast and declining thereafter to levels somewhat above postabsorptive concentrations.[9, 10] Both the immediate and long-term increases in circulating levels of glucagon may reflect the persistently low blood glucose concentrations seen in fasting persons.

Somewhat surprisingly, circulating concentrations of growth hormone, the one hormone that might, for reasons given later, be thought to be intimately associated with the fasting state, change little during the performance of a fast.

Changes in Blood Substrate Concentrations. During the transition from the postabsorptive to the fasted state, a number of changes in blood substrate concentrations are also seen (Fig. 1–2). Most prominent is the decline in circulating blood glucose from approximately 80–90 mg/dl to 50–60 mg/dl within the first three days of the fast, where it remains for the duration of the fast. In contrast, plasma free fatty acid concentrations promptly increase, reaching levels as high as 2 mM/L of plasma in some patients within 10 days of the fast and remaining high for the duration of the study. As might be expected in a metabolic state characterized by hypoinsulinemia and elevated plasma free fatty acid concentrations, circulating blood β-hydroxybutyric and acetoacetic acid concentrations promptly increase, reaching peaks after 21 days and remaining at these levels for the duration of the fast.

The changes in plasma amino acid levels during the transition from the postabsorptive

of dietary carbohydrate. Because triiodothyronine levels also appear to be linked closely to dietary carbohydrate intake, it is not surprising that T_3 concentrations also decrease during the same period, albeit somewhat more slowly.

Figure 1–2. Blood substrate response to prolonged fasting. Note the decline in glucose and the prompt increase in β-hydroxybutyric, acetoacetic, and free fatty acid concentrations.

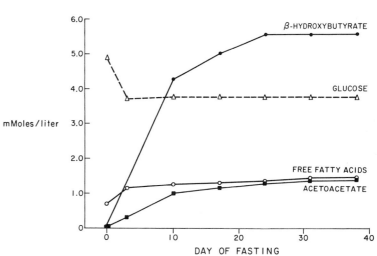

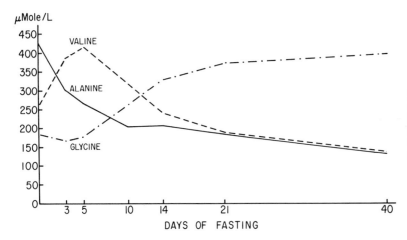

Figure 1–3. Plasma amino acid response to prolonged fasting. Note the decline in alanine, the increase in the branched chain amino acids, here exemplified by valine, and the unexplained rise of glycine (and threonine).

state to the prolonged-fasted state are shown in Figure 1–3. The glucogenic amino acids, here exemplified by alanine, promptly decrease at the outset of the fast, reach a nadir by day 21 of about 100 μM/liter of plasma, and remain low for the duration of the fast. In contrast, the branched-chain amino acids, here exemplified by valine, rise following initiation of the fast, reach a peak at days 5 to 7, and decline thereafter. In part, the rise in branched-chain amino acids may be attributable to two approximately concurrent events: (1) a fall in circulating insulin concentrations, resulting in either a decrease in incorporation of the amino acids into muscle or an increase in muscle proteolysis, and (2) a rise in plasma glucagon concentrations, which may be associated with increased hepatic proteolysis.[11–13] In contrast to glucogenic and branched-chain amino acids, levels of glycine and threonine initially decline and then gradually increase throughout the fasting period; the reason for this activity is at present unknown.

Changes in Urinary Ketoacid and Nitrogen Excretion. Total urinary nitrogen excretion is shown in Figure 1–4 in overweight but otherwise normal subjects undergoing a prolonged therapeutic fast. The primary nitrogenous component early in the fast is urea, with only a small amount of ammonia being excreted each day. However, with progression of the fast, urinary urea nitrogen excretion falls to approximately 1–2 gm/day, whereas urinary ammonia nitrogen excretion increases from approximately 0.5 to 2.5 gm/day. Because urinary urea nitrogen excretion reflects hepatic gluconeogenesis, which is an energy-requiring process, and ammonia nitrogen excretion reflects renal ammoniagen-

esis and gluconeogenesis, glucose production by the kidney equals or exceeds that by the liver late in the fast.

Urinary ketoacid excretion in individuals undergoing prolonged fast is shown in Figure 1–5. One should note the prompt and dramatic increase in urinary β-hydroxybutyric acid and acetoacetic acid excretion, which reflects their production in excess of

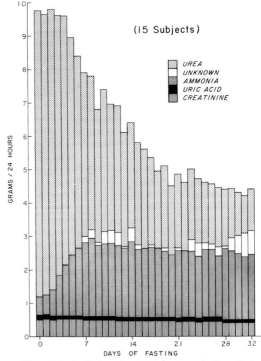

Figure 1–4. Daily urinary nitrogen excretion during prolonged fasting. Note the sharp diminution in urea (reflecting hepatic gluconeogenesis) and the prompt increase in ammonia (reflecting renal gluconeogenesis and ammoniagenesis) nitrogen excretion.

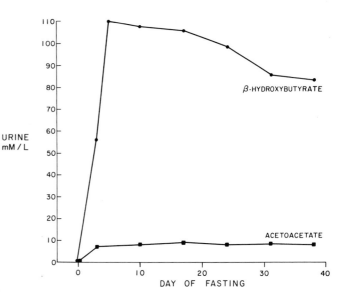

Figure 1–5. Note the prompt increases in urinary excretion of β-hydroxybutyric acid and the lesser excretion of acetoacetic acid during the performance of a prolonged fast.

metabolic needs by the liver, and their prompt excretion in the urine. In turn, ketoacid excretion necessitates a concomitant and stoichiometric increase in excretion of ammonia nitrogen to titrate the increased organic acid load. Thus, with progression of a therapeutic fast, there is a growing need to titrate the small but significant amount of ketoacid excreted in the urine using ammonia nitrogen derived primarily from glutamine.[14] It should be pointed out that although peak urinary ketoacid excretion occurs between days 7 and 10 of the fast, and blood levels of β-hydroxybutyrate and acetoacetate plateau at about the 21st day of the fast, hepatic production of these fuels, an energy-generating process, is maximal (ca. 130 gm/day) 24 to 48 hours following the initiation of the fast.[15] As we shall see later, the apparent discrepancies among maximal hepatic β-hydroxybutyric and acetoacetic acid production, ketonuria, and circulating concentrations of these important water-soluble fuels are due to their initial peripheral utilization early in the fast with a gradual decline later.[16]

Changes in Body Weight During a Fast and Refeeding. During the first week of a complete fast, and coincident with a fall in circulating insulin concentrations, most subjects manifest a weight loss of 5 to 10 lb. As seen in Figure 1–6, weight loss after that period (and well beyond the 21 days shown) proceeds at a much lower rate, approximately ½ lb/day. If following completion of a five- to six-week fast the subjects are allowed to eat *ad lib.*, weight gain approaching 20 pounds in a single week is common. This

weight gain is accompanied by massive pedal edema, and for this reason, following completion of a three- to six-week fast, participants are now routinely put on a 1200-calorie, low-sodium (high-potassium) diet for three weeks. On this regimen, a weight gain of approximately 4 lbs. during the first week is usual.

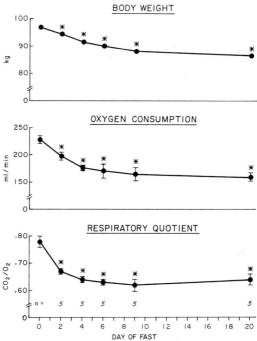

Figure 1–6. Note the gradual decrease in body weight, the characteristic decline in oxygen consumption, and the equally characteristic fall in the respiratory quotient during the performance of a prolonged fast.

Changes in Indirect Calorimetric Measurements. As reported by Benedict[17] in 1915, oxygen consumption falls by approximately 20 to 30 per cent during a fast (see Fig. 1–6). The reason for this decline is not well understood but may be related to the decrease in triiodothyronine levels noted elsewhere (see Fig. 1–1). Certainly, one might have theoretically expected oxygen consumption in fasting subjects to have increased along with their greater dependence on fat for energy.

As might be predicted, with this progressive increased reliance on fat for energy generation, the basal respiratory quotient (VCO_2 production/VO_2 consumption) declines to between 0.6 and 0.7, reflecting increased utilization not only of fat but also of β-hydroxybutyric and acetoacetic acids.[17, 18]

Changes in C_3 and C_4 During a Prolonged Fast. C_3 is a component of the alternative complement system, which includes factor D, factor B, and properdin. This system is activated by a number of factors, such as immune complexes, aggregated IgA, and endotoxin. Cleavage of C_3 by either the classical or the alternative pathway results in the formation of two molecules, C_{3a} (important in chemotaxis and C_{3b} (important in opsonization). As can be seen in Figure 1–7, serum C_3 levels decline modestly during the performance of a fast.

C_4, which along with C_1 and C_2 is a component of the classical complement pathway, does not change significantly during the performance of the fast. C_4 is important in viral neutralization.

Changes in Circulating Immunoglobulin Concentrations During a Prolonged Fast. Circulating concentrations of IgG (molecular weight: 150,000 daltons), the most abundant immunoglobulin, do not change significantly during the performance of a fast (Fig. 1–8). Four subclasses of IgG have been identified, of which IgG_1 and IgG_3 are capable of activating the classical complement pathway upon formation of immune complexes and of reacting with IgG receptors on monocytes and polymorphonuclear leukocytes.

Circulating concentrations of immunoglobulin IgA (molecular weight: 160,000 daltons) increase significantly in fasting subjects by day 6 and remain low thereafter. Both serum IgA and secretory IgA appear to be involved in the defense against respiratory tract infections.

Circulating concentrations of immunoglobulin IgM (molecular weight: 900,000 daltons), important in the early immune response, increase modestly but significantly in individuals undergoing a prolonged fast.

Changes in Circulating Blood Proteins. As seen in Figure 1–9, circulating concentrations of albumin and total protein decrease only slightly after 27 days of total starvation.

Fuel Depots

In a normal 70-kg individual, there are approximately 100 to 150 gm of mobilizable carbohydrate, primarily in the form of glucose and liver glycogen. Although there are

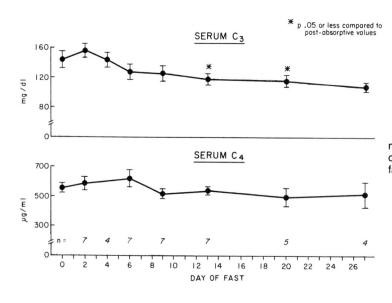

Figure 1–7. Serum C_3 levels fall modestly but C_4 concentrations do not change during the performance of a fast.

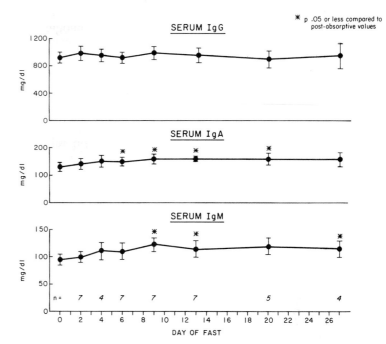

Figure 1–8. Although circulating serum concentrations of both IgA and IgM increase significantly during the fast, circulating serum concentrations of IgG do not change.

300 to 400 gm more of carbohydrate in the form of muscle glycogen, this source is not readily available to the rest of the body and is used by muscle only during periods of exercise and stress. Thus, readily available quantities of carbohydrate total approximately 400 to 600 calories, or less than one-third of a day's supply of energy for a normal individual. It should be pointed out that for every gram of liver or muscle glycogen, 3 or 4 ml more of water are required to permit storage of this particular fuel in body tissues. Hence, the energy density of glycogen is relatively low.

In the same individual, there are approximately 6 kg of potentially metabolizable pro-

tein, representing approximately 24,000 calories. However, because virtually all of this protein is in the form of functioning tissues such as muscle, enzymes, and blood proteins, the individual cannot sustain a loss in total body protein content greater than 2 kg without significantly compromising his or her ability to function normally (e.g., breathing, coughing). Finally, as with glycogen, approximately 3 to 4 ml of water are required to accompany each gram of protein retained in the body. Thus, protein also is relatively inefficient in terms of energy density.

In contrast to both carbohydrate and protein, adipose tissue is only 10 per cent water by weight. Thus, 1 gm of adipose

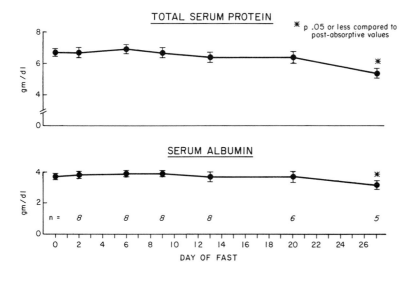

Figure 1–9. Only after approximately 4 weeks of fasting is a significant decline in total serum protein and albumin observed.

tissue yields close to the theoretical 9 calories obtained by the oxidation of 1 gm of pure triglyceride. The 15 kg of adipose tissue present in a 70-kg normal individual therefore represent the primary source of readily available, mobilizable, expendable energy.

Thus, it should be clear that protein, especially in muscle, is the rate-limiting tissue with respect to survival in starving humans, because it is already subserving and fulfilling essential functional roles. Utilization of this tissue for energy production, as seen in a severely traumatized person can only lead to impaired biochemical and physical functioning and hence to decreased survival. As will become evident, the fasting individual is somehow able to accommodate to this state of decreased dietary intake and to minimize the loss of protein even under the most adverse conditions.

The Metabolic Transition from the Postabsorptive State to the Briefly Fasted State

As seen in Figure 1–10, the primary consumer of glucose in the postabsorptive and briefly fasted states is the brain, which oxidizes approximately 150 gm of glucose into CO_2 and water. Initially, this requirement for glucose is met by hepatic glycogenolysis, but because mobilizable hepatic glycogen totals only 70 to 90 gm, less than one-third of a day's supply of energy, gluconeogenesis, which is an energy-requiring process, must initially supplement and later supplant glycogenolysis as the primary endogenous source of glucose. Toward this end, approximately 16 gm of glycerol, derived from hydrolysis of triglycerides, are shuttled to the liver in the company of approximately 70 to 90 gm of amino acids, which are in turn largely derived from peripheral tissues. As hepatic glycogen stores become depleted, muscle proteolysis initially increases, as evidenced by urinary 3-methylhistidine excretion, to meet this increased demand (Fig. 1–11). One should note, however, that the energy requirements of the body are being met primarily by the utilization of free fatty acids. Twenty-four to 48 hours following initiation of the fast, hepatic ketogenesis, an energy-generating process, is already proceeding at a maximal rate of approximately 130 gm per day.[15] However,

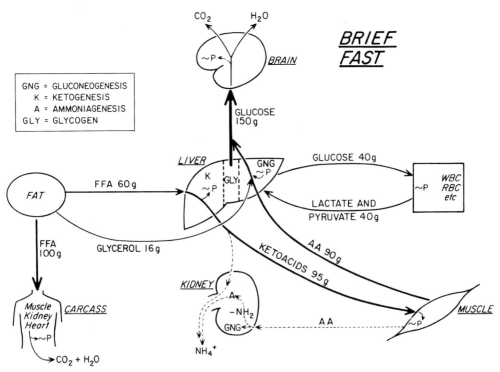

Figure 1–10. The metabolic adaptations observed in subjects during the performance of a brief (1–3 day) fast. Note the rather large quantities of amino acids being mobilized from peripheral tissues.

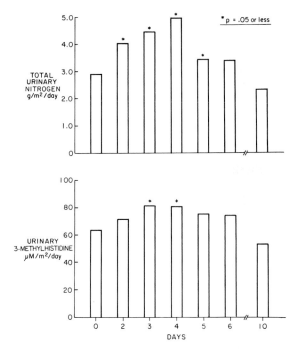

because the rest of the body, including muscle, is capable of utilizing these water-soluble, fat-derived glucose equivalents (4.5 calories/gm), blood concentrations of these substrates do not increase for several days.[19, 20]

In summary, amino acid mobilization, primarily from muscle, proceeds at an accelerated rate early in the fast, which if continued would result in a rapid depletion of functioning tissue. Later, however, further mechanisms are called into play that obviate the necessity for increased mobilization of muscle tissue in order to provide gluconeogenic precursors, such as alanine, and there appears to be a growing reliance on β-hydroxybutyric and acetoacetic acids for energy generation.

Metabolic Changes in Prolonged-Fasted Humans

With prolongation of the fasting period to three or more weeks, additional metabolic adaptations are observed that ensure the survival of the fasting subject (Fig. 1–12). First, as noted earlier, urinary excretion of nitrogen falls dramatically to approximately one-third

Figure 1–11. These data were obtained from individuals who had been placed on a 3-methylhistidine-free, balanced, 2500-calorie equilibration diet for 4 to 7 days prior to the initiation of a fast. Note the significant increase in total urinary nitrogen excretion and urinary 3-methylhistidine excretion by days 3 and 4 of the fast and the subsequent decline thereafter of both.

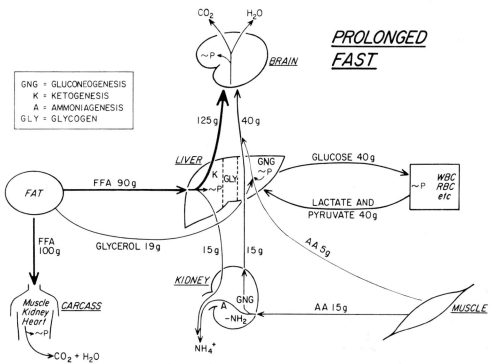

Figure 1–12. The metabolic changes observed in individuals undergoing a prolonged fast. Note the marked diminution in amino acid mobilization from peripheral tissues and the reliance on fat for energy generation.

to one-fourth that seen in the postabsorptive state. Because glucogenic amino acids represent the primary substrate for both hepatic and renal gluconeogenesis, the fall in urinary nitrogen excretion, which now largely reflects a decline of glucose production from the liver, together with the previously noted decline in circulating blood glucose concentrations could mean that the central nervous system might be deprived to a significant extent of this fuel. However, coincident with the decline in peripheral amino acid mobilization (and the subsequent decrease in conversion of these amino acids to glucose), the peripheral consumption of β-hydroxybutyric and acetoacetic acids, which is significant early in the fast, decreases markedly.[15] The decrease in peripheral utilization of these fat-derived glucose equivalents permits their blood concentrations to rise, in turn facilitating their utilization by the central nervous system, since both β-hydroxybutyric and acetoacetic acids can easily penetrate the blood-brain barrier. Indeed, Owen and colleagues[21] showed that 60 to 80 per cent of the fuel requirement of the brain in prolonged-fasted subjects is being met by the utilization of these ketoacids. Thus, most of the total hepatic ketoacid production is taken up by the central nervous system. However, the small amount (1 to 2 per cent of total hepatic production) of these fuels that is excreted in the urine requires renal ammoniagenesis to maintain acid-base relationships; for this reason, urinary ketoacid excretion and urinary ammonia excretion are virtually equivalent on a millimole per millimole basis.

Because the primary substrate for renal ammoniagenesis is glutamine, which is mainly synthesized in muscle,[22] it has recently become clear that ketonuria, renal ammoniagenesis, and muscle proteolysis are all intimately linked with respect to the protein conservation evidenced by individuals undergoing prolonged therapeutic fasts. It would therefore be predicted that in those situations in which renal ammoniagenesis was obviated, muscle proteolysis, at least as reflected by urinary nitrogen excretion and in particular by ammonia nitrogen excretion, should be significantly diminished. We and others[23] have found that the administration of sodium bicarbonate (150 mEq/day for three to five days) to individuals undergoing a prolonged fast does significantly reduce ammonia nitrogen excretion. In addition, the administration of glucose meals to pro-

longed-fasted subjects (37.5 gm every six hours for seven days) also markedly curtails hepatic ketogenesis and, in turn, significantly diminishes the need for renal ammoniagenesis.[24]

In summary, protein conservation in prolonged-fasted subjects is linked to the process of ketogenesis and the provisioning of the brain with adequate quantities of fuel. However, the need to titrate the small amounts of β-hydroxybutyric and acetoacetic acids that are excreted in the urine in turn necessitates muscle proteolysis and *de novo* synthesis of glutamine within muscle to provide the substrate for renal ammoniagenesis. Thus, for maximal protein conservation, prolonged-fasted individuals should theoretically produce only those amounts of β-hydroxybutyric and acetoacetic acids required by the central nervous system so that none is lost in the urine.

Sites of Regulation of Nitrogen Metabolism in Prolonged-Fasted Individuals

Protein mobilization, as reflected by urinary nitrogen excretion data, falls from approximately 70–90 gm in the postabsorptive state to about 20–25 gm in the prolonged-fasted state (see Fig. 1–12). How is this remarkable diminution in protein utilization accomplished?

Inspection of Figure 1–12 suggests that protein mobilization and utilization could be regulated at two anatomical sites, liver and muscle. First, the remarkable decrease in urea nitrogen excretion observed could reflect a markedly diminished hepatic capacity to convert glucogenic amino acids into glucose. In order to address this possibility, Felig and associates[25] elected to quantitatively assess the capacity of the liver to convert amino acids into glucose. They were aware that studies of perfused rat livers showed alanine to be a preferred gluconeogenic precursor,[26] and for this reason, they elected first to determine the rate at which the splanchnic bed, particularly the liver, of postabsorptive, briefly fasted, and prolonged-fasted individuals removed alanine from the systemic circulation.[25] They reported that the fractional extraction of arterial alanine was approximately 50 per cent in the postabsorptive state, 75 per cent after a three-day fast, and 50 per cent in a prolonged fast. These data suggested that the capacity of the liver of fasting subjects to extract alanine was normal. They then challenged individuals prior to and after a prolonged fast with 10 gm of L-alanine and were able to show that there was a prompt increase in blood glucose concentrations in both groups, with the fasted subjects showing the greater rise.[27] Incidentally, although plasma glucagon levels were not measured in that study, circulating concentrations of this hormone were almost certainly elevated in both postabsorptive and prolonged-fasted subjects. The importance of this observation is that glucagon is a potent stimulator of hepatic glycogenolysis, and the glucose rise observed when individuals were given 10 gm of L-alanine intravenously could have reflected hepatic glycogenolysis rather than hepatic gluconeogenesis. Fortunately, they also elected to perform a "cold" L-alanine infusion coupled to a tracer quantity of uniformly ^{14}C-labelled L-alanine. These researchers were able to show prompt incorporation of labelled L-alanine into glucose, thus providing convincing evidence that the livers of both postabsorptive and prolonged-fasted subjects were quite capable of processing alanine into glucose.[28]

Because the liver appeared to be fully functional with respect to hepatic gluconeogenesis, attention was then directed toward the second potential site of regulation, i.e., muscle. If amino acid release was significantly diminished during the performance of a fast, a marked diminution of substrate availability for hepatic gluconeogenesis could result, thus accounting for the diminution in urinary nitrogen excretion. Felig and colleagues[29] performed forearm studies in individuals prior to and after a prolonged (five to six weeks) fast, and they determined that amino acid release from the forearm muscle bed was dramatically curtailed after the fast and indeed that the decrease was commensurate with the remarkable diminution in urinary urea nitrogen excretion observed. Thus, the protein conservation, as reflected by a pronounced decrease in urinary urea nitrogen excretion, was attributable to a decrease in amino acid release from muscle.[29]

In the preceding description, emphasis is placed on the observation that the diminution of forearm amino acid release reported by Felig and colleagues[29] accounted for the decrease in urinary urea nitrogen excretion, the latter reflecting a commensurate reduction in hepatic gluconeogenesis. Earlier, reference was made to the observation that urinary excretion of ammonia nitrogen increased from approximately 0.5 gm/day in the postabsorptive state to 2.5 gm/day during a prolonged fast. These data suggested that the kidney was extracting more glutamine (13–15 gm/day versus 2–3 gm/day), the primary substrate for renal ammoniagenesis, and that muscle, the primary source of glutamine in humans,[22] was producing the quantity of glutamine required for this renal process. Indeed, Finley and co-workers[30] subsequently reported that glutamine release from forearm muscle beds in prolonged-fasted individuals was significantly higher than that in the same subjects when they were in the postabsorptive state. If one extrapolates the amount of glutamine release from forearm muscle to that of the whole body, the amount of glutamine released in prolonged-fasted individuals could easily account for the glutamine required for renal ammoniagenesis.

It should be emphasized that glutamine is synthesized within muscle[22] and that, in prolonged-fasted individuals, it must be synthesized using amino acids derived from muscle proteolysis. Muscle proteolysis must therefore proceed at a rate sufficient to provide adequate amounts of glutamine for renal ammoniagenesis so that titration of the organic acids, β-hydroxybutyric and acetoacetic acids, can be accomplished. Thus, if one could shut off ketogenesis in prolonged-fasted individuals, renal ammoniagenesis and urinary ammonia nitrogen excretion should fall. As previously noted, the administration of glucose meals to prolonged-fasted individuals does result in a marked diminution in urinary ammonia nitrogen excretion.

In summary, in prolonged-fasted individuals, protein conservation is compromised to the extent that body protein (i.e., muscle) must be broken down to provide sufficient quantities of amino acids to ensure adequate synthesis of glutamine, which in turn will be used for renal ammoniagenesis. At present, we know little about the signal by which this metabolic dialogue between muscle and kidney takes place. How does muscle know that it must produce more glutamine in a fasted individual?

The Hormonal Regulation of Nitrogen Metabolism in Prolonged-Fasted Individuals

Concurrent with the period in which the mechanism involved in the regulation of nitrogen metabolism in fasting individuals was first addressed by the metabolic unit of the Joslin Research Laboratory, hormonal mechanisms were first considered. The hormones studied included cortisol, growth hormone, glucagon, insulin, and triiodothyronine.

Cortisol. Investigators have long considered cortisol to be a permissive hormone, the presence of which is required in order for mobilization of amino acids from peripheral tissues to take place.[31] For this reason, Owen and associates[32] elected to study the effects of cortisone acetate injections in subjects who had fasted for five to six weeks. They were able to show that the administration of this hormone (100 mg twice a day) did not affect total urinary nitrogen balance, although there were a decrease in urinary ammonia nitrogen and an increase in urea nitrogen excretion. The researchers concluded that the glucocorticoids, specifically cortisone acetate, had a permissive but not a regulatory effect with respect to protein conservation.

Growth Hormone. At first glance, growth hormone appeared to be an ideal candidate for the title of "fasting hormone," i.e., the hormone that would set in motion all of the previously described metabolic changes observed in starving individuals. When administered to postabsorptive subjects, it produces an increase in circulating β-hydroxybutyric acid and acetoacetic acid concentrations and a decrease in urinary urea nitrogen excretion, metabolic changes characteristic of individuals undergoing a prolonged fast.[33, 34] For these reasons, Felig and colleagues[35] administered 5 mg of growth hormone intramuscularly every 12 hours for several days to subjects who had fasted for five to six weeks. They determined that, as expected, there was a prompt increase in circulating β-hydroxybutyric acid and acetoacetic acid concentrations and a significant decline in urinary urea nitrogen excretion. However, owing to the marked ketonemia, an equally marked ketonuria was observed. This latter phenomenon, in turn, necessitated increases in renal ammoniagenesis and urinary ammonia nitrogen excretion. On balance, there was no change in total nitrogen excretion, because the decrease in urinary urea nitrogen excretion was offset by the increase in ammonia nitrogen excretion. Felig and colleagues[35] concluded that growth hormone, like cortisol, did not appear to have an important regulatory role with respect to the protein conservation manifested by individuals undergoing a prolonged fast.

Glucagon. As previously noted, circulating concentrations of glucagon, a potent stimulator of hepatic gluconeogenesis, increase during days 3 to 5 of the fasting period in both normal and overweight subjects, declining thereafter to levels somewhat higher than postabsorptive concentrations (see Fig. 1–1).[9, 10] Studies were subsequently performed to answer the question, "Why are circulating plasma glucagon concentrations elevated at a time when hepatic gluconeogenesis, from a protein conservation point of view, should be suppressed?" One possible explanation is that because circulating glucose levels have fallen (see Fig. 1–2), the modestly but persistently elevated glucagon concentration is an attempt to at least maintain, if not increase, circulating glucose levels in order to ensure that the brain gets an adequate supply of glucose. A second possibility is that in the non-eating or fasting subject, the modestly elevated concentrations of glucagon are essential for preserving the capability of the subject's liver to process gluconeogenic precursors (e.g., lactate, amino acids) into glucose efficiently. The third possibility is that glucagon is directly acting on peripheral tissues (i.e., muscle) to curtail mobilization of amino acids, particularly alanine.

In order to explore these issues, Marliss and colleagues[9] infused glucagon into prolonged-fasted individuals at three dose rates (10 mg/24 hours for two days, 1 mg/24 hours for two days, and 0.1 mg/24 hours for two days). As expected, at the two higher infusion rates, there were marked increases in urinary urea and total nitrogen excretion and in circulating glucose and insulin concentrations, and a pronounced decrease in circulating amino acid concentrations, with the glucogenic amino acids showing the greatest fall. In contrast, at the lowest infusion rate (0.1 mg/24 hours for two days), which resulted in a physiologic elevation of glucagon concentration, urinary urea nitrogen excretion actually decreased, and circulating levels of glucose, insulin, free fatty acids, β-hydroxybutyric acid, and acetoacetic acid did not change. Because these results were somewhat surprising, it was elected to perform another study in which 0.1 mg/24 hours would be infused for a total of four days to permit better documentation of changes in urinary nitrogen excretion in general and urea nitrogen excretion in particular.[36] In addition, it was elected to determine the half-life of alanine 24 hours after the start of the glucagon infusion. This latter test was performed in order to determine whether the glucagon infusion had affected the liver's capacity to remove alanine from the systemic circulation. Prolongation, after glucagon infusion, of the half-life of alanine (50 μCi of L-^{14}C-U-alanine in an IV bolus) beyond that measured in a control group would certainly lend support to this possibility. On the other hand, a shortened alanine half-life would suggest increased hepatic extraction of this amino acid.[36]

During this study, as in the previously described inquiry, circulating glucose, insulin, β-hydroxybutyric acid, acetoacetic acid, and free fatty acid levels did not change significantly. Plasma glucagon concentrations were elevated significantly over basal levels during the glucagon infusion, whereas circulating levels of amino acids, primarily the glucogenic amino acids, fell modestly. In addition, a significant diminution in urinary urea nitrogen excretion was observed; however, concomitant with that diminution was an increase in urinary ammonia nitrogen excretion, presumably necessitated by the increased ketonuria induced by the administration of glucagon. Interestingly, glutamine concentrations which were not previously measured, fell (see Fig. 1–13). These data suggest that the administration of glucagon resulted in a significant increase in urinary excretion of β-hydroxybutyric and acetoacetic acids, which in turn necessitated greater utilization of glutamine by the kidney for titration of the larger organic acid load. In addition, since the half-life of alanine was found to be significantly prolonged over that in a control group, the glucagon infusion apparently decreased the capacity of the liver to convert alanine into glucose. Finally, the decline in circulating plasma alanine concentrations observed in the face of a lower hepatic capacity to process alanine suggests that peripheral formation of alanine was similarly diminished.[36] The elevated circulating plasma glucagon concentrations seen in subjects undergoing a prolonged fast may therefore play a significant role in the protein conservation also manifested by these subjects.

Insulin. Insulin, in both humans and animals, has long been considered the dominant hormone with respect to the stimulation of protein synthesis and the inhibition of muscle proteolysis.[31, 37–41] The large outpouring of amino acids from the forearm tissue of diabetic patients in ketoacidosis[42]

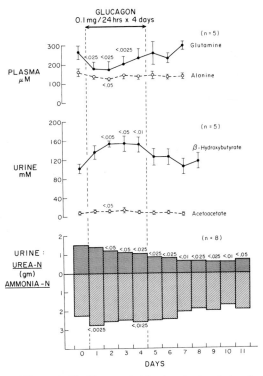

Figure 1–13. Changes in blood and urine during the infusion of glucagon (0.1 mg/24 hrs × 4 days). Note the progressive decline in urinary urea nitrogen excretion during the infusion and the prompt increase in ammonia nitrogen excretion in response to the equally prompt increase in excretion of β-hydroxybutyric acid and acetoacetic acids. Note also the decline in circulating glutamine and alanine concentrations.

can be rapidly reversed by the administration of insulin. When Pozefsky and associates[43] infused insulin in physiologic concentrations into the forearm muscle beds of postabsorptive normal subjects, they observed a significant diminution in the amino acid efflux from that tissue. Other investigators have demonstrated increased glutamate uptake following forearm instillation of physiologic quantities of insulin.[44] Results of these two studies suggest that insulin is capable of immediately modifying amino acid egress from muscle and presumably both encourages protein synthesis and inhibits muscle proteolysis. In contrast to the relatively dramatic immediate effect of insulin in postabsorptive subjects, when 20 units of crystalline zinc insulin are infused into prolonged-fasted individuals, only a small diminution in urinary urea nitrogen excretion is observed.[45] However, it is reasonable to expect that in individuals already maximally conserving nitrogen, the systemic infusion of small quantities of insulin would have only a minimal effect on nitrogen balance. Parenthetically, during the study, circulating blood glucose concentrations fell below 20 mg/dl, whereas circulating levels of β-hydroxybutyric and acetoacetic acids as well as free fatty acids remained at or above basal values. These higher circulating levels suggest that neither ketogenesis nor lipolysis was significantly affected by the insulin infusion, which raised systemic insulin concentrations by approximately 10 μU/ml over basal values. Finally, we have recently infused insulin directly into the forearm muscle beds of prolonged-fasted individuals and have noted no significant impact on amino acid efflux from forearm muscle tissue, thus indicating that maximal protein conservation probably had already taken place.[46]

On the basis of the preceding discussion, it still seems reasonable to conclude that insulin is the dominant factor responsible for curtailing amino acid efflux from the forearm muscle beds of prolonged-fasted subjects; however, other observations suggest that this hypothesis may not be entirely true. It is somewhat surprising that circulating insulin concentrations fall during the performance of a fast, at a time when (1) maximal restraint of amino acid efflux from muscle is desired and, with the exception of glutamine, is accomplished and (2) normal or even elevated insulin concentrations might be expected. Although it might be argued that this decline in circulating insulin concentrations facilitates free fatty acid mobilization from adipose tissue, thus enabling the transition from a mixed fuel economy to a fuel economy predominantly based on fat, the decline might also be expected to result in increased amino acid mobilization from peripheral tissues. In addition, we have recently begun to quantitate urinary C-peptide excretion in subjects undergoing a prolonged fast. We have determined that urinary C-peptide excretion in these subjects, after 21 days of fasting, approaches that seen in type I insulin-dependent diabetic subjects (5–8 μg/24 hours). This finding suggests that either there is a remarkable increase in muscle sensitivity to insulin in prolonged-fasted individuals or that insulin does not play the dominant role in the amino acid metabolism of these subjects that it does in postabsorptive subjects. Obviously, questions remain to be answered with respect to insulin and its role in protein conservation in fasted subjects.

Triiodothyronine. In the early 1920s, thyroid hormone was administered to individuals on a high-carbohydrate, low-protein diet, resulting in a marked increase in total urinary nitrogen excretion approximately one week later.[47] Because we and other investigators have reported that the concentrations of triiodothyronine (T₃) decline during the performance of a fast (see Fig. 1–1),[48–50] we wondered whether this decrease in thyroid hormone might in fact be closely related to the decrease in nitrogen excretion observed to occur simultaneously. For this reason, we gave 15 μg of T₃ every six hours for two days to six subjects prior to and after three weeks of fasting. The results are shown in Figures 1–14 and 1–15.

It can be seen that in the postabsorptive state, the administration of 15 μg of T₃ had relatively little effect on either blood or urine substrate concentrations. In addition, no significant changes in urinary 3-methylhistidine excretion were observed during or following the administration of T₃ (see Fig. 1–14). Finally, urinary ammonia and urea nitrogen excretion were not affected.

The participants were then fasted for 21 days, during which circulating T₃ levels de-

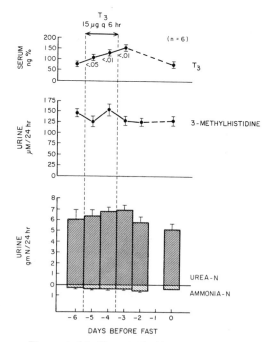

Figure 1–14. Changes in blood and urine in overweight but otherwise normal subjects receiving 15 μg of T₃ q6h for 2 days in the fed state. Note the increase in circulating T₃ concentrations and the lack of change in urinary nitrogen and 3-methylhistidine excretion.

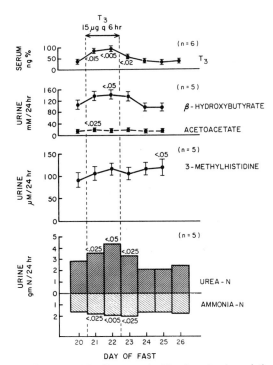

Figure 1–15. Changes in blood and urine of the same individuals in Figure 1–14, who has now fasted for 21 days and are undergoing the same protocol. Note the prompt return of circulating T_3 concentrations to postabsorptive levels and the increase in urinary excretion of urea and ammonia nitrogen. Urinary excretion of β-hydroxybutyric acid increases during the period of T_3 administration. Note, however, that despite the increase in urinary nitrogen excretion, there is no change of urinary 3-methylhistidine excretion, suggesting that muscle proteolysis is not the source of the nitrogen lost during the time of T_3 administration. Two days following cessation of T_3 administration, however, urinary 3-methylhistidine excretion is increased significantly. This increase may represent repletion, using muscle-derived amino acids, of depleted splanchnic stores of protein.

clined (see Fig. 1–15). Beginning on the 21st day, however, all six participants were given 15 μg of T_3 every six hours for two days, and their circulating T_3 levels were successfully restored to postabsorptive concentrations (see Fig. 1–15). Circulating glucose concentrations, which had declined during the fast, did not change during the period of T_3 administration. Insulin concentrations were similarly unaffected.

Urinary excretion of β-hydroxybutyric and acetoacetic acids increased significantly during the study period and declined following cessation of T_3 administration. Urinary excretion of both urea and nitrogen ammonia nitrogen increased significantly during T_3 administration and gradually returned to control levels following cessation of T_3

administration. Of great interest, urinary 3-methylhistidine excretion continued to increase following cessation of T_3 administration, reaching significant levels three days later (see Fig. 1–15).

In order to ascertain the source of the higher amount of nitrogen excreted in the urine, we performed forearm studies in the six fasted participants prior to and after 48 hours of T_3 administration when forearm blood flow was found to have increased by approximately 50 per cent. A small but significant decrease in arterial β-hydroxybutyric acid concentration, but not in acetoacetic acid concentration, was observed. Thus, a significant decrease in the arterial β-hydroxybutyric acid:acetoacetic acid ratio was documented, suggesting that the mitochondria in muscle were in a relatively more reduced state before the participants received T_3. Efflux of free fatty acids from the forearm increased significantly, whereas that of alanine did not change significantly, following T_3 administration (-6.7 ± 13 versus -12 ± 36 nM/100 ml forearm tissue/minute). Of interest, glutamine efflux from the forearm increased in five of the six subjects from -147 ± 32 to -394 ± 319 nM/100 ml forearm tissue/minute, but owing to the variability of the response, the statistical significance of this increase was not achieved. Arterial glutamine levels decreased from 429 ± 33 to 379 ± 35 μM/L by the second day of T_3 administration.

The preceding results suggest that the decline of T_3 levels during fasting is essential for conservation of protein, because restoration of T_3 to normal pre-fasting levels results in a prompt and significant increase in urinary nitrogen excretion. Because fasting levels of insulin and glucagon were not affected by administration of T_3 in physiologic doses, it appears that the conservation of nitrogen in prolonged-fasted individuals requires the precise interaction of both insulin and T_3, a finding that is consistent with the *in vitro* findings of Tata and associates.[51] It is interesting that the major portion of the greater nitrogen loss was in the form of urea, implying increased availability to the liver of glucogenic substrates. Increase in urinary excretion of 3-methylhistidine was not parallel to the increase in urinary excretion of ammonia and urea nitrogen, so skeletal muscle breakdown probably did not provide this substrate to the liver. Thus, the glucogenic substrate supporting enhanced urinary ammonia and urea nitrogen excretion were most likely derived from hepatic proteolysis.

Finally, the increases in clearance of creatinine and β-hydroxybutyric and acetoacetic acids and the concomitant increase in urinary ammonia nitrogen excretion suggest that T_3 also directly or indirectly affects renal metabolism and renal perfusion. Because glutamine, derived from muscle, is the primary substrate for renal ammoniagenesis, the increase in glutamine efflux from forearm muscle bed was directly or indirectly triggered by the administration of T_3. Thus, at present, it appears that the decline of T_3 observed in prolonged-fasted individuals is a necessary concomitant to protein conservation.

Regulation of Muscle Amino Acid Metabolism in Fasting Humans: Role of the Redox State

As previously noted, shortly after the initiation of a therapeutic fast, circulating insulin concentrations decline markedly in both normal and overweight individuals and remain low for the duration of the fasting period. At the same time, there is a marked decrease in urinary nitrogen excretion and, late in the fast, a marked diminution of amino acid release from forearm muscle bed, with the exception of glutamine. Thus, protein conservation evidenced by individuals undergoing a prolonged fast takes place in the presence of lowered concentrations of insulin. Because in the postabsorptive state the metabolic effects of insulin are a direct

function of its circulating concentrations, it was somewhat surprising to find that insulin levels declined at a time when protein conservation, presumably insulin-mediated, was taking place. These findings suggested that protein conservation might be mediated by both hormonal and nonhormonal mechanisms. In view of the latter possibility, the potential regulatory role played by the redox state of various tissues in fasting individuals, but especially that of muscle, was considered,[52] and over the past eight years this hypothesis has slowly gained support.[53-56]

In 1971, Owen and colleagues[16] reported that there was little or no utilization of β-hydroxybutyric and acetoacetic acids by forearm muscle tissues in fasting individuals. It appeared that acetoacetic acid entered forearm muscle and then left this tissue as β-hydroxybutyric acid. This observation suggested that forearm muscle tissue might be in a more reduced state than arterial blood with respect to muscle mitochondria. In order to evaluate this possibility, a brief survey was done of studies already performed at Joslin Research Laboratory.[52] In this survey, a number of important assumptions were made. First, it was assumed that the arterial β-hydroxybutyric acid/acetoacetic acid ratio represented the average or net redox state of the whole body of a fasting subject. Second, it was assumed that any change in the arterial ratio of these substrates after passage through a given tissue, as indicated by the venous ratio, reflected the redox state of that tissue relative to arterial blood. With these assumptions, Table 1–1 was constructed.

Table 1–1. BLOOD β-HYDROXYBUTYRATE (β-OH) AND ACETOACETATE (AcAc) AND LACTATE (L) AND PYRUVATE (P) VALUES AND/OR RATIO BEFORE (ARTERIAL) AND AFTER (VENOUS) PASSAGE THROUGH VARIOUS TISSUES OF THE FASTING HUMAN

TISSUE	VESSEL	β-OH VALUE (mM)	AcAc VALUE (mM)	RATIO β-OH/AcAc
Muscle	Artery	5.291	1.515	3.49
	Vein	5.378	1.345	4.00
Splanchnic bed + kidney	Artery	6.480	1.420	4.56
	Hepatic vein	6.815	1.600	4.26
	Renal vein	6.210	1.467	4.23
Brain	Artery	6.670	1.170	5.70
	Jugular vein	6.630	1.110	5.97
Muscle	Artery			L/P 13.9
	Vein			19.2

These observations suggested that in fasting subjects, muscle mitochondria, as reflected by the β-hydroxybutyric acid:acetoacetic acid ratio, and cytosol, as reflected by the lactic acid:pyruvic acid ratio, were, of those tissues studied, the most reduced. As discussed earlier, because this muscle tissue is rate-limiting with respect to hepatic gluconeogenesis, there was a possibility that muscle redox state and total body protein conservation were related. In 1978, we reviewed additional studies conducted by this laboratory, in which nitrogen retention or conservation was affected experimentally, and attempted to establish whether a consistent relationship existed between muscle redox state and nitrogen metabolism in fasting subjects.[53]

In these subjects, the β-hydroxybutyric acid/acetoacetic acid ratios in arterial blood and in blood draining forearm muscle tissue were compared and were related to urinary urea nitrogen excretion prior to and after (1) a prolonged fast, (2) four days of glucagon infusion (0.1 mg/day) in fasted subjects, (3) a 24-hour insulin infusion (crystalline zinc insulin, 20 U/day) in fasted subjects, (4) ingestion of a protein meal by a prolonged-fasted subject, (5) administration of 15 μg of T3 every six hours for two days to fasted subjects, and (6) infusion of hydrocortisone hemisuccinate, 200 mg/day for two days, in fasted subjects (Fig. 1–16).[53]

Compared with findings in the postabsorptive state, after 21 days of a complete fast, the blood β-hydroxybutyric acid/acetoacetic acid ratio increased following passage through forearm tissue. This increase was coincident with a marked decrease in urinary urea nitrogen excretion. An increase in the blood β-hydroxybutyric acid/acetoacetic acid ratio was also observed following passage through the forearm muscle bed during the glucagon and insulin infusion studies, again coincident with a significant decrease in urinary urea nitrogen excretion. Following the ingestion of a protein meal by a subject who had fasted for six weeks, there was a dramatic increase in the β-hydroxybutyric acid/acetoacetic acid ratio. In contrast to the previous findings, in individuals who received triiodothyronine and hydrocortisone, the blood β-hydroxybutyric acid:acetoacetic acid ratio decreased after passing through the forearm muscle bed at the same time that urinary urea nitrogen excretion increased. These data suggest that in those

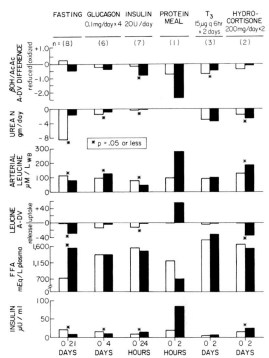

Figure 1–16. Hormone-substrate-redox interrelationships. *Vertical open bars* represent control period, and *solid bars* experimental period values. *Top panel,* arterial–deep venous β-hydroxybutyric acid:acetoacetic acid ratio differences across forearm muscle bed. These ratio differences are construed merely as reflecting the direction of the redox state of forearm muscle relative to that in arterial blood. The various conditions included in this study are shown at the top of the figure, and the measured parameters—urinary urea nitrogen excretion, arterial leucine concentration, arterial–deep venous leucine concentration differences, free fatty acid concentrations, and circulating insulin levels—are shown on the side. See text for more detailed explanation. Urine collections were not performed during the protein meal study.

experimental conditions in which the blood β-hydroxybutyric acid:acetoacetic acid ratio increased (i.e., tissue[s] was relatively more reduced), a decrease in urinary urea nitrogen excretion was observed. In contrast, in those experimental situations in which the blood β-hydroxybutyric acid/acetoacetic acid ratio decreased (i.e., tissue[s] was relatively more oxidized), an increase in urinary urea nitrogen excretion was observed.[53]

The next issue addressed was the determination of the theoretical link between muscle redox state and release of amino acids from forearm muscle tissue of fasting individuals. We had previously observed that in those situations in which forearm tissue became relatively more reduced, there was a decrease in the release of the branched-chain amino acids (insulin infusion studies) from muscle or an increase in removal by that tissue of the branched-chain amino acids (protein meal). In addition, in those clinical situations in which arterial branched-chain amino acid concentrations were elevated (diabetic ketoacidosis, three to five day fast, trauma), a marked increase in urinary urea nitrogen excretion was also observed. Conversely, in those situations in which branched-chain amino acid levels were low (prolonged fast, glucose and/or insulin infusion studies), urinary urea nitrogen excretion was low. Thus, a consistent association between the branched-chain amino acids and protein mobilization and utilization appeared to be present in humans.[53]

An examination of the metabolic pathways involving the branched-chain amino acids, particularly leucine, suggested that the low Km of the enzymes responsible for the oxidative decarboxylation of the ketoanalogs of these amino acids and the apparent inability of muscle to accumulate these amino acids ensure that circulating concentrations of the amino acids remain close to intracellular concentrations. Thus, a potentially highly responsive system is present that has one important rate-limiting site—the oxidative decarboxylation of the deaminated ketoanalogs, which, in turn, requires the availability of oxidized NAD and which may therefore be potentially rate-limiting. Thus, in fasted individuals in whom free mitochondrial and cytosolic NAD concentrations are low owing to the almost exclusive use of fat and β-hydroxybutyric and acetoacetic acids for energy generation, decreased concentrations of the product(s) of the oxidative decarboxylation step might be the signal to inhibit or suppress catabolism. In this model, therefore, two conditions must be present: low free mitochondrial and cytosolic NAD concentrations and low concentrations of branched-chain amino acids and/or their intermediates. Finally, an intact or non-disordered hormone-fuel milieu must also be present for this sequence to take place.

As noted previously, it is presumed that the reduced state of muscle mitochondria and cytosol in fasting individuals is largely, if not entirely, due to the exclusive utilization of fat for energy generation purposes. That is, the stepwise degradation of fatty acids is encouraged by decreasing insulin concentrations and in turn results in the generation of reduced NAD or decreased free or oxidized NAD concentrations. It should be noted that the reduced total body redox states of fasting and of diabetic ketoacidosis are distinguished by the modulating role played by insulin in the former but not in the latter state. Thus, (1) the gradual decrease in insulin concentrations, which ensures reliance on fat utilization, appears to be the first step toward protein conservation taken by fasting subjects and (2) insulin's role in fasting subjects is quite different from that in postabsorptive subjects, in whom free NAD is not rate-limiting and protein synthesis and inhibition of muscle proteolysis are associated with increased concentrations of insulin.

Simultaneous with the falling circulating insulin levels, a number of metabolic changes occur that together bring about the rapid development of this more reduced total body redox state in fasting persons. Adipose tissue rapidly becomes resistant to even low concentrations of insulin, lipolysis then proceeds quickly, and circulating concentrations of free fatty acids rise to as high as 2000 μEq/L of plasma. Hepatic ketogenesis is then accelerated, and the end-products, β-hydroxybutyric and acetoacetic acids, become available for use initially by the entire body but later only by the brain. After five to six weeks of fasting (and as if complementing adipose tissue resistance to insulin), muscle and, to a lesser extent, liver appear to remain more or less sensitive to changes in the concentration of this hormone.

In summary, the gradual decrease of circulating insulin concentration in fasting subjects, the gradual development of adipose tissue resistance to insulin, and the persistent sensitivity of muscle and hepatic tissues to the low concentrations of insulin appear to permit a greater utilization and/or conversion of fat to energy and accompany the orderly entry of the fasting human into a more reduced state.

REFERENCES

1. Foss, M. C., Vlachokosta, F. V., Cunningham, L. N., and Aoki, T. T.: Restoration of glucose homeostasis in insulin-dependent diabetic subjects. Diabetes, 31:46–52, 1982.
2. Vlachokosta, F. V., Asmal, A. C., Ganda, O. P., and Aoki, T. T.: The effect of strict control with the artificial β-cell on plasma lipid levels in insulin-dependent diabetes mellitus. Diabetes Care, 6:351–355, 1983.
3. Aoki, T. T., Vlachokosta, F. V., Foss, M. C., and Meistas, M. T.: Evidence for restoration of hepatic

glucose processing in type I diabetes mellitus. J. Clin. Invest., 71:837–839, 1983.

4. Wahren, J., Felig, P., Cerasi, E., and Luft, R.: Splanchnic and peripheral glucose and amino acid metabolism in diabetes mellitus. J. Clin. Invest., 51:1870–1878, 1972.

5. Wahren, J., Felig, P., and Hagenfeldt, L.: Effect of protein ingestion on splanchnic and leg metabolism in normal man and patients with diabetes mellitus. J. Clin. Invest., 57:987–999, 1976.

6. Felig, P., Wahren, J., and Hendler, R.: Influence of oral glucose ingestion on splanchnic glucose and gluconeogenic substrate metabolism in man. Diabetes, 24:468–475, 1975.

7. Aoki, T. T., Brennan, M. F., Müller, W. A., Soeldner, J. S., Alpert, J. S., Saltz, S. B., Kaufman, R. L., Tan, M. H., and Cahill, G. F., Jr.: Amino acid levels across normal forearm muscle and splanchnic bed after a protein meal. Am. J. Clin. Nutr., 29:340–350, 1976.

8. Felig, P., Wahren, J., and Hendler, R.: Influence of maturity-onset diabetes on splanchnic glucose balance after oral glucose ingestion. Diabetes, 27:121–126, 1978.

9. Marliss, E. B., Aoki, T. T., Unger, R. H., Soeldner, J. S., and Cahill, G. F., Jr.: Glucagon levels and metabolic effects in fasting man. J. Clin. Invest., 49:2256–2270, 1970.

10. Aguilar-Parada, E., Eisentraut, A. M., and Unger, R. H.: Effects of starvation on plasma pancreatic glucagon in normal man. Diabetes, 18:717–723, 1969.

11. Exton, J. H., and Park, C. R.: Control of gluconeogenesis in liver. I. General features of gluconeogenesis in the perfused livers of rats. J. Biol. Chem., 242:2622–2636, 1967.

12. Mallette, L. E., Exton, J. H., and Park, C. R.: Effects of glucagon on amino acid transport and utilization in the perfused rat liver. J. Biol. Chem., 244:5724–5728, 1969.

13. Exton, J. H., Mallette, L. E., Jefferson, L. S., Wong, E. H. A., Friedman, N., Miller, T. B., and Park, C. R.: The hormonal control of hepatic gluconeogenesis. Rec. Prog. Horm. Res., 26:411–461, 1970.

14. Pitts, R. F.: Renal production and excretion of ammonia. Am. J. Med., 36:720–742, 1964.

15. Reichard, G. A., Jr., Owen, O. E., Haff, A. C., Paul, R., and Bortz, W. M.: Ketone-body production and oxidation in fasting obese humans. J. Clin. Invest., 53:508–515, 1974.

16. Owen, O. E., and Reichard, G. A., Jr.: Human forearm metabolism during progressive starvation. J. Clin. Invest., 50:1536–1545, 1971.

17. Benedict, F. G.: A Study of Prolonged Fasting. Carnegie Inst. Wash. Publ. 203, 1915.

18. Owen, O. E., Trapp, V. E., Reichard, G. A., Jr., Mozzoli, M. A., Smith, R., and Boden, G.: Effects of therapy on the nature and quality of fuels oxidized during diabetic ketoacidosis. Diabetes, 29:365–372, 1980.

19. Cahill, G. F., Jr., Herrera, M. G., Morgan, A. P., Soeldner, J. S., Steinke, J., Levy, P. L., Reichard, G. A., Jr., and Kipnis, D. M.: Hormone-fuel interrelationships during fasting. J. Clin. Invest., 45:1751–1769, 1966.

20. Cahill, G. F., Jr.: Starvation in man. N. Engl. J. Med., 282:668–675, 1970.

21. Owen, O. E., Morgan, A. P., Kemp, H. G., Sullivan, J. M., Herrera, M. G., and Cahill, G. F., Jr.: Brain metabolism during fasting. J. Clin. Invest., 46:1589–1595, 1967.

22. Marliss, E. B., Aoki, T. T., Pozefsky, T., Most, A. S., and Cahill, G. F., Jr.: Muscle and splanchnic glutamine and glutamate metabolism in postabsorptive and prolonged-starved man. J. Clin. Invest., 50:814–817, 1971.

23. Hannaford, M. C., Leiter, L. A., Josse, R. G., Goldstein, M. D., Marliss, E. B., and Halperin, M. L.: Protein wasting due to acidosis of prolonged fasting. Am. J. Physiol., 243(Endocrinol. Metab. 6):E251–E256, 1982.

24. Aoki, T. T., Müller, W. A., Brennan, M. F., and Cahill, G. F., Jr.: Metabolic effects of glucose in brief and prolonged fasted man. Am. J. Clin. Nutr., 28:507–511, 1975a.

25. Felig, P., Owen, O. E., Wahren, J., and Cahill, G. F., Jr.: Amino acid metabolism during prolonged starvation. J. Clin. Invest., 48:584–594, 1969.

26. Ross, B. D., Hems, R., and Krebs, H. A.: The rate of gluconeogenesis from various precursors in the perfused rat liver. Biochem. J., 102:942–951, 1967.

27. Felig, P., Marliss, E., Owen, O. E., and Cahill, G. F., Jr.: Role of substrate in the regulation of hepatic gluconeogenesis in fasting man. Adv. Enzyme. Reg., 7:41–46, 1969.

28. Felig, P., Marliss, E., Pozefsky, T., and Cahill, G. F., Jr.: Amino acid metabolism in the regulation of gluconeogenesis in man. Am. J. Clin. Nutr., 23:986–992, 1970.

29. Felig, P., Pozefsky, T., Marliss, E., and Cahill, G. F., Jr.: Alanine: key role in gluconeogenesis. Science, 167:1003–1004, 1970.

30. Finley, R. F., Vignati, L., and Aoki, T. T.: Increased glutamine release from muscle during fasting in man. Clin. Res., 26:836a, 1978.

31. Cahill, G. F., Jr., Aoki, T. T., and Marliss, E. B.: Insulin and muscle protein. In Steiner, D. F., and Freinkel, N. (eds.): Handbook of Physiology, Section 7: Endocrinology, Vol. 1: Endocrine Pancreas. Baltimore, Maryland, The Williams & Wilkins Company, 1972, pp. 563–577.

32. Owen, O. E., and Cahill, G. F., Jr.: Metabolic effects of exogenous glucocorticoids in fasted man. J. Clin. Invest., 52:2596–2605, 1973.

33. Henneman, P. H., Forbes, A. P., Moldawer, M., Dempsey, E. F., and Carroll, E. L.: Effects of human growth hormone in man. J. Clin. Invest., 39:1223–1238, 1960.

34. Smith, C. K., and Long, C. N. H.: Effect of cortisol on the plasma amino nitrogen of eviscerated adrenalectomized-diabetic rats. Endocrinology, 80:561–566, 1967.

35. Felig, P., Marliss, E. B., and Cahill, G. F., Jr.: Metabolic response to human growth hormone during prolonged starvation. J. Clin. Invest., 50:411–421, 1971.

36. Aoki, T. T., Müller, W. A., Brennan, M. F., and Cahill, G. F., Jr.: Effect of glucagon on amino acid and nitrogen metabolism in fasting man. Metabolism, 23:805–814, 1974.

37. Manchester, K. L.: Oxidation of amino acids by isolated rat diaphragm and the influence of insulin. Biochim. Biophys. Acta, 100:295–298, 1965.

38. Wool, I. G., Stirewalt, W. S., Kurihara, K., Low, R. B., Bailey, P., and Oyer, D.: Mode of action of insulin in the regulation of protein biosynthesis in muscle. Recent Prog. Hormone Res., 24:139–208, 1968.

39. Wool, I. G., Castles, J. J., Leader, D. P., and Fox, A.: Insulin and the function of muscle ribosomes. In Steiner, D. F., and Freinkel, N. (eds.): Handbook of Physiology, Vol. 1, Endocrine Pancreas.

Baltimore, Maryland, The Williams & Wilkins Company, 1972, pp. 385–394.

40. Manchester, K. L.: Insulin and protein synthesis. *In* Biochemical Actions of Hormones, Vol. 1. New York, Acad. Press, 1970, pp. 267–320.

41. Manchester, K. L.: The control by insulin of amino acid accumulation in muscle. Biochem. J., *117*:457–465, 1970.

42. Aoki, T. T., Assam, J.-P., Manzano, F. M., Kozak, G. P., and Cahill, G. F., Jr.: Plasma and cerebrospinal fluid amino acid levels in diabetic ketoacidosis before and after corrective therapy. Diabetes, *24*:463–467, 1975.

43. Pozefsky, T., Felig, P., Tobin, J. D., Soeldner, J. S., and Cahill, G. F., Jr.: Amino acid balance across tissues of the forearm in postabsorptive man. Effects of insulin at two dose levels. J. Clin. Invest., *48*:2273–2282, 1969.

44. Aoki, T. T., Brennan, M. F., Müller, W. A., Moore, F. D., and Cahill, G. F., Jr.: Effect of insulin on muscle glutamate uptake. J. Clin. Invest., *51*:2889–2894, 1972.

45. Aoki, T. T., and Cahill, G. F., Jr.: Metabolic effects of insulin, glucagon, and glucose in man: clinical applications. *In* DeGroot, L. J., Cahill, G. F., Jr., Odell, W. D., Martini, L., Potts, J. T., Jr., Nelson, D. H., Steinberger, E., and Winegard, A. T. (eds.): Endocrinology, Vol. 3. New York, San Francisco and London, Grune & Stratton, 1979, pp. 1843–1854.

46. Finley, R. J., Vignati, L., and Aoki, T. T.: Effects of insulin and exercise on forearm metabolism in fasting man. Clin. Res., *26*:414A, 1978.

47. Deuel, H. J., Jr., Sandiford, K., Sandiford, I., and Boothby, W. M.: Deposit protein: the effect of thyroxin on the deposit protein after reduction of the nitrogen excretion to a minimal level by a prolonged protein-free diet. J. Biol. Chem., *67*:XXIII–XXIV, 1926.

48. Vignati, L., Finley, R. J., Haag, S., and Aoki, T. T.: Protein conservation during prolonged fast: a function of triiodothyronine levels. Trans. Assoc. Am. Phys., *91*:169–179, 1978.

49. Portnay, G. I., O'Brian, J. T., Bush, J., Vagenakis, A. G., Azizi, F., Arky, R. A., Ingbar, S. H., and Braverman, L. E.: The effect of starvation on the concentration and binding of thyroxine and triiodothyronine in serum and on the response to TRH. J. Clin. Endo. Metab., *39*:191–194, 1974.

50. Vagenakis, A. G., Burger, A., Portnay, G. I., Rudolph, M., O'Brian, J. T., Azizi, F., Arky, R. A., Nicod, P., Ingbar, S. H., and Braverman, L. E.: Diversion of peripheral throxine metabolism from activating to inactivating pathways during complete fasting. J. Clin. Endo. Metab., *41*:191–194, 1975.

51. Tata, J. R., Ernster, L., and Lindberg, D.: The action of thyroid hormone at the cell level. Biochem. J., *86*:408–428, 1963.

52. Aoki, T. T., Toews, C. H., Rossini, A. A., Ruderman, N. B., and Cahill, G. F., Jr.: Glucogenic substrate levels in fasting man. Adv. Enz. Reg., *13*:329–336, 1975.

53. Aoki, T. T., Finley, R. J., and Cahill, G. F., Jr.: The redox state and regulation of amino acid metabolism in man. Biochem. Soc. Symp., *43*:17–29, 1978.

54. Buse, M. G., Weigand, D. A., Peeler, D., and Hedden, M. P.: The effect of diabetes and the redox potential on amino acid content and release by isolated rat hemidiaphragms. Metabolism, *29*:605–616, 1980.

55. Tischler, M. E.: Is regulation of proteolysis associated with redox-state changes in rat skeletal muscle? Biochem. J., *192*:963–966, 1980.

56. Tischler, M. E., and Fagan, J. M.: Relationship of the reduction-oxidation state to protein degradation in skeletal and atrial muscle. Arch. Biochem. Biophys., *217*:191–201, 1982.

CHAPTER 2

Hormone-Substrate Interrelationships: The Cellular Reactions

NAJI N. ABUMRAD
MICHAEL CALDWELL

The minute-to-minute control of substrate concentration *in vivo* is maintained by three complex and communicating systems: the nervous system, the endocrine system, and a system of various local chemical modulators.

The nervous system can transmit messages from one area of the body to another by an elaborate arrangement of nerves. At the nerve ending, messages are transmitted to either the ganglia or the target organs via chemical substances, synthesized in the nerve cell, known as neurotransmitters. Such substances include acetylcholine, norepinephrine, histamine, serotonin, and γ-amino-butyric acid.

The endocrine system can also transmit messages from one area of the body to another via chemical substances known as hormones. Hormones are released by the endocrine glands into the circulation. When they reach their target organs, they bind to specific recognition sites known as receptors. The resulting hormone-receptor complex activates certain cellular processes that lead to a biologic response characteristic of that particular hormone.

The third system consists of a wide variety of chemical substances that are released by the tissues and serve locally to modulate the effects of hormones and neurotransmitters, enhancing or suppressing their actions. For example, the prostaglandins are released locally in response to certain stimuli,[1, 2] and the "autocoids" are a group of substances released in response to inflammation. All these compounds can alter the sensitivity of target cells and thus change the biologic response.

In addition to these three systems, circulating substrates themselves (glucose, amino acids, free fatty acids, ketone bodies, etc.) can carry important instructions to individual cells or groups of cells. Moreover, the concentrations of various ions (calcium, phosphorous, sodium, potassium, and chloride) and of certain trace elements (iron, zinc, iodine, vanadium, molybdenum, aluminum, fluorine, mercury, manganese, and arsenic) also serve important regulatory functions. This chapter discusses some of the factors that determine cellular sensitivity to hormones and neurotransmitters and explores how hormone-receptor interactions maintain the constancy of the "internal milieu" of the body.

CELLULAR ACTION OF HORMONES

Synthesis

Most of our understanding of peptide hormone synthesis has been derived from studies of parathyroid hormones.[3-5] Peptide hormone precursors are synthesized on the rough endoplasmic reticulum (RER), and are carried to the Golgi complex either by direct transfer through the cisternae of the ER or via transition elements.[3] In the membrane

This work was supported by JDF grant #82R564 and NIH grants #R01 AM 30515 and AM 20593. The authors would like to thank Rose Hornsby for excellent secretarial assistance.

channels of the ER, various endo- and exo-peptidase enzymes split the pre-hormone precursor, changing it to a prohormone and eventually to its final form.[5] In the Golgi complex, the hormone is packaged into secretory granules; it is then transported to the periphery of the cell and released to the extracellular space by a process of exocytosis (Fig. 2–1).

Precursor proteins have been identified for a number of peptide hormones, including insulin, parathyroid hormone (PTH), growth hormone (GH), prolactin, thyroid-stimulating hormone (TSH), and adrenocorticotropin hormone (ACTH).[3–7] The importance of the sequence of pre-prohormone to prohormone to hormone is not yet clear. There is considerable evidence supporting a transport function for the prehormones,[3, 6] but the significance of the prohormone in cellular transport is unknown.

Secretion

Secretion of polypeptide hormones is stimulated by signals that are highly specific for each hormone. These signals generally result from changes in the circulating levels of various substrates, such as glucose and amino acids. Certain hormones, such as glucocorticoids and thyroid hormones, may stimulate release of other hormones. The actions of these stimulating factors may also be modified by various substances. For example, the catecholamines may alter secretory activity of pancreatic hormones through action on adrenergic receptors.[8–10] Prostaglandins,[11] calcium,[12] and beta-endorphins[13] may act either as primary stimulating factors or as modulating factors. Several lines of evidence suggest that the prostaglandin E (PGE) series stimulates glucagon secretion.[1, 2] Lowered extracellular calcium levels, in addition to stimulating PTH release, inhibit the release of most polypeptide hormones.[3] Recent evidence indicates that beta-endorphins can selectively stimulate aldosterone secretion with a potency similar to that of an equimolar dose of ACTH.[13] The exact mechanism by which these stimuli cause hormone secretion is not well understood. In many instances there is evidence to suggest that cyclic AMP acts as a second messenger in this coupling of biosynthetic and secretory processes.[12]

In contrast to the cells responsible for peptide hormone synthesis, those responsible for synthesis of steroid hormones

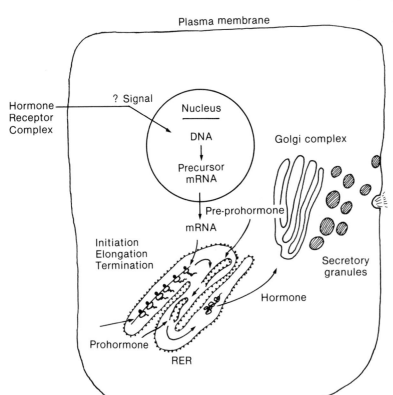

Figure 2–1. Schematic representation of polypeptide hormone secretion. The signal reaching the nucleus initiates transcription of DNA to form precursor mRNA, which after several steps of excision and rejoining forms mRNA. In the rough endoplasmic reticulum (RER), the mRNA acts as a template for protein synthesis, resulting in pre-prohormone. This hormone is transported to the Golgi complex, is packaged into secretory granules, and leaves the cell by a process of exocytosis.

have little capacity to store preformed hormone.[14, 15] Thus, the signals for hormone release activate steroid biosynthesis[16] rather than cause release of preformed steroids.[14, 15] In the case of cortisol synthesis, within two to three minutes, ACTH activates a membrane-bound adenylate cyclase, leading to phosphorylation of several enzyme systems[14, 15] that convert cholesterol to pregnenolone, a rate-limiting step in steroid biosynthesis.[17]

Once secreted, the majority of polypeptide hormones circulate to target cells in the free form. Steroid and thyroid hormones are transported in the blood bound to carrier proteins.[18, 19] The biologic importance of this binding process is not yet clear, but it has been postulated that bound hormone serves as a reservoir from which free hormone is subsequently released.[18, 20] These carrier proteins may also serve in the clearance of endogenously produced or exogenously administered steroid compounds.[17, 19] Finally, binding proteins may add selectivity to the hormone-receptor complex and may be necessary for the subsequent expression of biologic response,[21] as in the case of aldosterone's action on the target cell.[22]

STEROID HORMONE ACTIONS

The major classes of steroid hormones secreted by the adrenal gland and gonads are the glucocorticoids, mineralocorticoids, androgens, estrogens, and progestins. The majority of these hormones are bound to plasma proteins. More than 98 per cent of the androgens bind either to albumin, as in the case of dehydroepiandrostenedione (DHEA),[19] or to a testosterone-estradiol–binding globulin, as in the case of testosterone.[19] Cortisol is 90 to 93 per cent protein-bound, and 80 per cent of it binds to corticotropin-binding globulin (CBG).[18, 20] In contrast, aldosterone is only 50 to 55 per cent protein-bound, with the majority bound to albumin and less than 10 per cent to CBG.[17] The non-bound hormones diffuse freely and rapidly into all cells, and once in the cytoplasm, they bind to specific proteins or receptors. The hormone-receptor complex is then activated and translocated to the nucleus, where it binds to specific sites on chromatin and initiates synthesis of specific messenger RNA (mRNA) and proteins.[21, 22] Steroid receptors have been identified in many mammalian tissues, a finding that is consistent with their widespread action. In general, these receptors behave as 4-S or 5-S (Svedberg) proteins during density gradient centrifugation in the presence of high ionic salt gradients (0.4 M KCl). Activation of the receptor complex usually results in a change in the sedimentation rate.[21–23] For example, when the estrogen-receptor complex is activated, it changes from a 4-S to a 5-S species.[23]

Estrogen receptors are 4-S proteins that have been identified in the uterus and in estrogen dependent tissues, such as anterior pituitary and mammary glands.[23] Progesterone receptors, also 4-S proteins, are present predominantly in female reproductive tissues.[24] Whereas the activity and concentration of estrogen receptors depend primarily on the presence of estrogen, those of progesterone depend on both estrogen and progesterone availability as well as the timing of the estrous cycle.[24, 25] Recently, antibodies against purified forms of both estrogen[26] and progesterone[27] receptors have been raised. These antibodies are clinically important because they provide an immunochemical method for determining the number of estrogen and progesterone receptors present in human breast cancer, and thus they help to predict the response of mammary tumors to various ablative procedures.[28, 29]

Aldosterone receptors are 4-S proteins that have been identified in the kidneys, bladder, gut, and parotid glands.[22] They bind both glucocorticoids and mineralocorticoids, in proportion to their natriuretic action. For example, mineralocorticoids bind with high specificity at physiologic concentrations, where glucocorticoids bind less specifically and require greater concentrations for binding.[21, 22]

At present, little is known about the nature of receptors, and most of the current available knowledge concerns progesterone receptors. In experiments using "hybrid" chromatin, O'Malley and colleagues[30, 31] showed that the progesterone receptor consists of two subunits. The B-subunit serves to bind the receptor to DNA, recognizing specific sites determined by the acidic non-histone proteins. The A-subunit can bind to DNA in a non-specific fashion, but its main function is to initiate DNA transcription. In order for this sequence to occur, some communication must occur between the B- and A-subunits, but this has not yet been delineated.[30, 31]

The binding of the hormone-receptor complex to chromatin results in modulation of gene expression. In most instances, this binding initiates synthesis of a specific mRNA, which in turn leads to synthesis of the specific proteins, expressing the action of the hormone.[30] For example, glucocorticoids initiate transcription of the specific mRNA required for the formation of tyrosine aminotransferase, glutamine synthetase, and other enzymes[30, 32] that carry out the biologic responses characteristic of these hormones. However, steroid binding does not always cause stimulation of mRNA synthesis. In certain situations, mRNA formation is suppressed by the hormone-receptor complex. For example, glucocorticoids inhibit the formation of the mRNA specific for corticotropin in pituitary cells, and thus are responsible for the negative feedback that occurs between steroids and ACTH.[33]

The exact mechanism by which the hormone-receptor complex affects mRNA synthesis remains unclear, but evidence suggests that it may exert its influence at several steps in the synthetic process. Alteration may occur at the level of transcription, when a high-molecular-weight precursor of mRNA is synthesized from a DNA template. It can also occur at the post-transcriptional level, when the precursor mRNA is changed to its mature form.[30, 35] This latter maturation process involves excision and rejoining of mRNA segments, followed by modification of both ends of the molecule. The mature mRNA enters the cytoplasm, where it directs the process of translation. By pairing with the anticodons of acylated transfer RNA at the ribosomes, it causes assembly of amino acids into the appropriate proteins.[30, 34] Currently, no experimental evidence exists to suggest that the hormone-receptor complex affects protein synthesis at the post-translational level, i.e., at the steps of peptide bond cleavage, glycosylation, phosphorylation, and folding of the processed polypeptide chains.

THYROID HORMONE ACTIONS

Thyroxine (T_4) represents more than 80 per cent of the circulating iodothyronines. The remaining 20 per cent consists of nearly equal amounts of triiodothyronine (T_3) and reverse T_3 (rT_3), with very small amounts of monoiodotyrosine (MIT) and diiodotyrosine (DIT) detected in the circulation.[35] Eighty per cent of circulating T_3 and 90 per cent of reverse T_3 result from the deiodination of T_4 in extrathyroidal tissues such as in the liver

and kidney.[36] Like steroid hormones, most of the thyroid hormones are bound to protein carriers. Seventy per cent bind to thyroxin-binding globulin (TBG), 20 per cent to albumin, and the rest to thyroxin-binding prealbumin.[35]

Free hormone enters the cell by diffusion, and once in the cytoplasm, most of T_4 is converted to the more active T_3 by an NADP-linked deiodinase.[35] In contrast to steroid hormones, thyroid hormones do not require cytoplasmic receptors for translocation to the nucleus. Instead, T_3 binds directly to high-affinity, low-capacity receptors in the nucleus that have been identified as nonhistone, acidic chromatin proteins.[37–39] High concentrations of these nuclear protein receptors are found in various thyroid responsive tissues, such as the liver, kidney, and pituitary gland, whereas low concentrations are found in unresponsive tissues, such as the spleen and testis.[37] Thyroid receptors have also been identified on the cell plasma membrane and on inner mitochondrial membranes. Binding of thyroxin to its plasma membrane receptors leads to an acceleration of amino acid transport.[38] The function of mitochondrial receptors is not clear. They might, however, play a role in electron transport into the mitochondria and ATP synthesis.[40]

The mechanism by which nuclear binding of T_3 alters mRNA and protein synthesis is still under investigation. T_3 binding may affect RNA polymerase, thus altering transcription, or it may influence certain post-transcriptional steps.[37, 38] Like steroids, T_3 must be continuously present to elicit a biologic response.[38] For example, the stimulatory effect on oxygen consumption varies directly with circulating hormone concentration. It increases markedly in hyperthyroid states and is abnormally low in hypothyroidism.[41] Part of this calorigenic response has been ascribed to enhanced synthesis and activity of the Na^+-K^+-ATPase. This osmotic pump consumes ATP in order to maintain intracellular sodium homeostasis[42, 43] and thus may generate a significant portion of the thyroid hormone's calorigenic effects.

The actions of thyroid hormones vary both with species and with tissue type. In certain species, including humans, T_3 stimulates synthesis of the mRNA specific for the mitochondrial enzyme α-glycerol dehydrogenase (α-GPD) and its cytosolic counterpart, malic enzyme, both of which are important in free fatty acid synthesis. α-GPD can be used as an indicator of thyroid function because, like oxygen consumption, α-GPD concentration varies directly with the amount of circulating hormone.[37, 38] T_3 also stimulates the mRNA specific for alpha$_2$-macroglobulin synthesis by the liver and for growth hormone synthesis by the pituitary.[44] These actions of T_3 are produced synergistically with cortisol and androgens, illustrating the point that, *in vivo*, cells respond to a mixture of environmental stimuli.

PEPTIDE HORMONE ACTIONS

Hormone-Receptor Interactions

The search for peptide hormone target sites is an area of biology that keeps generating much interest and effort. The most important methodologic advance in this field has been the use of radioactively labeled hormones to locate receptors.[45-47] Receptors for polypeptide hormones, growth factors, and a variety of naturally occurring ligands are now known to be an integral part of the plasma membranes of hormone-sensitive cells. The description of these receptors, however, remains operational, resting on the functional characteristics of hormone binding.[46-48] These characteristics include the degree of specificity and affinity for the corresponding hormone, the saturability of the receptors, and the rapidity with which binding is reversed.

Receptor Specificity

Receptors are defined first by their biologic and structural specificity. Specificity can be studied using the labeled hormone and its natural analogues or chemically modified derivatives. It is measured by the degree of displacement of the labeled hormone bound to its receptors when varying concentrations of the corresponding unlabeled hormone are added. At high and nonphysiologic concentrations of the hormone, the residual radioactivity that remains associated with the receptor is considered a measure of "nonspecific" binding. Specific binding is determined by substracting "nonspecific" binding from total binding. Thus, at physiologic concentrations of unlabeled hormones, the higher the specific binding, the higher the sensitivity of the receptor for the hormone.[46-50] Natural antibodies to insulin receptors have been identified in certain patients with a rare dis-

ease characterized by insulin resistance and acanthosis nigricans.[51, 52] These antibodies have provided an important tool for probing the insulin receptor's biologic specificity and structure.[48]

Studies of human lymphocytes in culture indicate that insulin receptors may be localized to specialized areas on the cell surface called "coated pits."[53] These invaginations of the plasma membrane provide an excellent example of the structural specificity that is undoubtedly very important in hormone-receptor action.

Hormone Regulation of Receptor Affinity: The Concept of Negative Cooperativity

The quantitative aspects of hormone-receptor interactions are complex and subject to controversy. Early observations on receptor affinity and number, made in both experimental animals and humans, suggested that hormone-receptor binding was a simple and reversible bimolecular reaction.[48, 54-57] Hormones would interact with a specific target site on sensitive cells to form a transient hormone-receptor complex (H-R). This complex would soon dissociate, releasing both the hormone (H) and its receptor (R):

$$(H) + (R) \rightarrow (H\text{-}R) \rightarrow (H) + (R).$$

Many of the early studies, however, were conducted at unphysiologically low temperatures (24°C) and may not represent *in vivo* conditions. More recent work, especially by DeMeyts and colleagues[58] on the reversibility of hormone-receptor binding at 37°C, indicates that the process is more complex. These investigators found that the addition of unlabeled insulin accelerated the rate of dissociation of labeled hormone from its receptor (see Fig. 2–2).[57] Furthermore, increasing the concentration of the labeled hormone during the incubation period also accelerated subsequent dissociation in a dose-dependent manner.[59-61] They suggest that an initial rapid phase of dissociation occurs, followed by a more prolonged phase during which there is incomplete reversal of the hormone-receptor complex. This slower phase of dissociation would result from the receptors undergoing conformational changes, such that binding of the ligand becomes tighter.[58, 62] These conformational changes are caused by the interaction of the hormone with the receptor and thus provide

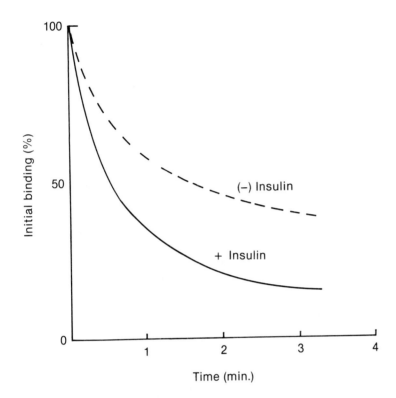

Figure 2–2. Representative rate of dissociation of ¹²⁵I-labeled insulin from isolated cells (e.g., adipocytes, hepatocytes, endothelial cells). The solid line represents rate of dissociation in the presence of insulin, and the dotted line represents the rate of dissociation in the presence of buffer alone.

a mechanism by which the ligand can regulate its own receptors.[50, 54] Hence, in the presence of excess hormone, rapid dissociation occurs. As the concentration of the hormone decreases, binding to the receptor becomes tighter. This form of interaction between the receptor and its hormone has been termed *negative cooperativity*.[58] DeMeyts and colleagues[62] were subsequently able to partially identify the region of the insulin molecule responsible for this cooperative effect. They accomplished this goal through the use of more than 20 naturally occurring analogues of the hormone. This site is distinct from both the sites responsible for hormone-receptor binding and those responsible for biologic potency.[62] These experiments offered the first explanation for the nonlinear Scatchard plots customarily obtained from the study of different hormones.[63] They indicated that the nonlinear plot does not necessarily result from multiple classes of receptors, but instead might result from a dose-dependent change with affinity of the individual receptors for insulin.

The precise mechanism by which negative cooperativity occurs is still not well understood. Recently, Ginsberg and associates[64] and Olefsky and colleagues[65] accumulated evidence that implicates site-site interactions in this phenomenon. Their data

imply that information is transmitted from one receptor to another via chemical mediators. These substances are released in the plasma membrane as a result of the interaction between hormone and receptor; this interaction would modulate subsequent dissociation rates. This situation is consistent with the "floating-receptor" hypothesis.[66–68] Other investigators suggest that the insulin molecule contains several moieties capable of binding to two distinct subsites on the insulin receptor. This multiple binding would cause more of the labeled ligand to dissociate.[59, 63]

Although it has been best investigated for insulin,[69–71] negative cooperativity has been claimed for a number of other receptor systems, including those for thyrotropin-releasing hormone, beta-adrenergic substances,[72] epidermal growth factor, and nerve growth factor.[59, 73] Even the binding of lectins and leukoagglutinins to lymphocytes[74, 75] and the binding of thrombin to platelets[76] may exhibit negative cooperativity.

The negative cooperativity model, however, is not yet universally accepted. It remains a controversial and thoroughly investigated concept. Critics of the model claim that the demonstration of enhanced dissociation rate of labeled hormone in the presence of excess unlabeled hormone is not definite proof. Many situations have been described in which enhanced dissociation of ligand from its receptor occurs without evidence of negative cooperativity.[77] For example, the dissociation of ^{125}I-TSH to cultured thyroid cells gives a linear Scatchard plot (i.e., no negative cooperativity), yet it is markedly enhanced by increasing concentrations of unlabeled TSH.[77] Moreover, negative cooperativity has been described for many inert substances.[65, 78, 79] For example, insulin stimulates the dissociation of ^{125}I bound to talc.[78]

Although the negative cooperativity theory has opponents, the interest and research it continues to stimulate furthers our understanding of the structure-activity relationships of different polypeptide hormones, particularly that of insulin.

Hormone Regulation of Receptor Number: Down-Regulation and Up-Regulation

A more chronic form of negative cooperativity has been described for insulin, growth hormone, thyrotropin-releasing hormones, gonadotropins, glucagon, and catecholamines. Termed *down-regulation*, this process involves an inverse relationship between hormone concentration and total receptor number, not affinity. This finding indicates that receptors are not static but instead are dynamic molecules whose concentration and affinity can be regulated by many factors.

The chronic regulation of insulin receptors has been the most extensively studied. Roth and co-workers[46] and Kahn and associates[80] accumulated *in vivo* and *in vitro* evidence showing that obesity, which is frequently associated with hyperinsulinemia, is characterized by a decrease in the number of insulin receptors on all cells. Weight reduction results in an improvement of glucose tolerance, a reversal to a euinsulinemic state, and an increase to normal levels in the number of cell receptors for insulin (*up-regulation*).[46, 80, 89] Similarly, more recent studies demonstrated an increased number of insulin receptors on hepatocytes from diabetic rats.[82] An increase in insulin binding and in its ability to stimulate glucose transport and metabolism in isolated soleus muscle preparations has also been described in streptozocin diabetes.[83]

Studies utilizing antibodies against insulin receptors have identified two subgroups of patients with insulin resistance and acanthosis nigricans.[84] The type A syndrome described in a group of young females is characterized by a marked decrease in the number of receptors.[48, 84] In the second subgroup, or type B syndrome, patients present with evidence of other immunologic diseases, such as systemic lupus erythematosus and ataxia telangiectasia. The binding defect in this group is caused by a decrease in receptor affinity rather than by a change in receptor number.[48, 84] A generalized autoimmune defect causes this lower affinity, but the number and structure of insulin receptors remained normal. These studies and others demonstrate that certain antireceptor antibodies decrease the affinity of the hormone-receptor complex and others decrease the total number of receptors.

The functional significance of negative cooperativity, down-regulation, and up-regulation of receptors is the subject of considerable speculation. Changing the receptor number or affinity might have buffering effects on the hormone's action on sensitive cells. Thus, when less insulin is available, a compensatory increase in receptor number and affinity, without changes in specificity, would occur and would delay the subsequent deleterious effects of hormone absence. Conversely, the decreased receptor number found in the peripheral tissues of overweight individuals might blunt the effects of circulating hyperinsulinemia. The enhanced affinity of the hormone to its receptor, which occurs in the latter phase of dissociation (see Fig. 2–2), may represent a preliminary step in the internalization of the hormone-receptor complex. Once internalized, the complex might induce changes in DNA and RNA synthesis, which in turn cause the trophic effects of many hormones, especially insulin, and possibly stimulate the synthesis of more hormone receptors.

Concept of Spare Receptors

The full biologic effect of a certain hormone becomes manifest with only a small percentage of the receptors occupied. For example, less than one per cent of testicular Leydig cell receptors can elicit a maximal steroidogenic response.[85] This situation is analogous to that previously described by Stephenson in drug-responsive tissues.[86] He proposed that a maximal drug response can occur with only a small number of the total receptors occupied. These findings led other investigators to propose the concept of "spare receptors" for polypeptide hormones.[55, 87]

The biologic significance of spare receptors is not totally understood. Excess receptors might allow variation in the nature and degree of biologic response. For example, lipolysis is inhibited in isolated adipocytes with less than two per cent of insulin receptors occupied. The requirements for stimulation of glycolysis and glucose oxidation, however, are approximately two per cent and five per cent, respectively.[87, 88] In certain situations, however, almost complete receptor occupancy is required for maximal biologic effect, as is the case for insulin stimulation of amino acid transport into adipocytes[87, 88] and for ACTH effect on mineralocorticoid synthesis from isolated adrenal tissue.[89] Thus, when hormone receptors are abundant, as shown in Figure 2–3, any change in the number of receptors induces a change in hormone sensitivity without changing the maximal biologic response. When no "spare receptors" exist, any decrease in receptor number would diminish the maximal potential biologic response.

Internalization of the Hormone-Receptor Complex: Long-Term Effects of the Hormones

Generally, the mechanism by which most of polypeptide hormones function is based on the assumption that binding to a cell membrane receptor causes specific cellular events to occur. As previously discussed, at 37°C the formation of the hormone-receptor complex is followed first by a very rapid dissociation phase and then by slow and incomplete loss of the complex.[50, 90, 91] During the latter stage, two kinds of responses can be elicited. An acute short-term response, which does not depend on the magnitude of receptor occupancy, can occur. Examples of such a response are the known acute effects of insulin, stimulation of glucose into muscle and fat cells, inhibition of lipolysis, and promotion of glycogen storage and triacylglycerol synthesis. A more chronic response, which depends on the continued presence of the hormone-receptor complex and affects more general processes like cell growth and differentiation, can also occur. Evidence exists that the chronic re-

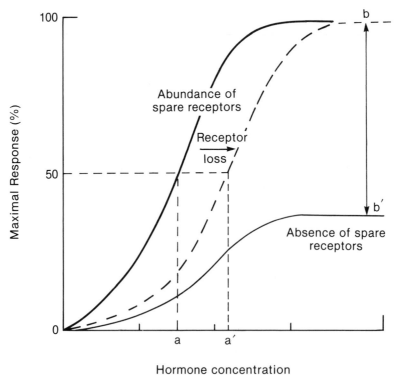

Figure 2–3. Biologic significance of spare receptors. When hormone receptors are abundant, any decrease in the receptor curve induces change in hormone sensitivity but not in the maximal hormone responsiveness. Under these conditions, more hormone is required to elicit the same responsiveness; e.g., more hormone is required to achieve 50 per cent maximal response (a' > a). In the absence of spare receptors, any decrease in receptor number diminishes the maximal biologic response (from b to b').

sponse requires internalization of the hormone-receptor complex, a process utilizing contractile elements in the cytoplasm and Golgi apparatus.

Investigation of the hormone-receptor internalization process has concerned ferritin-LDL in human fibroblasts[92] and ferritin-EGF in A-431 cells.[93] Indirect evidence for internalization of insulin receptor complex has been produced in many cell systems.[94–97] For example, specific binding sites for insulin have been identified on the smooth and rough endoplasmic reticulum,[98] the Golgi fractions,[99] and nucleic membranes.[100] Internalization and intracellular organelle binding have been demonstrated for several other polypeptides, including epidermal growth factor, nerve growth factor, growth hormone, prolactin, parathyroid hormone, gonadotropins, and thyrotropins.[93, 99–104] Many of these hormones are similar in their mechanism of action, eliciting both rapid and delayed responses in sensitive cells.

Epidermal growth factor (EGF), a 5000–molecular weight protein produced by the submaxillary glands of the mouse, deserves special mention. It is a potent mitogen in a number of cell systems. Recently, receptors for EGF have been identified in lysosomes[105] and isolated nuclei.[106] EGF has been shown to enter rat pituitary cells and accumulate in the nuclei, suggesting that EGF might mediate certain actions of these cells.[106] Nerve growth factor (NGF), a 26,500–molecular weight protein, is necessary for the development and maturation of the sympathetic nervous system and sensory ganglia. It has both rapid and delayed effects and has been found to act at intracellular sites.[106, 107] Recent observations indicate that NGF induces migration of its receptors from the cell surface to the nucleus.[108–110] In contrast to insulin, NGF, and EGF, growth hormone, and prolactin have only long-term effects that require protein and RNA synthesis for expression. Evidence indicates that the action of these latter hormones is mediated by internalization of hormone-receptor complexes.

The "Second Messenger" Theory: Acute Effects of Hormones

The acute effects of polypeptide hormones, as already mentioned, are not mediated by internalization of the hormone-receptor complex. The mechanism by which signals are transmitted from the cell membrane to intracellular sites, however, is poorly understood. Several polypeptide hormones, such as glucagon, ACTH, and thyrotropin, activate the adenylate cyclase enzyme complex found in the plasma membrane of target cells. This activation generates the intracellular second messenger, cyclic AMP (cAMP), which then elicits many of the actions of these hormones.[111, 112] Other hormones, such as the catecholamines, cholecystokinins, and angiotensins, alter the distribution of free intracellular calcium. This alteration then induces various intracellular responses.[113] Still other polypeptides, including growth hormone, prolactin, and insulin, appear to utilize neither cAMP nor calcium as second messenger, and the mechanism by which they effect acute responses remains poorly understood.

Activation of Adenylate Cyclase

Of hormone-receptor effector systems investigated, that of glucagon has provided the most information. Studies show that the adenylate cyclase of the glucagon system is located at or near the intracellular surface of the plasma membrane. This enzyme is magnesium-dependent, is inhibited by calcium, and is stimulated by fluoride in addition to glucagon.[104] Lefkowitz and colleagues recently observed that beta-adrenergic receptors exert their effect on this adenylate cyclase in a fashion similar to that of glucagon.[115] Recently, the mechanism by which the occupied receptor communicates with adenylate cyclase has been investigated. Some theories propose that the hormone-receptor complex induces phosphorylation of a plasma membrane kinase, which then activates the adenylate cyclase.[116] Little experimental evidence supports this theory; however, if the theory is true, the process is analogous to the events leading to glycogenolysis in the liver: Glucagon stimulates adenylate cyclase, which then leads to a series of phosphorylations.[117]

Bennett and colleagues,[118] on the other hand, suggest that adenylate cyclase activation depends on the fluidity of plasma membrane. These investigators showed that cholera toxin stimulates the adenylate cyclase system like glucagon.[118] They also found that these effects were not prevented by inhibitors of protein synthesis; however, they were temperature dependent, suggesting they occurred only when the plasma membrane lipids were in a fluid state, allowing fast lateral diffusion.[118–120] This theory predicts that hormones must form a specific hormone-receptor complex, which diffuses laterally along the cell membrane until it physically connects with the catalytic subunit of adenylate cyclase. While only speculative, this "mobile receptor" hypothesis is simple and explains many of the poorly understood features of the glucagon-receptor and beta-adrenergic–receptor adenylate cyclase systems. It also accounts for a large number of spare receptors present when only a small number is required to elicit a response. For example, it is known that the receptor number on the cell membrane is at least 100 to 1000 times that of adenylate cyclase units. Because of their mobility, only a small percentage of these receptors need to be occupied in order to elicit a response. Moreover, this theory explains how more than one polypeptide hormone can activate the same adenylate cyclase system.

The current theory of adenylate cyclase activation involves regulatory proteins that are present on both the receptor and the adenylate cyclase complex and that can bind guanine nucleotides. Using beta-adrenergic agonists, Lefkowitz and colleagues showed that formation of the agonist-receptor complex causes conformational changes in the receptor (R), which lead to transient binding of a nucleotide regulatory protein (N) (Fig. 2–4). When guanine nucleotide diphosphate (GDP) is bound to N, the hormone, receptor regulatory protein complex (H-R-N), is in a high-affinity state.[115, 120, 121] However, when the H-R-N complex reacts with guanine nucleotide triphosphate (GTP), it reverts to a low-affinity state.[115] Thus the transformation of the H-R-N complex from a low- to a high-affinity state is regulated by the presence of GTP.

In contrast, when the regulatory subunit of the adenylate cyclase binds GTP, the enzyme changes from inactive to active form. The active adenylate cyclase complex is then capable of converting ATP to AMP.[115] Adenylate cyclase is deactivated when GTP is cleaved to GDP by GTPase enzyme, which is tightly bound to the regulatory protein of the enzyme.[122] This model might account for the marked stimulation of adenylate cyclase by cholera toxin.[118, 120] Cholera toxins are known to inhibit the GTPase activity of the nucleotide regulatory protein.[115] A similar model for GTP-dependent activation of glucagon-sensitive adenylate cyclase was previ-

ously demonstrated by Rodbell.[123, 124] Thus, GTP is the physiologic regulator of the cyclase. Present evidence indicates that various hormones modulate the action of GTP by affecting the speed with which it is bound or released from the regulatory subunit of the adenylate cyclase enzyme.[115, 123, 124]

cAMP-Dependent Protein Kinase
(see Figure 2–4)

The discovery of cyclic AMP was a historic event in the understanding of hormone action. While investigating how epinephrine stimulates glycogenolysis in hepatocytes, Sutherland and Rall[111, 112] identified a heat-stable compound that was generated when ATP and magnesium ions were added to liver fractions treated with epinephrine. This substance was later identified to be 3',5' cyclic adenosine monophosphate (cAMP). The enzyme catalyzing the formation of AMP was later found to be adenylate cyclase. Subsequent studies showed that another enzyme, phosphodiesterase, inactivates cAMP by converting it to 5' AMP (see Fig. 2–3).

The second messenger, cAMP, has been shown to function in many cell systems. It is involved in the action of glucagon, beta-adrenergic hormones, PTH, antidiuretic hormone (ADH), calcitonin, luteinizing hormones, ACTH, lipotropin, prostaglandins, TSH, melanocyte-stimulating hormone (MSH), and follicle-stimulating hormone (FSH). All these hormones act in acute ways by promoting intracellular cyclic AMP accumulation, which leads the activation of cAMP-dependent protein kinases. Like cAMP, these enzymes are present in all eukaryocytes and act by phosphorylating (transferring a phosphate group from ATP to a serine or threonine residue) various protein substrates.[125] The phosphorylated protein retains some of the high energy of the nucleoside triphosphate bond.

Besides functioning as mediators of cAMP action, protein kinases mediate the effect of many other molecules, such as calcium, heme, and cyclic guanine nucleotides. These regulatory functions imply that protein kinases possess certain structural, thermodynamic, and kinetic properties.

Protein kinases have two structural domains: a regulatory domain and a catalytic domain. Each of these domains is divided into two subunits.[126–128] Two distinct cAMP-dependent protein kinases have been iden-

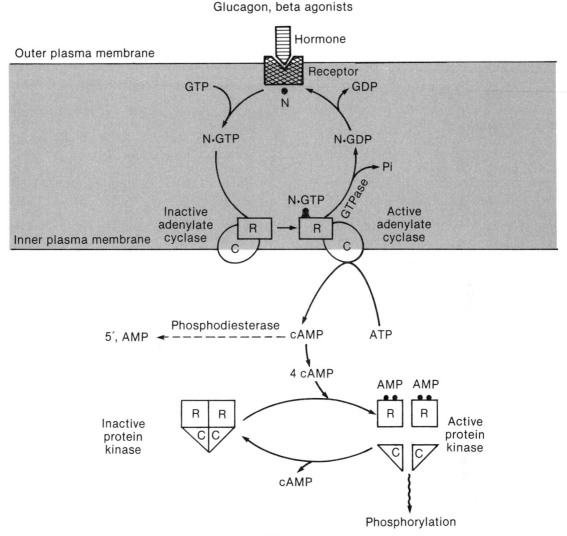

Figure 2–4. Activation of adenylate cyclase and AMP-dependent protein kinase by glucagon or beta-adrenergic agonist. GTP, guanine nucleotide triphosphate; GDP, guanine nucleotide diphosphate; N, nucleotide regulatory protein; ATP, adenosine triphosphate; R, regulatory subunit; C, catalytic subunit.

tified, type I and type II.[129] These isoenzymes vary with both species and tissue. The catalytic subunits are similar, with molecular weights of 39,000 to 42,000, but the regulatory subunits differ. Type I kinases have regulatory subunits of 49,000 molecular weight, and type II kinases have subunits of 54,000 to 56,000 molecular weight.[129] In both types, the regulatory subunit contains discrete regions having two distinct binding sites for cAMP.[128] Although the functional significance of duplicate binding sites remains unclear, recent observations suggest cooperativity between the two sites; it appears that site 2 must be occupied if activation of the catalytic subunit is to occur.

In the absence of cAMP, the regulatory and catalytic subunits have a high affinity for each other. Because regulatory subunits inhibit the action of the catalytic subunits, protein kinases are inactive when cAMP is not bound.[129, 130] The formation of cAMP leads to activation of the protein kinases. Present evidence indicates that when two moles of cAMP bind to each of the two regulatory subunits of protein kinases, a transient ternary nucleotide is formed on the holoenzyme. This new enzyme complex subsequently dissociates, yielding the active form of protein kinase.[129, 130, 131] This activated enzyme can now catalyze the transfer of a phosphate group.

Protein kinase activity has been measured in several crude tissue extracts after treatment of these tissues or of the animal with various hormones and substrates.[132–135] Activity is measured in the presence and absence of cAMP, yielding a protein kinase activity ratio (activity minus cAMP divided by activity plus cAMP). Although these measurements have several pitfalls,[135] they provide quantitative and qualitative information regarding cAMP activity under various hormonal conditions *in vivo*. In addition, these measurements allow investigation of non–cAMP-dependent mechanisms of protein kinase regulation. For example, they have helped to demonstrate that cAMP does not mediate alpha-agonist effects in the liver.[136] This demonstration led to the discovery of cAMP-independent protein kinase, which exists side by side with cAMP-dependent enzyme and functions similarly to catalyze the transfer of phosphate groups.

cGMP-Dependent Protein Kinase

Protein kinases that are dependent on cyclic GMP (cGMP) have been identified in many mammalian and invertebrate tissues.

The regulation of these enzymes differs from that of cAMP-dependent protein kinases. Although both types of kinases demonstrate similar substrate specificity, phosphorylation occurs 10 to 15 times faster when catalyzed by a cAMP-dependent kinase.[137, 138] Combined with the fact that levels of both types of protein kinases in the cells are low, these observations led Lincoln and Corbin[136] to propose that the cGMP-dependent kinase has limited functional significance.

Activated protein kinases induce a series of phosphorylation-dephosphorylation reactions that lead to changes in cell function, stimulating some processes and inhibiting others.[138] This type of regulation was first shown for skeletal muscle glycogen metabolism. Fisher and Krebs[139] showed that the conversions of phosphorylase kinase b (inactive form) to phosphorylase kinase a (active form) and of phosphorylase b (inactive form) to phosphorylase a (active form) were achieved by a cAMP-stimulated phosphorylation, as shown in Figure 2–5. Since this discovery, protein phosphorylation has been implicated in the regulation of many cellular functions, including glycogenolysis, gluconeogenesis, and amino acid and lipid metabolism.[140] Other functions mediated by

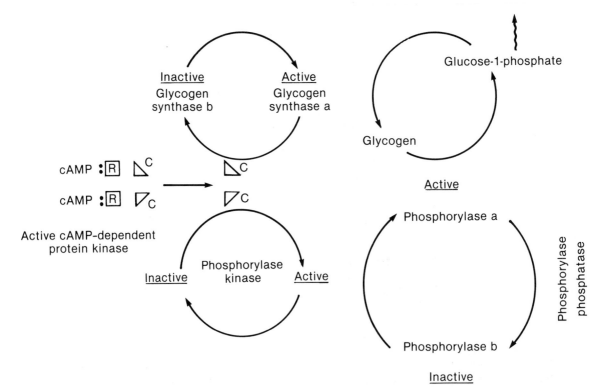

Figure 2–5. Phosphorylation-dephosphorylation reactions responsible for muscle glycogen breakdown leading to formation of glucose-1-phosphate.

phosphorylation include membrane transport,[141, 142] protein synthesis,[143] muscle cell contraction,[141] regulation of acetylcholine receptors, gene expression, viral cell transformation, and brain function.[142]

Phosphoprotein Phosphatases

The discovery of many of the hormone-induced cell processes mediated by cAMP-activated protein kinases led to an interest in several phosphoprotein phosphatases. These phosphatases function to dephosphorylate the enzymes and proteins acted on by the cAMP-dependent protein kinases[144] as follows:

$$ATP + Mg^{++} + protein \xrightarrow{\text{protein kinase}}$$
$$Protein = P + ADP = Mg^{++}$$

$$Protein = P + H_2O \xrightarrow{\text{phosphatase}} Protein + Pi$$

Several of these phosphatases have been isolated from hepatocytes, including the phosphoprotein phosphatases, which dephosphorylate glycogen synthase b, phosphorylase a, activated phosphorylase kinase b, phosphorylated histones, and others.[144–146] These enzymes, with molecular weights of 35,000 to 200,000, also consist of two subunits, catalytic and regulatory, and are under hormonal regulation.[114]

Other Second Messengers (Fig. 2–6)

By employing adrenergic agonists, Ahlquist[147] demonstrated two types of adrenergic receptors, subsequently identified as alpha and beta receptors. In some tissues, the physiologic responses to these receptors differ, whereas in others they are the same.

Beta receptors have been further subdivided into beta$_1$ receptors, which affect primarily the heart and fat cells, and beta$_2$ receptors, which affect both the bronchi and blood vessels.[148] The biologic effects of beta receptors are mediated through stimulation of adenylate cyclase, which subsequently increases intracellular cAMP. This increase in turn stimulates the cAMP-dependent protein kinase[117, 121] in a fashion similar to that already described for glucagon.

Alpha receptors are also subdivided into two populations. The alpha$_1$ receptors are located on target cells, and the presynaptic alpha$_2$ receptors are present on the sympathetic nerve endings.[149] In most tissues, the cellular location of these receptors has not been well identified. Present evidence, however, indicates that alpha$_1$ receptors mediate most alpha-adrenergic responses, whereas alpha$_2$ receptors cause feedback inhibition of catecholamine secretion.[149] The mechanism by which alpha-adrenergic responses are effected is not very clear. Generally, these responses are not mediated by changes in cAMP. However, alpha-agonists, as shown by Chan and Exton,[150] Jakobs and colleagues[151] and Cherrington and colleagues[152] can inhibit, stimulate, or have an effect on cAMP production. This is largely a function of the tissue studied but also may depend on the study conditions.

No substantial evidence implicates cGMP as a mediator of alpha-adrenergic response. Although earlier studies indicated that alpha$_1$-adrenergic effects in parotid glands, muscle, and platelets were caused by an increase in cGMP,[153] further work showed that these effects were actually mediated by an increase in intracellular calcium.[154, 155] This finding was supported by the fact that the actions of alpha$_1$ agonists could reproduce calcium ions and the ionophore A23187,[156] and that alpha$_1$-adrenergic effects could be inhibited by the calcium chelator EDTA.[157, 158]

Alpha$_1$-adrenergic receptors increase intracellular calcium concentration by two mechanisms. They stimulate the influx of extracellular Ca^{++} by opening plasma membrane "gates," and they increase the release of calcium from intracellular stores. For example, in the liver, calcium is released from mitochondrial stores during alpha-adrenergic stimulation of glycogenolysis.[60, 160] Calcium stores in the sarcoplasmic reticulum are mobilized when smooth muscle is induced to contract under the influence of alpha$_1$ agonists.[156, 161] In both situations, increased cytosolic Ca^{++} induces the biologic response. On the basis of such observations, Exton postulated that a second messenger is not necessary to mediate alpha-adrenergic effects, because the alpha$_1$ receptor can be directly linked to Ca^{++} "gates" in the plasma membrane.[162]

Jones and Michell[163] and Kirk and colleagues[164] recently established an association between alpha-adrenergic stimulation and phosphatidylinositol breakdown in parotid glands, platelets, and other tissues. Subsequently, it was proposed that enhanced Ca^{++} release stimulates a calcium-sensitive

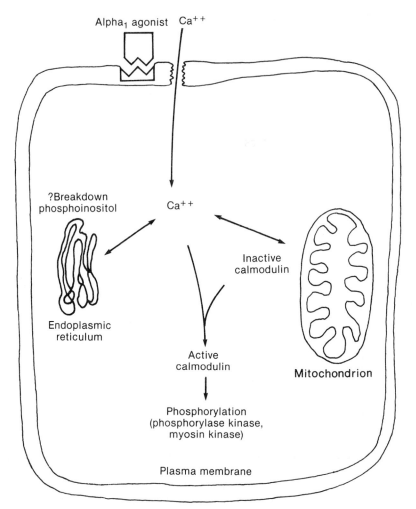

Figure 2–6. Alpha$_1$-agonist–mediated cellular response. Cytoplasmic calcium levels increase as a result of increased influx of calcium from extracellular sources and extrusion from endoplasmic reticulum and mitochondrial sources. Intracellular calcium activates inactive calmodulin, causing phosphorylation of enzymes similar to that shown in Figure 2–5.

plasma membrane enzyme that catalyzes the breakdown of membrane phosphatidylinositol and formation of di- and tri-phosphoinositides.[164] In turn, such processes would alter membrane permeability, allowing greater influx of calcium and other ions and thus accentuating biologic effects of alpha agonists.[163, 164]

Calmodulin

If calcium is to function as a mediator of hormone action, the cell must be able to regulate its concentration of this ion. The free cytosolic concentration of Ca^{++} is at least 100,000-fold lower than the extracellular concentration (1 mM). A number of mechanisms exist for maintaining intracellular homeostasis despite active and passive Ca^{++} entry; these have recently been summarized for the myocardial cell by Braunwald.[165] Cellular membranes have specialized enzyme systems that can return cytosolic Ca^{++} to the extracellular space or sequester it in internal storage compartments. These include the energy-dependent, membrane-bound Ca^{++} ATPases and the non–energy-dependent Na^+-Ca^{++} exchange system. Necessary for the function of these enzymes and for the maintenance of nanomolar calcium concentrations is the calcium-binding protein calmodulin, which has been found in most animal and plant tissues studied.[166] Calmodulin is a heat stable molecule with a molecular weight of approximately 17,000.

Calcium-Calmodulin Binding

The ability of calmodulin to bind to calcium was first recognized by Teo and Wang.[167] Calmodulin binds Ca^{++} at four distinct sites. One of these sites is specific for Ca^{++}; the others can bind Mg^{++}, Mn^{++}, Sr^{++}, Co^{++}, and K^+, although with less affinity than Ca^{++}.[166-169] The binding of calcium to calmodulin triggers conformational changes in the protein.[166] These changes allow the formation of one-to-one stoichiometric complexes with various cellular enzymes controlled by calmodulin, such as phosphorylase kinase, cyclic nucleotide phosphodiesterases, adenylate cyclase, myosin light-chain kinases, and ATPases.[167-169] The continued presence of calcium is needed to maintain this interaction. The presence of Ca^{++} chelators, such as EDTA[170] and the phenothiazines, inhibits the interaction between calmodulin and these enzymes.[171]

The initiation of smooth muscle contraction and platelet aggregation are among calmodulin's major functions.[141] The calmodulin-Ca^{++} complex activates actomyosin ATPase, which generates the ATP needed for contractile activity. Calmodulin-Ca^{++} also activates myosin kinase by catalyzing the transfer of phosphate (Pi) from ATP.[141] Pi in turn phosphorylates a light chain of myosin, which permits interaction with actin and leads to contraction of the muscle cell or to platelet aggregation.[141, 172]

In addition to its roles in muscle contractility and platelet aggregation, calcium-bound calmodulin has an important role in regulating the cytoskeleton, a network of elements important in all aspects of cell movement.[173] During mitosis, calmodulin associates with the polar regions of the spindle fiber apparatus, causing micro-assembly of microtubules.[174] Microtubular elements are responsible for flagellar and ciliary motility and chromosomal movement.[175] Calmodulin interaction with these elements enhances actin binding and facilitates microtubular contractility.[175]

Other functions of calmodulin include stimulation of Ca^{++}-dependent phosphodiesterase, the soluble enzyme that hydrolyzes both cAMP and cGMP.[176] In some cell types, like those of the brain, adrenal medulla, and pancreatic islets, calmodulin also stimulates adenylate cyclase. Recent studies demonstrate that calmodulin exerts this latter effect at the catalytic subunit of adenylate cyclase.[177]

Calmodulin-Dependent Phosphorylation-Dephosphorylation

Calmodulin regulates the activities of enzymes that are also controlled by cAMP-dependent protein kinase. Calmodulin has been shown to regulate directly three kinases—myosin, phosphorylase, and glycogen synthase kinases.[178] The most important of calmodulin's roles, however, is in mediating calcium-dependent regulation of the enzyme phosphorylase kinase in muscle.[179] This enzyme, whether activated by calcium-calmodulin binding or by cAMP, triggers a sequence of events that ultimately lead to glycogenolysis, as shown in Figure 2–4 for the liver. The glucose formed intracellularly equilibrates rapidly with the extracellular compartment; thus, the glucose formed from glycogen is released into the circulation. In muscle, the same sequence of reactions occur, except that this tissue lacks glucose-6-phosphatase, so any increase in glycogen breakdown will instead result in enhanced glycolysis.

Simultaneous with the activation of the phosphorylase b enzyme, cAMP-dependent protein kinase phosphorylates the active form of glycogen synthase to inactivate it (see Fig. 2–4).[180]

Other activities of calmodulin that may be shared by cAMP-dependent protein kinases include the release of arachidonic acid in platelets and the activation of calcium transport systems across membranes.[181] Wong and Cheung[181] have recently demonstrated a calmodulin-dependent, three-fold stimuation in the formation of arachidonic acid from phosphatidylcholine in platelets. This stimulation was due to activation of phospholipase A_2 in a calcium-dependent manner.[181] Studies on purified human erythrocyte Ca^{++}-ATPase system showed that lack of calmodulin deactivates the system and allows accumulation of calcium in the intracellular compartments.[182] Calmodulin and cAMP-dependent protein kinase can independently phosphorylate and activate Ca^{++}-ATPase enzymes in myocardial sarcoplasmic reticulum.[183] The same phenomenon was described for skeletal muscle sarcoplasmic reticulum.[184] The net result is internal sequestration of calcium and maintenance of free cytosolic calcium concentration at physiologic levels.

Among enzymes important in cellular function that are regulated by calmodulin is a calmodulin-dependent kinase that phosphorylates tyrosine and tryptophan hydroxylases, the rate-limiting enzymes for the synthesis of dopamine and serotonin, respectively.[185] The list also includes proteins Ia and Ib, two neuronal proteins that are usually clustered at presynaptic terminals of neurons and are responsible for enhanced neurotransmitter release.[186] In addition, recent observations have suggested that calmodulin and cAMP-dependent protein kinases can also independently modulate the number of muscarinic receptors on the synaptic membranes.[187]

The physiologic significance of many of the effects of calcium-activated calmodulin remains to be elucidated. By sharing many of the systems it regulates with cAMP, however, calmodulin seems to link the functions of the two main second messengers identified for polypeptide hormones, namely calcium and cAMP.

INSULIN

An important polypeptide hormone that does not appear to use calcium or cAMP as a second messenger is insulin. Since the discovery of insulin approximately 60 years ago, many investigators have devoted considerable effort in attempting to unravel the mechanism or mechanisms by which this hormone modulates target cell metabolism. The literature on this subject is vast and, in the absence of any generally acceptable hypothesis, tends to be rather confusing and conflicting.

Insulin has both short-term and long-term effects. The short-term effects can be observed a few minutes after the association of the hormone with the receptor. These include stimulation of glucose uptake into muscle and fat cells; inhibition of basal and stimulated lipolysis; inhibition of gluconeogenesis and stimulation of glycogen synthesis, which result in a net decrease in glucose release; and, last but not least, promoting of triglyceride formation. These events are usually accompanied by stimulation of Na^+-K^+-ATPase and acceleration of the flux of calcium and other cations. Changes in cyclic nucleotides also occur in some tissues. Long-term effects of insulin involve changes in protein synthesis and degradation, cell growth, replication, and differentiation.

The understanding of insulin's action has been one of the most confusing topics in hormone physiology. Many agents have been implicated, and several mechanisms have been proposed. For example, the observation that insulin causes diminution in the concentration of cAMP and a transient increase in cGMP in fat and liver cells has been offered as an explanation for insulin's action.[188] The changes in these cyclic nucleotides, however, are observed only when the cells are incubated with other hormones; they do not occur basally.[189] Moreover, insulin exerts no effects on the levels of cyclic nucleotides in muscle cells.[190] Calcium has been implicated as a key element in the action of insulin,[191] yet the available data suggest that insulin increases cytoplasmic calcium under certain conditions[192] and decreases it under other conditions.[193] Similarly, hydrogen peroxide has been proposed to act as a second messenger.[194]

The mechanism of insulin stimulation of glucose transport in fat cells has been the subject of much intensive research recently. The findings have been reproduced by different laboratories and are generally accepted. Interpretation of the data, however, is a matter of dispute. We will discuss the findings here briefly, because it is possible that they will help in the future to elucidate the mechanism of action of insulin on the many transport systems it activates. The first important observation in this connection was made by Seals and Jarrett.[195] They showed that plasma membranes isolated from fat cells pretreated with insulin possessed higher glucose transport activity.[196] This increase in activity was later shown to be due to an apparent increase in the number of glucose transporters in the membrane. Membranes from insulin-treated cells possessed more binding sites for the glucose transport inhibitor cytochalasin.[197] Cytochalasin binds specifically to the glucose transporter and can be thus used to quantitate it. Subsequently, Cushman and Wardzala[198] and Suzuki and Kono[199] found independently that as insulin increased the number of transporter molecules in the plasma membrane, it simultaneously decreased their number in an intracellular depot tentatively identified as the Golgi apparatus. This finding led to the formulation of the "translocation hypothesis" for insulin action on hexose transport. According to this theory, the transporter molecules are recycled between the plasma membrane and an intracellular depot. Insulin produces translocation of transporter molecules from this depot into the cell membrane. Translocation leads to an increase in glucose transport activity. When insulin levels decrease, the glucose transporters are returned to the intracellular compartment, possibly by endocytosis.

The mechanism by which insulin bound to its membrane receptor produces this translocation of transporter from the Golgi into the plasma membrane is not clear. The translocation theory is supported by an impressive amount of experimental evidence. It is still questioned, however, by some, notably Czech,[200, 201] who suggests that the apparent translocation of transporter could be a result of artifacts in membrane fractionation techniques.

Understanding of the insulin receptor complex has progressed rapidly over the past five years, as a result of refinement in affinity purification methodology[202] and development of affinity cross-linking procedures.[203] When these methods were combined with use of antibodies directed against insulin receptors,[48, 51, 52] new models for insulin receptors, which were directly linked to the biologic action of this hormone, were proposed.

Recently, Czech and colleagues[204, 205] proposed the receptor to be composed of a disulfide-linked heterotetramer (β-S-S-α)-S-S-(α-S-S-β), with each half of this complex composed of one alpha and one beta subunit linked by disulfide bonds. Reduction of the disulfide bond linking the two halves will not result in loss of function; however, reduction of the bonds connecting the alpha and beta subunits together will result in loss of receptor activity.[204, 205] More complex models have since been presented. Kasuga and colleagues[206–208] have recently observed that the addition of insulin to either whole cells or solubilized plasma membranes increases the extent of autophosphorylation of the receptor on a tyrosine residue. These authors raised the possibility that the receptor itself was a protein kinase. Using monoclonal antibodies against highly purified receptors to the insulin receptor, Roth and Cassel have most recently established that the highly purified insulin receptor preparation retained kinase activity, and that the beta subunit of the insulin receptor is phosphorylated by this kinase activity and has an ATP binding site.[209] In this fashion, insulin receptor is itself a kinase as well as a substrate for phosphorylation.

Combining the results described makes it possible to regard the insulin receptor as consisting of two subunits, an alpha subunit that binds insulin and a beta subunit that has a kinase activity. Autophosphorylation could then induce a cascade of activities resulting in the various effects of insulin. If true, this theory is analogous to that originally suggested by Benjamin and Singer[210] and later by Brownsey and colleagues.[211] These authors, however, surmised the existence of the plasma membrane–bound protein kinase on the inner surface of the membrane; the activation of the receptor with insulin would then result in kinase phosphorylation in a cascade fashion.[212] This model does not necessitate the existence of a second messenger to explain the mechanism of action of insulin on the target cell. By analogy, epidermal growth factor (EGF) receptor has also been found to be a protein kinase.[213, 214] In all these situations, however, this kinase activity of the receptor may not be sufficient to induce all the effects of the hormone on the target cell, a condition well-proven for EGF receptors.[214] Thus, it remains to be determined whether the kinase activity of the receptor is necessary and sufficient to account for all the biologic activities of insulin.

In 1979, Larner and colleagues[215] extracted a chemical mediator from hindlimb muscles of rats that was capable of eliciting three of the important functions of insulin—namely, inhibition of cAMP-dependent protein kinase, stimulation of glycogen synthase phosphoprotein phosphatase, and activation of pyruvate dehydrogenase. A similar mediator (molecular weight 1000 to 1500) was isolated by Jarett and colleagues[216] from adipocytes, skeletal muscle, and hepatoma cells. This peptide was capable of simulating insulin's action and phosphorylating the same protein substrates. Larner and colleagues[217] further proposed that the interaction of insulin with its receptor initiated rapid redistribution of membrane phospholipids from the outer to the inner layer of plasma membrane, thus creating pores. The pores allow interaction between the insulin-receptor complex and oligopeptide molecules present on the inner surface of the membrane, resulting in rapid internalization of the oligopeptides in free form in the cytoplasm.[217] The model also proposed subsequent recycling of the peptide via lysosomes and Golgi apparatus and back to the cell membrane, thus restoring the membrane's composition and function.[217]

Czech[200] has further extended the concepts of Jarett and Larner and colleagues by proposing that insulin binding to the membrane receptor results in activation of membrane-bound protease enzyme, which releases a small (2000 molecular weight) hydrophilic peptide that acts as a mediator of one or more enzymes. Such mediators would also be formed when the receptor binds to anti-insulin receptor antibody. These mediators have been found to stimulate pyruvate dehydrogenase[200] or even calcium uptake[218] when added to mitochondria. They also stimulate glycogen synthase when added to cell suspensions and stimulate RNA synthesis when added to isolated nuclei.[218] Implicit in the understanding of this and other models is the assumption of the existence of different chemical mediators that phosphorylate different enzyme systems, or the presence of a cascade pattern of phosphorylation reactions identical to those described for cAMP-dependent protein kinases. The full scientific acceptance of these models awaits time and further investigation.

REFERENCES

1. Giugliano, D., Torella, R., and D'Onofrio, F.: Prostaglandins and the alpha cell. Prostaglandins Med., 6:283–297, 1981.
2. Robertson, R. P.: Prostaglandins as modulators of pancreatic islet function. Diabetes, 28:943–948, 1979.
3. Habener, J. F., and Potts, J. T., Jr.: Biosynthesis of parathyroid hormone. N. Engl. J. Med., 299:580–585, 1978.
4. Dorner, A. J., and Kemper, B.: Conversion of pre-parathyroid hormone to proparathyroid hormone by dog pancreatic microsomes. Biochemistry, 17:5550–5555, 1978.
5. Habener, J. F., Potts, J. T., Jr., and Rich, A.: Pre-proparathyroid hormone: Evidence for an early biosynthetic precursor of proparathyroid hormone. J. Biol. Chem., 251:3893–3899, 1976.
6. Shields, D., and Blobel, G.: Cell-free synthesis of fish preproinsulin, and processing by heterologous mammalian microsomal membranes. Proc. Natl. Acad. Sci. U.S.A., 74:2059–2063, 1977.
7. Jackson, R. C., and Blobel, G.: Post-translational cleavage of presecretory proteins with an extract of rough microsomes from dog pancreas containing signal peptidase activity. Proc. Natl. Acad. Sci. U.S.A., 74:5598–5602, 1977.
8. Gerich, J. E., Karam, J. H., and Forsham, P. H.: Stimulation of glucagon secretion by epinephrine in man. J. Clin. Endocrinol. Metab., 37:479–481, 1973.
9. Rizza, R. A., Cryer, P. E., Haymond, M. W., and Gerich, J. E.: Adrenergic mechanisms for the effects of epinephrine on glucose production and clearance in man. J. Clin. Invest., 65:682–689, 1980.
10. Altszuler, N., Steele, R., Rathgeb, I., et al.: Glucose metabolism and plasma insulin level during epinephrine infusion in the dog. Am. J. Physiol., 212:677–682, 1967.
11. Ligumsky, M., Goto, Y., Debas, H., and Yamada, T.: Prostaglandins mediate inhibition of gastric acid secretion by somatostatin in the rat. Science, 219:301–303, 1983.
12. Karl, R. C., Zawalich, W. S., Ferrendelli, J. A., et al.: The role of Ca^{2+} and cyclic adenosine 3′, 5′-monophosphate in insulin release induced in vitro by the divalent cation ionophore A23187. J. Biol. Chem., 250:4575–4579, 1975.
13. Gullner, H. G., and Gill, J. R., Jr.: Beta endorphin selectively stimulates aldosterone secretion in hypophysectomized, nephrectomized dogs. J. Clin. Invest., 71:124–128, 1983.
14. Brown, M. S., Kovanen, P. T., and Goldstein, J. L.: Receptor-mediated uptake of lipoprotein-cholesterol and its utilization for steroid synthesis in the adrenal cortex. Recent Progr. Horm. Res., 35:215–257, 1979.
15. Hilton, J. G., Weaver, D. C., Muelheims, G., Glaviano, V. V., and Wegria, R.: Perfusion of the isolated adrenals in situ. Am. J. Physiol., 192:525–530, 1958.
16. Pedersen, R. C., Brownie, A. C., and Ling N.: Proadrenocorticotropin/endorphin-derived peptides: Coordinate action on adrenal steroidogenesis. Science, 208:1044–1046, 1980.
17. Baxter, J. D., and MacLeod, K. M.: The molecular basis for hormone action. In Bondy, P. K., and Rosenberg, L. E. (eds.): Metabolic Control and Disease. Philadelphia, W. B. Saunders Co., 1979, pp. 104–160.
18. Westphal, U.: Steroid-Protein Interactions. New York, Springer-Verlag, 1971.
19. Forest, M. G., Rivarola, M. A., and Migeon, C. T.: Percentage binding of testosterone, androstenedione and dehydroisoandrosterone in human plasma. Steroids, 12:323–343, 1968.
20. Chen, P. S., Jr., Mills, I. H., and Bartter, F. C.: Ultrafiltration studies of steroid-protein binding. J. Endocrinol., 23:129–137, 1961.
21. Higgins, S. J., Baxter, J. D., and Rousseau, G. G.: Nuclear binding of glucocorticoid receptors. In Baxter, J. D., and Rousseau, G. G. (eds.): Glucocorticoid Hormone Action. New York, Springer-Verlag, 1979, pp. 315–316.
22. Anderson, N. S., and Fanestil, D. W.: Biology of mineralocorticoid receptors. In O'Malley, B. W., and Birnbaumer, L. (eds.): Receptors and Hormone Action. New York, Academic Press, 1978, Vol. II, p. 323–351.
23. Gorski, J., Toft, D., Shyamaia, G., et al.: Hormone receptors: Studies on the interaction of estrogen with the uterus. Recent Progr. Horm. Res., 24:45–80, 1968.
24. Leavitt, W. W., Tong, J. C., Yung, S. D., Betsy, D. C., and Thomas, C. A.: Biology of progesterone receptors. In O'Malley, B. S., and Birnbaumer, L. (eds.): Receptors and Hormone Action. New York, Academic Press, 1978, Vol. II, p. 157–188.
25. Catt, K. J., Harwood, J. P., Clayton, R. N., Davies, T. F., Chan, V., Katikineni, M., Nøzu, K., and Dufou, M. L.: Regulation of peptide hormone receptors and gonadal steroidogenesis. Recent Progr. Horm. Res., 36:557–662, 1980.
26. Vedeckis, W., Schrader, W. T., and O'Malley, B. W.: The chick oviduct progesterone receptor. In

Litwack, G. (ed.): Biochemical Actions of Hormones. New York, Academic Press, 1978, Vol. 5, pp. 322–372.

27. Greene, G. L., Fitch, F. W., and Jensen, E. V.: Monoclonal antibodies to estrophilin: Probes for the study of estrogen receptors. Proc. Natl. Acad. Sci. U.S.A., 77:157–161, 1980.

28. McGuire, W. L.: Physiological principles underlying therapy in breast cancer. *In* McGuire, W. L. (ed.): Breast Cancer. Vol. 1: Current Approaches to Therapy. Edinburgh, Churchill Livingstone, 1977, pp. 1–56.

29. Leclercq, G., and Heuson, J. C.: Therapeutic significance of sex-steroid hormone receptors in the treatment of breast cancer. Perspectives in cancer research. Eur. J. Cancer, 13:1205–1215, 1977.

30. O'Malley, B. W., Schwartz, R. J., and Schrader, W. T.: A review of regulation of gene expression by steroid hormone receptors. J. Steroid Biochem., 7:1151–1159, 1976.

31. Baxter, J. D., and Ivarie, R.: Regulation of gene expression by glucocorticoid hormones: studies of receptors and responses in cultured cells. *In* O'Malley, B. W., and Birnbaumer, L. (eds.): Receptors and Hormone Action. New York, Academic Press, 1978, Vol. II, p. 252–297.

32. Palmiter, R. D., Moore, P. B., and Mulvhill, E. R.: A significant lag in the induction of ovalbumin messenger RNA by steroid hormones: A receptor translocation hypothesis. Cell, 8:557–572, 1976.

33. Nakamura, M., Nakanishi, S., Sueokas, S., Imura, H., and Numa, S.: Effects of steroid hormones on the levels of corticotropin mRNA activity in cultured mouse–pituitary tumour cells. Eur. J. Biochem., 86:61–66, 1978.

34. Palade, G.: Intracellular aspects of the process of protein synthesis. Science, 189:347–358, 1975.

35. Robbins, J., Cheng, S. Y., Gershengorn, M. C., Glinoer, D., Cahnmann, H. J., and Edelnoch, H.: Thyroxine transport proteins of plasma. Molecular properties and biosynthesis. Recent Progr. Horm. Res., 34:477–519, 1978.

36. Kaplan, M. M., Tatro, J. B., Breitbart, R., and Larsen, P. R.: Comparison of thyroxine and 3,3′,5′-triiodothyronine metabolism in rat kidney and liver homogenates. Metabolism, 28:1139–1146, 1979.

37. Eberhardt, N. W., Apriletti, J. W., and Baxter, J. B.: The molecular biology of thyroid hormone action. *In* Litwak, G. (ed.): Biochemical Actions of Hormones. New York, Academic Press, 1980, Vol. 7, pp. 311–394.

38. Oppenheimer, J. H.: Thyroid hormone action at the cellular level. Science, 203:971–979, 1979.

39. Blake, C. C. F., and Oakley, S. J.: Protein DNA and protein hormone interactions in prealbumin: A model of the thyroid hormone nuclear receptor. Nature, 268:115–120, 1977.

40. Stocker, W. W., Samaha, F. J., and DeGroot, L. J.: Coupled oxidative phosphorylation in muscle of thyrotoxic patients. Am. J. Med., 44:900–909, 1968.

41. Hoch, F. L.: Thyrotoxicosis as a disease of mitochondria. N. Engl. J. Med., 266:446–454, 1962.

42. Lo, S. C., August, T. R., Liberman, U. A., et al.: Dependence of renal (Na+ and K+)-ATPase activity on thyroid status. J. Biol. Chem., 251: 7826–7833, 1976.

43. Folke, M., and Sesteft, L.: Thyroid calorigenesis in isolated perfused rat liver: Minor role of active Na-K transport. J. Physiol., 269:407–419, 1977.

44. DeGroot, L. J., Rue, P., Robertson, M., Bernal, J., and Scherberg, N.: Triiodothyronine stimulates nuclear RNA synthesis. Endocrinology, 101: 1690–1700, 1977.

45. Berson, S. A., and Yalow, R. S.: Assay of plasma insulin in human subjects by immunological methods. Nature, 184:1648–1649, 1959.

46. Roth, J., Kahn, C. R., Lesniak, M. A., et al.: Receptors for insulin, NSILA-s, and growth hormone: Application to disease states in man. Recent Progr. Horm. Res., 31:95–139, 1975.

47. Freychet, P., Roth, J., and Neville, D. M., Jr.: Insulin receptors in the liver: Specific binding of ^{125}I-insulin to the plasma membrane and its relation to insulin bioactivity. Proc. Natl. Acad. Sci. U.S.A., 68:1833–1837, 1971.

48. Kahn, C. R., Baird, K. L., Filier, J. S., Grunfeld, C., Harmon, J. T., Hamson, L. J., Karlsson, F. A., Kasuga, M., King, G. L., Lang, U. C., Poskalny, J. M., and Van Obberghen, E.: Insulin receptors, receptor antibodies, and the mechanism of insulin action. Recent Progr. Horm. Res., 37:477–538, 1981.

49. Bolton, A. E., and Hunter, W. N.: The labeling of proteins to high specific radioactivities by conjugation to a ^{125}I-containing acylating agent. Biochem. J., 133:529–539, 1973.

50. Gavin, J. R., 3rd, Roth, J., Neville, D. M., et al.: Insulin-dependent regulation of insulin receptor concentrations. A direct demonstration in cell culture. Proc. Natl. Acad. Sci. U.S.A., 71:84–88, 1974.

51. Jarrett, D. B., Roth, J., Kahn, C. R., et al.: Direct method for detection and characterization of cell surface receptors for insulin by means of ^{125}I-labeled autoantibodies against the insulin receptor. Proc. Natl. Acad. Sci. U.S.A., 73:4115–4119, 1976.

52. Kahn, C. R., Baird, K., Filier, J. S., and Jarrett, D. B.: Effects of autoantibodies to the insulin receptor on isolated adipocytes. Studies of insulin binding and insulin action. J. Clin. Invest., 60:1094–1106, 1977.

53. Willingham, M. C., Maxfield, F. R., and Pastan, I. H.: α-2 Macroglobulin binding to the plasma membrane of cultured fibroblasts: Diffuse binding followed by clustering in coated regions. J. Cell Biol., 82:614–625, 1979.

54. Freychet, P.: Interactions of polypeptide hormones with cell membrane specific receptors: Studies with insulin and glucagon. Diabetologia, 12:83–100, 1976.

55. Birnbaumer, L., and Phol, S. L.: Relation of glucagon-specific binding sites to glucagon-dependent stimulation of adenylyl cyclase activity in plasma membranes of rat liver. J. Biol. Chem., 248:2056–2061, 1973.

56. Rodbard, D.: Mathematics of hormone-receptor interaction. I: Basic principles. *In* O'Malley, B. W., and Means, A. R. (eds.): Receptors for Reproductive Hormones. New York, Plenum, 1973, pp. 342–358.

57. Stadie, W. C., Haugaard, N., and Vaughn, M.: The quantitative relation between insulin and its biological activity. J. Biol. Chem., 200:745–751, 1953.

58. DeMeyts, P., Bianco, A. R., and Roth, J.: Insulin interactions with its receptors: Experimental evidence for negative cooperativity. Biochem. Biophys. Res. Commun., 55:154–161, 1973.

59. DeMeyts, P.: Cooperative properties of hormone

receptors in cell membranes. J. Supramol. Struct., 4:241–258, 1976.

60. DeMeyts, P., Bianco, A. R., and Roth, J.: Site interactions among insulin receptors: Characterization of negative cooperativity. J. Biol. Chem., 241:1877–1888, 1976.

61. DeMeyts, P., Roth, J., Van Obberghen, E., and Waelbroeck, M.: Hormonal control of affinity of polypeptide hormone receptors by negative cooperativity and dissociation rate modulation. In James, V. H. T. (ed.): Proceedings of the 5th International Congress on Endocrinology, Hamburg, 1976. Excerpta Medica, Vol. 1, 1977, pp. 578–581.

62. DeMeyts, P., Van Obberghen, E., and Roth, J.: Mapping of the residues responsible for the negative cooperativity of the receptor-binding region of insulin. Nature, 273:504–509, 1978.

63. Schwarz, G.: Some general aspects regarding the interpretation of binding data by means of a Scatchard plot. Biophys. Struct. Mech., 2:1–12, 1976.

64. Ginsberg, B. H., Kahn, C. R., Roth, J., and DeMeyts, P.: Insulin-induced dissociation of its receptor into subunits, possible molecular concomitant of negative cooperativity. Biochem. Biophys. Res. Commun., 73:1068–1074, 1976.

65. Olefsky, J. M., and Chang, H.: Further evidence for functional heterogeneity of adipocyte insulin receptors. Endocrinology, 104:462–466, 1979.

66. Boeynaems, J. M., and Dumont, J. E.: The two-step model of ligand-receptor interaction. Mol. Cell. Endocrinol., 7:33–47, 1977.

67. DeHalen, C.: The non-stoichiometric floating receptor model for hormone sensitive adenylate cyclase. J. Theor. Biol., 582:383–400, 1976.

68. Jacobs, S., and Cuatrecasas, P.: The mobile receptor hypothesis and "cooperativity" of hormone binding: Application to insulin. Biochem. Biophys. Acta, 433:482–495, 1976.

69. Pollet, R. J., Standaert, M. L., and Haase, B. A.: Insulin binding to the human lymphocyte receptor. Evaluation of the negative cooperativity model. J. Biol. Chem., 252:5828–5834, 1979.

70. Donner, D. B.: Regulation of insulin binding to isolated hepatocytes: Correction for bound hormone fragments linearizes Scatchard plots. Proc. Natl. Acad. Sci. U.S.A., 77:3176–3180, 1980.

71. Kahn, C. R., Goldfine, I. D., Neville, D. M., Jr., and DeMeyts, P.: Alterations in insulin binding induced by changes in vivo in the levels of glucocorticoids and growth hormone. Endocrinology, 103:1054–1066, 1978.

72. Limbird, L. E., DeMeyts, P., and Lefrowitz, R. J.: β-Adrenergic receptors: Evidence for negative cooperativity. Biochem. Biophys. Res. Commun., 64:1160–1168, 1975.

73. DeLisi, C.: Physical chemical and biological implications of receptor clustering. In DeLisi, C., and Blumenthal, R. (eds.): Development in Cell Biology. Physical and Chemical Aspects of Cell Surface Events in Cellular Regulation. New York, Elsevier/North Holland, 1979, Vol. 4, pp. 261–292.

74. Faguet, G. B.: Leukoagglutinin binding to human lymphocytes: Experimental support for negative cooperativity. Am. J. Physiol., 237:E207–E213, 1979.

75. Sandvig, K., Olsnes, S., and Pihl, A.: Kinetics of binding of the toxic lectins abrin and ricin to

surface receptors of human cells. J. Biol. Chem., 251:3977–3984, 1976.

76. Tollefsen, D. M., and Majerus, P. W.: Evidence for a single class of thrombin-binding sites of human platelets. Biochemistry, 15:2144–2149, 1976.

77. Verrier, B., Fayet, G., and Lissitzyk, S.: Thyrotropin-binding properties of isolated thyroid cells and their purified plasma membranes. Relation of thyrotropin-specific binding to adenylate-cyclase activation. Eur. J. Biochem., 42:355–365, 1974.

78. Cuatrecasas, P., and Hollenberg, M. D.: Binding of insulin and other hormones to non-receptor materials: Saturability, specificity and apparent "negative cooperativity." Biochem. Biophys. Res. Commun., 62:31–41, 1975.

79. Sandrig, K., Olsnes, S., and Pihl, A.: Interactions between Abrus, lectins and Sephadex particles possessing immobilized desialylated fetuin. Model studies of the interaction of lectins with cell surface receptors. Eur. J. Biochem., 88:307–313, 1979.

80. Kahn, C. R., Megyesi, K., Bar, R. S., et al.: Receptors for peptide hormones. New insights into the pathophysiology of disease states in man. Ann. Rev. Intern. Med., 86:205–219, 1977.

81. Bar, R. S., Harrison, L. C., Muggeo, M., Gorden, P., Kahn, C. R., and Roth, J.: Regulation of insulin receptors in normal and abnormal physiology in humans. Adv. Intern. Med., 24:23–52, 1979.

82. Kasuga, M., Akanuma, Y., Iwamoto, Y., and Kosaka, K.: Insulin binding and glucose metabolism in adipocytes of streptozotocin-diabetic rats. Am. J. Physiol., 235:E175–E182, 1978.

83. Marchand-Brustel, B., and Freychet, P.: Effect of fasting and streptozotocin diabetes on insulin binding and action in the isolated mouse soleus muscle. J. Clin. Invest., 64:1505–1515, 1979.

84. Bar, R. S., Muggeo, M., Kahn, C. R., Gorden, P., and Roth, J.: Characterization of insulin receptors in patients with the syndromes of insulin resistance and acanthosis nigricans. Diabetologia, 18:209–216, 1980.

85. Mendelson, C., Dufau, M. L., and Catt, K. J.: Gonadotropin binding and stimulation of cyclic adenosine 3'5'monophosphate and testosterone production in isolated Leydig cells. J. Biol. Chem., 250:8818–8823, 1982.

86. Stephenson, R. P.: A modification of receptor theory. Br. J. Pharmacol., 11:379–393, 1956.

87. Kono, T., and Barnham, F. W.: The relationship between insulin-binding capacity of fat cells and the cellular response to insulin. J. Biol. Chem., 246:6210–6216, 1971.

88. Kono, T., and Barnham, F. W.: Effects of insulin on the levels of adenosine 3',5'-monophosphate and lipolysis in isolated rat epididymal fat cells. J. Biol. Chem., 248:7417–7426, 1973.

89. Douglas, J., Saltman, S., Fredlund, P., et al.: Receptor binding of angiotensin II and antagonists. Correlation with aldosterone production by isolated adrenal glomerulosa cells. Circ. Res., 38(Suppl.2):108–112, 1976.

90. Kahn, C. R., and Baird, K. L.: The fate of insulin bound to adipocytes: Evidence for comparmentalization and processing. J. Biol. Chem., 253:4900–4906, 1978.

91. Gorden, P., Carpentier, J. L., Freychet, P., and Orci, L.: Receptor linked ^{125}I-insulin degradation

is mediated by internalization. Clin. Res., 27:485, 1979.

92. Anderson, R. G. W., Goldstein, J. L., and Brown, M. S.: Localization of low density lipoprotein receptors on plasma membrane of normal human fibroblasts and their absence in cells from a familial hypercholesterolemia homozygote. Proc. Natl. Acad. Sci. U.S.A., 73:2434–2438, 1976.

93. Haigler, H., Ash, J. F., Singer, S. J., and Cohen, S.: Visualization by fluorescence of the binding and internalization of epidermal growth factor in human carcinoma cells A-431. Proc. Natl. Acad. Sci. U.S.A., 75:3317–3321, 1978.

94. Blackard, W. G., Guzelian, P. S., and Small, M. F.: Down regulation of insulin receptors in primary cultures of adult rat hepatocytes in monolayer. Endocrinology, 103:548–553, 1978.

95. Mott, D. M., Howard, B. V., and Bennett, P. H.: Stoichiometric binding and regulation of insulin receptors on human diploid fibroblasts using physiologic insulin levels. J. Biol. Chem., 254:8762–8767, 1979.

96. Olefsky, J. M., Marshall, S., Bernhau, P., Saekow, M., Heidenreich, K., and Green, A.: Internalization and intracellular processing of insulin and insulin receptors in adipocytes. Metabolism, 31:670–690, 1982.

97. Fambrough, D. M., and Devereotes, P. N.: Newly synthesized acetylcholine receptors are located in the Golgi apparatus. J. Cell Biol., 76:237–244, 1978.

98. Kahn, C. R.: Membrane receptors for hormones and neurotransmitters. J. Cell Biol., 70:261–286, 1976.

99. Bergeron, J. J., Posner, B. I., Josefsberg, Z., and Sikstrom, R.: Intracellular polypeptide hormone receptors: The demonstration of specific binding sites for insulin and hGH in Golgi fractions isolated from the liver of female rats. J. Biol. Chem., 253:4058–4066, 1978.

100. Goldfine, I. D., Smith, G. J., Wong, K. Y., et al.: Cellular uptake and nuclear binding of insulin in cultured human lymphocytes: Evidence for potential intracellular site of insulin action. Proc. Natl. Acad. Sci. U.S.A., 74:1368–1372, 1977.

101. Kaplan, J.: Polypeptide-binding membrane receptors: Analysis and classification. Science, 4490:14–20, 1979.

102. Ansorge, S., Bohley, P., Kirschke, H., et al.: Metabolism of insulin and glucagon: Breakdown of radioiodonated insulin and glucagon in rat liver cell fractions. Eur. J. Biochem., 19:283–288, 1971.

103. Ascoli, M., and Puett, D.: Degradation of receptor-bound human choriogonadotropin by murine Leydig tumor cells. J. Biol. Chem., 253:4892–4899, 1978.

104. Gorden, P., Carpentier, J. L., Freychet, P. O., and Orci, L.: Internalization of polypeptide hormones: Mechanism, intracellular localization and significance. Diabetologia, 18:263–274, 1980.

105. Carpenter, G., and Cohen, S.: ^{125}I-labeled human epidermal growth factor binding, internalization and degradation in human fibroblasts. J. Cell Biol., 71:159–171, 1976.

106. Johnson, L. K., Vlodavsky, I., Baxter, J. D., and Gospodarowicz, D.: Nuclear accumulation of epidermal growth factor in cultured rat pituitary cells. Nature, 287:340–343, 1980.

107. Mobley, W. C., Server, A. C., Ishii, D. N., Riopelle, R. J., and Shooter, E. M.: Nerve growth factor. N. Engl. J. Med., 297:1096–1104, 1977.

108. Schwab, M. E.: Ultrastructural localization of a nerve growth factor–horseradish peroxidase (NGF-HRP) coupling product after retrograde axonal transport in adrenergic neurons. Brain Res., 130:190–196, 1977.

109. Goldfine, I. D.: Interaction of insulin, polypeptide hormones, and growth factors with intracellular membranes. Biochim. Biophys. Acta, 650:53–57, 1981.

110. Andres, R. Y., Jeng, I., and Bradshaw, R. A.: Nerve growth factor receptors: Identification of distinct classes in plasma membranes and nuclei of embryonic dorsal root neurons. Proc. Natl. Acad. Sci. U.S.A., 74:2785–2789, 1977.

111. Sutherland, E. W., and Rall, T. W.: Fractionation and characterization of a cyclic adenine ribonucleotide formed by tissue particles. J. Biol. Chem., 232:1077–1091, 1975.

112. Sutherland, E. W., and Rall, R. W.: The relation of adenosine 3′,5′-phosphate and phosphorylase to the actions of catecholamines and other hormones. Pharmacol. Rev., 12:265–299, 1960.

113. Exton, J. H.: Mechanisms involved in alpha-adrenergic effects of catecholamines on liver metabolism. J. Cyclic Nucleotide Res., 5:277–287, 1979.

114. Birnbaumer, L., and Iyengar, R.: Coupling of receptors adenylate cyclase. In Nathanson, J. A., and Kebabian, J. W. (eds.): Cyclic Nucleotides. Handbook of Experimental Pharmacology. New York, Springer-Verlag, 1982, Vol. 58, pp. 144–168.

115. Lefkowitz, R. J., Caron, M. G., Michel, T., and Stadel, J. M.: Mechanisms of hormone receptor-effector coupling: The β-adrenergic receptor and adenylate cyclase. Fed. Proc., 41:2665–2670, 1982.

116. Najjar, V. A., and Constantopoulos, A.: The activation of adenylate cyclase. I. A postulated mechanism for fluoride and hormone activation of adenylate cyclase. Mol. Cell Biochem., 2:87–93, 1973.

117. Exton, J. H., and Park, C. R.: Control of gluconeogenesis in liver. II. Effects of glucagon, catecholamines and adenosine 3′,5′-monophosphate on gluconeogenic intermediates in the perfused rat liver. J. Biol. Chem., 244:1424–1433, 1969.

118. Bennett, V., O'Keefe, E., and Cuatrecasas, P.: Mechanism of action of cholera toxin and the mobile receptor theory of hormone-receptor–adenylate cyclase interactions. Proc. Natl. Acad. Sci. U.S.A., 72:33–37, 1975.

119. Bennett, V., and Cuatrecasas, P.: Mechanism of activation of adenylate cyclase by Vibrio cholerae enterotoxin. J. Memb. Biol., 22:29–52, 1975.

120. Bennett, V., and Cuatrecasas, P.: Mechanism of action of Vibrio cholerae enterotoxin. Effects on adenylate cyclase of toad and rat erythrocyte plasma membrane. J. Memb. Biol., 22:1–28, 1975.

121. Lefkowitz, R. J.: β-Adrenergic receptors: Recognition and regulation. N. Engl. J. Med., 295:323–328, 1976.

122. Cassel, D., Levkovitz, H., and Selinger, Z.: The regulatory GTPase cycle of turkey erythrocyte adenylate cyclase. J. Cyclic Nucleotide Res., 3:393–406, 1977.

123. Rodbell, M.: The role of nucleotide regulatory components in the coupling of hormone receptors and adenylate cyclase. In Folco, G., and Pavletti, R. (eds.): Molecular Biology and Pharmacology of Cyclic Nucleotides. Amsterdam, Elsevier/North Holland, 1977, Vol. 1, p. 1–16.

124. Rodbell, M.: The role of hormone receptors and

GTP-regulatory proteins in membrane transduction. Nature, 284:17–22, 1980.

125. Greengard, P.: Phosphorylated proteins as physiological effectors. Science, 199:146–152, 1978.

126. Carlson, G. M., Bechtel, P. J., and Graves, D. J.: Chemical and regulatory properties of phosphorylase kinase and cAMP-dependent protein kinase. Adv. Enzymol., 50:41–115, 1979.

127. Corbin, J. D., Keely, S. L., and Park, C. R.: The distribution and dissociation of cAMP-dependent protein kinase in adipose, cardiac and other tissues. J. Biol. Chem., 250:218–225, 1975.

128. Hoffman, F.: Apparent constants for the interaction of regulatory and catalytic subunit of cAMP-dependent protein kinase I and II. J. Biol. Chem., 255:1559–1564, 1980.

129. Builder, S. E., Beavo, J. A., and Krebs, E. G.: The mechanism of activation of bovine skeletal muscle protein kinase by adenosine, 3',5'-monophosphate. J. Biol. Chem., 225:3514–3519, 1980.

130. Corbin, J. D., Soderling, T. R., and Park, C. R.: Regulation of adenosing 3',5'-monophosphate–dependent protein kinase. I. Characterization of the adipose tissue enzyme in crude extracts. J. Biol. Chem., 248:1813, 1973.

131. Soderling, T. R., Corbin, J. D., and Park, C. R.: Regulation of adenosine 3',5'-monophosphate–dependent protein kinase. II. Hormonal regulation of the adipose tissue enzyme. J. Biol. Chem., 248:1822–1829, 1973.

132. Keely, S. L., Corbin, J. D., and Park, C. R.: Regulation of adenosine 3',5'-monophosphate–dependent protein kinase: Regulation of the heart enzyme by epinephrine, glucagon, insulin, and 1-methyl-3-isobutyl-xanthine. J. Biol. Chem., 250:4832–4840, 1975.

133. Palmer, W. K., McPherson, J. M., and Walsh, D. A.: Critical controls in the evaluation of cAMP-dependent protein kinase activity ratios as indices of hormonal action. J. Biol. Chem., 255:2663–2666, 1980.

134. Benjamin, W. B., and Singer, I.: Actions of insulin, epinephrine and dibutyrylcyclic adenosine 3',5'-monophosphate dependent and independent mechanisms. Biochemistry, 14:3301–3309, 1975.

135. Lincoln, T. M., Dills, W. L., Jr., and Corbin, J. D.: Purification and subunit composition of cGMP-dependent protein kinase from bovine lung. J. Biol. Chem., 252:4269–4275, 1977.

136. Lincoln, T. M., and Corbin, J. D.: Hypothesis: On the role of the cAMP and cGMP-dependent protein kinase in cell function. J. Cyclic Nucleotide Res., 4:3–14, 1978.

137. Krebs, E. G., Love, D. S., Bratvold, G. E., et al.: Purification and properties of rabbit skeletal muscle phosphorylase b kinase. Biochemistry, 3:1022–1033, 1964.

138. Krebs, E. G.: Protein kinases. Curr. Top. Cell. Regul., 5:99–133, 1972.

139. Fischer, D., and Kreb, H.: Concerted regulation of glycogen metabolism and muscle contraction. In Weiland, O., Helmreich, E., and Holzer, H. (eds.): Metabolic Interconversion of Enzymes. New York, Springer-Verlag, 1976.

140. Huang, H. P., et al.: In Miami Winter Symposium. New York, Academic Press, 1979, Vol. 16, pp. 449–470.

141. Adelstein, R. S., and Eisenberg, E.: Regulation and kinetics of actin-myosin ATP interaction. Ann. Rev. Biochem., 49:921–956, 1980.

142. Krebs, E. G., and Beavo, J. A.: Phosphorylation-

143. Jefferson, L. S., Flaim, K. E., and Peavy, D. E.: Effect of insulin on protein turnover. In Brownlee, M. (ed.): Diabetes Mellitus Biochemical Pathology. New York, Garland STPM Press, 1981, Vol. IV, pp. 133–177.

144. Lee, E. Y. C., Millgren, R. L., Killilea, S. D., and Axelward, J. H.: Properties and regulation of liver protein phosphatases. In Esmann, V. (ed.): Regulatory Mechanisms of Carbohydrate Metabolism. New York, Pergamon, 1978, pp. 327–346.

145. Brandt, H., Lee, E. Y. C., Killilea, S. D.: A protein inhibitor of rabbit liver phosphorylase phosphatase. Biochem. Biophys. Res. Commun., 63:950–956, 1975.

146. Khandelwal, R. L., and Zinman, S. M.: Purification and properties of a heat-stable protein inhibitor of phosphoprotein phosphatase from rabbit liver. J. Biol. Chem., 253:560–565, 1978.

147. Ahlquist, R. P.: A study of adrenotropic receptors. Am. J. Physiol., 153:586–600, 1948.

148. Silverberg, A. B., Shah, S. D., Haymond, M. W., and Cryer, P. E.: Norepinephrine: Hormone and neurotransmitter in man. Am. J. Physiol., 234:E252–E256, 1978.

149. Langer, S. Z.: Presynaptic regulation of catecholamine release (commentary). Biochem. Pharmacol., 23:1793–1800, 1974.

150. Chan, T. M., and Exton, J. H.: α-Adrenergic-mediated accumulation of adenosine 3',5'-monophosphate in calcium-depleted hepatocytes. J. Biol. Chem., 252:8645–8651, 1977.

151. Jakobs, K. H., Saur, W., and Schultz, G.: Reduction of adenylate cyclase activity in lysates of human platelets by the alpha-adrenergic component of epinephrine. J. Cyclic Nucleotide Res., 2:381–392, 1976.

152. Cherrington, A. D., Assimacoupaulous, F. D., Harper, S. C., et al.: Studies on the α-adrenergic activation of hepatic glucose output. II. Investigation of the roles of adenosine 3':5'-monophosphate and adenosine 3':5'-monophosphate-dependent protein kinase in the actions of phenylephrine in isolated hepatocytes. J. Biol. Chem., 251:5209–5218, 1976.

153. Pointer, R. H., Butcher, F. R., and Fain, J. N.: Studies on the role of cyclic guanosine 3',5'-monophosphate and extracellular Ca^{2+} in the regulation of glycogenolysis in rat liver cells. J. Biol. Chem., 251:2987–2992, 1976.

154. Schutz, G., Schutz, K., and Hardman, J. G.: Effects of norephinephrine on cyclic nucleotide levels in the ductus deferens of the rat. Metabolism, 24:429–437, 1975.

155. Van de Werve, G., Hue, L., and Hersh, G.: Hormonal and ionic control of the glycogenolytic cascade in rat liver. Biochem. J., 162:135–142, 1977.

156. Somlyo, A. P., and Somlyo, A. V.: Vascular smooth muscle. II. Pharmacology of normal and hypertensive vessels. Pharmacol. Rev., 22:249–353, 1970.

157. Burgess, G. M., Claret, M., and Jenkinson, D. H.: Effects of catecholamines, ATP and ionophore A23187 on potassium and calcium movement in isolated hepatocytes. Nature, 279:544–546, 1979.

158. Marier, S. H., Putney, J. W., Jr., and Van de Wall, C. M.: Control of calcium channels by membrane receptors in the rat parotid gland. J. Physiol., 279:141–151, 1978.

159. Blackmore, P. F., Brumley, F. T., Marks, J. L., and

Exton, J. H.: Studies on α-adrenergic activation of hepatic glucose output. Relationship between α-adrenergic stimulation of calcium efflux and activation of phosphorylase in isolated rat liver parenchymal cells. J. Biol. Chem., 253:4851–4858, 1978.

160. Blackmore, P. E., Dehavy, J. P., and Exton, J. H.: Studies on α-adrenergic activation of hepatic glucose. J. Biol. Chem., 254:6945–6950, 1979.

161. Hurwitz, L., and Suria, A.: The link between agonist action and response in smooth musle. Ann. Rev. Pharmacol., 11:303–326, 1971.

162. Exton, J. H.: Mechanism involved in α-adrenergic effects of catecholamines. In Kunos, G. (ed.): Adrenoceptors and Catecholamine Action. New York, John Wiley & Sons, 1981, Vol. 1. pp. 117–129.

163. Jones, L. M., and Michell, R. H.: Stimulus-response coupling alpha-adrenergic receptors. Biochem. Soc. Trans., 6:673–688, 1978.

164. Kirk, C. J., Verrinder, T. R., and Hems, R. A.: Rapid stimulation by vasopressin and adrenaline of inorganic phosphate incorporation into phosphotidylinositol in isolated hepatocytes. F.E.B.S. Lett., 83:267–271, 1977.

165. Braunwald, E.: Mechanism of action of calcium channel blocking agents. N. Engl. J. Med., 307:1618–1626, 1982.

166. Klee, C. B., Crouch, T. H., and Richman, P. G.: Calmodulin. Ann. Rev. Biochem., 49:489–515, 1980.

167. Teo, T. S., and Wang, J. H.: Mechanism of activation of a cyclic adenosine 3′,5′-monophosphate phosphodiesterase from bovine heart by calcium ions. J. Biol. Chem., 248:5950–5955, 1973.

168. Watterson, D. M., Van Eldik, U. J., Smith, R. E., et al.: Calcium-dependent regulatory protein of cyclic nucleotide metabolism in normal and transformed chicken embryo fibroblasts. Proc. Natl. Acad. Sci. U.S.A., 73:2711–2715, 1976.

169. Jarrett, H. W., and Kyle, J.: Human erythrocyte calmodulin. J. Biol. Chem., 254:8237–8244, 1979.

170. Cohen, S., et al.: Identification of the Ca^{2+}-dependent modulator protein as the fourth subunit of rabbit skeletal muscle phosphorylase kinase. F.E.B.S. Lett., 92:287–293, 1978.

171. Weiss, B., Prozialeck, W., Cimino, M., Barnette, M. S., and Wallace, T. L.: Pharmacological regulation of calmodulin. Ann. N.Y. Acad. Sci., 356:319–345, 1980.

172. Klee, C. B., Crouch, T. H., and Richman, P. G.: Calmodulin. Ann. Rev. Biochem., 49:489–515, 1980.

173. Martin, F., Gabrion, J., and Cavadore, J. C.: Thyroid myosin filament assembly-disassembly is controlled by myosin light chain phosphorylation dephosphorylation. F.E.B.S. Lett., 131:235–238, 1981.

174. Adelstein, R. S., and Klee, C. B.: Purification and characterization of smooth muscle myosin light chain kinase. J. Biol. Chem., 256:7501–7509, 1981.

175. Welsh, M. J., Dedman, J. R., Brinkley, B. R., and Means, A. R.: Calcium-dependent regulator protein: Localization in mitotic apparatus of eukaryotic cells. Proc. Natl. Acad. Sci. U.S.A., 75:1867–1871, 1978.

176. Wells, J. N., and Hardman, J. G.: Cyclic nucleotide phosphodiesterases. Adv. Cyclic Nucleotide Res., 8:119–143, 1977.

177. Salter, R. S., Krinks, M. K., Klee, C. B., and Neer, E. J.: Calmodulin activates the isolated catalytic unit of brain adenylate cyclase. J. Biol. Chem., 256:9830–9833, 1981.

178. Schulman, H., and Greengard, P.: Ca^{2+} dependent protein phosphorylation system in membranes from various tissues, and its activation by calcium dependent regulator. Proc. Natl. Acad. Sci. U.S.A., 75:5432–5436, 1978.

179. Chrisman, T. D., and Exton, J. H.: Activation of endogenous phosphorylase kinase in liver glycogen pellet by cAMP-dependent protein kinase. J. Biol. Chem., 255:3270–3272, 1980.

180. Soderling, T. R., Srivastava, A. K., Bass, M. A., and Khatra, B. S.: Phosphorylation and inactivation of glycogen synthase by phosphorylase kinase. Proc. Natl. Acad. Sci. U.S.A., 76:2536–2540, 1979.

181. Wong, P. Y., and Cheung, W. Y.: Calmodulin stimulates human platelet phospholipase A_2. Biochem. Biophys. Res. Commun., 40:473–480, 1979.

182. Gietzen, K., Tejcra, M., and Wolf, H. U.: Calmodulin affinity chromatography yields a functional purified erythrocyte $(Ca^{2+} + Mg^{2+})$-dependent adenosine triphosphatase. Biochem. J., 189:81–88, 1980.

183. Tada, M., Yamamoto, T., and Tonomura, T.: Molecular mechanism of active calcium transport by sarcoplasmic reticulum. Physiol. Rev., 58:1–79, 1978.

184. Hoil, W. H., and Heilmeyer, L. M. G., Jr.: Evidence for the participation of a Ca^{2+}-dependent protein kinase and protein phosphotase in the regulation of the Ca^{2+} transport ATPase of the sarcoplasmic reticulum. 2. Effect of phosphorylase kinase and phosphorylase phosphatase. Biochemistry, 17:766–772, 1978.

185. Yamauchi, T., Nakata, H., and Fujisawa, H.: A new activator protein that activates tryptophan 5-monooxygenase and tyrosine 3-monooxygenase in the presence of Ca^{2+}, calmodulin-dependent protein kinases. J. Biol. Chem., 256:5404–5409, 1981.

186. DeLorenzo, R. J.: Phenytoin: Calcium- and calmodulin-dependent protein phosphorylation and neurotransmitter release. Adv. Neurol., 27:399–414, 1980.

187. Burgoyne, R. D.: The loss of muscarinic acetylcholine receptors in synaptic membranes under phosphorylating conditions is dependent on calmodulin. F.E.B.S. Lett., 127:144–148, 1981.

188. Fain, J. N.: Hormonal regulation of lipid mobilization from adipose tissue. Biochem. Action Horm., 7:119–204, 1980.

189. Wong, E. H. A., and Loten, E. G.: The antilipolytic action of insulin on adrenocorticotropin-stimulated rat fat cells. Eur. J. Biochem., 115:17–22, 1981.

190. Tarui, S., Saito, Y., Fujimoto, M., et al.: Effects of insulin on diaphragm muscle independent of the variation of tissue levels of cyclic AMP and cyclic GMP. Arch. Biochem. Biophys., 174:192–198, 1976.

191. Clausen, T., and Marlen, B. R.: The effect of insulin on the washout of [^{45}Ca] calcium from adipocytes and soleus muscle of the rat. Biochem. J., 164:251–255, 1977.

192. Kissebah, A. H., Clarke, P., Vydelingum, N., et al.: The role of calcium in insulin action. III. Calcium distribution in fat cells; its kinetics and the effects of adrenaline, insulin and procaine-HCl. Eur. J. Clin. Invest., 5:339–349, 1975.

193. Hope-Gill, H., et al.: The effects of insulin on adipocyte calcium flux and the interaction with the effects of dibutyryl cyclic AMP and adrenaline. Horm. Metab. Res., 7:194–196, 1975.

194. May, J. M., and de Haen, C.: The insulin-like effect of hydrogen peroxide on pathways of lipid synthesis in rat adipocytes. J. Biol. Chem., 254:9017–9021, 1979.

195. Seals, J. R., and Jarett, L.: Activation of pyruvate dehydrogenase by direct addition of insulin to an isolated plasma membrane/mitochondria mixture: Evidence for generation of insulin's second messenger in a subcellular system. Proc. Natl. Acad. Sci. U.S.A., 77:77–81, 1980.

196. Jarett, L., and Smith, R. M.: The natural occurrence of insulin receptors on adipocyte plasma membranes as demonstrated with monomeric ferritin-insulin. J. Supramol. Struct., 6:45–59, 1977.

197. Jarett, L., and Smith, R. M.: Effect of cytochalasin B and D on groups of insulin receptors and on insulin action in rat adipocytes. J. Clin. Invest., 6:571–579, 1979.

198. Cushman, S. W., and Wardzala, L. J.: Potential mechanism of insulin action on glucose transport in the isolated rat adipose cell. Apparent translocation of intracellular transport systems to plasma membrane. J. Biol. Chem., 255:4758–4762, 1980.

199. Suzuki, K., and Kono, T.: Evidence that insulin causes translocation of glucose transport activity to the plasma membrane from an intracellular storage site. Proc. Natl. Acad. Sci. U.S.A., 77:2542–2545, 1980.

200. Czech, M. P.: Insulin action and the regulation of hexose transport. Diabetes, 29:399–409, 1980.

201. Czech, M. P.: Insulin action. Am. J. Med., 70:142–150, 1981.

202. Jacobs, S., Hazun, E., and Cuatrecasas, P.: The subunit structure of rat liver insulin receptor: Antibodies directed against the insulin receptor subunit. J. Biol. Chem., 255:6937–6940, 1980.

203. Pilch, P. F., and Czech, M. P.: Interaction of cross-linking agents with the insulin effector system of isolated fat cells. J. Biol. Chem., 254:3375–3381, 1979.

204. Massague, J., Pilch, P. F., and Czech, P. M.: Electrophoretic resolution of three major insulin receptor structures with unique subunit stoichiometrics. Proc. Natl. Acad. Sci. U.S.A., 77:7137–7141, 1980.

205. Czech, M. P., and Massaque, J.: Subunit structure and dynamics of the insulin receptor. Fed. Proc., 4:2719–2723, 1982.

206. Kasuga, M., Karlsson, F. A., and Kahn, C. R.: Insulin stimulates the phosphorylation of the 95,000-dalton subunit of its own receptor. Science, 215:185–187, 1982.

207. Kasuga, M., Zick, Y., Blithe, D. L., Crettaz, M., and Kahn, C. R.: Insulin stimulates tryrosine phosphorylation of the insulin receptor in a cell-free systen. Nature (London), 298:667–669, 1982.

208. Kasuga, M., Zick, Y., Blithe, D. L., Karlsson, F. A., Häring, H. U., and Kahn, C. R.: Insulin stimulation of phosphorylation of the beta subunit of the insulin receptor. J. Biol. Chem., 257:9891–9894, 1982.

209. Roth, R. A., and Cassell, D. J.: Insulin receptor: Evidence that it is a protein kinase. Science, 219:299–301, 1983.

210. Benjamin, W. B., and Singer, I.: Actions of insulin, epinephrine and dibutyryl cyclic adenosine 3',5'-monophosphate on fat cell protein phosphorylations. Cyclic adenosine 3',5'-monophosphate dependent and independent mechanisms. Biochemistry, 14:3301–3309, 1975.

211. Brownsey, R. W., Belsham, G. J., and Denton, R. M.: Evidence that the activation of acetyl-CoA carboxylase by insulin involves c-AMP independent phosphorylation. Biochem. Soc. Trans., 2:232, 1977.

212. Denton, R. M., Brownsey, R. W., and Belsham, G. J.: A partial view of the mechanism of insulin action. Diabetologia, 21:347–362, 1981.

213. Cohen, S., Carpenter, G., and King, L., Jr.: Epidermal growth factor–receptor–protein kinase interactions. J. Biol. Chem., 255:4834–4842, 1980.

214. Cohen, S., Ushiro, H., Stoscheck, C., and Chinkers, M.: A native 170,000 epidermal growth factor receptor–kinase complex from shed plasma membrane vesicles. J. Biol. Chem., 257:1523–1531, 1982.

215. Larner, J., Galasko, G., Cheng, K., DePaoli-Roach, A., Huang, L., Daggyi, P., and Kellog, J.: Generation by insulin of a chemical mediator that controls protein phosphorylation and dephosphorylation. Science, 206:1408–1410, 1979.

216. Jarett, L., Kiechle, F. L., and Parker, J. C.: Chemical mediator or mediators of insulin action: Response to insulin and mode of action. Fed. Proc., 41:2736–2741, 1982.

217. Larner, J., Cheng, K., Schwartz, C., Kikuchi, K., Tamura, S., Creacy, S., Dubler, R., Galasko, G., Pullin, C., and Katz, M.: A proteolytic mechanism for the action of insulin via oligopeptide mediator formation. Fed. Proc., 41:2724–2729, 1982.

218. Seals, J. R., and Czech, M. P.: Production by plasma membranes of a chemical mediator of insulin action. Fed. Proc., 41:2730–2735, 1982.

CHAPTER 3

Carbohydrate Metabolism and Requirements

ROBERT R. WOLFE

The beneficial effect of infused glucose as a nutrient has been documented repeatedly by nitrogen balance studies. The N-sparing effect of infused glucose may stem both from the suppression of endogenous glucose production (thereby sparing gluconeogenic amino acids) and from the direct oxidation of the infused glucose (thereby competing with the oxidation of amino acids). Separate quantification of these processes is desirable in determining the optimal glucose infusion rate in clinical settings. Determination of the infusion rate required to maximally suppress endogenous glucose production allows examination of the relationship of risk to benefit in situations in which the maximal rate of oxidation is exceeded and fat deposition occurs. It is important to understand the role of insulin in directing the metabolic response to infused glucose, both in the range of the moderate (two- to four-fold) increases in insulin elicited by glucose infusion at a brisk rate and in the higher ranges that result from exogenous insulin infusion. Finally, because the plasma glucose concentration (or urinary excretion) is generally the only parameter of glucose metabolism easily observed by the clinician, the utility of plasma glucose measurements should be maximized by an understanding of the factors involved in the regulation of plasma glucose concentration during glucose infusion.

GLUCOSE PRODUCTION

Under normal circumstances, many physiologic control mechanisms ensure that there is a relatively close matching of the uptake of glucose by tissues and the appearance of glucose in the blood stream. Peripheral mechanisms involved in the regulation of glucose uptake and oxidation will be considered later; the regulation of glucose production is of primary importance in the regulation of the plasma glucose concentration.

During periods of fasting, the body relies on endogenous glucose production to replace the glucose taken up and catabolized by glucose-dependent tissues. The primary organs responsible for glucose production are the liver and the kidneys. Although other tissues, such as muscle, may be able to synthesize glucose-6-phosphate (g-6-P), the enzyme glucose-6-phosphatase, which is necessary to convert g-6-P to glucose, can be found in significant quantities only in the liver and kidney. The liver's relative contribution to total glucose production is far in excess of the kidney's, but in certain situations, such as starvation, the kidney may contribute significantly.[1] Glycogenolysis in the liver and gluconeogenesis in the liver and kidneys are the two primary processes of glucose production.

Glycogen Metabolism

Glycogen exerts a neglible osmotic pressure and can be degraded on demand. In contrast to most tissues, in which glycogen can be broken down to provide energy locally via glycolysis, liver tissue makes little direct use of its stored glycogen.[2] The liver consumes mostly fatty acids for energy.[3] Instead, glycogen is stored in the liver when glucose is abundant (such as immediately after a meal) and released into the circulation during fasting.

Following the ingestion of a high-carbohydrate meal, a significant portion of the absorbed glucose is taken up by the liver.[4] If the blood glucose level exceeds approximately 150 mg/dl, the liver becomes an organ of net uptake.[5] When the liver is relatively depleted of glycogen,[6] as would be expected to be the case at mealtime, most of the glucose uptake by the liver is directed to glycogen synthesis. It appears that rather than glycogen synthesis being "pushed" as a consequence of an elevated hepatic concentration of hexose monophosphates, glucose stimulates glycogen synthesis by activating the last enzyme of the pathway (glycogen synthetase). The net result is a "pull" mechanism whereby the concentrations of intermediary metabolites, including glucose-6-phosphate, are lowered by the liver.[2] The stimulation of glycogen synthetase results from the direct action of glucose rather than from the high insulin levels secondary to the hyperglycemia.[7]

Whereas the storage of glucose seems to be stimulated directly by excess glucose in the blood, glycogenolysis (the breakdown of glycogen) is under hormonal control. Hormones released in response to hypoglycemia or stress stimulate glycogenolysis at increased rates and tend to inhibit glycogen synthesis. Glucagon-stimulated glycogenolysis is one of the most sensitive and reproducible metabolic effects of hormones on any tissue.[8] Other hormones that stimulate glycogenolysis are epinephrine, norepinephrine, vasopressin, and angiotensin II. In the first few hours after a meal, glycogenolysis can account for as much as 50 per cent of total glucose production, but by 24 hours of fasting, most of the liver glycogen is depleted.[8] Following stress, glycogen depletion is more rapid, even though hyperglycemia is evident.[9]

The central nervous system also plays a role in the regulation of glycogen metabolism. When branches of the splanchnic nerve that innervate the liver are stimulated, the activities of glycogenolytic enzymes are increased more rapidly than after the injection of pharmacologic quantities of epinephrine.[10] Sympathetic stimulation also inhibits glycogen synthetase activity, thereby decreasing glycogen formation.[10] The locus of control of glucose homeostasis within the central nervous system has been under investigation since more than 100 years ago, when Claude Bernard found that puncture of the fourth ventricle resulted in glycosuria. Current studies suggest that the hypothalamus is the most important area of control of glucose homeostasis in CNS. Stimulation of the ventromedial hypothalamus is accompanied by acute rises in glucose, glucagon, and epinephrine and by the suppression of insulin secretion; stimulation of the lateral hypothalamus is followed by a decrease in blood glucose levels.[10]

Gluconeogenesis

Gluconeogenesis refers to the new formation of glucose from noncarbohydrate precursors. Gluconeogenesis is a complex reaction sequence comprising many intermediate steps; it involves some reactions of glycolysis in reverse and some additional reactions that overcome the energy barriers, preventing a direct reversal of glycolysis. The pathways of gluconeogenesis from various precursors are summarized in Figure 3–1.

Cori Cycle

Lactate is an important glucose precursor in resting humans, and in some circumstances it is the primary gluconeogenic precursor. Because much of the lactate is derived from plasma glucose via glycolysis, the resynthesis of glucose from lactate is a cyclic reaction. This cycle was originally described by Cori[11] and is commonly called the Cori cycle. Resynthesis of glucose from lactate in the liver is an important route of lactate disposal, for although other tissues can also dispose of lactate, animals with surgical hepatectomies developed lactic acidosis. When the ability of a tissue to completely catabolize substrates to CO_2 and H_2O is limited (for example, during the partly anaerobic conditions in exercising muscle), the Cori cycle maintains a supply of fuel (glucose) that can provide a certain amount of energy anaerobically. The "net" glucose formation does not increase via the Cori cycle, and in that sense it may be considered a waste of energy, as energy is required to resynthesize the glucose from lactate. However, energy to resynthesize the glucose comes from fat oxidation in the liver,[12] so that the Cori cycle results in a transfer of energy from adipose tissue to muscle, with glucose and lactate serving as the "currency." The resting rate of Cori cycle activity in normal humans has been determined to account for approximately 15 per cent of the total glucose production in fasting.[13]

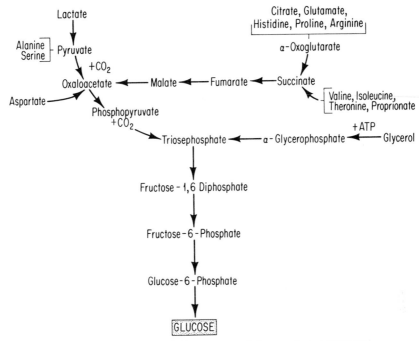

Figure 3–1. Pathways of gluconeogenesis from various precursors.

Gluconeogenesis from Alanine

Alanine and glutamine account for 50 to 60 per cent of the total amino acids released from muscle. In non-acidotic conditions, little glutamine is taken up by the kidney; rather, it is taken up by the mucosal cells of the small intestine and is converted to alanine.[15] Alanine is thus presented to the liver in far greater quantities than any other amino acid and is the major amino acid involved in gluconeogenesis. Alanine is known to be released from muscle in greater quantity than is present in muscle protein, but controversy exists regarding its origin. It has been suggested that pyruvate resulting from the glycolytic catabolism of glucose is transaminated and that the resulting alanine is released into the bloodstream, where it travels to the liver for reincorporation into glucose.[16] According to this proposal, alanine functions in a metabolic cycle analogous to the Cori cycle, in that no new "net" glucose is produced. The α-NH_2 group required for the transamination of pyruvate is derived from amino acids that are oxidized by muscle, including the branched-chain amino acids valine, leucine, and isoleucine, as well as aspartate and glutamate. The role of this process has been suggested to be the transfer of ammonia from muscle to liver in the nontoxic form of alanine.

The physiologic role of the glucose-alanine cycle is not clear. At most, the cycle accounts for a small percentage of glucose production at rest. During exercise, it becomes more important.[17] During starvation, most of the carbons in alanine released by muscle are derived from amino acids, rather than from glucose.[18] Much of the gluconeogenesis from alanine (and also from lactate, since alanine and lactate are in rapid equilibration) in this circumstance represents the "net" synthesis of glucose rather than a cyclic process.

Renal Gluconeogenesis

The precise contribution of renal gluconeogenesis to total glucose production is open to controversy. It is agreed that under most conditions the contribution is not more than 20 per cent of the total, and some investigators have placed the figure much lower. Prolonged starvation is the one circumstance in which the kidney assumes a more significant role in gluconeogenesis.[1] Metabolic acidosis is probably the major factor increasing renal gluconeogenesis during starvation. Under acidotic conditions, glutamine uptake by the kidney is increased by an unknown mechanism. Glutamine is converted to glutamate in the kidney (via the enzyme glutaminase), and then glutamate is converted to d-oxoglutarate and to glucose. Glutaminase activity is inhibited by glutamate, and thus the accumulation of glutamate leads to increased formation of ammonia from glutamine rather than formation of glutamate. The ammonia passes into the renal tubular fluid, enabling the kidney to buffer H^+ ions and thereby permitting more acid to be secreted.

Control Mechanisms for Gluconeogenesis

Rate control of gluconeogenesis is exerted primarily through certain "bottlenecks" of the reaction chain. These include: (1) availability of substrates (precursors) and the conversion of certain starting materials to the first intermediate step, (2) conversion of pyruvate to PEP, and (3) conversion of fructose-diphosphate to fructose-6-phosphate. All controlling steps therefore occur at points where metabolic alternatives are available. At the initiating step, the alternative to the degradation of the precursor is its nondegradation. Gluconeogenesis is only one of many potential fates of pyruvate, including the TCA cycle and use for synthetic purposes. Finally, at the fructose-diphosphate step, the alternative to gluconeogenesis is the TCA cycle and eventual oxidation.

Substrate Availability. Regulation of the supply of substrates to the liver is a factor in regulating the rate of total gluconeogenesis as well as the relative contribution of a particular precursor to gluconeogenesis.[19] The entry of lactate, pyruvate, and glycerol into the liver does not appear to be under hepatic control. Amino acid uptake by the liver, on the other hand, is influenced by several hormones, but it is not clear whether these are direct effects on transport. Once the precursor is in the liver cell, the rate of gluconeogenesis depends on the rate at which the starting material is degraded. The control mechanism might be via the activity of the initiating enzymes.

Conversion of Pyruvate to PEP. The pathway of the conversion of pyruvate to PEP is shown in Figure 3–2. There are several potential sites of control of this conversion:

1. Entry of pyruvate into the mitochondria is a potential control point that is influenced by glucagon, epinephrine, and cortisol.[20]

2. Pyruvate carboxylase is an enzyme responsible for converting pyruvate to oxaloacetate. Pyruvate carboxylase is activated by high concentrations of acetyl-CoA, thus directing pyruvate away from oxidation and toward gluconeogenesis. Many other factors may also be involved in the regulation of pyruvate carboxylase.[19]

3. The pyruvate dehydrogenase enzyme complex competes with pyruvate carboxylase for pyruvate; consequently, regulation of

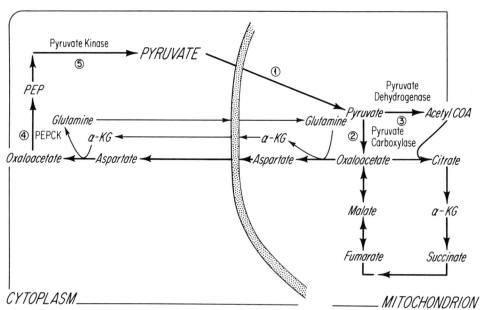

Figure 3–2. Potential sites of regulation of pyruvate to PEP: 1, pyruvate entry into mitochondrion; 2, pyruvate carboxylase; 3, pyruvate dehydrogenase; 4, phosphoenolpyruvate carboxykinase (PEPCK); 5, pyruvate kinase.

pyruvate dehydrogenase is important in determining the eventual fate of pyruvate. The control of pyruvate dehydrogenase is not completely understood, but it involves a phosphorylation-dephosphorylation sequence in which phosphorylation decreases the enzyme activity, with a resulting decrease in the amount of pyruvate directed to oxidation.[12]

4. Oxaloacetate in the cytosol is converted by PEP carboxykinase (PEPCK) to PEP. There does not appear to be a mechanism for short-term control, because the enzyme does not exist in interconvertible forms with differing activities.[20] However, long-term adaptations in gluconeogenesis (e.g., starvation, diabetes) may be mediated through alterations in the rate of synthesis of PEPCK. Cortisol stimulates synthesis, as do hormones acting through the cyclic AMP "second messenger" system (glucagon, epinephrine). Activity of PEPCK is increased in fasting and experimental diabetes.[12]

5. If the liver is in the gluconeogenic mode, it would be desirable to have pyruvate kinase activity low so that any PEP formed would be directed back toward glucose instead of being reconverted to pyruvate. It is clear that a certain amount of such "futile cycling" does occur during active gluconeogenesis (see later), but there may be some suppression of pyruvate kinase during gluconeogenesis.

Conversion of Fructose-Diphosphate (FDP) to Fructose-6-Phosphate (F-6-P). The direction of the net flux between FDP and F-6-P is determined by the relative activities of phospho-fructokinase and fructose-diphosphatase (FDPase). Conditions resulting in the stimulation of one enzyme tend to inhibit the other. For example, in conditions requiring a high rate of glycolysis (such as anoxia), PFK is stimulated by AMP, ADP, and Pi. On the other hand, FDPase is inhibited by AMP, and the subsequent accumulation of FDP potentiates the inhibitory action. Total inhibition of one enzyme never occurs, though, so there is always a certain amount of "futile cycling" (see later).

Futile Cycles

Until the 1970s, it was generally thought that "glycolytic" enzymes were completely suppressed during active gluconeogenesis. Over the past several years, however, it has become evident that this is not the case. For example, during active gluconeogenesis in both kidney and liver tissue, the appearance of ^{14}C from labeled glucose (as well as from other compounds that enter the pathway at different sites) in certain products implies the continued operation of glycolysis. Many of the glycolytic and gluconeogenic reactions are readily reversible and are common to both pathways. The movement of a radiolabeled isotope against the net flux of unlabeled substrate in such a reaction is called an exchange reaction and is not accompanied by energy dissipation. Whereas exchange reactions cause the biochemist methodologic headaches, they are of little physiologic significance. The key steps in glycolysis and gluconeogenesis, however, are unique to each path and are irreversible. When two opposing metabolic pathways are catalyzed by separate enzymes, cyclic reactions occur whereby ATP is hydrolyzed without any change in the reactants. There are three such cycles in the glycolytic/gluconeogenic pathways: (1) the glucose cycle (glucose → G6P → glucose), (2) the fructose-6-phosphate cycle (F6P → FDP → F6P), and (3) the phosphoenol-pyruvate cycle (pyruvate → PEP → pyruvate) (Fig. 3–3).[21] The glucose cycle and the F-6-P cycle are catalyzed by a pair of irreversible enzymes, but the PEP cycle is a complex sequence that differs according to the gluconeogenic precursor. These cycles were originally considered to be useless, energy-wasting reactions and thus were termed *futile cycles*. However, it now appears that under certain circumstances there may be two possible physiologic roles for futile cycles: thermogenesis and amplification of the control over the net flux of substrates at each reaction exerted by allosteric enzyme modification.

Evidence that futile cycling can play an important role in thermogenesis was first obtained from the flight muscles of bees.[22] For a bee to fly, its muscle temperature must be maintained at about 30°F; during the winter, only bees capable of maintaining a high rate of futile cycling in muscle can maintain such a temperature and fly. The importance of the thermogenic aspect of futile cycling in human physiology remains to be proven. The most satisfactory teleologic explanation of futile cycling is that it provides an amplification of control of substrate uptake and utilization.[21] For example, if both PFK activity and FDPase activity are always high, a small percentage of change in the activity of either enzyme could greatly change the magnitude of the flux between F-6-P and FDP and could

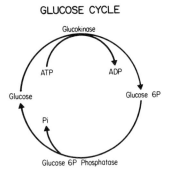

GLUCOSE CYCLE

FRUCTOSE 6P CYCLE

PEP CYCLE

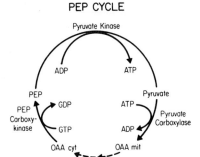

Figure 3–3. Potential futile cycles.

even reverse its direction. Optimal amplification will occur when the cycling is considerably larger than the net flow.[21] For example, if the forward rate of a reaction is 100 arbitrary units and the reverse rate is 80, the net flux forward is 20. A reciprocal change in each rate of only 5 per cent (to 105 and 76, respectively) will result in a 45 per cent increase in net flux. If the forward rate is only 20 units and the reverse rate 0, on the other hand (no futile cycling), a 5 per cent change in the forward rate will result in a 5 per cent change in the total net flux. In the other extreme, if the forward reaction rate is

1000 units and the reverse 980 units, a 5 per cent reciprocal changes in reaction rate (to 1050 and 931, respectively) will increase net flux by 600 per cent. It can be seen from these examples that the larger the individual reaction rates relative to the net flow, the smaller the percentage change in each reaction rate necessary to elicit a given change in the net flow.

Hormonal Control of Gluconeogenesis

Glucagon, epinephrine, and norepinephrine all stimulate hepatic gluconeogenesis via the adenyl cyclase–cAMP "second messenger" system. In this system, the hormone binds to a receptor on the cell surface that is part of adenyl cyclase, the enzyme involved in the formation of cAMP. Adenyl cyclase converts ATP to cAMP and inorganic phosphate (P).[23] The concentration of cAMP within the cell is determined by both the rate of conversion of ATP to cAMP (by adenyl cyclase) and also by the rate of destruction of cAMP (by phosphodiesterase). Phosphodiesterase is inhibited by methylxanthines such as caffeine, with the result that intrahepatic cAMP concentrations rise substantially.

A doubling of hepatic cAMP concentrations stimulates gluconeogenesis maximally.[20] The stimulation that occurs so rapidly after a rise in cAMP action consists of: (1) stimulation of the transport of certain amino acids across the plasma membrane of hepatic cells; (2) reduction of pyruvate dehydrogenase activity, which thereby increases the amount of pyruvate converted to oxaloacetate by pyruvate carboxylase; and (3) activation of a step at the level of PEP carboxykinase.[20]

On the basis of *in vitro* studies, it has been suggested that gluconeogenesis is stimulated by increased availability and oxidation of fatty acids (FFA), and the effect of glucagon on gluconeogenesis is via alterations in hepatic fat metabolism. However, there is little evidence that FFA, either *in vivo* or *in vitro* (in physiologic quantities), increases gluconeogenesis.[24] In fact, elevated FFA levels exert a direct inhibitory effect on glucose production.[25] Elevation of FFA levels will stimulate glucose production only if the original level was so low that availability of energy substrate was the limiting factor in determining the rate at which glucose is produced. The glucocorticoids play a role in the stimulation of gluconeogenesis, but the specific nature of the role is not clear. Glucocorticoids can influence the precursor supply to the liver by stimulating the release of amino acids peripherally. A direct stimulatory effect of glucocorticoids on the rate of synthesis of gluconeogenic enzymes, for example, PEPCK, has also been described.[2] However, the role most generally ascribed to glucocorticoids is that they exert a "permissive action" on gluconeogenesis. Thus, adrenal-deficient animals may have normal rates of gluconeogenesis in fed states but are unresponsive to the hormonal stimulation for increased rates of gluconeogenesis during fasting or other conditions when the tissue level of cAMP is increased by another hormone such as glucagon.

Insulin inhibits gluconeogenesis. Insulin can lower the cAMP concentrations in the liver within a few minutes, and it has been proposed that the inhibitory effect of insulin on gluconeogenesis and glycogenolysis is the result of the lowering of cAMP, because the inhibition of glucose release from the liver is closely linked to a fall in cAMP concentration.[26] However, several experiments indicate that the key to the mechanism of action of insulin may not be related to cAMP. A currently attractive theory is that insulin triggers the release of membrane-bound Ca^{++} into the cytoplasm, which in turn leads to an increased mitochondria uptake of Ca^{++}; the increased cytoplasmic and mitochondrial Ca^{++} concentrations are purported to mediate the actions of insulin.[26]

METABOLISM OF GLUCOSE

Three principal aspects of glucose metabolism will be considered: (1) glycolysis, (2) the oxidation of pyruvate to acetyl-CoA for entrance into the TCA cycle, and (3) the hexose monophosphate shunt.

Glycolysis and Pyruvate Oxidation

Glycolysis involves the anaerobic breakdown of glucose to pyruvate and lactate and occurs in the cytosol of all tissues. With the exception of the end-products and the rate at which glycolysis proceeds, the reactions in glycolysis are the same regardless of whether oxygen is present or not. When oxygen is not available, NADH that is formed during glycolysis cannot readily be oxidized. In this case, the oxidation of NADH that is formed allows glycolysis to proceed. The overall equation for glycolysis to lactate is:

$$\text{Glucose} + 2\,\text{ADP} + \text{Pi} \rightarrow$$
$$2\,\text{lactate} + 2\,\text{ATP} + 2\,H_2O.$$

The specific steps are shown in Figure 3–4. Only highlights of control points will be considered here.

$$(1)\ \text{Glucose} + \text{ATP} \xrightarrow{\text{mg H}} \text{Glucose-6-phosphate}$$

This reaction is catalyzed by the enzyme hexokinase. Hexokinase has a high affinity for glucose, thereby enabling cells to take up glucose and immediately convert it to glucose-6-phosphate even when the plasma concentration of glucose is low. The phosphorylation of glucose is important because it is essentially an irreversible reaction, thus trapping the glucose inside the cell unless the specific enzyme necessary to convert glucose to glucose-6-phosphate (glucose-6-phosphatase) is present. Glucose-6-phosphatase is present in significant quantities only in the liver; in other tissues, therefore, once the glucose is taken up from plasma, it is rapidly converted to glucose-6-phosphate and must be either metabolized for energy or stored.

In addition to hexokinase, the liver possesses a second enzyme, called glucokinase, that catalyzes the conversion of glucose to glucose-6-phosphate. Glucokinase normally plays an important role in enabling the liver to clear glucose from the blood at an accelerated rate. In addition to being the first intermediate in the pathway of glycolysis,

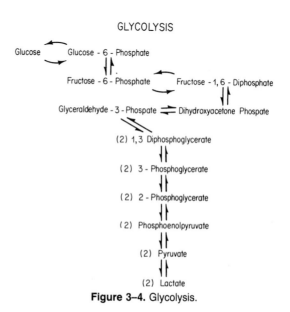

Figure 3–4. Glycolysis.

glucose-6-phosphate is important because it is at a key point in other metabolic pathways as well, including the hexose monophosphate shunt, glycogen synthesis, and gluconeogenesis.

(2) Fructose-6-phosphate + ATP →
$\qquad$ Fructose-1,6-diphosphate

The conversion of fructose-6-phosphate to fructose-1,6-diphosphate is catalyzed by phosphofructokinase (PFK). PFK is an inducible enzyme whose activity is considered to be of prime importance in the regulation of glycolysis.

(3) Glyceraldehyde-3-phosphate + NAD^+ + Pi →
$\qquad$ 1,3-diphosphoglycerate + NADH + H^+

The enzyme responsible for the oxidation reaction, glyceraldehyde-3-phosphate dehydrogenase, is NAD-dependent. The energy released in the oxidation is captured in the form of a high-energy phosphate bond, which subsequently results in the formation of ATP when 1,3-diphosphoglycerate is converted to 3-phosphoglycerate.

(4) Phosphoenolpyruvate + ADP →
$\qquad$ Pyruvate + ATP

This step is catalyzed by the enzyme pyruvate kinase. At this point in glycolysis, 2 net mol of ATP have been generated for 1 mol of glucose oxidized. Once pyruvate is formed, the redox state of the tissue determines whether the pyruvate is reduced to lactate by lactate dehydrogenase or enters the TCA cycle. Although the state of oxygenation of the tissues is clearly an important issue in determining the fate of pyruvate, other factors may also play a role. For example, a high rate of glycolysis, regardless of the state of oxygenation, will result in accelerated lactate release. However, in this case pyruvate release will also increase, leaving the lactate/pyruvate ratio relatively constant.

Pyruvate Oxidation

If adequate NAD^+ is available when pyruvate is formed, pyruvate will enter the TCA cycle. In order to enter the TCA cycle, pyruvate must first be transported into the mitochondria and converted to acetyl-CoA. This process is catalyzed by several enzymes collectively referred to as the pyruvate dehydrogenase complex. Once acetyl-CoA is formed, it can enter the TCA cycle, where-

upon it is oxidized. Complete oxidation of 1 mol of glucose yields 38 mol of ATP, which represents about one-half the energy liberated in the process. The remainder of the energy is released as heat. The considerable discrepancy between the amount of energy obtained from the complete aerobic oxidation of glucose and the amount obtained from the anaerobic glycolysis emphasizes the importance of the availability of oxygen.

Hexose Monophosphate Shunt (Pentose Phosphate Pathway)

This additional pathway for glucose oxidation occurs in certain tissues. Since a major function of shunt is the provision of NADPH, which is required for processes such as fatty acid and steroid synthesis, it is not surprising to find the monophosphate shunt occurring in liver and adipose tissue. The net reaction is as follows:

3 glucose-6-P + 6 $NADP^+$ → 3 CO_2 +
$\quad$ 2 glucose-6-P + glyceraldehyde-3-phosphate +
$\qquad$ 6 NADPH + 6 H^+

REGULATION OF GLUCOSE UTILIZATION

Physiologically, several considerations beyond the metabolic pathways play roles in determining the rate at which glucose is metabolized. Although the concentration of glucose in the blood is normally regulated within narrow limits (see later), the rate of glucose uptake and oxidation in various tissues can vary greatly. Following a high carbohydrate meal, glucose is the major fuel of the body; after several hours of fasting, only about 25 per cent of total CO_2 production is from glucose oxidation.[13] Certain tissues, most notably the brain and erythrocytes, depend on glucose for energy and have a relatively constant rate of uptake of glucose under most conditions. An exception to this is in prolonged starvation, during which the brain adapts to the use of ketone bodies for energy; however, this is a special situation that is not relevant to the day-to-day regulation of glucose utilization when nutrition is available. Therefore, even though the brain and erythrocytes may account for greater than 50 per cent of glucose uptake in fasting, they probably do not play a significant role in the fluctuations in the rate of glucose oxidation observed in different physiologic states. The liver plays an important role in the disposition of a glucose load,[4] but because much of this glucose uptake is converted to glycogen rather than CO_2, the liver is not a site where the rate of glucose oxidation varies much either. The muscle mass, on the other hand, exerts a profound influence on the overall rate of glucose utilization of the individual. Because muscle constitutes approximately 40 per cent of the body mass, any change in the rate of glucose uptake by muscle will significantly affect the overall rate of glucose uptake of the individual. In the postabsorptive human at rest, it is debatable whether the muscle takes up any glucose at all,[27] but in hyperglycemia or during exercise, the rate of glucose utilization by the muscle can increase several-fold. Considerable attention has been focused on the regulation of glucose utilization by the muscle, but as with many aspects of carbohydrate metabolism, the issue is not settled.

Muscle Uptake of Glucose—Entry into the Cell

The rate of entry of glucose into the muscle cell is a rate-limiting step of glucose metabolism. Glucose is rapidly phosphorylated to G-6-P once inside the cell, so the intracellular concentration of glucose is lower than the extracellular concentration, and movement of glucose into the cell occurs down its concentration gradient. Glucose diffusion is facilitated by a carrier-transport system that, when combined with glucose, renders the glucose sufficiently lipid-soluble to move through the cell membrane. No energy is expanded in this process, so it is considered a passive (as opposed to active) transport mechanism. The rate of glucose uptake increases in muscle as the blood level of glucose increases, and for any blood concentrations of glucose, insulin increases the ability of the muscle cell to take up glucose. Insulin works on the surface of the cells by binding to specific receptors, which then initiate its action.[28] The maximal metabolic effect of insulin can apparently be elicited when only two per cent of the insulin receptors are filled.[26] The mechanism whereby insulin stimulates glucose transport may involve membrane phosphorylation,[26] but the details are not clear.

Muscle glucose uptake and utilization are increased significantly during exercise, and bed rest causes decreased forearm glu-

cose uptake during glucose infusion.[29] It has been confirmed that during bed rest it is the lack of physical activity that impairs glucose uptake rather than the disruption of the vertical plane.[29] Muscle glucose uptake in exercise is caused by an increased sensitivity to the action of insulin,[30] which perhaps is due to an increase in binding to receptors.[31] For this reason, exercise has generally proved useful in helping diabetics control their blood glucose concentration and may also be useful in "insulin-resistant" stress patients. Conversely, many of the alterations in glucose metabolism seen in hospitalized patients may be related to their inactivity.

Influence of FFA on Glucose Utilization

Whereas it is generally accepted that insulin regulates muscle glucose utilization by controlling the rate of entry of glucose, there is an alternative explanation originally described as the *glucose–fatty acid cycle*[32] and later updated and renamed the *glucose–ketone–fatty acid cycle*.[18] The cornerstone of the theory is that free fatty acids (FFA) inhibit glucose utilization. Because insulin inhibits lipolysis and thereby reduces the circulatory levels of FFA in the plasma, a low level of insulin (e.g., during fasting) releases that inhibition and results in a high FFA level. The high FFA level in turn inhibits glucose utilization, and because the rate of uptake of glucose is thus reduced, a given blood concentration of glucose can be maintained at a reduced rate of glucose production. The further fall in glucose production that occurs with prolonged fasting is ascribed to the ketosis that develops. The ketones are proposed to compete with glucose as energy substrates in the brain, thereby further reducing the need for glucose production. Thus, this theory focuses on peripheral mechanisms influencing the rate of glucose production secondarily as a consequence of changes in plasma glucose concentration.

In vitro evidence for the glucose–ketone–fatty acid hypothesis includes the fact that in the heart, diaphragm, and soleus muscle, fatty acid oxidation inhibits glucose utilization by inhibiting glucose transport, conversion of F-6-P to FDP (by decreasing the activity of phosphofructokinase), and the conversion of pyruvate to acetyl-CoA (by decreasing pyruvate dehydrogenase activity). In contrast to these findings, it should be noted that some experiments with the perfused hindlimb of the rat have generally failed to demonstrate an inhibitory effect of fatty acids on glucose utilization,[33] although recent evidence indicates that glucose uptake may be inhibited by FFA in that preparation as well.[34]

In vivo, the proposed effects of FFA and ketones on glucose clearance and oxidation have not been demonstrated. Whereas it is true that there is generally an inverse relationship between the plasma level of FFA and the rate of glucose utilization, this relationship can be explained by the fact that the factors that control fatty acid mobilization (e.g., hormones) may influence glucose utilization as well. Figure 3–5 shows the results from an experiment in conscious dogs in which the concentrations of insulin and glucagon were pharmacologically maintained at a constant during the infusion of either a lipid emulsion (Liposyn) plus heparin to raise fatty acid levels or beta-hydroxybutyrate to raise ketone levels. Neither procedure directly affected the ability of the animal to oxidize glucose, as reflected by the percentage of glucose uptake oxidized (determined by means of uniformly labeled ^{14}C-glucose)[35] nor the rate of clearance of glucose from the blood. Rather than indirectly affecting glucose production via peripheral effects on glucose clearance and thus plasma concentration, it seems more likely that ketones and FFA exert direct inhibitory effects on the ability of the liver to produce glucose. In the isolated perfused dog liver, elevation of either ketones or fatty acid levels in the pefusion medium causes a fall in glucose production.[25] *In vivo*, the direct effect of ketones and FFA to suppress glucose production can be demonstrated independently of changes in hormones and in sympathetic activity.[35, 36] Thus, although there are many significant interactions between glucose, FFA, and ketones, they do not appear to be so much through peripheral effects on the oxidation of the other substrates but as through direct effects on the rate of glucose production.

Influence of Lactate on Glucose Metabolism

Lactate is the product of the anaerobic metabolism of glucose (see Fig. 3–4), and as such is considered by many to be a metabolic dead end. However, recent studies have shown that lactate plays an active role in the overall energy metabolism of the individual, both as an energy substrate and as a regulator. The crucial point to remember when applying knowledge of metabolic pathways to the *in vivo* organism is that *in vivo*, many tissues and organs are functioning simultaneously, and not all tissues behave the same

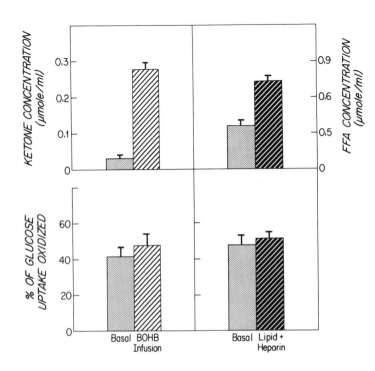

Figure 3–5. Effect of the infusion of lipid emulsion (Liposyn) plus heparin or BOH butyrate (BOHB) on the ability of the conscious dog to oxidize glucose, as reflected by the percentage of glucose uptake oxidized. Glucose kinetics and oxidation were determined by means of U-^{14}C-glucose. (*From* Shaw, J. H. F., and Wolfe, R. R.: Glucose-fatty acid interactions: kinetic evaluation using stable and radioisotopes. In press; and Shaw, J. H. F., and Wolfe, R. R.: The influence of β-hydroxybutyrate infusion on glucose and free fatty acid metabolism in vivo: a kinetic study. Am. J. Physiol., in press, with permission.)

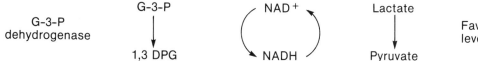

Figure 3–6. Effect of lactate on glucose oxidation.

biochemically. Lactate plays an active role in the regulation of glucose oxidation in several tissues. Lactate reduces glyceraldehyde-3-phosphate dehydrogenase activity, which converts glyceraldehyde-3-phosphate to 1,3-diphosphoglyceric (1,3 DPG) acid in the glycolytic chain. The mechanism appears to involve both a direct lactate effect of the enzyme, and a reduction in NAD^+ availability, owing to the competition illustrated in Figure 3–6.

GLUCOSE METABOLISM DURING PARENTERAL NUTRITION

In the normal human, the concentration of plasma glucose is regulated quite closely. Teleologically, this can be explained on the one hand by the constant need for a certain amount of glucose for glucose-dependent tissue (brain, erythrocytes) and on the other hand by the detrimental effects of extreme hyperglycemia (e.g., hyperosmotic coma). The mechanisms responsible for the regula-

tion of plasma glucose concentration during a glucose infusion are of fundamental importance to the entire metabolic response to parenteral nutrition.

Two processes can minimize changes in plasma glucose concentration during a glucose infusion: (1) reduction of glucose production and (2) enhanced ability to clear glucose from the bloodstream. During the first few hours of glucose infusion, the primary operative mechanism is the suppression of glucose production. This response can occur independently of changes in insulin concentration, as shown in Figure 3–7. In one case, glucose was infused in normal volunteers and glucose production was measured isotopically. In the second study, the glucose infusion was repeated, but the insulin (and glucagon) response was blocked by the constant infusion of somatostatin, insulin, and glucagon. Despite the absence of an insulin response, total glucose production, gluconeogenesis from alanine, and urea production were all suppressed to the same extent when the hormones were controlled

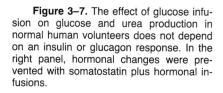

Figure 3–7. The effect of glucose infusion on glucose and urea production in normal human volunteers does not depend on an insulin or glucagon response. In the right panel, hormonal changes were prevented with somatostatin plus hormonal infusions.

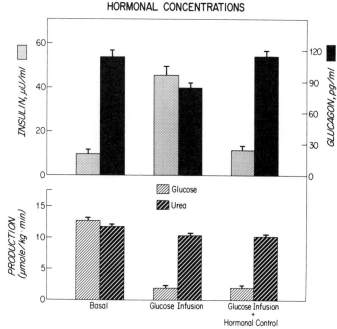

as when there was an insulin response. In the initial response to a glucose infusion, glucose clearance is not affected by the insulin response. However, after several hours of glucose infusion, the insulin becomes effective in stimulating glucose clearance. Because glucose clearance is increased, early hyperglycemia will subside to some extent after a time. Once the peripheral adaptation of the glucose infusion occurs, the rate of glucose infusion can be progressively increased to higher and higher rates without markedly elevating the blood glucose level any further.

The clinical significance of the suppressive effect of infused glucose on glucose production is evident. If the rate of gluconeogenesis from amino acids is suppressed, that amount of nitrogen (with the carbon skeletons) will be available for reincorporation into protein rather than for excretion as urea. Because the liver is very sensitive to the infused glucose, relatively small amounts of infused glucose (100 gm/day) can effectively spare a significant amount of nitrogen. Higher rates of glucose infusion can suppress glucose production to an even greater extent, but once the glucose infusion rate is greater than the endogenous production rate (about 250 gm/day in normal volunteers), little further benefit in terms of suppression of glucose production can be expected.

To understand the response to infused glucose, it is important to realize that the rate of gluconeogenesis cannot be suppressed below zero. Once enough glucose is given to achieve the maximal suppression of gluconeogenesis, the justification of administering glucose at rates in excess of that amount must reside in the ability of the body to oxidize the infused glucose, since equal benefit in terms of sparing the body from providing gluconeogenic precursors can be achieved with lower infusion rates. Figure 3–8 shows the rate of glucose oxidation in five postoperative (nonseptic) patients given TPN (glucose and amino acids) at progressively increasing rates. Each value for glucose oxidation was obtained after two days of continuous glucose infusion at that rate. The rate of oxidation was determined with the primed-constant infusion of U-^{13}C-glucose. The important points to be made from these data are that even during the 4 mg/kg·min infusion, less than half of the infused glucose was directly oxidized; the percentage of infused glucose that was oxidized fell at an infusion rate of 9.0 mg/kg·min, only 61.6 per cent of CO_2 production was from the direct oxidation of glucose. The percentage of CO_2 from glucose did not rise in a parallel manner with the glucose oxidation rate, because CO_2 production also rose as the glucose infusion rate increased. The data shown in Figure 3–8 are from a small sampling of patients, but the data from other studies are comparable. Thus, in cancer patients given glucose infusion rates ranging from 4.0 to 7.4 mg/kg·

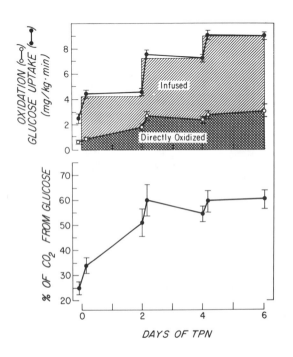

Figure 3–8. Glucose oxidation during total parenteral nutrition in five general surgical patients.

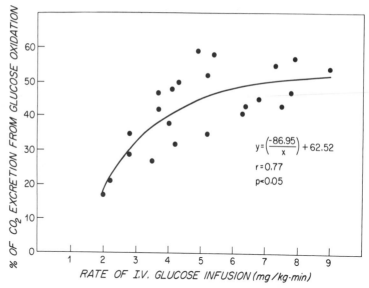

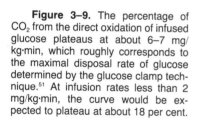

Figure 3–9. The percentage of CO_2 from the direct oxidation of infused glucose plateaus at about 6–7 mg/kg·min, which roughly corresponds to the maximal disposal rate of glucose determined by the glucose clamp technique.[51] At infusion rates less than 2 mg/kg·min, the curve would be expected to plateau at about 18 per cent.

$$y = \left(\frac{-86.95}{x}\right) + 62.52$$

$$r = 0.77$$

$$p < 0.05$$

min, the percentage of CO_2 from glucose oxidation ranged from 37 to 62 per cent, with the average being 50.2 per cent.[38] The percentage of CO_2 resulting from the direct oxidation of infused glucose also reaches a plateau around 60 per cent in burn patients, regardless of infusion rate (Fig. 3–9). Recent studies using indirect calorimetry and different glucose infusion rates have confirmed the results of earlier isotopic studies.[39, 40]

Insulin is commonly given during a high-dose glucose infusion in order to minimize the resulting hyperglycemia. Although insulin may have a direct action to inhibit protein breakdown, extra insulin has little effect on the oxidation of infused glucose (Fig. 3–10). This point is amplified by the fact that when data from a large number of isotopic studies are considered, there appears to be no relationship between the ability of tissues to clear glucose from the blood and the subsequent oxidation of the glucose.

The lack of correlation between glucose clearance and oxidation is not surprising. Less than 50 per cent of glucose uptake at any time is oxidized to CO_2 and water. There is every reason to expect that adaptation to high glucose loads will occur in the other pathways involved with the disposal of glucose, particularly lipogenesis. Indirect lines of evidence, including results of body compositional studies[41] and hepatic biopsy data,[42] support the concept that during prolonged glucose infusions the glucose that is not oxidized is converted to fat.

From the N excretion data from the pa-

tients whose results are shown in Figure 3–8, we calculated that 16 per cent of $\dot{V}CO_2$ came from protein during the 9 mg/kg·min infusion; thus, 22 per cent of $\dot{V}CO_2$ was coming from fat oxidation, even though glucose was being infused at a rate in excess of the metabolic rate. This might appear to be in conflict with the fact that during the 9 mg/kg·min infusion, the respiratory quotient (RQ) was well in excess of 1,[1, 13] which would indicate

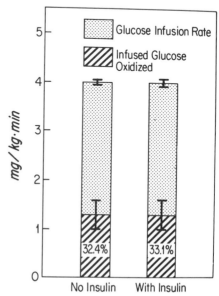

Figure 3–10. The direct oxidation of glucose is not affected by the infusion of extra insulin. (*From* Wolfe, R. R., Allsop, J. R., and Burke, J. F.: Glucose metabolism in man: response to intravenous glucose infusion. Metabolism, *28*:210, 1979, with permission.)

that all energy was being derived from carbohydrate. However, it must be remembered that the RQ reflects net oxidation only. The high RQ during the glucose infusion can be explained by the conversion of infused glucose to fat. This point can be clarified by examining the stoichiometry of triglyceride (TG) synthesis from glucose, assuming that the TG is composed of equimolar amounts of palmitic, stearic, and oleic acids[43]:

$$13.5\ C_6H_{12}O_6 + 3\ O_2 \rightarrow C_{55}H_{104}O_6 + 26\ CO_2 + 29\ H_2O$$
$$9728\ kcal \rightarrow 8184\ kcal;\ therefore\ \Delta E = 1544\ kcal$$
$$(4.0\ kcal/gm) \rightarrow (9.5\ kcal/gm);\ therefore\ \Delta E = -.63\ kcal/gm\ glucose$$

During the 9 mg/kg·min infusion, 5.9 mg/kg·min (32.7 µmole/kg·min) of glucose was not oxidized. If it is assumed that all of this was directed to fat (to obtain a maximal value), then 32.7 µmole glucose + 7.26 µmole $O_2 \rightarrow$ 4.42 µmole TG + 62.9 µmole CO_2 + 70.2 µmole H_2O. Thus, 5.9 mg/kg·min glucose $\rightarrow$ 2.08 mg/kg·min TG, and $\Delta E = -3.93$ kcal/kg·min.

From this discussion, it is clear how an RQ can be in excess of 1 even when there is a significant rate of fat oxidation (in an absolute sense). For the example cited, 22 per cent of $\dot{V}CO_2$ could not be accounted for by glucose or protein oxidation and thus was due to fat oxidation. Twenty-two per cent of total $\dot{V}CO_2$ (180 µmole/kg·min) = 39.6 µmole/kg·min.
Thus:

$$\frac{39.6\ \text{µmole/kg·min } CO_2 \text{ from fat oxidation}}{52\ \text{µmole } CO_2 \text{ produced from /µmole TG oxidation of FA}} = \begin{array}{l} .76\ \text{µmole TG/kg·min oxidized} \\ .65\ \text{mg TG/kg·min oxidized} \end{array}$$

$$\frac{.65\ \text{mg TG/kg·min/oxidized}}{2.08\ \text{mg/kg·min synthesized}} = 31\%\ \text{of TG synthesized was subsequently oxidized}$$

Therefore, the net rate of fat synthesis would be: 2.08 mg/kg·min −0.65 mg/kg·min = 1.43 mg/kg·min. Whereas this is a maximal rate of fat synthesis from the infused glucose, calculation of the rate of conversion of glucose to fat purely from the indirect calorimetry data as described by Elwyn and Kinney[44] yields a value of 1.01 mg/kg·min. Since the fundamental assumptions used to derive the two figures for TG synthesis are different and yet the two values are relatively close, it is reasonable to assume that the true value is in the same range. The important point revealed by the isotopic data that cannot be appreciated from the indirect calorimetry data is the rate of oxidation of fat occurring at the same time that net fat synthesis is occurring. Thus, even though glucose was not infused at a rate in excess of caloric requirement and a large quantity was converted to fat, certain tissues continued to rely on fat as their oxidative substrate. We have recently confirmed this conclusion in dogs infused simultaneously with ^{14}C-glucose and ^{13}C-palmitic acid.[35] This observation establishes a rationale for providing the calories in TPN in the form of both glucose and fat. Administering fat simultaneously with glucose might be anticipated to reduce the efficiency of oxidation of the infused glucose according to the glucose–fatty acid cycle originally proposed by Randle and colleagues,[32] but as discussed previously, in vivo experiments have shown this not to be the case.[35]

The preceding argument establishes that there is a maximal rate of glucose infusion beyond which beneficial effect cannot be expected. When the optimal rate is exceeded, detrimental side effects occur. The high rate of fat synthesis cited previously is associated with fatty livers.[42] The increased energy required for TG synthesis from carbohydrate contributes to an increased metabolic rate, and because of the high RQ of TG synthesis, CO_2 production increases to a much greater extent than the $\dot{V}O_2$. This process of glucose conversion to fat prior to oxidation is accompanied by a greater production of CO_2 and H_2O, as well as a higher consumption of O_2, than if the glucose had been directly oxidized. This is because additional substrate carbon and hydrogen must be oxidized to provide the energy needed for fat synthesis. Also, because of the high respiratory quotient (RQ) of fat synthesis (8.7), a disproportionate amount of CO_2 is excreted relative to the O_2 consumed, leading to a high RQ (as high as 1.3 in some patients). The result may be a significant ventilatory load to a patient with pre-existent respiratory impairment.[45] Further, the water load imposed on the subject (primarily infused, but also from the conversion of glucose to fat) may contribute to pulmonary edema. In this light it is interesting that body composition studies utilizing neutron activation and ^3H_2O have shown that weight gain over two weeks of TPN with glucose and amino acids is essentially attributable to gain in total body water.[41]

Clinical Implications

Extrapolation from the quantitative aspects of glucose oxidation leads to the conclusion that the primary N-sparing effects of infused glucose are in terms of its suppressive effects on glucose production. From direct measurements of glucose production during graded glucose infusions, the maximal N sparing (relative to glucose infusion rate) would be predicted to occur with the infusion of glucose at the rate 1 mg/kg/min, because at that rate production is most efficiently suppressed. Although higher rates of glucose infusion should result in greater N sparing than during the 1 mg/kg/min infusion, any additional N sparing would be modest because there is a limit to the extent to which glucose production can be suppressed. Glucose given in excess of the amount required for most efficient suppression of production is not readily oxidized for energy production. Nitrogen balance data in normal volunteers given two doses of glucose infusion for ten days are consistent with the results predicted from our isotopic data.[46] Volunteers infused with glucose at the rate of approximately 1.3 mg/kg/min had a decrease in the rate of nitrogen excretion from 6.1 to 2.4 gm N/m^2 day. Increasing the glucose rate 450 per cent (to approximately 7 mg/kg/min) had a further modest effect on N excretion, in that the control value of 6.3 gm N/m^2 day was reduced to 1.6 gm N/m^2 day.[46] Thus, changes in nitrogen excretion rate can be approximately predicted from the degree of suppression of endogenous glucose production.

The fact that plasma glucose concentration is regulated primarily through modulation of glucose production enables the clinician to infer useful information about the effect of a given glucose infusion on nitrogen balance from the simple measurement of plasma glucose concentration. The infusion rate that causes plasma glucose concentration to rise in excess of 15 mg/dl is the rate beyond which further suppression of endogenous production cannot be anticipated. The infusion of insulin in that setting would effectively lower the concentration of glucose but would have no further effect on glucose production (beyond that resulting from the endogenous insulin already released in response to the glucose infusion, assuming that pancreatic islet function is normal). Thus, if a patient becomes hyperglycemic during a glucose infusion, it is likely that glucose production is maximally suppressed, glucose is being wasted, and little "benefit" (in terms of nitrogen balance) can be anticipated from a further increase in the glucose infusion rate.

It should be noted that beneficial effects of high doses of glucose associated with large doses of insulin have been reported in catabolic patients.[47] Although this finding remains to be substantiated on a widespread basis, particularly in noncatabolic patients, it is important to realize that if high-dose insulin + glucose exerts an effect of N balance, the effect is almost certainly due to the direct effects of insulin on protein metabolism, rather than to the effects of the glucose. The high-dose glucose is needed to cover the insulin in order to prevent hypoglycemia. Thus, the same (or worse) detrimental side effects of glucose overdose discussed previously will occur if high-dose insulin is added to the glucose infusion. Possible beneficial effects of insulin must therefore be weighed against the side effects that will occur secondary to the large amounts of glucose that must be given with the insulin.

Response to Trauma

The term *insulin resistance* has been widely used to describe glucose metabolism in the trauma patient. Although this phrase is rarely defined, *insulin resistance* generally is used to describe a situation in which insulin is not functioning normally in terms of its stimulation of glucose uptake. Consequently, the blood level of glucose rises, stimulating a further elevation in the insulin level, which still fails to stimulate uptake of glucose. Thus, the "insulin-resistant" patient will have elevated plasma glucose and insulin concentrations, with insulin usually being elevated to a greater extent than glucose.

Although the clinical finding of hyperglycemia in association with an elevated plasma insulin concentration is frequently observed in trauma patients, the preceding picture of insulin resistance seems to be an oversimplification of what is happening in such a patient. The first point to consider is that the important action of incremental rises in endogenous insulin secretion above the basal level is to suppress hepatic glucose production, in addition to the stimulation of peripheral glucose uptake. In terms of the suppression of basal glucose production by insulin, most trauma patients are "insulin resistant"; i.e., glucose production is elevated above the normal rate even though insulin concentration is normal or even elevated.[48, 49] The source of the newly produced glucose may vary, depending on the particular circumstance. In shock, glycogenolysis may increase the glucose output of the liver, even in the fact of marked hyperglycemia. Glycogen stores are rather quickly exhausted, though, and in the "high-flow" state of response to trauma (when no glucose is infused), the increased glucose production originates mainly from amino acids and lactic acid. Much of the glucose production from lactic acid represents increased activity of the Cori cycle, and thus "new" glucose is not generated. The primary source (other than glycogen) of precursors for the production of "new" glucose (gluconeogenesis) is protein that is broken down into amino acids. There are two possibilities to explain the relationship between protein metabolism and gluconeogenesis after trauma. One is that an elevated rate of protein catabolism may result in an increased supply of gluconeogenic precursors (amino acids) to the liver, which then drives gluconeogenesis. The other possibility is that hormonally mediated stimulation of gluconeogenesis (e.g., via adrenalin and glucagon) may indirectly result in an increased rate of net protein catabolism, because amino acids are directed away from re-incorporation into protein and towards glucose production.

As referred to previously, a common manifestation of hepatic "insulin resistance" is a failure of exogenously injected or infused glucose to suppress endogenous glucose production. However, a lack of suppressibility of glucose production by glucose is not a universal finding in the trauma patient, even in the burn patient, whose basal rate of glucose production is elevated by more than 100 per cent.[49] Why, on the one hand, the rate of basal glucose production is elevated but, on the other hand, glucose production is suppressed by exogenously infused glucose has not been conclusively explained. An exaggerated insulin response to the infused glucose is a likely explanation.[49] Regardless, the ability of infused glucose to suppress endogenous production provides the basis for providing more than the normal amount of glucose to injured patients. If basal glucose production is elevated to 6 mg/kg · min and infused glucose is effective in suppressing endogenous production, then as much as 5 or 6 mg/kg · min glucose can be infused into the patient without actually altering the total amount of glucose appearing in plasma.

In the physiologic steady state, glucose uptake equals the rate of glucose production. It therefore follows that since most trauma patients have elevated rates of glucose production, they likewise have increased rates of glucose uptake.[49] However, an increased rate of uptake does not necessarily reflect an enhanced ability of the tissues to take up glucose, because glucose uptake increases proportionately as blood glucose concentration rises, independent of any change in the ability of the tissues to take up glucose (e.g., insulin effect).[50] This may be because most glucose uptake occurs in non–insulin-sensitive tissues, and the rate of uptake is to a large extent determined by the diffusion gradient for glucose. Thus, in evaluating the ability of tissues to take up glucose, it is convenient to correct the rate of glucose uptake for the prevailing plasma concentration. The resulting value (the glucose clearance rate) is an index of the ability of tissues to take up glucose. Even the basal glucose clearance rate, however, is usually normal or elevated in burn patients.[49] Nonetheless, these patients may have "insulin resistance" in the traditional sense of the term—insulin does not stimulate glucose uptake in insulin-sensitive tissues as effectively as in normal volunteers.

When glucose was infused at the rate of 4 mg/kg · min (without insulin) into normal volunteers and burned patients, endogenous glucose production was suppressed to a similar extent in each group.[49] The insulin response to the glucose infusion was not enough to stimulate the ability of tissues to take up glucose in either the patients or the volunteers, and thus hyperglycemia ensued. However, if insulin was infused into the volunteers in conjunction with the glucose infusion, the hyperglycemia could be controlled (Fig. 3–11). This is because the peripheral concentration of insulin reached a high enough level to stimulate the ability of the tissues to take up glucose. The same effect could be achieved with insulin infusion

Figure 3–11. *Top panel,* When glucose was infused at 4 mg/kg·min in normal controls and burn patients, the basal glucose concentration was maintained if exogenous insulin was administered. In this experiment, 10.3 ± 1.68 U of insulin was required over 2 hours in the burn patients, as opposed to 1.9 ± 0.10 U over 2 hours in the controls. *Bottom panel,* Representative examples of the manner in which the insulin was infused. Resulting plasma insulin concentrations after 2-hour insulin and glucose infusions were 94.3 ± 8.9 µU/ml in burn patients and 53.2 ± 12.3 µU/ml in controls, indicating a higher rate of insulin clearance in the burn patients. (*From* Wolfe, R. R., Durkot, M. J., Allsop, J. R., and Burke, J. F.: Glucose metabolism in severely burned patients. Metabolism, 28:1031–1039, 1979, with permission.)

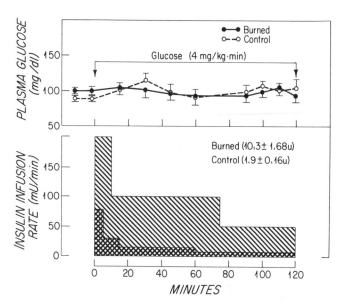

in burned patients, but on the average, approximately five times the amount of infused insulin was required to increase the glucose clearance comparably. Thus, there would appear to be peripheral "insulin resistance" in burned patients, meaning a decreased responsiveness to the stimulatory action of infused insulin on glucose uptake. Here again, though, there are two components to the "insulin resistance." Although five times as much infused insulin was required in burned patients as in controls, the resulting plasma insulin concentration was only doubled in the burned patients. This means that infused insulin is cleared from the bloodstream approximately three times faster in burned patients than in controls. Even so, a higher plasma concentration of insulin was required in burn patients to elicit a similar increase in glucose clearance in controls. These results are consistent with a more recent study in which the "euglycemic insulin clamp" technique was used.[51] The principle of the method is similar to that shown in Figure 3–11, except that a fixed insulin infusion rate is used, the glucose is varied appropriately to maintain euglycemia, and the amount of glucose infused is used as the index of the amount of "insulin resistance." In this study, it was found that the maximal rate of glucose disposal is reduced in burned patients and that peripheral insulin resistance appears to occur in skeletal muscle.

Thus, the responsiveness to insulin is diminished both at the liver and peripherally. Nonetheless, the term "insulin resistance" may not be appropriate for describing the situation in the trauma patient, because it implies that insulin is without effect. In fact, several lines of evidence give indirect support to the concept that peripheral insulin resistance may not be related to any real deficiency in the action of insulin on glucose transport, but rather may be due to a block in the metabolism of glucose once it enters the cell. For example, the insulin resistance of isolated fat cells from obese mice is due to a reduction in the activity of one or more intracellular enzymes involved in glucose metabolism.[52] The hexose transport system in these cells is fully sensitive to activation of insulin under conditions in which glucose utilization is not. The possibility that the same phenomenon may occur after trauma is suggested by the high intracellular glucose concentrations observed in burned rats,[53] which indicate that glucose has entered the cell but that its metabolism, once inside the cell, is limited. Support for the concept that insulin-stimulated glucose uptake in the trauma patient is limited by the ability to metabolize glucose is provided by the observation that patients with peripheral insulin resistance oxidize a lower percentage of basal glucose uptake.[49] Further, the severely burned patient oxidizes a smaller percentage of infused glucose than normal.[49] Finally, the glucose clamp study cited previously also concluded that the peripheral resistance to insulin in burn injury is related to a postreceptor defect.[51]

The evidence that infused glucose can effectively suppress glucose production in burn patients, as well as the fact that burn patients have elevated rates of glucose production, provides the rationale for infusing glucose at rates up to about 6 mg/kg·min. However, the data discussed in relation to a limit of the maximal glucose disposal rate due to a postreceptor defect in glucose oxidation indicates that glucose should not be infused into burned patients in excess of this amount.

REFERENCES

1. Owen, O. E., Felig, P., Morgan, A. P., Wahren, J., and Cahill, G. F., Jr.: Liver and kidney metabolism during prolonged starvation. J. Clin. Invest., 48:574, 1969.
2. Hers, H. G.: The control of glycogen metabolism in the liver. Ann. Rev. Biochem., 45:167–189, 1976.
3. Krebs, H. A.: Some aspects of the regulation of fuel supply in omnivorous animals. Adv. Enzyme Regul., 10:397, 1972.
4. Felig, P., Wahren, J., and Hendler, R.: Influence of oral glucose ingestion on splanchnic glucose and gluconeogenic substrate metabolism in man. Diabetes, 24:468, 1975.
5. Bergman, R. N.: Integrated control of hepatic metabolism. Fed. Proc., 36:265, 1977.
6. Stalmans, W., De Wulf, H., Hue, L., and Hers, H. D.: The sequential inactivation of glycogen phosphorylase and activation of glycogen synthetase in liver after the administration of glucose to mice and rats. The mechanism of hepatic threshold to glucose. Eur. J. Biochem., 41:127, 1974.
7. Hems, D. A.: Short-term hormonal control of hepatic carbohydrate and lipid catabolism. F.E.B.S. Letters, 80:237, 1977.
8. Cahill, G. F., Jr.: Starvation in man. N. Engl. J. Med., 282:668, 1970.
9. Filkins, J. R., and Cornell, R. P.: Depression of hepatic gluconeogenesis and the hypoglycemia of endotoxic shock. Am. J. Physiol., 227:778, 1974.
10. Frohman, L. A.: The hypothalamus and metabolic control. In Ioachim, H. (ed.): Pathobiology Annual. New York, Appleton-Century-Crofts, 1971.
11. Cori, C. F.: Mammalian carbohydrate metabolism. Physiol. Rev., 11:143, 1931.
12. Exton, J. H.: Gluconeogenesis. Metabolism, 21:945, 1975.
13. Wolfe, R. R., Allsop, J. R., and Burke, J. F.: Glucose metabolism in man: response to intravenous glucose infusion. Metabolism, 28:210, 1979.
14. Bortz, W. M., Paul, P., Haff, A. G., and Holmes, W. L.: Glycerol turnover and oxidation in man. J. Clin. Invest., 51:1537, 1972.
15. Windmueller, H. G., and Spaeth, A. E.: Intestinal metabolism of glutamine and glutamate from the lumen as compared to glutamine from blood. Arch. Biochem. Biophysiol., 171:662, 1975.
16. Felig, P.: The glucose-alanine cycle. Metabolism, 22:179, 1973.
17. Wolfe, R. R., Wolfe, M. H., Nadel, E. R., and Shaw, J. H. F.: Amino acid–urea interactions in exercising humans. J. Appl. Physiol., 56:221, 1984.
18. Newsholme, E. A.: Carbohydrate metabolism in vivo: Regulation of blood glucose level. Clin. Endocrinol. Metab., 5:543, 1976.
19. Krebs, H.: Gluconeogenesis. Proc. R. Soc. Lond., Ser. B, 159:545, 1964.
20. Exton, J. H., Mallete, L. E., Jefferson, L. S., Wong, E. H., Friedman, N., Miller, T. B., Jr., and Park, C. R.: The hormonal control of hepatic gluconeogenesis. Recent Prog. Hormone Res., 26:411, 1970.
21. Katz, J., and Rognstad, R.: Futile cycles in the metabolism of glucose. Curr. Top. Cell. Regul., 10:237, 1976.
22. Newsholme, E. A., Crabtree, B., Higgins, S. J., Thornton, S. D., and Start, C.: The activities of fructose diphosphatase in flight muscle from the bumble bee and the role of this enzyme in heat generation. Biochem. J., 128:89, 1972.
23. Newholme, E. A., and Gevers, W.: Control of glycolysis and gluconeogenesis in liver and kidney cortex. Vitam. Horm., 25:1, 1967.
24. Williamson, J. R., Browning, E. T., and Scholz, R.: Control mechanisms of gluconeogenesis and ketogenesis. I. Effects of oleate on gluconeogenesis in perfused rat liver. J. Biol. Chem., 244:4607, 1969.
25. Shaw, J. H. F., and Wolfe, R. R.: The effect of free fatty acids and ketone bodies on glucose production in the perfused dog liver. J. Surg. Res., 37:437, 1984.
26. Czech, M. P.: Molecular basis of insulin action. Ann. Rev. Biochem., 46:359, 1977.
27. Andres, R., Cader, G., and Zierler, K. L.: The quantitatively minor role of carbohydrate in oxidative metabolism by skeletal muscle in intact man in the basal state. Measurements of oxygen and glucose uptake and carbon dioxide and lactate production in the forearm. J. Clin. Invest., 35:671, 1956.
28. Cuatrecasas, P.: Insulin-receptor interactions in adipose tissue cells: Direct measurement and properties. Proc. Nat. Acad. Sci. USA, 68:1264, 1971.
29. Lipman, R. L., Raksin, P., Love, T., Teirbwasser, T., Lecong, R. R., and Schnure, J. J.: Glucose intolerance during decreased physical activity in man. Diabetes, 21:101, 1972.
30. Wolfe, R. R., Nadel, E. R., and Shaw, J. H. F.: Effect of exercise on glucose homeostasis in man with insulin and glucagon clamped. In Knuttgen, H., Vogel, J. A., and Poortmans, J. (eds.): Biochemistry of Exercise. Champaign, Ill., Human Kinetics, 1983, pp. 707–713.
31. Kiovisto, V., Soman, V., Nadel, F., et al.: Exercise and insulin: studies on insulin binding, insulin mobilization and counterregulatory hormone secretion. Fed. Proc., 39:1481, 1980.
32. Randle, P. J., Garland, P. B., Hales, C. N., and Newsholme, E. A.: The glucose and fatty acids cycle. Its role in insulin sensitivity and the metabolic disturance of diabetes mellitus. Lancet, 1:785, 1963.
33. Goodman, M. N., Berger, M., and Ruderman, N. B.: Glucose metabolism in rat skeletal muscle at rest. Effect of starvation, diabetes, ketone bodies and free fatty acids. Diabetes, 23:881–888, 1974.
34. Rennie, M., and Holloszy, J. O.: Inhibition of glucose uptake and glycogenolysis by availability of oleate in well oxygenated perfused skeletal muscle. Biochem. J., 168:161, 1977.
35. Shaw, J. H. F., and Wolfe, R. R.: Glucose–fatty acid interactions: Kinetic evaluation using stable and radioisotopes. In press.
36. Shaw, J. H. F., and Wolfe, R. R.: The influence of β-hydroxybutyrate infusion on glucose and free fatty acid metabolism in vivo: a kinetic study. Am. J. Physiol., 247:E756, 1984.

37. Wolfe, R. R., and Shaw, J. H. F.: In vivo interaction between plasma FFA levels and glucose production during adrenergic blockade and hormonal control in the conscious dog. Am. J. Physiol., 246:E181, 1984.

38. Holroyde, C. P., Meyers, R. N., Smith, R. D., Putnam, R. C., Paul, P., and Reichard, G. A.: Metabolic response to total parenteral nutrition in cancer. Cancer Res., 37:3109, 1977.

39. DeFronzo, R. A., Jacot, E., Jequier, E., Moeder, E., Wharen, J., and Felber, J. P.: The effect of insulin on the disposal of intravenous glucose. Results from indirect calorimetry and hepatic and femoral venous catheterization. Diabetes, 30:1000, 1981.

40. Thieband, D., Schutz, Y., Acheson, K., Jacot, E., DeFronzo, R. A., Felber, J. P., and Jequier, E.: Energy cost of glucose storage in human subjects during glucose-insulin infusion. Am. J. Physiol., 244:E216, 1983.

41. Hill, G. L., Bradley, J. A., Smith, R. C., Smith, A. H., McCarthy, I. D., Oxby, C. B., Burkinshaw, L., and Morgan, D. B.: Changes in body weight and body protein with intravenous nutrition. J.P.E.N., 3:215, 1979.

42. Jeejeebhoy, K. N., Langer, B., Tsallas, G., Shu, R. C., Kiksis, A., and Anderson, G. H.: Total parenteral nutrition at home: Studies in patients surviving 4 months to 5 years. Gastroenterology, 71:943, 1976.

43. Merrill, A. L., and Watt, B. K.: Energy value of foods. Agriculture Handbook No. 74, Washington, D.C., U.S. Government Printing Office, March, 1955.

44. Elwyn, D. H., and Kinney, J. M.: A unique approach to measuring total energy expenditure by indirect calorimetry. In Kinney, J. M., Munro, H. M., and Buskirk, E. (eds.): First Ross Conference on the Assessment of Energy Metabolism in Health and Disease. North Chicago, Ill., Abbott Products, 1981.

45. Askanazi, J., Nordenstrom, J., Rosenbaum, S. H., Elwyn, D. H., Hyman, A. L., Carpentier, Y. A., and Kenney, J. M.: Nutrition for the patient with respiratory failure: Glucose vs. fat. Anesthesiology, 54:373–377, 1981.

46. O'Connell, R. C., Morgan, A. P., Aoki, T. T., et al.: Nitrogen conservation in starvation: Graded responses to intravenous glucose. J. Clin. Endocrinol. Metab., 39:555–559, 1974.

47. Allizon, S. P.: Effect of insulin on metabolic response to injury. J.P.E.N., 4:175–179, 1980.

48. Long, C. L., Spencer, J. L., and Kinney, J. M.: Carbohydrate metabolism in man: Effect of elective operations and major trauma. J. Appl. Physiol., 31:110–116, 1971.

49. Wolfe, R. R., Durkot, M. J., Allsop, J. R., and Burke, J. F.: Glucose metabolism in severely burned patients. Metabolism, 28:1031–1039, 1979.

50. Cherrington, A. D., Williams, P. E., and Harris, M. S.: Relationship between the plasma glucose level and glucose uptake in the conscious dog. Metabolism, 27:787–791, 1978.

51. Black, P. R., Brooks, D. C., Bessey, P. Q., Wolfe, R. R., and Wilmore, D. W.: Mechanisms of insulin resistance following injury. Ann. Surg., 192:420–435, 1982.

52. Czech, M. P., Richardson, D. K., and Smith, C. I.: Biochemical basis of fat cell insulin resistance in obese rodents and man. Metabolism, 26:1057–1078, 1977.

53. Frayn, K. N.: The site of insulin resistance after injury. Endocrinology, 101:312–314, 1977.

CHAPTER 4

Lipid Metabolism in Parenteral Nutrition

BRUCE M. WOLFE
DENISE M. NEY

Lipids are organic substances that are relatively insoluble in water but soluble in organic compounds such as ether, chloroform, and benzene. Lipids are responsible for a wide range of metabolic and structural functions. Pertinent to parenteral nutrition, they are a major source of metabolic fuel, providing utilizable energy for a wide range of metabolic processes and a source of essential fatty acids. Lipids function as the primary source of stored energy in mammals. An average 70-kg male contains approximately 12.5 kg of fat consisting of approximately 112,500 kcal.[1] Lipids are a particularly efficient form of energy storage as a result of their high energy content (9 kcal/gm) and anhydrous state in stored fat. Structural functions of lipids include being an essential component of cell membranes, padding critical organs, and insulating against heat loss. Lipids are precursors of the regulatory compounds, the prostaglandins. Certain nutrients essential to body metabolism, such as vitamins A, D, E, and K, are lipids.

The major classes of lipids found in plasma include triacylglycerols, phospholipids, cholesterol and cholesterol esters, and free fatty acids. The lipid content of human plasma is summarized in Table 4–1.

TERMINOLOGY AND CLASSIFICATION

Fatty Acids

Fatty acids consist of carboxyl groups with hydrocarbon chains, represented by the formula R—COOH. In mammals, the hydrocarbon chain is usually straight, contains an even number of carbon atoms, and may contain no double bonds (saturated fatty acid) or one or more double bonds (unsaturated fatty acid). The nomenclature and classification of fatty acids is a function of the number of carbon atoms and the number and position(s) of the double bonds. Fatty acids with six to ten carbons are termed *medium-chain fatty acids*, whereas fatty acids with 12 to 26 carbons are *long-chain fatty acids*. In the "n" numbering system, the total number of carbon atoms is given first, followed by a colon,

Table 4–1. LIPID CONTENT OF HUMAN PLASMA

LIPID	PLASMA CONTENT (mg/dl) Mean	Range
Total lipid	570	360–820
Triacylglycerol	142	80–180*
Total phospholipid†	215	123–390
Lecithin		50–200
Cephalin		50–130
Sphingomyelins		15–35
Total cholesterol	200	107–320
Free cholesterol (nonesterified)	55	26–106
Total fatty acids‡	—	200–800
Free fatty acids (nonesterified)	12	6–16*

*Varies with nutritional state.
†Analyzed as lipid phosphorus; mean lipid phosphorus is 9.2 mg/dl (range 6.1–14.5 mg/dl); lipid phosphorus × 25 = phospholipid as lecithin (4% phosphorus).
‡Of total fatty acids (such as stearic acid), 45% are triacylglycerols, 35% phospholipids, 15% cholesterol esters, and less than 5% free fatty acids.
(*Modified from* Martin, D., Mayes, P., and Rodwell, V. (eds.): Harper's Review of Biochemistry, 19th ed. Los Altos, Lange Medical Publications, 1983, p. 195, with permission.)

Table 4–2. COMMON FATTY ACIDS

NUMERICAL DESIGNATION	COMMON NAME	SYSTEMATIC NAME
2:0	Acetic	Ethanoic
4:0	Butyric	*n*-Butanic
6:0	Capnoic	*n*-Hexanoic
14:0	Myristic	*n*-Tetradecanoic
16:0	Palmitic	*n*-Hexadecanoic
18:0	Stearic	*n*-Octadecanoic
18:1n9	Oleic	9-Octadecenoic
18:2n6	Linoleic	9,12-Octadecadienoic
18:3n3	Linolenic	9,12,15-Octadecatrienoic
20:4n6	Arachidonic	5,8,11,15-Eicosatetraenoic
22:5n3	None	5,8,11,14,17-Eicosapentaenoic

the total number of double bonds, "n," and the number of carbon atoms between the terminal noncarboxyl carbon and the closest double bond.* Thus, oleic acid (18:1n9) contains 18 carbon atoms, and 1 double bond, 9 carbons from the terminal carbon. Examples of common fatty acids are given in Table 4–2. Humans cannot synthesize fatty acids with double bonds between the ninth carbon and the terminal carbon of the fatty acid chain. Thus, linoleic acid (18:2n6) and linolenic acid (18:3n3) are essential fatty acids that must be supplied in the diet. The prostaglandin precursor, arachidonic acid (20:4n6), can be synthesized from linoleic acid.

The unesterified long-chain fatty acids (free fatty acids; FFA) constitute the smallest but most metabolically active component of plasma lipids. These hydrophobic molecules are solubilized in plasma by the formation of an albumin-FFA complex. The FFA content of plasma can be determined by a newly developed microfluorometric method.[2] At present, this method is not generally available clinically, but it has the potential for incorporation into automated systems for plasma analysis. Separation of specific fatty acids for identification and quantitation requires thin-layer, gas-liquid, or high-performance liquid chromatography.

Glycerides (Acylglycerols)

Most fatty acids in mammals exist as fatty acid esters of glycerol and are known as acylglycerols or glycerides. One, two, or three of the hydroxyl groups of glycerol may be esterified to form monoglycerides, diglyc-

erides, or triglycerides (Fig. 4–1). Triglycerides are quantitatively the predominant form of dietary, storage, and transport lipid. Plasma triglyceride levels may be quantitated by enzymatic fluorometric methods widely available in automated analytical procedures.[3]

Phospholipids

Phospholipids may be derived from glycerol (phosphoglycerides) or sphingosine. In phosphoglycerides, two hydroxyl groups of glycerol are esterified to fatty acids and one to phosphoric acid (see Fig. 4–1). The phosphoric acid may be esterified to a nitrogen-containing moiety such as choline, forming the phospholipid lecithin, to serine or ethanolamine, forming cephalin phospholipids, or to inositol.

The essential feature of phospholipid structure is that these lipids have both a hydrophobic (fatty acid) end and a hydro-

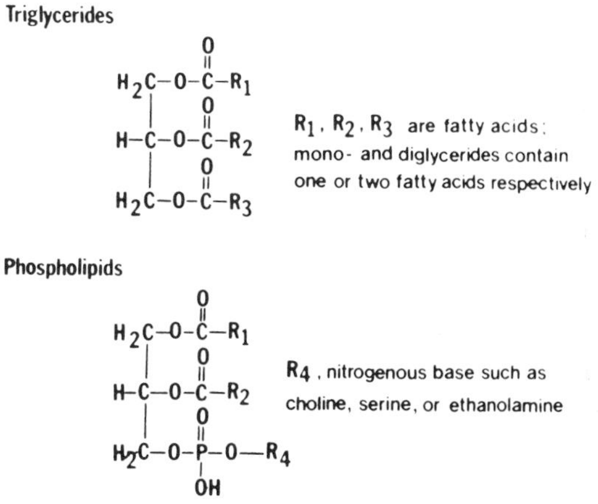

Figure 4–1. Chemical structure of triglycerides and phospholipids.

---

*For further discussion of the "n" numbering system, see *Clinical Nutrition*, Vol. 1, Chapter 2.

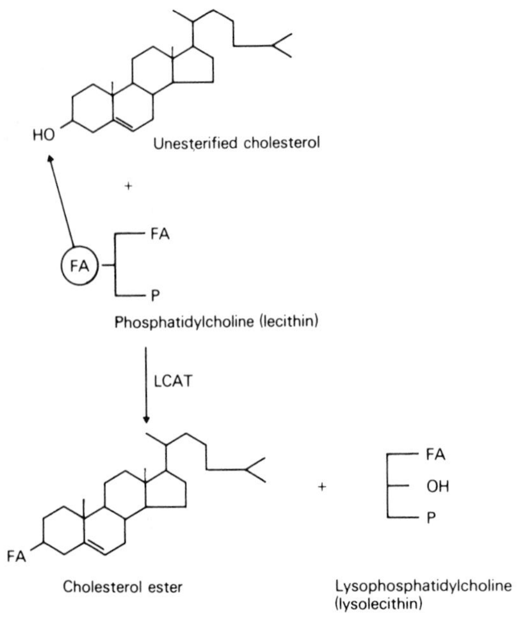

Figure 4–2. The esterification of plasma cholesterol by the enzyme lecithin:cholesterol acyl transferase (LCAT). (*From* Simons, L., and Gibson, J.: Lipids: A Clinician's Guide. Balgowlah, Australia, ADIS Press, 1980, p. 12, with permission.)

philic (phosphoryl) end. This feature allows interaction between both fat-soluble and water-soluble interfaces, making phospholipids ideal emulsifying agents and essential components of cell membranes. The commercial intravenous fat emulsions contain 1.2 per cent egg yolk phospholipid in order to emulsify the 10 or 20 per cent lipid component. Phospholipids are not generally available as an energy source and will be retained even in starvation to maintain membrane integrity.

Essential fatty acids and other nutrients are necessary for the synthesis of the phospholipid lecithin. Lecithin and protein are needed to assemble lipoprotein particles in order to transport lipid from the liver to the periphery. Thus, essential fatty acid deficiency is associated with fatty liver.[4]

Lecithin is one of the major phospholipids found on the surface of lipoprotein particles. It interacts with the enzyme lecithin:cholesterol acyltransferase (LCAT) to esterify free cholesterol from the tissue for transport in plasma lipoproteins, as shown in Figure 4–2.

Sterols

Sterols are derived from complex cyclic compounds composed of three six-member

carbon rings and one five-member carbon ring. Cholesterol is the predominant sterol in humans and is widely distributed in all cells of the body. Cholesterol is a precursor to bile acids and steroid hormones as well as an important constituent of cell membranes, especially in nervous tissue.

The greater part of plasma cholesterol is in the esterified form and is transported as lipoprotein complexes. Free or unesterified cholesterol exchanges readily between tissues, particularly high-density lipoprotein (HDL) particles, because of the action of LCAT.

Other lipids that occur in humans but are not considered in this chapter include glycolipids and the fat-soluble vitamins, A, D, E, and K.

NORMAL FAT METABOLISM

Digestion and Absorption

Digestion and absorption of lipids have been described in detail in the first volume of this work (Chapter 2). Briefly, dietary lipids are composed of approximately 150 gm/day of long-chain triglycerides, 4 to 8 gm/day of phospholipids (predominantly lecithin), and 300 to 600 mg/day of cholesterol.[5]

Biliary lipids, including bile salts, lecithin, and cholesterol, play an important role in lipid digestion and absorption. The liver secretes between 7 and 22 gm of lecithin per day into the bile.[5] Lecithin and bile salts interact to form lecithin-coated emulsions of dietary lipids, which promote hydrolysis of lipids by pancreatic lipases. Hydrolytic products of pancreatic lipase include long-chain fatty acids, 2-monoglycerides, and 1-lysolecithin, which are dispersed in bile salt micelles for absorption into the intestinal mucosa. Within the mucosa cell, long-chain triglycerides are resynthesized, specific apoproteins are synthesized, and triglycerides are packaged in chylomicron lipoprotein particles composed of a triglyceride core and a phospholipid and apoprotein surface coat. The chylomicrons are then secreted into the lymph and transported into blood via the thoracic duct.

Lipid Transport—Lipoproteins

Combination with solubilizing agents is necessary for transport of lipids through the aqueous medium of the lymph and plasma.

Table 4–3. COMPOSITION AND CLASSIFICATION OF THE MAJOR
HUMAN PLASMA LIPOPROTEINS

FEATURE	CHYLOMICRONS	LIPOPROTEINS		
		VLDL	*LDL*	*HDL*
Density (gm/ml)	< 1.006	< 1.006	1.006–1.063	1.063–1.21
Electrophoretic mobility	Origin	*Prebeta*	*Beta*	*Alpha*
Composition (weight percentage)				
Triglyceride	85–90	50–55	6–10	3–6
Cholesterol ester	3–4	14–16	35–45	12–18
Unesterified (free) cholesterol	2–3	6–8	8–12	2–4
Phospholipid	6–8	16–20	20–25	25–30
Protein	1–2	8–10	18–22	47–52

(*From* Simons, L., and Gibson, J.: Lipids: A Clinician's Guide. Balgowlah, Australia, ADIS Press, 1980, p. 2, with permission.)

This is done by combination of the lipid with specific proteins or apoproteins and phospholipids to form lipoprotein particles. The general structure of a lipoprotein particle consists of a hydrophobic core of triglyceride and cholesterol ester surrounded by a surface coat of apoproteins, phospholipids, and free cholesterol.

Lipoproteins are classified into four categories according to ultracentrifugal flotation and electrophoretic mobility. The ultracentrifugal terminology—chylomicron, very-low-density lipoprotein (VLDL), low-density lipoprotein (LDL), and high-density lipoprotein (HDL)—is used in this chapter. The lipoprotein categories vary with respect to lipid and protein composition and are summarized in Table 4–3.

Specific proteins or apoproteins are associated with the various categories of lipoproteins (see Table 4–4). These apoproteins are primarily synthesized in the liver and intestine. Current research has focused on the apoprotein composition of the lipoproteins, as specific apoproteins have been demonstrated to direct the metabolism of lipoprotein particles via interaction with key enzymes and receptors.[6] It has recently been demonstrated that the apoprotein composition of plasma differs with total parenteral nutrition,[7, 8] providing a new insight into the metabolism of intravenously supplied lipids.

Chylomicrons and VLDL

Chylomicron and VLDL particles have a rapid turnover, are composed primarily of triglyceride, and function in the transport of triglyceride to peripheral tissues. Chylomicrons, synthesized in the intestine, are the major transport form of *dietary* fat, as reflected in high blood triglyceride concentrations during the absorptive phase of digestion. VLDL is derived principally from the liver and transports triglyceride derived from *endogenous* sources. Thus, although VLDL and chylomicrons share many metabolic and physical properties, they vary in the *origin* of the transported triglyceride.

LDL and HDL

The low-density and high-density lipoproteins are the major cholesterol-transporting lipoproteins. LDL is involved in the transfer of cholesterol to the periphery, and HDL is important in the transport of cholesterol from the periphery to the liver for degradation and excretion. Approximately 60 per cent of the LDL lipid is cholesterol, and it represents about 70 per cent of the total plasma cholesterol in humans.[9] LDL particles result from the catabolism of VLDL and may also be secreted directly by the liver. The HDL molecule, which contains approximately 50 per cent protein and 50 per cent lipid, is composed primarily of the phospholipid lecithin and also esterified cholesterol. HDL levels have been shown to vary inversely with cardiovascular disease risk.[10]

Table 4–4. APOPROTEIN COMPOSITION OF
HUMAN PLASMA LIPOPROTEINS

LIPOPROTEIN FRACTION	MAJOR APOPROTEIN(S)
Chylomicrons	B, E, A-I, A-IV, C
Chylomicron remnants	B, E
VLDL	B, E, C
LDL	B
HDL	A-I, A-II, C, E

(*Adapted from* Mahley, R. W.: Atherogenic hyperlipoproteinemia. The cellular and molecular biology of plasma lipoproteins altered by dietary fat and cholesterol. Med. Clin. North Am., 66:375–403, 1982, with permission.)

Lipoprotein-X (Lp-X)

In addition to the four major lipoprotein classes, an abnormal lipoprotein particle deserves comment. Lp-X has a flotation density similar to that of LDL but a very different lipid and protein composition. This abnormal lipoprotein is characterized by an unusually high proportion of phospholipid and free cholesterol and by a low protein content.[9] Lp-X is found in plasma of patients with biliary obstruction[11] and familial LCAT deficiency[12] and has also been observed in neonates,[13] adults,[14] and rats[15] receiving fat emulsion–supplemented parenteral nutrition. Several authors suggest that the particle arises from fat emulsion–supplied phospholipid, which leaches free cholesterol associated with membranes to form a lipoprotein particle that is slowly cleared from the plasma.[14, 15] The formation and metabolism of Lp-X is discussed further later.

Lipoprotein Metabolism and Lipid Clearance

The clearance of plasma triglyceride contained in chylomicron and VLDL particles occurs as a result of the action of lipoprotein lipase. This enzyme is located on the endothelial cells of the capillaries in adipose tissue, skeletal muscle, heart, and, to a lesser extent, other organs, including spleen, lung, and renal medulla. The activity of lipoprotein lipase varies in different tissues according to the nutritional and hormonal state. For example, starvation increases muscle lipoprotein lipase activity and decreases adipose lipase activity, and the fed state causes the opposite response in muscle and adipose lipoprotein lipase activity.[16] The net effects of this tissue specificity for lipoprotein lipase would be to assure an energy source for muscle during starvation and to facilitate fat storage with feeding.

The presence of apoprotein C-II on chylomicrons and VLDL particles is required for the activation of lipoprotein lipase. Chylomicron particles acquire apo C-II and apo E, which are not synthesized to an appreciable degree by the intestine, through transfer from the HDL fraction when chylomicrons enter the general circulation.[17] Triglyceride hydrolysis via lipoprotein lipase occurs at the plasma capillary wall interface and results in the release of FFA and glycerol. The glycerol is transported in the blood and taken up primarily by the liver, and the FFAs enter the adjacent muscle or adipose cells, where they are either oxidized for energy or re-esterified for storage (Fig. 4–3).

As the triglyceride core of chylomicrons and VLDLs is depleted, the particles shrink and transfer excess surface materials, including free cholesterol, phospholipids, and apoproteins, to the HDL fraction. The depleted chylomicron, now known as a chylomicron remnant, retains its cholesterol ester and apoproteins B and E. The chylomicron remnant is rapidly taken up by the liver via apo E receptor–mediated endocytosis (see Fig. 4–3). The triglyceride-depleted VLDL particle is converted to a cholesterol ester–rich LDL particle by means of exchange reactions with HDL and the action of LCAT.

Administration of heparin stimulates the release of lipoprotein lipase from the walls of the capillaries into the circulation and is accompanied by a more rapid clearing of lipemia. Plasma "post–heparin lipase activity" is frequently used as an indicator of lipoprotein-triglyceride hydrolyzing capacity. However, this estimation is not completely reliable, owing to problems with assay standardization and specificity.[9]

Oxidation of Lipids

Free fatty acids diffuse freely across cell membranes and are rapidly taken up from plasma by a variety of tissues for use as an energy source. The rate of FFA uptake increases as the plasma FFA to albumin molar ratio increases.[18] The fatty acids are activated in the cytosol by the formation of long-chain acyl-CoA and then transported into the mitochondria in association with carnitine for oxidation. Inside the mitochondria, the carnitine is removed from the acyl-carnitine, and the resulting acyl-CoA undergoes beta oxidation.

Beta oxidation occurs only in the mitochondria and is controlled primarily by the availability of acyl-CoA and oxidized cofactors. The term *beta oxidation* refers to the process whereby acyl-CoA molecules are reduced two carbons at a time to form acetyl-CoA units. A total of five high-energy phosphate bonds are synthesized for *each* of the first seven acetyl-CoA molecules formed by the beta oxidation of, for example, palmitate. Each acetyl-CoA may then enter the citric acid cycle for complete oxidation to carbon dioxide and water, which would yield 12

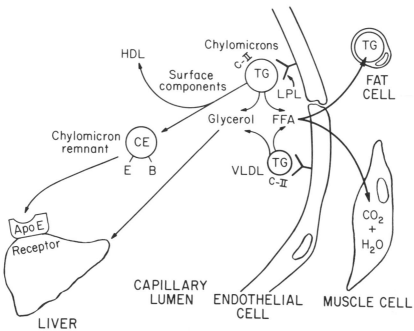

Figure 4–3. Delivery of plasma triglyceride contained in chylomicron and VLDL particles to target tissues. Triglycerides (TG) contained in chylomicron and VLDL particles are hydrolyzed by the enzyme lipoprotein lipase (LPL), which is attached to the endothelial cells of the capillary lumen. Apo C-II is required as an activator of LPL. Glycerol and free fatty acids (FFA) are released as a result of TG hydrolysis. The glycerol is taken up primarily by the liver, and the FFA's enter adjacent muscle or fat cells for oxidation or storage. The TG-depleted chylomicron is converted to a chylomicron remnant via transfer of surface components to HDL particles. The cholesterol ester–rich chylomicron remnant (CE) is rapidly taken up by the liver via Apo E receptor mediated endocytosis. The apoproteins responsible for the interactions (C-II, B, and E) are indicated. (*Adapted from* Brown, M. S., Kovanen, P. T. and Goldstein, J. L.: Regulation of plasma cholesterol by lipoprotein receptors. Science, 212:628–635, 1981.)

more high-energy phosphate bonds for *each* molecule of acetyl-CoA. The acetyl-CoA units may also be diverted to ketone body synthesis.

The liver is the primary site of ketone body synthesis. Increased lipolysis, such as occurs during starvation or with limited glucose availability, results in an increased diversion of fatty acids to ketones and decreased oxidation via the citric acid cycle.[19] During starvation, 80 per cent of the fatty acids catabolized in the liver yield ketone bodies.[20] The primary ketones, beta hydroxybutyrate and acetoacetic acid, are released from the liver, taken up by extrahepatic tissues in proportion to their circulating concentration, and converted back to acetyl-CoA for oxidation in the citric acid cycle. Because they cross the mitochondrial membranes without carnitine, ketone bodies are more readily utilized in muscle than are fatty acids. Liver has no activating enzymes for ketone bodies and therefore does not compete with other tissues for their use. As described in Chapter 1, during starvation, ketosis is a mechanism whereby the central nervous system, which does not take up fatty acids, may derive energy from stored fat.

Triglycerides with medium-chain fatty acids differ from triglycerides with long-chain fatty acids in both their absorption and metabolism. Medium-chain fatty acids do not require chylomicron formation and are delivered directly to the liver in association with albumin. They also do not require carnitine to enter the mitochondria for oxidation and are oxidized more rapidly than long-chain fatty acids.[21, 22] Presumably as the result of rapid beta oxidation, ketosis is associated with provision of medium-chain triglycerides.[23, 24]

The utilization of glycerol released from the hydrolysis of triglycerides depends upon whether tissues possess the necessary activating enzyme, glycerokinase. Muscle and adipose tissue have low or no amounts of this enzyme, whereas liver, kidney, and intestine contain significant amounts. Glycerokinase converts glycerol to glycerol-3-phosphate, which can be esterified with fatty acids to form triglycerides, can be oxidized to carbon dioxide and water, or can act as a gluconeogenic precursor (the only gluconeo-genic potential possessed by triglyceride) in the liver and kidney.

Lipid Storage and Mobilization

Carbohydrate metabolism and lipid metabolism are very interrelated. Lipid is stored when carbohydrate or energy supplies are adequate, and triglyceride hydrolysis predominates when energy is inadequate. Insulin is of major importance in lipid metabolism.

During the fed state, insulin increases the activity of lipoprotein lipase and hence the availability of fatty acids for triglyceride synthesis in adipose tissue. It also increases the permeability of adipose tissue to glucose, enabling adipose tissue to form the glycerol-3-phosphate needed for triglyceride synthesis. Triglyceride hydrolysis occurs continually in adipose tissue, but the adipose cells cannot reutilize the glycerol released because of lack of the enzyme glycerokinase. The formation and hydrolysis of triglyceride in adipose tissue create what is often called the glucose–fatty acid cycle (Fig. 4–4).[25] If glucose is not available to the adipose cell, fatty acids will be released into the blood.

The rates of formation and hydrolysis of

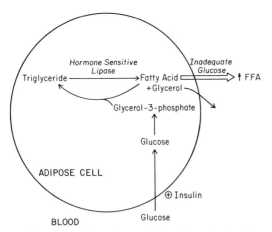

Figure 4–4. The glucose–fatty acid cycle describes the relationship of glucose availability to the formation of hydrolysis of triglyceride in adipose tissue. Insulin is required for glucose entry into the adipose cell so that formation of glycerol-3-phosphate may occur. Glycerol-3-phosphate acts to re-esterify fatty acids released from stored triglyceride by action of the enzyme hormone-sensitive lipase. Glycerol is released from adipose to be used by other tissues that possess the enzyme glycerokinase. Decreased glucose availability or increased activity of hormone sensitive lipase may result in increased release of free fatty acids (FFA) from adipose tissue.

triclycerides are regulated not only by glucose and insulin availability, as already discussed, but also by catabolic hormones. The key enzyme for promoting hydrolysis of triclyceride from adipose is hormone-sensitive lipase. Insulin inhibits the activity of this enzyme, and epinephrine, norepinephrine, glucagon, adrenocorticotropic hormone, and thyroid-stimulating hormone enhance its action. The net effect of this stimulation is an accelerated release of FFA from adipose tissue for use as an energy source.

Epinephrine, which is released in response to stress,[26] has been shown to have potent lipolytic effects in humans. The epinephrine threshold for lipolytic effects is less than the epinephrine stimulation encountered during exercise, myocardial infarction, or surgical stress.[27] Thus, lipid mobilization is more sensitive to increases in plasma epinephrine than is the depletion of glycogen stores, which is also mediated by epinephrine.

Role of the Liver

The liver interacts with adipose tissue and muscle to play a central role in lipid metabolism. The long-chain triglycerides, unlike other nutrients, bypass the liver when they enter the circulation. The bypass is thought to reflect low liver lipoprotein lipase levels and to spare fatty acids for use by extrahepatic tissue. In humans, the liver is the predominant site of *de novo* fatty acid synthesis from carbohydrate and other precursors. Triglyceride synthesized in the liver is transported into the plasma as VLDL for storage in adipose tissue or for use as an energy source. The liver is also the only site for the production of ketone bodies.

The liver plays a major role in cholesterol metabolism, because it is a major site for LDL and HDL synthesis and catabolism. In addition, the only major pathway for cholesterol excretion involves bile acid synthesis in the liver and excretion of cholesterol in bile.

Summary

The fate of ingested and absorbed or intravenously infused lipids can be seen from the preceding considerations to depend upon many factors. The actions of lipoproteins are necessary for transport and uptake of lipids by tissues. The decision to oxidize or store lipid depends on the nutritional and hormonal state. The oxidation of fatty acids depends on the availability of oxygen and intermediates such as carnitine. Finally, the storage or mobilization of fat from adipose tissue is determined by carbohydrate availability and the action of hormones such as insulin and epinephrine.

ARACHIDONIC ACID METABOLITES

Prostaglandins are a group of potent regulatory compounds derived from unsaturated fatty acids. In humans, although linoleic and linolenic acids may be prostaglandin precursors, the prostaglandins that are derived from the metabolism of arachidonic acid are quantitatively and functionally the most important prostaglandins. These prostaglandins contain two double bonds in the hydrocarbon side-chain and are referred to as the "2" series. The fatty acid eicosapentaenoic acid (EPA), which contains five double bonds, gives rise to prostaglandins containing three double bonds in the hydrocarbon side-chain, referred to as the "3" series. Arachidonic acid occurs in humans primarily as a component of cell membrane phospholipids. The arachidonic acid is derived primarily by synthesis from linoleic acid. Dietary sources may also contribute small amounts. The synthesis of prostaglandins from arachidonic acid ("2" series) is schematically outlined in Figure 4–5. A variety of stimuli release arachidonic acid from membrane phospholipids. Arachidonic acid is then metabolized under the action of one of two enzymes. The first pathway, catalyzed by lipoxygenase, leads to the synthesis of a variety of compounds known as leukotrienes. Alternatively, cyclooxygenase may catalyze conversion to unstable endoperoxides, first prostaglandin G_2 (PGG$_2$) and subsequently PGH$_2$. One of several individual prostaglandin synthetases then acts on PGH$_2$ to form more stable, active compounds. A total of five such compounds have been described.

PGE$_2$

The primary functional role of PGE$_2$ appears to be in mediating inflammation, either systemically or locally. PGE$_2$ stimulates muscle protein degradation *in vitro*.[28] It has been suggested that accelerated protein break-

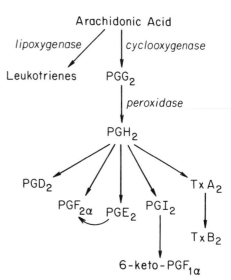

Figure 4–5. Metabolism of arachidonic acid. Arachidonic acid is metabolized by the action of one of two enzymes. Lipoxygenase stimulates leukotriene synthesis, and cyclooxygenase stimulates synthesis of prostaglandins and related compounds. The actions of these specific compounds are described in the text. PG, prostaglandin; PGI$_2$, prostacyclin; TxA$_2$ thromboxane A$_2$.

down in muscle is mediated by stimulation of PGE$_2$ released by human leukocytic pyrogen.[29] PGE$_2$ also possesses vasodilator and bronchodilator properties, although it is not a major mediator of vessel or bronchial tone.

PGF$_{2\alpha}$

This prostaglandin is similar to PGE$_2$ and may arise from breakdown of PGH$_2$ or PGE$_2$. PGF$_{2\alpha}$ has a similar capacity to stimulate protein degradation, but it is a vasoconstrictor.

PGI$_2$ (Prostacyclin)

PGI$_2$ is produced in the endothelial cells of blood vessel walls. Its primary actions are vasodilation and inhibition of platelet aggregation. Its metabolic breakdown product, 6-keto-PGF$_{1\alpha}$, is more stable. Thus, measurement of 6-keto-PGF$_{1\alpha}$ is used as a quantitative estimate of PGI$_2$ production.

TxA$_2$ (Thromboxane A$_2$)

TxA$_2$ is synthesized and released from platelets. It is a potent vasoconstrictor and stimulates platelet aggregation. Its stable metabolite, TxB_2, is an inactive compound.

PGD₂

This prostaglandin is released from pulmonary mast cells and is a potent bronchoconstrictor. Its other actions include vasoconstriction and inhibition of platelet aggregation.

The balance between the synthesis rates of vasoactive prostaglandins is a major factor in determining local vascular tone and hemodynamics in specific vascular beds, particularly the lungs.[30] The balance between PGI_2 and TxA_2 determines the behavior of platelets and the extent of aggregation at the site of endothelial injury, which is thought to play a major role in the genesis of atherosclerotic disease.[31, 32]

The leukotrienes have a variety of properties, including a role in mediating allergic responses, such as bronchoconstriction, and a role in inflammation.

The availability of prostaglandin precursors as the result of dietary variations may have an impact on prostaglandin synthesis and action. Studies of essential fatty acid deficiency in animals have demonstrated decreased tissue levels of prostaglandins.[33] Some manifestations of essential fatty acid deficiency have been reversed by infusion of PGE_2,[34] but not all manifestations of essential fatty acid deficiency have been reversible by prostaglandin infusion alone.[35] Enhanced platelet aggregation and associated thrombosis have been reported in human essential fatty acid deficiency.[36]

Feeding a diet high in EPA, found primarily in certain fish, has been thought to explain the lack of atherosclerotic disease and the increased tendency for bleeding seen among Eskimos.[32] The explanation for this phenomenon appears to be that the PGI_3 derived from EPA is similar in activity to PGI_2 with regard to inhibition of platelet adhesiveness, whereas thromboxane A_3 (TxA_3) possesses considerably less potency as a platelet aggregator than TxA_2. Finally, increased PGI_2 production, as evidenced by increased 6-keto-$PGF_{1\alpha}$ excretion, has been demonstrated among normal subjects receiving infusion of an emulsion of safflower oil, which is high in linoleic acid.[37] Evidence indicating that the availability of precursor fatty acids may have an impact on prosta-

glandin-mediated disease states in humans during total parenteral nutrition with fat emulsion infusion is described later.

FAT METABOLISM IN STRESS

Exercise

The metabolism of energy substrates in exercise is of substantial interest because of many of the similarities in the metabolic settings of exercise and stress induced by injury or sepsis. During exercise, fatty acids are increasingly mobilized from fat stores and taken up by skeletal muscle. Associated with these findings are an increased concentration of free fatty acids in the circulation and concomitant increases in fatty acid uptake.[38] In sustained exercise, fatty acids are the predominant source of fuel for skeletal muscle. Despite this increased uptake of fatty acids by muscle, it has been believed by many that a high-fat diet with associated nutritional ketosis impairs the capacity for endurance exercise. The studies of Phinney and colleagues,[39] however, have demonstrated that a physiologic adaptation to a low-carbohydrate, high-fat (ketogenic) diet occurs over a period of up to four weeks in normal subjects. Such adapted subjects demonstrate reversal of initial negative nitrogen balance after one week of a high-fat diet (Fig. 4–6),[39] and no compromise of exercise endurance occurs in well-trained athletes.[40] The demonstration of an interval required for adaptation to the high-fat diet by normal subjects is of critical importance in interpreting many clinical studies that have been done of the efficacy of fat emulsion infusions.

Trauma and Sepsis

Studies in humans have generally indicated that the responses to trauma and sepsis vary primarily according to the severity, with septic states tending to be more severe. Thus, for the purpose of this discussion, trauma and sepsis will be considered a single source of metabolic stress.

Reliance on fat as a major source of energy in the injured human was recognized in the early studies by Moore of the metabolic response to injury.[41] More recently, techniques such as indirect calorimetry and iso-

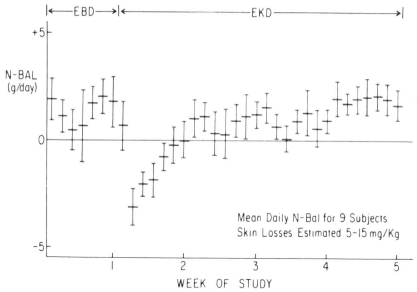

Figure 4–6. Daily nitrogen balance in normal subjects fed oral high fat (ketogenic) diet for 4 weeks. Intake determined by weighed portion intake, with food aliquots assessed for nitrogen by Kjeldahl analysis. Excretion measured by complete urine and stool collections plus estimated cutaneous and exercise-induced losses. Initial negative nitrogen balance was followed by adaptation to the high-fat diet and nitrogen equilibrium in the second week of feeding. EBD, eucaloric balanced diet; EKD, eucaloric ketogenic diet. Values shown are mean ± SEM, n = 9. (*From* Phinney, S. O., Bistrian, B. R., Wolfe, R. R., and Blackburn, G. L.: The human metabolic response to chronic ketosis without caloric restriction: Physical and biochemical adaptation. Metabolism, 32:727–768, 1983, with permission.)

tropic turnover studies have demonstrated reliance on endogenous fat for as much as 80 per cent of energy supply in the injured human receiving minimal nutrient intake.[42] These observations demonstrate the capacity for endogenous fat to serve as a major energy source for the stressed human. A variety of abnormalities of lipid metabolism may be induced by increasingly severe states of stress. Fatty acid mobilization from fat stores is increased, and unlike the normal, starving, or exercising human, this increased mobilization of fatty acids is not substantially inhibited by glucose infusion.[42, 43] The hypersecretion of catecholamines and glucagon induced by stress appears to override the inhibitory stimulus of insulin in producing this fat mobilization. The turnover and uptake of free fatty acids are also accelerated in stress. Fatty acid oxidation, however, may not be increased to the same extent as is fatty acid mobilization in both animals and humans.[42, 44]

Beta oxidation of fatty acids is a prerequisite for ketone formation. One manifestation of the limitation to fatty acid oxidation in stress is the consistent finding of a lack of ketosis in both animals[44] and humans.[45, 46, 47] The alternate pathway for fatty acids taken up by the liver but not oxidized is re-esteri-

fication to triglyceride and subsequent VLDL formation. It therefore appears that a "futile cycle," involving mobilization of fat from peripheral fat stores, transport to the liver, and resynthesis of fat for transportation back to fat stores, may occur in stressed humans. The lack of ketosis may be a manifestation of the limited oxidation of fatty acids in the liver and suggests that there may be a limit to the extent to which stored fat can contribute to meeting energy requirements in stressed humans.

Carnitine

Recognition of limitations to the rate of fatty acid oxidation and of the potential for carnitine deficiency to occur in patients fed carnitine-free total parenteral nutrition has led to investigation of the role of potential carnitine deficiency in impaired fatty acid metabolism, as reviewed by Tao and Yoshimura.[48] Carnitine may be synthesized in humans from lysine and methionine, although carnitine is also present in the normal human diet. Congenital states of carnitine deficiency are well-established and produce abnormal fat metabolism. Clinical manifestations may include lipid storage myopathy of both skeletal and cardiac muscle, and fatty liver storage with hepatic dysfunction.[49, 50] Plasma concentrations of carnitine may fall rapidly in patients receiving TPN despite persistence of normal concentrations in red blood cells, skeletal muscle, and liver. Depressed carnitine levels in liver and heart have been reported in premature infants who receive more than 15 days of TPN[51] and in adults on long-term total parenteral nutrition.[52] Addition of carnitine to total parenteral nutrition solutions has produced improved nitrogen balance and diminished hepatic fat deposition in rats[53] and improved nitrogen retention in piglets.[54] Evidence that carnitine deficiency is responsible for observed limitations of fatty acid oxidation in the stressed human remains to be generated, and the potential therapeutic role for carnitine infusion in humans has yet to be investigated.

INTRAVENOUS FAT EMULSIONS

Composition

The commercially available fat emulsions are aqueous dispersions composed of a neutral triglyceride such as soybean or safflower oil, egg yolk phospholipid for use as an emulsifying agent, and glycerin to achieve isotonicity with plasma. The preparations contain emulsified fat particles similar in diameter (0.4 to 1.0 μ) to naturally occurring chylomicrons. Of the four brands currently marketed in the United, States, three utilize soybean oil and one safflower oil. All of the manufacturers offer 10 and 20 per cent lipid concentratins with similar caloric densities.

The fatty acid compositions of the soybean and safflower oil preparations differ (Table 4–5). The safflower oil emulsions contain 77 per cent linoleic acid and only a trace of linolenic acid, whereas the soybean oil emulsions contain 49 to 60 per cent linoleic acid and six to nine per cent linolenic fatty acid.[55] Both soybean and safflower oil emulsions have been shown to be effective as energy sources and in reversing essential fatty acid deficiency. Safflower oil fat emulsions have been reported to be cleared more slowly from the plasma than the soybean oil preparations.[56] An isolated case of linolenic acid deficiency associated with neurologic abnormalities has been recently reported in a young child who received safflower oil emulsion for five months.[57] The linolenic acid deficiency responded to the infusion of a soybean oil emulsion but resulted in lower linoleic acid levels. Further research is needed to determine the optimum balance of fatty acids, especially linoleic and linolenic acids, in the intravenous fat emulsion preparations.

Metabolism and Clearance

Intravenous fat emulsions behave as chylomicrons carrying exogenous triglyceride; however, the composition and metabolism of emulsion particles differs somewhat from those of chylomicron particles. Fat emulsion particles contain less protein and cholesterol and more phospholipid and triglyceride than chylomicrons synthesized by the small intestine. Like chylomicrons, emulsion particles acquire apoprotein C-II and other apoproteins from the HDL fraction.[17, 58] This acquisition results in activation of lipoprotein lipase and subsequent hydrolysis of intravenous triglyceride particles in the capillary beds of muscle and especially adipose tissue[59] and rapid uptake of FFA by the surrounding tissues.

The kinetics for triglyceride hydrolysis and FFA uptake from artificial fat emulsions are similar to that from chylomicrons.[60] Kinetic studies have demonstrated a zero-order reaction at high and a first-order reaction at low concentrations of triglycerides in plasma. The zero-order reaction is interpreted as a maximal elimination capacity operating above a "critical concentration" of plasma triglyceride. The first-order reaction reflects a fractional removal rate that operates at triglyceride concentrations below the "critical concentration." The maximal elimination capacity can be influenced by both nutritional state and physiologic state. Fasting and abdominal surgery have been noted to increase the maximal elimination capacity, and abdominal surgery was also noted to increase the fractional removal rate of artificial fat emulsions from the bloodstream.[60]

The fate of the intravenous fat emulsion particle after triglyceride hydrolysis differs from that of the chylomicron. From 60 to 90 per cent of the fat emulsion–associated phospholipid is metabolized by an unknown, possible LCAT-associated pathway.[13] The remainder of the phospholipid rapidly forms single phospholipid bilayer vesicles, which acquire equimolar amounts of free cholesterol from peripheral cell membranes to form Lp-X.[13, 14] Thus, in this case, Lp-X seems to be

Table 4–5. COMPOSITION OF COMMERCIAL INTRAVENOUS FAT EMULSIONS

CONTENTS	INTRALIPID		LIPOSYN		McGAW IV FAT EMULSION		TRAVAMULSION	
	10%	*20%*	*10%*	*20%*	*10%*	*20%*	*10%*	*20%*
Oil (%)	Soybean 10	Soybean 20	Safflower 10	Safflower 20	Soybean 10	Soybean 20	Soybean 10	Soybean 20
Fatty acid content (%)								
Linoleic	54	50	77	77	49–60	49–60	56	56
Oleic	26	26	13	13	21–26	21–26	23	23
Palmitic	9	10	7	7	9–13	9–13	11	11
Linolenic	8	9	0.1	0.1	6–9	6–9	6	6
Stearic	—	—	2.5	2.5	3–5	3–5	—	—
Egg yolk phospholipids (%)	1.2	1.2	1.2	1.2	1.2	1.2	1.2	1.2
Glycerin (%)	2.25	2.25	2.5	2.5	2.21	2.21	2.25	2.25
Calories/ml	1.1	2.0	1.1	2.0	1.1	2.0	1.1	2.0
Osmolarity (mOsm/L)	280	330	300	340	280	315	270	300
pH	5.5–9.0	5.5–9.0	8.0	8.3	6.0–7.9	6.0–7.9	5.5–9.0	5.5–9.0
Container size (ml)	50, 100, 500	100, 500	50, 100, 200, 500	200, 500	250, 500	250	500	500

(*From* Dirks, I.: Intravenous fat emulsion as a component of TPN. Nutr. Supp. Serv. 4:41–49, 1984, with permission.)

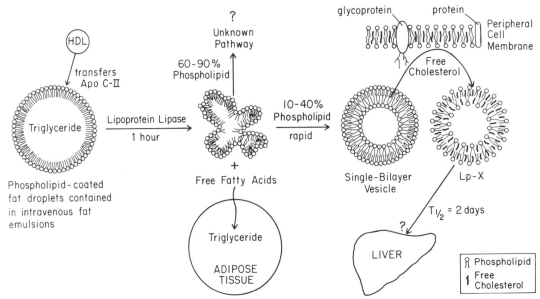

Figure 4–7. Suggested metabolism of intravenous fat emulsions. The phospholipid-coated fat droplets contained in intravenous fat emulsions acquire Apo C-II by transfer from the HDL fraction, resulting in activation of lipoprotein lipase and subsequent hydrolysis of triglyceride. The released free fatty acids are rapidly taken up by adipose and other tissues. Between 60 and 90 per cent of the intravenous phospholipids are also rapidly removed from plasma by an unknown pathway. The remainder of the phospholipids form single bi-layer vesicles, which rapidly extract free cholesterol from peripheral cell membranes to form the Lp-X particle. Lp-X is cleared slowly from the circulation with first-order kinetics and a half-life of approximately 2 days. Lp-X is not converted to other lipoproteins. It is speculated that the liver may clear Lp-X from the blood. (*Adapted from* Untracht, S.: Intravascular metabolism of an artificial transporter of triacylglycerols. Alterations of serum lipoproteins resulting from total parenteral nutrition with Intralipid. Biochim. Biophys. Acta, *711*:176–192, 1982, with permission.)

formed as a result of the intravascular metabolism of intravenous fat emulsions, and unlike chylomicrons, Lp-X does not transfer surface components to the HLD fraction. Lp-X has been characterized as containing 66 per cent phospholipid, 28 per cent cholesterol, all unesterified, and 5 per cent protein, predominantly albumin and Apo-C.[13, 14] Kinetic studies indicate that the Lp-X particle is removed from the circulation as a unit, with a half-life of approximately two days.[14] It has been proposed that the liver is responsible for eliminating Lp-X from the blood. This suggested metabolism of intravenous fat emulsions is shown in Figure 4–7.

Associated Changes in Plasma Lipids

The increase in plasma lipids associated with infusion of fat emulsions occurs in two forms. The first form includes an increase in plasma triglycerides and FFA associated with saturation of the action of lipoprotein lipase and peripheral uptake of fatty acids. The second form includes the increase in plasma free cholesterol and phospholipids associated with accumulation of the Lp-X particle. After the cessation of lipid-supplemented total parenteral nutrition, plasma levels of triglycerides and FFA are cleared in a matter of hours, but plasma levels of Lp-X are usually cleared within two to four days.[13, 14] Thus, the clearance of Lp-X is slower than that of plasma triglyceride. Overall, the degree of lipemia is a primary function of the rate of lipid infusion.

Most of the human lipid–supplemented TPN studies demonstrate a significant increase in mean plasma cholesterol levels and a variable effect on plasma triglyceride and FFA levels. Plasma cholesterol, triglyceride, and FFA levels from four normal human subjects infused with a soybean fat emulsion are shown in Figure 4–8. Note the consistent, gradual increase in plasma cholesterol from 150 mg/dl at 1 day to 400 mg/dl at eight days and the varying increase in plasma triglyceride and FFA levels after fat emulsion infusion. Figure 4–9 further demonstrates the tremendous individual variation in plasma triglyceride levels in response to fat emulsion infusion.

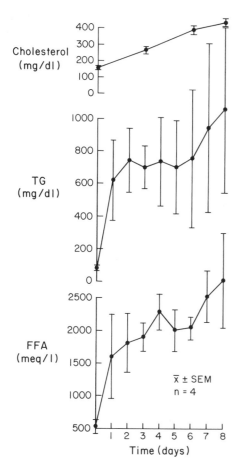

nents to HDL particles, whereas chylomicrons do. Lp-X is also a very poor substrate for LCAT.[62]

The significance of alterations in tissue lipids during intravenous fat infusion are unknown. Results of animal studies suggest that fat emulsions may promote a progressive efflux of cholesterol from atherosclerotic plaque.[63, 64] In view of the number of patients receiving home TPN, it is interesting to speculate on the long-term effects of parenteral nutrition on atherogenesis. Formulation of a fat emulsion in which the phospholipid surfactant is more rapidly metabolized may result in a reduction in fat emulsion–associated lipemia and warrants further research.

Effects of Heparin

Heparin has been demonstrated to decrease triglyceride concentration in the blood during alimentary lipemia[65] and intravenous lipid infusion.[66] Following heparin injection, lipoprotein lipase activity is increased in plasma but diminished in tissue.[67] Heparin is thought to stimulate release of lipoprotein lipase from endothelial cells into the circulation. Thus, at triglyceride concentrations be-

Figure 4–8. Serum or blood concentration of cholesterol, triglyceride (TG), and free fatty acids (FFA) of normal human subjects who received a continuous infusion of amino acids plus fat emulsion (3 g/kg/day) for 8 days. Cholesterol concentration rose predictably and steadily, as did FFA. TG concentration varied considerably among the subjects.

A multicenter study has compared the use of Intralipid 10% and Intralipid 20%.[61] The researchers noted a significantly greater increase in plasma cholesterol concentration in patients receiving the 10 per cent soybean fat emulsion. Patients in both groups received equivalent amounts of triglyceride, but the group receiving the 20 per cent lipid infusion received a smaller amount of phospholipid. It is suggested that higher levels of phospholipid infusion may be associated with elevations of plasma cholesterol and formation of the Lp-X particle.

Long-term infusions of fat emulsions have also been associated with a decrease in HLD concentration[8] and LCAT activity.[14] One explanation is that HDL and LCAT are synthesized more slowly during TPN, because fat emulsions do not donate surface compo-

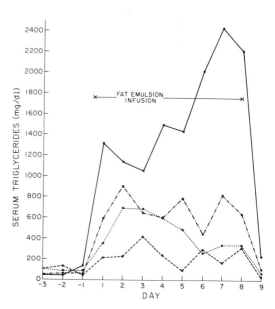

Figure 4–9. Triglyceride concentration in serum of individual normal human subjects receiving amino acids plus 3 g/kg/day of fat emulsion intravenously. All subjects had normal triglyceride and other lipid concentrations and no evidence of glucose intolerance after an overnight fast. The marked variability of the clearance rate of intravascular fat despite identical infusion rates among "normal" subjects is demonstrated.

low utilization of maximal enzyme capacity, the change in distribution favoring circulating activity increases exposure of circulatory triglyceride to enzyme, and triglyceride hydrolysis is enhanced. In contrast, at high triglyceride concentrations with maximal enzyme utilization, redistribution of enzyme by heparin has little effect.[65] This hypothesis would explain, in part, the variable clinical results observed as to the effect of heparin on triglyceride clearance from plasma.[68–70]

Brennan and Moore[71] have shown, in normal humans receiving intravenous fat emulsion, that heparin-stimulated triglyceride clearance produces equivalent increases of circulating free fatty acids and glycerol, demonstrating that the chemical form of the lipid has changed but clearance of total lipid components is not affected. Owing to the risk of induction of complications specific to fatty acid toxicity (discussed later), routine addition of heparin to fat emulsion infusions as a "clearing factor" is not recommended.[71, 72]

CLINICAL APPLICATION OF INTRAVENOUS FAT EMULSIONS

Essential Nutrients

A clinical syndrome primarily consisting of a diffuse dermatitis[73] and occasional hemolytic anemia,[74] enhanced platelet aggregation,[36] diminished wound healing,[75] and hepatic dysfunction secondary to fatty metamorphosis[4] may be induced by feeding oral[76, 77] or intravenous[78, 79] diets deficient in essential fatty acids (linoleic and linolenic acids). Biochemical alterations consist of elevations of the concentrations of saturated fatty acids in plasma and tissue, decreases of the essential fatty acids, and appearance of an abnormal fatty acid—5,8,11-eicosatrienoic acid (20:3n9). The ratio of this fatty acid to arachidonic acid (20:4n6) is termed the *triene/tetraene ratio*. A ratio of greater than 0.4 indicates essential fatty acid deficiency.[80] Quantitation of specific fatty acids, however, appears preferable to expression of the ratio when possible. Provision of fat-free TPN induces biochemical evidence of a deficiency state in two to three weeks.[4]

This syndrome occurs primarily in the presence of minimal-fat or fat-free feeding, rather than in global starvation, because mobilization of essential fatty acids from fat depots prevents a deficiency state. Thus, essential fatty acid intake sufficient to prevent or treat a deficiency state is expressed as the percentage of total energy intake. Barr and colleagues[79] reported prevention of essential fatty acid deficiency in TPN patients through inclusion of 3.2 per cent of total energy as soybean oil emulsion. Lesser intakes of safflower oil emulsions prevent lineoleic acid deficiency[80] but may produce linolenic acid deficiency.[57, 82] Providing approximately 10 per cent of energy intake as soybean or safflower oil emulsion to patients receiving TPN should assure prevention of fatty acid deficiency.

Intravenous Fat Emulsion as an Energy Source

Metabolism of Fat Emulsions in Stress

Clearance. The capacity for clearance of exogenous intravenous fat emulsion from the bloodstream may be affected by stress. Several studies have reported accelerated lipid clearance following lipid infusion in patients with moderate, generally nonseptic stress.[83–85] More severely stressed patients, however, particularly those with sepsis, may demonstrate impaired lipid clearance.[85, 86] Factors affecting lipid clearance in sepsis include observed hyperlipidemia in patients with gram-negative sepsis[87, 88] associated with evidence of depressed lipoprotein lipase activity in muscle and increased fatty acid synthesis activity in the liver.[89] Thus, the accelerations of fatty acid mobilization, fatty acid synthesis in the liver, and fatty acid re-esterification in the liver may all contribute to the appearance of diminished triglyceride clearance during sepsis. Continuous as opposed to intermittent lipid infusion has been associated with increased net lipid clearance in neonates.[90] Lipid clearance may be expected to increase with increased duration of fat emulsion infusion because of stimulation of peripheral lipoprotein lipase activity.[91]

Oxidation of Fat Emulsions. The extent to which stress affects the oxidation of intravenously infused fat emulsions has generated considerable controversy. Isotopic studies in animals have demonstrated that variable portions of the fat emulsions are directly oxidized to CO_2, although the utilization of exogenous fat has been demonstrated to be decreased in septic rats.[92] A lack of correlation between clearance rates and fat utilization using isotope studies in humans has demonstrated that disappearance of triglyceride from the plasma cannot be used as a measure of fat utilization.[93] Carpentier and associates[93] and Nordenström and colleagues[94, 95] have demonstrated direct oxidation of isotopically labeled fat emulsions in traumatized and septic patients and have concluded that fat emulsions are an effective source of energy in these patients. Nanni and co-workers[96] have also presented metabolic evidence of utilization of infused fat emulsions in septic patients, supporting the concept that intravenous lipids can be used to increase oxidative metabolism. In contrast, Goodenough and Wolfe[43] have found that the contributions of glucose and fat to total energy production in burn patients were similar in subjects fed a predominantly glucose mixture and those fed a mixture of glucose and fat, suggesting that fat mobilization, stimulated by the stress response, continues despite the infusion of exogenous lipid and that the exogenous lipid contributes only a small amount of the energy produced by these patients. Goodenough and Wolfe[43] concluded that the primary effect of exogenous lipid infusion in severely stressed patients is to maintain fat storage. The issue of the relative contributions of endogenous fat and exogenous fat to energy supply in stressed patients who are stimulated to mobilize fat requires further study.

The impact of infused lipid on glucose metabolism in stressed patients is also controversial. Both an increase and a decrease in the rate of glucose oxidation have been reportedly stimulated by exogenous lipid infusion.[96, 97]

Impact of Intravenous Fat Emulsion on Protein Metabolism

Determination of the impact of infusion of fat emulsion on protein metabolism is an appropriate endpoint for the study of the efficacy of such infusion because essentially all the elements for recovery from illness or injury depend on active new protein synthesis. The relationship between provision of effective energy sources and protein metabolism has been known for many years.[98] For an exogenous energy source to be effective in modulating protein metabolism, oxidation to provide utilizable energy is required. Because most patients receiving parenteral nutrition have not exhausted their fat stores, consideration of the impact of exogenous fat on protein metabolism in patients who are

stimulated to mobilize and oxidize endogenous fat is appropriate.

The essential interchangeability of glucose and fat in the diet of healthy animals and humans, with the exception of a transient interval of "adaptation" to the fat diet, has been extensively demonstrated.[40, 98] Studies of intravenous infusion of fat emulsions in normal humans have demonstrated the requirement for the presence of adequate amino acid intake in order for fat to be an effective energy source. Intravenous fat emulsion given alone does not appear to improve protein sparing over that afforded by endogenous fat.[99] In contrast, normal subjects provided with adequate intravenous amino acid intake, and similar caloric infusion as either fat emulsion or glucose, show essentially zero nitrogen balance following the first four days of infusion (Fig. 4–10).[100] Infusion of a mixture of amino acids and glucose in normal subjects similarly produces zero nitrogen balance.[101] Thus, results of the studies of the impact on protein metabolism of intravenous glucose and fat as calorie sources parallel closely results of the studies of the impact of oral feeding.

The effectiveness of intravenous fat emulsion in supporting protein metabolism in both stressed animals and stressed humans has been studied extensively, including comparisons with the effectiveness of glucose. Several studies provided total energy in excess of estimated energy expenditure and substituted approximately 40 to 50 per cent of the glucose calories with lipid calories. The majority of these studies found that the substitution of fat for glucose had no impact on nitrogen balance.[95, 102–104] MacFie and co-workers,[105] using total body nitrogen determination by neutron activation, found an increase in body nitrogen in gastrointestinal surgical patients infused with a mixture of glucose and fat calories but no increase in body nitrogen in similar patients infused with glucose as the sole energy source.[105]

Studies in which lipid has served as the predominant or exclusive energy source have shown an impact on nitrogen economy similar to that of glucose infusion in both monkeys and humans.[106–108] In contrast, both Freund and colleagues[109] and Souba and associates,[110] studying stressed rats, found that glucose was superior to infused fat as an energy source for nitrogen balance; and Long and co-workers,[111] studying severely stressed patients, found that urea nitrogen excretion was inversely related to carbohydrate intake

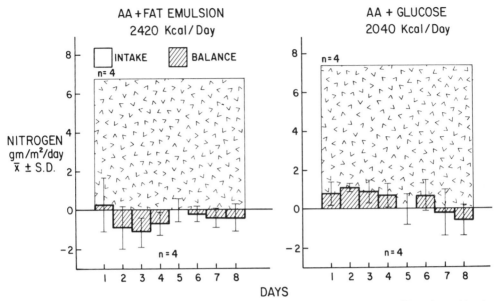

Figure 4–10. Daily nitrogen balance ($\times \pm$ SD) in normal volunteer subjects infused with amino acids plus either fat emulsion or glucose. Nitrogen balance is slightly negative initially during fat emulsion infusion, but nitrogen equilibrium is established on the fifth day of infusion. There is no statistical difference of nitrogen balance for days 5–8 between provisions of fat emulsion and glucose.

and was not affected by fat infusion at any level of carbohydrate intake. Thus, in these more severely stressed patients, fat was believed to have had no impact on protein metabolism.[111] Woolfson and colleagues[112] found amino acids plus glucose to be marginally more protein-sparing than glucose plus sorbitol and fat emulsion in stressed patients. As described previously, Goodenough and Wolfe[43] concluded that the primary effect of exogenous fat emulsion infusion in stressed patients receiving glucose at approximate maximal oxidation capacity is to spare fat stores.

The results of all of the study protocols involving infusion of mixtures of glucose and fat are difficult to interpret, because most studies comparing the efficacy of substitution of a portion of glucose intake with fat have provided 1.5 times the resting energy expenditure. Elimination of 40 to 50 per cent of glucose calories with or without substitution with fat may have no effect on nitrogen balance in this situation.[113]

It is concluded that, for most patients, mixtures of glucose and fat as energy sources in parenteral nutrition are effective in supporting protein metabolism. The primary issue that remains to be resolved is the extent to which fat should be added to glucose in stressed patients receiving glucose in appropriate doses to achieve maximum oxidation. Fat should be provided to all patients to

ensure avoidance of essential fatty acid deficiency. Decisions regarding the percentage of calories to be infused as fat above this minimum probably should be based on considerations other than the impact on protein metabolism.

Complications of Intravenous Fat Emulsion

Pulmonary Complications

Consideration of potential pulmonary complications of infusion of intravenous fat emulsion is appropriate in view of the widespread recommendation for increasing proportions of fat as a nonprotein energy source in patients with respiratory compromise. Historically, concern that hypertriglyceridemia and associated elevations of circulating free fatty acids might cause pulmonary damage arose following description of the fat embolism syndrome in patients with multiple trauma, particularly skeletal trauma. The finding of fat associated with pulmonary hemorrhage in the lungs of autopsy specimens of trauma patients with respiratory failure led to the conclusion that embolization of marrow fat from the site of long-bone fractures was a major cause of this pulmonary damage.[114] In rabbits, infusion of a preparation of fat produced pulmonary arteriolar obstruction and right ventricular failure, and infusion of free fatty acids caused intraparenchymal hemorrhage.[114] More recent studies have demonstrated that the amount of fat embolization that occurs from either fractures or intramedullary fixation of fractures is minimal[115] and that the cause of post-traumatic adult respiratory distress syndrome is a complex process involving pulmonary endothelial injury, neutrophil aggregation, and a series of complex chemical reactions. The use of free fatty acids as an agent for production of an animal model for the study of acute respiratory distress syndrome, however, has persisted.[116] Finally, it was recognized, prior to consideration of the use of intravenous fat emulsions, that circulating hypertriglyceridemia may interact with red cell membranes and produce an oxygen diffusion defect.[117] More detailed studies of the effect of hypertriglyceridemia on red cell membranes has shown a loss of cholesterol from the membrane and associated diminished oxygen diffusion capacity.[118]

Several investigators have identified accumulation of lipid in the lungs or pulmonary vasculature at autopsy of neonates given intravenous lipids.[119–121] Lipid-laden macrophages have been recovered from tracheal aspirates from newborn infants receiving intravenous fat emulsion infusion.[122] The potential for the serum of neonates to agglutinate the fat emulsion may contribute to this phenomenon.[123, 124] It is difficult, if not impossible, to determine the extent to which the lipid deposits may have contributed to the severe respiratory distress experienced by these neonates as a result of intravenous lipid infusion. Further difficulty in interpreting the significance of these findings arises from the demonstration that the interval between death and postmortem examination is a factor in the extent of formation of intravascular fat globules in the lungs and other tissues, raising some question as to whether all of the fat droplets recovered at postmortem examination were in fact present *in vivo*.[125] Nevertheless, hypoxemia in premature infants secondary to intravenous lipid infusion has been demonstrated.[126]

Infusion of fat emulsion into normal adult patients produced a pulmonary oxygen diffusion gradient in some but not all subjects.[127, 128] The diffusion gradients were not severe and apparently could be easily overcome by increased ventilation, because no change in PaO_2 occurred in these subjects or in normal volunteers infused with 3 gm/kg of fat emulsion daily for eight days.[129] No

defect in pulmonary diffusion capacity could be demonstrated by carbon monoxide diffusion or by xenon-133 perfusion/diffusion scan in convalescing burn patients.[130] It is apparent that whatever pulmonary impairment may be induced by fat emulsion infusion in relatively healthy adults is minor and of no clinical significance. Determination of the impact of fat emulsion infusion on patients with severe respiratory insufficiency, however, is exceedingly difficult, owing to the complex nature of the pulmonary lesions in these patients.

Several recent studies in animals suggest that although fat emulsion infusion has minimal impact on the function of healthy lungs, it may cause substantial impairment of previously injured lungs. The changes in damaged lungs appear to be secondary to alterations in prostaglandin synthesis and balance. Hunt and colleagues[131] demonstrated a fall in PaO_2 with fat emulsion infusion in rabbits with oleic acid–injured lungs but not in rabbits with uninjured lungs. The fall in PaO_2 was blocked by administration of indomethacin, an inhibitor of prostaglandin synthesis. Hageman and associates[132] repeated this study and demonstrated that increases in the vasodilator prostaglandins PGE_2 and 6-keto-$PGF_{1\alpha}$, as well as the fall in PaO_2, were induced by fat emulsion infusion. Both the PaO_2 decrease and the vasodilating prostaglandin increases were blocked by indomethacin (Fig. 4–11).[132] In both of these studies, the indomethacin did not affect the extent of hypertriglyceridemia, leading to the conclusion that the hypoxemia was not a direct result of the triglycerides but rather was prostaglandin-mediated. The explanation offered for the hypoxemia was that obliteration of hypoxia-induced pulmonary arterial vasoconstriction resulted in perfusion of damaged (unventilated) pulmonary tissue. Fat emulsion infusion may modulate the extent of pulmonary arterial hypertension and associated hypoxemia by altering the synthesis rates of dilating and constricting prostaglandins in sheep.[133] The capacity of FFA such as oleic acid for producing the pulmonary microvascular permeability lesion associated with acute respiratory distress syndrome is well established.[116, 134] The role of prostaglandins in production of this vascular permeability is less certain.[135] Prostaglandin-induced platelet aggregation[136, 137] or increased leukocyte chemotaxis[138] following fat emulsion infusion could play a potentiating role. Lipoxygenase products of arachidonic acid

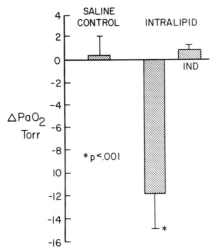

Figure 4–11. Changes of PaO₂ in rabbits with oleic acid–damaged lungs following infusion of saline control or intravenous fat emulsion (4 ml 10%/kg over 1 hr). A statistically significant decrease of PaO₂ of 12 ± 1.5 torr occurred following the fat emulsion infusion. Pretreatment with indomethacin (IND) blocked the decrease in PaO₂ and the associated increases in vasodilating prostaglandins. Data are mean ± SEM, n = 5. (*From* Hageman, J. R., McCulloch, K., Gora, P., Olsen, E. K., Pachman, L., and Hunt, C. E.: Intralipid alterations in pulmonary prostaglandin metabolism and gas exchange. Crit. Care Med., *11*:794–798, 1983, with permission, Williams & Wilkins Co.)

metabolism (see Fig. 4–5) may also mediate the increase in pulmonary capillary permeability.[139] Although depression of respiratory function has limited fat emulsion infusion in neonates, adults with respiratory failure appear less prone to manifestation of prostaglandin-mediated pulmonary impairment.[140, 141]

Hepatic Complications

Hepatic complications of TPN have included hepatic dysfunction associated with fatty metamorphosis, cholestasis, and, rarely, cirrhosis with hepatic failure.[142] The nature and extent of nonprotein energy provision in TPN has been thought to play a major role in the development of at least the fatty metamorphosis.[143] The fatty metamorphosis has generally been attributed to overfeeding of glucose. However, alterations of lipid metabolism induced by stress, as well as lipid infusion itself, may also contribute to fatty metamorphosis. The metabolic alterations induced by stress, discussed previously, lead to endogenous mobilization of fatty acids from fat stores and increased hepatic free fatty acid re-esterification in the

liver. Accumulation of hepatic triglyceride as little as 24 hours after endotoxin infusion in rabbits has been demonstrated.[144] Additional exogenous fat provision may potentiate the accumulation of hepatic fat in stress.

Deposition of hepatic lipid may also occur in unstressed patients receiving intravenous fat emulsions. Accumulation of fat in the reticuloendothelial system of the liver occurs particularly when the threshold for triglyceride clearance by lipoprotein lipase is exceeded.[145, 146]

Experimental evidence in rats indicates that provision of intravenous amino acids and nonprotein calories as either 100 per cent glucose or 100 per cent fat produces fatty metamorphosis of the liver.[147, 148] Amino acids with hypocaloric glucose infusion avoided development of fatty liver, but only a mixture of glucose and fat provided sufficient energy to accomplish nutritional repletion while avoiding development of fatty liver.[148] Rats receiving calories as 100 per cent glucose developed depressed linolate concentration in hepatocytes.[147] Fatty acid deficiency has been associated with fatty liver in both experimental animals and humans.[149] Depression of the rate of lipoprotein synthesis in the liver occurs in protein deficiency states and presumably contributes to hepatic fat accumulation in the presence of both excessive glucose intake (with accelerated hepatic lipogenesis) and excessive exogenous lipid infusion.

The development of cholestasis with hyperbilirubinemia particularly in neonates may be a more deleterious development associated with parenteral nutrition than simple hepatic fatty metamorphosis. Salvian and Allardyce[150] conducted a randomized study comparing the effects of parenteral nutrition regimens composed of varying portions of glucose and fat on liver function parameters and hepatic morphology. They found that the high-carbohydrate infusions produced increased fatty liver but that elevations in the concentration of bilirubin, alkaline phosphatase, and cholesterol occurred primarily in the groups receiving intravenous fat. Of greatest concern was the finding of periportal inflammation and bile duct proliferation limited to those patients who received intravenous fat emulsion.[150] In a subsequent report, progressive cholestatic jaundice occurred in ten of 18 patients receiving lipid emulsion in a dose of 3 gm/kg/day, whereas evidence of cholestasis appeared in only one of 17 patients infused with a dose of 1 gm/kg/day.[151]

A mechanism for the induction of cholestasis by fat emulsion infusion was not established by these studies. The significance of the association of lipoprotein-X in patients infused with intravenous fat emulsion and in patients with cholestasis due to bile duct occlusion, for example, remains to be investigated.

Effects of Fat Emulsions on Immune Function

Infection is a major cause of morbidity and mortality among patients who require parenteral nutrition. Enhancement of immune function is therefore one of the major purposes of providing parenteral nutrition. Considerable evidence has accumulated indicating that, in addition to supporting immune function by promoting protein synthesis, fat emulsion infusion may affect immune function directly.

Blockade of the reticuloendothelial system (RES) impairs clearance of particulate matter, including bacteria from the circulation, thereby increasing the risk of systemic infection.[152] When the lipoprotein lipase system is saturated, the RES becomes a major site of fat emulsion clearance from plasma.[60] Demonstration of the accumulation of lipid or lipid-associated pigment in the RES cells of the liver, lung, and spleen[145, 153] has led to concern regarding possible RES dysfunction following fat emulsion infusion. Clearance of ^{125}I-labeled microaggregated human serum albumin was not affected by a single bolus of fat emulsion infusion in minimally stressed patients,[154] but lipid infusion in mice increased mortality associated with controlled bacterial infusion (Fig. 4–12).[155] Impairment of RES function *in vivo* by fatty (oleic) acid infusion indicates that accumulation of triglyceride in the RES cells following plasma clearance may not be the entire explanation for impairment of RES function associated with fat emulsion infusion.[156]

Evidence for and against induction of abnormalities of white blood cell (WBC) function by intravenous lipid has been reported. Both *in vitro* incubation of WBC with fat emulsion[155, 157] and *in vivo* infusion in humans inhibit leukocytic chemotaxis.[158–160] Pretreatment of patients with heparin prevents impairment of monocytic chemotaxis by fat infusion.[160] The mechanism of protection by heparin was unclear. Fat emulsion may inhibit the synthesis of complement (C_2),[161, 162] phagocytosis,[154, 157] bacteriocidal capacity,[154] and lymphoproliferation.[163]

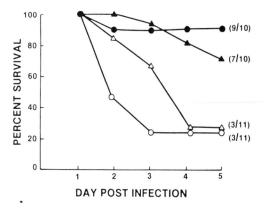

Figure 4–12. Effect of lipid emulsion on survival of AKR/J mice infected with type III GBS. Strain 0136C alone (●), or 0136C + lipid (○); strain IIIN alone (▲), or IIIN + lipid (△). (*From* Fischer, G. W., Wilson, S. R., Hunter, K. W., et al.: Diminished bacterial defense with Intralipid. Lancet, 2:819, 1980.)

In contrast to the preceding studies, the study by Helms and co-workers[164] found no effect of fat emulsion on cell-mediated immunity, and that by Palmblad and associates[165] found no functional impairment of WBC following fat infusion in humans. Siegel and colleagues[166] reported variable results in red cell and neutrophil immune adherence in patients after fat infusion.

Evidence of a direct impact of fatty acids on immune function has included interference with phagocytic activity of Kupffer cells,[167] impairment of lymphocyte transformation,[168] and inhibition of chemotaxis by palmitic (but not oleic) acid[169] in addition to the RES blockade already discussed.[156] Thus, the net effect of providing heparin with fat emulsion infusion to stimulate intravascular hydrolysis to free fatty acids and glycerol cannot be predicted. Heparin protects against fat-induced impairment of chemotaxis but may stimulate other adverse effects on the immune system by increasing fatty acid concentration. Arachidonic acid metabolites (leukotrienes and prostaglandins) are known to affect WBC function,[170, 171] but the impact of fat intake on the extent of arachidonic acid metabolite–mediated alteration of immune function remains to be clarified.

Despite the concern regarding impairment of immune function raised by these and other reports, only one study has evaluated the impact of fat emulsions on the *in vivo* response to an infectious challenge,[155] and no study has provided evidence for or against an actual impact of fat emulsion infusion on infectious morbidity or mortality in humans. Such data would be exceedingly difficult to generate because of the multiplicity of factors predisposing patients who require parenteral nutrition to infectious complications. Therefore, no conclusions can be reached regarding clinical management of patients from the preceding studies of specific aspects of immune function.

Fat Emulsions and Pancreatitis

An association between acute pancreatitis and hyperlipemia has been established.[172, 173] The incidence of hyperlipemia in patients with pancreatitis has varied from four to 53 per cent in various reports.[174] Persistence of the hyperlipemia following resolution of the pancreatitis suggests that the pancreatitis is the result of the hyperlipemia, rather than that hyperlipemia is secondary to pancreatitis.[175] Additional evidence that hyperlipemia may cause pancreatitis includes successful prevention of recurrence by feeding a low-fat diet[173] and induction of manifestations of pancreatitis in alcoholic patients by lipid feeding.[176]

Speculation that hyperlipemia secondary to intravenous fat emulsion infusion may precipitate acute pancreatitis has led to several investigations of a possible relationship. No evidence of exocrine pancreatic stimulation has been found in normal subjects,[177] or in patients with pancreatic fistulas.[178] Although isolated cases of pancreatitis precipitated by fat emulsion infusion have been reported,[179, 180] such cases apparently are rare. Intravenous fat emulsions have been successfully used in rats[181] and in humans[182] with pancreatitis, with no evidence of adverse effects. It is concluded that use of fat emulsions should be avoided in patients with a history of associated hyperlipemia and pancreatitis but that otherwise fat emulsions may be used with caution in pancreatitis patients.

Other Complications of Intravenous Fat Emulsions

A clinical syndrome termed *fat overload syndrome*, variably consisting of hyperlipemia, hemolytic anemia, thrombocytopenia with associated coagulopathy, respiratory impairment, and hepatic and renal dysfunction, was a major cause for withdrawal of cottonseed oil emulsion from the United States market in the past. This syndrome has been reported following soybean oil emulsion in isolated cases.[183, 184] Individual components of this syndrome have been reported

more frequently. Hemolytic anemia associated with fat emulsion infusion has been described.[185, 186] This complication may be due to the action of free fatty acids on red cell membranes rather than to a direct effect of the infused triglyceride.[187, 188] Thrombocytopenia appears to be a rare complication of soy lipid emulsions.[189] Thrombotic complications have been attributed to fat emulsions (particularly, increased free fatty acid concentration),[190] but reports of the effect of fat emulsions on platelet function have been conflicting.[191–193] Allergy has been reported rarely,[194] as has induction of bacteremia secondary to contamination of the fat emulsion infusion units.[195]

Potential cardiovascular complications of fat emulsions have been investigated. Using a fat emulsion perfusion, Grimes and Abel[196] produced a negative inotropic effect on the left ventricle of dogs on cardiopulmonary bypass.[196] Abel and colleagues[197] subsequently demonstrated that significant decreases in cardiac output and increases in pulmonary capillary wedge pressure occur in postoperative aortocoronary bypass patients given high-dose fat emulsion infusion but not lower-dose infusions.[197] Jarnberg and associates[198] found no hemodynamic effect of fat infusion in critically ill patients. Sinus bradycardia has been attributed to fat emulsion infusion.[199]

Free fatty acids may produce more serious cardiac complications through induction of thrombosis with infarction,[200] extension of infarction,[201] or induction of arrhythmia.[202–204]

Free Fatty Acid Toxicity

Fat emulsion infusion increases the free fatty acid concentration in the blood. The increase may be potentiated by stress or heparin. Thus, consideration of the potential toxicity of free fatty acids, apart from the triglycerides, that constitute fat emulsions is appropriate. The role of free fatty acids in the development of pulmonary, immune, hematologic, or cardiovascular complications of fat emulsion infusion have been discussed. Fatty acids compete for albumin binding sites with free tryptophan[205] and bilirubin[206, 207] such that induction of hepatic coma by tryptophan or brain injury by bilirubin in neonates may be potentiated. Elevated free fatty acid concentrations may impair carbohydrate metabolism.[208] Owing to the present clinical inability to monitor free fatty acid concentrations, fat emulsion infusion, particularly with heparin, must be given with considerable caution in patients with impairment of one of the organ systems just listed.[72]

Summary

The preceding discussion of complications of intravenous fat emulsion infusion implies that the safety of such infusions may be of major concern. In fact, clinical experience has shown that adverse reactions that are clearly attributable to the fat emulsion infusion have been distinctly uncommon. Wretlind[209] reported only eight cases of suspected adverse reaction for 1.6 million infusion units of Intralipid in Sweden, and Hansen and co-workers[210] reported minor complications of Intralipid infusion in two of 133 adult and eight of 159 pediatric patients. It must be emphasized that these very low complication rates generally do not consider the potential impact of fat emulsions on conditions such as respiratory and hepatic failures or the induction of sepsis or pancreatitis, because all of these conditions have multiple causes, and often one cannot determine the extent to which intravenous fat may have contributed to a given organ failure. As TPN is increasingly applied to critically ill patients, consideration of the impact of the feeding on existing organ failure assumes greater importance. Until these issues are more accurately resolved, limiting the rate of fat emulsion infusion so that intravascular accumulation of triglyceride or free fatty acids is avoided would appear to ensure an acceptably low incidence of adverse reactions to fat emulsion infusion.

CLINICAL IMPLICATIONS

Once a decision to provide intravenous nutritional support has been made, the approximate percentages of energy intake to be provided as fat and carbohydrate must be determined. Considerations in this decision include: (1) the vascular access (central *versus* peripheral venous administration); (2) assurance of avoidance of essential fatty acid deficiency; (3) the efficacy of fat in supporting protein synthesis; (4) potential complications of fat emulsion infusion; and (5) cost.

The availability of 20 per cent fat emulsions makes possible delivery of modest protein and energy intake in 3.7 L/day using a solution of three per cent amino acids plus five per cent glucose. This formulation pro-

vides 73 per cent of nonprotein energy as fat. The percentage of energy given as fat can be reduced to 47 per cent by using 10 per cent glucose, well within the manufacturer's recommendation that fat not constitute more than 60 per cent of nonprotein energy intake. Induction of phlebitis and thrombosis of the peripheral veins may occur with the more concentrated solution, but continuous fat emulsion infusion may afford a degree of protection to the veins.[211] It is thus possible to avoid the hazards of central venous cannulation in both pediatric and adult patients. For patients with no specific contraindication to either central or peripheral venous access, this decision is based on consideration of the efficacy, complications, and cost of the greater fat emulsion proportion required for peripheral venous administration.

Patients receiving parenteral nutrition through central venous catheters may receive sufficient nutrients in minimal volume without fat intake. As discussed previously, providing a minimum of 10 per cent of energy as fat will avoid development of essential fatty acid deficiency. This amount should be provided to all patients receiving parenteral nutrition as a minimum, and greater fat intake should be provided if fatty acid deficiency is suspected.

As already reviewed, the comparative efficacy of fat *versus* glucose in supporting protein metabolism has been extensively studied and debated. It appears that patients with minimal stress but inability to accept gastrointestinal feeding do equally well with the higher fat intake required for peripheral venous administration as with centrally administered high-glucose formulations, provided that peripheral venous access can be maintained. Patients with critical or septic illness may not benefit from the higher fat intake, perhaps because of ongoing stimulation of endogenous fat mobilization and the limitations of fatty acid oxidation. In addition, patients with critical illness may be more prone to potentiation of impaired pulmonary, hepatic, or immune function with high fat intake. Further studies are required to clarify the importance of provision of more than 10 per cent of energy as fat for critically ill patients.

The issue of cost of parenteral nutrition is discussed in Chapter 19. Fat emulsions are more expensive to produce, and thus increasing replacement of glucose with fat in parenteral nutrition increases the cost. For example, the cost of providing 10 per cent of energy as fat in TPN is less than the cost of providing 60 per cent of energy as fat in peripheral parenteral nutrition. The extent of this cost difference may vary among hospitals because contracts for nutritional components vary. Also, the pitfalls of comparing patient charges as opposed to real or total cost to the hospital must be considered (Chapter 19). Higher complication rates may occur among patients with central venous catheters, raising their total cost, for example. Nevertheless, increasing fat intake in parenteral nutrition may be expected to increase cost, a consideration that cannot be ignored.

REFERENCES

1. Moore, F. D., and Brennan, M. F.: Surgical injury: Body composition, protein metabolism, and neuroendocrinology. *In* ACS Manual of Surgical Nutrition. Philadelphia, W. B. Saunders Co., 1975, pp. 174–180.
2. Miles, J., Glasscock, R., Aikens, J., Gerich, J., and Haymond, M.: A microfluorometric method for the determination of free fatty acids in plasma. J. Lipid Res., 24:96–99, 1983.
3. Kessler, G., and Lederer, H.: The fluorometric measurement of triglycerides—automation in analytical chemistry. *In* Skeggs, L. T. Jr. (ed.): Technicon Symposia, 1965. New York, Mediad, Inc., 1966, p. 341.
4. Richardson, T. J., and Sgoutas, D.: Essential fatty acid deficiency in four adult patients during total parenteral nutrition. Am. J. Clin. Nutr., 28:258–263, 1975.
5. Carey, N., Small, D., and Bliss, C.: Lipid digestion and absorption. Ann. Rev. Physiol., 45:651–677, 1983.
6. Mahley, R. W.: Atherogenic hyperlipoproteinemia—the cellular and molecular biology of plasma lipoproteins altered by dietary fat and cholesterol. Med. Clin. North Am., 66:375–403, 1982.
7. Ney, D., Lefevre, M., and Schneeman, B. O.: Alteration of high density lipoprotein (HDL) composition with fat-free total parenteral nutrition in the rat. Fed. Proc., 43:796, 1984.
8. Badimon, J., Fleming, R., Patton, J., and Mao, S.: Changes of plasma levels of apolipoproteins A-I, A-II, and B and their isoforms in patients with intestinal failure receiving long term parenteral nutrition. Gastroenterology, in press.
9. Simons, L. A., and Gibson, J. C.: Lipids: A Clinicians' Guide. Baltimore, University Park Press, 1980, p. 1–5.
10. Gordon, T., Castelli, N. P., Hjortland, M. C., Icannel, W. B., and Dawber, T. R.: High density lipoprotein as a protective factor against coronary heart disease. Am. J. Med., 62:707–714, 1977.
11. Hamilton, R. L., Havel, R. J., Kane, J. P., Blaurock, A. E., and Salta,, T.: Cholestasis: Lamellar structure of the abnormal human serum lipoprotein. Science, 172:475–478, 1971.
12. McConathy, W. J., Alaupovic, J. P., Curry, M. D., Magnani, H. N., Torsvik, H., Berh, R., and Gjone, E.: Identification of lipoprotein families in familial lecithin cholesterol acyltransferase deficiency. Biochim. Biophys. Acta, 326:406–418, 1973.
13. Griffin, E., Breckenridge, W. C., Kuksis, A., Bryan, M. H., and Angel, A.: Appearance and characterization of lipoprotein X during continuous Intralipid infusions in the neonate. J. Clin. Invest., 64:1703–1712, 1979.
14. Untraucht, S.: Alterations of serum lipoproteins resulting from total parenteral nutrition with Intralipid. Biochim. Biophys. Acta, 711:176–192, 1982.
15. Innis, S. M., and Boyd, M.: Cholesterol and bile acid synthesis during total parenteral nutrition with and without lipid emulsion in the rat. Am. J. Clin. Nutr., 38:95–100, 1983.
16. Freedland, R. A., and Briggs, S.: A Biochemical Approach to Nutrition. New York, Halsted Press, 1977, pp. 29–37.
17. Havel, R. J., Kane, J. P., and Kashyap, M. L.: Interchange of apolipoproteins between chylomicrons and high density lipoproteins during alimentary lipemia in man. J. Clin. Invest., 52:32–38, 1973.
18. Spector, A. A., Steinberg, D., and Tanaka, A.: Uptake of free fatty acids by Ehrlich ascites tumor cells. J. Biol. Chem., 240:1032–1041, 1965.
19. McGarry, J. D., and Foster, D. W.: Regulation of hepatic fatty acid oxidation and ketone body production. Ann. Rev. Biochem., 49:395–420, 1980.
20. Krebs, H. A., Wallace, P. G., Hems, R., and Freedland, R. A.: Rates of ketone body formation in the perfused rat liver. Biochem. J., 112:595–600, 1969.
21. Birkhahn, R. H., and Border, J. R.: Alternate or supplemental energy sources. J.P.E.N., 5:24–31, 1981.
22. Schwabe, A. D., Bennett, L. R., and Bowman, L. P.: Octanoic acid absorption and oxidation in humans. J. Appl. Physiol., 19:335–337, 1964.
23. Bach, A., Guisard, D., Metais, P., et al.: Metabolic effects following a short and medium chain triglyceride load in dogs. Nutr. Metab., 14:203–209, 1972.
24. Sailer, D., and Muller, M.: Medium chain triglycerides in parenteral nutrition. J.P.E.N., 5:115–119, 1981.
25. Randel, P. J., Hales, C. N., Garland, P. B., and Newsholme, E. A.: The glucose fatty-acid cycle. Lancet, 1:785–789, 1963.
26. Wilmore, D. W., Long, J. M., and Skreen, R. A.: Catecholamines, mediator of the metabolic response to thermal injury. Ann. Surg., 180:653, 1974.
27. Galster, A. D., Clutter, W. E., Cryer, P. E., Collins, J. A., and Bier, D. M.: Epinephrine plasma thresholds for lipolytic effects in man. J. Clin. Invest., 67:1729–1738, 1981.
28. Rodemann, H. P., and Goldberg, A. L.: Arachidonic acid, prostaglandin E_2 and $F_{2\alpha}$ influence rates of protein turnover in skeletal and a cardiac muscle. J. Biol. Chem., 257:1632–1638, 1982.
29. Baracos, V., Rodemann, H. P., Dinarello, C. A., and Goldberg, A. L.: Stimulation of muscle protein. Degradation and prostaglandin E_2 release of leukocytic pyrogen (interleukin-1). N. Engl. J. Med., 308:553–558, 1983.
30. Brigham, K. L., Newman, J. H., Snapper, J. R., and Ogletree, M. L.: Metabolites of arachidonic

acid in the pathophysiology of the pulmonary circulation. *In* Oates, J. A. (ed.): Prostaglandins and the Cardiovascular System. New York, Raven Press, 1982, pp. 357–366.

31. Moncada, S., and Vane, J. R.: Arachidonic acid metabolites and the interactions between platelets and blood vessel walls. N. Engl. J. Med., *300*:1142–1147, 1979.

32. Moncada, S.: Biology and therapeutic potential of prostacyclin. Stroke, *14*:157–168, 1983.

33. VanDorp, D.: Recent developments in the biosynthesis and the analyses of prostaglandins. Ann. N.Y. Acad. Sci., *180*:181–199, 1971.

34. Ziboh, V. A., and Hsia, S. L.: Effects of prostaglandin E₂ on rat skin: Inhibition of sterol ester biosynthesis and clearing of scaly lesions in essential fatty acid deficiency. J. Lipid Res., *13*:458–467, 1972.

35. Kupiecki, F. P., Sekhar, N. C., and Weeks, J. R.: Effects of infusion of some prostaglandins in essential fatty acid–deficient and normal rats. J. Lipid Res., *9*:602–605, 1968.

36. Lamberth, E. L., Jr., and Frolich, J. C.: Essential fatty acids: Prostaglandins. *In* Meng, H. C., and Wilmore, D. W. (eds.): Fat Emulsions in Parenteral Nutrition. Chicago, American Medical Association, 1975, pp. 14–18.

37. Epstein, M., Lifschitz, M., and Rappaport, K.: Augmentation of prostaglandin production by linoleic acid in man. Clin. Sci., *63*:565–571, 1982.

38. Wahren, J., Hagenfeldt, L., and Feug, P.: Glucose and free fatty acid utilization in exercise. Israel J. Med. Sci., *11*:551–559, 1975.

39. Phinney, S. D., Bistrian, B. R., Wolfe, R. R., and Blackburn, G. L.: The human metabolic response to chronic ketosis without caloric restriction: Physical and biochemical adaptation. Metabolism, *32*:757–768, 1983.

40. Phinney, S. D., Bistrian, B. R., Evans, W. J., Gervino, E., and Blackburn, G. L.: The human metabolic response to chronic ketosis without caloric restriction: Preservation of submaximal exercise capability with reduced carbohydrate oxidation. Metabolism, *32*:769–776, 1983.

41. Moore, F. D.: Metabolic Care of the Surgical Patient. Philadelphia, W. B. Saunders Co., 1959, pp. 35–36.

42. Nördenstrom, J., Carpentier, Y. A., Askanazi, J., Robin, A. P., Elwyn, D. H., Hensle, T. W., and Kinney, J. M.: Free fatty acid mobilization and oxidation during total parenteral nutrition in trauma and infection. Ann. Surg., *198*:725–735, 1983.

43. Goodenough, R. D., and Wolfe, R. R.: Effect of total parenteral nutrition on free fatty acid metabolism in burned patients. J.P.E.N., *8*:357–360, 1984.

44. Neufeld, H. A., Pace, J. G., Kaminski, M. V., Sobocinski, P., and Crawford, D. J.: Unique effects of infections or inflammatory stress on fat metabolism in rats. J.P.E.N., *6*:511–521, 1982.

45. O'Donnell, T. F., Clowes, G. H. A., Blackburn, G. L., et al.: Proteolysis associated with a deficit of peripheral energy fuel substrates in septic man. Surgery, *80*:192–200, 1976.

46. Birkhahn, R. H., Long, C. L., Fitkin, D. L., Busnardo, A. C., Geiger, J. W., and Blakemore, W. S.: A comparison of the effects of skeletal trauma and surgery on the ketosis of starvation in man. J. Trauma, *21*:513–519, 1981.

47. Harris, R. L., Frenkel, R. A., Cottam, G. L., and Baxter, C. R.: Lipid mobilization and metabolism after thermal trauma. J. Trauma, *22*:194–198, 1982.

48. Tao, R. C., and Yoshimura, N. N.: Carnitine metabolism and its application in parenteral nutrition. J.P.E.N., *4*:469–486, 1980.

49. Mitchell, M. E.: Carnitine metabolism in human subjects. III. Metabolism in disease. Am. J. Clin. Nutr., *31*:645–659, 1978.

50. Chapoy, P. R., Angelini, C., Brown, W. J., Stiff, J. E., Shug, A. L., and Cederbaum, S. D.: Systemic carnitine deficiency—a treatable inherited lipid-storage disease presenting as Reye's syndrome. N. Engl. J. Med., *303*:1389–1394, 1980.

51. Penn, D., Schmidt-Sommerfeld, E., and Pascu, F.: Decreased tissue carnitine concentrations in newborn infants receiving total parenteral nutrition. J. Pediatr., *98*:976–978, 1981.

52. Worthley, L. I. G., Fishlock, R. C., and Snoswell, A. M.: Carnitine deficiency with hyperbilirubinemia, generalized skeletal muscle weakness and reactive hypoglycemia in a patient on long-term total parenteral nutrition: Treatment with intravenous L-carnitine. J.P.E.N., *7*:176–180, 1983.

53. Tao, R. C., Peck, G. K., and Yoshimura, N. N.: Effect of carnitine on liver fat and nitrogen balance in intravenously fed growing rats. J. Nutr., *111*:171–177, 1981.

54. Bohles, H., Segerer, H., and Fekl, W.: Improved N-retention during L-carnitine supplemented total parenteral nutrition. J.P.E.N., *8*:9–13, 1984.

55. Dirks, I.: Intravenous fat emulsion as a component of TPN. Nutr. Supp. Serv., *4*:41–49, 1984.

56. Cooke, R. J., and Burckhart, G. J.: Hypertriglyceridemia during the intravenous infusion of a safflower oil–based fat emulsion. J. Pediatr., *103*:959–961, 1983.

57. Holman, R. T., and Johnson, S. B.: Linolenic acid deficiency in man. Nutr. Rev., *40*:144–147, 1983.

58. Connelly, P. W., and Kuksis, A.: Effect of core composition and particle size of lipid emulsions on apolipoprotein transfer of plasma lipoproteins in vivo. Biochim. Biophys. Acta, *666*:80–89, 1981.

59. Scow, R. O., Hamosch, M., Blanchete-Mackie, E. J., et al.: Uptake of blood triglyceride by various tissues. Lipids, *7*:497–505, 1972.

60. Hallberg, D.: Elimination of exogenous lipids from the blood stream. Acta Physiol. Scand., *65*(Suppl. 254):5–23, 1965.

61. Flaim, L.: Unpublished data. Cutter Labs, Berkeley, Ca., 1982.

62. Patsch, J. R., Soutar, A. K., Morrisett, J. D., Gotto, A. M., Jr., and Smith, L. C.: Lipoprotein-X: A substrate for lecithin:cholesterol acyltransferase. Eur. J. Clin. Invest., *7*:213–217, 1977.

63. Stafford, W. W., Day, C. E.: Regression of atherosclerosis effected by intravenous phospholipid. Artery, *1*:106–114, 1975.

64. Maurukas, J., and Thomas, R. G.: Treatment of experimental atherosclerosis in the rabbit with L,D, alpha (dimyristoyl) lecithin. J. Lab. Clin. Med., *56*:30–37, 1960.

65. Boberg, J., and Hallberg, D.: Studies on the elimination of exogenous lipids from the blood stream. Acta Chir. Scand., *137*:749–755, 1971.

66. Somani, P., Leathem, W. D., and Barlow, A. L.: Safflower oil emulsion: Single and multiple infusions with or without added heparin in normal human volunteers. J.P.E.N., *4*:307–311, 1980.

67. Payza, A. N., Eiber, H. B., and Walters, S.: Studies with clearing factor V. Proc. Soc. Exp. Biol., 125:188–192, 1967.
68. Dhanireddy, R., Hamosh, M., Sivasubramanian, K. N., Chowdhry, P., Scanlon, J. W., and Hamosh, P.: Postheparin lipolytic activity and Intralipid clearance in very low-birth-rate infants. J. Pediatr., 98:617–622, 1981.
69. Benderly, A., Rosenthal, E., Levi, J., and Brook, G.: Effect of heparin on lipoprotein profile during parenteral fat infusions. J.P.E.N., 7:37–39, 1983.
70. Coran, A. G., Edwards, B., and Zaleska, R.: The value of heparin in the hyperalimentation of infants and children with fat emulsion. J. Pediatr. Surg., 9:725–732, 1974.
71. Brennan, M. F., and Moore, F. D.: Intravenous fat and glycerol: Effect of heparin. Surg. Forum., 24:57–58, 1973.
72. Jung, R. T., Shetty, P. S., and James, W. P. T.: Heparin, free fatty acids and an increased metabolic demand for oxygen. Postgrad. Med. J., 56:330–332, 1980.
73. Holman, R. T.: Significance of essential fatty acids in human nutrition. Lipids, 1:215–226, 1976.
74. Terry, B. E., and Wixom, R. L.: Hemolytic anemia associated with essential fatty acid deficiency in a normal man on long-term TPN. In Meng, H. C., and Wilmore, D. W. (eds.): Fat Emulsion in Parenteral Nutrition. Chicago, American Medical Association, 1975, pp. 18–24.
75. Caldwell M. D., Jonsson, H. T., and Othersen, H. B.: Essential fatty acid deficiency in an infant receiving prolonged parenteral alimentation. J. Pediatr., 81:894–898, 1972.
76. Wiese, H. F., Hansen, A. E., and Adam, D. J. D.: Essential fatty acids in infant nutrition. I. Linoleic acid requirement in terms of serum di-, tri- and tetraenoic acid levels. J. Nutr., 66:345–360, 1958.
77. Holman, R. T., Johnson, S. B., Mercuri, O., Itarte, H. J., Rodrigo, M. A., and De Tomas, M. E.: Essential fatty acid deficiency in malnourished children. Am. J. Clin. Nutr., 34:1534–1539, 1981.
78. Goodgame, J. T., Lowry, S. F., and Brennan, M. F.: Essential fatty acid deficiency in total parenteral nutrition: Time course of development and suggestions for therapy. Surgery, 84:271–277, 1978.
79. Barr, L. H., Dunn, G. D., and Brennan, M. F.: Essential fatty acid deficiency during total parenteral nutrition. Ann. Surg., 193:304–311, 1981.
80. Holman, R. T.: The ratio of trienoic:tetraenoic acids in tissue lipids as a measure of essential fatty acid requirement. J. Nutr., 70:405–410, 1960.
81. Biuins, B. A., Rapp, R. P., Record, K., Meng, H. C., and Griffen, W. O., Jr.: Parenteral safflower oil emulsion (Liposyn 10%): Safety and effectiveness in treating or preventing essential fatty acid deficiency in surgical patients. Ann. Surg., 191:307–315, 1980.
82. Apelgren, K. N., Miller, R. A., Livermore, T. A., and Rombeau, J. L.: Evaluation of a new intravenous fat emulsion. Current Surg., 36:438–440, 1979.
83. Robin, A. P., Nördenstrom, J., Askanazi, J., Elwyn, D. H., Carpentier, Y. A., and Kinney, J. M.: Plasma clearance of fat emulsion in trauma and sepsis: Use of a three-stage lipid clearance test. J.P.E.N., 4:505–510, 1980.
84. Blasier, R., Dahn, M., and Kirkpatrick, J.: Exogenous lipid clearance in sepsis. Surg. Forum, 32:116–118, 1981.

85. Lindholm, M., and Rossner, S.: Rate of elimination of the Intralipid fat emulsion from the circulation in ICU patients. Crit. Care Med., 10:740–746, 1982.
86. Park, W., Paust, H., and Schroder, H.: Lipid infusion in premature infants suffering from sepsis. J.P.E.N., 8:290–292, 1984.
87. Gallin, J. I., Kaye, D., and O'Leary, W. M.: Serum lipids in infection. N. Engl. J. Med., 281:1081–1086, 1969.
88. Infection and serum-lipids (annotation). Lancet, 2:1409–1410, 1969.
89. Lanza-Jacoby, S., Lansey, S. C., Cleary, M. P., et al.: Alterations in lipogenic enzymes and lipoprotein lipase activity during gram-negative sepsis in the rat. Arch. Surg., 117:144–147, 1982.
90. Kao, L. C., Cheng, M. H., and Warburton, D.: Triglycerides, free fatty acids, free acids/albumin molar ratio, and cholesterol levels in serum of neonates receiving long-term lipid infusions: Controlled trial of continuous and intermittent regimens. J. Pediatr., 104:429–435, 1984.
91. Forget, P. P., Fernandes, J., and Begemann, P. H.: Utilization of fat emulsion during total parenteral nutrition in children. Acta Paediatr. Scand., 64:377–384, 1975.
92. Chen, W. J.: Utilization of exogenous fat emulsion (Intralipid) in septic rats. J.P.E.N., 8:14–17, 1984.
93. Carpentier, Y. A., Nördenstrom, J., Askanazi, J., et al.: Relationship between rates of clearance and oxidation of ^{14}C-intralipid in surgical patients. Surg. Forum, 30:72–74, 1979.
94. Nordenström, J., Carpentier, Y. A., Askanazi, J., et al.: Metabolic utilization of intravenous fat emulsion during total parenteral nutrition. Ann. Surg., 196:221–231, 1982.
95. Nordenström, J., Askanazi, J., Elwyn, D. H., et al.: Nitrogen balance during total parenteral nutrition. Ann. Surg., 197:27–33, 1983.
96. Nanni, G., Siegel, J. H., Coleman, B., et al.: Increased lipid fuel dependence in the critically ill septic patient. J. Trauma, 24:14–30, 1984.
97. Das, J. B., Joshi, I. D., and Philippart, A. I.: Depression of glucose utilization by Intralipid in the post-traumatic period: An experimental study. J. Pediatr. Surg., 15:739–745, 1980.
98. Munro, H. N.: Carbohydrate and fat as factors in protein utilization and metabolism. Physiol. Rev., 31:449–488, 1951.
99. Brennan, M. F., Fitzpatrick, G. F., Cohen, K. H., et al.: Glycerol: Major contributor to the short-term protein sparing effect of fat emulsion in normal man. Ann. Surg., 182:386–394, 1975.
100. Wolfe, B. M., Culebras, J. M., Sim, A. J. W., et al.: Substrate interaction in intravenous feeding. Ann. Surg., 186:518–540, 1977.
101. Clarke, D.: The effect of fat infusion on protein metabolism. Acta Chir. Scand (Suppl.), 507:475–484, 1981.
102. Elwyn, D. H., Kinney, J. M., Gump, F. E., et al.: Some metabolic effects of fat infusions in depleted patients. Metabolism, 29:125–132, 1980.
103. Yeo, M. T., Gazzaniga, A. B., Bartlett, R. H., et al.: Total intravenous nutrition: Experience with fat emulsions and hypertonic glucose. Arch. Surg., 106:792–796, 1973.
104. Askanazi, J., Nordenström, J., Rosenbaum, S. H., et al.: Nutrition for the patient with respiratory failure: Glucose vs. fat. Anesthesiology, 54:373–377, 1981.
105. MacFie, J., Smith, R. C., and Hill, G. L.: Glucose

or fat as a nonprotein energy source? A controlled clinical trial in gastroenterological patients requiring intravenous nutrition. Gastroenterology, 80:103–107, 1981.

106. Wannemacher, R. W., Jr., Kaminski, M. V., Neufeld, H. A., et al.: Protein-sparing therapy during pneumococcal infection in rhesus monkeys. J.P.E.N., 2:507–518, 1981.

107. Wannemacher, R. W., Kaminski, M. V., Dinterman, R. E., and McCabe, T. R.: Use of lipid calories during pneumococcal sepsis in the rhesus monkey. J.P.E.N., 6:100–105, 1982.

108. Jeejeebhoy, K. N., Anderson, G. H., Nakhooda, A. F., et al.: Metabolic studies in total parenteral nutrition with lipid in man. J. Clin. Invest., 57:125–136, 1976.

109. Freund, H., Yoshimura, N., and Fischer, J. E.: Does intravenous fat spare nitrogen in the injured rat? Am. J. Surg., 140:377–383, 1980.

110. Souba, W. W., Long, J. M., III, and Dudrick, S. J.: Energy intake and stress as determinants of nitrogen excretion in rats. Surg. Forum, 29:76–77, 1978.

111. Long, J. M., III, Wilmore, D. W., Mason, A. D., et al.: Effect of carbohydrate and fat intake on nitrogen excretion during total intravenous feeding. Ann. Surg., 185:417–422, 1977.

112. Woolfson, A. M. J., Heatley, R. V., and Allison, S. P.: Insulin to inhibit protein catabolism after injury. N. Engl. J. Med., 300:14–17, 1979.

113. Chock, E., Wolfe, B. M., and Yamahata, W.: Comparison of glucose, fat emulsions, and glycerol in total parenteral nutrition. J.P.E.N., 5:578, 1981.

114. Peltier, L. F.: Fat embolism III. The toxic properties of neutral fat and free fatty acids. Surgery, 40:665–670, 1956.

115. Manning, J. B., Bach, A. W., Herman, C. M., et al.: Fat release after femur nailing in the dog. J. Trauma, 23:322–326, 1983.

116. Slotman, G. J., Machiedo, G. W., Casey, K. F., et al.: Histologic and hemodynamic effects of prostacyclin and prostaglandin E_1 following oleic acid infusion. Surgery, 92:93–100, 1982.

117. Martin, G. J., and Hueper, W. C.: Biochemical studies of atheromatous animals. Proc. Soc. Exp. Biol., 49:452–455, 1942.

118. Bagdade, J. D., and Ways, P. O.: Erythrocyte membrane lipid composition in exogenous and endogenous hypertriglyceridemia. J. Lab. Clin. Med., 75:53–60, 1970.

119. Levene, M. I., Wigglesworth, J. S., and Desai, R.: Pulmonary fat accumulation after Intralipid infusion into the preterm infant. Lancet, 2:815–818, 1980.

120. Hertel, J., Tygstrup, I., and Anderson, G. E.: Intravascular fat accumulation after Intralipid infusion in the very low-birth-weight infant. J. Pediatr., 100:975–976, 1982.

121. Dahms, B. B., and Halpin, T. C.: Pulmonary arterial lipid deposit in newborn infants receiving intravenous lipid infusion. J. Pediatr., 97:800–805, 1980.

122. Recalde, A. L., Nickerson, B. G., Vegas, M., et al.: Lipid-laden macrophages in tracheal aspirates of newborn infants receiving intravenous lipid infusions. Pediatr. Pathol., 2:25–34, 1984.

123. Hulman, G., Pearson, H. J., Frazer, I., et al.: Agglutination of Intralipid by sera of acutely ill patients. Lancet, 2:1426–1427, 1982.

124. Hulman, G., Pearson, H. J., Fraser, I., et al.: Agglutination of Intralipid by serum. Lancet, 1:985–986, 1983.

125. Allardyce, D. B.: The postmortem interval as a factor in fat embolism. Arch. Pathol., 92:248–253, 1971.

126. Pereira, G. R., Fox, W. W., Stanley, C. A., et al.: Decreased oxygenation and hyperlipidemia during intravenous fat infusions in premature infants. Pediatrics, 66:26–30, 1980.

127. Greene, H. L., Hazlett, D., and Demaree, R.: Relationship between Intralipid-induced hyperlipidemia and pulmonary function. Am. J. Clin. Nutr., 29:127–135, 1976.

128. Sundstrom, G., Zaunder, C. W., and Arborelius, M., Jr.: Decrease in pulmonary diffusing capacity during lipid infusion in healthy men. J. Appl. Physiol., 34:816–820, 1973.

129. Wolfe, B. M.: Unpublished data, 1977.

130. Wilmore, D. W., Moylan, J. A., Helmkamp, G. M., et al.: Clinical evaluation of a 10% intravenous fat emulsion for parenteral nutrition in thermally injured patients. Ann. Surg., 178:503–513, 1973.

131. Hunt, C. E., Gora, P., and Inwood, R. J.: Pulmonary effects of Intralipid: The role of Intralipids as prostaglandin precursor. Prog. Lipid Res., 20:199–204, 1981.

132. Hageman, J. R., McCulloch, K., Gora, P., et al.: Intralipid alterations in pulmonary prostaglandin metabolism and gas exchange. Crit. Care Med., 11:794–798, 1983.

133. McKeen, C. R., Brigham, K. L., Bowers, R. E., et al.: Pulmonary vascular effects of fat emulsion infusion in unanesthetized sheep. J. Clin. Invest., 61:1291–1297, 1978.

134. Eiermann, G. J., Dickey, B. F., and Thrall, R. S.: Polymorphonuclear leukocyte participation in acute oleic-acid-induced lung injury. Am. Rev. Respir. Dis., 128:845–850, 1983.

135. Jacobs, E. R., and Bone, R. C.: Mediators of septic lung injury. Med. Clin. North Am., 67:701–715, 1983.

136. Bergentz, S. E., Gelin, L. E., and Rudenstam, C. M.: Intravascular aggregation of blood cells following intravenous infusion of fat emulsions. Acta. Chir. Scand., 120:115–120, 1960.

137. Rinaldo, J. E., and Rogers, R. M.: Adult respiratory distress syndrome: Changing concepts of lung injury and repair. N. Engl. J. Med., 306:900–909, 1982.

138. Wedmore, C. V., and Williams, T. J.: Control of vascular permeability by polymorphonuclear leukocytes in inflammation. Nature, 289:646–650, 1981.

139. Brigham, K. L., and Ogletree, M. L.: Effects of prostaglandins and related compounds on lung vascular permeability. Bull. Europ. Physiopath. Resp., 17:703–722, 1981.

140. Van Deyk, K., Hempel, V., Munch, F., et al.: Influence of parenteral fat administration on the pulmonary vascular system in man. Int. Care Med., 9:73–77, 1983.

141. Jarnberg, P., Lindholm, M., and Eklund, J.: Lipid infusion in critically ill patients. Acute effects on hemodynamics and pulmonary gas exchange. Crit. Care Med., 9:27–31, 1981.

142. Wolfe, B. M., Beer, W. H., Hayashi, J. T., et al.: Experience with home parenteral nutrition. Am. J. Surg., 146:7–14, 1983.

143. Sheldon, G. F., Scott, R. P., and Sanders, R.: Hepatic dysfunction during TPN. Arch. Surg., 113:504, 1978.

144. Hirsch, R. L., McKay, D. G. Travers, R. I., and Skraly, R. K.: Hyperlipidemia, fatty liver, and bromsulfophthalein retention in rabbits injected

intravenously with bacterial endotoxins. J. Lipid Res., 5:563–568, 1964.

145. Thompson, S. W., II: Hepatic toxicity of intravenous fat emulsion. *In* Meng, H. C., and Wilmore, D. W. (eds.): Fat Emulsions in Parenteral Nutrition. Chicago, American Medical Association, 1975, pp. 90–95.

146. Jacobson, S., Ericsson, J. L. E., and Obel, A.: Histopathological and ultrastructural changes in the human liver during complete intravenous nutrition for seven months. Acta. Chir. Scand., 137:335–349, 1971.

147. Stein, T. P., Buzby, G. P., Leskiw, M. J., et al.: Protein and fat metabolism in rats during repletion with total parenteral nutrition (TPN). J. Nutr., 111:154–165, 1981.

148. Buzby, G. P., Mullen, J. L., Stein, T. P., et al.: Manipulation of TPN caloric substrate and fatty infiltration of the liver. J. Surg. Res., 31:46–54, 1981.

149. Jeejeebhoy, K. N., Langer, B., Tsallas, G., et al.: Total parenteral nutrition at home: Studies in patients surviving 4 months to 5 years. Gastroenterology, 71:943–953, 1976.

150. Salvian, A. J., and Allardyce, D. B.: Impaired bilirubin secretion during total parenteral nutrition. J. Surg. Res., 28:547–555, 1980.

151. Allardyce, D. B.: Cholestasis caused by lipid emulsions. Surg. Gynecol. Obstet., 154:641–647, 1982.

152. Lanser, M. E., and Saba, T. M.: Neutrophil-mediated lung localization of bacteria: A mechanism for pulmonary injury. Surgery, 90:473–481, 1981.

153. Koga, Y., Swanson, V. L., and Hays, D. M.: Hepatic "intravenous fat pigment" in infants and children receiving lipid emulsion. J. Pediatr. Surg., 10:641–648, 1975.

154. Jarstrand, C., Berghem, L., and Lahnborg, G.: Human granulocyte and reticuloendothelial system function during Intralipid infusion. J.P.E.N., 2:663–670, 1978.

155. Fischer, G. W., Wilson, S. R., Hunter, K. W., et al.: Diminished bacterial defense with Intralipid. Lancet, 2:819–820, 1980.

156. Spratt, M. G., and Kratzing, C. C.: Oleic acid as a depressant of reticuloendothelial activity in rats and mice. J. Reticuloendothel. Soc., 17:135–140, 1975.

157. English, D., Roloff, J. S., Lukens, J. N., et al.: Intravenous lipid emulsions and human neutrophil function. J. Pediatr., 99:913–916, 1981.

158. Nordenström, J., Jarstrand, C., and Wiernik, A.: Decreased chemotactic and random migration of leukocytes during Intralipid infusion. Am. J. Clin. Nutr., 32:2416–2422, 1979.

159. Wiernik, A., Jarstrand, C., and Julander, I.: The effect of Intralipid on mononuclear and polymorphonuclear phagocytes. Am. J. Clin. Nutr., 37:256–261, 1983.

160. Fraser, I., Neoptolemos, J., Darby, H., et al.: The effects of Intralipid and heparin on human monocyte and lymphocyte function. J.P.E.N., 8:381–384, 1984.

161. Strunk, R. C., Kunke, K. S., Kolski, G. B., et al.: Intralipid alters macrophage membrane fatty acid composition and inhibits complement (C_2) synthesis. Lipids, 18:493–500, 1983.

162. Kolski, G. B., and Strunk, R. C.: Soybean oil emulsion induces a selective and reversible inhibition of C_2 production by human mononuclear phagocytes. J. Immunol., 126:2267–2271, 1981.

163. Ladisch, S., Poplack, D. G., and Blaese, R. M.: Inhibition of human lymphoproliferation by intravenous lipid emulsion. Clin. Immuno. Immunopathol., 25:196–202, 1982.

164. Helms, R. A., Herrod, H. G., Burckart, G. J., et al.: E-rosette formation, total T-cells, and lymphocyte transformation in infants receiving intravenous safflower oil emulsion. J.P.E.N., 7:541–545, 1983.

165. Palmblad, J., Brostrom, O., Lahnborg, G., et al.: Neutrophil functions during total parenteral nutrition and Intralipid infusion. Am. J. Clin. Nutr., 35:1430–1436, 1982.

166. Siegel, I., Liu, T. L., Zaret, P., et al.: Parenteral fat emulsions and immune adherence: The effects of triglycerides on red cells and neutrophil immune adherence in vitro and in vivo. J.A.M.A., 251:1574–1579, 1984.

167. DiLuzio, N. R., and Wooles, W. R.: Depression of phagocytic activity and immune response by methyl palmitate. Am. J. Physiol., 206:939–943, 1964.

168. Mertin, J., and Hughes, D.: Specific inhibitory action of polyunsaturated fatty acids on lymphocyte transformation induced by PHA and PPD. Int. Arch. Allergy Appl. Immunol., 48:203–210, 1975.

169. Hawley, H. P., and Gordon, G. B.: The effects of long chain free fatty acids on human neutrophil function and structure. Lab. Invest., 34:216–222, 1976.

170. Rouzer, C. A., Scott, W. A., Cohn, Z. A., et al.: Mouse peritoneal macrophages release leukotriene C in response to a phagocytic stimulus. Proc. Natl. Acad. Sci., 77:4928–4932, 1980.

171. Stenson, W. F., and Parker, C. W.: Prostaglandins, macrophages, and immunity. J. Immunol., 125:1–5, 1980.

172. Cameron, J. L., Capuzzi, D. M., Zuidema, G. D., et al.: Acute pancreatitis with hyperlipidemia: The incidence of lipid abnormalities in acute pancreatitis. Ann. Surg., 177:483–489, 1973.

173. Farmer, R. G., Winkelman, E. I., Brown, H. B., et al.: Hyperlipoproteinemia and pancreatitis. Am. J. Med., 54:161–165, 1973.

174. Wang, C., Adlersberg, D., and Feldman, E. B.: Serum lipids in acute pancreatitis. Gastroenterology, 36:832–840, 1959.

175. Cameron, J. L., Capuzzi, D. M., Zuidema, G. D., et al.: Acute pancreatitis with hyperlipidemia: Evidence for a persistent defect in lipid metabolism. Am. J. Med., 56:482–487, 1974.

176. Cameron, J. L., Zuidema, G. D., and Margolis, S.: A pathogenesis for alcoholic pancreatitis. Surgery, 77:754–763, 1975.

177. Edelman, K., and Valenzuela, J. E.: Effect of intravenous lipid on human pancreatic secretion. Gastroenterology, 85:1063–1066, 1983.

178. Grundfest, S., Steiger, E., Selenkoff, P., et al.: The effect of intravenous fat emulsions in patients with pancreatic fistula. J.P.E.N., 4:27–31, 1980.

179. Buckspan, R., Woltering, E., and Waterhouse, G.: Pancreatitis induced by intravenous infusion of a fat emulsion in an alcoholic patient. South. Med. J., 77:251–252, 1984.

180. Noseworthy, J., Colodny, A. H., and Eraklis, A. J.: Pancreatitis and intravenous fat: An association in patients with inflammatory bowel disease. J. Pediat. Surg., 18:269–272, 1983.

181. Raasch, R. H., Hak, L. J., Benaim, V., et al.: Effect

of intravenous fat emulsion on experimental acute pancreatitis. J.P.E.N., 7:254–256, 1983.

182. Silberman, H., Dixon, N. P., and Eisenberg, D.: The safety and efficacy of a lipid-based system of parenteral nutrition in acute pancreatitis. Am. J. Gastroenterol., 77:494–497, 1982.

183. Taylor, R. F., and Buckner, C. D.: Fat overload from 10% soybean oil emulsion in a marrow transplant recipient. West. J. Med., 136:345–349, 1982.

184. Belin, R. P., Bivins, B. A., Jona J. Z., et al.: Fat overload with a 10% soybean oil emulsion. Arch. Surg., 111:1391–1393, 1976.

185. Marks, L. M., Patel, N., and Kurtides, E. S.: Hematologic abnormalities associated with intravenous lipid therapy. Am. J. Gastroenterol., 73:490–495, 1980.

186. McGrath, K. M., Zalcberg, J. R., Slonim, J., et al.: Intralipid induced hemolysis. Br. J. Haematol., 50:376–378, 1982.

187. Bagdade, J. D., and Ways, P. O.: Erythrocyte membrane lipid composition in exogenous and endogenous hypertriglyceridemia. J. Lab. Clin. Med., 75:53–60, 1970.

188. Greisman, S. E.: Ability of human plasma to lyse homologous erythrocytes pretreated with fatty acid. Proc. Soc. Exp. Biol. (N.Y.), 98:778–780, 1958.

189. Lipson, A. H., Pritchard, J., and Thomas, G.: Thrombocytopenia after Intralipid infusion in a neonate. Lancet, 2:1462–1463, 1974.

190. Hoak, J. C., Connor, W. E., and Warner, E. D.: Thrombogenic effects of albumin-bound fatty acids. Arch. Pathol., 81:136–139, 1966.

191. Kapp, J. P., Duckert, F., and Hartmann, G.: Platelet adhesiveness and serum lipids during and after Intralipid infusions. Nutr. Metab., 13:92–99, 1971.

192. Van Way, C. W., III, Dunn, E. L., and Hamstra, R. D.: The effect of intravenous safflower oil emulsion on the clotting mechanism. Am. Surg., 49:460–464, 1983.

193. Burnham, W. R., Heptinstall, S., Cockbill, S. R., et al.: Blood platelet behavior during infusion of an Intralipid-based intravenous feeding mixture. Postgrad. Med. J., 58:152–155, 1982.

194. Kamath, K. R., Berry, A., and Cummins, G.: Acute hypersensitivity reaction to Intralipid. N. Engl. J. Med., 304:360, 1981.

195. Jarvis, W. R., Highsmith, A. K., Allen, J. R., et al.: Polymicrobial bacteremia associated with lipid emulsion in a neonatal intensive care unit. Pediatr. Infect. Dis., 2:203–208, 1983.

196. Grimes, J. B., and Abel, R. M.: Acute hemodynamic effects of intravenous fat emulsion in dogs. J.P.E.N., 3:40–44, 1979.

197. Abel, R. M., Fisch, D., and Grossman, M. L.: Hemodynamic effects of intravenous 20% soy oil emulsion following coronary bypass surgery. J.P.E.N., 7:534–540, 1983.

198. Jarnberg, P., Lindholm, M., and Eklund, J.: Lipid infusion in critically ill patients. Crit. Care Med., 9:27–31, 1981.

199. Sternberg, A., Gruenevald, T., Deutsch, A. A., et al.: Intralipid-induced transient sinus bradycardia. N. Engl. J. Med., 304:422–423, 1981.

200. Connor, W. E., Hoak, J. C., and Warner, E. D.: Massive thrombosis produced by fatty acid infusion. J. Clin. Invest., 42:860–866, 1963.

201. Opie, L. H., Tansey, M., and Kennelly, B. M.: Proposed metabolic vicious circle in patients with large myocardial infarcts and high plasma-free fatty-acid concentrations. Lancet, 2:890–892, 1977.

201. Kurien, V. A., and Oliver, M. F.: A metabolic cause for arrhythmias during acute myocardial hypoxia. Lancet, 1:813–815, 1970.

202. Kurien, V. A., and Oliver, M. F.: A metabolic cause for arrhythmias during acute myocardial hypoxia. Lancet, 1:813–815, 1970.

203. Most, A. S., Capone, R. J., and Mastrofrancesco, P. A.: Free fatty acids and arrhythmias following acute coronary artery occlusion in pigs. Cardiovasc. Res., 10:198–205, 1976.

204. Lantigua, R. A., Amatruda, J. M., Biddle, T. L., et al.: Cardiac arrhythmias associated with a liquid protein diet for the treatment of obesity. N. Engl. J. Med., 303:735–738, 1980.

205. Fischer, J. E.: Amino acids in hepatic coma. Dig. Dis. Sci., 27:97–102, 1982.

206. Thiessen, H., Jacobsen, J., and Brodersen, R.: Displacement of albumin-bound bilirubin by fatty acids. Acta Paediatr. Scand., 61:285–288, 1972.

207. Andrew, G., Chan, G., and Schiff, D.: Lipid metabolism in the neonate. II. The effect of Intralipid on bilirubin binding in vitro and in vivo. J. Pediatr., 88:279–284, 1976.

208. Schalch, D. S., and Kipnis, D. M.: Abnormalities in carbohydrate tolerance associated with elevated plasma nonesterified fatty acids. J. Clin. Invest., 44:2010–2020, 1965.

209. Wretlind, A.: Development of fat emulsions. J.P.E.N., 5:230–235, 1981.

210. Hansen, L. M., Hardie, W. R., and Hidalgo, J.: Fat emulsion for intravenous administration. Ann. Surg., 184:80–88, 1976.

211. Fujiwara, T., Kawarasaki, H., and Fokalsrud, E. W.: Reduction of postinfusion venous endothelial injury with Intralipid. Surg. Gynecol. Obstet., 158:57–65, 1984.

CHAPTER 5

Protein Metabolism and Parenteral Nutrition

T. P. STEIN, Ph.D.

Deficiencies in protein metabolism are extremely common in many life-threatening illnesses. The aim of nutritional support is to preserve the body's protein metabolism or, when necessary, to restore it to its premorbid state by providing the optimal nutrition. The reason for the emphasis on protein metabolism is that proteins are the "machinery" of the body. It is a dynamic system; more than 300 gm of new protein are made every day (Fig. 5–1). If the ability to make protein is compromised by either malnutrition or disease, function is usually correspondingly impacted. Malnourished patients do not heal as well after surgery and are more susceptible to infection, and as a consequence, their hospitalization is prolonged.[112, 113, 160]

It is therefore important to assess the amount and functional capacity for a patient. Unfortunately, there is no simple way of quantitatively assessing a patient's protein status. "High-tech" methods such as neutron activation analysis and nuclear magnetic resonance may be usable as research methods, but they are too cumbersome and expensive for routine use.[35] Nutritional assessment, pa-

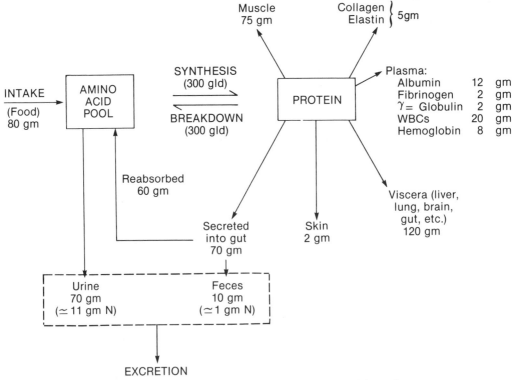

Figure 5–1. Estimated daily protein synthesis by a 70-kg male.

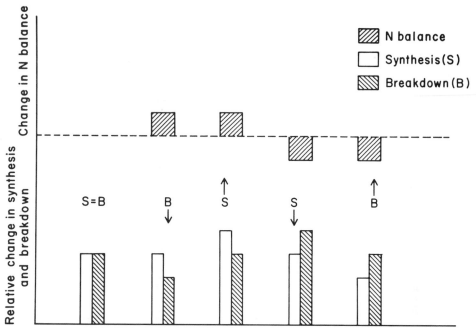

Figure 5–2. The relationship between protein synthesis, protein breakdown, and nitrogen balance.

tient history, and evidence of recent changes in weight (see Chapter 10) give a satisfactory qualitative estimate of a patient's overall protein status. Clinical assessment is the only realistic way of assessing a patient's protein status at present.

The much maligned, classic nitrogen balance technique is still the best method for detecting sudden changes. In assessing nitrogen losses, it is important to include losses from malabsorption and fistulas as well as feces and urine. Any change from a neutral or positive total nitrogen balance to a negative nitrogen balance is indicative of a problem in protein metabolism and cannot be allowed to continue for more than a few days. The body has no significant quantity of "reserve proteins."

As well as being a very important objective for designing optimal TPN mixtures, measurements of parameters related to protein metabolism provide good, easily measurable assays of how (relatively) good a TPN formulation is. Examples of such parameters are nitrogen balance, protein synthesis, and protein breakdown. Nitrogen balance is a particularly useful "endpoint."

The more compromised the patient, the more important it is to optimize the TPN regimen, because the less tolerance there is to suboptimal mixtures. However, a change to positive balance can occur via either an increase in protein synthesis or a decrease in

protein breakdown, so the mechanism cannot be inferred unless synthesis or breakdown is also measured (Fig. 5–2).

Factors that can be varied to improve the utilization of TPN include the route and timing of the TPN as well as the actual composition of the TPN mixture (Table 5–1). The improvements attributable to any one factor are not likely to be very great; they may be as little as ten per cent. A ten per cent improvement in the tolerance to nutrition of

Table 5–1. PARAMETERS THAT CAN BE VARIED TO IMPROVE THE EFFICIENCY OF TPN

Chemical parameters	Calorie source
	Amount of calories
	Amount of amino acids
	Amino acid pattern
	Cal:N ratio
Mechanical parameters	Route
	Central
	Portal
	Peripheral
	Intragastric
	Jejunal
	Timing
	Continuous
	Cyclic
Utilization parameters	Insulin level
	Respiratory quotient (RQ)
	Glucose tolerance
	Fat tolerance

a severely compromised patient is likely, however, to be important. Consider a patient with enough metabolic capacity to meet 70 per cent of the body's need from a given TPN solution. Giving more TPN will not improve matters, because the capacity to process that particular mixture has already been exceeded; but a series of additive 10 per cent improvements in TPN utilization could well increase the liver's effective capacity to a point where it could meet the body's needs. Much research is currently being directed toward this goal.

GENERAL PRINCIPLES

To some extent, the more calories given, the better the nitrogen retention. However, retention also depends on the calorie/nitrogen ratio. This makes for a highly complex situation that is compounded by human heterogeneity and disease-related effects. Making matters a little simpler, though, is the fact that evolution has equipped humankind with an ability to accommodate to a wide range of diets. For metabolically healthy individuals, all that is required, therefore, is a rough estimate. However, the more metabolically compromised the patient, the narrower the tolerance range and, unfortunately, the harder it becomes to determine this range accurately.

The options for formulating TPN solutions are in theory infinite but in practice rather limited. There are certain boundary conditions, which can be summarized as follows.

First, the RDA for amino acids is about 0.8 gm/kg/day of a balanced amino acid mixture, so less should not be given (see *Clinical Nutrition*, Vol. I, Chapter 10). The upper limit is reached in severely burned patients, in whom it has been suggested that protein requirements can be as high as 2.5 gm/kg/day of nitrogen for adults and 4.8 gm/kg/day of amino acids for children.[3] A conservative approach in giving amino acids to critically ill patients is generally advisable because excess amino acids are toxic.[120]

Second, the results of enteral experiments, which also apply equally to TPN, have shown that the optimal calorie:N ratio is between 100 and 225:1, with 150 ± 25 being an acceptable median.[50]

Third, because of the limited solubility of some of the amino acids, the amount of fluid given can be a limiting factor. Final TPN amino acid concentrations of greater than 60 gm/L ($\approx$10 gm N) are difficult to formulate if they are to contain adequate calories. Moreover, too much fluid cannot be given. Three liters per day places an upper limit on amino acids of about 180 gm/day ($\approx$ 30 gm/day N).[53]

Fourth, it has not been shown that a depleted or stressed patient is any better off in a positive nitrogen balance of +6 than in a balance of +3. The important objective is to make sure the patient is not in negative nitrogen balance.

Source of Calories

The question of which is the best calorie source—glucose, glucose plus fat, or fat—for protein metabolism has been a subject of much interest in recent years. The issues are not whether the nonprotein calories should be given exclusively as fat or carbohydrate, but rather which one—if either—should be the dominant calorie source, and whether clinical status should have any influence on the choice of calorie source.

There are cogent arguments in favor of giving most of the calories as glucose (with enough fat to prevent essential fatty acid deficiency) or as fat. The arguments in favor of glucose are: (1) it is much cheaper than a fat emulsion; (2) neonates appear not to tolerate well a high proportion of calories as fat; (3) allergic reactions to the fat emulsion can occur; at the Graduate Hospital in Philadelphia, the frequency was about one per cent in a sample of more than 800 patients (author's unpublished observations); (4) carbohydrates are the normal major calorie source; and (5) the effect of very high dosages of synthetic chylomicrons on the blood vessels is not known. Conceivably, this last factor could be a potentially serious problem for patients on long-term TPN at home, because the high lipid TPN doses may predispose them to thrombosis and atherosclerosis even more than would high-fat enteral diets.

The arguments in favor of giving most calories as fat are: (1) it can be given via a peripheral vein because of its lower osmolarity; (2) it does not promote insulin release; (3) it does not lead to essential fatty acid deficiency; (4) it is a means of giving calories to glucose-intolerant patients; and (5) there appears to be a preference for at least some of the calories to be as fat in stressed states.

Irrespective of the route of administration, substituting lipid for carbohydrate leads to a temporary (three to four days) increase in the urinary N excretion.[114] Jeejeebhoy and colleagues[77] found, in a study of patients with adequate hepatic functional capacity, that glucose and fat were, after an initial adjustment period, equally effective in promoting positive nitrogen balance. Wolfe and associates[162, 163] also found glucose and fat to be equivalent in healthy subjects, as did Bark and co-workers[11] and Dworkin and colleagues[48] in postoperative patients. In contrast, others have reported that in (stressed) injured humans and rats, glucose calories are significantly more effective than fat calories in promoting nitrogen anabolism (Fig. 5–3).[4, 60, 92, 136, 149]

The reason for the discrepant results is that parenteral fat emulsions are particularly prone to accumulate in the liver, leading to the paradoxical situation of depletion of the endogenous fat stores and simultaneous accumulation of infused fat in the liver (Fig. 5–4). If some of the infused fat is deposited in the liver, it is not available for oxidation by the other tissues in the body. The apparent "decreased effectiveness" of fat calories in stressed patients is due to the tendency of such patients to accumulate fat in the liver secondary to decreased liver functional capacity. Hence, the apparent greater effectiveness of the use of exogenous glucose in stressed states.[149] This problem may be unique to current fat emulsions.

Although fat may be more prone to become deposited in the liver, excess glucose can also lead to hepatomegaly.[24, 107, 142] Indeed, hepatomegaly is the more common clinical finding because glucose is usually the major parenteral calorie source. (The non–protein-related aspects of hepatic lipid metabolism during TPN are discussed in Chapter 4.) Usually, however, glucose or fat is not given alone. A considerable amount of animal and human experimental data have shown that glucose plus fat is better than either glucose or fat alone. There does seem to be a consensus, based on a variety of parameters, that the optimal calorie source is a mixture of glucose plus fat, but the precise ratio is not known.[26, 50, 96, 117, 144, 157]

Animal experiments suggest that to exceed 50 per cent fat is to increase the likelihood of fat deposition from accumulation of the infused lipid in the liver.[26, 144] In rats, under isocaloric conditions, fat is more prone to become deposited in the liver with Intralipid than with glucose.[144] The incidence of fat deposition in the liver is minimized by giving a mixed calorie regimen, with about a third of the calories from fat (Fig. 5–5).[26] The reason that a mixed calorie source is better than a single calorie source is that the use of mixed calorie sources decreases the possibility of fat deposition in the liver due to the

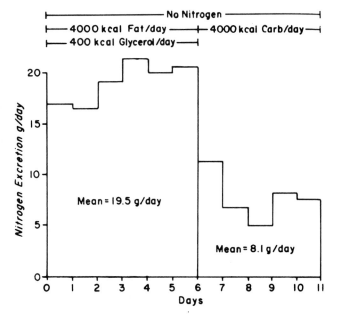

Figure 5–3. Difference in N retention between isocaloric glucose and fat in a severely stressed (burned) patient. (*From* Long, J. M., Wilmore, D. W., Mason, A. D., and Pruit, B. A., Jr.: Effect of carbohydrate and fat on nitrogen excretion during total intravenous feedings. Ann. Surg., *185*:417–421, 1977, with permission.)

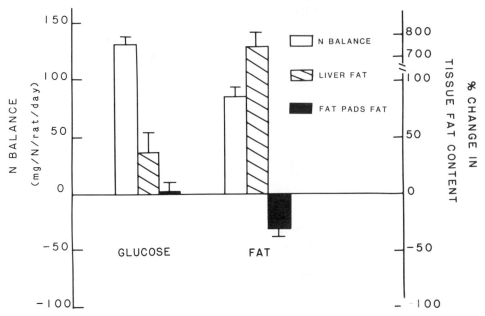

Figure 5–4. Mechanism for the apparent "decreased caloric effectiveness" of parenteral fat calories. Some of the infused fat is retained in the liver and is therefore not available for use by other tissues. (*From* Stein, T. P., Presti, M. E., Leskiw, M. J., Torosian, M. H., Settle, R. G., Buzby, G. P., and Schuster, M. D.: Comparison of glucose, LCT and LCT plus MCT as calorie sources in parenterally nourished rats. Am. J. Physiol., *246*:E277–E287, 1984, with permission.)

overloading of the metabolic pathways for handling either glucose or fat. Not unexpectedly, a mixed calorie source is closer to the composition of a normal diet than either an all-glucose or all-fat source.

The problem of calorie source becomes more complicated for the stressed patient. In

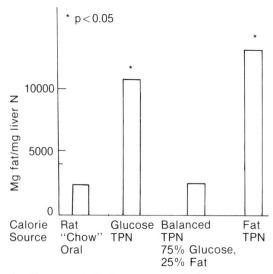

Figure 5–5. Both an excess of glucose and fat calories lead to extensive fat accumulation in the liver. In contrast, a balanced mixture given either orally or parenterally does not cause hepatomegaly. (*From* Stein, T. P., Buzby, G. P., Leskiw, M. J., Giandominico, A. L., and Muller, J. L.: Protein and fat metabolism in rats during repletion with parenteral nutrition (TPN). J. 'Nutr., *111*:154–167, 1981.)

formulating TPN regimens for severely stressed patients, optimizing nitrogen retention becomes one of many factors to consider; other factors include glucose tolerance, renal insufficiency, liver status, and fluid intolerance. Nordenstrom and associates[117] suggested that for some severely septic or injured patients, especially those who are glucose intolerant, up to 75 per cent of the nonprotein calories of a *moderate energy* intake can be given as fat. Because of the potential for fat accumulation in the liver, care should be taken that energy intake is not excessive.

There appears to be a shift in the preferred substrate from glucose to endogenous fat in the septic state. Fat metabolism seems to be very different in the septic state. Energy expenditure studies by Askanazi and colleagues[6] showed that fat is well oxidized by septic patients. A follow-up study by Stoner and associates[153] showed that as the severity of the sepsis increased, so did the amount of fat oxidized, whereas the glucose oxidative capacity decreased.

In acutely septic rats, nitrogen retention actually decreased with parenteral glucose. If some fat was added to the infusate, nitrogen retention continued to increase (Fig. 5–6). In the rats given the fat-free parenteral regimen, there was extensive mobilization of endogenous fat. In control, nonseptic rats, there was, as expected, no mobilization of endogenous fat when a high glucose dosage

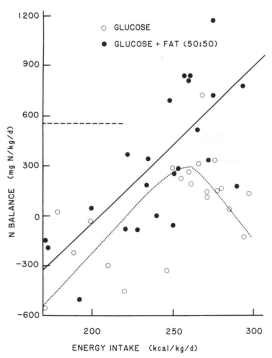

Figure 5–6. Nitrogen retention as a function of non-protein calorie source in septic rats given either glucose (○) or a 50:50 mixture of glucose plus LCT (●) as their non-protein calorie source. There is an unknown methodologic error in the determination of N balance in parenterally fed rats, which leads to the overestimation of N retention by about 550 mg N/kg/day. A true positive N balance, which is an apparent N balance > 550 mg N/kg/d, is indicated by the broken line at 550 mg N on the Y axis. (*Modified from* Stein, T. P., Ang, S. D., Schluter, M. D., Leskiw, M. J., and Nusbaum, M.: Whole body protein turnover in metabolically stressed patients with cancer as measured with [15N] glycine. Biochem. Med., 30:59–77, 1983.)

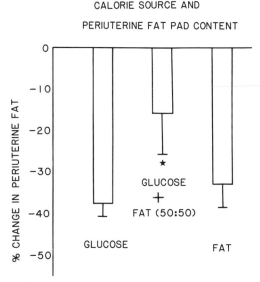

Figure 5–7. Percentage change in lipid content of the periuterine fat pads in the rats given the low-calorie regimen (series II). Glucose plus LCT has a lipid sparing effect. * p < 0.05 vs. either glucose or fat. (*Adapted from* Stein, T. P., Ang, S. D., Schluter, M. D., Leskiw, M. J., and Nusbaum, M.: Whole-body protein turnover in metabolically stressed patients with cancer as measured with [15N] glycine. Biochem. Med., 30:59–77, 1983.)

was given. Replacing some of the glucose with fat spared endogenous fat and promoted nitrogen retention in septic rats (Fig. 5–7).[151]

All of these findings indicate that there is a demand for a substantial proportion of the calories as fat in the septic state if valuable body protein is to be conserved. What is the mechanism, and why the preference for fat?

The differences between the septic (stressed) and nonseptic (unstressed) states may be related to differences in the hormonal milieu. Many studies have shown that catecholamine levels are elevated in sepsis, and catecholamines stimulate lipid mobilization. A high plasma glucose concentration and the associated elevated insulin level inhibit peripheral lipid mobilization in the unstressed state. In the septic state, the effect of glucose on the inhibition of lipid mobilization is negated because the catecholamines stimulate

lipolysis and the tissues become insulin resistant.

The simplest explanation is teleologic. A severely ill patient or animal is unable to forage for food. Unless it can shift its energy metabolism to using endogenous fat, it will starve, because nearly all of a mammal's energy reserves are fat. The utilization of endogenous fat as the fuel source is associated with protein and energy sparing. When fat is the predominant calorie source, protein turnover proceeds at a lower rate in unstressed humans and rats but not in septic rats because of the need to be able to make maximal use of the body's protein systems to combat the sepsis.[151]

Adaptation to a lipid-based metabolism requires a decrease in glucose utilization, which in the normal (nonparenterally fed) state is accomplished initially by the utilization of glycogen and gluconeogenesis from amino acids with progressively increasing reliance on endogenous fat. As fat utilization increases, gluconeogenesis decreases, and protein conservation occurs. Gluconeogenesis is subject to product inhibition; hence, as glucose utilization decreases, glucose accumulates and gluconeogenesis decreases.

The mechanism is similar to that operating in the response to starvation, except that the hormones involved are different. In starvation, insulin drops and glucagon increases, stimulating lipid mobilization. In severe stress, the catecholamines and corticosteroids are dominant; there is peripheral insulin resistance, and catecholamine-stimulated lipolysis occurs. The insulin resistance decreases glucose uptake. In addition, fatty acids, or some metabolite derived from fatty acids, inhibits glucose utilization, which in turn decreases gluconeogenesis and spares protein. Thus, giving hypercaloric glucose at a time when the animal's natural response is to minimize glucose utilization is not likely to result in optimal glucose utilization.[151]

In summary, if protein metabolism (as determined by N retention) is used as the criteria, parenteral glucose and parenteral fat are not always equally effective as calorie sources. For nonstressed states, it is unlikely that either an all-fat or an all-glucose regimen will be given, and giving a mixture ($\approx$ 70 per cent glucose, $\approx$ 30 per cent fat) avoids problems. For the septic state, however, and possibly other severely stressed states, the optimal ratio of glucose to fat is not known. In view of the findings of Stoner and colleagues,[153] the optimal ratio could well be one in which fat is the dominant calorie source.

Quantity and Quality of Amino Acids

As already stated, the effectiveness of amino acid utilization depends on the amount of calories given as well as the amino acid pattern. In general, the same rules apply as for amino acids given enterally. If an amino acid is essential for enteral feedings, it is equally essential for parenteral feedings. Table 5–2 lists the essential and nonessential amino acids.

Because egg protein has the highest biologic availability coefficient, most general-purpose amino acid formulations have used egg protein composition as a frame of reference.[5] In formulating "balanced" amino acid solutions, manufacturers of parenteral solutions have also had to consider some nonphysiologic factors, such as cost, poor solubility of some of the amino acids, stability factors, and compatibility with lipid emulsions. Within these constraints is a myriad of possible amino acid combinations. Some of the early solutions were very high ($\approx$ 35 per cent) in the cheapest amino acid, glycine. They were not as well utilized as better-balanced solutions.[158] There are no "super

Table 5–2. ESSENTIAL, SEMI-ESSENTIAL, AND NONESSENTIAL AMINO ACIDS IN PARENTERAL NUTRITION

Essential amino acids	Leucine
	Isoleucine
	Valine
	Lysine
	Threonine
	Methionine
	Phenylalanine
	Tryptophan
	Histidine
Semi-essential amino acids	Cystine
	Tyrosine
Nonessential amino acids	Glycine
	Arginine
	Proline
	Glutamic acid
	Aspartic acid
	Serine
	Alanine

high" glycine solutions on the market at present, although most amino acid solutions available in the United States still contain a disproportionately larger amount of glycine than either egg or milk protein. Recent developments aimed at improving amino acid formulations have concentrated mainly on the essential amino acids.

Not all commercially available solutions are equal in ability to promote net nitrogen retention. As is to be expected, deficiencies in the essential amino acids such as methionine have a marked negative impact on N retention.[79, 80] The nonessential amino acids are also important, however. For example, Roche and co-workers[126] compared Azonutril, Totamine, and Vamine, and found N retention to be best with Vamine (Fig. 5–8; Table 5–3). The three solutions had about the same proportions of the essential amino acids and about equal amounts of the branched-chain amino acids, but they differed in the nonessential amino acids. The researchers suggested that the high arginine content in Azonutril (16 per cent) may have been deleterious because arginine interferes with lysine metabolism, as reported by Wretlind.[168] However, too little arginine is also deleterious, because in its absence, immune function is compromised.[9] Vamine, on the other hand, has much more glutamate.

Whether these (small) differences in N balance among the various formulations available are of any clinical significance is not clear. Perhaps they are not, but it would

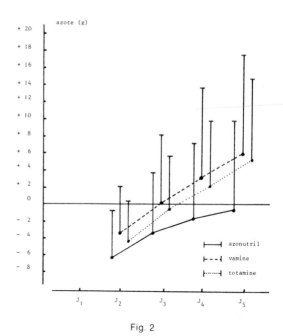

Fig. 2

Bilans azotés cumulés
(my ± SEM)

Figure 5–8. Differences in cumulative N retention in postoperative patients given Vamine, Azonutril and Totamine. (*From* Roche, A., Fabre, P., Crozat, R. P., Desplantez, J., and Sabathie, M.: Etude comparative de trois solutions d'acides amines de synthèse: Azonutril 25, Totamine concentré glucidique et Vamine en réanimation digestive post-opèratoire. A propos de 120 malades. Ann. Anesth. Franc., *4*:331–338, 1981, with permission.)

Table 5–3. AMINO ACID COMPOSITION OF AZONUTRIL, TOTAMINE, AND VAMINE*

COMPOSITION	AZONUTRIL (per 500 ml)	TOTAMINE (per 1000 ml)	VAMINE (per 1000 ml)
Total N (gm)	12.5	12.4	9.4
Essential amino acids			
L-Isoleucine	2.55	5.57	3.90
L-Leucine	6.95	8.00	5.25
L-Lysine	9.75	4.80	3.85
L-Methionine	4.70	3.00	1.90
L-Phenylalanine	6.25	6.67	5.45
L-Threonine	2.50	2.93	3.00
L-Tryptophan	1.30	1.47	1.00
L-Valine	6.25	6.05	4.25
Semi-essential amino acids			
L-Arginine	12.50	8.00	3.30
L-Histidine	2.50	2.50	2.40
Nonessential amino acids			
L-Alanine	4.75	5.33	3.00
L-Aspartic acid	2.00	2.67	4.05
L-Cysteine	0.75	1.33	1.40
L-Glutamic acid	2.50	2.67	9.00
Glycine	4.50	9.33	2.10
L-Ornithine	1.70	2.38	
L-Proline	4.00	5.33	0
L-Serine	0.65	2.67	3.10
L-Tyrosine	0.13	0.40	7.50
L-Citrulline	1.50	0	0.50
			0
Total essential amino acids	40.25	39.42	28.60
Total amino acids	77.25	82.00	64.95

*In the comparative study by Roche and co-workers,[126] isonitrogenous amounts were given to each patient (see also Fig. 5–7). Quantities are in grams.

seem that in situations in which other factors are equal, it would be better to use the formulation that gives the best N retention.

The status of arginine is particularly interesting. In rodents, arginine has both metabolic and immune effects. The role of arginine as a stimulant of thymic function appears to be independent of its nutritional role. This independence is important, because anything that will facilitate the immune state in a depleted patient is likely to be of benefit.[10] Whether supplemental arginine can improve N retention in stressed rats is not clear; two studies[125, 131] report that it does and one[10] that it does not. Whether or not there is a slight improvement in N retention is probably not as important as the potential for immunologic improvement.[10]

Unfortunately for the customer, there are few good comparative studies in humans of the different manufacturers' products available. Part of the reluctance of investigators to perform such studies is no doubt due to the continual reformulation of the solutions. A useful approach for qualitatively comparing amino acid formulations is that developed by Yoshimura of McGaw Laboratories (N. Yoshimura, personal communication). It involves comparison against a high-quality reference protein (egg white). The parameters used are as follows:

1. *A/E Ratio.* The A/E ratio compares the amount of an essential amino acid present in the test mixture (A) with the amount present in the reference mixture (egg protein [E]). The less deviation, the better the formulation.

2. *Essential amino acid content.* Egg protein has a relatively high proportion (43.4 per cent) of essential amino acids, and a good amino acid solution should have a similar proportion.

3. *Amino acid score.* The FAO/WHO reference protein is used as the standard. The ratio sample/standard is computed for each amino acid and multiplied by 100, and the lowest percentage is taken as the score. A protein can be considered poor if the lowest score for an essential amino acid is below about 85.

4. *Branched-chain amino acid content.* The percentage of amino acids in the test mixture is compared with that in egg protein. As is discussed in more detail later in this chapter and in Chapter 35, numerous studies have shown that the branched-chain amino acids improve N retention and stimulate protein synthesis. Thus, there is no reason to give

less than is present in egg protein, and on some occasions there may be advantages to giving more.

5. *Completeness of the amino acid pattern.* Not all amino acid solutions contain all of the amino acids present in egg protein. Specifically, some have less, or a poorer distribution, of the nonessential amino acids. The role of the nonessential amino acids in TPN mixtures has not been extensively investigated. Enteral studies indicate that a balanced mixture is better than assuming that all nonessential amino acids are equal and then giving the two cheapest ones (alanine and glycine) as "fillers." What is unknown is whether the omission of one or two or the use of "fillers" is of any consequence.

6. *E/T ratio.* The ratio of essential amino acids (E) to total amino acid N (T) in the mixture to that in egg protein is another useful point of comparison.

Table 5–4 summarizes the amino acid composition of 4 of the most popular solutions available in North America, gives the composition of egg protein for comparison, and supplies some of the ratios described previously. Not included in Table 5–4 are most of the many different solutions available in Europe and Japan, because there are so many and their formulae are frequently being changed; nevertheless, the same principles of use apply. Table 5–5 lists some "special factors" that should be considered in evaluating mixtures.

Is there a need for disease-specific amino acid formulations? Decades of patient research in the first half of this century have established that eight amino acids are essential and the rest are nonessential for healthy adults and children (see Table 5–2). By *nonessential* is meant that they can be synthesized *in vivo* at a satisfactory rate to meet demand. Maintenance of amino acid homeostasis is a highly complicated sum of many metabolic pathways. In the diseased, the neonate, the elderly, and other individuals whose metabolism is not as complete as that of a typical healthy young adult, some of these processes may become limiting. Synthetic capacity for a nonessential amino acid may become inadequate because of disease, malnutrition, or increased demand, making a normally nonessential amino acid into an essential one. An example of a marginal essential amino acid is histidine.[13, 83]

Most likely, humankind is heterogeneous with respect to nonessential amino acid biosynthesis, and the threshold for in-

Table 5–4. AMINO ACID COMPOSITIONS OF SOLUTIONS AVAILABLE IN NORTH AMERICA AND COMPARISON WITH HIGH-QUALITY REFERENCE (HENS' EGG PROTEIN)

COMPOSITION	EGG PROTEIN %W/W	VAMINE %W/W	AMINOSYN %W/W	FREAMINE %W/W	TRAVENOL %W/W
Essential amino acids					
L-Isoleucine	6.414	5.575	7.313	7.157	4.775
L-Leucine	8.552	7.505	9.464	9.340	6.187
L-Lysine	6.220	5.504	7.313	7.521	5.787
L-Methionine	3.013	2.716	4.015	5.459	5.787
L-Phenylalanine	5.637	7.791	4.445	5.822	6.187
L-Tryptophan	1.555	1.430	1.721	1.577	1.788
L-Threonine	4.956	4.289	5.305	4.124	4.187
L-Valine	7.094	6.076	8.030	6.793	4.587
Semi-essential amino acids					
L-Arginine	6.317	4.718	9.894	9.825	10.351
L-Histidine	2.332	3.431	3.011	2.911	4.375
Nonessential amino acids					
L-Alanine	7.191	4.289	12.905	7.278	20.701
L-Proline	4.082	11.580	8.747	11.524	4.187
Glycine	3.401	3.002	12.905	14.435	20.701
L-Serine	8.066	10.722	4.302	6.065	.000
L-Tyrosine	4.082	.715	.631	.000	.400
L-Glutamic acid	11.953	12.866	.000	.000	.000
L-Aspartic acid	7.000	5.790	.000	.000	.000
L-Cysteine	2.332	2.001	.000	.170	.000
E/T	3.19	3.04	3.00	3.04	2.34
% Essential AA W/W	43.44	40.89	47.61	47.49	39.28
% Branched-chain AA W/W	22.06	19.16	24.81	23.29	15.55

(Data courtesy of Dr. N. Yoshimura, McGaw Laboratories, Inc., Glendale, California.)

Table 5–5. "SPECIAL FACTORS" TO BE CONSIDERED IN EVALUATING AMINO ACID SOLUTIONS FOR GENERAL USE

AMINO ACID COMPONENTS	COMMENT
Methionine	Toxic in some patients.
Phenylalanine	Toxic in some patients (hepatic encephalopathy).
Too little branched-chain amino acid content	May become limiting in stress.
Glutamic/aspartic acid	Infusion alone can cause nausea, flushing. Omission can lead to excessive use of filler amino acids.
Tyrosine	Very poor solubility. Can be made from phenylalanine *in vivo*.
Arginine	Needed for immunocompetence, prevention of hyperammonemia. Arginine N poorly retained.
Alanine	A cheap filler?
Glycine	A cheap filler? Excess may cause hyperammonemia. If too little, may become limiting.
Cysteine	Important in pediatric nutrition.

sufficient synthetic capacity very likely varies markedly from person to person.[14] An increased demand could well lead to a need for more of a nonessential amino acid than there is synthetic capacity for; the particular amino acid would then no longer be nonessential. A corollary of this change is that the degradative capacity for an essential amino acid may be reduced in metabolically compromised patients. Therefore less of the amino acid should be given in order to prevent a toxic build-up. This aspect has been explored by Fischer[52] in his studies on hepatic encephalopathy (see Chapter 35).

Should different combinations or amounts of amino acids therefore be given for different disease and stress states? The rationale for devising disease-targeted formulations depends on: (1) knowing what the metabolic differences from normal are at a biochemical level; (2) deciding what a desirable sequence of events would be; and (3) designing an amino acid mixture to favor such a course.

The areas where this approach has been tried are trauma/sepsis, renal failure, and liver failure. The results are discussed in the appropriate chapters in this text. It is worth pointing out, however, that any successes with solutions targeted at renal or hepatic failure have not (yet) correlated with detectable changes in protein metabolism or N retention.[110] Rather, their beneficial effects are more in the direction of preventing toxic metabolites of amino acids from accumulating and thereby interfering with other body functions.[1, 83]

These specific formulations are, therefore, discussed in detail in the appropriate chapters. From the viewpoint of protein metabolism, the subject matter of this chapter, only the "trauma" solutions have made any claims to improve protein synthesis or breakdown or nitrogen retention and are therefore discussed later in this chapter as well as in Chapter 27.

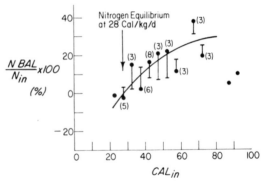

Figure 5–9. Apparently biphasic response of N retention to calorie dosage in depleted patients. The first phase represents replacement of lost protein. The second phase most probably represents synthesis of proteins involved in storage and vascularization of the newly synthesized fat resulting from the excess of calories. (*From* Peters, C., and Fischer, J. E.: Studies on calorie to nitrogen ratio for total parenteral nutrition. Surg. Gynecol. Obstet., *151*:1–8, 1980, by permission of Surgery Gynecology & Obstetrics.)

The Calorie:Nitrogen Ratio

Protein synthesis is an energy-intensive process. If energy is limited, protein synthesis is impaired. The question is, How much energy should be given to permit the optimal use of a balanced amino acid mixture? The intake of nutrients providing nonprotein energy sources increases the degree of nitrogen retention up to a certain point. Most studies have concluded that there is an optimal ratio somewhere between 100 and 200 nonprotein calories per gram of nitrogen, with 135 to 185 being considered best for unstressed patients and a slightly lower ratio (130 cal/gm N) for severely stressed states.[21, 47, 50, 122, 135] The experimental data in this area are not extensive, and there is much scatter in the data. Fortunately, the human organism is quite adaptable, so a precise match to the ideal ratio is not necessary. If a slight excess is given, it can be disposed of via brown adipose tissue thermogenesis.

Higher calories/nitrogen (cal:N) ratios improve N retention. As the calorie intake is increased from a very low level, nitrogen balances improve rapidly, suggesting a high avidity for N, especially in malnourished patients.[21, 50, 122, 135] As the caloric input goes beyond a certain point, however, it becomes progressively harder to obtain substantial increases in N retention, although there is still some increase. The response is best described as biphasic (Fig. 5–9).

Much interest has been focused on just what and where this increased N retention is. There is no doubt that the steep part of

the curve reflects the repletion of body protein, but the less steep curve found at the higher calorie intakes is more controversial. Most likely it represents the ancillary protein need to store the newly synthesized fat and supply it with vasculature. This is not the type of protein that is needed, and some of the fat tends to accumulate in the wrong place, such as the liver.

Increased N retention with higher cal:N ratios is found at all energy levels. Figure 5–10 illustrates the relationship between caloric intake and N balance at different amino acid dosages in depleted and stressed patients. There are two important conclusions to be drawn from it. First, the more calories given, the more N retained. The steeply ascending part of the curve most likely represents repletion of lean body mass; the flatter parts at high calorie-to-protein ratios reflect mostly the proteins necessary to store and provide a vasculature structure for the newly synthesized fat. Second, stressed patients have a greater need for amino acids than nonstressed patients. Notice that at the lower cal:N ratios, N retention is worse in stressed patients, but as N intake is increased, N retention becomes better. The implication is that without adequate energy, amino acids cannot be effectively utilized.

Does Giving More TPN Increase Protein Synthesis Proportionately?

It is intuitively obvious that protein synthesis and protein accretion cannot proceed optimally if too little TPN is given, but the

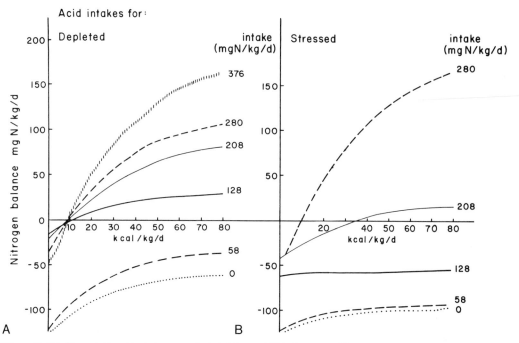

Figure 5–10. The relationship between caloric intake and N balance at different amino acid dosages for depleted *(A)* and stressed *(B)* patients. (*Modified from* Bozetti, F.: Parenteral nutrition in surgical patients. Surg. Gynecol. Obstet., *142*:16–25, 1976; by permission of Surgery, Gynecology & Obstetrics; data from Elwyn,[50] Messing and Bernier,[105] Peters and Fischer,[122] and Smith et al.[133])

converse, whether more is better, is not so apparent. For example, is there a ceiling beyond which "pumping in" more of a balanced TPN mix no longer causes a progressive increase in protein anabolism?

Stein and Ang[149] studied eight malnourished patients who required TPN because of inflammatory bowel disease or a gastrointestinal malignancy. As the TPN rate increased, protein synthesis and accretion increased up to a point corresponding to about the patients' calculated energy requirements and then "plateaued out" (Fig. 5–11). Thus, overaggressive TPN does not lead to further improvement in protein balance, probably because the necessary metabolic pathways become saturated. The plateau phenomenon occurred at about the calorie level corresponding to the calculated TPN dosage.

There are two interrelated reasons for this saturation phenomenon. First, the capacity to metabolize parenteral glucose is limited; when that limit is exceeded, glucose is converted to fat, resulting in the deposition of fat in the liver and increased carbon dioxide production.[6, 7, 49] The maximal capacity for effective glucose utilization is about 7 mg/kg^{-1}/$min.^{-1}$ This comes to about 700 gm glu-

Figure 5–11. The effect of increasing TPN on the protein synthesis rate in depleted patients. (*From* Stein, T. P., and Ang, S. D.: Effect of increasing TPN on protein metabolism. J.P.E.N., *7*:525–529, 1983, with permission.)

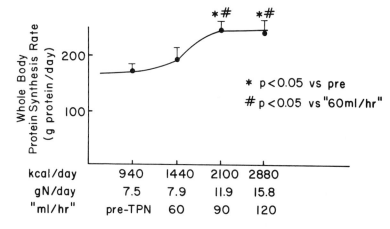

kcal/day	940	1440	2100	2880
gN/day	7.5	7.9	11.9	15.8
"ml/hr"	pre-TPN	60	90	120

* p < 0.05 vs pre
# p < 0.05 vs "60ml/hr"

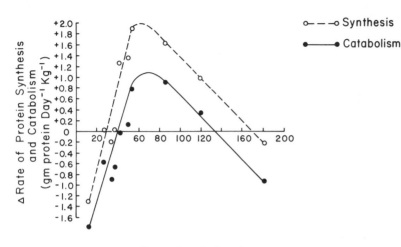

○ — —○ Synthesis

●———● Catabolism

Figure 5–12. Relationship between the whole-body protein synthesis rate and the change in serum insulin level (post-TPN–pre-TPN). The study group consisted of malnourished patients with localized esophageal carcinoma. (Burt, M. E., Stein, T. P., Schwabe, J. G., and Brennan, M. F.: Effect of total parenteral nutrition on protein metabolism in man. Cancer, *53*:1246–1252, 1984, with permission.)

cose for a 70-kg patient per day, or 2800 kcal/day[6, 130, 135, 164, 165] for a patient who has a healthy liver. Undoubtedly, the capacity decreases as hepatic status worsens. By monitoring the patient's respiratory quotient one can avoid this problem. An RQ of greater than 0.97 indicates fat deposition in the liver secondary to excess glucose (see Chapter 11).

Second, as has long been suspected, serum insulin levels are important in modulating the effectiveness of TPN. A recent study by Burt and colleagues[25] suggests why. Protein metabolism was studied by two independent methods, ^{15}N glycine for protein synthesis and 3-methylhistidine for protein breakdown. Increased protein synthesis and turnover occurred only if the change in the serum insulin level following the institution of TPN fell within a range of 20 to 120 units (Fig. 5–12). Changes outside that range resulted in no change in protein synthesis.

Likewise, TPN decreased protein breakdown only if the serum insulin was within this range (Fig. 5–13). These findings may explain why all patients do not respond equally well to the same dosage of TPN. The observations are not entirely unexpected. Some insulin is needed to promote glucose and amino acid utilization, but with too much insulin, resistance occurs and substrate utilization is impaired.

It is not just the extra energy that cannot be used; excess amino acids have no effect either. The study by Stein and Ang[149] was done at a constant calorie:nitrogen ratio in nonstressed patients. Increasing the protein intake does not increase the protein synthesis rate in either healthy young men[147] or severely burned patients.[166] Wolfe and associates[166] gave burned patients 40.8 kcal/kg/day and protein at either 1.4 gm/kg/day (cal:N ratio = 182:1) or 2.2 gm/kg/day (cal:N ratio

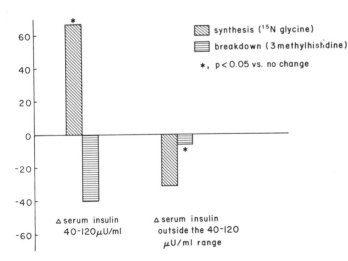

▨ synthesis (^{15}N glycine)

▤ breakdown (3 methylhistidine)

*, p < 0.05 vs. no change

Figure 5–13. Relationship between the change in serum insulin levels (pre-TPN–post-TPN) and protein breakdown. Protein synthesis was measured with [^{15}N] glycine (see Fig. 5–11) and protein breakdown with 3-methylhistidine. *(Replotted from* Burt, M. E., Stein, T. P., Schwabe, J. G., and Brennan, M. F.: Effect of total parenteral nutrition on protein metabolism in man. Cancer, *53*:1246–1252, 1984, with permission.)

= 115:1) in a crossover study. There was no difference in the protein synthesis rate at the two protein intake levels.

Nitrogen balance studies in severely burned patients have suggested, however, that N requirements could go as high as 2.5 gm/kg/day and even higher in children,[3] who have correspondingly increased caloric needs. These patients, though, have very large nonmetabolic nitrogen losses because of protein losses from their wounds, rather than from protein breakdown and oxidation, so much of the increased N requirement is to replace these losses.

Wolfe and associates[166] concluded that "there is a limitation to the extent to which nutrition alone can optimize protein synthesis in the burned patient." We suggest that this conclusion is generally applicable. In other words, *there is a limit to the extent to which nutrition alone can optimize protein metabolism, and this limit is approached when the patient is receiving calculated energy requirements with a balanced amino acid mixture at a reasonable calorie:nitrogen ratio.*

The Effect of Stress on Protein and Calorie Requirements

Protein and calorie requirements are increased by stress. Protein metabolism in stressed states is different from that in nonstressed patients for reasons that are not fully understood. There is a relationship between the severity of the stress and the degree of hypermetabolism. The response to stress appears to involve a general set of responses common to all stresses. The definition of *stress* includes severe trauma, sepsis, and the ultimate stress, a major burn.[161] The changes in protein metabolism are part of the general response.

Figure 5–14 summarizes the calorie and nitrogen requirements and their relationship to the degree of injury. Because it is a summary of similar figures published by others, it should serve as only a first step in formulating an appropriate TPN mix. The second step is to adjust the formulation to meet the patient's specific requirements. The aim should be to get the patient in positive N balance with an RQ in the range of 0.92 to 0.97 when glucose is the sole nonprotein caloric source and 0.83 to 0.88 when a solution of 70 per cent glucose, 30 per cent fat is being used (Fig. 5–15).

Some hypermetabolic patients, because of their inability to handle the calories, will remain in negative N balance. It is probably better to leave them in negative N balance rather than to exceed their capacity for nutrient processing, thereby forcing lipogenesis in the liver and eventual liver damage. Attention should be directed elsewhere as to why such patients are in negative balance (e.g., sepsis, fistulas, gastrointestinal losses, presence of a tumor), and appropriate steps taken to correct the underlying medical prob-

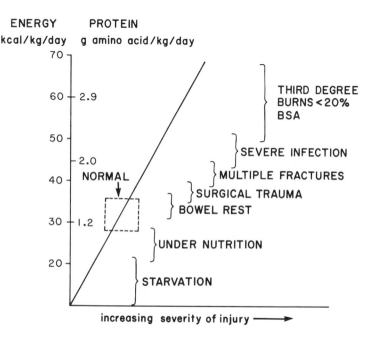

Figure 5–14. The effect of stress and injury on calorie and nitrogen requirements. The administration of these amounts of nutrients presupposes adequate renal and hepatic function. (*Modified from* Elwyn, D. H.: Nutritional requirements of adult surgical patients. Crit. Care Med., 8:9–20, 1980.)

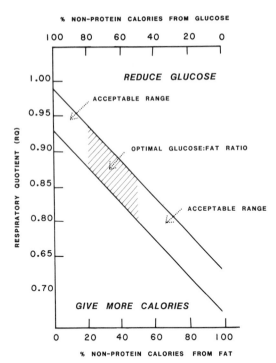

Figure 5–15. Relationship between respiratory quotient and substrate utilization. The area between the parallel lines represents the calculated range of adequate input of calories and their effective utilization. The shaded area is the range for an optimal mixture of glucose and fat.

lem. For such patients, nutrition is literally nutritional support pending the resolution of the primary problem. A small negative N balance, although not desirable, is better than a large one and allows time to attend to the primary problem.

Route of Administration of Nutrients

Nutrients can be given either enterally or parenterally, with the parenteral nutrients given either via a central venous line or peripherally (see Table 5–1). Enteral feeding is generally believed to be a more efficient route for nutritional support than direct intravenous administration of nutrients. Most likely the higher efficiency is due to the greater latitude for tolerance in nutrient composition. If the TPN nutrient mix is balanced and not excessive, no difference in net N retention is found between the enteral and parenteral routes.[101]

The theoretic advantages of the enteral route, which have been discussed extensively in Clinical Nutrition, Volume 1, are that with enteral feeding about 30 per cent of the

metabolic work in processing nutrients is done by the gut. Enteral nutrients must pass through first the gut and then the liver before interacting with the tissues. With TPN, greater reliance is placed on the liver; so the weaker the liver, the closer the TPN solution has to match the patient's needs and the more likely is a mismatched formulation to cause problems. In general, the sicker the patient, the narrower the tolerance range.

Hence the attractiveness of routes of administration that mimic enteral nutrition (prehepatic route) or the bolus feeding of normal life (cyclic TPN). In theory, portal venous (prehepatic) infusion should be the metabolically superior parenteral alternative to standard central venous TPN, because the former partially simulates the normal route of enteral substrate absorption. Experimentally, the results are mixed.

Increased weight gain[88] and improved glucose tolerance[103, 104, 123] as well as better nitrogen retention[88] have been reported to occur with enteral and prehepatic feeding than with central venous infusions in humans and rats.[85] In one rat study, portal vein feeding appeared to be superior; there were small but significant increases in nitrogen retention and serum albumin and transferrin levels over values seen with the intragastric route, with central venous infusion producing intermediate values (Fig. 5–16).[20]

This difference in nitrogen retention was not reproduced, however, in an analogous study by Fairman and colleagues[51] of parenterally nourished monkeys. Prehepatic infusion and superior vena cava infusion were equally effective in maintaining protein synthesis. Neither did they find any marked differences between the prehepatic and SVC routes as far as nitrogen balance and plasma hormonal levels were concerned. The accuracy of such studies is greatest with rats and least with humans, and "in between" with monkeys; hence, a small difference might not have been detectable.

Thus, the apparent ("biochemical") advantages of the prehepatic route are, *in vivo*, probably of marginal significance. There is also some risk with the prehepatic route; phlebitis or thrombosis of the hepatic vein could cause serious problems in the blood supply to the liver. It therefore seems unlikely that prehepatic intravenous infusions of nutrients will become popular because of the clinical difficulties associated with such regimens.

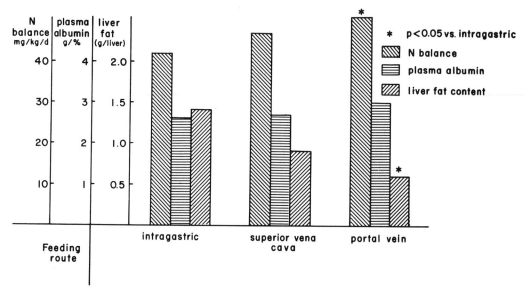

Figure 5–16. The effect of route of administration on nitrogen balance, plasma albumin, and liver fat content in parenterally fed rats. (*Replotted from* Boraas, M. C., Buzby, G. P., Stein, T. P., Zinsser, K. R., and Mullen, J. L.: Comparison of intragastric, prehepatic, and central venous TPN in the rat. Submitted for publication.)

Cyclic TPN

Another approach that was also designed to mimic the more natural situation of bolus feeding is cyclic TPN. Maini and coworkers[98] hypothesized that cyclic hyperalimentation may simulate normal enteral feeding more closely by allowing the development of a postabsorptive state with a fall in insulin levels and more serum protein repletion. It would appear desirable to allow a period daily during which lipogenic signals could be diminished and lipolysis could occur. Cyclic TPN in theory allows for the development of a postabsorptive state, facilitating the mobilization and utilization of calories stored as fat during the standard or hypertonic dextrose–amino acid infusion.[98]

As with prehepatic feeding, the theory is valid, but none of the published studies has documented any improvement over the N retention achieved with the standard continuous regimens in humans. The advantages appear to involve a decrease in the metabolic burden on the liver, as evidenced by a lower incidence of elevated liver enzymes.[56, 78, 80] Cyclic TPN requires much more catheter care than continuous TPN, detracting greatly from its theoretic attractiveness for the hospitalized patient. Not surprisingly, therefore, there has been no great enthusiasm for cyclic TPN for hospitalized patients. However, for the patient on home TPN, cyclic TPN is the method of choice; it allows the patient to feed himself at night and have a normal life during the day (see Chapter 39). The real advantage of cyclic TPN is not at the biochemical level but in the quality of life.

Minerals and Supplements

Amino acids and energy are not the only nutrients needed for protein anabolism. For the chemically pure nutrients given parenterally, an extensive list of cofactors, vitamins, and minerals is essential for protein synthesis. It is not commonly realized how strikingly the omission of some of these items affects protein metabolism. The results of omitting sodium, phosphorus, or potassium from the TPN mix are almost as bad as those of starvation (Fig. 5–17).[50]

TPN may even potentiate any incipient deficiencies in trace minerals. For example, with enteral nutrition, zinc deficiency is very rare, and it takes several weeks of starvation to produce symptoms attributable to zinc deficiency. With zinc-free TPN, however, zinc deficiency can be produced within a matter of weeks, with an adverse effect on protein synthesis. It has been argued that most of the lesions attributed to amino acid deficiency in kwashiorkor are actually due to the concomitant zinc deficiency.[69]

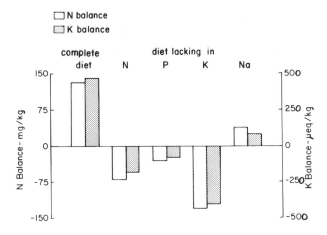

Figure 5–17. The effect of eliminating various non-protein components on N and K balance in depleted patients. (*From* Elwyn, D. H.: Nutritional requirements of adult surgical patients. Crit. Care Med., 8:9–20, 1980.)

There is a good correlation between the insulin level and the negative nitrogen balance.[167] Wolman and colleagues[167] suggested that insulin may be the missing link connecting protein metabolism with zinc metabolism. However, the role of zinc is ubiquitous in many enzyme systems, so which ones become limiting in zinc deficiency and impair protein synthesis is not yet known. Because prophylaxis is easier than trace metal analyses, minerals are now added routinely to hyperalimentation solutions (see Chapter 14).

TPN AND DISEASE-RELATED CHANGES IN PROTEIN METABOLISM

Malnutrition

In the early phases of starvation, muscle is the source of most of the urinary nitrogen loss. About 40 per cent of total body protein is muscle, so although a five per cent loss of muscle protein would have a marked effect on urine N excretion ($\approx$40 gm N), the actual effect on muscle tissue is small. Loss of a small proportion of muscle protein is not serious. A patient resting in bed does not need as much muscle as an ambulatory person. Prolonged undernutrition, however, inevitably results in the loss of protein from other more important sites, and this loss will eventually interfere with vital functions. The resultant weakness of respiratory muscles, for example, renders a patient more prone to pneumonia. Diminished visceral protein synthesis leads to hypoalbuminemia, edema, and hypogammaglobulinemia. The effects of starvation on the tissues are the predicted ones of progressively diminished functional capacity.

In the patient in whom the malnutrition is due solely to a lack of means of administering nutrients, TPN invariably remedies the underlying nutritional problem with minimal complications. This achievement ranks as one of the major advances in medicine in this century.

Repletion of such "healthy" patients is achieved by giving the calculated amount of calories and a balanced amino acid solution with a calorie:N ratio in the range of 150 ± 25:1. The nonprotein calories are calculated using the Harris-Benedict equation and 10 to 15 kcal/kg/day are added, bringing the total to about 35 kcal/day and about 1.3 gm/day of a balanced amino acid mixture for a non-stressed patient.[50] As long as the essential fatty acid requirement is met, it matters little whether most of the nonprotein calories are given to these "healthy" patients as fat or glucose. As is to be expected, muscle, the primary source of N loss, is the major beneficiary of repletion with TPN.[137]

Figure 5–18, which is compiled from a variety of sources, describes the changes in protein synthesis, protein breakdown, and nitrogen balance associated with starvation and refeeding. The initial response to starvation is a fall in the rate of protein synthesis, with either no change or a slight increase in protein breakdown. Reducing protein syn-

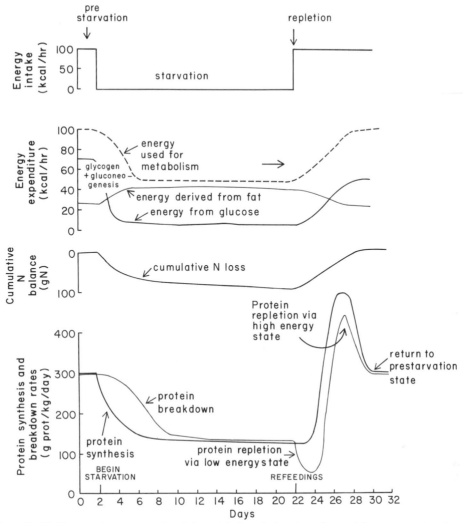

Figure 5–18. Changes in energy and protein metabolism during starvation and the response to refeeding.

thesis spares energy, and leaving protein breakdown unchanged provides the necessary amino acids for gluconeogenesis. As glucose utilization is replaced by fat mobilization, the need for amino acids drops, and protein breakdown is reduced correspondingly. The subject has adapted to undernutrition.

The first response to refeeding is a decrease in protein breakdown.[127] This is the most economical means, in terms of energy, of replacing lost protein. Decreasing protein breakdown allows protein to accumulate. Then, after a few days, the body switches into the high-energy repletion state, which is associated with an increase in protein synthesis and a smaller increase in protein breakdown.[25, 68, 108, 144] Growth is also associated with a higher turnover rate (high energy state).[99, 109, 121] The chronic low-energy state is

stable and not necessarily "unhealthy." Undernourished children grow poorly, but they survive to reproduce if the degree of undernutrition is not great.

One point that should receive comment is why the plasma albumin level, an excellent indicator of malnutrition, is a poor index of protein repletion.[57, 104, 159] Because albumin is an early indicator of malnutrition, the corollary is that it is one of the last proteins to be restored to the premorbid level. Usually, patients are weaned from TPN as soon as possible and put on an enteral diet, so the final stages of the repletion occur with enteral feeding. Sometimes the plasma albumin level drops even after TPN is begun, probably because most patients experience some fluid retention. Any increase in distribution space would tend to dilute the body albumin pools. Two separate studies have shown that TPN increases the plasma albumin synthesis rate by as much as twofold (Fig. 5–19).[132, 142] Presumably, breakdown is increased proportionately, since the actual concentration does not change. The actual serum concentration does not increase until nutrition status is back to near normal, as is to be expected for an early indicator–late recovery protein. For depleted cancer patients, in whom it may not be possible to completely replete protein stores, the final step in albumin repletion is not usually seen.[102, 115, 116]

Protein Sparing

Blackburn and colleagues[18, 19, 54] made the beguiling suggestion that the postoperative N loss could be decreased by giving amino acids instead of the customary five per cent dextrose. The tradition of giving D5W goes back to the Second World War studies of Gamble,[62] who demonstrated the nitrogen-sparing effect of dextrose. The argument for amino acids is that infused glucose stimulates insulin production, which in turn limits lipolysis, thereby decreasing the availability of such endogenously derived energy sources as free fatty acids and ketones and necessitating the use of amino acids for energy. Giving amino acids (or fat) would not stimulate insulin release.

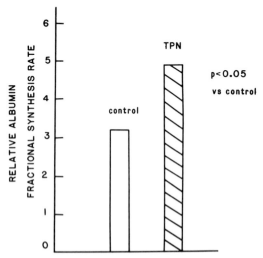

Figure 5–19. Improvement in the plasma albumin fractional synthesis rate in depleted patients given TPN. (*From* Stein, T. P., Buzby, G. P., Gertner, M. H., Hargrove, W. C., Leskiw, M. J., and Mullen, J. L.: Effect of parenteral nutrition on protein synthesis and liver fat metabolism in man. Am. J. Physiol., *239*:G280–G287, 1980, with permission.)

Follow-up studies showed that there was indeed a decrease in N loss, although the difference was not very large.[70, 72] Greenberg and co-workers[70] found that amino acids alone, with lipid, and with glucose were equivalent in nitrogen sparing, but if calories (glucose) alone were given, nitrogen balance was significantly worse. The inference is that most traumatized patients had some endogenous energy reserves available and so amino acids became limiting before energy. In other words, there is a requirement for protein, and the utilization of this protein does not appear to be contingent on the presence of other substrates or hormonal levels in the plasma. There does seem to be a calorie component to the (small) protein-sparing effect. Garden and associates[63] compared 400 kcal/day as glucose with 268 kcal/day as amino acids and observed no statistically significant protein-sparing effect. The mechanism of the protein sparing is increased protein synthesis, because muscle protein breakdown as measured by 3-methylhistidine excretion is unaffected by whether glucose, fat, or amino acids are given.[87]

There is another aspect of protein sparing with amino acid solutions. Some patients, specifically obese patients, do not need the calorie part of TPN. Protein-sparing therapies are discussed in detail in Chapter 10. The discussion here is restricted to the effect of protein-sparing therapies on protein metabolism. The aim of protein sparing is to have the patient use endogenous fat for energy while maintaining nitrogen homeostasis. The rationale is that an obese patient given amino acids but little energy will be forced to draw on endogenous lipid for energy. Because this is a normal physiologic response, it should occur without complications. Some glucose (≈400 kcal) has to be given to supply energy to tissues such as the brain, which are obligate glucose utilizers and take a long time to adapt to ketone bodies.

Experimentally, this rationale appears to be plausible. Figure 5–20 shows the effect of restricting calories but not protein on a morbidly obese patient. In the study whose results are illustrated, protein synthesis was hardly affected by the severe reduction of calories.[64] If amino acids were omitted as well as calories, however, protein synthesis was much reduced and the subject went into negative N balance.

On the basis of the encouraging results obtained with protein sparing, protein sparing with amino acids is worth considering in

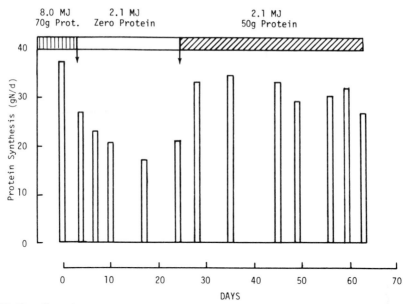

Figure 5–20. The effect of protein sparing (enteral) on protein synthesis in an obese patient. Note that omission of exogenous calories had little effect on protein synthesis. (*From* Garlick, P. J., Clugston, G. A., and Waterlow, J. C.: Influence of low energy diets on whole body protein turnover in obese subjects. Am. J. Physiol., *238*:E235–E244, 1980, with permission.)

devising a TPN regimen for obese patients. Weight loss in itself often leads to an improvement in the patient's status. Such patients need to be closely monitored, and at the first signs of any problems (e.g., negative N balance, elevated liver enzymes), a standard TPN regimen should be instituted and optimized as described previously. The gain of a few pounds by an already obese patient is just a minor side effect of an otherwise satisfactory TPN regimen. The additional weight loss problem can be handled separately after the major problem has been resolved. Even so, the tendency to gain weight can be minimized by making sure that the respiratory quotient (RQ) stays within acceptable limits.

Trauma, Sepsis, and Burns

As pointed out previously, many aspects of the metabolic responses of protein metabolism to trauma, sepsis, and major burns are similar, being part of a generalized response to stress.[161] Severe injury causes an increase in net protein breakdown (increased N excretion in the urine) in well-nourished subjects. Many years ago, Cuthbertson[42] discovered that the increased nitrogen excretion that occurred after severe injury was more than that to be expected from the quantity of

protein damaged by the injury. It was assumed that the enhanced N excretion was due to an increase in protein catabolism (breakdown).

Tracer studies with labeled amino acids revealed the unexpected findings that the increased net protein breakdown is due to an increase in synthesis and a larger increase in protein breakdown, rather than just a simple increase in protein breakdown or a decrease in protein synthesis.[15, 16, 76, 81, 90, 91, 110, 133, 140] In other words, protein turnover is increased. A decrease in protein synthesis is found at other times.[41, 82, 119, 140] Table 5–6 lists the potential changes in protein metabolism following stress, including such mild stresses as vaccination,[65] growth (a change from the status quo), and the relationship to nutrition.[36, 68, 109]

In order to understand why it is so important to pay attention to an injured patient's protein status, it is necessary to briefly review the role of protein turnover in determining how effectively the body is able to respond to severe stress. As pointed out previously, the body's proteins are in a continual state of flux. Most of the proteins made are visceral (enzymes, circulating proteins, hormones, etc.), with the balance being skeletal muscle proteins. Protein turnover is an energy-intensive process and may account for about 20 per cent of the total rest energy

Table 5–6. LEVELS OF HUMAN PROTEIN AND ENERGY METABOLISM AND THEIR RELATIONSHIP TO NUTRITIONAL STATUS, DIET, AND CLINICAL STATUS

RELATIVE PROTEIN TURNOVER RATE AND ENERGY EXPENDITURE	CLINICAL STATE	MAJOR FUEL SUBSTRATES	NITROGEN BALANCE	COMMENT
150 (high)	Hypermetabolic	CHO	↓ ↓	Most efficient and fastest response to stress/change in protein status
	Stress response	CHO	↓ ↓	
	Repletion	CHO	↑ ↑ ↑	
	Normal growth	CHO	↓ ↓	
100 (normal)	Normal	Oral food	⟷	Normal state
	Maintenance TPN	CHO	⟷	Glucose system
	Repletion TPN	Fat	↑	Repletion with fat
70 (low)	Chronic undernutrition	Any oral food	⟷	Minimal nutrition for stable protein metabolism
	Stunted growth	Any oral food	↑	Minimal nutrition for stable protein metabolism
	Adaptation to starvation	Glycogen, gluconeogenesis, fat	↓	Survival with starvation
	TPN	CHO	↓	Undernutrition
	TPN	Fat	⟷	Stable
50 (very low)	Starvation	Any, including endogenous protein	↓	Terminal if prolonged

expenditure.[146] Teleologically, therefore, protein turnover must carry with it some very significant advantage(s) to justify this amount of energy utilization, or evolutionary pressures would have selected a more energy-efficient alternative.

The rates of metabolic pathways are governed by the activities of key enzymes, and enzyme level is a major, if not the major, determinant in long-term regulation.[84, 160] The greater the importance of a particular protein in the regulation of metabolism, the faster its rate of turnover.[67, 146] In contrast, the proteins with no regulatory role, such as actin, myosin, and collagen, have very slow turnover rate (Fig. 5–21). Very rapid turnover provides a means of metabolic control.

Rapid protein turnover also enables a limited pool to be used with optimal efficiency. For example, the liver consists mainly of several hundred different proteins, most of which are enzymes. The functional role of the liver is to maintain metabolic hemostasis by processing exogenous nutrients, to provide glucose and keto acids for other tissues during fasting, and to detoxify and excrete a multitude of waste products. The workload on the liver (and therefore its rate of protein synthesis) varies considerably with relation to meals, nutritional state, presence of stress or disease, and rate of release of metabolic

end-products from other tissues. Speed of response to changed circumstances is essential; hence, most liver proteins have fast turnover rates, whereas muscle proteins have much slower turnover rates.

Optimal levels of all possible enzyme systems are not maintained all the time; rather, those that are not immediately needed are maintained at relatively low lev-

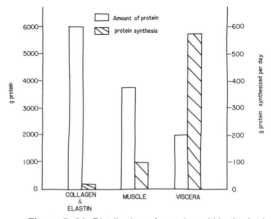

Figure 5–21. Distribution of proteins within the body and their relative contributions to the whole-body protein synthesis rate. Note the inverse relationship between protein quantity and protein turnover. (*From* Stein, T. P.: Nutrition and protein turnover, a review. J.P.E.N., 6:444–454, 1982, with permission.)

els. As a result of the rapid turnover process, the concentration of a particular enzyme system can be rapidly increased if required through changes in the relative synthesis and breakdown rates. Concomitantly, when high levels of other enzymes are no longer required, they can be rapidly diminished through a decrease in the synthesis rate or an increase in the breakdown rate, so that the total protein pool need not be expanded. Neither must it be forgotten that in land mammals there is an advantage to compactness. The weight has to be carried around and increases energy demands, in turn leading to greater need for food—a potential problem when food supplies are limited.

According to these arguments, the more rapid the turnover rate, the more flexible and the better prepared the system is for coping with perturbations of the normal steady state. There is, therefore, some advantage to a temporary increase in protein turnover following a metabolic stress. Increasing the turnover rate is a way of providing for a rapid increase in protein concentration, if and when needed, without taking up more space or tying up (scarce) amino acids.

The actual degree of increase is about 40 to 60 per cent above normal (see Table 5–6). For the patient in a well-nourished state, the transition to a "high-energy–high-turnover" state is regulated by hormones, particularly the catecholamines.[153, 161] As expected, there is increased synthesis of the acute-phase proteins, secretory proteins, proteins involved in leukocytic activity, and, if there is a wound, proteins involved in wound healing.[12, 124] As long as the stress persists and nutritional status does not become limiting, the protein turnover rate is elevated. If nutrition is mildly limiting, some of the low-priority proteins (e.g., muscle) are cannibalized to supply amino acids for higher-priority proteins.

We can therefore distinguish three sets of proteins within the body, according to their response to stress. First, proteins involved in the dynamic response (enzymes, immunoglobulins, acute phase proteins, etc.), respond via an increase in turnover; increasing turnover is a way of facilitating rapid changes in concentration without taking up more space. Second, proteins that supply amino acids have no real role in the metabolic response to stress; examples are structural proteins and proteins involved in muscle work, such as actin and myosin. Decreasing synthesis, like increasing break-down, frees up amino acids but in a energetically "cheap" way. Third, the inert structural proteins, like collagen, show little if any response to the stress. If the patient is malnourished, the "high-energy" response described above cannot be made.

There is also a "low-energy" response to stress and changed circumstances (see Table 5–6). Malnourished patients do not show the characteristic N loss after trauma, and although they are prone to more serious complications, they usually recover. In these patients protein synthesis is decreased after trauma.[32, 119, 134, 140] Decreased protein synthesis is a metabolically "cheap" way of redistributing protein; proteins that are catabolized are not replaced; other required proteins are allowed to accumulate through decreases in breakdown rate. It is a passive response rather than dynamic as the high-energy response is. The mildly undernourished patient responds via the low-energy pathway and, from the limited available evidence (or lack thereof), appears to do as well as the well-nourished patient.

If nutritional status is limiting, the two tissues that show a decrease in protein synthesis are first muscle and then lung. The finding that lung is affected as well as muscle is significant, in that pulmonary complications are common in malnourished, traumatized, and septic patients. A lung that cannot maintain a normal rate of protein turnover has a diminished ability to respond to an insult (bacterial infection) or increased workload (Fig. 5–22).[140]

The preceding paragraphs contain the rationale for the emphasis given to the status of protein metabolism in a patient. Proteins are the machinery of the body. Recovery from stress, disease, or injury is effected by the proteins within the body. The role of nutrition is to ensure that the ability to provide the necessary proteins is not limited for the want of amino acids, energy, or a micronutrient.

The Role of TPN

The biochemical changes associated with injury and how the response is affected by nutritional status have been extensively investigated. The conclusion is that the increased N loss after trauma in a previously well-nourished patient is not usually serious, provided that it does not extend beyond five to six days, because adequate reserves of

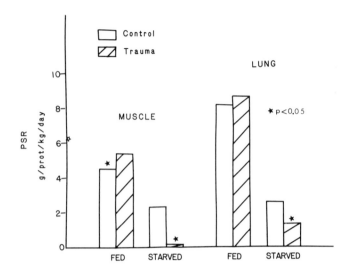

Figure 5–22. The effects of nutritional status and trauma on protein synthesis in the skeletal muscle and lung of traumatized rats.[23] Units are %/day of the protein pool. (*), $P < 0.05$ vs. control; (★), p. < 0.05 for fed vs. starved. (*From* Stein, T. P.: Nutrition and protein turnover, a review. J.P.E.N., 6:444–454, 1982, with permission.)

protein and energy are available. Muscle, by virtue of its large size and relative unimportance, is the major site of the protein reserve, although there are no specific reserve proteins *per se*.

If the negative N balance continues beyond five or six days, however, more aggressive nutritional intervention is called for, because of the increasing likelihood that the injury requirements will force the body to mobilize proteins of greater physiologic importance, such as immunologic proteins and lung proteins.[31, 71] The situation is different with the severely malnourished patient, because this step has already been taken. The next event is a continuing series of choices between ever higher priority functions, and the consequent losses of functional capacity increase the chances of a complication or even an adverse outcome. Examples of such choices are synthesis of circulating proteins *versus* provision of proteins for wound healing or, worse, lung protein synthesis, which would thereby compromise pulmonary function.[140] There is no question that for these patients, aggressive nutritional support is essential and should be instituted as soon as possible to minimize body protein loss.

Although it has long been known that the poorly nourished patient has a higher incidence of complications than a well-nourished patient, there has as yet been no definitive study showing that giving a few days of TPN to undernourished patients is enough to "build them up for surgery" and to reduce the incidence of subsequent complications.[22, 74, 112] It seems intuitively obvious that this might be the case, and because there is no

reason to suspect harmful effects, the preoperative build-up of depleted patients for surgery is not uncommon. At the very least, it should provide them with protein to lose postoperatively.

Some seriously injured patients cannot be fed enterally and therefore need TPN. The TPN provides the materials (amino acids, energy) for healing, which sometimes is enough. In other patients, the role of TPN is different. TPN keeps the patient alive during a prolonged illness, prevents further wasting away of the patient's protein, and provides time for other therapies to take effect. An example is a patient with prolonged sepsis. Without the nutrition to prevent wasting during the course of a prolonged illness, the patient would most likely die. Yet TPN does not cure the patient; it provides time through "nutritional support" for other measures to take effect. In this sort of patient, it is important not to expect more from TPN than preventing the body protein from wasting away and keeping the patient alive.

Can Varying the Amino Acid Pattern Improve Nitrogen Metabolism in the Injured Patient?

The trauma/stress-related nitrogen loss in the adequately nourished patients continues to encourage efforts aimed at decreasing the loss. The kinetic studies of protein metabolism already described suggested that amino acids become limiting before energy. The next step would be to determine which amino acid(s). Several investigators proposed that one (leucine) or all of the branched chain amino acids (leucine, isoleucine and valine) are the limiting amino acids and that consequently there would be a benefit to giving patients with trauma or sepsis more of these amino acids.[17, 29, 33, 59, 77, 90, 111] The discussion here is limited to the effects of supplemental branched-chain amino acids (BCAAs) on protein metabolism; clinical studies are discussed in detail in Chapter 35.

If the demand for branched-chain amino acids is increased relative to that for the other 17 amino acids, the BCAAs will become limiting. The excess of the other 17 amino acids must be promptly degraded to urinary nitrogen and CO_2. This hypothesis explains the increased urinary N excretion found after trauma. An imbalanced mix of free amino acids is highly toxic if allowed to accumulate.[120]

Why would there be an increased need for the branched-chain amino acids after injury? Four arguments have been advanced supporting the administration of additional amino acids to severely injured patients.[97] They are as follows:

1. Branched-chain amino acids, particularly leucine, promote protein synthesis.[2]

2. If more branched-chain amino acids were given, the amount of low-priority (mainly muscle) protein breakdown needed to supply high-priority processes with the branched-chain amino acids would be decreased. The BCAAs might become the limiting amino acids because they are mainly oxidized by skeletal muscle. At times of stress, when energy demands by other tissues are at a maximum, muscle, which is a low-priority tissue, may oxidize more of the BCAAs derived from protein breakdown for energy than in the nonstressed state.[72] There is some evidence that a circulating 33-residue polypeptide is involved in regulating the amount of muscle protein broken down.[34] The peptide may be related to leukocytic pyrogen (interleukin-1), which has been shown to stimulate muscle proteolysis via the enhanced release of prostaglandin E_2.[9]

3. The theoretical argument in favor of giving more of the BCAAs is that the amount of branched-chain amino acids slipping through (lost) into the degradative/oxidative pathways is increased by the overall increase in amino acid flux.[55]

4. There may be a concomitant increase in demand for BCAAs by other tissues.

Animal and human studies have been promising. With BCAA infusions, nitrogen retention and protein synthesis are improved in rats,[17, 58, 61, 89, 129] and nitrogen balance becomes positive a little earlier in injured humans (Fig. 5–23). Most likely the mechanism in humans is a stimulation of protein synthesis, since protein breakdown was unaffected

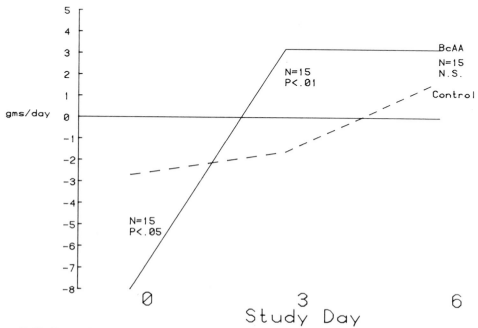

Figure 5–23. N retention becomes positive earlier when a solution enriched with branched-chain amino acids is given to traumatized patients. (*From* Cerra, F. B., Upson, D., Angelico, R., Wiles, C., III, Lyons, J., Faulkenbach, L., and Paysinger, J.: Branched chains support postoperative protein synthesis. Surgery, *92*:192–199, 1982.)

and protein synthesis was increased in similar experiments with rats. However, the clinical studies have not as yet documented an improvement in morbidity and mortality, which is the "bottom line." One must bear in mind, though, that if the magnitude of the improvement is only about 10 per cent, it might be very difficult to detect in studies on small, heterogenous populations. It is, however, a most important first step to have demonstrated that a solution devised from a theory of the mechanism of the response to trauma does indeed show the predicted effects at a biochemical level.

It is also conceivable that the sparing of protein by supplemental branched-chain amino acids is of biochemical interest only and that the protein sparing found has little if any clinical significance.

TPN and Nitrogen Metabolism in the Cancer Patient

In any discussion of TPN and nitrogen metabolism in the cancer patient, there are two questions of interest. What is the effect of the tumor on the host's protein metabolism? and What is the effect of TPN on this tumor-host relationship?

N Metabolism in the Cancer Patient

The current theories of the role of protein turnover in the living organism explain why it is important to maintain protein homeostasis, but not why many cancer patients die from protein depletion or how to prevent them from doing so. Unlike other clinical situations, where the trend has been toward aggressive nutritional intervention, there have been serious reservations about giving TPN to cancer patients because nutrition may not only correct the malnutrition but also disproportionately benefit the tumor.

Most studies of how a tumor affects protein metabolism in the host have been done with tumor-bearing rats or mice. The tumor grows while the host wastes away.[94] Mider[107] described the tumor as functioning as a nitrogen and energy trap. From the emaciated appearance of some cancer patients, it is obvious that the same host-wasting phenomenon occurs in humans.

However, the relevance of rodent tumor models to the human situation may not be quite so simple. It is not difficult to envisage

that a 30-gm tumor on a 200-gm rat will kill the rat; the tumor constitutes 15 per cent of the rat's total body weight. But how does a 300-gm tumor kill a 70,000-gm man? After all, many men carry around 20 to 30 kg (or more) of extra fat and adipose tissue for years.

Beyond the well-known observations that many cancer patients are protein depleted, little is known about the effect of the tumor on the host's protein metabolism. Cancer patients are often malnourished and have significant weight loss, so one might predict that protein turnover would be correspondingly decreased.

In the absence of a tumor, the whole-body protein synthesis rate is decreased in undernourished states. Three separate studies concluded that some cancer patients apparently have an anomalously high protein turnover rate.[28, 118, 143] A confounding variable in these three studies was that the subjects were not just healthy individuals who happened to be carrying a tumor; they were also very sick. Other possibly tumor-induced metabolic complications were present, such as anorexia, metastases, and liver involvement. There is also some doubt as to whether the model used for estimating turnover rates applies to seriously ill patients with metabolic complications.

In a later study by Burt and colleagues[25] of patients with esophageal tumors, care was taken to exclude patients with liver insufficiency. Elevated protein turnover rates, relative to fed non–tumor-bearing adults, were not found. A study by Glass and co-workers[66] also failed to document evidence of increased protein turnover in patients with rectal tumors; removal of the tumor appeared to have little effect on the rest of the body's protein metabolism.

Direct measurements of human gastrointestinal tumor fractional synthesis rates showed that tumor protein synthesis rates were a little higher than those in other visceral tissue, but not by the order of magnitude needed to affect the whole-body rate (Fig. 5–24).[141] Neither was there any evidence of an increased muscle protein synthesis rate in humans.[95, 142] In rats, muscle synthesis is actually reduced because of the demands of the tumor (Fig. 5–25).[139] Thus, on balance, it seems reasonable to conclude that the presence of a tumor does not lead to an increase in the whole-body protein synthesis rate beyond the small, and probably undetectable,

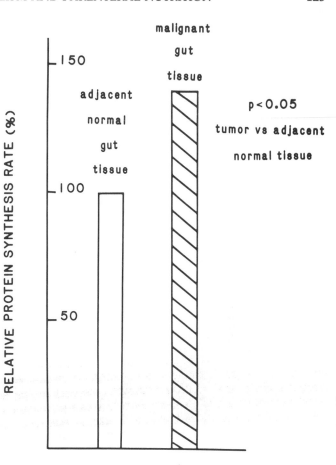

Figure 5–24. Relative relationship between the protein synthesis rates of a gastrointestinal tumor and of the adjacent normal tissue. The tumor has a slightly faster turnover rate, but it is not enough to cause any major additive change in the whole-body rate. (*Based on* Stein, T. P., Leskiw, M. J., Oram-Smith, J. C., and Wallace, H. W.: Changes in protein synthesis after trauma: Importance of nutrition. Am. J. Physiol., *223*:348–355, 1976.)

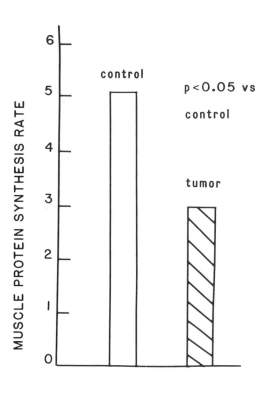

Figure 5–25. Reduced rate of protein synthesis in muscle of tumor-bearing rats caused by tumor sequestration of nutrients that in the absence of the tumor would have gone to muscle. (*Data from* Stein, T. P., Leskiw, M. J., Oram-Smith, J. C., Miller, E. E., and Wallace, H. W.: The effect of a tumor on the host's protein metabolism. Cancer Res., *36*:3936–3940, 1976.)

increase that is to be expected from adding the tumor synthesis rate to the whole-body rate. The apparently high rates reported in some studies are most likely due to methodologic problems of the tracer techniques used.[28, 121, 143, 148]

Obviously, however, a tumor does affect body protein metabolism. The effect may not be a simple additive one of the tumor plus the host's protein synthesis. If the host is unaware of the presence of a tumor, the appetite-controlled nutritional intake will be inadequate for the host plus tumor, resulting in the slow deprivation of the host. Eventually the tumor's amino acid and energy demands on the undernourished host's weakened liver may exceed the liver's capacity to handle the combined workload from the tumor-host system. At what point this occurs will depend on the health of the liver. When it occurs, the host must make other metabolic arrangements to ensure a semblance of nitrogen hemostasis. The obvious one is for the individual tissues to do more of their own amino acid processing rather than rely on the liver for this function, i.e., to decrease the metabolic load on the liver. When this compartmentation occurs, the one amino acid pool model used for calculating turnover rates is no longer valid. The greater the degree of compartmentation, the higher the apparent rate of protein synthesis.[143] Rather, what is being measured is the degree to which the liver has abdicated its role to the other tissues. It is therefore not surprising to find a good correlation between an elevated protein turnover rate in a cancer patient and a poor prognosis, but no correlation with tumor size.[148]

It does not have to be a tumor to cause this effect; any stress on a compromised patient can exceed the liver's capacity and cause apparently elevated turnover rates. As is to be expected, the higher the apparent turnover rate (the greater the shortfall in liver metabolic capacity), the poorer the prognosis (Fig. 5–26).[148]

The Effect of TPN

The critical question here is, which does the TPN benefit, the tumor or the host? This subject is covered in detail in Chapter 26. The discussion here is limited to the effects of TPN on protein metabolism in cancer patients.

In rats, the benefit of TPN is clearly to the tumor: the tumor grows faster and kills

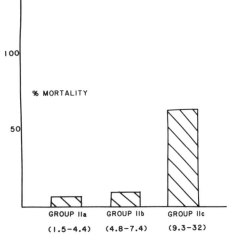

Figure 5–26. As the apparent elevated whole-body protein synthesis rate obtained using [¹⁵N] glycine as the tracer increases, mortality increases correspondingly. Whole-body protein synthesis rates are in parentheses, because the assay actually measures the degree of hepatic insufficiency in such patients; hence, the correlation between the apparent "protein synthesis rate" (degree of hepatic dysfunction) and mortality. (*From* Stein, T. P., Ang, S. D., Schluter, M. D., Leskiw, M. J., and Nusbaum, M.: Whole-body protein turnover in metabolically stressed patients with cancer as measured with [¹⁵N] glycine. Biochem. Med., *30*:59–77, 1983, with permission.)

the host in a shorter time.[45, 138] In humans, the situation may or may not be different. Human tumors are relatively small; they do not amount to 20 per cent of the total body weight, as in some rodent models, and most are much more slower-growing even when consideration is given to the longer human lifespan.

Yet the same biochemical relationships between the host and tumor are found. In the malnourished patient with a GI tract tumor, the tumor is deprived of nutrients along with the host, although the tumor is likely to be more effective in competing for available nutrients. But when TPN is instituted, human gastrointestinal tumors take up a disproportionate amount of the infused amino acids (Fig. 5–27). Thus, when additional exogenous amino acids are provided in the early stages of repletion, the tumor competes more effectively for the essential amino acids than the adjacent normal tissue.[145]

Again there is the question of whether a biochemical result translates into a phenomenon of clinical importance. This biochemical advantage to the tumor has to be balanced against the fact that (1) the TPN also feeds the host's tissues and (2) if something is not

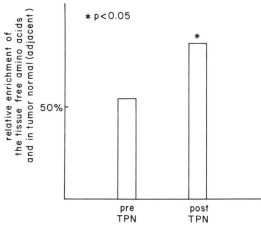

Figure 5–27. Increased avidity of human tumors for parenterally administered amino acids. The free amino acid concentrations in tumor were compared with those in adjacent nonmalignant tissue. Pre-TPN, there was no difference. Post-TPN, the tumor tissue was much more enriched in essential amino acids than the normal tissue. Specimens were obtained from patients undergoing surgical removal of a gastrointestinal tumor.

done about repleting the host, death from starvation is inevitable.

The immediate response to TPN in the malnourished cancer patient appears to be beneficial to the host. There is a net gain of protein by most patients, and there is often a marked improvement in immunologic status.[23, 40] An exception is patients receiving aggressive chemotherapy or radiotherapy. For reasons that are not fully understood, however, non-cancer patients can be repleted better than nutritionally matched cancer patients. In terms of Table 5–6, it would appear that cancer patients could be put into the low energy repletion state but not the "normal" state.[115, 116]

Protein makes up a small percentage (20 per cent) of body weight. An increase of 300 to 400 gm in protein when there are simultaneous changes of kilogram size in fat and water can be very hard to detect by whole-body studies, but such a gain can be of considerable physiologic importance. TPN does restore nutritional indices, function, and well-being in many cachectic cancer patients before, during, and after therapy.[37, 38, 46]

But as Brennan[23] pointed out, these are statistical summaries, with about one-third of the patients showing no improvement. The reason for the apparent demarcation between those patients who do improve and those who do not is not known. Possibly, the nonresponders are, as suggested by Burt and colleagues,[25] those patients whose change in serum insulin levels falls outside

the 20 to 120 unit range (see Fig. 5–12). Probably their RQs are also greater than one.

A study of the incidence of complications from surgery in esophageal and gastric neoplasia showed a decrease in complications in patients given TPN.[73, 74] Most likely, the explanation for this is restoration of the patient's protein status, which permits a normal response to the stress of the therapeutic regimen. Thus, once the effects of surgery are over, there should be no short-term difference between patients given postoperative TPN and control patients, and none is found.[23] By "short-term" is meant up until time of discharge, but not after.

There is controversy as to whether the long-term effect of TPN is to the tumor or the host. As pointed out, a human gastrointestinal tumor's protein metabolism does appear biochemically to benefit a little more than the host in the short run (see Fig. 5–25). Does this advantage translate into a long-term advantage? The only answer at this time is "Perhaps."

Some eleven studies of the effect of TPN as an adjunct to chemotherapy have been performed. (For details see Chapter 26.) In none of them did TPN improve survival. In fact, in one of the best studies, of patients with metastatic colon cancer, decreased survival was reported with TPN.[116] The interpretation of these results has been disputed, because although patients were randomized, retrospective analyses showed a nonrandom distribution, with the TPN group having a higher incidence of liver involvement. If allowance is made for this and other inhomogeneities in the study, the statistical significance of the result disappears—but the trend is still there. Could it be that the preferential uptake of TPN-originated amino acids by the tumor does in fact lead to a stronger tumor? It is a real possibility.

In summary, the problem of whether the benefit of TPN is to the tumor's or the host's protein metabolism is not resolved; the available data are conflicting. Nevertheless, from this uncertainty some inferences can be made. The primary effect is the correction of any underlying malnutrition. Many cancer patients have been given total parenteral nutrition, but no spectacular remissions or increased survival times have been reported; there may be a small (adverse) stimulatory effect on the tumor. The current practice of using TPN as an adjunct—e.g., repleting debilitated patients so they can withstand surgery better[44]—seems reasonable, but us-

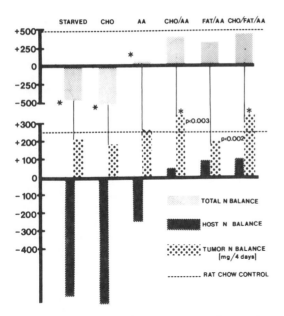

Figure 5–28. Effect of calorie source on tumor and host nitrogen metabolism in tumor-bearing rats. The rats were given one of six dietary regimens—starvation, glucose, amino acids, glucose plus amino acids, fat plus amino acids, and glucose plus fat plus amino acids. Tumor N uptake continued on all diets, with varying degrees of host N retention. Only the fat-based TPN (fat/AA) promoted positive host N balance without increased uptake in the tumor. P values denote significant levels between adjacent diets. (*From* Buzby, G. P., Mullen, J. L., Stein, T. P., Miller, E. E., Cobbs, C. L., and Rosato, E. F.: Host-tumor interaction and nutrient supply. Cancer, 45:2940–2948, 1980, with permission.)

ing it as adjuvant therapy—e.g., increasing tolerance or potentiating the effectiveness of chemotherapy[39, 43, 86]—is still uncertain, as is using TPN for just feeding undernourished cancer patients to improve the quality of life.[23, 40]

Outlook

Using TPN as described to influence the host-tumor relationship is a relatively unsophisticated first step, and one should not be surprised that the results to date have been disappointing. Numerous biochemical studies have documented subtle differences in the nutritional requirements of the tumor. Because TPN is a completely synthetic regimen using building blocks that can easily be varied, it offers the opportunity to selectively influence the protein metabolism in both tumor and host.

In theory, selective nutrition could be used to (1) selectively starve the tumor, (2) increase the tumor's vulnerability to chemotherapy, and (3) selectively strengthen the host. Some recent experiments with a rat tumor model have been promising. It has proved possible to shift the benefit of TPN away from the tumor to the host.[27] Tumors have an obligate requirement for glucose. If glucose is replaced with isocaloric fat, the host's tissues gain protein as well as with the glucose, but the tumor grows only half as well (Fig. 5–28).[27]

TPN has also been used to increase the susceptibility of a rat tumor to chemother-

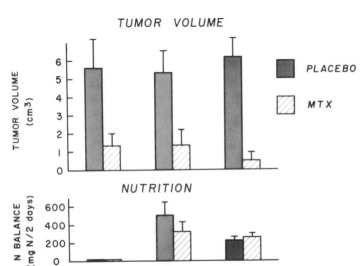

Figure 5–29. Enhanced tumor response of a rat tumor to chemotherapy with methotrexate (MTX) when the MTX treatment is given 2 hr. after beginning TPN to protein depleted rats.

apy.[153-155] This is done by exploiting the tumor's more avid uptake of amino acids relative to the host tissues. During the initial stages of refeeding a protein-depleted, tumor-bearing rat, the tumor, which is more aggressive, "turns on" its metabolism faster. At this time, which in the rat occurs within two hours of giving TPN or even amino acids alone, more tumor cells "turn on." Only active cells are vulnerable to chemotherapy. Thus, when a pulse of methotrexate was given, a greater decrease in tumor volume was found than in control animals who were not fed (Fig. 5–29).[153, 154] The mechanism appears to be via stimulation of tumor growth. After two hours, the percentage of cells in the S phase reverts to a random distribution, and the potentiating effect of TPN is no longer found.[155] The promise of these preliminary rat experiments suggests that TPN may have an important role in selectively preserving host protein, decreasing tumor nitrogen accretion, and possibly selectively increasing tumor tissue susceptibility to chemotherapy.[155]

REFERENCES

1. Abel, R. M., Beck, C. H., Jr., Abbott, W. M., et al.: Improved survival from acute renal failure following treatment with intravenous essential L-amino acids and glucose. N. Engl. J. Med., 288:695–703, 1973.
2. Adibi, S. A.: Roles of branched-chain amino acids in metabolic regulation. J. Lab. Clin. Med., 95:475–484, 1980.
3. Alexander, J. W., MacMillan, B. G., Stinnett, J. D., et al.: Beneficial effects of aggressive protein feeding in severely burned children. Ann. Surg., 192:505–517, 1980.
4. Allison, S. P.: Modifying nitrogen loss after injury. In Richards, J. R., and Kinney, J. M. (eds.): Nutritional Aspects of Care in the Critically Ill. Edinburgh, Churchill Livingstone, 1977, pp. 389–442.
5. Anderson, G. H., Patel, D. G., and Jeejeebhoy, K. H.: Design and evaluation by nitrogen balance and blood aminograms of an amino acid mixture for total parenteral nutrition of adults with gastrointestinal disease. J. Clin. Invest., 53:904–912, 1974.
6. Askanazi, J., Rosenbaum, S. H., Hyman, A. I., Silverberg, P. A., Milic-Emili, J., and Kinney, J. M.: Respiratory changes induced by the large glucose loads of total parenteral nutrition. J.A.M.A., 243:1444–1447, 1980.
7. Askanazi, J., Elwyn, D. H., Silverberg, P. A., Rosenbaum, S. H., and Kinney, J. M.: Respiratory distress secondary to a high carbohydrate load: A case report. Surgery, 87:596–598, 1980.
8. Baracos, V., Rodemann, H. P., Dinarello, C. A., and Goldberg, A. L.: Stimulation of muscle protein degradation and prostaglandin E_2 release by leukocytic pyrogen (interleukin-1). A mechanism for the increased degradation of muscle proteins during fever. N. Engl. J. Med., 308:553–559, 1983.
9. Barbul, A., Sisto, D. A., Wasserkrug, H. L., Yoshimura, N. N., and Efron, G.: Metabolic and immune effects of arginine in postinjury hyperalimentation. J. Trauma, 21:970–974, 1981.
10. Barbul, A., Wasserkrug, H. L., Penberthy, L. T., Yoshimura, N. N., Tao, R. C., and Efron, G.: Optimal levels of arginine in maintenance intravenous hyperalimentation. J.P.E.N., 8:281–284, 1984.
11. Bark, S., Holm, H., Hakansson, I., and Wretlind, A.: Nitrogen-sparing effect of fat emulsion compared with glucose in the postoperative period. Acta Chir. Scand., 142:423–427, 1976.
12. Beisel, W. R.: Magnitude of host responses to infection. Am. J. Clin. Nutr., 30:1236–1245, 1977.
13. Bergstrom, J., Furst, P., Josephson, B., and Noree, L. O.: Improvement of nitrogen balance in a uremic patient by the addition of histidine to essential amino acid solutions given intravenously. Life Sci., 9:787–794, 1970.
14. Bessman, S. P.: The justification theory: The essential nature of the non-essential amino acids. Nutr. Rev., 37:207–220, 1979.
15. Birkhahn, R. H., Long, C. L., Fitkin, D., Geiger, J. W., and Blakemore, W. S.: Effects of major skeletal trauma on whole body protein turnover in man measured by L-[1,^{14}C]-leucine. Surgery, 88:294–300, 1981.
16. Birkhahn, R. H., Long, C. L., Fitkin, D., Jeevanandam, M., and Blakemore, W. S.: Whole body protein metabolism due to trauma in man as estimated by N-^{15}N alanine. Am. J. Physiol., 241:E64–E71, 1981.
17. Blackburn, G. L., Moldawer, L. L., Usui, S., O'Keefe, S. D., Bothe, A., and Bistrian, B. R.: Branch chain amino acid metabolism during starvation, injury and sepsis. Surgery, 86:307–315, 1980.
18. Blackburn, G. L., Flatt, J. P., Clowes, G. H. A., Jr., et al.: Protein sparing during periods of starvation with sepsis or trauma. Ann. Surg., 177:588–596, 1973.
19. Blackburn, G. L., Flatt, J. P., Clowes, H. A., et al.: Peripheral intravenous feeding with isotonic amino acid solutions. Am. J. Surg., 125:447–454, 1973.
20. Boraas, M. C., Buzby, G. P., Stein, T. P., Zinsser, K. R., and Mullen, J. L.: Comparison of intragastric, prehepatic and central venous TPN in the rat. Submitted for publication.
21. Bozetti, F.: Parenteral nutrition in surgical patients. Surg. Gynecol. Obstet., 142:16–25, 1976.
22. Brandl, M., Tonak, J., and Rottler, H.: Influence of high caloric parenteral nutrition on catabolism and cellular immune competence in carcinoma patients. Aust. N.Z. J. Surg., 52:350–353, 1982.
23. Brennan, M. F.: Total parenteral nutrition in the cancer patient. N. Engl. J. Med., 305:375–382, 1981.
24. Burke, J. F., Wolfe, R. R., Mulhaney, C. J., et al.: Glucose requirements following burn injury: Parameters of optimal glucose infusion and possible hepatic and respiratory abnormalities following excessive glucose intake. Ann. Surg., 190:274–285, 1979.
25. Burt, M. E., Stein, T. P., Schwabe, J. G., and Brennan, M. F.: Effect of total parenteral nutri-

tion on protein metabolism in man. Cancer, 53:1246–1252, 1984.

26. Buzby, G. P., Mullen, J. L., Stein, T. P., and Rosato, E. F.: Manipulation of TPN caloric substrate and fatty infiltration of the liver. J. Surg. Res., 31:46–54, 1981.

27. Buzby, G. P., Mullen, J. L., Stein, T. P., Miller, E. E., Gobbs, C. L., and Rosato, E. F.: Host-tumor interaction and nutrient supply. Cancer, 45:2940–2948, 1980.

28. Carmichael, M. J., Clague, M. B., Keir, M. J., and Johnston, I. D. A.: Whole body protein turnover synthesis and breakdown in patients with colorectal carcinoma. Br. J. Surg., 67:736–739, 1980.

29. Cerra, F. B., Siegel, J. H., Coleman, B., et al.: Septic autocannibalism, a failure of exogenous nutrition support. Ann. Surg., 192:570–576, 1980.

30. Cerra, F. B., Upson, D., Angelico, R., Wiles, C., III, Lyons, J., Faulkenbach, L., and Paysinger, J.: Branched chains support postoperative protein synthesis. Surgery, 92:192–199, 1982.

31. Chandra, R. K., Chakraburty, S., and Chandra, S.: Malnutrition, humoral immunity and infection. Ind. J. Pediatr., 43:159–171, 1976.

32. Clague, M. B.: Turnover in pathological states. In Waterlow, J. C., and Stephen, J. M. L. (eds.): Nitrogen Metabolism in Man. London, Applied Science Publications, 1981, pp. 525–539.

33. Clowes, G. H. A., Heidman, M., Lindberg, B., et al.: Effect of parenteral alimentation on amino acid metabolism in septic patients. Surgery, 88:531–543, 1980.

34. Clowes, G. H. A., Jr., George, B. C., Villee, C. A., Jr., and Saravis, C. A.: Muscle proteolysis induced by a circulating peptide in patients with sepsis or trauma. N. Engl. J. Med., 308:545–552, 1983.

35. Cohn, S. H., Vartsky, D., Yasumura, S., Sawitsky, A., Zanzi, I., Vaswani, A., and Ellis, K. J.: Compartmental body composition based on total-body nitrogen, potassium and calcium. Am. J. Physiol., 239:E524–E530, 1980.

36. Conde, R., and Scornik, O. A.: Faster synthesis and degradation of liver protein during developmental growth. Biochem. J., 166:115–121, 1977.

37. Copeland, E. M., III, MacFadyen, B. V., Jr., and Dudrick, S. J.: Intravenous hyperalimentation in cancer patients. J. Surg. Res., 16:241–253, 1974.

38. Copeland, E. M., III, MacFadyen, B. V., Jr., Lanzotti, V. J., and Dudrick, S. J.: Intravenous hyperalimentation as an adjunct to cancer chemotherapy. Am. J. Surg., 129:167–173, 1975.

39. Copeland, E. M., III, MacFadyen, B. V., Jr., and Dudrick, S. J.: Effect of intravenous hyperalimentation on established delayed hypersensitivity in the cancer patient. Ann. Surg., 184:60–64, 1976.

40. Copeland, E. M., III, Daly, J. M., and Dudrick, S. J.: Nutrition as an adjuvant to cancer treatment in the adult. Cancer Res., 37:2451–2456, 1977.

41. Crane, C. W., Picou, D., Smith, R., and Waterlow, J. W.: Protein turnover in patients before and after elective orthopaedic operations. Br. J. Surg., 64:129–133, 1977.

42. Cuthbertson, D. P.: In Wilkinson, A. W., and Cuthbertson, D. (eds.): Metabolism and the Response to Injury. London, Pitman Medical, 1976, pp. 1–34.

43. Daly, J. M., Copeland, E. M., III, Guinn, E., and Dudrick, S. J.: Relationship of protein nutrition to tumor growth and host immunocompetence. Surg. Forum, 27:113–114, 1976.

44. Daly, J. M., Dudrick, S. J., and Copeland, E. M., III: Evaluation of nutritional indices as prognostic indicators in the cancer patient. Cancer, 43:925–931, 1979.

45. Daly, J. M., Reynolds, H. M., Rowlands, B. J., Dudrick, S. J., and Copeland, E. M., III: Tumor growth in experimental animals. Nutritional manipulation and chemotherapeutic response in the rat. Ann. Surg., 191:316–322, 1980.

46. Daly, J. M., Dudrick, S. J., and Copeland, E. M., III: Intravenous hyperalimentation: Effect on delayed cutaneous hypersensitivity in cancer patients. Ann. Surg., 192:587–592, 1980.

47. Dudrick, S. J., and Ruberg, R. L.: Principles and practice of parenteral nutrition. Gastroenterology, 61:901–910, 1971.

48. Dworkin, B., Daly, J., Massar, E., Alcock, N., Dudrick, S. J., and Copeland, E. M., III: Intravenously administered amino acids with either dextrose or lipid as nutritional support in surgical patients. Surg. Gynecol. Obstet., 156:577–581, 1983.

49. Elwyn, D. H., Kinney, J. M., Jeevanandam, M., et al.: Influence of increasing carbohydrate intake on glucose kinetics in injured patients. Ann. Surg., 190:117–127, 1979.

50. Elwyn, D. H.: Nutritional requirements of adult surgical patients. Crit. Care Med., 8:9–20, 1980.

51. Fairman, R. M., Crosby, L. O., Stein, T. P., Buzby, G. P., and Mullen, J. L.: Prehepatic total parenteral nutrition in the chair-adapted primate. J.P.E.N., 7:237–243, 1983.

52. Fischer, J. F.: The etiology of hepatic encephalopathy—nutritional implications. Acta Chir. Scand. [Suppl.] 507:50–68, 1981.

53. Fischer, J. E.: Nutritional support in the seriously ill patient. Curr. Prob. Surg., 17:466–531, 1980.

54. Flatt, J. P., and Blackburn, G. L.: The metabolic fuel regulatory system: Implications for protein sparing therapy during caloric deprivation and disease. Am. J. Clin. Nutr., 27:175–183, 1974.

55. Flatt, J. P.: Interactions between energy and protein metabolism in man. Z. Ernahrungswiss. [Suppl.] 23:58–71, 1979.

56. Fleming, R. C., and Magill, D. B.: Home parenteral nutrition: A primary therapy in patients with extensive Crohn's disease of the small bowel and malnutrition. Gastroenterology, 73:1077–1081, 1977.

57. Fosse, R. A., and Shizgal, H. M.: Serum albumin and nutritional status. J.P.E.N., 4:450–454, 1980.

58. Freund, H. R., Ryan, J. A., and Fischer, J. E.: Amino acid derangements in patients with sepsis: Treatment with branch chain amino acid rich infusions. Ann. Surg., 188:423–431, 1978.

59. Freund, H. R., Hoover, H. C., Atamian, S., and Fischer, J. E.: The effects of branched chain amino acids in decreasing muscle protein catabolism in vivo. Surgery, 83:611–618, 1979.

60. Freund, H. R., Yoshimura, N., and Fischer, J. E.: Does intravenous fat spare nitrogen in the injured rat? Am. J. Surg., 140:377–383, 1980.

61. Freund, H. R., Yoshimura, N., and Fischer, J. E.: The effect of branched chain amino acids and hypertonic glucose on post-injury catabolism in the rat. Surgery, 87:401–408, 1980.

62. Gamble, J. L.: Physiological information gained from studies on life raft ration. Harvey Lect., 42:247–273, 1946.

63. Garden, O. J., Smith, A., Harris, N. W. S., Shenkin, A., Sim, A. J. W., and Carter, D. C.: The effect of isotonic amino acid infusions on serum proteins and muscle breakdown following surgery. Br. J. Surg., 70:79–82, 1983.

64. Garlick, P. J., Clugston, G. A., and Waterlow, J. C.: Influence of low energy diets on whole body protein turnover in obese subjects. Am. J. Physiol., 238:E235–E244, 1980.

65. Garlick, P. J., McNurlan, M. A., Fern, E. B., Tomkins, A. M., and Waterlow, J. C.: Protein synthesis and breakdown after vaccination. Br. Med. J., 283:263–265, 1980.

66. Glass, R. E., Fern, E. B., and Garlick, P. J.: Whole-body protein turnover before and after resection of colorectal tumours. Clin. Sci., 64:101–108, 1983.

67. Goldberg, A. L., and Dice, J. F.: Intracellular protein degradation in mammalian and bacterial cells. Ann. Rev. Biochem., 43:845–869, 1974.

68. Golden, M. H. N., Waterlow, J. C., and Picou, D.: Protein turnover synthesis before and after recovery from protein-energy malnutrition. Clin. Sci., 53:473–477, 1977.

69. Golden, M. H. N., Golden, B. E., Harland, P. S. E. G., and Jackson, A. A.: Zinc and immunocompetence in protein-energy malnutrition. Lancet, 1:1226–1227, 1978.

70. Greenberg, G. R., Marliss, E. B., Anderson, G. H., et al.: Protein-sparing therapy in post-operative patients. N. Engl. J. Med., 294:1411–1416, 1976.

71. Gross, R. L., and Newberne, P. M.: Role of nutrition in immunologic function. Physiol. Rev., 60:188–302, 1980.

72. Groves, A. C., Woolf, L. I., Duff, J. H., and Finley, R. J.: Metabolism of branched-chain amino acids in dogs with *Escherichia coli* endotoxin shock. Surgery, 93:273–278, 1983.

73. Heatley, R. V., Williams, R. H. P., and Lewis, M. H.: Pre-operative intravenous feeding—a controlled trial. Postgrad. Med. J., 55:541–545, 1979.

74. Holter, A. R., and Fischer, J. E.: The effects of perioperative hyperalimentation on complications in patients with carcinoma and weight loss. J. Surg. Res., 23:31–34, 1977.

75. Hoover, H. C., Grant, J. P., Gorschboth, C., et al.: Nitrogen-sparing intravenous fluids in postoperative protein metabolism. N. Engl. J. Med., 293:172–175, 1975.

76. James, W. P. T.: The Cuthbertson Lecture: Protein and energy metabolism after trauma: Old concepts and new developments. Acta Chir. Scand. [Suppl.] 507:1–22, 1981.

77. Jeejeebhoy, K. N., Anderson, G. H., Nakooda, F., et al.: Metabolic studies in total parenteral nutrition with lipid in man. J. Clin. Invest., 57:125–136, 1976.

78. Jeejeebhoy, K. N., and Langer, B.: Total parenteral nutrition at home; studies in patients surviving four months to five years. Gastroenterology, 91:943–953, 1976.

79. Jurgens, P.: Parenteral nutrition studies four L-amino acid solutions in metabolically normal adults. J.P.E.N., 3:374–377, 1979.

80. Jurgens, P., Dolif, D., and Fondalinski, G.: Vergleichende ernahrungsstridien mit vier L-amino-saurelosungen bei 25 stoffwechselgesunden erwachsenen unter den bedingungen der totalen parenteralen ernahrung. Infusionther. Klin. Ernaehr., 5:141–154, 1978.

81. Kien, C. L., Young, V. R., Rohrbaugh, D. K., et al.: Increased rates of whole body protein synthesis and breakdown in children recovering from burns. Ann. Surg., 187:383–391, 1978.

82. Kien, C. L., Young, V. R., Rohrbaugh, D. K., and Burke, J. F.: Whole body protein synthesis and breakdown rates in children before and after reconstructive surgery of the skin. Metabolism, 27:27–34, 1978.

83. Kopple, J. D., Jones, M., Fukuda, S., et al.: Amino acid and protein metabolism in renal failure. Am. J. Clin. Nutr., 31:1532–1540, 1978.

84. Krebs, H. A.: Some aspects of the regulation of fuel supply in omnivorous animals. Adv. Enzyme Reg., 10:397–420, 1972.

85. Lanza-Jacoby, S., Sitren, H. S., Stevenson, N. R., and Rosato, F. E.: Changes in circadian rhythmicity of liver and serum parameters in rats fed a total parenteral nutrition solution by continuous and discontinuous intravenous or intragastric infusion. J.P.E.N., 6:496–502, 1982.

86. Lanzotti, V. C., Copeland, E. M., George, S. L., Dudrick, S. J., and Samuels, M. L.: Cancer chemotherapeutic response and intravenous hyperalimentation. Cancer Chemother. Rep., 59: 437–439, 1975.

87. Larsson, J., Liljedahl, S.-O., Schildt, B., Furst, P., and Vinnars, E.: Metabolic studies in multiple injured patients. Clinical features, routine chemical analyses and nitrogen balance. Acta Chir. Scand., 147:317–324, 1981.

88. Lickley, H. L., Track, N. S., Vranic, M., and Bury, K. D.: Metabolic responses to enteral and parenteral nutrition. Am. J. Surg., 135:172–176, 1978.

89. Lindberg, B., and Clowes, G. H. A.: The effects of hyperalimentation and infused leucine on amino acid metabolism in sepsis: An experimental study in vivo. Surgery, 90:278–291, 1981.

90. Lindsay D. B.: Amino acids as energy sources. Proc. Nutr. Soc., 39:53–59, 1980.

91. Long, C. L., Jeevanandam, M., Kim, B. M., and Blakemore, W. S.: Whole body protein synthesis and catabolism in septic man. Am. J. Clin. Nutr., 30:1340–1344, 1977.

92. Long, C. L., Birkhan, R. H., Geiger, J. W., and Blakemore, W. S.: Contribution of skeletal muscle protein in elevated rates of whole body protein catabolism in trauma patients. Am. J. Clin. Nutr., 34:1087–1093, 1981.

93. Long, J. M., Wilmore, D. W., Mason, A. D., and Pruitt, B. A., Jr.: Effect of carbohydrate and fat on nitrogen excretion during total intravenous feeding. Ann. Surg., 185:417–421, 1977.

94. Lowry, S. F., Goodgame, J. T., Norton, J. A., et al.: Effect of chronic protein malnutrition on host-tumor composition and growth. J. Surg. Res., 26:76–87, 1979.

95. Lundholm, K., Bylund, A-C., Holm, J., and Schersten, T.: Skeletal muscle protein metabolism in patients with malignant tumor. Europ. J. Cancer, 12:465–478, 1976.

96. Macfie, J., Smith, R. C., and Hill, G. L.: Glucose or fat as a nonprotein energy source. A controlled clinical trial in gastroenteral patients requiring

intravenous nutrition. Gastroenterology, *80*: 103–107, 1981.

97. Madsen, D. C.: Branched-chain amino acids: metabolic roles and clinical applications. *In* Johnston, I. D. (ed.): Advances in Clinical Nutrition. Lancaster, England, MTP Press, Ltd., 1982, pp. 3–23.

98. Maini, B., Blackburn, G. L., Bistrian, B. R., et al.: Cyclic hyperalimentation: An optimal technique for preservation of visceral protein. J. Surg. Res., *20*:515–525, 1976.

99. Maruyama, K., Sunde, M. L., and Swick, R. W.: Growth and muscle protein turnover in the chick. Biochem. J., *176*:573–582, 1978.

100. Matuchansky, C., Morichau-Beauchant, M., Druart, F., et al.: Cyclic (nocturnal) total parenteral nutrition in hospitalized adult patients with severe digestive diseases. Gastroenterology, *81*:433–437, 1981.

101. McArdle, A. H., Palmason, C., Morency, I., and Brown, R. A.: A rationale for enteral feeding as the preferable route for hyperalimentation. Surgery, *90*:616–623, 1981.

102. McCauley, R. L., and Brennan, M. R.: Serum albumin levels in cancer patients receiving total parenteral nutrition. Ann. Surg., *197*:305–309, 1983.

103. McIntyre, N., Holdsworth, C. D., and Turner, D. S.: Intestinal factors in the control of insulin secretion. J. Clin. Endocrinol. Metab., *25*: 1317–1324, 1965.

104. McIntyre, N., Turner, D. S., and Holdsworth, C. D.: The role of the portal circulation in glucose and fructose tolerance. Diabetologia, *6*:593–596, 1970.

105. Messing, B., and Bernier, J.-J.: Effects of two energy: nitrogen ratios in patients with gastroenterological disease and malnutrition. J.P.E.N., *4*:272–276, 1980.

106. Messing, B., Bitoun, A., and Galian, A.: Fatty liver during parenteral nutrition. Does it depend on the amount of calories given as glucose? Gastroenterol. Clin. Biol., *1*:1015–1025, 1977.

107. Mider, G. B.: Some tumour host relationships. Can. Cancer Conf., *1*:120–137, 1955.

108. Millward, D. J., Garlick, P. J., Nnanyelugo, D. O., and Waterlow, J. C.: The relative importance of muscle protein synthesis and breakdown in the regulation of muscle mass. Biochem. J., *156*:185–188, 1976.

109. Millward, D. J., Bates, P. C., Brown, J. G., Cox, M., and Rennie, M. J.: Protein turnover and the regulation of growth. *In* Waterlow, J. C., and Stephen, J. M. L. (eds.): Nitrogen Metabolism in Man. London, England, Applied Science Publishers, 1981, pp. 409–418.

110. Mirtallo, J. M., Schneider, P. J., Mavko, K., Ruberg, R. L., and Fabri, P. J.: A comparison of essential and general amino acid infusions in the nutritional support of patients with compromised renal function. J.P.E.N., *6*:109–113, 1982.

111. Moldawer, L. L., O'Keefe, S. J. D., Bothe, A., et al.: In vivo demonstration of nitrogen sparing mechanisms for glucose and amino acids in the injured rat. Metabolism, *29*:173–180, 1980.

112. Mullen, J. L., Buzby, G. P., Mathews, D. C., Smale, B. F., and Rosato, E. F.: Reduction of operative morbidity and mortality by combined preoperative and postoperative nutritional support. Ann. Surg., *192*:604–613, 1980.

113. Mullen, J. L.: Consequences of malnutrition in the surgical patient. Surg. Clin. North Am., *61*: 465–487, 1981.

114. Munro, H. N.: General aspects of the regulation of protein metabolism by diet and by hormones. *In* Mammalian Protein Metabolism. Munro, H. N., and Allison, J. B. (eds.): New York, Academic Press, Vol. 1, pp. 381–481.

115. Nixon, D. W., Lawson, D. H., Kutner, M., Ansley, J., Schwartz, M., Heymsfield, S., Chawla, R., Cartwright, T. H., and Rudman, D.: Hyperalimentation of the cancer patient with protein-calorie undernutrition. Cancer Res., *41*: 2038–2045, 1981.

116. Nixon, D. W., Moffitt, S., Lawson, D. H., Ansley, J., Lynn, M. J., Kutner, M. H., Heymsfield, S. B., Wesley, M., Chawla, R., and Rudman, D.: Total parenteral nutrition as an adjunct to chemotherapy of metastatic colorectal cancer. Cancer Treat. Rep., *65*(Suppl. 5):121–128, 1981.

117. Nordenstrom, J., Askanazi, J., Elwyn, D. H., Martin, P., Carpentier, Y. A., Robin, A. P., and Kinney, J. M.: Nitrogen balance during total parenteral nutrition. Ann. Surg., *197*:27–33, 1983.

118. Norton, J. A., Stein, T. P., and Brennan, M. F.: Whole body protein synthesis and turnover in normal man and malnourished patients with and without known cancer. Ann. Surg., *194*:123–181, 1981.

119. O'Keefe, S. J. D., Sender, P. M., and James, W. P. T.: "Catabolic" loss of body nitrogen in response to surgery. Lancet, 2:1035–1038, 1974.

120. Owen, O. E., Reichard, G. A., Boden, G., et al.: Interrelationships among key tissues in the metabolic utilization of substrates. *In* Katzen, H. M., and Mahler, R. I. (eds.): Advances in Modern Nutrition: Diabetes, Obesity, & Vascular Disease. New York, John Wiley & Sons, 1978, pp. 517–550.

121. Pencharz, P. B., Parsons, H., Motil, K., and Duffy, B.: Total body protein turnover in children: Is it a futile cycle? Med. Hypotheses, 7:155–160, 1981.

122. Peters, C., and Fischer, J. E.: Studies on calorie to nitrogen ratio for total parenteral nutrition. Surg. Gynecol. Obstet., *151*:1–8, 1980.

123. Piccone, V. A., LeVeen, H. H., Glass, P., et al.: Prehepatic hyperalimentation. Surgery, *87*:263–270, 1980.

124. Powanda, M. C.: Changes in body balances of nitrogen and other key nutrients: Descriptions and underlying mechanisms. Am. J. Clin. Nutr., *30*:1254–1268, 1977.

125. Pui, Y. M. L., and Fisher, H.: Factorial supplementation with arginine and glycine on nitrogen retention and body weight gain in the traumatized rat. J. Nutr., *109*:240, 1979.

126. Roche, A., Fabre, P., Crozat, R. P., Desplantez, J., and Sabathie, M.: Etude comparative de trois solutions d'acides amines de synthèse: Azonutril 25, Totamine concentré glucidique et Vamine en réanimation digestive post-opèratoire. À propos de 120 malades. Ann. Anesth. Franc., *4*:331–338, 1981.

127. Rose, D., Horowitz, G. D., Jeevanandam, M., Brennan, M. F., Shires, G. T., and Lowry, S. F.: Whole-body protein kinetics during acute starvation and intravenous refeeding in normal man. Fed. Proc., *42*:1070, 1983.

128. Rudman, D., Millikan, W. J., Richardson, T. J.,

Bixler, T. J., II, Stackhouse, W. J., and McGarrity, W. C.: Elemental balances during intravenous hyperalimentation of underweight adult subjects. J. Clin. Invest., 55:94–104, 1975.

129. Sakamoto, A., Moldawer, L. L., Palombo, J. D., Desai, S. P., Bistrian, B. R., and Blackburn, G. L.: Alterations in tyrosine and protein kinetics produced by injury and branched chain amino acid administration in rats. Clin. Sci., 64:321–331, 1983.

130. Sailer, D., and Muller, M.: Medium chain triglycerides in parenteral nutrition. J.P.E.N., 5:115–119, 1981.

131. Sitren, H. S., and Fisher, M.: Nitrogen retention in rats fed on diets enriched with arginine and glycine: I. Improved N retention after trauma. Br. J. Nutr., 37:195, 1977.

132. Skillman, J. J., Rosenoer, V. M., Smith, P. C., et al.: Improved albumin synthesis in postoperative patients by amino acid infusion. N. Engl. J. Med., 295:1037–1042, 1976.

133. Smith, M. F., Blackburn, G. L., Bistrian, B. R., and Griffin, R. E.: Beneficial effects of high nitrogen-calorie (N:Cal) ratios in intravenous hyperalimentation (IVH). Surg. Forum, 31:63–64, 1977.

134. Smith R., and Williamson, D. H.: Biochemical effects of human injury. Trends Biochem. Sci., 8:142–146, 1983.

135. Smith, R. C., Burkinshaw, L., and Hill, G. L.: Optimal energy and nitrogen intake for gastroenterological patients requiring intravenous nutrition. Gastroenterology, 82:445–452, 1982.

136. Souba, W. W., Long, J. M., and Dudrick, S. J.: Energy intake and stress as determinants of nitrogen excretion in rats. Surg. Forum, 29:76–78, 1978.

137. Starker, P. M., Askanazi, J., Lasala, P. A., Elwyn, D. H., Pump, F. F., and Kinney, J. M.: The effect of parenteral nutrition repletion on muscle, water and electrolytes. Ann. Surg., 198:213–217, 1983.

138. Steiger, E., Oram-Smith, J. C., Miller, E., Kuo, L., and Vars, H. M.: Effect of nutrition on tumor growth and tolerance to chemotherapy. J. Surg. Res., 18:455–461, 1975.

139. Stein, T. P., Leskiw, M. J., Oram-Smith, J. C., Miller, E. E., and Wallace, H. W.: The effect of a tumor on the host's protein metabolism. Cancer Res., 36:3936–3940, 1976.

140. Stein, T. P., Leskiw, M. J., Oram-Smith, J. C., and Wallace, H. W.: Changes in protein synthesis after trauma: Importance of nutrition. Am. J. Physiol., 233:348–355, 1977.

141. Stein, T. P., Mullen, J. L., Oram-Smith, J. C., Rosato, E. F., and Hargrove, W. C.: Relative rates of tumor, normal gut, liver and fibrinogen protein synthesis. Am. J. Physiol., 234:E648–E652, 1978.

142. Stein, T. P., Buzby, G. P., Gertner, M. H., Hargrove, W. C., Leskiw, M. J., and Mullen, J. L.: Effect of parenteral nutrition on protein synthesis and liver fat metabolism in man. Am. J. Physiol., 239:G280–G287, 1980.

143. Stein, T. P., Buzby, G. P., Rosato, E. F., and Mullen, J. L.: Effects of parenteral nutrition on protein synthesis in adult cancer patients. Am. J. Clin. Nutr., 34:1484–1489, 1981.

144. Stein, T. P., Buzby, G. P., Leskiw, M. J., Giandomenico, A. L., and Mullen, J. L.: Protein and fat metabolism in rats during repletion with parenteral nutrition (TPN). J. Nutr., 111:154–167, 1981.

145. Stein, T. P., Buzby, G. P., and Leskiw, M. J., and Mullen, J. L.: Parenteral nutrition and human gastrointestinal tumor protein metabolism. Cancer, 49:1476–1480, 1982.

146. Stein, T. P.: Nutrition and protein turnover, a review. J.P.E.N., 6:444–454, 1982.

147. Stein, T. P., Settle, R. G., Howard, K. A., and Diamond, C. E.: Protein turnover and physical fitness in man. Biochem. Med., 29:207–213, 1983.

148. Stein, T. P., Ang, S. D., Schluter, M. D., Leskiw, M. J., and Nusbaum, M.: Whole-body protein turnover in metabolically stressed patients with cancer as measured with [^{15}N] glycine. Biochem. Med., 30:59–77, 1983.

149. Stein, T. P., and Ang, S. D.: Effect of increasing TPN on protein metabolism. J.P.E.N., 7:525–529, 1983.

150. Stein, T. P., Presti, M. E., Leskiw, M. J., Torosian, M. H., Settle, R. G., Buzby, G. P., and Schluter, M. D.: Comparison of glucose, LCT and LCT plus MCT as calorie sources in parenterally nourished rats. Am. J. Physiol., 246:E277–E287, 1984.

151. Stein, T. P., Fried, R. C., Torosian, M. H., Leskiw, M. J., Leonard, J. M., and Buzby, G. P.: Effect of calorie source (glucose, LCT, MCT) on protein and energy metabolism in septic rats. Am. J. Physiol., in press.

152. Stoner, H. B.: An integrated neuro-endocrine response to injury. In Wilkinson, A. W., and Cuthbertson, D. (eds.): Metabolism and the Response to Injury. Tunbridge Wells, Pitman, 1976, p. 194.

153. Stoner, H. B., Little, R. A., Frayn, K. N., Elebute, A. E., Tresadern, J., and Gross, E.: The effect of sepsis on the oxidation of carbohydrate and fat. Br. J Surg., 70:32–35, 1983.

154. Torosian, M. H., Mullen, J. L., Miller, E. E., Zinsser, K. R., Stein, T. P., and Buzby, G. P.: Enhanced tumor response to cycle-specific chemotherapy by parenteral amino acid administration. J.P.E.N., 7:337–345, 1983.

155. Torosian, M. H., Mullen, J. L., Miller, E. E., Wagner, K. M., Stein, T. P., and Buzby, G. P.: Adjuvant, pulse total parenteral nutrition and tumor response to cycle-specific and cycle-nonspecific chemotherapy. Surgery, 94:291–299, 1983.

156. Torosian, M. H., Tsou, K. C., Daly, J. M., Mullen, L. J., Stein, T. P., Miller, E. E., and Buzby, G. P.: Alteration of tumor cell kinetics by pulse total parenteral nutrition. Cancer, 53:1409–1415, 1984.

157. Tulikoura, I., and Huikuri, K.: Changes in nitrogen metabolism in catabolic patients given three different parenteral nutrition regimens. Acta Chir. Scand., 147:519–524, 1981.

158. Tweedle, D. E.: Metabolism of amino acids after trauma. J.P.E.N., 4:165–172, 1980.

159. Waterlow, J. C.: The assessment of protein nutrition and metabolism in the whole animal, with special reference to man. In Munro, H. N. (ed.): Mammalian Protein Metabolism. New York, Academic Press, 1969, Vol. 3, pp. 325–390.

160. Waterlow, J. C., Garlick, P. J., and Millward, D. J.: Protein Turnover in Mammalian Tissues and the Whole Body. Amsterdam, Elsevier–North Holland, 1978.

161. Wilmore, D. W.: Alterations in protein, carbohydrate, and fat metabolism in injured and septic patients. J. Am. Coll. Nutr., 2:3–13, 1983.

162. Wolfe, B. M.: Substrate-endocrine interactions and protein metabolism. J.P.E.N., 4:188–194, 1980.

163. Wolfe, B. M., Culebras, J. M., Sim, A. J. W., et al.: Substrate interaction in intravenous feeding. Comparative effects of carbohydrate and fat on amino acid utilization in fasting man. Ann. Surg., 186:518–540, 1977.
164. Wolfe, R. R., Allsop, J. R., and Burke, J. F.: Glucose metabolism in man: Responses to intravenous glucose infusion. Metabolism, 28:210–220, 1979.
165. Wolfe, R. R., O'Donnell, T. F., Jr., Stone, M. D., et al.: Investigation of factors determining the optimal glucose infusion rate in total parenteral nutrition. Metabolism, 29:892–900, 1980.
166. Wolfe, R. R., Goodenough, R. O., Burke, J. F., and Wolfe, M. H.: Response of protein and urea kinetics in burn patients to different levels of protein intake. Ann. Surg., 197:163–171, 1983.
167. Wolman, S. L., Anderson, G. H., Marliss, E. B., and Jeejeebhoy, K. N.: Zinc in total parenteral nutrition: Requirements and metabolic effects. Gastroenterology, 76:458–467, 1979.
168. Wretlind, A.: Complete intravenous nutrition. Nutr. Metab., 14(Suppl.):1–57, 1972.

CHAPTER 6

Fluids, Electrolytes, and Body Composition

JORGE E. ALBINA
GEORGE MELNIK

The ability to deliver total parenteral nutrition has added a new dimension to fluid and electrolyte management. Classically, fluid and electrolyte therapy was directed mainly to the maintenance or restitution of the volume and composition of the extracellular fluid. Total parenteral nutrition (TPN) is concerned with the provision of elements for the conservation or repletion of the cellular compartment while also preserving the extracellular environment. As a consequence, the physical, chemical, and functional anatomy of all body compartments has to be considered when planning and delivering nutrition by vein. Patients receiving intravenous nutrition frequently have disturbances in body composition, alterations in the normal control mechanisms that guard the constancy of this composition, and a loss of the ability to regulate intake, a basic link in the homeostatic control chain.

In the early years of total parenteral nutrition, significant morbidity was related to lack of information regarding the requirements for intracellular electrolytes and trace elements. Our current knowledge permits reasonable estimations of these requirements, although our understanding is incomplete, as shown by the recent description of metabolic bone disease in long-term TPN,[1] new trace element deficiency states,[2] and the publication of sophisticated body composition studies in humans that reveal wide gaps in our understanding of the effects of intravenous nutrition on compositional changes in disease.

This chapter outlines the normal composition of the body, the changes brought about by starvation and injury, and the effects of intravenous feedings on the size and structure of the diverse compartments, mainly as related to their electrolyte constituents.

BODY COMPOSITION

The development of isotope dilution techniques and *in vivo* total body element analysis has provided a thorough knowledge of the anatomy of body minerals and their functional distribution in health and disease. The measurement of naturally occurring (^{40}K) or externally induced radioactivity for elemental analysis *in vivo*[3, 4] is developing rapidly. Because the results obtained by these methods do not substantially differ from those obtained by tracer dilution, the terminology used and results obtained by Moore and colleagues[5] using tracer dilution are used in this discussion.

Total Body Water

Water constitutes over one-half of body weight in normal individuals, and it functions as a structural component, a medium for chemical reactions, and a vehicle for interchange between the body cells and organs. Several substances are currently available for indirect measurement of total body water (TBW) by the dilution technique.[5-8] Deuterium oxide, tritium oxide, antipyrine, and N-acetyl-4-amino-pyrine have been used as markers, yielding values similar to those obtained through desiccation.[9]

Table 6–1 shows TBW as determined by diverse methods in males and females of different ages. Table 6–2, compiled by

Table 6–1. TOTAL BODY WATER (PERCENTAGE OF BODY WEIGHT) IN NORMAL HUMANS

| SUBJECTS | TOTAL BODY WATER BY VARIOUS METHODS* | | | | | |
	D_2O + AP (No.)	D_2O (No.)	SG (No.)	AP (No.)	HTO (No.)	Mean (All Methods) (No.)
Children						
0–1 mo.	75.7 (20)	—	—	—	—	—
1–12 mo.	64.5 (15)	—	—	—	—	—
1–10 yr.	61.7 (24)	—	—	—	—	—
Adults†						
10–16 yr. M	—	59.0 (9)	—	58.5 (2)	—	58.9 (11)
F	—	57.3 (7)	—	—	—	57.3 (7)
17–39 yr. M	—	60.4 (39)	61.4 (106)	59.9 (96)	57.5 (7)	60.6 (248)
F	—	51.4 (19)	53.8 (23)	44.6 (19)	—	50.2 (61)
40–59 yr. M	—	55.4 (8)	55.3 (78)	54.3 (28)	51.8 (13)	54.7 (127)
F	—	46.9 (5)	46.9 (29)	44.6 (4)	—	46.7 (38)
60+ yr. M	—	54.1 (3)	—	51.0 (17)	—	51.5 (20)
F	—	46.2 (5)	—	45.1 (9)	—	45.5 (14)

*D_2O = deuterium oxide; AP = antipyrine and its derivatives; SG = specific gravity; HTO = tritium oxide; No. = number of subjects.

†M = male; F = female.

(Adapted from Edelman, I. S., and Leibman, J.: Anatomy of body water and electrolytes. Ann. J. Med., 27:256, 1959.)

Table 6–2. TOTAL BODY WATER (TBW) BY SEX AND AGE

SEX	AGE GROUP (YEARS)	NO. SUBJECTS	MEAN BODY WT (KG)	MEAN TBW (L)	95% CONFIDENCE LIMITS OF MEAN AS % OF MEAN	RATIO (%) TBW (L) TO WEIGHT (KG)
Male	16–30	63	71.75	42.26	± 16	58.9
	31–60	56	73.57	40.24	± 17	54.7
	61–90	13	69.42	35.82	± 16	51.6
Female	16–30	54	60.89	30.99	± 13	50.9
	31–90	34	62.62	28.36	± 21	45.2

Predicted normal:

Males: $\dfrac{\text{TBW in L}}{\text{body wt in kg}} \times 100 = 79.45 - 0.24\ (\text{wt}) - 0.15\ (\text{age})$

Females: $\dfrac{\text{TBW in L}}{\text{body wt in kg}} \times 100 = 69.81 - 0.2\ (\text{wt}) - 0.12\ (\text{age})$

(*From* Randall, H. T.: Water, electrolytes and acid base balance. *In* Goodhart, R. S., and Shils, M. E. (Eds.): Modern Nutrition in Health and Disease. 6th ed. Philadelphia, Lea & Febiger, 1980, p. 356 with permission; data from Moore, F. D., Olsen, K. H., McMurrey, J. D., Parker, H. Y., Ball, M. R., and Boyden, C. M.: The Body Cell Mass and Its Supporting Environment. *In* Body Composition in Health and Disease. Philadelphia, W. B. Saunders, 1963.)

Randall[11] from data by Moore and colleagues,[5] also shows the effect of age and sex on total body water. From these data, it can be appreciated that TBW in normal young adult males averages approximately 55 ± 5 per cent of body weight. In females of comparable age it constitutes about 50 ± 5 per cent of body weight. The difference is explained by the larger ratio of water-free neutral fat to muscle in females. The progressive decrease of TBW with age is also apparent; this is also regarded as a consequence of the reduction in lean tissues and a relative expansion of body fat with aging. The reciprocal relation of TBW, body fat, and age has been consistently shown in a number of studies using different measuring techniques.[4, 12]

Moore and colleagues[5] derived regression equations for the prediction of TBW from body weight, age, and sex (see Table 6–2). Values calculated from these equations are useful in clinical practice, although the rather wide confidence limits of these estimates have to be kept in mind in any attempt to predict TBW in individual subjects.

Body fat, exclusive of the protoplasmic cellular elements in adipose tissue and its supportive connective component, constitutes the anhydrous phase of body weight. All measures of body water that are computationally related to body weight vary in relation to body fat. Evidently, different body fat contents in different individuals diminish the standardizing value of total body weight as a nutritional and metabolic frame of reference.

Total body water is kept constant by mechanisms that regulate fluid intake and output. This balance results in the maintenance of body weight within two per cent from day to day.[11] In patients on total parenteral nutrition, the mechanism that regulates intake, thirst, is bypassed by the intravenous infusion. Therefore, careful monitoring of clinical signs, urine output, and body weight are required to restore or maintain a normal state of hydration.[13]

The body experiences a daily turnover of about six per cent of its total water. Water entering the system comes from food, fluids or intravenous solutions, from the oxidation of hydrogen in carbohydrates, fat, and protein, and from the liberation of water bound to macromolecules.

Oxidation of foodstuffs in a normal diet provides about 20 to 25 gm of electrolyte-free water per 100 calories.[14, 15] In addition, tissue breakdown adds fluid to the total body pool. Lysis of 1 kg of lean tissue frees approximately 750 ml of intracellular water.[15] In the severely catabolic patient, this mechanism may add over 500 ml of water to the total body pool every day.[15] Normal kidney function disposes of this fluid and of the electrolytes and other solutes contained in it. If antidiuretic forces are in effect, this mechanism may not operate, and total body water will be expanded.

Oxidation of substrates contained in TPN solutions can also add to the body water pool, as seen in Table 6–3. Thus, approximately 500 ml of water from substrate oxidation can be derived from a representative total parenteral nutrition regimen, assuming all nutrients are oxidized for energy. In the presence of normal renal function, this volume of water from substrate oxidation will be easily managed. In critically ill patients with major fluid shifts and antidiuretic tendencies, dilutional hyponatremia may result.

Water losses from the body occur through the urine, stool, skin, and lung. Insensible water loss through vaporization from lung and skin amounts to approximately 800 to 1000 ml/day (0.6 ml/kg/hr in the afebrile patient in a thermally neutral environment).[16] This volume contains a very small amount of electrolytes and may be considered a free water loss. Fever or a warm environment may induce sweating with increased water and concomitant sodium losses. Additional external losses may occur from gastroenteric suction, wounds, and burns.

Redistribution of fluid in patients suffering from ileus and burns constitutes volume lost from functional body water. This phenomenon, "third spacing" of fluid following traumatic injury, was first described by Blalock[17] in 1930. Without changes in total body water, a fraction of the extracellular fluid is sequestered in the injured area after trauma, or in the gut during ileus, resulting in a decrease in circulating plasma volume

Table 6–3. CONTRIBUTION TO TBW FROM OXIDATION OF TPN SOLUTION SUBSTRATES

Intake (70% glucose, 30% fat, 90 gm amino acids)	40 kcal/kg
Water from carbohydrate oxidation	346 ml
Water from fat oxidation	100 ml
Water from protein oxidation	37 ml
Total water	483 ml

and functional extracellular water. Shires and associates[18] demonstrated that the degree of reduction of the functional extracellular fluid space is linearly related to the magnitude of trauma.

Minimal urine output is determined by the amount of substrate to be excreted and the patient's ability to concentrate the urine. Minerals, urea, and other metabolic waste materials constitute the main solutes to be excreted. This quantity can vary with different metabolic states and feeding regimens. In starvation, ketone bodies, urea, and electrolytes represent the major substrates requiring water for excretion. In this setting, feedings of small doses of carbohydrates reduce substantially the obligatory water loss by abolishing ketosis, decreasing urea production, and conserving sodium. Figure 6–1 shows the relationship between glomerular filtration rate, total solutes, urine output, and minimal urinary volume. High-protein feedings may result in a high production and excretion of nitrogen waste products and an increase in solute load. Hyperglycemia with glycosuria will also increase the minimal water loss.

Murray and co-workers[13] distinguished water balance from fluid balance. Water balance must take into consideration all the different fractions of intake and output mentioned previously. Some of these fractions (e.g., insensible and fecal water losses) are generally not measured outside the research setting. Fluid balance, which considers sensible water intake and output corrected with an estimate of insensible losses, is generally acceptable for clinical management. Frequent weighing of the patient combined with good intake and output records will result in a reasonably adequate accounting of water balance.[11] Day-to-day changes in body weight will closely reflect changes in total body water.[16]

Body Fluid Compartments

Body water is described as occupying two major compartments: intracellular and extracellular.

Intracellular Fluid

Intracellular water (ICW) is that portion of TBW contained within cell membranes. It represents between 50 and 55 per cent of TBW (30 and 33 per cent of body weight) in normal healthy adults.[5] There is an inverse relationship between ICW and total body fat and age: a leaner, younger, more muscular individual has a higher ICW/TBW ratio than an elderly female or an obese subject. Pitts[19] pointed out that intracellular water is neither a continuous nor a homogeneous phase and that it includes the fluid content of different populations of cells, probably with diverse water contents and chemical structures. Even within one cell, ionic distribution may vary among the different intracellular compartments and organelles; for example, it is known that magnesium and calcium are concentrated in the mitochondria[20, 21] and that sodium may be accumulated in the cell nucleus.[22] Despite these variations, the concept of a single intracellular compartment is useful in describing the organization of water in the whole organism.[10]

Extracellular Fluid

The extracellular water (ECW) compartment includes plasma and lymph water, interstitial water, transcellular fluids, and water contained in noncellular support structures such as tendons, dermis, fascia, collagen, and bone. Although conceptually extracellular water is a well-defined space (all water not contained in cells), its measurement is difficult with present methodology.[5, 8, 10, 19]

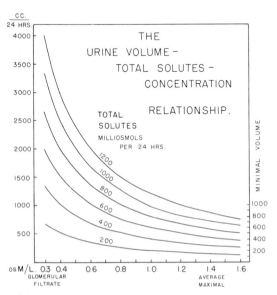

Figure 6–1. The relationship between glomerular filtration rate, total solutes, urine output, and minimal urinary volume. (From Gamble, J. L.: Chemical Anatomy, Physiology, and Pathology of Extracellular Fluid. Cambridge, Harvard University Press, 1964, p. 49, with permission.)

Moore and colleagues[5] believed biologic validation of the extracellular volume to be impossible. According to Edelman and Leibman,[10] "The heterogeneity of the extracellular space makes it unlikely that any dilution method will be suitable for accurate definition of all the nonintracellular water and electrolytes."

Extracellular water can therefore be estimated only from the space of distribution of substances that are excluded from cell water. Large molecules, generally saccharides that do not enter cells, are also precluded by their size from penetrating and equilibrating in all extracellular fluid in a reasonable time and yield rather low values for extracellular water.[5, 6, 10] In contrast, small anions like chloride and bromide with rapid equilibration times do permeate cell membranes to some extent and consequently have larger spaces of distribution. For clinical purposes, extracellular volume can be estimated as being approximately 20 to 23 per cent of body weight in the healthy individual.[11, 15]

The intercellular space has to be conceived as nonhomogeneous, with various types and concentrations of macromolecules, such as proteins and carbohydrates, in different tissues. The intermolecular spaces in such gels may differ markedly among tissues, thus modifying the local permeability for the different markers, with the smaller solutes gaining access to smaller spaces between and within the larger structural molecules.

The difficulties in the quantification of extracellular volume should be remembered when one is considering that intracellular water is not measurable by dilution techniques but is derived from total body water minus extracellular water.

Electrolytes

Extracellular Ions. The intracellular and extracellular fluid compartments have greatly different mineral contents. The extracellular fluid contains about 1500 mEq of sodium at concentrations between 138 and 145 mEq/L.[15] Neutron activation analysis[23] and isotope dilution studies[8] measure different body sodium contents. Although the first method detects all body sodium, the second method measures only "exchangeable sodium," the fraction of total body sodium that equilibrates rapidly with the injected isotope and is equal to approximately 65 per cent of total body sodium. Of the exchangeable sodium, 85 per cent is within the extracellular fluid and 15

per cent is contained within cells and other nonaqueous sites, mainly adsorbed to bone crystals.[10] Five to 10 per cent of total body sodium is held in bone, does not rapidly exchange with the radioactive sodium tracer, and is referred to as *residual sodium*. Total body sodium varies considerably with body build, as a function of extracellular fluid; females and obese individuals have smaller extracellular fluid and therefore proportionately less total body sodium.

The total body chloride content of the average adult male is approximately 2,300 mEq.[5] Chloride is mainly an extracellular anion found in low concentration in bone and in high concentration in some components of connective tissue such as collagen. Intracellular chloride is high in red blood cells and gastric mucosa.[11]

Bicarbonate, which is generated by the hydration of carbon dioxide, and protein constitute the other quantitively important extracellular anions. The difference in concentrations of soluble proteins in plasma and interstitial fluid is due mainly to the relative difficulty with which large molecules pass through the capillary endothelium and the subsequent removal of them from the interstitium by lymphatic flow. The gradient in protein content between plasma and interstitial fluid determines differences in electrolyte concentration in both spaces, as explained by the Gibbs-Donnan equilibrium.[19]

Because of its low molecular weight and high concentration in plasma, albumin is responsible for most of the plasma colloid-osmotic pressure. Although clinically important in the regulation of intravascular volume as the major determinant of effective osmotic pressure, serum albumin represents only 0.2 per cent of total plasma osmolarity, with the electrolytes being responsible for most of the remainder.[24] Only 38 to 45 per cent of total body albumin is intravascular.[25] This protein exerts a low colloid-osmotic pressure in interstitial fluid because it is diluted in the larger extravascular space.

Intracellular Ions. Whereas sodium and chloride are mainly extracellular ions, potassium is located almost completely in the intracellular space.[10] Total body exchangeable potassium content is approximately 2,900 to 3,300 mEq, when measured by ^{42}K dilution.[5] In addition, total body potassium can be derived from the measurement of the radioactivity of naturally occurring ^{40}K, which represents 0.0118 per cent of total body potassium.[3, 4] (See articles by Goode[4] and Moore[26] for discussions of the technique and interpretative difficulties of the method.)

Total exchangeable potassium represents 85 to 95 per cent of total body potassium as measured by ^{40}K counting.[10] The intracellular location of potassium at a rather constant concentration and its relationship with intracellular protein allowed Moore and colleagues[5] to derive the concept of the body cell mass. As defined by these researchers, *body cell mass* is the compartment of body composition containing the oxygen-exchanging, potassium-rich, glucose-oxidizing, work-performing tissue. It is a pure culture of living cells and a logical reference entity for the consideration of the energy conversion of foodstuffs, oxygen requirements, carbon dioxide production, and work performance.[5]

Anatomically, the body cell mass consists of all cellular components of the body and represents about 35 per cent of body weight in the normal subject. Compositionally, it is defined by intracellular water, intracellular protein, and intracellular potassium, since total body potassium, as pointed out before, is over 90 per cent intracellular. Only about 60 mEq of the almost 3,200 mEq of total body potassium are located in the extracellular space.

Kinney and associates[27] found a good correlation between energy expenditure and exchangeable potassium. This relationship was nonlinear, with a tendency for energy expenditure to plateau at higher levels of exchangeable potassium. The authors interpreted this result as being a consequence of the nonhomogeneous nature of the body cell mass as related to resting energy expenditure. A visceral compartment with constantly active metabolism and a muscle compartment with low resting energy utilization contain most of the exchangeable potassium. At rest, the higher the ratio of muscle mass to visceral cell mass, the lower the change in energy expenditure with increases in exchangeable potassium.

A key assumption of Moore's calculations regarding the body cell mass is a constant relationship of intracellular potassium to nitrogen at a ratio of approximately 3 mEq of potassium per gram of nitrogen. This assumption is shared by other methods of determining body composition.[3, 28] Moore[26] states that when new intracellular protein is synthesized, potassium and nitrogen are deposited in this ratio, and that when protein is lost as a result of starvation, the losses of potassium and nitrogen maintain the aforementioned stable proportion. According to this relationship, changes in total body potassium can be equated with changes in the size of the body cell mass.[28]

Flear and colleagues[29] proposed that the potassium content of cells is determined by the cellular anions whose charges are not balanced by sodium ions. Sodium ion concentration itself is regulated by membrane pump activity. Studies in muscle have shown that potassium and other monovalent ions exist in both free and bound forms.[30] Free ions exist in concentrations that are determined by Gibbs-Donnan equilibrium. The bound fraction equilibrates with the free ions and is apparently associated with the contractile proteins.

Scribner and Burnell[31] proposed the concepts of total body potassium capacity and content. As defined by these authors, *total body potassium capacity* is determined by all anions outside the extracellular space that are capable of holding or binding potassium ions. Protein constitutes the largest component of this capacity. Glycogen has also been shown to hold 0.34 gm of potassium per gm.[32, 33] *Total body potassium content*, on the other hand, reflects the degree to which the potential potassium-holding capacity is saturated. With this interpretation, several compositional alterations can be associated with a decrease in total body potassium. Both potassium content and its binding capacity can be reduced concurrently, resulting in a small but normally composed body cell mass. Alternatively, potassium content can be reduced out of proportion with a reduction in capacity, resulting in an unsaturated capacity that would avidly retain potassium on refeeding. The importance of this distinction to interpretation of studies reporting changes in total body potassium in starvation and refeeding is discussed later.

Nichols and co-workers have associated the potassium capacity concept with Ling's[35] view of muscle function.[35] According to Ling's hypothesis, ions and water within cells are not in free solution. Ions are mostly adsorbed to macromolecules whose affinity for different elements is determined by the energy state of the tissue. In conditions of high ATP production and content, proteins have fixed charges with high potassium-binding affinity. A relative lack of energy substrates would result in a decrease in the number of sites occupied by potassium and an increased affinity of the macromolecules for sodium. The potassium capacity concept, whether related or not to the energy states of the cells, serves to view changes of total body potassium from a different perspective.

Summary

Total body water and its subdivision into intracellular water and extracellular water constitute a good basis for the description of body composition in health and disease. Intracellular fluid (the potassium space) defines the size of the active body cell mass. Extracellular fluid (the sodium and chloride spaces) defines the internal milieu in which the cells live.

Although considered for this discussion as two independent volumes, extracellular fluid and intracellular fluid extensively and rapidly interchange, as do the solutes dissolved in them. Exogenous intake of water and solutes, as well as the production of metabolic intermediates by the cells, add continuously to the differential composition and osmolalities of either or both fluid compartments. These differences are not tolerated by the body in health and are dispelled by rapid homeostatic responses. No osmolality gradient between intracellular and extracellular fluids persists for any extended period. Water and solute shifts rapidly reinstate equilibrium. The presence of nondiffusible solutes like organic phosphates, proteins, and other metabolic substrates and intermediates (most of which behave as anions at physiologic pH) in the cellular compartment constrain cations like potassium and magnesium to the intracellular phase, thus distributing them asymmetrically according to the Gibbs-Donnan equilibrium. This action is counterbalanced by the pump-driven motion of sodium toward the extracellular fluid. Although the sodium pump activity seems *prima facie* essential for cell volume regulation, pump inhibition with ouabain or ethacrinic acid does not result in progressive cell swelling or cell wall disruption.[29] Other factors may help maintain cell volume regulation, such as the degree of ionic binding to protein[11] and the charge of the intracellular matrix material.[29] The intracellular organic ion milieu is complex and poorly understood. The regulation of intracellular metabolite content within low and constant concentrations by variations in enzyme activity and substrate uptake and disposal avoids the changes in cell volume that would result if these concentrations were to vary widely.[29, 36]

STARVATION AND INJURY

The water and electrolyte content of the body and their distribution are deeply affected by starvation and injury. According to Moore,[37] "The common denominators of disease are three in number: loss of body cell mass, gain in extracellular water and oxidation of fat. The rate at which these three occur and the balance between them determine the clinical picture observed in a variety of disease states." It is difficult to separate the starvation component from independent, disease-related changes in body composition induced by injury or disease. The changes in water and electrolytes brought about by simple starvation have been well described. Although different in magnitude, the qualitative changes induced by starvation in lean and obese subjects are very similar, and data from studies in both groups can be reviewed together.[32, 38]

In acute starvation, rapid weight loss parallels increased water loss[39] and exceeds what can be predicted from caloric deprivation alone.[40] The water deficit is thought to result from increased urine output[41] and has been shown by isotope dilution techniques to be equal to the weight loss during the first two weeks of fasting.[39] Spark and associates[42] have proposed that the increased urine output may be secondary to an initial expansion of plasma volume brought about by a fluid shift from the gastrointestinal tract. Others have failed to detect an increase in urinary volume and have proposed an increase in insensible water loss during early starvation in obese subjects.[43, 44] In either case, most of the weight loss in the first few days of starvation is accounted for by a negative water balance. The deficit is marked in the first four to five days, and then rapidly diminishes, and after ten days of fasting, the daily water loss becomes relatively constant.[32]

The Extracellular Fluid in Starvation

Most of the early water loss in starvation originates from the extracellular fluid. There is a decrease in plasma volume during the first ten days of fasting, which may be in the order of 14 to 20 per cent of the original volume.[32] The magnitude of the initial loss of extracellular fluid has been estimated as being about 1.6 L in the first two days of fasting and a total of approximately 2 L after five days of starvation.[45] The total water loss after a one-month fast in lean subjects is approximately 7 L, as determined in balance studies.[32]

If fasting continues, the loss of extracellular fluid is reduced markedly. Water and sodium are conserved, and the catabolism of the body cell mass results in a proportionally high extracellular water content in the starving individual.[15] Spark suggested that the hypoalbuminemia of prolonged fasting results in a diminished plasma volume, triggering reflex mechanisms that result in water and sodium conservation. Others have found an increased plasma volume in starving subjects.[46]

Sodium metabolism is altered during starvation. In the first few days of fasting, a brisk natriuresis is the rule. During the first day, sodium losses are usually between 50 and 250 mEq.[41, 42, 48] After eight to ten days, sodium excretion decreases to very low levels (1 to 15 mEq/day) and remains low during the remainder of the fast.[32, 42, 47, 49] Lean subjects lose about 350 mEq of sodium in a 15-day fast. The mechanism for the initial sodium loss is not known. It is probably not related to ketone body excretion,[16, 50] although this mechanism may be operational in the early fast, before maximum urinary ammonium production is reached.[32] Spark and associates[42] discussed the possibility of an altered sensitivity of the kidney to mineralocorticoids and proposed that glucagon may modulate this differential sensitivity. They observed increased natriuresis in fed subjects infused with glucagon in doses that resulted in plasma levels similar to those found by others during starvation.[51, 52, 53]

After the first week or two of fasting, the sodium content of the urine is substantially decreased, as pointed out before. Total exchangeable sodium remains virtually unchanged in prolonged starvation, although there is a small, continuing negative water balance.[39] Smith and Drenick[39] found a decrease in total body water in obese subjects after prolonged fasting. The observation of lower total body water content with constant exchangeable sodium and plasma sodium concentrations was interpreted by the authors as evidence of a stable extracellular fluid volume. They proposed that sodium has to move either into bone or to the intracellular space to account for the observed changes in total body water and exchangeable sodium during fasting.[39]

The constant volume of the extracellular fluid during starvation represents an increase in the fraction of total body water that is extracellular, although the body cell mass and fat deposits are diminishing during starvation. The constancy of the extracellular fluid was observed by Keys and associates,[46] who measured the thiocyanate space in normal volunteers during semistarvation. They found this space to represent in these circumstances 34 per cent of body weight. After refeeding, it decreased to a mean of 23.5 per cent of body weight.

The mechanism for sodium and water conservation in prolonged fasting is unknown. Changes in aldosterone and other hormones have not been consistently documented.[32] Potassium depletion with an intracellular sodium shift has been proposed as a potential mechanism, because a potassium chloride load during fasting results in an increased sodium excretion.[16]

The Intracellular Fluid in Starvation

During starvation, major changes also occur in the intracellular water compartment. The oxidation of cell substrates results in net production of free water in the amounts discussed previously. In addition, water normally bound to macromolecules such as glycogen and protein is free to diffuse to the extracellular fluid after these compounds are metabolized. Glycogen is deposited in the liver and muscle, with 3 to 4 gm of water per gram of polysaccharide.[54] Liver glycogen catabolism frees approximately 400 ml of electrolyte-free water in the first two to three days of fasting, whereas muscle glycogen utilization can be calculated to release 600 to 700 ml of water during this period.[32] Water bound to protein amounts to 3 ml/gm of protein.[32] Knowledge of nitrogen excretion during the fast allows for the calculation of the amount of water freed by protein catabolism. Gamble[16] and associates[55] pointed out that the oxidation of cellular protein requires the removal of intracellular water to maintain the cell's protein/volume ratio and requires additional water loss to excrete the end-products of protein metabolism.

Initial losses of potassium during a fast parallel those of sodium.[16] The origin of this excreted potassium is obviously mainly intracellular, since the extracellular potassium pool is small and the concentration of this ion in plasma does not change greatly during fasting.[46] Because lean tissue contains approximately 60 mEq of potassium per kg, a one-month fast will result in a loss of approximately 300 mEq of potassium. Balance studies performed during fasts confirm these calculations. Lean subjects lose 30 to 40 mEq/day over the initial ten days of fasting. Deficits at the end of one month of fasting amount to between 450 and 500 mEq, and at that time, daily potassium loss continues at a rate of 10 to 15 mEq per day.[42, 48, 56]

Starvation is characterized by a low total body potassium. This has been equated with a loss of body cell mass. Although the previous discussion of total body potassium supports this concept, the extent of the losses may not agree with the degree of body cell mass catabolism. Gamble and co-workers[55] studied children who fasted for four to 15 days. Over the duration of the fast, there was a decrease in the ratio of potassium lost to nitrogen lost in the urine. The mean ratio of potassium loss to nitrogen loss for the 15 days was 3.11 mEq of potassium per gram of nitrogen, remarkably close to the potassium/nitrogen ratio found in muscle tissue. When the data are analyzed for consecutive three-day periods, they show a K/N ratio of 4.2 in the first three days and a decrease to 2.68 during the last three days. This observation would agree with a mixed loss of muscle and nonmuscle lean tissue, the latter having a lower potassium/nitrogen ratio.[57] Potassium losses during a short-term fast could therefore be explained by a loss of lean body mass without a selective potassium depletion. These studies, as well as others showing that during prolonged fasting the ratio of potassium loss to nitrogen loss resembles the potassium/nitrogen ratio of tissue, have supported the concept that potassium losses quantify lean body mass deficits. Despite this, the variability in the experimental data justified the statement by Keys and colleagues[46] that "There are enough discrepancies to make this explanation highly questionable."

Abbott and co-workers[58, 59] performed metabolic balance studies on normal subjects who underwent short-term fasts and on surgical patients receiving diverse amounts of postoperative nutrition. Normal subjects lost an average of 5.6 mEq of potassium per gram of nitrogen while receiving a small number of calories and no potassium or nitrogen. The excess potassium loss was not explained.

Those patients who underwent surgery also had a very high potassium loss compared with nitrogen output (K/N = 4.5 to 6).

Urinary potassium losses during fasting can be modified by several factors. Sodium supplemention during fasting results in a higher potassium loss, whereas nitrogen output remains unchanged.[16, 49, 56] The provision of potassium during starvation magnifies sodium losses and reduces potassium excretion, changing the K/N ratio to less than 2.[16] The progressive potassium conservation that is seen in prolonged fasting and that has been attributed to a decreased lean body mass breakdown with starvation adaptation[60–62] could be secondary to a decreased sodium ion presentation to the distal tubule for exchange with potassium,[48] because sodium supplementation reverses potassium conservation. It has also been reported that potassium intake prior to a fast can modulate potassium excretion.[54]

These data point out that although potassium losses in starvation generally parallel body cell mass wasting, they are not an infallible index of tissue catabolism and that, to a certain extent, potassium losses in starvation are determined by factors different from those that affect protoplasmic losses. This concept is also substantiated by the finding that on refeeding, potassium balance returns to equilibrium or positivity much earlier than nitrogen balance.

As will be discussed later, changes in total body potassium have been equated with efficacy of nutritional support in short- and long-term studies. For this premise to be valid, potassium loss or gain has to reliably measure the body cell mass. If factors other than changes in the body cell mass can modulate total body potassium, the validity of this concept is questionable.

For this reason, the origin of the potassium losses seen in malnutrition and injury needs to be analyzed and correlated with changes in the body cell mass. If intracellular potassium can be depleted independently of cellular protein losses, then it could be expected to increase independently of protein accretion on refeeding.

Smith and Waterlow[63] described a decrease in total body potassium in malnourished children who had a mean total body potassium content of 27.9 ± 3.0 mEq/kg on admission to the hospital and of 38.9 ± 2.8 mEq/kg on recovery from malnutrition. These authors showed a significant correlation between total body potassium and muscle potassium when this latter value was expressed per DNA phosphorus. As indirect evidence of intracellular potassium depletion, they observed that those subjects with low total body potassium had difficulty excreting a load of ammonium chloride.

Frenk and co-workers[64] studied the water and electrolyte composition of muscle in 22 children suffering from malnutrition. Most subjects had diarrhea, and 30 per cent presented with edema. Muscles were characterized by an increased water content with normal potassium content. There was a marked decrease in muscle potassium in the edematous children. The ratio of potassium to noncollagenous nitrogen was less than that found in normal children. Alleyne and colleagues[65] have shown a good correlation between total body potassium and creatinine excretion, suggesting no differential loss of potassium in malnutrition.

Nichols and associates[66] studied children with edematous protein-calorie malnutrition who were fed a baseline diet (0.7 gm protein, 70 kcal, and 4 mEq potassium per kg per day) for two weeks and then a high-protein, high-calorie diet (3 gm protein and 120 kcal per kg per day) with similar potassium supplements. No change in weight, creatinine excretion, or serum protein levels was observed during the administration of the baseline diet. The repletion diet resulted in an increase in body weight, muscle mass, body fat, and serum albumin. Muscle biopsies performed at admission and at the time of diet changeover showed a low initial muscle potassium (whether expressed per muscle wet weight or per dry, fat-free weight) and no increase in muscle potassium until ten days after the high-protein, high-calorie diet was started. Water content of muscle was high at admission and declined during refeeding. The lack of change in muscle potassium with the maintenance diet was interpreted by the authors as an absence of a differential potassium deficiency in muscle or, using Scribner and Burnell's[31] terminology, an absence of desaturation of the muscle potassium capacity. When the subjects were fed a diet that resulted in growth, muscle potassium content increased when expressed in relation to muscle fat-free wet weight; there was no change in muscle potassium in relation to muscle fat-free dry weight. These last two findings probably indicate an increase in the potassium capacity of the muscle.

Balance studies have shown that potassium retention on refeeding is greater than would be predicted from growth of normal tissues. Alleyne and co-workers[67] investigated whether the reduced total body potassium seen in malnourished children represented a loss of tissues that contain potassium or whether it was due to a low potassium content of the remaining tissues by measuring total body potassium by ^{40}K and muscle potassium in muscle biopsies. They observed a very constant level of muscle potassium over a wide range of total body potassium values. Only those children with a total body potassium below 30 mEq/kg body weight showed a significantly decreased muscle potassium. These results were interpreted as showing a decreased muscle potassium capacity at higher levels of total body potassium and a decreased content with total body potassium less than 30 mEq/kg.

SUMMARY

At least in malnourished children and within a wide range of total body potassium contents, changes in total body potassium follow changes in body protein, or total body potassium capacity, without a desaturation of this capacity. Increases in body potassium seen on refeeding probably reflect increases in potassium capacity and are a good index of lean body mass growth.

Fluid and Electrolytes in Injury

Acute injury is followed by characteristic fluid and electrolyte distortions that tend to maintain plasma volume and tissue perfusion. Sodium retention and water retention are mediated by alterations of kidney function that are both hormonal (aldosterone, ADH, renin-angiotensin) and local (peritubular, capillary hemodynamic autoregulation, and redistribution of renal blood flow). The formation of "third spaces" in injured areas or in the gastrointestinal tract distort normal body composition even more, as discussed before. The combination of these factors with the other changes induced by injury-associated starvation results in complex alterations in body composition.

Bergstrom[68, 69] and colleagues[70] have pioneered the needle biopsy technique for the study of muscle composition in humans. They have shown increases in extracellular fluid and in muscle sodium content after trauma, burns, and sepsis that correlate with the severity of the insult. In addition, they observed a decrease in muscle potassium after trauma, concluding that this change was associated with increased muscle protein breakdown and did not represent a reduction of the intracellular potassium concentration, with maintenance of the capacity/content ratio.

Lehr and associates[71] studied total exchangeable potassium by ^{40}K counting in a group of patients suffering from a variety of disease processes. They also measured total body water by titrated water dilution and extracellular space by ^{82}Br distribution. They found a reduction of total body potassium in patients who were starved or had high-output gastrointestinal fistulas or Crohn's disease. These second and third groups had larger decreases in total body potassium. Because no changes were found in total body water or in extracellular water, the authors concluded that the intracellular potassium concentration was reduced in patients with fistulas or Crohn's disease. Their findings disagreed with previously discussed information regarding the relative expansion of extracellular fluid in disease and starvation.

Cunningham and co-workers[72] compared muscle electrolytes in normal subjects and critically ill patients. They described an increased intracellular sodium content in the muscles of critically ill subjects with no changes in intracellular potassium. Nichols and colleagues[73] studied the changes in muscle composition that occurred in rhesus monkeys suffering a sublethal infection with *Salmonella typhimurium*. They observed a reduction in intracellular potassium concentration that correlated with an increase in muscle fiber content of water and sodium.

EFFECTS OF NUTRITIONAL SUPPORT ON BODY COMPOSITION

The changes in body composition during intravenous nutrition of patients suffering from injury and starvation have been studied in a variety of ways, including metabolic balances,[74] muscle biopsy,[75] and total body element contents by dilution techniques or whole body counting.[76–78] Analysis of results is difficult owing to patient heterogeneity,

inadequate or nonexistent controls, poor definition of data, and a lack of consideration of the shortcomings and limitations of the methodology given in many of the publications on this topic. We will briefly analyze the landmark publications in this area and formulate some tentative conclusions.

In general terms, adequate total parenteral nutrition results in weight gain. A knowledge of the composition and compartmental distribution of this gain is important to evaluate the efficacy of nutritional support. Some of the compositional changes observed during intravenous feedings are similar to those induced by oral refeeding of starved subjects. We will first discuss those alterations that are known to occur during oral feeding of fasting or starving individuals and then those changes that occur during intravenous nutrition.

Changes Induced by Oral Feeding

Gamble[16] demonstrated that carbohydrates fed during a fast to normal volunteers resulted in decreased urinary water and sodium losses. Because carbohydrate feeding also resulted in diminished ureagenesis and reduced urea excretion, these results were partially explained by a concurrent reduction in nitrogen excretion. Ketosis and ketonuria were also abolished by carbohydrate feedings, therefore decreasing obligatory water loss. The reduction in sodium excretion by carbohydrate feedings went unexplained. It is remarkable that the maximal sodium conservation occurred with a glucose load that produced only half the maximal nitrogen sparing.

Bloom[50, 79] and Bloom and Mitchell[47] studied water and sodium conservation during refeeding in obese subjects who had fasted for varying periods. When 600 calories were provided in the form of glucose after 72 to 192 hours of fasting, there was an almost complete cessation of sodium excretion in the urine. Weight loss promptly stopped, and if sodium was given with the carbohydrate meal, the subjects retained sodium and showed a weight gain that persisted for several days. When refed protein and fat rather than glucose (also at the level of 600 kcal/day), the subjects continued to lose weight and showed no decrease in sodium excretion. The authors speculated that the effects of glucose feeding on sodium excreted "must be related to some finite range of change in carbohydrate metabolism, not to the presence or absence of carbohydrate. In other words, this phenomenon must be related to an excess of carbohydrate in the metabolic mixture greater than can be provided from normal protein catabolism."[79]

Veverbrants and Arky[44] obtained comparable results when they studied obese subjects at the end of a three-day fast. Feeding carbohydrate at a level of 600 kcal/day resulted in a weight gain of almost half a kilogram and a marked reduction in urinary sodium. When this dose of carbohydrate was given after the subjects consumed a 2340-calorie diet daily for one week, a prompt natriuresis resulted. This finding suggests that the transition from fed to starved state and back to fed state, rather than the absolute amount of carbohydrate given, determined the level of sodium excretion. When fat was substituted isocalorically for carbohydrate at the end of a fast, no sodium-sparing effect was evoked. Protein feeding had a delayed effect in reducing sodium excretion. Katz and associates[80] obtained similar results when fasting obese volunteers interrupted their fast by eating 500 calories of carbohydrate or, alternatively, a protein-fat mixture. Carbohydrate refeeding resulted in a marked reduction of sodium and urea excretion and the correction of the ketosis of fasting. The protein-fat meal also resulted in a decreased sodium output, but this effect occurred later and was quantitatively smaller than that seen with carbohydrate feedings. Of interest was the observation that the protein meal induced higher urea excretion but did not alleviate ketosis. The need for fixed base to accompany ketone bodies and the requirement for extra water diuresis to solubilize urea have been proposed as mechanisms to explain the water and sodium diuresis of fasting.[16] The data of Katz and associates[80] appear to contradict this hypothesis.

Boulter and co-workers[81] isocalorically substituted fat for carbohydrates in a 1500-calorie diet. When the daily carbohydrate intake was reduced to 50 grams or less, they observed a marked increase in urinary sodium comparable with that seen in fasting experiments. After five days of a low-carbohydrate diet, sodium output decreased and a positive sodium balance was observed. Isocaloric substitution of protein for carbohydrate failed to modify urinary sodium excretion. A study reported by Garnett and Nahmtas[82] followed sodium excretion after a short fast in normal, nonobese subjects. Refeeding with 25 grams of glucose resulted in a 35 per cent decrease in sodium excretion.

Several hypotheses have been offered to explain the natriuresis of fasting and the antinatriuresis of refeeding. Changes in aldosterone secretion have been found to be both associated[41, 83] and not related[44, 80, 85] to these phenomena. Spark and associates[42, 86] have proposed that aldosterone has variable potency in diverse metabolic circumstances, with subnormal activity during fasting and supranormal activity during refeeding. In support of this hypothesis, they reported that a large dose of aldosterone antagonist (1200 mg of spironolactone) abolished the antinatriuresis of refeeding,[81] whereas normal therapeutic doses were not effective.[86]

Glucagon has also been postulated to be involved in the regulation of sodium conservation and excretion. The antinatriuresis of glucose refeeding has been reported to be abolished by glucagon,[42] and the provision of glucagon to fed individuals increases sodium excretion.[52, 53]

The potential involvement of insulin in the regulation of sodium excretion was explored by Hoffman and colleagues.[87] These investigators fed 100 grams of carbohydrate to normal volunteers after an overnight fast or after a 72-hour fast. In both cases, there was an increase in circulating insulin, but whereas interrupting the 72-hour fast resulted in a marked decrease in urinary sodium and potassium, giving carbohydrate after an overnight fast produced an increase in sodium and potassium excretion. In contrast, DeFronzo and co-workers[88, 89] found that insulin consistently decreased sodium excretion in humans independent of any changes in aldosterone, blood glucose, glomerular filtration rate, and renal plasma flow.

In summary, refeeding in fasting or starved individuals with carbohydrate results in a reduction of sodium and water excretion, and when sodium is provided simultaneously, the subjects can gain weight rapidly through expansion of extracellular space. The mechanism for this phenomenon has not been elucidated.

Changes Induced by Intravenous Nutrition

A similar response to high-calorie, high-carbohydrate intravenous feedings has been described. Randall[11] reported a weight gain of two to four per cent over initial weight when patients were started on total parenteral nutrition. Other authors have reported increases in extracellular fluid in patients on total parenteral nutrition.[90] An increase in extracellular fluid was calculated by Heymsfield and associates[91] when they refed cachectic patients intravenously. In general terms, the response to high-calorie, high-volume intravenous nutrition could be predicted from the degree of starvation of the patient prior to the institution of therapy. Heymsfield and associates[91] stressed the changes in cardiovascular function that follow starvation. A rapid increase in extracellular fluid in a patient with reduced cardiac reserve can result in overt heart failure.

When injury is added to simple starvation, strong antidiuretic tendencies occur. It is predictable that patients who are both starved and injured will respond to high-carbohydrate feedings with expansion of the extracellular compartment. The result of short-term studies on the effects of body composition of total parenteral nutrition should be interpreted in this light. The volume, electrolyte content, and calorie source of TPN solutions may determine changes in body composition and compartmental distribution that are probably independent of any nutritional effect.

The results of TPN have been evaluated using both balance studies and body composition analysis. Positive nitrogen balance with adequate TPN has been extensively documented. Balances of other elements have been less frequently reported. Rudman and co-workers[74] conducted balance studies in underweight subjects fed intravenously with glucose as the main calorie source. These studies were conducted over six-day periods, and different elements were withdrawn or added, one at a time, to the nutrient solution during succeeding periods. Several points of interest can be derived from this work:

1. A complete mixture, containing a calorie source, nitrogen, potassium, sodium, and phosphorus, was necessary for positive nitrogen balance.

2. When nitrogen was deleted from the diet, the balances of the other elements became negative.

3. At all levels of nitrogen intake, the ratio of retention of nitrogen and the other elements was constant (nitrogen 1 gm, phosphorus 0.08 gm, potassium 3.1 mEq, sodium 3.5 mEq, chloride 2.7 mEq).

4. According to the authors, the ratios of N/P/K demonstrated that the retained elements went mainly toward forming protoplasm.

5. Sodium and chloride retention showed a concurrent expansion of the extracellular fluid space.

6. Extracellular fluids increased by 0.8 gm per gm of protoplasm formed.

7. Calculations from the previous observations suggested that weight gain during TPN consisted of 35 to 50 per cent protoplasm, 35 to 50 per cent extracellular fluid, five to 25 per cent adipose tissue, and less than one per cent bone.

8. Potassium withdrawal resulted in an expansion of extracellular fluid without changes in intracellular fluid volume.

9. Infusions without sodium resulted in a large decrease of extracellular fluid volume with marked expansion of the calculated adipose tissue stores.

It has to be kept in mind that actual water balances during this study were not reported and that the above-mentioned changes in body compartments were derived from calculations. It is also of interest that nitrogen retention improved substantially with each stepwise increase in nitrogen infusion. Because of the shortness of the study periods and the lack of information regarding changes in total body urea, this improvement in nitrogen balance may have been related to the mass effect of increased protein intake.

The reported gain of 3 mEq of potassium per gram of nitrogen matched very closely the values used by Moore[5] for the intracellular potassium/nitrogen ratio. This ratio resembles the composition of muscle and is higher than that of nonmuscle lean body mass.[3] The measured K/N balance ratio does not leave room for any expansion of extracellular nitrogen, which represents about 40 per cent of total body nitrogen as calculated from K/N and total body nitrogen data from Cohn and associates.[3]

Other investigators using different techniques for measuring body composition have reported similar findings. Shoemaker and associates[92] studied five patients on glucose-based total parenteral nutrition receiving 60 to 80 kcal/kg/day. Although they found an expanded extracellular fluid compartment (7.2 ± 1.2 L above predicted) and a decreased intracellular compartment (5.4 ± 0.7 L below expected) at the start of the study, the authors observed that two to five weeks of TPN resulted in an average weight gain of 1 kg with a mean decrease of extracellular fluid of

2.4 L and increases in total body water and intracellular fluid of 1.2 and 3.7 L, respectively. In a later publication, the same group reported similar results in nine patients before and after total parenteral nutrition.[93] They found a 27 per cent increase in intracellular water after two to three weeks of total parenteral nutrition.

As previously mentioned, all calculations of intracellular fluid are derived from total body water and extracellular water measurements. The assumptions made in the calculations of extracellular water in critically ill subjects make the absolute values given for intracellular water tentative. Changes in the cellular penetration of extracellular fluid markers (radiolabeled bromide in this case) due to illness and/or refeeding can markedly distort the results.

Shizgal[76, 77] and Spanier and Shizgal[94] calculated the ratio of extracellular fluid to intracellular fluid from total exchangeable sodium and total exchangeable potassium. When approximately 50 kcal/kg/day were delivered to their patients for about two weeks, increases in body cell mass, as assessed by calculated total exchangeable potassium, were detected without major changes in extracellular space. These studies and others[95, 96] utilized total body potassium as an index of body cell mass. Changes in total body potassium were thus interpreted as changes in protoplasmic mass. This approach has been questioned.

In a series of papers, Jeejeebhoy and colleagues[78, 92, 98] reported their measurements of total body potassium by ^{40}K and of total body nitrogen by neutron activation analysis in patients receiving TPN for different periods of time. Feeding regimens were not described beyond a statement that a glucose and fat mixture constituted the energy source.[78] The patients reported in these studies either received a short-term (less than 40 days) course of TPN or were on home total parenteral nutrition and were studied for up to 33 months after initial baseline determinations. The patient population was heterogeneous regarding weight loss and diagnosis. In the short-term studies,[97, 98] a small increment in total body potassium above the error of the measurement was detected. Although some patients had changes in total body nitrogen, no correlation was found between these changes and those in total body potassium. The authors concluded that the increase in lean body weight, as estimated by anthropometry, reflected a gain of water

and potassium but not of nitrogen and that, therefore, the cellular potassium content must have changed independently of nitrogen.

The long-term home TPN patients[78] had a reportedly different response. There was a mean increase of total body nitrogen of 30 per cent and an increase in body weight of ten per cent, with little change in total body potassium. The discordance between changes in total body nitrogen and total body potassium in some patients was remarkable. Some of the patients had total body nitrogen gains above 500 grams, which if converted to cell mass should have resulted in marked changes in body weight. Some of the same patients lost weight while on the study. Gains of nitrogen in extracellular compartment or major changes in body fat and water would be needed to explain these results. It is unfortunate that nutrient balances were not reported, because 60 per cent of the patients had short-bowel syndrome and would be expected to have increased fecal fluid and mineral losses.

Jeejeebhoy and colleagues[78, 97, 98] contended that malnourished patients may have increased intracellular water volume and correspondingly augmented total body potassium. Under this assumption, refeeding would result in loss of fluid and reduction of cell volume and potassium content. The elevation of the nitrogen/potassium ratio seen during refeeding was interpreted as secondary to the restoration of nonmuscle lean body mass with little rebuilding of the muscle compartment. Cohn and associates,[99] however, using neutron activation analysis and a mathematical compartmental model derived by Burkinshaw and colleagues,[57] found no changes in nonmuscle lean body mass in patients with cancer and severe weight loss. Muscle is generally believed to be the main source of nitrogen loss in starvation and after trauma, whereas the protein losses from the viscera are proportionately smaller under these circumstances.[100] Even if maximal reduction of visceral size and protein stores were considered, the amounts of nitrogen gain in several individual patients of the Jeejeebhoy studies appear to be too large to be satisfactorily explained by rebuilding of these tissues.

Other authors have used whole-body potassium analysis and muscle biopsies to evaluate the response to TPN. Goode[4] presented a detailed discussion of the use of total body potassium as an indicator of nutritional status. He stated that this determination is an invalid index of the body cell mass in those conditions in which intracellular potassium content has changed. Among other circumstances in which this concentration can be altered he listed hyperaldosteronism, acid-base changes, diabetes, the immediate postoperative period, and shock. Data obtained by this method in rapidly changing clinical situations or in short-term studies should therefore be interpreted carefully.

Bocking and associates[95] measured exchangeable potassium by ^{42}K dilution in 13 patients on total parenteral nutrition with hypertonic dextrose and amino acids and in 12 patients who received 60 per cent of their calorie supply as intravenous fat emulsion and 40 per cent as dextrose, with similar amino acid intake. The study population was heterogeneous, including patients with cancer, burns, and sepsis. The authors observed a maintenance of total exchangeable potassium at calorie intakes of approximately 32 to 34 kcal/kg/day. The two calorie sources, glucose and glucose with fat, were equally effective in maintaining or increasing total body potassium. The group of septic and burned patients had a decrease in total body potassium. All patients in this group received less than 30 kcal/kg/day. No correlation was found between protein intake and changes in total body potassium.

King and associates[101] studied 15 consecutive patients suffering a variety of critical illnesses, including cancer and enterocutaneous fistulas. All of them had lost weight and eight were septic. These patients were on total parenteral nutrition, receiving between 34 and 64 total kcal/kg/day for 11 to 26 days. All patients were judged to be improved clinically, and they maintained weight during the study. Muscle biopsies were performed before and after the course of nutritional support. Muscle biopsies were also obtained in eight normal subjects as controls. In whole muscle, the authors found a high correlation between total nitrogen and fat-free dry solids. Water content per fat-free dry weight was higher before TPN in patients than in normal controls, and it did not change after TPN. No difference was found in the ratio of potassium to fat-free dry weight between patients and controls, and no changes were seen after total parenteral nutrition. Extracellular water was increased in the patients before and after TPN. It was concluded that the changes observed proba-

bly reflected an increase in muscle extracellular fluid and that total parenteral nutrition did not change intracellular water. The authors stated that this last finding was not surprising in view of persistent sepsis in half of the study patients.

Hill and co-workers[102] studied 25 patients who were critically ill and on total parenteral nutrition for at least 14 days, receiving an average of 38.1 nonprotein kcal/kg/day and nitrogen at 0.3 gm/kg/day. The patients were selected on the basis of receiving 14 days of intravenous nutrition, consenting to a muscle biopsy, and showing weight gain during the study. Neutron activation analysis was used to determine multi-element body composition. Muscle biopsies were performed and the specimens analyzed for electrolyte content. The subjects had an average weight gain of 2.6 kg, which was interpreted as being mainly secondary to an increase in extracellular water. The patients also showed a significant increase in total body potassium. There was an increase in total body nitrogen of 30 gm over the 14 days of the study; this increase represented approximately 750 gm of lean body mass. The authors interpreted the observed increase in total body potassium as a normalization of intracellular potassium, because the pre-TPN muscle biopsies showed a decrease in intracellular potassium concentration.

The same group reported their findings in 20 surgical patients receiving total parenteral nutrition for 11 to 40 days at 31 to 72 kcal/kg/day.[103] They confirmed the results of the previous study, namely, weight gain representing increased total body water and minimal changes in total body nitrogen as determined by neutron activation analysis. They found no correlation between daily change in total body nitrogen and caloric intake.

A further study from the same group compared intravenous nutrition with glucose alone versus intravenous nutrition utilizing fat emulsions to provide 60 per cent of nonprotein calories.[104] The patients once again represented a heterogeneous population. Results showed that those subjects receiving dextrose had an increase in body weight comparable with that of patients receiving fat emulsions as a calorie source. The glucose group gained total body water with minimal changes in total body protein, whereas the fat emulsion group gained a smaller amount of water and had a significant increase in total body nitrogen.

McPhee and colleagues[105] studied 16 gastroenterologic patients receiving TPN for two weeks. Two groups of patients received comparable amounts of calories and nitrogen, but one of the study groups received 30 units of insulin per 1006 kcal of nutrient solution. The two groups of patients had similar increases in body weight, body fat, and body water. Total body protein was maintained to the same extent. Those patients receiving insulin demonstrated a significant increase in total body potassium.

Smith and associates[106] reported the result of a prospective study providing two levels of energy intake as glucose through the intravenous route to gastroenterologic patients. A group receiving an average of 40 kcal/kg/day maintained energy balance but lost body protein. The maintenance of body weight was due to water retention. A second group of patients, receiving a higher calorie intake, increased body fat, protein, and water. The authors concluded that a high calorie intake was needed to promote lean tissue synthesis.

Starker and co-workers[90] reported a prospective study of total parenteral nutrition and preoperative repletion in malnourished patients undergoing major abdominal surgery. Each patient received one week of intravenous nutrition prior to operation, with a caloric intake calculated to be approximately 1.5 times estimated resting energy expenditure. One group of patients responded with reductions in extracellular fluid and weight loss and a rise in serum albumin, and there was only one complication in 16 surgical procedures. A second group of patients showed weight gain, fluid retention, and decrease in serum albumin; in this group, eight patients developed a total of 15 postoperative complications. The authors proposed that the response to preoperative nutrition may be an important factor in assessing operative risk and mortality.

Conclusions

From the previous data, some conclusions can be drawn and new questions arise. Increases in body cell mass seem to relate to the provision of a complete nutrient mix and an adequate caloric intake. The extent of malnutrition and the nature and severity of the disease process probably modify the response to nutritional support.

The reported increases in total body potassium without concurrent changes in total body nitrogen or in muscle composition may represent changes in whole-body glycogen stores[67] or in the activities of cellular membrane pumps. Alterations of cell membrane function have been described in malnutrition,[107] and some evidence suggests that these alterations can be reversed during refeeding. Curreri and associates[108] showed that burn patients had abnormally high red blood cell intracellular sodium and that a hypercaloric diet promoted its normalization within three to five days.

Lastly, it would be extremely informative if studies of body compositional changes induced by intravenous feeding using whole-body element analysis would also report nutrient balances. Data from whole body element analysis have wide confidence limits, and small differences in element retention, of potential clinical significance in short-term studies, can probably be better detected with careful balance records.

REFERENCES

1. Bone disease resulting from total parenteral nutrition (editorial). Nutr. Rev., 39:268, 1981.
2. Abumrad, N. N., Schneider, A. J., Steel, D., et al.: Amino acid intolerance during prolonged total parenteral nutrition reversed by molybdate therapy. Am. J. Clin. Nutr., 34:2551, 1981.
3. Cohn, S. H., Vartsky, D., Yasumura, S., Sawitsky, A., Zanzi, I., Vaswani, A., and Ellis, K. J.: Compartmental body composition based on total body nitrogen, potassium and calcium. Am. J. Physiol., 239:E524, 1980.
4. Goode, A.: Total body potassium as an index of nutritional status. In Karran, S. J., and Alberti, K. G. M. M. (eds.): Practical Nutritional Support. New York, John Wiley & Sons, 1980.
5. Moore, F. D., Olsen, K. H., McMurrey, J. D., Parker, H. V., Ball, M. R., and Boyden, C. M.: The Body Cell Mass and Its Supporting Environment. In Body Composition in Health and Disease. Philadelphia, W. B. Saunders, 1963, pp. 3–11.
6. Edelman, I. S., Olney, J. M., James, A. H., et al.: Body composition: studies in the human being by the dilution principle. Science, 115:447, 1952.
7. Edelman, I. S., and Moore, F. D.: Body water, water distribution and water kinetics as revealed by the use of deuterium oxide. J. Clin. Invest., 30:637, 1951.
8. Moore, F. D.: Determination of total body water and solids with isotopes. Science, 104:157, 1946.
9. Pace, N., Kline, L., Schachman, H. K., and Hartenist, M.: Studies on body composition. IV: Use of radioactive hydrogen for measurement in vivo of total body water. J. Biol. Chem., 168:459, 1947.
10. Edelman, I. S., and Leibman, J.: Anatomy of body water and electrolytes. Am. J. Med., 27:256, 1959.
11. Randall, H. T.: Water, electrolytes and acid base balance. In Goodhart, R. S., and Shils, M. E. (eds.): Modern Nutrition in Health and Disease,

6th ed. Philadelphia, Lea & Febiger, 1980, pp. 355–394.

12. Novak, L. P., Hyatt, R. E., and Alexander, J. F.: Body composition and physiologic function of athletes. J.A.M.A., *205*:764, 1968.

13. Murray, R. L., Schaffel, N. A., Geiger, J. W., Long, C. L., and Blakemore, W. S.: Body composition changes in the critically ill patient: Emphasis on water balance. J.P.E.N., *3*:219, 1979.

14. Darrow, D. C., and Pratt, E. L.: Fluid therapy—Relation to tissue composition and the expenditure of water and electrolytes. J.A.M.A., *143*:365, 1950.

15. Moore, F. D.: Metabolic Care of the Surgical Patient. Philadelphia, W. B. Saunders, 1959, pp. 5–24.

16. Gamble, J. L.: Chemical Anatomy, Physiology and Pathology of the Extracellular Fluid, 6th ed. Cambridge, Harvard University Press, 1960.

17. Blalock, A.: Experimental shock: The cause of low blood pressure caused by muscle injury. Arch. Surg., *20*:959, 1930.

18. Shires, E. T., Williams, J., and Brown, W.: Acute changes in extracellular fluids associated with major surgical procedures. Ann. Surg., *154*:803, 1961.

19. Pitts, R. F.: Physiology of the Kidney and Body Fluids, 3rd ed. Chicago, Year Book Medical Publishers, 1974, pp. 22–43.

20. Carafoli, E., Rossi, C. S., and Lehninger, A. L.: Cation and anion balance during active accumulation of calcium and magnesium by isolated mitochondria. J. Biol. Chem., *239*:3055, 1964.

21. Vasington, F. D., and Murphy, J. V.: Calcium uptake by rat kidney mitochondria and its dependence on respiration and phosphorylation. J. Biol. Chem., *237*:2670, 1962.

22. Alfrey, V. G., Meudt, R., Hopkins, J. W., and Mirsky, A. E.: Sodium dependent transport reactions in the cell nucleus and their role in protein and nucleic acid synthesis. Proc. Natl. Acad. Sci. U.S.A., *47*:907, 1961.

23. Hill, G. L., and Beddoe, A. H.: In vivo neutron activation in metabolic and nutritional studies. I: Introduction. J. Clin. Surg., *1*:270, 1982.

24. Chinard, F. P.: Body water: Compartments and distribution. *In* Clinical Fluid and Electrolyte Management (II). Oklahoma, Veterans Adm. Dept. of Med. and Surg., 1981, pp. 18–41.

25. Rothschild, M. A., Oratz, M., and Schreiber, S. S.: Albumin synthesis (I). N. Engl. J. Med., *286*:748, 1972.

26. Moore, F. D.: Energy and the maintenance of the body cell mass. J.P.E.N., *4*:228, 1980.

27. Kinney, J. M., Lister, J., and Moore, F. D.: Relationship of energy expenditure to total exchangeable potassium. Ann. N.Y. Acad. Sci., *110*:711, 1963.

28. Spanter, A. H., and Shizgal, H. M.: Caloric requirements of the critically ill patient receiving intravenous hyperalimentation. Am. J. Surg., *133*:99, 1977.

29. Flear, C. T. G., Bhattacharya, S. S., and Singh, C. M.: Solute and water exchanges between cells and extracellular fluids in health and disturbances after trauma. J.P.E.N., *4*:98, 1980.

30. Hinke, J. A. M., Caille, J. P., and Gayton, D. C.: Distribution and state of monovalent ions in skeletal muscle based on ion electrode, isotope and diffusion analyses. Ann. N. Y. Acad. Sci., *204*:274, 1973.

31. Scribner, B. H., and Burnell, J. H.: Interpretation of the serum potassium concentration. Metabolism, *5*:468, 1956.

32. Drenick, E. J.: The effects of acute and prolonged fasting and refeeding on water, electrolyte and acid-base metabolism. *In* Maxwell, M. H., and Kleeman, C. R. (eds.): Clinical Disorders of Fluid and Electrolyte Metabolism, 3rd ed. New York, McGraw-Hill Book Co., N.Y. 1980.

33. Fenn, W. O.: The deposition of potassium and phosphate with glycogen in rat liver. J. Biol. Chem., *128*:297, 1939.

34. Nichols, B. L., Alvarado, J., Hazlewood, C. F., and Viteri, F.: Clinical significance of muscle potassium depletion in protein-calorie malnutrition. J. Pediatr., *80*:319, 1972.

35. Ling, G.: A Physical Theory of the Living State: The Association Induction Hypothesis. Blaisdell, N.Y., 1962, pp. 438–448.

36. Atkinson, D. E.: Limitation of metabolite concentration and the conservation of solvent capacity in the living cell. *In* Horecker, B. L., and Stadman, E. R. (eds.): Current Concepts in Cellular Regulation, Vol. 1. New York, Academic Press, 1969.

37. Moore, F. D.: Clinical implications of research on body composition. N. Y. Acad. Sci., *110*:814, 1963.

38. Levenson, S. M., Barbul, A., and Seifter, E.: Some biochemical, endocrinologic and immunologic changes and adaptations following starvation. *In* Richards, J. R., and Kinney, J. M. (eds.): Nutritional Aspects of Care in the Critically Ill. Edinburgh, Churchill-Livingstone, 1972.

39. Smith, R., and Drenick, E. J.: Changes in body water and sodium during prolonged starvation for extreme obesity. Clin. Sci., *31*:437, 1966.

40. Benedict, F. G.: A study of prolonged starvation. Carnegie Institute Publ. 203, Washington, D.C., 1915.

41. Rapoport, A., From, G. L., and Husdan, H.: Metabolic studies in prolonged fasting. I. Inorganic metabolism and kidney function. Metabolism, *14*:31, 1965.

42. Spark, R. F., Arky, R. A., Boulter, P. R., Saudek, C. D., and O'Brian, J. T.: Renin, aldosterone and glucagon in the natriuresis of fasting. N. Engl. J. Med., *292*:1335, 1975.

43. Bloom, W. L.: Fasting as an introduction to the treatment of obesity. Metabolism, *8*:214, 1959.

44. Veverbrants, E., and Arky, R. A.: Effects of fasting and refeeding. I. Studies on sodium, potassium and water excretion on a constant electrolyte and fluid intake. J. Clin. Endocrinol. Metab., *29*:55, 1969.

45. Winkler, A. W., Danowski, T. S., Elkington, J. R., and Peters, J. P.: Electrolyte and fluid studies during water deprivation and starvation in human subjects and the effect of ingestion of fish or carbohydrate and of salt solutions. J. Clin. Invest., *23*:807, 1944.

46. Keys, A., Brozek, J., Heuschel, A., Nickelson, O., and Taylor, H. L.: The Biology of Human Starvation, Vol. 1. Minneapolis, University of Minnesota Press, 1950, pp. 273–285.

47. Bloom, W. L., and Mitchell, W.: Salt excretion of fasting patients. Arch. Intern. Med., *106*:321, 1960.

48. Weinsier, R. L.: Fasting. A review with emphasis on the electrolytes. Am. J. Med., *50*:233, 1971.

49. Magoe, H.: Changes in blood volume during ab-

solute fasting with and without sodium chloride administration. Metabolism, 17:133, 1968.

50. Bloom, W. L.: Carbohydrates and water balance. Am. J. Clin. Nutr., 20:157, 1967.

51. O'Brian, J. T., Saudek, C. D., Spark, R. F., et al.: Glucagon induced refractoriness to exogenous mineralocorticoid. J. Clin. Endocrinol. Metab., 38:1147, 1974.

52. Saudek, C. D., Boulter, P. R., Spark, R., et al.: Glucagon: The natriuretic hormone of starvation? Clin. Res., 20:556, 1972.

53. O'Brian, J. T., Saudek, C. D., Spark, R. F., et al.: Glucagon: A potent mineralocorticoid antagonist. Clin. Res., 21:499, 1973.

54. Heymsfield, S. B., McManus, C., Stevens, V., and Smith, J.: Muscle mass: Reliable indicator of protein-energy malnutrition severity and outcome. Am. J. Clin. Nutr., 35:1192, 1982.

55. Gamble, J. L., Ross, S. G., and Tisdall, G.: The metabolism of fixed base during fasting. J. Biol. Chem., 57:633, 1923.

56. Drenick, E. J., Blahd, W. H., Singer, F. R., and Lederer, M.: Body potassium content in obese subjects and potassium depletion during prolonged fasting. Am. J. Clin. Nutr., 18:278, 1966.

57. Burkinshaw, L., Hill, G. L., and Morgan, D. B.: Assessment of the distribution of protein in the human body by in vivo neutron activation analysis—Nuclear activation techniques in the life sciences. International Atomic Energy Agency - Sm. 227 - 39, Vienna, 1979.

58. Abbott, W. E., Levey, S., and Krieger, H.: Metabolic changes in surgical patients in relation to water, electrolytes, nitrogen and caloric intake. In Moore, F. D. (ed.): Metabolism in Post-Traumatic State. New York, Grune & Stratton, 1960.

59. Abbott, W. E., and Albertsen, K.: The effect of starvation, infection and injury on the metabolic processes and body composition. Ann. N. Y. Acad. Sci., 110:941, 1963.

60. Cahill, G. F., Jr., Owen, O. E., and Morgan, A. P.: The consumption of fuels during complete starvation. Adv. Enzymol., 6:143, 1968.

61. Felig, P., Marliss, E., Owen, O. E., and Cahill, G. F., Jr.: Blood glucose and gluconeogenesis in fasting man. Arch. Intern. Med., 123:293, 1969.

62. Owen, O. E., Morgan, A. P., Kemp, H. G., et al.: Brain metabolism during fasting. J. Clin. Invest., 46:1589, 1967.

63. Smith, R., and Waterlow, J. C.: Total exchangeable potassium in infantile malnutrition. Lancet, 1:147, 1960.

64. Frenk, S., Metcoff, J., Gomez, F., et al.: Intracellular composition and homeostatic mechanisms in severe chronic infantile malnutrition. Pediatrics, 20:105, 1957.

65. Alleyne, G. A., Viteri, F., and Alvarado, J.: Indices of body composition in infantile malnutrition: Total body potassium and urinary creatinine. Am. J. Clin. Nutr., 23:875, 1970.

66. Nichols, B. L., Alvarado, J., Hazlewood, C. F., and Viteri, F.: Clinical significance of muscle potassium depletion in protein-calorie malnutrition. J. Pediatr., 80:319, 1972.

67. Alleyne, G. A., Millward, D. J., and Scullard, G. H.: Total body potassium, muscle electrolytes and glycogen in malnourished children. J. Pediatr., 76:75, 1970.

68. Bergstrom, J.: Muscle electrolytes in man. Scand. J. Clin. Lab. Invest., 14(Suppl. 68):1, 1962.

69. Bergstrom, J., Alvestrand, A., Furst, P., et al.: Influence of severe potassium depletion and subsequent repletion with potassium on muscle electrolytes, metabolytes and amino acids. Clin. Sci., 51:589, 1976.

70. Bergstrom, J., Furst, P., Chao, L., et al.: Changes in muscle water and electrolytes with severity of trauma. Acta Chir. Scand. (Suppl.) 494:139, 1979.

71. Lehr, L., Schober, O., Hundeshagen, H., et al.: Total body potassium depletion and the need for preoperative nutritional support in Crohn's disease. Ann. Surg., 196:709, 1982.

72. Cunningham, J. N., Carter, N. W., Rector, F. C., and Seldon, D. W.: Resting transmembrane potential difference of skeletal muscle in normal subjects and severely ill patients. J. Clin. Invest., 50:49, 1971.

73. Nichols, B. L., Bilbrey, G. L., Hazlewood, C. F., et al.: Sequential changes in body composition during infection. Am. J. Clin. Nutr., 30:1439, 1977.

74. Rudman, D., Millikan, W. J., Richardson, T. J., et al.: Elemental balances during intravenous hyperalimentation of underweight adult subjects. J. Clin. Invest., 55:94, 1975.

75. King, R. F. J. G., Collins, J. P., Morgan, D. B., and Hill, G. L.: Muscle chemistry of critically ill surgical patients and the effects of a course of intravenous nutrition. Br. J. Surg., 65:495, 1978.

76. Shizgal, H. M.: Total body potassium and nutritional status. Surg. Clin. North Am., 56:1185, 1976.

77. Shizgal, H. M.: Body composition and nutritional support. Surg. Clin. North Am., 61:729, 1981.

78. Mernagh, J. R., McNeill, K. G., Harrison, J. E., and Jeejeebhoy, K. N.: Effect of total parenteral nutrition in the restitution of body nitrogen, potassium and weight. Nutr. Res., 1:149, 1981.

79. Bloom, W. L.: Inhibition of salt excretion by carbohydrate. Arch. Intern Med., 109:26, 1962.

80. Katz, A. L., Hillingworth, D. R., and Epstein, F. H.: Influence of carbohydrate and protein on sodium excretion during fasting and refeeding. J. Lab. Clin. Med., 72:93, 1968.

81. Boulter, P. R., Spark, R. F., and Arky, R. A.: Effect of aldosterone blockade during fasting and refeeding. Am. J. Clin. Nutr., 11:329, 1962.

82. Garnett, E. S., and Nahmtas, C.: The effect of glucose on the urinary excretion of sodium and hydrogen ion in man. Clin. Sci. Molec. Med., 47:589, 1974.

83. Haag, B. L., Reidenberg, M. M., Shuman, C. R., and Channick, B. J.: Aldosterone, 17-OH-corticosteroids, 17-ketosteroids and fluid and electrolyte responses to starvation and selective refeeding. Am. J. Med. Sci., 254:652, 1967.

84. Frege, N. S., Weinberg, J. M., Ross, B. D., et al.: Stimulation of sodium transport by glucose in the perfused kidney. Am. J. Physiol., 233:F235, 1977.

85. Gersing, A., and Bloom, W. L.: Glucose stimulation of salt retention in patients with aldosterone inhibition. Metabolism, 11:329, 1962.

86. Boulter, P. R., Spark, R. F., and Arky, R. A.: Dissociation of the renin-aldosterone system and refractoriness to the sodium retaining action of mineralocorticoids during starvation in man. J. Clin. Endocrinol. Metab., 38:248, 1974.

87. Hoffman, R. S., Martino, J. A., Wahl, G., et al.: Fasting and refeeding. Metabolism, 20:1065, 1971.

88. DeFronzo, R. A., Cooke, C. R., Andress, R., Faloona, G. R., and Davis, P. J.: The effect of

insulin on renal handling of sodium, potassium, calcium, and phosphate in man. J. Clin. Invest., 55:845, 1975.

89. DeFronzo, R. A., Goldberg, M., and Agus, Z. S.: The effects of glucose and insulin on renal electrolyte transport. J. Clin. Invest., 58:83, 1976.

90. Starker, P. M., Lasala, P. A., Askanazi, J., Gump, F. E., Forse, R. A., and Kinney, J. M.: The response to total parenteral nutrition. A form of nutritional assessment. Ann. Surg., 198:720, 1983.

91. Heymsfield, S. B., Bethel, R. A., Ansley, J. D., Gibbs, D. M., Felner, J. M., and Nutter, D. O.: Cardiac abnormalities in cachectic patients before and during nutritional repletion. Am. Heart J., 95:584, 1978.

92. Shoemaker, W. C., Bryan-Brown, C. W., Quigley, L., Stahr, L., Elwyn, D. H. and Kark, A. E.: Body fluid shifts in depletion and post-stress states and their correction with adequate nutrition. Surg. Gynecol. Obstet., 136:371, 1973.

93. Elwyn, D. H., Bryan-Brown, C. W., and Shoemaker, W. C.: Nutritional aspects of body water dislocations in postoperative and depleted patients. Ann. Surg., 182:76, 1975.

94. Spanier, A. H., and Shizgal, H. M.: Caloric requirements of the critically ill patient receiving intravenous hyperalimentation. Am. J. Surg., 133:99, 1977.

95. Bocking, J. K., Holliday, R. L., Reid, B., Mustard, R., and Duff, J. H.: Total exchangeable potassium in patients receiving TPN. Surgery, 88:551, 1980.

96. Bernard, R. W., and Stahl, W. R.: Total body potassium measurements as a guide to intravenous alimentation. Ann. Surg., 178:559, 1973.

97. Jeejeebhoy, K. N., Baker, J. P., Wolman, J. P., Wesson, D. E., Langer, B., Harrison, J. E., and McNeill, K. G.: Critical evaluation of the role of clinical assessment and body composition studies in patients with malnutrition and after TPN. Am. J. Clin. Nutr., 35:1117, 1982.

98. McNeill, K. G., Harrison, J. E., Mernagh, J. R., Stewart, S., and Jeejeebhoy, K. N.: Changes in body protein, body potassium and lean body mass during total parenteral nutrition. J.P.E.N., 6:106, 1982.

99. Cohn, S. H., Gartenhaus, W., Sawitsky, A., Rai, K., et al.: Compartmental body composition of cancer patients by measurement of total body nitrogen, potassium and water. Metabolism, 30:222, 1981.

100. Levenson, S. M., Crowley, L. V., and Seifter, E.: Starvation. In Ballinger, W. (ed.): Manual of Surgical Nutrition. Philadelphia, W. B. Saunders, 1975.

101. King, R. F. J. G., Collins, J. P., Morgan, D. B., and Hill, G. L.: Muscle chemistry of critically ill surgical patients and the effects of a course of intra-venous nutrition. Br. J. Surg., 65:495, 1978.

102. Hill, G. L., King, R. F. G. J., Smith, R. C., et al.: Multi-element analysis of the living body by neutron activation analysis—application to critically ill patients receiving intravenous nutrition. Br. J. Surg., 66:868, 1979.

103. Hill, G. L., Bradley, J. A., Smith, R. C., et al.: Changes in body weight and body protein with intravenous nutrition. J.P.E.N., 3:215, 1979.

104. Macfie, J., Smith, R. C., and Hill, G. L.: Glucose or fat as a nonprotein energy source? Gastroenterology, 80:103, 1981.

105. Macfie, J., Yule, A. G., and Hill, G. L.: Effect of added insulin on body composition of gastroenterologic patients receiving intravenous nutrition—a controlled clinical trial. Gastroenterology, 81:285, 1981.

106. Smith, R. C., Burkinshaw, L., and Hill, G. L.: Optimal energy intake for gastroenterological patients requiring intravenous nutrition. Gastroenterology, 82:445, 1982.

107. Kaplay, S. S.: Erythrocyte membrane Na and K activated triphosphatase in protein caloric malnutrition. Am. J. Clin. Nutr., 31:579, 1978.

108. Curreri, P. W., Wilmore, D. W., Mason, A. D., et al.: Intracellular cation alterations following major trauma: Effect of supranormal caloric intake. J. Trauma, 11:390, 1971.

CHAPTER 7

Parenteral Vitamin Therapy in Hospital Patients

DANIEL DEMPSEY
ROBERT E. HODGES

"As little as the modern clinician can afford to ignore the physiological significance of the proteins or of certain amino acids, just so little need he doubt the importance of the vitamins for human nutrition."

CASIMIR FUNK (1922)[1]

Modern parenteral vitamin therapy remains empirical. It is generally recognized that vitamins are essential dietary components, required in proper quantities for normal cell maintenance, function, and growth. Elucidation of clinical syndromes resulting from individual vitamin deficiencies is well known to clinicians in all branches of medicine. However, with the exceptions noted later, clinically overt vitamin deficiency syndromes are uncommon today. There is now a growing appreciation, based primarily on animal data, of the possible relevance of marginal vitamin deficiencies in hospitalized patients. Because essential vitamins often serve as enzyme cofactors in a variety of important metabolic pathways, suboptimal enzyme function may exist before overt clinical evidence of a vitamin deficiency appears. It is also possible that some malnourished patients may suffer adverse clinical consequences (e.g., inefficient substrate utilization, poor wound healing, sepsis, death) as a result of unrecognized vitamin deficiency.[2]

Unfortunately, there are few simple, reproducible, readily available laboratory tests to enable us to diagnose obscure vitamin deficiencies. Most tests used to assess the vitamin status of patients require special equipment and specially trained personnel.

There is little agreement among vitamin experts as to which test is of most value in diagnosing deficits of each vitamin.

These observations, together with the knowledge that vitamin toxicity can be avoided by conservative prescribing for hospitalized patients, have lead to the widespread use of IV vitamin preparations in standard total parenteral nutrition regimens. In this chapter we discuss the use of parenteral vitamin therapy in hospitalized patients.

VITAMIN METABOLISM

The digestion, absorption, transport, metabolism, and disposition of the 13 recognized vitamins has been discussed in part in other sections of this text. (See *Clinical Nutrition*, Vol. I, Chapter 6, pp. 84–126). It should be emphasized that continuous parenteral infusion of a multivitamin preparation into the central venous circulation is physiologically quite different from intermittent ingestion of foodstuffs. The gut and liver play important roles in modifying and storing orally ingested vitamins. The liver is the major storage site for several vitamins. A large percentage of biotin presented to the liver has been synthesized by gut bacteria, which are also important sources of vitamin K in normal humans. Furthermore, oral ingestion of vitamins assures that two important organs, the gut and liver, are the first tissues presented with these nutrients. Continuous infusion of vitamins into the central venous circulation presents approximately 25 per cent of the administered vitamins first to the kidney, the major excretory organ for water-soluble vitamins.

The relevance of these factors to parenteral vitamin requirements has yet to be demonstrated conclusively, but there is reason to suspect that parenteral requirements for vitamins may be quantitatively different from oral requirements.

The Fat-Soluble Vitamins

Vitamin A

The recommended daily dietary allowance of vitamin A is met by ingestion of plant caretenoids, which are then hydrolyzed by intestinal mucosal enzymes to vitamin A and three or more forms of pre-formed vitamin A—chiefly, retinyl esters and also retinol, and retinoic acid.[4, 5] Retinal and retinyl esters are transported from the gut via the thoracic duct lymph as components of chylomicrons. In the periphery, lipoprotein lipase reduces these particles to chylomicron remnants, still rich in vitamin A. These particles are then further metabolized in the liver, where retinol and retinyl esters are stored in hepatic parenchymal cells.[6] A small quantity of liver retinol is oxidized to retinal, which is promptly oxidized to retinoic acid.[7] Retinoic acid is transported in the portal circulation, rapidly metabolized in the liver, and excreted in the bile as free retinoic acid or as a glucuronide conjugate.[8] A small amount of retinoic acid is reabsorbed in an enterohepatic circulation.

Normally, vitamin A is mobilized from hepatic stores as retinol bound to a highly specific, liver-made protein, retinol-binding protein (RBP). A similar protein is present in cells and is called retinoic acid–binding protein. In vitamin A deficiency, serum RBP (and therefore serum retinol) falls. Zinc deficiency, on the other hand, interferes with RBP synthesis, as presumably does protein calorie malnutrition. The retinol-RBP complex may be catabolized in the kidney; if so, the unusually high levels of retinol in the serum of some patients with renal failure are accounted for. Biliary excretion and renal catabolism are therefore two routes of vitamin A degradation. Others may exist when previous dietary intake has been adequate. Early marginal vitamin A deficiency is unlikely to develop during brief periods of dietary deprivation, unless some superimposed clinical condition (e.g., sepsis, protein deficiency) interferes with the normal transport of active forms of this vitamin from storage sites to the target organs.

Food content of vitamin A is measured in retinol equivalents (RE). Most parenteral preparations provide vitamin A as retinol acetate. It is important to realize that as much as half of the vitamin A originally added to a newly formulated bag or bottle of TPN is apparently destroyed after two to three hours through the effects of sunlight and possibly adsorption on the plastic IV tubing.[9] Whether hepatic processing of parenterally infused retinol is necessary for biologic activity has not been elucidated.

Vitamin A is essential for normal visual cycle activity of the human retina. It is also necessary for normal growth, reproduction, and immunity.[7] A major role of vitamin A in glycoprotein synthesis is considered likely.[10]

Vitamin D

Vitamin D acts as a hormone to promote intestinal calcium and phosphate absorption and to regulate calcium release from bone.[11] Requirements of vitamin D are minimal in people with adequate exposure to sunlight, the ultraviolet component of which activates skin 7-dehydrocholesterol to vitamin D_3 (cholecalciferol), the major dietary form of vitamin D. Vitamin D_3 is doubly hydroxylated, first in the liver, $25(OH)D_3$, and then in the kidney, to the biologically active form (25-dihydroxy-D_3). Most parenteral vitamin supplements contain vitamin D_2, the active end-product being 1,25-dihydroxy,D_2. In chickens, D_3 is ten times more potent than D_2, but in rats (and presumably in humans) they are of equal potency.

Recently, the long-term parenteral administration of vitamin D has been implicated in the etiology of TPN-associated metabolic bone disease.[12, 13] This syndrome is characterized by bone pain, sometimes with pathologic fractures in patients receiving long-term (several months') TPN. Osteomalacia is diagnosed by radiography. The pathophysiology of this syndrome remains elusive. Serum levels of the active vitamin D metabolite (1,25-dihydroxy-D_3) may be low or normal. Serum investigators have reported definite improvement in both the symptoms and the radiologic findings after deletion of vitamin D from the parenteral formulae.[13] In affected patients regular exposure to sunlight assumes great importance, and calcium supplementation may have to be increased. The important role of calcium as an enzyme cofactor and intracellular modulator makes vitamin D deficiency highly undesirable.

Vitamin E

Vitamin E protects membranes from damage by virtue of its antioxidant activity.[14] It also appears to play an important role in selenium and sulfur amino acid metabolism[15] and possibly in liver microsomal enzyme systems.[16] There are many biologically active forms of this vitamin, referred to as *tocopherols*. Clinical manifestations of vitamin E deficiency are extremely difficult to produce even after months or years of depletion, because of significant tissue storage the presence of vitamin E in a wide variety of foodstuffs. Diverse symptoms have been produced in laboratory animals fed vitamin E–free diets. Most parenteral vitamin preparations contain enough alpha-tocopherol to provide satisfactory vitamin E activity.

Vitamin K

Vitamin K is not usually added to commercially available parenteral vitamin preparations. It controls the hepatic synthesis of at least four coagulation factors (II, VII, IX, and X) via a microsomal membrane-bound, vitamin K–dependent carboxylase system.[17] Deficiency of this enzyme in hospitalized patients is most commonly manifested as prolongation of the prothrombin time. It is sometimes seen in patients receiving TPN who have little or no oral intake, are jaundiced, or are being treated with antibiotics. All of these factors interfere with vitamin K synthesis or assimilation. Vitamin K is the only vitamin routinely administered intramuscularly to TPN patients, although intravenous administration should be possible.

The Water-Soluble Vitamins

The B Vitamins

Vitamin B_1 (Thiamine).[18] Thiamine pyrophosphate is an important enzyme cofactor

in the Krebs' cycle (pyruvate dehydrogenase and alpha-ketoglutarate dehydrogenase) and the phosphogluconate pathway (transketolase). As with most water-soluble vitamins, tissue storage of vitamin B_1 is minimal.[1] Biochemical deficiency can be demonstrated within a few weeks of cessation of thiamine intake, at which time a carbohydrate load results in abnormal elevations of plasma pyruvate. Anorexia and weight loss follow. It is likely that inefficient utilization of carbohydrate occurs in thiamine-deficient TPN patients. Anaphylactoid reactions have been reported very rarely after intravenous B_1 administration.

Vitamin B_2 (Riboflavin).[19] Cellular growth and repair cannot occur without this vitamin, which is an integral part of several oxidative enzyme systems necessary for electron transport (succinic dehydrogenase, glutathione reductase, and amino acid oxidase, to name a few) and, therefore, for efficient production of cellular energy.

Niacin. *Nicotinamide*, the biologically active form of niacin, is an intricate part of the coenzymes NAD(H) and NADP(H), which are essential for normal glycolysis, fat synthesis, and energy production from oxidative phosphorylation.[20] Dietary tryptophan may be converted in the liver to niacin metabolites (about 60 mg of dietary tryptophan being equivalent to 1 mg niacin). The relative importance of parenterally infused tryptophan in meeting the requirements for niacin of patients receiving TPN is unclear.

Pantothenic Acid. Panthothenic acid is another water-soluble vitamin that plays a critical role in intermediary metabolism. It forms the backbone of coenzyme A, a crucial factor in the tricarboxylic acid (TCA) cycle (Krebs' cycle). It may also be significant as part of the acyl carrier protein necessary for fat synthesis[21] and probably is important in the maintenance of normal immune function.[22]

Vitamin B_6 (Pyridoxine). Pyridoxine is the vitamin most intimately involved in amino acid metabolism, acting as a cofactor for numerous enzymes (transaminases, decarboxylases, synthetases, etc.).[23] Pyridoxine is necessary in some way for the synthesis and/or catabolism of all the amino acids.[24] Whether protein synthesis and degradation are normal in patients with mild pyridoxine deficiency is unknown. Pyridoxine is also essential for normal heme synthesis and glycogen phosphorylase activity. Some drugs commonly used in hospitalized patients, such as, isoniazid and anticonvulsants, are vitamin B_6 antagonists and must be given with B_6 supplements, lest manifestations of overt deficiency symptoms (e.g., peripheral neuropathy) appear.

Folic Acid. Folic acid is transformed to numerous compounds (folates), which serve as coenzymes in a variety of one-carbon transfer reactions involved in purine biosynthesis and amino acid metabolism.[25] DNA synthesis is abnormal in folate-deficient animals.[26] Although abnormal protein synthesis due to folate deficiency has not been demonstrated, abnormally high urinary excretion of an amino acid metabolite (FIGLU from histidine) is commonly used to detect dietary deficiency of folic acid.

Vitamin B_{12} (Cyanocobalamin). Vitamin B_{12} serves as a coenzyme catalyst for numerous vital cellular reactions.[27] It is crucial for the biologic activation of folates necessary for DNA synthesis; this fact explains why the hematologic pictures of folate and B_{12} deficiencies are morphologically indistinguishable. Vitamin B_{12} is also necessary for normal carbohydrate and protein metabolism, because it is involved in the formation of succinate from methylmalonate and in the synthesis of the amino acid methionine. Whether the neurologic symptoms of pernicious anemia are due in part to abnormal lipoprotein metabolism in the myelin sheath is speculative. Dietary deficiency of vitamin B_{12} is rather unusual owing to excess consumption and a rather frugal enterohepatic circulation. The latter factor, along with tissue storage, may explain the remarkably long period of inadequate intake necessary to produce the hematologic changes of B_{12} deficiency. The activity of enterohepatic circulation in patients given B_{12} parenterally has not been adequately investigated, but patients with pernicious anemia can sometimes remain in apparent good health for several years without supplemental B_{12}.

Biotin. Biotin is required, along with ATP and magnesium, for normal activity of the numerous carboxylase enzyme systems involved in carbohydrate (e.g., pyruvate carboxylase), fat (acetyl COA carboxylase) and protein metabolism.[28] Although it is possible that significant derangements in protein and energy metabolism may exist in hospitalized patients who have marginal deficiency, overt clinical symptoms and signs of biotin deficiency are distinctly unusual. A recent report describes two patients receiving biotin-free TPN, both of whom developed a clinical syndrome responsive to intravenous supplements of biotin.

Vitamin C

The human and the guinea pig are two mammals incapable of endogenous synthesis of sufficient vitamin C (ascorbic acid) to meet normal metabolic requirements. Although the optimal daily intake of vitamin C is debated, the vitamin is undoubtedly necessary for normal collagen formation and wound healing. It may also be necessary for normal hematopoiesis and for certain immune functions.[29]

"Probable" Vitamins

Several food substances possess one or another known biologic activity that has not as yet been demonstrated to be essential in the human diet.

Carnitine is an example. It serves as a carrier molecule for long-chain fatty acid transport across the inner mitochondrial membrane.[30] Under normal conditions, a dietary intake of carnitine is unnecessary. Whether this is true in situations that increase carnitine catabolism or inhibit its synthesis is speculative. Such a situation might be the hypermetabolism of sepsis.[31]

Choline is a structural part of lecithin and a precursor to the neurotransmitter acetylcholine. Animals fed a choline-deficient diet develop a fatty liver and renal insufficiency. Choline requirements may be elevated in certain hospitalized patients, but whether choline deficiency plays a role in the etiology of TPN-associated hepatic steatosis is unknown.[32]

Inositol, a substance structurally similar to glucose, is important for normal cell membrane function and lipoprotein synthesis.[33] Dietary deficiency is lethal in female gerbils, which develop intestinal lipodystrophy, weight loss, and dermatitis when fed an inositol-deficiency diet. The American Academy of Pediatrics has recommended that inositol be added to synthetic infant formulae,[33] but this substance is not added to standard parenteral nutrition solutions.

THE IMPORTANCE OF VITAMIN NUTRITURE IN HOSPITALIZED PATIENTS

Energy Substrate Utilization

Even a cursory review of a standard biochemistry text reminds the reader of the vital role that vitamins play in the transformation of foodstuffs into energy. Optimal organ function depends on an adequate cellular supply of utilizable energy. Many clinicians fail to recognize that the mere infusion of glucose or fat into the gut or the central venous circulation does not ensure optimal cellular ultilization of these fuel sources. Many rate-limiting enzymes are involved in the biochemical conversion of "food" into "energy," and vitamin cofactors are required for optimal function. Several examples of this concept are available: Animal and human data show that thiamine deprivation for a short time produces unrecognized glucose intolerance.[34, 35] This occurs several weeks before the onset of overt thiamine deficiency (i.e., beri-beri). Thiamine status may be assessed by examining the erythrocyte activity of the enzyme transketolase before and after the addition of supplemental thiamine to the reaction. A 25 per cent increase in transketolase activity, measured by the accumulation of D-ribose-5-phosphate, indicates biochemical thiamine deficiency.[36] Similarly, riboflavin nutriture may be assessed by determining erythrocyte glutathione reductase activity.[37]

Although the kinetics of other enzyme-vitamin-substrate reactions may vary, it is possible that patients with multiple deficiencies utilize exogenous and endogenous energy substrates somewhat inefficiently. It is interesting that patients with kwashiorkor frequently exhibit abnormally low levels of vitamins A, B_1, B_2, C, D, and E.[38] Children with this disorder do not gain weight when fed large excesses of nonprotein calories.[39] Similar observations have been made in protein-deficient rats, suggesting inefficient utilization of exogenous energy sources. One hypothesis regarding the reduction of postoperative complications with aggressive preoperative nutritional support suggests that such therapy may replenish depleted intracellular energy stores. That the clinical effectiveness of TPN might be due in part to correction of unrecognized vitamin deficits is intriguing.

Nitrogen Dynamics

Data on protein synthesis and degradation in vitamin deficiency is sparse in animals and nonexistent in humans. Nevertheless, the intimate relationship between an adequate energy supply and optimal net protein synthesis,[40, 41] together with a direct involvement of several vitamins that govern amino acid metabolism, provides reason for further experimentation in this area. Evidence has repeatedly shown that protein deficiency has an adverse effect on the recovery of seriously ill patients. This finding makes the possible relationship between adequate vitamin nutriture and the "protein status" of the host clinically relevant to designing an anabolic nutritional regimen.[42]

It is possible that specific vitamin deficiencies interfere with normal net protein synthesis. B-complex vitamins are generally thought to be necessary for normal utilization of dietary protein.[43] Pyridoxine deficiency interferes with amino acid transport and interconversions in various tissues.[44] Growing animals deficient in riboflavin, pyridoxine, pantothenate, or any other essential nutrient fail to gain total body protein. In some instances, liver protein increases, suggesting an "internal redistribution" of total body nitrogens.[45] In burn patients, abnormalities in vitamin C metabolism seem to parallel the changes in nitrogen metabolism.[46]

Whether protein deficiency predisposes to certain vitamin deficiencies is unclear. Vitamin deficiencies are common in protein-deficient children. Vitamin A absorption is impaired in patients with kwashiorkor, despite the administration of supplemental pancreatic enzymes and bile salts.[38] Protein synthesis in intestinal mucosal cells is markedly depressed in vitamin A–deficient rats.[45] The relevance of this observation and the increased risk of gastric stress ulceration in burn patients with hypovitaminosis A is unknown.[47]

Wound Healing

The essence of an uneventful surgical recovery is normal wound healing. This process occurs relatively unimpeded in most severely malnourished individuals because of a high biologic priority afforded wound healing. However, it has been demonstrated conclusively that wound disruptions and anastomotic dehiscences are more common in hospitalized patients with nutritional deficits.[48] Much animal and human research has been done concerning the impact of protein-calorie malnutrition on wound healing.

Studies on vitamins and wound healing have focused primarily on vitamins A and C in laboratory animals. It has been shown in rats that supplemental vitamin A corrects the impaired wound healing seen with experimental diabetes.[49] This improvement is associated with an increased inflammatory response and hydroxyproline content in the wound. In addition, diabetic animals supplemented with vitamin A show less lymphocytopenia, less thymic atrophy, and more adrenal hypertrophy than pair-fed controls. Supplemental vitamin A has been shown to be helpful in ameliorating the impaired wound healing associated with irradiation.[50] A beneficial influence on the healing of colon anastomosis in vitamin A–deficient rats has recently been suggested.[51]

It may be that an intake of vitamin A that is adequate for healthy rats becomes inadequate during severe stress, resulting in rapid weight loss, poor wound healing, relative hypoglycemia, and death. These changes are largely reversible when animals are given supplements of vitamin A following surgical stress.[52]

Ascorbic acid, iron, and alpha-ketoglutarate, among other nutrients, are necessary for normal collagen synthesis. Wounds in vitamin C–deprived animals appear to have abnormal collagenous substance. Vitamin C deficiency is associated with poor wound healing and a demonstrable abnormality in fibroblastic rough endoplasmic reticulum in guinea pigs.[53] Human studies lag behind this experimental animal work, and there is insufficient evidence at this time to warrant routine clinical use of larger doses of vitamins A and C to promote wound healing.

Immune Function

Overwhelming sepsis accounts for an increasingly large share of in-hospital deaths. Malnutrition is a significant risk factor for septic complications and subsequent death.[54] Unfortunately, the adverse effects of vitamin deprivation on the multiple components of the normal host defense responses are frequently ignored.[55–59] Deficiencies of vitamins A, C, B_1, B_6, and E and pantothenate are associated with impairment of immune func-

tion. Ongoing infection leads to increased urinary wastage of B_1, C, and niacin. Vitamin A–deficient animals show an increased susceptibility to infection but a normal humoral antibody response. The increased vulnerability to bacterial pathogens seen in these animals appears to reflect an impairment in leukocyte phagocytosis related in part to a decrease in nonspecific opsonins. Activity of the reticuloendothelial system is also abnormal in vitamin A–deficient rats.[57] Ascorbic acid deprivation results in both diminished phagocyte function and macrophage migration,[58] whereas thiamine deficiency impairs lymphocyte proliferation. Humoral antibody response is impaired by vitamin C and/or pyridoxine deficiency. Phagocytosis is also abnormal in B_6–deficient animals. Deficiencies of folate, pyridoxine, and vitamin A consistently impair cell-mediated immunity and T cell–dependent antibody responses.

At present, the data remain scanty, and an argument for the routine use of large vitamin supplements in hospitalized patients cannot be defended. More studies are needed in surgical patients, elderly patients, patients requiring extended hospitalization, and patients with compromised vital organ function.

Parenteral Vitamin Therapy of Hospitalized Patients

Many hospitalized patients are at high risk for development of vitamin malnutrition unless they are given vitamins parenterally. Parenteral vitamin therapy is now routine in patients receiving total parenteral nutrition. Before, when vitamin-free TPN was given, clinically overt vitamin deficiencies were reported.[60, 61] It is reasonable to recommend routine parenteral feeding for patients who must be starved for seven or more days, because biochemically significant deficiencies may develop in normal individuals after a week or two of vitamin deprivation[62] and because vitamin requirements may be increased in some hospitalized patients.[63] To understand the rationale for these recommendations, it is important to appreciate (1) the importance of vitamin-dependent processes to normal convalescence, (2) the difficulty in assessing vitamin status, and (3) the low risk of vitamin toxicity.

The Assessment of Vitamin Nutriture

History, physical examination, and specialized laboratory tests are utilized to assess nutritional status in hospitalized patients.

The majority of vitamin deficiencies cannot be detected until clinical signs and symptoms appear. One study of 80 elderly nursing home residents reported a very high incidence (95 per cent) of physical signs, largely mucocutaneous, most of which improved after routine vitamin supplements were given.[64] Unfortunately, when physical signs of a vitamin deficiency are present, they are often subtle and nonspecific.[65] Mild angular stomatitis may be due to a deficiency of riboflavin, pyridoxine, or niacin. Deficiencies of thiamine, pyridoxine, or pantothenate may present as an insidious peripheral neuropathy that could be missed by a casual observer.

The history is useful in identifying those patients at risk for vitamin deficiencies. Important risk factors include age, malabsorption, infection, length of hospitalization, adequacy of pre-hospital diet, and abuse of alcohol or drugs. Low vitamin levels, especially of the B group, C, and D, are common in elderly patients.[66] Routine supplementation with commercially available vitamin tablets reportedly is associated with improvement in vitamin levels and weight gain in old people.[67] Malabsorption (from mucosal disease, gastrointestinal surgery, or bacterial overgrowth) may result in a cumulative negative balance of vitamins A, D, E, K, and B_{12}. Infection increases metabolic demands and may be associated with increased requirements for many vitamins.[52] An inadequate pre-hospital diet is often followed by prolonged periods of enforced in-hospital dietary restriction (e.g., for testing or "bowel rest"). Furthermore, hospitalized patients eating *ad libitum* often consume less than the recommended allowances for thiamine, riboflavin, and vitamin C.[68] In one study, several hospital meals were found to be devoid of vitamin C by the time they were consumed by the patients.[69]

The preceding clinical clues are useful in identifying individual patients at risk for vitamin deficiencies. The ideal biochemical test for the assessment of vitamin status would be a sensitive, specific, simple, and inexpensive means of identifying those patients with suboptimal biochemical processes related to an inadequate cellular supply of individual vitamins. Such a test would also be useful in following the response to therapy (i.e., vitamin supplementation), and should mirror tissue supply rather than recent intake. As with other aspects of nutritional assessment, the ideal test of vitamin status does not exist.

There are basically two types of laboratory tests for assessment of vitamin status: those that measure the level of vitamin in an easily accessible body fluid (urine or blood) and those that assay a vitamin-dependent function (e.g., enzyme activity).[70, 71] or a physiologic function (electroencephalography in B_6 deficiency). Unfortunately, the relationship between vitamin levels as assayed by current techniques and whole-body vitamin status remains elusive. Although a reasonably good correlation has been shown between serum and tissue levels for vitamins A, E, and C and folate, data to support such a relationship for many other vitamins are scanty. Subnormal serum and urine vitamin levels are generally believed to represent an ongoing negative vitamin balance, which puts the patient at risk for clinical or biochemical deficiency. The time required to develop a clinically significant vitamin deficiency depends on the vitamin, intake, metabolic demands, and tissue stores. Generally, a low vitamin level means that the patient is at risk for developing a clinically significant biochemical deficiency. Low vitamin levels in blood or urine may reflect a vitamin deficiency in organs that usually depend on whole-body stores. In ill hospitalized patients, both vitamin levels and tissue stores may become depleted. Currently utilized laboratory tests for the assessment of vitamin status are summarized in Table 7–1, and standards for commonly used tests are given in Table 7–2.

It is important to interpret the results of these tests in the context of each case. Urinary vitamin levels are generally low in deficient subjects. However, spuriously high values can result from recent vitamin intake, infection, antibiotics, and negative nitrogen balance. Blood levels may also reflect recent vitamin intake or drug use (e.g., oral contraceptives and vitamin A). Enzyme activity measurement is a sensitive test for vitamin deficiency, but at present it can be used only for thiamin and riboflavin. The clinician must also be mindful that some vitamin assays analyze only one biochemically active vitamin metabolite; this fact is particularly important in assessing vitamin D status, since

Table 7–1. ESTABLISHED LABORATORY PROCEDURES USED IN ASSESSMENT OF VITAMIN NUTRITURE

VITAMIN	GENERAL PROCEDURE(S)	SPECIAL PROCEDURE(S)	POTENTIAL PROCEDURE(S)
A	Serum retinol measurement	Serum retinol-binding protein measurement	HPLC analyses of serum retinol or urinary metabolites of vitamin A
C	Serum ascorbate measurement	Leukocyte ascorbate measurement Saturation test Urinary ascorbate measurement	HPLC analysis of serum or urinary ascorbate
D	Serum calcium and phosphorus measurement Serum alkaline phosphatase measurement	Radiographic examinations Serum 25-(OH) or 1,25-(OH)$_2$ measurement	Radioassays
E	Serum vitamin E measurement	Erythrocyte hemolysis test Erythrocyte vitamin E measurements	HPLC analyses of serum
Thiamine	Urinary thiamine measurement Erythrocyte transketolase activity measurement	Blood thiamine measurement Thiamine load test	HPLC analysis of urinary thiamine or thiamine metabolites Radioassays
Riboflavin	Urinary riboflavin measurement Erythrocyte glutathione reductase activity measurement	Plasma riboflavin measurement Erythrocyte riboflavin measurement Riboflavin load test	Radioassays
B$_6$	Urinary vitamin B$_6$ measurement Erythrocyte transaminase activity measurement	Erythrocyte and serum vitamin B$_6$ measurements Tryptophan load test Urinary 4-pyridoxic acid measurement	HPLC measurement of urinary 4-pyridoxic acid, xanthurenic acid, and vitamin B$_6$
Folic acid	Serum folacin measurement Erythrocyte folacin measurement	Radioassays Formiminoglutamic acid (FIGLU) and amino-imidazolecarboxamide (AIC) excretion test	
K	Prothrombin test	Clotting factors tests	
B$_{12}$	Serum vitamin B$_{12}$ measurement Schilling test	Methylmalonate excretion test Urinary AIC excretion test Erythrocyte vitamin B$_{12}$ measurement	
Niacin	Urinary N-methylnicotinamide measurement Urinary 2-pyridone measurement Pyridone/N-methylnicotinamide ratio determination	Erythrocyte nicotinamide mononucleotide measurement	
Pantothenic acid	Urinary pantothenic acid excretion test	Blood pantothenic acid measurement	Radioassays Coenzyme A–dependent blood enzyme measurements
Biotin		Urinary biotin measurement	Blood biotin measurement Biotin-dependent blood enzymes measurements

(Modified from Sauberlich, H. E.: Laboratory procedures used in vitamin nutritional assessment. *In* Levenson, S. M. (ed.): Nutritional Assessment—Present Status, Future Directions and Prospects. Columbus, OH, Ross Laboratories, 1981, pp. 65–67, with permission.)

many commercially available vitamin preparations contain vitamin D$_2$, which will not be measured by assays of vitamin D$_3$.

Although some of the currently available assays (e.g., for vitamins A, E, and C) are easy to perform and quite reproducible, other tests (e.g., for vitamins B$_1$, B$_2$, and D) are difficult and yield variable results. Most are expensive in terms of equipment (spectrophotometry, fluorometry, high-performance

Table 7–2. STANDARDS FOR COMMONLY USED TESTS FOR ASSESSMENT OF VITAMIN STATUS

VITAMIN	TEST	DEFICIENT VALUE	MARGINAL VALUE	ACCEPTABLE VALUE
A	Serum measurement (mcg/100 ml)	< 10	10–19	≥ 20
C	Serum measurement (mg/100 ml)	< 0.20	0.20–0.29	≥ 0.30
Thiamine	Urinary measurement (mcg/gm creatinine)	< 27	27–65	≥ 66
	Transketolase (TK) stimulation (%)	> 20	16–20	0–15
Riboflavin	Urinary measurement (mcg/gm creatinine)	< 27	27–79	≥ 80
	Glutathione reductase (GSSR) stimulation (%)	> 40	20–40	< 20
Folic acid	Serum measurement (ng/ml)	< 3.0	3.0–5.9	≥ 6.0
	RBC measurement (ng/ml)	< 140	140–159	≥ 160
B_{12}	Serum measurement (pg/ml)	< 150	150–200	≥ 200
B_6	Urinary measurement (mcg/gm creatinine)		< 20	≥ 20
	Plasma pyridoxal measurement (ng/ml)	< 5.0	5–8	≥ 8.0
E	Serum measurement (mg/100 ml)	< 0.50	0.50–0.70	> 0.70
Niacin	Urinary 2-pyridone/N'-methylnicotinamide ratio determination		< 1.0	1.0–4.0
Pantothenic acid	Urinary measurement (mg/gm creatinine)		< 2.0	≥ 2.0

(Modified from Sauberlich, H. E.: Laboratory procedures used in vitamin nutritional assessment. *In* Levenson, S. M. (eds.): Nutritional Assessment—Present Status, Future Directions and Prospects. Columbus, OH, Ross Laboratories, 1981, pp. 65–67, with permission.

liquid chromatography) and/or technician time (microbiologic assays). Research and development of more readily available and accurate techniques must be supported by the conviction that such tests are clinically useful. Many studies have shown that early protein-calorie malnutrition is associated with a measurable increase in hospital morbidity and mortality, which can probably be reduced by the appropriate use of enteral or parenteral protein, and calories, and essential nutrients.[72, 73] Whether such is the case with any or all of the marginal vitamin deficiencies remains to be demonstrated. The importance of many vitamins in substrate utilization, wound healing, and host defenses suggests that hospitalized patients with deficiencies in these nutrients will be at higher risk for complications or death. Testing this hypothesis in a clinically relevant animal model and in a well-designed clinical study should provide valuable data.

These caveats notwithstanding, there is a substantial body of data to suggest that the vitamin nutriture of many hospitalized patients requiring parenteral nutrition is suboptimal (Table 7–3). Whether commonly used parenteral vitamin doses are adequate to correct these deficiencies or to prevent further deterioration in vitamin levels is

problematic (Table 7–4). Nichoalds and colleagues[63] studied 45 adult surgical patients requiring TPN and found the baseline population means for vitamins A, E, and folate to be low. After two weeks of a daily regimen providing 4200 IU vitamin A, 2.1 IU vitamin E, and 0.6 mg folate, the mean levels of these nutrients had normalized.

In 39 adults requiring TPN for postoperative complications, Stromberg and associates[74] found a prevalence of low values for deficiencies of vitamins A, E, and folate to be 74, 35, and 31 per cent of the population, respectively. Parenteral vitamin therapy with daily doses of 2500 IU vitamin A, 30 IU vitamin E, and 0.2 mg folate for a mean of 17 days had the following results: 100 per cent normalization of vitamin E status, improved vitamin A levels in only nine of 29 patients (31 per cent), and normalized folate levels in only five of 12 patients (42 per cent).

Lowry and co-workers studied 40 cancer patients receiving TPN and found a substantial number of low baseline levels for vitamin A (29 per cent), vitamin C (28 per cent), and folate (9 per cent). The same group subsequently investigated the effect of parenteral vitamin therapy in 75 cancer patients receiving 97 courses of TPN of varying length (7 to 35 days).[76] They administered daily doses of

Table 7–3. PREVALENCE OF LOW VITAMIN LEVELS IN TPN AND NON-TPN PATIENTS*

REFERENCE	A	D	E	Thiamine	Riboflavin	Niacin	C	Folate	B_{12}	Biotin	Pantothenate	Pyridoxine	COMMENTS
Nichoalds et al.[63]	15/45	—	11/45	—	NL (10) Normal 10/45	—	NL (19) Normal 19/45	15/45	High 18/45	—	—	—	Data from 45 TPN surgical patients; mean levels only reported; baseline mean levels of vitamin A and E and folate were low
Stromberg et al.[74]	29/36	—	14/29	1/?	0/27	—	—	14/17	0/16	—	—	0/24	Data from 39 adult patients on TPN for postoperative complications
Lowry et al.[8]	10/35	2/14	—	—	—	—	7/18	3/34	0/39	—	—	—	Data from 40 adult malnourished patients on TPN, 36 with cancer
Kirkemo et al.[76]	15/74	6/9	—	—	—	—	17/97	10/62	2/85	—	—	—	Data from 97 courses of TPN in 75 adult cancer patients
Bradley et al.[77]	—	—	—	4/15	0/16	—	4/24	4/11	—	—	—	1/16	Data from 26 critically ill surgical patients on TPN; tissue levels measured
Dempsey et al.[78]	8/31	25/28	13/35	1/27	5/27	0/17	8/35	19/30	1/35	8/16	4/23	5/28	Data from 35 surgical patients on TPN
Lemoine et al.[79]	—	—	—	129/515	61/562	—	82/576	—	—	—	—	130/530	Data from 656 non-TPN hospital inpatients

*Prevalence expressed as number of low values/number of patients in whom level measured.

Table 7–4. INFLUENCE OF PARENTERAL VITAMIN THERAPY ON VITAMIN LEVELS IN TPN PATIENTS*

REFERENCE	A	D	E	Thiamine	Riboflavin	Niacin	C	Folate	B12	Biotin	Pantothenate	Pyridoxine
Nichoalds et al.[73]†												
Dose 1	D 10, R 17		D 7, R 17	—	M 9	—	M 10	D 7, R 16	M 9	—	—	—
Dose 2				—	M 14	—	M 16	M 3, R 5, D 7	M 16	—	—	M 24
Stromberg et al.[74]‡	M 4, R 9, D 23	—	M 14, R 14	M 33?, R 1, D 2	M 27	—	—		M 16	—	—	
Kirkemo et al.[76]‖	M 59, R 12, D 3	M 2, R 6, D 1			—	—	M 80, R 17	M 52, R 10	M 83, R 2	—	—	—
Bradley et al.[77]**	—	—	—	M 11, R 4	M 16	—	M 20, R 4	M 7, R 4	—	—	—	M 15, R 1
Dempsey et al.[78]††												
Dose 1	M 19, R 2, D 2	M 0, R 1, D 19	M 11, R 3, D 10	M 11, R 0, D 1	M 11, R 1, D 1	M 7, R 0, D 0	M 21, R 0, D 3	M 3, R 3, D 12	M 23, R 0, D 0	M 4, R 1, D 1	M 8, R 0, D 3	M 13, R 0, D 0
Dose 2	M 3, R 2, D 2	M 2, R 0, D 7	M 8, R 2, D 0	M 9, R 0, D 1	M 8, R 2, D 0	M 5, R 0, D 0	M 5, R 3, D 2	M 0, R 0, D 7	M 9, R 0, D 1	M 1, R 2, D 1	M 5, R 2, D 0	M 6, R 2, D 2

*M = maintained (level remained normal or high); R = repleted (low baseline level increased to normal range); D = depleted (low baseline remained low or normal baseline became low).

†Mean vitamin levels only presented in this study. Treatment of two dose levels were given for 14 days each. Dose 1 consisted of: vitamin A, 3300 IU; E, 1.65 IU: riboflavin, 3.3 mg; C, 465 μg; folate, 300 μg; B12, 30 μg. Dose 2 consisted of: vitamin A, 4200 IU; E, 2.10 IU; riboflavin, 4.2 mg; C, 210 μg; folate, 600 μg; B12, 15 μg.

‡Treatment course variable; mean 17 days. Daily dose consisted of: vitamin A, 2500 IU: E, 30–35 IU; thiamine, 1.2 mg; riboflavin, 1.8 mg; folate, 0.2 mg; B12, 2 μg; pyridoxine, 2 mg.

§Author: please supply information.

‖Summary of 97 courses of TPN in 75 cancer patients treated for seven to 60 days. Daily dose consisted of: vitamin A, 2664 IU; D, 245 IU: C, 437 mg; B12, 15 mg; folate, 1 mg.

**Daily dose: Author: please supply information.

††Ten-day treatment course. Daily dose 1 identical to AMA suggestions for parenteral vitamin formulation (see Table 7–6). Daily dose 2 consisted of: vitamin A, 10,000 IU; D, 1000 IU: E, 5 IU: thiamine, 50 mg; riboflavin, 10 mg; niacin, 100 mg; C, 500 mg; folate, 400 μg; B12, 5 μg; biotin, 60 μg, pantothenate, 25 mg; pyridoxine, 15 mg.

2664 IU vitamin A, 245 IU vitamin D, 0.8 mg folate, and 436 mg vitamin C. This dosage led to normalization of low baseline vitamin A and C and folate levels in 80, 100, and 100 per cent of cases, respectively. However, levels of vitamin D (i.e., serum 25 (OH)D$_3$) continued to deteriorate, and none of the low baseline levels were normalized.

Dempsey and colleagues[78] assayed 12 vitamins in 35 adult general surgical patients requiring TPN and found a particularly high prevalence of low levels of vitamin E (37 per cent), D$_3$ (89 per cent), folate (63 per cent), and biotin (50 per cent).[78] Interestingly, there was a poor correlation between vitamin status (as measured by vitamin levels or by the number of abnormal vitamin levels per patient) and nutritional status (as measured by percentage of ideal body weight, serum albumin, or nitrogen balance). After ten days of TPN containing one of two commercially available vitamin preparations, there was suboptimal improvement in low vitamin levels. Only 31 per cent of baseline low values increased to normal, whereas 78 per cent of the low post-treatment levels represented measurements that were low at baseline. The higher dosage level appeared to lead to a significantly greater relative increase in vitamin A, C, and B$_6$ levels.

Although there were no reports of overt vitamin toxicity in any of the patients in the previously cited studies, judicious prescribing of parenteral vitamin therapy is necessary

Table 7–6. SUGGESTED FORMULATIONS FOR INTRAVENOUS USE IN ADULTS AND IN CHILDREN AGE 11 YEARS OR MORE

VITAMINS	RDA ADULT RANGE	MULTIVITAMIN FORMULATION FOR IV USE
A (IU)	4,000–5,000*	3,330
D (IU)	400	200
E (IU)	12–15	10.0
Ascorbic acid (mg)	45	100.0
Folacin ($\geqq$g)	400	400.0
Niacin (mg)	12–20	40.0
Riboflavin (mg)	1.1–1.8	3.6
Thiamine (mg)	1.0–1.5	3.0
B$_6$ (pyridoxine) (mg)	1.6–2.0	4.0
B$_{12}$ (cyanocobalamin) (μg)	3	5.0
Pantothenic acid (mg)	5–10†	15.0
Biotin (μg)	150–300†	60.0

*Assumes 50 per cent intake as carotene, which is less available than vitamin A.

†RDA not established; this amount considered adequate in usual dietary intake.

(From: Multivitamin preparations for parenteral use—a statement by the Nutrition Advisory Group. J.P.E.N., 3:258–262, 1979, with permission.)

because of this possibility. It is well known that excessive doses of vitamin A may produce liver damage and intracranial hypertension, and indiscreet consumption of vitamin D is associated with hypercalcemia. In addition to these direct vitamin "toxicities," there are several other mechanisms whereby intravenous vitamins may be harmful (Table 7–5).

Recommendations

Total parenteral nutrition is a new and highly effective modality for providing nutritional support to selected hospitalized patients. Although it remains to be demonstrated conclusively that vitamin malnutrition is associated with poor clinical outcome, the routine use of parenteral vitamin supplements can safely improve vitamin status in many of these patients. Table 7–6 shows the recommendations of the Nutrition Advisory Group of the American Medical Association for parenteral vitamin requirements. It is reasonable to administer these vitamin dosages to all adult patients receiving TPN or taking nothing by mouth for more than five days. Much work remains to be done before parenteral vitamin therapy can be tailored to the individual TPN patient or even to demonstrate that such tailoring is beneficial. Enthu-

Table 7–5. MECHANISMS OF VITAMIN TOXICITY

MECHANISMS	EXAMPLE/COMMENT
Direct toxicity	Vitamin A, vitamin D (see text).
Exacerbation of disease	Niacin may lead to histamine release, which may exacerbate asthma or peptic ulcer disease.
Masking of disease	Folate may mask hematologic signs of B$_{12}$ deficiency.
Withdrawal deficiency	Large doses of vitamins probably induce enzymes necessary for their own degrading, e.g., vitamin C.
Vitamin-drug interaction	Vitamin C may interfere with enteral iron absorption. Acidification of urine from vitamin C may alter renal drug excretion.

(From Aldaheff, L., Gualtieri, T., and Lipton, M.: Toxic effects of water-soluble vitamins. Nutr. Rev., 42:33–40, 1984, with permission.)

siasm for the therapeutic potential of vitamin preparations in malnourished hospitalized patients should be tempered by an awareness of several facts: (1) we are only beginning to explore the links between malnutrition and clinical outcome, (2) early vitamin deficiency is difficult to diagnose, and (3) a potential for toxicity exists.

REFERENCES

1. Funk, D.: The Vitamins (trans. H. E. Dubin). Baltimore, Williams & Wilkins, 1922, p. 156.
2. Detsky, A. S., Barker, J. P., Mendelson, R. A., Wolman, S. L., Wesson, D. E., and Jeejeebhoy, K. N.: Evaluating the accuracy of nutritional assessment techniques applied to hospitalized patients: Methodology and comparisons. J.P.E.N., 8:153–159, 1984.
3. Swendseid, M. E., Schick, G., Vinyard, E., and Drenick, D. J.: Vitamin excretion studies in starving obese subjects. Some possible interpretations for vitamin nutriture. Am. J. Clin. Nutr., 17:272–276, 1965.
4. Goodman, D. C., Blomstrand, B., Huang, H. S., and Shiratori, T.: The intestinal absorption and metabolism of vitamin A and β-carotene in man. J. Clin. Invest., 45:1615–1623, 1966.
5. Olson, J. A.: The absorption of beta-carotene and its conversion into vitamin A. Am. J Clin. Nutr., 9:1–11, 1961.
6. Linder, M. C., Anderson, G. H., and Ascarelli, I.: Quantitative distribution of vitamin A in Kupffer cell and hepatocyte populations of rat liver. J. Biol. Chem., 246:5538–5540, 1971.
7. Lui, N. S. T., and Roels, O. A.: Vitamin A and carotene. In Goodhart, R. S., and Shils, M. E. (eds.): Modern Nutrition in Health and Disease. Philadelphia, Lea & Febiger, 1980, pp. 142–159.
8. Fidge, N. H., Shiratori, T., Ganguly, J., and Goodman, D. S.: Pathways of absorption of retinal and retinoic acid in the rat. J. Lipid Res., 9:103–109, 1968.
9. Hartline, J. V., and Zachman, R. D.: Vitamin A delivery in total parenteral nutrition solution. Pediatrics, 58:448–451, 1976.
10. Wolf, G., and DeLuca, H. F.: Recent studies on some metabolic functions of vitamin A. In DeLuca, H. F., and Suttie, J. W. (eds.): The Fat Soluble Vitamins. Madison, The University of Wisconsin Press, 1969, pp. 257–265.
11. Fraser, D. R.: The physiological economy of vitamin D. Lancet, 1:969–972, 1983.
12. Klein, G. L., Ament, M. E., Bluestone, R., et al.: Bone disease associated with total parenteral nutrition. Lancet, 2:1041–1044, 1980.
13. Shike, M., Sturtridge, W. C., Cherk, S. T., et al.: A possible role of vitamin D in the genesis of parenteral-nutrition–induced metabolic bone disease. Ann. Intern. Med., 95:560–568, 1981.
14. Horwitt, M. K.: Vitamin E. In Goodhart, R. S., and Shils, M. E. (eds.): Modern Nutrition in Health and Disease. Philadelphia, Lea & Febiger, 1980, pp. 181–191.
15. Scott, M. L.: Studies on Vitamin E and related factors in nutrition and metabolism. In DeLuca, H. F., and Suttie, J. W. (eds.): The Fat Soluble Vitamins. Madison, The University of Wisconsin Press, 1969, pp. 355–367.
16. Carpenter, M. P., and Howard, C. N., Jr.: Vitamin E, steroids and liver microsomal hydroxylations. Am. J. Clin. Nutr., 27:966–979, 1974.
17. Esmon, C. T., Sadowski, J. A., and Suttie, J. W.: A new carboxylation reaction. The vitamin K dependent incorporation of $H_{12}CO_3$ into prothrombin. J. Biol. Chem., 250:4744–4748, 1975.
18. Gubler, C. J., Fujiwara, M., and Dreyfus, P. M. (eds.): Thiamine. New York, John Wiley & Sons, 1976.
19. Rivlin, R. S. (ed.): Riboflavin. New York, Plenum Press, 1975.
20. Darby, W. J., McNutt, K. W., and Todhunter, E. N.: Niacin. In Hegsted, D. M. (ed.): Present Knowledge in Nutrition. Washington, D.C., The Nutrition Foundation, 1976, pp. 162–174.
21. Pugh, E. L., and Wakil, S. J.: Studies on the mechanism of fatty acid synthesis. XIV. The prosthetic group of acyl carrier protein and its mode of attachment of the protein. J. Biol. Chem., 240:4727–4733, 1965.
22. Hodges, R. E., Bean, W. B., Ohlson, M. A., and Bleiler, R. E.: Factors affecting human antibody response. III. Immunologic responses of men deficient in pentothenic acid. Am. J. Clin. Nutr., 11:85–93, 1962.
23. Fasella, P.: Pyridoxal phosphate. Ann. Rev. Biochem., 36:185–210, 1967.
24. Gershoff, S. N.: Vitamin B_6. In Hegsted, D. M. (ed.): Present Knowledge in Nutrition. Washington, D.C., The Nutrition Foundation, 1976, pp. 149–161.
25. Blakely, R. L.: The Biochemistry of Folic Acid and Related Pteridines. New York, John Wiley & Sons, 1969.
26. Menzies, R. C., Crossen, P. E., Fitzgerald, P. H., and Gunz, F. W.: Cytogenetic and cytochemical studies on marrow cells in B_{12} and folate deficiency. Blood, 28:581–594, 1966.
27. Arnstein, H. V., and Wrighton, R. J. (eds.): The Cobalamins. London, J & A Churchill, 1971.
28. Bonjour, J. P.: Biotin in man's nutrition and therapy—a review. Int. J. Vitamin Nutr. Res., 47:107–118, 1977.
29. Hodges, R. E.: Ascorbic acid. In Hegsted, D. M. (ed.): Present Knowledge in Nutrition, Washington, D.C., The Nutrition Foundation, 1976, pp. 119–130.
30. Mitchell, M. E.: Carnitine metabolism in human subjects—normal metabolism. Am. J. Clin. Nutr., 31:293–306, 1978.
31. Rebouche, C. J., and Engel, A. G.: Carnitine metabolism and deficiency syndromes. Mayo Clin. Proc., 58:533–540, 1983.
32. Appel, J. A., and Briggs, G. M.: Choline. In Goodhart, R. S., and Shils, M. E. (eds.): Modern Nutrition in Health and Diseases. Philadelphia, Lea & Febiger, 1980, pp. 282–286.
33. Committee on Nutrition: Commentary on breast feeding and infant formulas, including proposed standards for formulas. Pediatrics, 57:278–285, 1976.
34. Brin, M.: Recent information on thiamine nutritional status in selected countries. In Gubler, C. J., Fujiwara, M., and Dreyfus, P. M. (eds.): Thiamine. New York, John Wiley & Sons, 1976.

35. Horwitt, M. K., and Kreisler, O.: The determination of early thiamine deficient states by estimation of blood lactic and pyruvic acids after glucose administration and exercise. J. Nutr., *108*:421, 1978.

36. Gubler, C. J.: Biochemical changes in thiamine deficiency. *In* Gubler, C. J., et al. (eds.): Thiamin. New York, John Wiley & Sons, 1976, pp. 121–141.

37. Bamji, M. S.: Glutathione reductase activity in red blood cells and riboflavin nutritional status in humans. Clin. Chim. Acta, *26*:263, 1969.

38. Viteri, F., Behar, M., Arroyave, G., and Scrimshaw, N. S.: Clinical aspects of protein malnutrition. *In* Munro, H. N. (ed.): Mammalian Protein Metabolism. New York, Academic Press, 1964, Vol. 2, pp. 523–568.

39. Himms-Hagen, J.: Current status of non-shivering thermogenesis. *In* Kinney, J. (ed.): Assessment of Energy Metabolism in Health and Disease. Columbus, OH, Ross Laboratories, 1980, pp. 92–104.

40. Calloway, D., and Spector, H.: Nitrogen balance as related to caloric and protein intake in active young men. Am. J. Clin. Nutr., *2*:405, 1954.

41. Platt, B. S., Heard, C. R. C., and Stewart, R. J. C.: Experimental protein-calorie deficiency. *In* Munro, H. N. (ed.): Mammalian Protein Metabolism. New York, Academic Press, 1964, Vol. 2, pp. 446–522.

42. Stinnett, J. D.: Proteins and amino acids—prospects for nutritional therapy in infection. *In* Fischer, J. E. (ed.): Relevance of Nutrition to Sepsis. Columbus, OH, Ross Laboratories, 1982, pp. 104–109.

43. Munro, H. N.: An introduction to nutritional aspects of protein metabolism. *In* Munro, H. N. (ed.): Mammalian Protein Metabolism. New York, Academic Press, Vol. 2, 1964, pp. 3–39.

44. Christensen, H. N.: Free amino acids and peptides in tissues. *In* Munro, H. N. (ed.): Mammalian Protein Metabolism. New York, Academic Press, 1964, Vol. 1, pp. 105–124.

45. Munro, H. N.: General aspects of the regulation of protein metabolism by diet and by hormones. *In* Munro, H. N. (ed.): Mammalian Protein Metabolism. New York, Academic Press, 1964, Vol. 1, pp. 381–481.

46. Lund, C. C., Levenson, S. M., and Green, R. W.: Ascorbic acid, thiamine, riboflavin, and nicotinic acid in relation to acute burns in man. Arch. Surg., *55*:557, 1947.

47. Rai, K., and Courtemanche, A. D.: Vitamin A assay in burned patients. J. Trauma, *15*:419, 1975.

48. Rhoads, J. E., and Alexander, C. E.: Nutritional problems of surgical patients. Ann. N.Y. Acad. Sci., *63*:268, 1955.

49. Seifter, E., Rettura, G., Stratford, F., et al.: Impaired wound healing in streptozotocin diabetes. Ann. Surg., *194*:42, 1981.

50. Seifter, E., Rettura, G., Stratford, F., et al.: Vitamin A inhibits some aspects of systemic disease due to local irradiation. J.P.E.N., *5*:288, 1981.

51. Proceedings of the European Society for Parenteral and Enteral Nutrition, 1983, Abstract 36.

52. Levenson, S. M., Hopkins, B. S., Waldron, M., and Sefter, E.: Vitamin requirements of seriously injured patients with and without sepsis. *In* Fischer, J. E. (ed.): Relevance of Nutrition to Sepsis. Columbus, OH, Ross Laboratories, 1982, pp. 111–116.

53. Peacock, E. E.: Structure, synthesis, and interaction of fibrous protein and matrix. *In* Peacock, E. E.: Wound Repair. Philadelphia, W. B. Saunders, 1984.

54. Scrimshaw, N. S., Taylor, C. E., and Gordon, J. E.: Interactions of Nutrition and Infection. Monograph Series No. 57. Geneva, World Health Organization, 1968.

55. Stinnet, J. D., and Alexander, J. W.: Nutrition as related to host defense and infection. *In* Richards, J. R., and Kinney, J. M. (eds.): Nutritional Aspects of Care in the Critically Ill. London, Churchill-Livingstone, 1977, pp. 557–569.

56. Axelrod, A. E.: Immune process in vitamin deficiency states. Am. J. Clin. Nutr., *24*:265–271, 1971.

57. Jenks, J. S., Michalek, A. V., Howard, L. J., Saba, T. M., and Blumenstock, F. A.: Altered reticuloendothelial function in vitamin A deficiency (abstract 23). *In* Proceedings of the American Society for Parenteral and Enteral Nutrition, 1984.

58. Ganguly, R., Durieux, M. F., and Waldman, R. H.: Macrophage function in vitamin C–deficient guinea pigs. Am. J. Clin. Nutr., *29*:762, 1976.

59. Beisel, W. R.: Single nutrients and immunity. Am. J. Clin. Nutr., *35*:417–468, 1982.

60. Ibbotson, R. M., Colvin, B. T., and Colving, M. P.: Folic acid deficiency during intensive therapy. Br. Med. J., *2*:145, 1975.

61. Kramer, J., and Goodwin, J. A.: Wernicke's encephalopathy. Complications of intravenous hyperalimentation. J.A.M.A., *238*:2176, 1977.

62. Moran, M. R., and Greene, H. L.: The B vitamins and vitamin C in human nutrition. Am. J. Dis. Child., *133*:192, 1979.

63. Nicholalds, G. E., Meng, H. C., and Caldwell, M. D.: Vitamin requirements in patients receiving total parenteral nutrition. Arch. Surg., *112*:1061–1064, 1977.

64. Taylor, G. F.: A clinical survey of elderly people from a nutritional standpoint. *In* Exton-Smith, A. N., and Scott, D. L. (eds.): Vitamins in the Elderly. Bristol, John Wright & Sons, 1969, pp. 51–56.

65. Bamji, M. S.: Laboratory tests for the assessment of vitamin nutritional status. *In* Briggs, M. H. (ed.): Vitamins in Human Biology and Medicine. Boca Raton, FL, CRC Press, 1981, pp. 1–28.

66. Brin, M.: Biochemical methods and findings in USA surveys. *In* Exton-Smith, A. N., and Scott, D. L. (eds.): Vitamins in the Elderly. Bristol, John Wright & Sons, 1968, pp. 25–33.

67. Gounelle, H.: In Exton-Smith, A. N., and Scott, D. L. (eds.): Vitamins in the Elderly. Bristol, John Wright & Sons, 1968, pp. 47–48.

68. Brown, A. M.: Dietary intakes of elderly female patients in hospital. *In* Exton-Smith, A. N., and Scott, D. L. (eds.): Vitamins in the Elderly. Bristol, John Wright & Sons, 1968, pp. 93–97.

69. Eddy, T. P.: The problem of retaining vitamins in hospital food. *In* Exton-Smith, A. N., and Scott, D. L. (eds.): Vitamins in the Elderly. Bristol, John Wright & Sons, 1968, pp. 86–92.

70. Baker, H., Frank, O., and Hutner, S. H.: Vitamin analyses in medicine. *In* Goodhart, R. S., and Shils, M. E.: Modern Nutrition in Health and Disease. Philadelphia, Lea & Febiger, 1980, pp. 611–640.

71. Sauberlich, H. E.: Laboratory procedures used in vitamin nutritional assessment. *In* Levenson, S. M. (ed.): Nutritional Assessment—Present Status, Future Directions and Prospects. Columbus, OH, Ross Laboratories, 1981, pp. 65–67.

72. Mullen, J. L., Buzby, G. P., Matthews, D. C., et al.:

Reduction of operative morbidity and mortality by combined preoperative and postoperative nutritional support. Ann. Surg., *192*:604, 1980.

73. Muller, J. M., Dienst, C., Brenner, U., and Pichlmaier, G.: Preoperative parenteral feeding in patients with gastrointestinal carcinoma. Lancet, *1*:68–71, 1982.

74. Stromberg, P., Shenkin, A., Campbell, R. A., Spooner, R. J., Davidson, J. F., and Sim, A. J.: Vitamin status during total parenteral nutrition. J.P.E.N., *5*:295–299, 1981.

75. Lowry, S. F., Goodgame, J. T., Maher, M. M., and Brennan, M. F.: Parenteral vitamin requirements during intravenous feeding. Am. J. Clin. Nutr., *31*:2149–2158, 1978.

76. Kirkemo, A. K., Burt, M. E., and Brennan, M. F.: Serum vitamin level maintenance in cancer patients on total parenteral nutrition. Am. J. Clin. Nutr., *35*:1003–1009, 1982.

77. Bradley, J. A., King, R. F., Schjorah, C. J., and Hill, G. L.: Vitamins in intravenous feeding: A study of water soluble vitamins and folate in critically ill patients receiving intravenous nutrition. Br. J. S., *64*:84–86, 1977.

78. Dempsey, D. T., Oberlander, J., Crosby, L., et al.: Vitamin deficiencies in general surgical patients. Surg. Forum, *34*:84–87, 1983.

79. Lemoine, A., LeDevehat, C., Codaccioni, J. L., Monges, A., Bermond, P., and Salkeld, R. M.: Vitamin B_1, B_2, B_6 and C status in hospital inpatients. Am. J. Clin. Nutr., *33*:2595–2600, 1980.

80. Alhadeff, L., Gualtieri, T., and Lipton, M.: Toxic effects of water-soluble vitamins. Nutr. Rev., *42*:33–40, 1984.

81. Multivitamin preparations for parenteral use—a statement by the Nutrition Advisory Group. J.P.E.N., *3*:258–262, 1979.

CHAPTER 8

Trace Minerals

NOEL W. SOLOMONS

THE ESSENTIAL TRACE MINERALS

The *trace minerals* are a subgroup of the trace elements that occur in the human body. *Trace elements* can be defined as those elements that constitute less than 0.01 per cent of the total body of a human, i.e., less than 7 gm in a 70-kg man. The nutritional aspects of this class of elements has recently been reviewed in detail.[1] The trace elements of biologic importance in mammalian systems are listed in Table 8–1. Not all of these trace elements are minerals, and not all trace minerals listed have been confirmed as essential nutrients in humans. Nutritional deficiency syndromes in humans have been recognized, however, for iron, zinc, copper, selenium, chromium, and molybdenum.

Although trace minerals are diverse in their biochemical and physiologic functions in biology, several generalizations can be made. Most trace minerals, for instance, express their biologic roles as part of *metalloenzymes*, that is, enzymes with stoichiometric

Table 8–1. TRACE ELEMENTS OF BIOLOGIC IMPORTANCE IN MAMMALS

Iron*
Zinc*
Copper*
Manganese*
Selenium*
Chromium*
Cobalt*†
Iodine*
Fluorine
Molybdenum*
Vanadium
Nickel
Silicon
Tin
Lithium

*Definitely essential in humans.
†Note: cobalt is essential *only* as a component of vitamin B$_{12}$.

amounts of one or more trace minerals firmly bound to the protein and required for maximal enzymatic activity.[2] Trace minerals, however, can also participate in metabolism as soluble ionic cofactors (e.g., Zn, Mn) or in specialized, non-protein organic molecules (e.g., Cr). A common feature of many trace minerals is their inefficient absorption from dietary sources. Substantial differences exist, therefore, between the amounts that must be ingested daily, i.e., the Recommended Dietary Allowances, and the amounts that must be absorbed daily to replace normal losses, i.e., requirements for absorption (parenteral requirement). With sufficiently large oral intakes or heavy environmental exposures, moreover, most of the trace mineral nutrients can become toxic to the human organism. An important further generalization, bearing directly on the mission of this text, is the fact that concentrations of trace minerals in parenteral nutrition solutions are variable and often extraordinarily low, such that intravenous delivery of the calories and protein required by a patient undergoing total parenteral nutrition (TPN) is not sufficient to meet the situational nutritional requirements of that individual for one or another trace mineral nutrient.[3]

GENERAL CONSIDERATIONS REGARDING TRACE MINERAL NUTRITURE AND DEFICIENCY DURING TOTAL PARENTERAL NUTRITION

It is an axiom in clinical nutrition that, in addition to reduced intake and impaired absorption, decreased utilization, increased loss, or excessive metabolic demand for a given nutrient can precipitate clinical deficiency states.[4] In a given patient, several mechanisms often act in concert. With total parenteral nutrition, issues of gastrointestinal absorption are moot, although they emerge when, for instance, a patient is maintained parenterally but is permitted an oral intake as well. Figure 8–1 illustrates four possible mechanisms by which a low circulating concentration of a trace mineral nutrient might develop: (1) through deficient intake, (2) through enhanced loss, (3) through redistribution from the vascular space to tissues, and (4) through a deficient maintenance of the circulating binding protein. In the latter two instances, a low serum level need not signify a total-body deficit. However, in both instances, utilization of the nutrient at certain sites may be compromised by the internal redistribution. It has recently become clear that even when steps are taken to ensure an adequate intake of a nutrient, reactions in the nutrient solution may cause the mineral to precipitate or to be "complexed" to a form that is not biologically available to the host.

Although the full-blown manifestations of iatrogenic deficiencies of a trace mineral can be dramatic, such deficiency states are rarely an urgent concern in the patient on TPN.* In fact, if a patient is nutritionally replete before parenteral therapy (as a patient

---

*By virtue of the involvement of Cr and Mo deficiency syndromes with the central nervous system and state of consciousness, and of Se deficiency with the myocardium, acute deficiency of these three minerals during TPN theoretically presents the greatest threat to life.

with acute abdominal trauma) and the expected interval to full restoration of oral alimentation is relatively brief, a period of negative trace mineral balance poses little hazard to the patient or recovery. However, the complex surgical conditions and chronic medical disorders for which TPN is prescribed may themselves precondition nutrient depletion; patients with such conditions often begin TPN with severe total-body trace mineral deficits. These same conditions, moreover, may increase losses or may create excessive metabolic demands for a given nutrient. In patients with trauma, burns, or extensive infections or inflammation, a massive catabolic loss not only of macronutrients but also of micronutrients, including trace minerals, will be seen. On the other hand, the processes of rapid cell proliferation or hyperplasia attendant on tissue repair and nutritional repletion may require amounts of one or another minerals greatly in excess of those for normal maintenance and turnover. In acute TPN, therefore, a positive balance with respect to trace minerals is often desirable.

Growth unquestionably requires a positive nutrient balance. Thus, whenever infants or children are on TPN, sufficient amounts of trace minerals to replace deficits, permit growth, and foster normal accumulation must be provided. The only sign of a nutrient deficiency in a child receiving an apparently "adequate" total parenteral intake may be the failure to resume or to maintain the

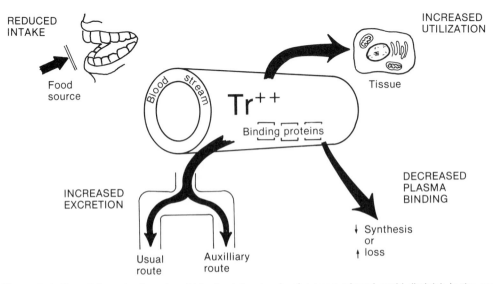

Figure 8–1. Potential mechanisms by which circulating levels of a trace mineral could diminish in the context of total parenteral nutrition (see text). (*From* Solomons, N. W.: Mineral deficiencies. *In* Paige, D. M. (ed.): Manual on Clinical Nutrition. Pleasantville, N. J., Nutrition Publications, Inc., p. 34.2, with permission.)

expected growth velocity. Under this circumstance, the limiting nutrient—be it vitamin or mineral—should be identified and its deficiency should be expediently corrected.

QUANTITATIVE ASPECTS OF TRACE MINERAL CONTENTS OF INTRAVENOUS PRODUCTS USED IN TOTAL PARENTERAL NUTRITION

The various solutions that constitute daily TPN regimens contain, by virtue of contamination in processing or as a consequence of intrinsic features of the constituents, some specific content of trace minerals. This content can range from undetectable levels to amounts in excess of the recommended daily parenteral requirements. Theoretically, at least, it would be important to ascertain how much of a given element was already in an intravenous nutritional regimen before rational exogenous adjustment with additives could be made.

Over the last one and one-half decades, copious information on trace mineral concentrations in intravenous preparations has been published.[3-18] Representative values are summarized in Table 8–2. Geography would appear to be a major determinant of trace mineral content of solutions. Protein hydrolysates were formerly in fashion during the early years of TPN; they tend to contain more iron and zinc than the crystalline amino acid solutions that have supplanted them in current usage. Contact with rubber tubing and stoppers was found to provide contaminant zinc to parenteral solutions.[7] In practice, exact calculations of supplementary additive dosages of trace minerals are not based on the intrinsic mineral content of each solution in the TPN regimen, but when glaring examples of elevated mineral concentrations are apparent (such as the chromium content in German solutions),[14] the physician should be aware of the situation and should plan mineral delivery accordingly.

IRON

Biochemical and Physiologic Role

The predominant function of iron is oxygen transport, in which it serves as the ligand in the hemoglobin of red cells. Each molecule of hemoglobin contains four atoms of iron. It has recently been appreciated,

however, that iron deficiency, *even before the onset of anemia*, can impair cognitive function,[19, 20] muscle metabolism,[21] and immune defense[22] by virtue of its involvement in other metalloproteins (respiratory chain cytochromes) and in metalloenzymes (e.g., cellular dehydrogenases). The erythron requires from 1.5 to 2.5 gm of iron in the nonanemic state. Additional reserves of iron are 1000 mg in the normally iron-replete man and 300 to 500 mg in the menstruating woman.[23] This storage iron is distributed equally among reticuloendothelial tissue in bone marrow, spleen, and liver; striated muscle tissue; and hepatocytes. The daily loss of iron in adult males is about 1 mg, and in fertile women it averages 2 mg.[24] Thus, in the absence of bleeding or other forms of excessive iron loss, the stores of a healthy individual should suffice for up to a year or more. Some factors common to TPN or disease states that predispose to its use, such as the reduced turnover of intestinal cells in the non-alimented gut and the secondary amenorrhea of severe inanition, would theoretically tend to *reduce* basal iron losses.

Assessment of Iron Status

Modern clinical chemistry has permitted the fairly precise, graded assessment of an individual as anemic, iron-depleted but not anemic, or iron-sufficient. Assessment of iron status involves the use of hemoglobin, transferrin (or total iron-binding capacity) saturation, free erythrocyte protoporphyrin, and serum ferritin determinations (Table 8–3).[25] Refinements can be added by evaluating the morphology of red cells. The assessment of iron status by laboratory means, however, becomes problematic in patients undergoing TPN. Anemia can be caused by a number of nutritional factors other than iron deficiency in diseases for which TPN is employed. The diseases themselves may also produce bone marrow hypoplasia. In sum, anemia is not a specific sign of iron deficiency in this situation. Because transferrin saturation depends on the concentration of protein as well as the quantity of circulating iron, protein deficiency will artifactually raise the percentage of saturation even in the face of iron deficiency. Serum ferritin has been related to the amount of iron in deposits.[26] However, tumors and inflammatory conditions produce elevations of ferritin. A recent survey indicated that laboratory indices of iron status

Table 8–2. CONCENTRATIONS OF VARIOUS TRACE MINERALS IN INTRAVENOUS SOLUTIONS COMMONLY USED IN TPN

SOLUTION	COMMERCIAL SOURCE	COUNTRY OF ORIGIN	Iron	Zinc	Copper	Manganese	Selenium	Chromium	Molybdenum
Amigen	Baxter	U.S.A.	1.16[11]	1.19[11]	0.62[11]	—	—	—	—
	Baxter	Israel	—	2.83–4.01[5]	0.40–0.50[5]	—	—	—	—
			—	4.0[6]	—	—	—	—	—
Aminofusin 800	Pfimmer	New Zealand	—	—	—	—	< 0.002[16]	—	—
Aminofusin 850	Pfimmer	Australia	—	1.17[3]	0.051[3]	—	—	—	—
Aminofusin L1000	Pfimmer	Australia	—	0.61[3]	0.044[3]	—	—	—	—
Aminofusin forte	Pfimmer	Australia	—	0.86[3]	0.137[3]	—	—	—	—
Aminofusin L600	Pfimmer	New Zealand	—	—	—	—	< 0.002[16]	—	—
Aminosol		Germany	—	0.03–0.20[5]	0.030–0.050[5]	—	—	0.018–0.105[15]	—
	Abbott Laboratories	U.S.A.	—	—	—	—	—	—	—
AmiU (essential)	—	Japan	—	0.02[9]	0.010[4]	—	—	—	—
Casein hydrolysate, 8%	—	U.S.A.	—	< 2.1[4]	—	—	—	—	—
FreAmine	McGaw Laboratories	U.S.A.	—	0.92–1.62[5]	0.05–0.08[5]	—	—	—	—
			—	< 4.0[4]	0.18[4]	—	—	—	—
			—	0.33–0.42[10]	—	—	—	—	—
FreAmine II	McGaw Laboratories	U.S.A.	0.030–0.066[11]	1.34–4.04[11]	0.009–0.011[11]	—	0.019[17]	—	—
		New Zealand	—	—	—	—	< 0.002[16]	—	—
Hyprotigen	—	U.S.A.	—	3.0–3.2[8]	0.023[8]	0.82[8]	—	—	—
Ispol, 12%	—	Japan	—	0.08[9]	—	—	—	—	—
Polynute	Cutter Laboratories, Inc.	U.S.A.	—	2.21–2.90[5]	0.10–0.20[5]	—	—	—	—
Protamine	Cutter Laboratories, Inc.	U.S.A.	0.76[11]	—	—	—	—	—	—
Protein hydrolysate, 7%	Cutter Laboratories, Inc.	U.S.A.	—	0.030[13]	—	—	—	—	—
Travamin	Travenol Laboratories, Inc.	U.S.A.	1.37[11]	0.95[11]	0.038[11]	—	—	—	—
			1.11[18]	—	—	—	—	—	—
Travasol	Travenol Laboratories, Inc.	U.S.A.	0.02–0.03[12]	0.01[12]	0.01[12]	0.01[12]	0.032[17]	—	0.02–0.03[12]
			0.043[18]	—	—	—	—	—	—
Travasol c̄ electrolytes	Travenol Laboratories, Inc.	U.S.A.	0.56–1.02[12]	0.15–0.25[12]	0.4[12]	0.06–0.1[12]	—	—	0.5[12]
Vamin-based regimen	Apoteksvarucentralen Vitrum AB	Sweden	—	—	—	—	0.003[7]	0.013[7]	0.003[7]
Vamin N	Vitrum AB	United Kingdom	—	—	—	—	—	0.006[14]	—

TRACE MINERAL COMPOSITION (MG/L)*

*Superscript numbers signify chapter references in which these data can be found.

Table 8–3. LABORATORY ASSESSMENT OF IRON STATUS

STATUS	LABORATORY VALUES			
	Serum Ferritin	Transferrin Saturation	Free Erythrocyte Protoporphyrin	Hemoglobin Concentration
Normal iron nutriture	Normal	Normal	Normal	Normal
Iron depletion without anemia	Low	Normal	Normal	Normal
Iron-deficient erythropoiesis without anemia	Low	Low	High	Normal
Iron deficiency anemia	Low	Low	High	Low

(Modified from Cook, J., and Finch, C. A.: Assessing the iron status of a population. Am. J. Clin. Nutr., 32:2115–2119, 1979.)

performed poorly in a population receiving TPN.[27]

When it is essential to have a diagnosis of iron status, a bone marrow aspiration may be the only recourse. Alternatively, the use of iron absorption tests with radiolabeled iron and whole-body counting might serve to indicate iron deficiency *when access to a sufficient segment of healthy small intestine is present.* In iron deficiency, the efficiency of isotopic uptake is increased.[28]

The clinical manifestations of iron deficiency include pallor, fatigue, exertional dyspnea, tachycardia, headache, listlessness, paresthesias, burning sensation on the tongue, and altered attention span. The first four symptoms are present with overt anemia, but it is believed that the remainder of the symptoms are due to iron deficiency at the tissue level.

Iron Deficiency During TPN

With normal rates of iron turnover, iron deficiency will develop only slowly even with no iron intake. However, iron deficiency is widespread in the U.S. population, especially among women of childbearing age. Moreover, acute or chronic hemorrhage is common in diseases that require TPN, such as cancer and inflammatory bowel disease. Thus, many individuals on TPN will be iron-depleted even early in the course and their iron status will not always be amenable to detection by laboratory means.

Total-body iron stores are normally regulated by the intestine.[28] There is no efficient mechanism for excretion of excess iron. Bypassing the gut with parenteral iron creates substantial risk of overloading the organism with iron and producing siderosis. Neither iatrogenic deficiency nor excess of iron is likely to develop in short-term TPN, but in the long-term, multi-year, home TPN situation, achieving a net mean daily intake of iron in a narrow range around 1 mg is a formidable challenge.

ZINC

Biochemical and Physiologic Role

The adult human body contains two to three grams of zinc. Zinc concentrations in most human tissues range from 50 to 200 $\mu g/gm$, but specific tissues such as pancreas, testis, and ocular retina are extraordinarily rich in zinc.[29] The biochemical functions of zinc fall into three categories: formation of metalloenzymes, RNA conformation, and membrane stabilization. In nature, over 70 metalloenzymes of zinc have been identified; some of the more common are carbonic anhydrase, alkaline phosphatase, alcohol dehydrogenase, and Zn-Cu superoxide dismutase. Because not all of the biochemical reactions subtended by zinc are rate-limiting in their respective pathways, the pathophysiologic manifestations of zinc deficiency cannot universally be explained in terms of deficient activity of one or another metalloenzyme.[30] In addition to enzymes in which stoichiometric amounts of zinc have been identified (zinc metalloenzymes), a number of enzymes show specific sensitivity to experimental and acquired zinc deficiency (zinc-dependent enzymes). Examples of such zinc-dependent enzymes are thymidine kinase[31] and nucleoside phosphorylase.[32] Zinc in an *ionic* form appears to play a role in the conformation of polyribosomes during protein synthesis.[33] Finally, a host of effects of the concentrations of circulating zinc on membrane stability of cells have been identified[34]; here, too, ionic zinc appears to be the important agent. The physiologic functions dependent on an adequate zinc nutriture in humans include: cell growth and proliferation, sexual maturation and reproduction, dark adaptation and night vision, gustatory acuity, wound healing, host immune defenses, and hemostasis.

Assessment of Zinc Status

No unequivocal diagnostic index to faithfully and reliably reflect human zinc status has been developed.[35, 36] The laboratory and clinical tests that have been reported in the literature are listed in Table 8–4. Not all of the indices listed are necessarily useful or valid; many require further validation. The problem with validation, of course, is that there is no "gold standard" of zinc nutriture assessment against which to measure the performance of the various parameters.

By far the most commonly used index of zinc nutriture is the circulating zinc concentration. Blood plasma and serum, a relatively accessible fluid, and atomic absorption spectrophotometry provide an accurate and precise method for quantifying zinc in biologic materials. Yet there is a host of pitfalls to the

assessment of zinc status using the plasma level of zinc.[35] The first problem is the fact that circulating zinc levels are loosely—but homeostatically—regulated. The remaining pitfalls are of a technical or situational nature. External contamination or hemolysis will artificially increase measured levels of zinc. Short-term (24 to 72 hours) fasting will also increase circulating zinc concentrations through release of the mineral from tissue catabolism. Even application of a tourniquet during the blood extraction increases apparent zinc concentration significantly.[37] Acute or chronic infection, corticosteroids, oral contraceptives, and pregnancy will artificially lower zinc levels. Plasma and serum zinc levels fall transiently following an ordinary meal. Zinc levels depend upon the availability of a circulating binding protein, specifically albumin. Hypoalbuminemia per se can account for a low zinc level. Despite these pitfalls, circulating zinc concentration does have a reasonable role to play in assessment of patients undergoing TPN when care is taken to avoid the technical errors, and when serial determinations beginning prior to the implementation of TPN are utilized.

Of the other static indices listed, leukocyte zinc content appears to show substantial promise as an index of zinc status.[38, 39] Presumably, however, leukocyte proliferation kinetics must be normal for the interpretation of white cell zinc to be valid. For evaluation of populations, hair zinc content may have a useful role, but in a given individual, studied at one point in time, it is of dubious utility.

A conceptually promising strategy for assessing zinc status is to use functional indices; that is, to assess distinct physiologic processes that are zinc-dependent. Taste acuity and dark adaptation are two reasonable indices that can reflect changes in zinc status. Not all impairments of either of these two parameters can a priori be ascribed to zinc deficiency. Newer functional tests have been suggested by recent investigations with experimental or acquired human zinc deficiency states. The oral zinc tolerance test[40] has promise, but the usually compromised intestinal function of the patient requiring TPN obviates its use. Tests of platelet aggregation[41] and delayed cutaneous hypersensitivity[42, 43] deserve further exploration.

A decade and a half of monitoring the trace mineral states of TPN patients has engendered several curious observations. The

Table 8–4. LABORATORY AND DIAGNOSTIC OPTIONS FOR ASSESSING ZINC STATUS

Circulating (plasma/serum) zinc concentration*
Red cell zinc content
Leukocyte zinc content
Platelet zinc content
Salivary zinc concentration
Hair zinc content
24-hour urine zinc excretion*
Urinary zinc/creatinine ratio

Serum alkaline phosphatase concentration*
Erythrocyte carbonic anhydrate concentration
Erythrocyte nucleoside phosphorylase concentration
Serum ribonuclease (RNAase) concentration

Taste acuity
Dark adaptation
Neutrophil/macrophage chemotaxis
In vitro red cell zinc-65 uptake
Oral zinc tolerance test†
Platelet aggregation tests†
Delayed cutaneous hypersensitivity response†

*Of particular utility in evaluation of TPN patients.
†Requires further experience and validation in humans.

first is the frequency with which alkaline phosphatase—a zinc metalloenzyme—is low in association with hypozincemia.[44, 45] In fact, in a South African patient for whom no access to zinc analyses was possible, alkaline phosphatase depression and restoration were the guides to the diagnosis and treatment of zinc deficiency.[46] Recently, Main and colleagues[47] have promoted the monitoring of urinary zinc excretion in TPN patients, on the basis of a large series of inflammatory bowel disease patients subjected to parenteral nutrition. These researchers observed that urinary zinc excretion increases when the zinc is supplied by a parenteral route, because of inefficient delivery to the tissues and a "spill-over" into the urine with low-molecular-weight chelating agents (such as amino acids). They suggest, in fact, that if zinc output is low (less than 1.3 mg/day) in a patient on TPN, the IV dose may be insufficient to cover the metabolic demands. Their notion is to provide incremental parenteral doses of zinc to permit a minimum overflow into the urine, thus ensuring adequate tissue delivery.[47] This postulation is an interesting concept that deserves further evaluation, but obviously, situations in which hyperzincuria was a factor in the development of zinc depletion cannot be evaluated by such a criterion.

Satisfactory management of zinc nutrition in TPN involves *serial* determinations of assessment indices. No single index is universally reliable, and the best strategy is to perform a battery of zinc status tests over the course of parenteral alimentation. The probability of a pre-existing zinc depletion or of a marginal zinc status is a further guide to the level of concern for zinc nutriture in a given patient. A number of diseases and clinical situations—many of which often require TPN intervention—predispose to zinc deficiency (Table 8–5).

If laboratory monitoring fails, the clinical recognition of frank zinc deficiency should not be missed. The clinical manifestations of zinc deficiency are listed in Table 8–6. Many are not specific to zinc. Hair loss, for instance, occurs in protein-energy malnutrition. Skin lesions are found in deficiencies of protein and energy, essential fatty acids, and biotin deficiency, as well as zinc. All can be seen in TPN patients. When any of the signs or symptoms become manifest in a patient undergoing TPN, a thorough diagnostic

Table 8–5. COMMON DISEASES AND SITUATIONS PREDISPOSING TO ZINC DEFICIENCY

Acrodermatitis enteropathica
Alcoholic cirrhosis
Alcoholic pancreatitis
Alcoholism
Anorexia nervosa
Celiac disease
Cystic fibrosis
Inflammatory bowel disease
Jejunoileal bypass
Nephrotic syndrome
Pancreatic insufficiency
D-Penicillamine administration
Pica
Pregnancy
Prematurity
Short-bowel syndrome
Sickle cell anemia
Thalassemia
Thermal burns
Uremia

work-up oriented to excluding zinc deficiency should be conducted.

Zinc Deficiency During TPN

The topic of zinc deficiency in patients on TPN has been discussed in several excellent reviews.[48–51] The first probable cases of TPN-induced zinc deficiency appeared close to 1970 but were not appropriately recognized. MacMahon and colleagues[52] reported zinc deficiency in a patient with malabsorption, but their subject had been receiving exclusive intravenous alimentation prior to investigation; the authors emphasized the

Table 8–6. CLINICAL MANIFESTATIONS AND CONSEQUENCES OF ZINC DEFICIENCY

Growth retardation
Hypogonadism
Hypospermia
Alopecia
Skin lesions
Diarrhea
Mental depression/apathy
Glucose intolerance
Night blindness
Impaired taste sensation/perception
Impaired wound healing
Impaired white cell chemotaxis
Impaired T-lymphocyte function
Cutaneous anergy

gastrointestinal issues, but the origin of the zinc depletion could have been the mode of feeding. Schlappner and co-workers[53] reported acute, papulopustular acne in a patient on prolonged TPN; in retrospect, it was possibly a manifestation of zinc deficiency. The first clear, clinical-pathophysiologic observation of TPN with zinc deficiency was made in 1975 by Kay and Tasman-Jones.[54-56]

In the early days of parenteral therapy, nitrogen sources came from both protein hydrolysates and mixtures of crystalline amino acids. The only zinc in parenteral regimens was the instrinsic contamination zinc in the materials used to make the mixtures. It was noted by several groups that circulating zinc levels declined gradually in the majority of unsupplemented adult patients in prospective studies.[57-60] In a recent study, however, a zero level of zinc supplementation was *not* associated with depression of zinc levels.[47] In infants requiring intensive care and parenteral nutrition, plasma zinc levels also show a steady decline.[61-63] Supplementation of infants with 400 µg/kg—but not with lesser dosages of zinc—prevented the decline in serum zinc in short-term TPN.[63] Metabolic balance study data also revealed zinc losses exceeding zinc intake in patients on TPN.[7, 64] From the standpoint, therefore, of zinc distribution and zinc economy, the stage was set for zinc deficiency to emerge in patients on TPN.

Over the past decade, case reports of overt clinical zinc deficiency with one or more signs or symptoms have been reported frequently in preterm neonates,[65-70] infants and children,[71-81] and adults.[13, 46, 82-101] The most common sign has been one or another variant of the skin lesions produced by acute zinc deficiency, often the scaly, hyperpigmented lesion over the acral surfaces of elbows and knees reminiscent of acrodermatitis enteropathica. Immune deficiencies have also been observed commonly in this setting. Even individuals with consciously supplemented TPN regimens have developed zinc deficiency.[80, 81] Patients with malignancies have higher parenteral zinc requirements than patients without cancer.[102]

Not only is the decreased delivery of zinc to the patient a significant etiologic factor, but there can be significant additional losses of zinc on the basis of the pathologic conditions that led to the indication for parenteral therapy. For instance, the patients studied by Kay and associates[54-56] had severe trauma and put out between 4000 and 20,000 µg of zinc in the urine daily, as opposed to the 400 to 600 µg normally excreted by the kidneys. Moreover, if amino acid mixtures are combined with the dextrose solutions *prior to heat sterilization*, Maillaird reaction products are formed; these complex with zinc when infused into patients and promote a major urinary excretion of the mineral.[103-105] Such a procedure is not common practice, but as TPN is extended to new regions of the world that are unfamiliar with the history of TPN technology, there is a possibility that this type of sterilization processing could be instituted, with unfortunate consequences for the patients. Even ordinary amino acids, however, specifically cysteine and histidine, promote zinc excretion in anesthetized dogs.[106] In humans, a correlation between the amount of amino acids infused and urinary zinc losses has been shown; a four-fold difference in zinc excretion has been observed in humans receiving different amino acid mixtures.[107, 108]

In certain disease conditions, a gastrointestinal loss of zinc can also predispose to zinc depletion. It has been noted that symptomatic zinc deficiency on TPN was most commonly reported in patients with Crohn's disease,[87] and large gastrointestinal zinc losses were documented in a patient population with this form of inflammatory bowel disease.[109] Patients with short-bowel syndrome are also prone to a fecal output of zinc greater than oral intake when feeding *ad libitum* by mouth; these zinc losses must be made up by parenteral infusion.[110] Other common situations predisposing to zinc deficiency on TPN are general malnutrition, pancreatic disease, and malabsorption syndromes.[101]

The studies of Wolman and associates[109] were enlightening in showing that negative zinc balance during TPN was associated with a lesser retention of nitrogen and a decreased secretion of insulin. Positive zinc balance affected both parameters favorably. Another concern is postoperative wound healing, in which zinc is necessary for tissue repair and accumulates in the site of wound closure.[111]

COPPER

Biochemical and Physiological Role

The adult human body contains about 80 to 200 mg of copper. The main site of copper storage, distribution, regulation, and excretion is the liver. Copper is transported in the circulation and delivered to tissues by the protein ceruloplasmin.[112] It is excreted with the bile into the fecal stream and thus eliminated from the body via the intestinal tract. Copper expresses the majority of its biochemical function as a component of copper metalloenzymes.[113] There is also some suggestion that a nonspecific effect of free copper or of ceruloplasmin-copper may play a role in certain functions, such as bone mineralization and antioxidant protection. Common cuproenzymes include: tyrosinase, lysyl oxidase, amine oxidases, cytochrome c oxidase, and Zn-Cu superoxide dismutase.[113] The common feature of cuproenzymes is their utilization of molecular oxygen or a derivative species to effect an oxidation reaction. As such, unlike zinc metalloenzymes, cuproenzymes almost universally govern the determinant step in a specific reaction sequence. Thus, the pathophysiology of copper deficiency can be explained almost entirely on the basis of defective copper enzyme activities.[114] The confirmed or suspected physiologic roles for copper in the human organism are manifold and are based on the known functions of cuproenzymes and on experimental copper-restriction studies in laboratory animals and humans. They include: erythropoiesis, leukopoiesis, skeletal mineralization, elastin and collage synthesis, myelin formation, catecholamine metabolism, oxidative phosphorylation, thermal regulation, antioxidant protection, cholesterol metabolism, lymphocyte function, cardiac function, and glucose metabolism.

Assessment of Copper Status

The laboratory assessment of copper status is as uncertain and fraught with pitfalls as that of zinc.[35] Because copper is much more toxic than iron or zinc when tissue accumulation is excessive, the assessment mandate in the TPN patient involves not only detecting conditions of copper *under*nutrition, but also situations of excess accumulation (*over*nutrition) as well. A list of laboratory and diagnostic options for assessing human copper status are listed in Table 8–7. Not all of the listed indices are necessarily useful or valid for detecting copper depletion or overload.

Table 8–7. LABORATORY AND DIAGNOSTIC OPTIONS FOR ASSESSING COPPER STATUS

Hemoglobin concentration
Packed red cell volume (hematocrit)
Reticulocyte count
White cell and differential counts

Circulating (plasma/serum) copper concentration
Serum ceruloplasmin concentration
Erythrocyte copper content
Hair copper content
24-hour urinary copper excretion

Erythrocyte superoxide dismutase content
Serum amine oxidase content
Leukocyte cytochrome c oxidase content

The clinical signs of human copper deficiency are listed in Table 8–8. As can be seen, hematologic manifestations—hypochromic anemia and neutropenia—are common. Laboratory detection of copper deficiency exploits this situation, using hematologic parameters as one line of diagnostic investigation. Of course, neither anemia nor neutropenia is a specific nutritional sign. The red cell changes are similar to those seen in iron deficiency, but the failure of a reticulocyte response to iron administration can be suggestive of copper depletion.

Static indices of copper have also been used, the most common being circulating copper concentrations. Once again, a homeostatic regulation of circulating copper levels is maintained. It is important to recognize that 94 per cent of circulating copper is in the form of ceruloplasmin.[115] Thus, whatever influences levels of ceruloplasmin will determine serum and plasma total copper levels as well. A number of pitfalls and limitations to the use of circulating copper levels are recognized.[35] External contamination during

Table 8–8. CLINICAL MANIFESTATIONS AND CONSEQUENCES OF COPPER DEFICIENCY

Microcytic, hypochromic anemia
Neutropenia
Skeletal demineralization*
Depigmentation of hair
Skin pallor
Vascular aneurysms*
Central nervous system abnormalities*
Growth retardation*
Hypotonia*
Hypothermia*

*Thus far reported only in acquired copper deficiencies in children.

obtaining, handling, or processing of the blood samples is to be avoided. Copper determinations are less sensitive to hemolysis than are zinc determinations, and they are not affected by application of a tourniquet during venipuncture.[37] Corticosteroid therapy tends to lower copper levels, but a number of conditions increase circulating copper/ceruloplasmin concentrations. These include: acute and chronic infections, pregnancy, oral contraceptive agents, and smoking. Hair copper content is a poor index of copper nutriture because of the adsorption of copper from the environment onto the hair.[116]

Experience with monitoring copper status via the *in vitro* activity of copper metalloenzymes has been accumulated over the years.[35] Particularly promising are two recent reports suggesting that the Zn-Cu superoxide dismutase activity of erythrocytes may prove to be a sensitive monitor of copper nutriture.[117, 118] An interaction with the state of zinc nutriture must be excluded however, because in TPN *both* zinc and copper nutriture can be precarious. Assessing overload states by noninvasive means is severely restricted. Liver biopsies provide a reliable marker but are much too hazardous and invasive for routine nutritional assessment. However, if suspicion that a prescription or dosing error in the copper additive of a patient on prolonged TPN is raised, the merits of tissue diagnosis—specifically, a liver biopsy—must be weighed.

The most common clinical signs in acquired human copper deficiency are anemia and neutropenia. In children, bone mineralization changes reminiscent of scorbutic bone disease are manifest, leading to the speculation that copper has a role in vitamin C metabolism in growing bone.[58] The bone disease can predispose to fractures,[119] and as with scurvy itself, a swelling deformity due to subperiosteal bleeding has been documented.[120] A number of the clinical manifestations of acquired copper deficiency are seen only in children and are analogous to the lesions of the inborn error of copper metabolism, Menkes' kinky hair syndrome. Of these, the vascular changes are the most potentially life-threatening. No corresponding vascular lesion has been reported in acquired copper deficiency in adults, but cardiac disease of various types can be produced in experimental copper deficiency in animals,[121, 122] a finding that may have implica-

tions for adult TPN patients. It has also been speculated that copper plays a role in human aortic aneurysm formation; the superimposition of prior marginal copper intakes with a copper-deficient TPN regimen might hasten the development of arterial wall defects of the major blood vessels.[123]

Copper Deficiency During TPN

The topic of copper deficiency in TPN has been reviewed.[48–51] Similar to the observation for zinc, circulating levels of copper were found to fall progressively when patients were followed prospectively with unsupplemented TPN.[13, 57, 78] Supplementation of infants on TPN with 20 or 40 µg/kg/day of copper did not affect the circulating concentrations of copper.[62]

The first documented case of TPN-associated copper deficiency was reported by Karpel and Peden[124] in an infant on long-term intravenous nutrition. Since then, overt manifestations of copper deficiency have been observed in preterm infants,[65, 119, 125] children,[75, 120, 126–130] and adults.[90, 126, 131–133] The most commonly observed signs of copper deficiency were anemia and neutropenia, with the skeletal lesions confined to premature and full-term infants, but the entire gamut of deficiency manifestations has been reported (see Table 8–8).

In a study of trauma patients, Askari and colleagues[134] found negative copper balance when crystalline solutions alone were given, but the addition of blood and blood products to the regimen tended to preserve copper balance. Gastric suction of patients on TPN is associated with excessive copper loss.[7] Four of eight TPN patients studied by Phillips and Garnys[64] were in negative copper balance, but Shike and associates[135] reported the maintenance of copper economy with a daily infusion of 0.25 mg.

As with zinc, the factor of amino acid infusion *per se* seems to have an influence on the renal excretion of copper, enhancing the urinary wasting of the mineral. Tyrala and co-workers[136] found that total excretion of amino nitrogen in the urine positively correlated with urinary copper output. The urinary levels of glycine, methionine, histidine, and lysine notably correlated with copper loss in urine. Similarly, a greater than expected contribution of urinary output was found in the daily excretion patterns of copper in the balance studies by Shike and associates.[135]

Certain physiologic conditions and disease states predispose to depletion of copper and frank copper deficiency when patients are placed on total intravenous nutrition. Notable is the situation of prematurity. It seems that the liver's capacity to synthesize or release copper into the circulation as ceruloplasmin is limited in the preterm infant, and copper levels do not spontaneously increase until the child reaches a postconceptional age corresponding to full-term maturity.[137, 138] Oral supplementation of preterm infants with copper is unable to influence the course of serum copper elevation.[137, 139] Burn patients also have increases in loss of copper, susceptibility to depletion, and copper requirement when alimented by vein.[140] The data of Lowry and colleagues[102] would also suggest that malignancies adversely effect copper nutriture, although circulating levels of copper may be elevated because of the effect of tumors on ceruloplasmin *per se.*

MANGANESE

Biochemical and Physiologic Role

Manganese is a component of two metalloenzymes, Mn-superoxide dismutase and pyruvate carboxylase. As such, it functions in antioxidant protection and in energy metabolism. There is abundant confirmation in mammalian species that manganese is important in the formation of connective tissue, presumably through an involvement in the attachment of the terminal carbohydrate moieties of mucopolysaccharides.[141] It is also postulated that the divalent Mn(II) ion functions as a soluble, ionic cofactor analagous to magnesium ion in certain metabolic reactions.[142]

No clear-cut, definitive instance of clinical manganese deficiency in a human subject has been reported. A *suggestive* case has been put forward by Doisy,[143] involving a young male experimental subject on a metabolic ward. The subject was given a vitamin K–deficient, purified diet from which manganese had inadvertently been omitted. He manifested marked hypocholesterolemia, changes in the rate of growth and pigmentation of hair and beard, dermatitis, and nausea, all of which resolved on his returning to a normal diet. The evidence for manganese

deficiency in this case report is not rigorous. It can be speculated that perhaps because magnesium may compensate for the ionic functions of manganese, and because nonmanganese forms of pyruvate carboxylase and superoxide dismutase are present in humans, clear deficiency symptoms may never emerge despite the absence of manganese from an oral or intravenous regimen.

Assessment of Manganese Status

Normal levels for manganese in plasma and serum and in red cells have been published. The reported means for healthy individuals vary from 0.5 to 13 μg/L.[144] The most reliable reported mean levels for concentrations in plasma and serum are 0.54,[145] 0.57,[144] and 0.59 μg/L.[146] Mean levels in whole blood range from 8.44 to 9.03 μg/L.[144, 147] However, to what extent whole-body nutriture is reflected by circulating or whole blood manganese levels is not known. It is believed, however, that excessive manganese accumulation in the body is manifested by a rise of whole blood concentrations above normal limits.[148]

The manganese-containing superoxide dismutase (Mn-SOD) can be distinguished from the copper-zinc variety by the former's insensitivity to inhibition by cyanide. In recent animal studies, dietary restriction of manganese produced tissue depression of Mn-SOD in one study of rats,[149] but not in another.[150] Hepatic levels of Mn-SOD were depressed profoundly, however, in mice and chicks subjected to dietary manganese restriction.[151] Unfortunately, the mangano-enzyme is found exclusively in mitochondria, and a biopsy material for humans that would be readily and noninvasively accessible, and at the same time rich in mitochondria, is elusive; this fact represents a major limitation to the exploration of Mn-SOD levels to assess manganese status of humans.[152]

Manganese Deficiency During TPN

Clinical manganese deficiency in a patient undergoing TPN has not been reported. Nonetheless, no one would seriously deny its essentiality in human nutrition nor omit it from a "complete" intravenous nutrient regimen. In one study, in which serum manganese levels were monitored in an eight-year-old girl after five months on TPN, concentrations were 12.1 µg/L, distinctly elevated for that laboratory.

In animals, manganese deficiency during gestation is extraordinarily teratogenic.[153] Specific teratogenesis in human fetuses due to dietary manganese deficiency has not been described, but with the advent of successful maintenance of pregnancy in women on long-term TPN,[154] the theoretic possibility that a manganese-free TPN regimen might produce damage to the fetus is an eventuality to be avoided.

SELENIUM

Biochemical and Physiologic Role

Selenium is involved in the protection of the cell from oxidant stress. Its antioxidant functions mimic to some extent the role of vitamin E in preventing the extension of lipid peroxidation in the membranes of cells and their intracellular organelles. In mammals, selenium is a constituent of the selenoenzyme glutathione peroxidase.[155, 156] This enzyme catalyzes the oxidation of glutathione with the simultaneous reduction of peroxides.

Assessment of Selenium Status

The laboratory indices used in the clinical assessment of selenium status are shown in Table 8–9. Normal plasma selenium levels are 5 to 15 µg/dl.[157] Erythrocyte glutathione peroxidase represents the most practical in-

Table 8–9. LABORATORY OPTIONS FOR ASSESSING SELENIUM STATUS

STATIC INDICES
    Plasma or serum selenium concentration
    Whole-blood selenium concentration
    Erythrocyte selenium concentration
    Erythrocyte glutathione peroxidase activity
    Platelet glutathione peroxidase activity
    Leukocyte glutathione peroxidase activity
    24-hour urine selenium excretion

FUNCTIONAL INDICES
    Erythrocyte selenium-75 uptake *in vitro*
    Erythrocyte fragility to antioxidant stress *in vitro*
    ? Breath excretion of ethane and pentane
    ? T-lymphocyte function tests

dex at present. A functional index of selenium status is the *in vitro* fragility of red cells in the presence of an oxidizing agent. A potential functional index, not yet fully developed and validated, is a breath analysis test in which the pulmonary excretion of ethane and pentane—the volatile hydrocarbon split-products formed by peroxidation of endogenous, unsaturated fatty acids—is determined.[158] Neither of the two functional indices mentioned differentiates between the deficiencies of selenium and vitamin E. Of the functional indicators listed, the uptake by red cells of radioselenium is perhaps the most specific of the functional assays of selenium status.

Selenium Deficiency During TPN

It has been noted in several studies that circulating selenium levels in patients undergoing TPN are lower on average than those of healthy control subjects.[16, 59, 159] A progressive fall in whole blood selenium levels was noted in a patient undergoing six weeks of TPN therapy.[59] Recent surveys have uncovered low selenium status in patients on long-term home TPN.[160, 161] Jacobson and Wester[7] observed a mean negative balance of −19 µg/24 hours in their subjects on a daily intravenous intake of 9 µg of selenium; the major route of obligatory excretion was in urine. Of the eight TPN patients studied by Phillips and Garnys[64] who received from 0 to 25 µg of selenium daily, four were in positive or neutral and four in negative selenium balance.

The first putative case of clinical selenium deficiency in a TPN patient was reported from southern New Zealand,[159] a region notorious for its hyposeleniferous environment. The patient had a plasma selenium level of 0.9 µg/dl and developed muscle tenderness and pain on active and passive motions of the limbs. The patient was treated for one week with 100 µg of selenium as selenomethionine, and the myositis symptoms regressed. Clearly, this patient had low selenium reserves. The fact that a controlled trial of selenium supplementation in New Zealand failed to associate selenium treatment with the relief of muscular complaints placed in doubt, however, the validity of skeletal muscle inflammation and necrosis as a component of the clinical syndrome of human selenium deficiency.[162] Nevertheless, Kien and Ganther[163] provided substantial evidence for a true association of myositis and selenium deficiency in an eight-year-old child with a familial form of chronic, secretory diarrhea. After 18 months on TPN, he developed muscle tenderness and elevation of muscle enzymes. Enzyme elevations and intermittent complaints of muscle pain and tenderness after exercise persisted ten months later. At 32 months into therapy, the clinical situation and objective evidence of low serum selenium levels prompted the institution of oral selenium at a dosage of 400 μg daily as whole yeast for 17 days, followed by intravenous supplementation with 42 μg of selenium from 34 months of TPN. The dosage was adjusted upward to 66 μg/day at 35 months, and to 97 μg at 39 months. Retrospective analyses of stored serum samples showed selenium levels to have been 0.3 to 0.7 μg/dl. Stored urine samples from the 14th to 16th month of TPN had no detectable amounts of selenium. At the beginning of intravenous selenium supplementation, the serum selenium concentration was 1.8 μg/dl, and the red cell glutathione peroxidase activity was one-tenth of normal. Both serum selenium level and erythrocyte glutathione peroxidase activity rose toward normal over five months with the incremental change in intravenous selenium administration. It was only with the 97 μg daily dosage, however, that muscle enzyme activity returned toward normal and muscular complaints disappeared. Another anomalous finding was an intense pallor of the fingernails and nailbeds, which appeared at 24 months of TPN and resolved after selenium supplementation. At no time were cardiac abnormalities detected. The persistence of diarrhea may have contributed to depletion of selenium and to the incomplete response to oral selenium in this patient.

That oral selenium supplementation *can* be effective, however, in some patients on TPN was shown by King and colleagues,[164] who treated a patient with multiple enterocutaneous fistulas secondary to necrotizing pancreatitis who had been on TPN for 14 months. Red cell selenium concentration and glutathione peroxidase activity were severely depressed, although no clinical manifestations of selenium deficiency were evident. An oral dosage of 400 μg of selenium daily for seven days followed by 100 μg for five days raised the erythrocyte glutathione peroxidase activity to 50 per cent of normal. After five months of the 100 μg dose, both the selenium concentration and the glutathione peroxidase activity of the patient's red cells were normal.

TPN-associated selenium deficiency manifested as cardiomyopathy has been demonstrated convincingly in two additional patients. Johnson and colleagues[165] reported on a 43-year-old man with extensive small bowel resections who had been on a home TPN regimen of crystalline amino acids, dextrose, and lipids for two years. He received supplements of zinc and copper, but not selenium. In the aftermath of a surgical intervention for a cholecystocolonic fistula, he experienced ventricular arrhythmias, cardiac dilatation, and pulmonary edema. Serum selenium levels and red cell glutathione peroxidase activity were only 10 per cent of normal. Oral supplementation with selenium tablets was instituted. The patient expired on the 48th hospital day, of circulatory failure. Postmortem examination of cardiac tissue revealed depressed selenium concentration and glutathione peroxidase activity. Fleming and associates[166] reported a similar occurrence in a 24-year-old man on home TPN for six years because of severe, chronic idiopathic pseudo-obstruction. He developed sudden onset of cardiac arrhythmias followed by cardiac dilatation and congestive heart failure. His electrocardiogram showed bifascicular heart block and low voltage, findings consistent with cardiomyopathy. He was discharged on digoxin but died at home two weeks after hospitalization. Whole blood selenium levels obtained two days before death were one-ninth of normal. Postmortem examination of tissue specimens showed glutathione activity and selenium concentrations to be depressed in heart, skeletal muscle, and liver, and the selenium content of the myocardium was one-sixth that of normal.

In addition to overt clinical syndromes, unsupplemented long-term home TPN regimens can produce several functional consequences of selenium deficiency in individuals who do not manifest frank signs and symptoms. Lane and co-workers[161] found, along with low plasma and erythrocyte selenium concentrations, a reduction in mean red cell glutathione peroxidase activity to one-half that of normal university students in nine patients receiving home TPN for from 1 to 27 months. Shils and associates[167] showed various abnormalities of T-lymphocyte function in seven patients on home TPN for three to ten years without specific supplementation with selenium. Plasma selenium levels were universally low, and neutrophil function was normal. Supplementation of the intravenous solutions with 50 to 99 μg of selenium daily restored normal T-lymphocyte activity patterns in the majority of the subjects with initially defective patterns.

Some degree of selenium depletion may pre-exist in the types of patients in which TPN is indicated. Malnourished children demonstrate low selenium status.[168, 169] Patients with cancer are also likely to have selenium deficiency.[170] The combination of disease and a TPN regimen that does not contain adequate selenium supplementation provides a setting for the development of clinical manifestations of selenium deficiency.

CHROMIUM

Biochemical and Physiologic Role

Chromium does not participate in any metalloproteins. Its main biologic action appears to be the potentiation of the action of insulin. Chromium presumably participates in the hormonal transmission of insulin at the level of the receptor cells in the form of a ternary organic complex known as glucose tolerance factor (GTF).[171] The precise chemical composition and structure of GTF has not been elucidated. Deficiency of chromium leads to impairment of glucose tolerance.[172] There is also recent evidence that chromium participates in the regulation of lipoprotein metabolism in humans.[173–174]

Assessment of Chromium Status

The indices used clinically to evaluate human chromium status are listed in Table 8–10. Hubert[175] has commented on the detection of chromium deficiency, specifically with relationship to plasma, hair, and urinary chromium determinations. Retrospective analysis of the published literature reveals that sample contamination and improper instrumental analysis, specifically with respect to atomic absorption spectrophotometric techniques,[176] have led to severe overestimation of chromium in biologic materials.[175] For instance, estimates of chromium in the circulation ranged between 10 and 1000 μg/L from 1948 to 1968. Recently, it has become

Table 8–10. LABORATORY OPTIONS FOR ASSESSING CHROMIUM STATUS

STATIC INDICES
 Plasma chromium concentration
 Serum chromium concentration
 Erythrocyte chromium content
 Whole-blood chromium content
 Hair chromium content
 24-hour urinary chromium excretion
 Chromium/creatinine ratio

FUNCTIONAL INDICES
 Urinary chromium excretion in response to glucose load
 Change in circulating chromium concentration in response to glucose load ("relative chromium response")
 Serial glucose tolerance tests (oral or IV) before and after chromium supplementation

clear that normal levels are less than 0.1 μ/L (or 1 μg/dl).[175] Table 8–10 lists approaches to the diagnostic assessment of chromium nutriture in man. The fact that all but the last index listed in this table depend upon accurate measurement of chromium makes their clinical application difficult at most centers.

Several of the indices are functional in nature. On the basis of the fact that chromium should normally be mobilized in the face of an insulin response to a glucose load, investigators have used the change in circulating chromium concentration[177–179] or the output of urinary chromium[178–181] after a standard carbohydrate challenge. The glucose tolerance test as a functional measure of chromium status is also popular,[178, 182, 183] but must be performed before and after chromium supplementation for full interpretation.

Chromium Deficiency During TPN

In the studies of Jacobson and Wester[7] in Sweden, the amount of chromium administered to the patients ranged from 19 to 57 μg/24 hours (mean 46 μg/24 hours). Three of the subjects were in positive chromium balance (range 1 to 10 μg/24 hours), and one subject, who was undergoing gastric suction, was in negative balance. Fell and colleagues[14] measured intravenous intakes and urinary output of chromium in three patients on TPN studied for five to 18 days. Daily intakes of the mineral ranged from 20 to 41 μg. All patients were in negative balance (omitting fecal and insensible losses) of from −2.6 to −9.1 μg/24 hours.

Jeejeebhoy and associates[184] found concentrations of serum chromium in patients on long-term home TPN, without specific supplementation, to range from 1.8 to 3.8 μg/L. The investigators assumed that these values were low, but current standards would consider them to be in the normal range.[175]

Two instances of clinical chromium deficiency in patients on long-term TPN have been reported. Jeejeebhoy and associates[184] reported on a woman who had undergone total enterectomy for a mesenteric artery thrombosis at age 34 and had subsequently been maintained on TPN. After 34 months on this regimen, weight loss of 5 kg was noted as well as elevated plasma glucose levels two hours following her nightly TPN infusion. She subsequently developed a peripheral sensory and motor neuropathy suggestive of diabetic neuropathy. She required insulin to control blood glucose levels. Blood and hair levels of chromium were low, and she was found to be in severe negative chromium balance. Infusion of 250 μg of chromium daily for two weeks normalized post-infusion glucose levels without the assistance of exogenous insulin. She recovered weight, and the peripheral neuropathy gradually abated.

Freund and co-workers[185] reported the case of a 45-year-old woman who also had undergone massive intestinal resection for mesenteric circulatory insufficiency. Blood glucose levels were initially normal, but five months into TPN, following a urologic operation, she went into hyperglycemic, hyperosmotic, nonketotic coma. Insulin therapy—20 to 30 units/day—maintained her blood glucose unevenly in the range of 72 to 581 mg/dl, with frequent glycosuria. She developed a metabolic encephalopathy resistant to a branched-chain amino acid–enriched formula. Serum chromium levels were found to be at the lower limit of normal, and daily intravenous infusions of 150 μg of chromium were begun. Glucose tolerance improved and insulin could be omitted. The patient's encephalopathy cleared completely and she regained weight.

Shapcott[186] has commented on these two cases, noting that after the initial administration of 3100 μg[184] and 9000 μg[185] of chromium, the patients could maintain glucose control without insulin and reduced their daily caloric intakes by 200 and 1000 kcal, maintaining weight recovery on about 2000 kcal of daily intake.

The metabolism of chromium was studied in the acute TPN situation by German anesthetists in 16 patients severely injured in traffic accidents and undergoing parenteral alimentation while on life-support systems and artificial ventilation in an intensive care unit. It should be remembered that intravenous solutions of German manufacture contain excessive amounts of chromium (see Table 8–2). Compared with the serum concentrations of the mineral in healthy controls (median, 0.62 μg/L), injured patients had high levels, ranging from 2 to 45 μg/L. The same investigators observed a chromium concentration of 8.8 μg/dl in an eight-year-old girl after only five months on TPN. This experience was further confirmed in three premature neonates, who over the first three to six days of TPN, which was begun two days after birth, showed a consistent rise in serum chromium concentration.[15]

Patients undergoing TPN also have excessive excretion of chromium in urine, not only in Germany, where the TPN solutions are chromium rich, but also in Scotland, where the TPN solutions are low in intrinsic chromium. In the German series of intensive care trauma patients,[15] urinary chromium excretion ranged from 10 to 400 μg/24 hours, with daily intakes of from 18.5 to 105 μg/L in the intravenous infusions. The mean output of chromium in the urine of five Scottish patients ranged from 13 to 71 μg/24 hours, compared with less than 5 μg/24 hours in patients not on TPN.[14] Intakes of chromium in the Scottish TPN solutions were in the range of 5 to 18 μg/L, leading the authors to conclude that the "increase in urinary Cr presents the effect of mobilization of Cr glucose tolerance factor in response to glucose infusion."[15]

MOLYBDENUM

Biochemical and Physiologic Role

Molybdenum is important in the oxidative metabolism of purines and sulfur-containing compounds into forms that can be excreted by the kidney. It is a constituent of three metalloenzymes in mammals: xanthine oxidase, sulfite oxidase, and aldehyde oxidase. Each metalloenzyme catalyzes a reaction involving the transfer of oxygen from water to an acceptor substrate that is being oxidized. Xanthine oxidase catalyzes the oxidation of hypoxanthine and xanthine in the degradation of purines derived from dietary or endogenous nucleic acids in the pathway that leads to the formation of uric acid.[187] Sulfite oxidase oxidizes the toxic anionic sulfur compound sulfite (SO_3^{--}) derived from organic sulfur compounds in the body such as cysteine and methionine to sulfate (SO_4^{--}), which is readily excreted by the kidneys.[187] Aldehyde oxidase catalyzes the hydroxylation of various heterocyclic nitrogen-containing compounds. A common feature of the mammalian molybdoenzyme is a molybdenum cofactor that is the core structure of the active holoenzyme.

Assessment of Molybdenum Status

The analytic determination of molybdenum in organic fluids and tissue matrices is difficult and not widely available. As with chromium, plasma and serum samples are easily contaminated during collection and handling. Neutron activation analysis (NAA) represents the method of choice, and in recent years a consensus has developed that normal circulating molybdenum levels are less than 1 µg/L. Some representative mean (± SD) values for healthy populations are: 0.58 /p, 0.21,[188] 0.59 ± 0.23,[189] and 0.55 ± 0.21[190] µg/L. NAA is an expensive, cumbersome technique not sufficiently available to be useful for routine clinical determinations. Obstructive and hepatocellular liver disease produces an elevation in serum molybdenum concentrations,[190] which would constitute a pitfall to the use of this index to assess molybdenum nutriture in certain patients undergoing TPN.

On the basis of work with inborn errors of molybdenum cofactor, a number of *in vivo* and *in vitro functional* indicators of molybdenum nutrition can be proposed.[191] Levels of xanthine oxidase, sulfite oxidase, and molybdenum cofactor can be measured in cultured fibroblasts or hepatic biopsy tissue. The urinary excretion pattern of sulfite, sulfate, and various organic sulfur compounds, and its response to load tests with methionine or sodium metabisulfite or to the elimination of sulfur amino acids, can characterize the *in vivo* activity of sulfite oxidase. The indications can be confirmed by examining the urinary metabolite pattern and repeating the load tests after supplementation with molybdenum. Similarly, the urinary excretion pattern

of xanthine, hypoxanthine, and uric acid, and blood levels of uric acid, either alone or in response to purine loading, would be indicative of xanthine oxidase status, which could be confirmed by repeating the evaluations following molybdenum supplementation. An *in vivo* load test for aldehyde oxidase involves monitoring the conversion of L-histidine to hydantoin-5-propionic acid and determining the latter metabolite's urinary concentration. In many respects, the functional indices are more accessible and reliable as measures of molybdenum status than determination of molybdenum in tissues or body fluids.

Molybdenum Deficiency During TPN

A case of molybdenum deficiency in a 24-year-old man with short-bowel syndrome secondary to Crohn's disease associated with parenteral nutrition has been reported.[187] The patient had been maintained on TPN for 12 months when he developed a syndrome of intermittent headache, night blindness, central scotomas, nausea, vomiting, tachycardia and tachypnea progressing to edema, disorientation, and coma. The syndrome was precipitated by crystalline amino acid solutions and was associated with a ten-fold rise in plasma methionine concentration and a three- to five-fold decrement in serum uric acid concentration. Sodium metabisulfite precipitated the same syndrome. Low urinary inorganic sulfate and high levels of urinary thiosulfate were seen as well as hypouricosuria. Urinary excretion values for xanthine and hypoxanthine were correspondingly high.

Administration of ammonium molybdate, 300 µg (163 µg of elemental Mo) daily in combination with a low-sulfur amino acid infusion mixture, reversed the clinical syndrome, increasing the serum levels and urinary output of uric acid. The metabolic alterations in this patient were characteristic of deficiencies of sulfite oxidase (disordered sulfur metabolism) and xanthine oxidase (hypouricemia, hypouricosuria), two molybdoenzymes. The sulfur amino acid intolerance produced the neurologic manifestations, a situation not dissimilar from the clinical pattern in hereditary sulfite oxidase deficiency.[191] It is unfortunate that no tissue or blood levels of molybdenum were measured and that the intrinsic concentration of molybdenum in the infusion solution was not reported. The possibility of a mild inborn error of molybdenum metabolism in this individual, stressed by his TPN regimen, cannot be ruled out. Such a hypothesis would explain the rarity of apparent cases of molybdenum deficiency uncovered in the 15 years of TPN therapy.

SUPPLEMENTARY AND THERAPEUTIC ADMINISTRATION OF TRACE MINERALS IN TOTAL PARENTERAL NUTRITION

In Great Britain and on the Continent, the inclusion of trace minerals in TPN regimens became a common practice early on.[192, 193] In the United States, approval from the Food and Drug Administration (FDA) for the use of intravenous trace elements lagged far behind. Moreover, despite (1) the low intrinsic content of trace minerals in the nutrient solutions used in TPN (see Table 8–2) and (2) recognition of negative balance with respect to trace minerals in the absence of supplements,[7, 64, 109, 110] determination of the precise dosages for intravenous delivery is still problematic. Two approaches have been used to determine the "parenteral requirement" for trace minerals. The first is to base the dosage on the dietary allowance and correct it by a factor of absorptive efficiency. The second is to determine experimentally the amount of minerals required to maintain positive or neutral nutrient balance in patients on TPN.

A committee of experts was convened by the American Medical Association (AMA) to develop preliminary recommendations for intravenous administration of trace minerals during TPN. They published suggested dosages for four elements: zinc, copper, manganese, and chromium (Table 8–11).[194] Recommendations for iron have been made by individual investigators.[193, 195] No formal recommendations have been made for selenium and molybdenum, although experience with their use as trace mineral additives in TPN is expanding.[196, 197] With FDA approval, a myriad of products has become available commercially in the past several years; partial listings of the trace mineral additives on the market are given in Tables 8–12 and 8–13.

The expert committee of the AMA was emphatic in recommending that the various additives be made as *single-entity* formulations.[194] Nevertheless, several multiple-element additive solutions—based largely on the relative proportions recommended by the AMA committee—have been marketed (see Table 8–13). The pros and cons of the use of single-entity and multiple-element formulations should be clearly understood. The committee urged the creation of only single-entity additives on the basis of a number of considerations, including: (1) the variation of individual requirements among patients and between age groups; (2) the fact that fixed-dosage multiple-element solutions might encourage the overdosage of several nutrients when the requirement for one or another was specifically elevated; (3) the intrinsic and variable natural contamination of different intravenous products used in TPN with different minerals; and (4) the theoretic necessity for the additives to complement the quantities of a given mineral already supplied

Table 8–11. SUGGESTIONS BY AMA EXPERT COMMITTEE FOR DAILY INTRAVENOUS INTAKE OF ZINC, COPPER, CHROMIUM, AND MANGANESE

| TYPE OF PATIENT | DAILY INTAKE | | | |
	Zinc	*Copper*	*Chromium**	*Manganese**
Pediatric patient	100 µg/kg†	20 µg/kg	0.14–0.2 µg/kg	2–10 µg/kg
Stable adult	2.5–4.0 mg	0.5–1.5 mg	10–15 µg	0.15–0.8 mg
Adult in acute catabolic state	Add 2.0 mg	NS	NS	NS
Stable adult with intestinal losses	Add 12.2 mg for each L of small intestinal fluid; add 17.1 mg for each L of stool or ileostomy output	NS	20 µg	NS

*NS = not specified.
†For premature infants, a daily intake of 300 µg/kg of zinc has been suggested.
(Data from American Medical Association: Guidelines for essential tract element preparation for parenteral use. J.A.M.A., 241:2051–2054, 1979.)

Table 8–12. COMMERCIAL SINGLE-ENTITY FORMULATIONS OF TRACE MINERAL ADDITIVES*

PRODUCT	MANUFACTURER	TYPE OF SALT	IONIC CONCENTRATION (mg/ml)	HOW SUPPLIED
Zinc				
Zinc chloride	Abbott Laboratories	Chloride	1.0	10-ml vial
Zinc sulfate	International Medication Systems, Ltd.	Sulfate	4.0	10-ml vial
Zinc sulfate	Lyphomed	Sulfate	5.0	5-ml vial
			1.0	10-ml and 30-ml vials
ZincTrace	USV Laboratories	Chloride	1.0	10-ml vial
Copper				
CopperTrace	USV Laboratories	Chloride	0.4	10-ml vial
Manganese				
MangaTrace	USV Laboratories	Chloride	0.1	10-ml vial
Selenium				
Selepen	Lyphomed	Selenious acid	0.04	10-ml vial
Chromium				
ChromeTrace	USV Laboratories	Chloride	0.004	10-ml vial
Molybdenum				
Molypen	Lyphomed	Ammonium molybdate	0.025	10-ml vial

*This is not an exhaustive listing of all formulations of trace mineral additives commercially available at the time of publication. Mention of a proprietary name does not constitute an endorsement, guarantee, or warranty of the product nor imply its approval to the exclusion of other products that may be suitable.

by the TPN regimen. Multiple-element formulas have, nonetheless, emerged and become popular for their simplicity of prescription by physicians and addition by pharmacy or nursing staff. To the extent that their convenience encourages a consciousness about trace mineral nutrition in TPN, they serve a useful purpose. In a large number of patients—those on home TPN with stable medical conditions—the combination of minerals approximates the nutritional requirements. However, a casual attitude toward the use of trace mineral additives could produce as many nutritional problems as were seen in the days before trace mineral supplementation became widespread.

A checklist of concerns regarding the administration of trace elements is presented in Table 8–14. When planning and prescribing a TPN regimen for a given patient and when trying to resolve any unexpected or unexplained problem occurring during TPN, the physician should run through such a checklist, addressing the questions sequentially. Both single-entity and multiple-element preparations have roles in parenteral

Table 8–13. COMMERCIAL MULTIPLE-ELEMENT FORMULATIONS OF TRACE MINERAL ADDITIVES*

PRODUCT	MANUFACTURER	IONIC CONCENTRATIONS (mg/ml)					HOW SUPPLIED
		Zinc	Copper	Chromium	Manganese	Iodine	
NEDH Formulation	Pentcal	1.5	0.5	0.005	0.2	0.028	10-ml vial
Multiple Trace Mineral Additive	International Medication Systems, Ltd.	4.0	1.0	0.01	0.5	—	1-ml select-a-jet syringe, 5-ml and 10-ml vials
M.T.E.-4	Lyphomed	1.0	0.4	0.004	0.1	—	3-ml, 10-ml, and 30-ml vials
M.T.E.-concentrated	Lyphomed	5.0	1.0	0.01	0.5	—	1-ml and 10-ml vials
P.T.E.-4 (pediatric)	Lyphomed	1.0	0.1	0.001	0.025	—	3-ml vial

*This is not an exhaustive listing of all formulations of trace mineral additives commercially available at the time of publication. Mention of a proprietary name does not constitute an endorsement, guarantee, or warranty of the product nor imply its approval to the exclusion of other products that may be suitable.

Table 8–14. CHECKLIST OF CONCERNS AND QUESTIONS REGARDING TRACE MINERAL ADDITIVE ADMINISTRATION

Need for an exogenous source	Is the patient likely to have sufficient reserves of a given trace mineral to sustain him/her through the expected course of parenteral nutrition?
Prior depletion	Is the patient likely to have a pre-existing depletion of a given trace mineral and to be in need of its specific repletion?
Maintenance requirement	Is the patient stable and without a condition(s) that would predispose to excessive trace mineral loss or retention?
Supramaintenance requirement	Does the patient's condition predispose to continuous loss of a given trace mineral? Is the patient catabolic? Is the patient anabolic?
Submaintenance requirement	Does the patient have a pre-existing whole-body excess of a trace mineral, or does his/her condition preclude the normal excretion of the trace mineral and predispose to its excessive accumulation?
Incompatibilities	Are there any interactions of a given trace mineral with other nutrients in the solution or with drugs given to the patient that might alter the bioavailability of that mineral?
Intrinsic mineral content	How much of a given trace mineral is delivered by the solutions in the TPN regimen as a native contaminant? Is this amount less than, equal to, or greater than the patient's estimated parenteral requirement for that mineral?
Nutrient overdose	What are the signs and symptoms of adverse or toxic reactions to a given trace mineral? Is the patient manifesting a toxicity or overload syndrome?

alimentation. Most often, both types must be used to provide routine maintenance levels for some nutrients while delivering individually adjusted doses of others. This practice is particularly necessary because the majority of trace mineral additive containers do not contain bacteriostatic agents and so must be discarded after a single use.

Common to all uses of trace minerals by a parenteral route are two concerns. The first is that direct, internal introduction of a mineral into the bloodstream bypasses the potential regulatory mechanism of the gut. The second is the possibility that the bioavailability of a mineral entering the peripheral circulation as an inorganic salt will not be utilized in metabolism with the same efficiency as that of a mineral introduced from the diet via the gastrointestinal tract, the portal vein, and the liver. The chemical forms may be altered by enteral passage, and infused, inorganic materials may be cleared and deposited in abnormal ways, making them potentially toxic to tissues and potentially less available for nutritional purposes. Minerals that are infused may also be cleared by the kidneys to a far greater extent than minerals taken up by normal absorptive processes. All of these possibilities are in some way factored into the long-term behavior of trace minerals in a chronic TPN regimen.

Iron

Iron is the most problematic of all trace minerals with respect to its parenteral administration. No commercial iron additive specifically designed for addition to TPN solution exists as yet. Iron dextran preparations (Imferon, Dextraron-50, Proferdex) have been used commonly to supply iron to TPN patients. They have been formulated, however, for treatment of iron deficiency and are concentrated solutions containing 50 mg/ml of elemental iron. When pre-existing iron depletion is present, or when acute blood loss has supervened, replacement therapy with "total-dose" parenteral iron therapy is indicated. Mathematical formulas for estimating the amount of iron necessary to replace the deficit for either situation, using body weight, hemoglobin concentration, and age as parameters, are available.[198] The total volume of iron dextran additive required to effect replacement can then be calculated, and daily administration continued until the calculated volume has been delivered. Formerly, up to 15 ml of iron dextran preparation was injected in a single treatment,[198] but currently the maximum approved single administration is 2 ml (100 mg of elemental iron). A test dose of 0.1 ml (5 mg of elemental iron) *must* be administered with each treatment. Satisfactory replacement of iron stores and hemoglobin levels in patients on TPN have been reported using iron dextran.[200, 201] An alternative route of administration is intramuscular, but the local pain, inflammation, and skin staining render it less desirable.

The turnover of iron by insensible losses has been calculated at 14 µg/kg for nonmenstruating individuals.[24] Daily maintenance doses ranging from 1.2 to 3.9 mg have been recommended.[193, 195] Menstruation will increase these requirements. Until recently, the only option to supply daily iron maintenance has been with iron dextran. Diluted stock solutions of iron dextran containing 0.5 mg/ml, stabilized with benzyl alcohol, have proved to be adequately stable.[202] Such dilution increases the precision of dosing. Theoretic objections to this approach are raised on two grounds, however: (1) the incorporation of iron from dextran into red cells—even in anemic individuals—is poor, around 39 per cent,[203] and (2) with the proliferation of independent TPN regimens, the occurrence of an anaphylactic reaction at home would be disastrous.[18] On an *experimental* basis, Sayers and colleagues[18] have tested ferrous citrate as an iron additive in TPN. They found it to be stable when diluted, transferrable to transferrin *in vitro,* and incorporated into new red cells with an efficiency of 81 per cent, twice that of iron dextran. At present, there are no commercial preparations of ferrous citrate, nor has it received FDA approval; it would require individual formation in a hospital pharmacy.

A confounding issue in iron bioavailability is the poor incorporation of iron into hemoglobin and its sequestration by the reticuloendothelial cells in chronic inflammation, such as Crohn's disease.[204] A theoretic objection to the intravenous delivery of iron is the potential for provoking gram-negative sepsis.[205] Infants treated with iron dextran[206, 207] or oral iron[208] seem more susceptible to disseminated bacterial infections. Some investigators have advocated the use of packed red blood cells in TPN patients to avoid the infusion of quantities of free iron that might favor bacterial proliferation.[205]

Improper adjustment of an iron dosage can lead eventually to an overload of the body with iron (nutritional siderosis). This is generally a benign situation, but concern that it might induce cirrhotic changes in the liver has been expressed. By far the most serious adverse reactions to parenteral iron are apparent in replacement therapy with full-strength iron dextran. Allergic reactions, including fatal anaphylaxis, and a host of systemic reactions are often observed.[199] The iron reserves of a newborn term infant are sufficient for expansion of the red cell mass for three to five months, and an iron-replete adult male has iron stores that would last for up to two years. In short courses of TPN in these classes of patients, therefore, routine administration of iron can potentially be omitted.

Zinc

Zinc for parenteral administration is available in both single-entity and multiple-element formulations (see Tables 8–12 and 8–13). Because the majority of zinc is transferred from the maternal compartment to the fetal compartment during the last trimester of pregnancy, daily parenteral zinc requirements for premature infants are high, 300 µg/kg.[194] For children up to five years of age, maintenance requirements for zinc are 100 µg/kg. For stable patients over five years of age, 2.5 to 4 mg of parenteral zinc is required for maintenance of balance. In tumor-bearing patients, requirements for parenteral zinc are 70 to 80 µg/kg.[102] Acute catabolic stress (fever, burns, etc.) produces an increase in intravenous zinc requirements of about 2 mg. The work of Wolman and associates[109] demonstrated the magnitude of zinc losses in intestinal fluids. Thus, the replacement of zinc in patients with active ileostomy or diarrheal losses while receiving TPN must be based on the volume of fluid excreted and the average zinc content of the fluid lost (see Table 8–11).

Once zinc deficiency is recognized in a patient on TPN, it must be corrected by supplying therapeutic doses of zinc. Dosages from 9 to 10 mg of zinc daily in the early repletion period have been used in adult patients with large zinc losses.[56] Both oral zinc (8 mg/day)[72] and intravenous zinc (1 to 16 mg/day)[74] have been used to initiate treatment of zinc deficiency in children and adolescents.

In one study, transient flushing, blurred vision, and sweating were seen when 10 mg of zinc were infused over a one-hour period.[87] Inadvertent overdosage with 23 mg/day of zinc in seven TPN patients in

Brazil produced asymptomatic hyperamylasemia.[209] The death of an elderly woman was precipitated by the acute infusion of 1.6 gm of zinc over 60 hours as a consequence of an error in home hemodialysis; she died 47 days later as a result of anemia, thrombocytopenia, cholestatic jaundice, and uremia.[210] Hyperamylasemia without pancreatitis was also observed in this case.

Copper

Copper is available in both single-entity and multiple-element additives (see Tables 8–12 and 8–13). The AMA expert committee has specified the parenteral requirements as 20 μg/kg in children and 0.5 to 1.5 mg in stable adults (see Table 8–11). Balance studies in tumor-bearing patients revealed a parenteral requirement of 50 to 60 μg/kg. The balance studies by Shike and colleagues[135] indicate that the parenteral copper requirement for the adult was closer to 0.3 mg, and that copper in excess of that amount was efficiently retained and accumulated by the body.

Treatment of TPN-induced copper deficiency with parenteral copper has been reported. Both Vilter and associates[131] and Pulmissano[132] achieved a rapid hematologic correction with daily administration of 1 mg of copper daily by the parenteral route. In a pediatric patient, reversal of symptoms was effected with a 35 μg/kg/day copper dosage added to the infusate. Dunlap and co-workers[126] used *oral* copper therapy (5 mg copper sulfate containing 1.25 mg of copper) with satisfactory resolution of symptoms; one patient had gastric irritation.

Massive introduction of copper into the circulation can produce fatal hemolysis and hepatic necrosis,[211, 212] but this is virtually impossible with commercial additives. No adverse reactions to the commonly used doses of parenteral copper have been reported. Because copper is excreted in the bile, its dosage should be modified or eliminated in patients with cholestatic conditions and biliary obstruction.

Manganese

Manganese for parenteral administration is available both in single-entity and multiple-element mineral additive preparations (see Tables 8–12 and 8–13). The AMA expert committee has recommended a pediatric dose of 2 to 10 μg/kg and an adult dose of 0.15 to 0.8 mg for routine maintenance.[194] Catabolic states and diarrheal fluid losses are not believed to increase the manganese requirement. Occasion for the use of "therapeutic" doses of manganese is unlikely to arise, given the absence of documentation of manganese deficiency in humans. On the other hand, because manganese is excreted by the biliary tract, cholestatic conditions or biliary obstruction might contraindicate the parenteral administration of this mineral. Industrial exposure to manganese has led to toxic neurologic and psychiatric disorders, but no such consequences of any dietary exposure have been reported. They are unlikely to occur with parenteral administration.

Selenium

Selenium for parenteral administration recently became available in a single-entity preparation (see Table 8–12). There is no recommendation for its maintenance administration by the AMA or any other collective authority. The manufacturers of Selepen recommend 20 to 40 μg daily. Experience in home parenteral nutrition at the Cleveland Clinic suggests that a daily intake of 120 μg of selenium maintained adequate selenium status.[196] Levander and colleagues[213] have shown the *dietary* requirement of selenium to be about 60 μg daily. With its high efficiency of absorption, 50 μg of parenteral selenium might be considered a reasonable maintenance dosage for a North American adult. Human populations seem to adapt to a wide range of selenium intakes, and the whole-body selenium pool will vary with the habitual dietary intake. In hyposeleniferous countries such as Finland and New Zealand, the parenteral requirement to maintain the customary selenium pool would be considerably less. It is perhaps this adaptive capacity that permits a wide range of parenteral maintenance doses to be effective in adult patients.

The manufacturer's recommended maintenance dosage for children is 3 μg/kg. By the time a child reaches 7 kg, at 6 months of age, his or her dosage requirement has already entered the adult range. Steiger and co-workers[196] have advocated the administration of selenium at 30 μg/L of infusate for infants and young children, and 14 μg/L for older children and adolescents, on the basis of experience at the Hospital for Sick Children in Toronto.

It has recently been shown that interactions within the TPN solutions can reduce the bioavailability of selenium by precipitating selenium in the elemental state.[214] The factors implicated in this phenomenon were copper and the high ascorbic acid content of MVI. Copper without high-dose vitamin C was not harmful. The newer formulation of the multivitamin additive, MVI-12, in which a five-fold reduction was made in ascorbic acid content, has a less deleterious influence on selenium availability when combined in TPN solutions.

Selenium deficiency has occurred in patients on TPN. At the Cleveland Clinic, evidence of low selenium status in a TPN patient is treated with an initial therapeutic dosage of 240 µg/day, which is increased in increments to 480 µg/day; doses as high as 720 µg/day have been used in this center.[196] In the case reports of TPN-induced selenium deficiency in the literature, oral selenium pills were used in two instances.[164, 165] In one, a daily dose of 100 µg of selenium reversed deficiency symptoms and signs.[164] Sterile selenomethionine (100 µg/day) administered parenterally has been used as a source of selenium,[162] but the organic compound cannot be recommended.

There are no commonly reported adverse reactions to intravenous selenium in the limited experience to date. Selenium toxicity is recognized in livestock and laboratory animals. The current additives contain inorganic selenium. Extreme caution should be used with regard to the infusion of "organic" selenium compounds such as selenomethionine. Although the seleno–amino acids are part of the normal diet, their retention in the body and distribution in tissues differs from those of inorganic selenium. Until understanding of the necessary balance of inorganic and organic selenium in human nutrition is greater, the prudent course is to use only the inorganic form of selenium in the approved commercial additives.

Chromium

Chromium for parenteral administration is available both in single-entity formulation and as part of multiple-element additives (see Tables 8–12 and 8–13). The AMA expert committee addressed chromium maintenance requirements (see Table 8–11).[194] For pediatric patients, the parenteral requirements are 0.14 to 0.20 µg/kg. For stable adults, the intravenous allowance is 10 to 15 µg, 20 µg for individuals with intestinal fluid losses. No increment for adults in acute catabolic states was specified. These allowances may be excessive, because Mertz[172] has recently calculated that the obligatory, insensible losses of chromium are on the order of 0.5 to 1.0 µg daily in adults. Therapeutic administration of chromium by the parenteral route was undertaken in the two well-documented cases of TPN-induced chromium deficiency.[184, 185] Dosages of 150 to 250 µg were used by the authors of these reports.

Adverse reactions to parenteral chromium are unknown, and the possibility for intoxication with parenteral administration of the mineral is minimal. European clinicians should be aware that TPN solutions manufactured on that continent often contain substantial amounts of chromium as incidental contamination, presumably from exposure to stainless steel during manufacture (see Table 8–2).[15] In these circumstances, exogenous supplementation with additives may not be necessary to maintain the parenteral requirements.

Molybdenum

Molybdenum is available only as a single-entity additive (see Table 8–12). No official recommendations for its parenteral administration have been developed. The manufacturer of Molypen recommends an adult daily dosage of 20 to 120 µg of molybdenum, and the calculation of a pediatric dosage "by extrapolation." Noting that the intrinsic content of molybdenum in TPN solutions of amino acids is 5 to 15 µg/L, Abumrad and colleagues[187] advised reticence in the routine administration of molybdenum to patients undergoing TPN. Thus, discretion should be used in determining whether a given patient requires conscious, daily supplementation with molybdenum.

CONCLUSION

A large number of trace minerals are essential for human nutrition. A diet—be it oral, enteral, or parenteral—would not be "nutritionally complete" unless it contained adequate amounts of the essential trace minerals. Until recently, trace minerals were not consciously added to TPN regimens. Variable amounts of the trace minerals are present in intravenous solutions as a result of incidental contamination or as intrinsic components of the starting materials. Nonetheless, individuals undergoing TPN are often in negative balance with respect to one or another trace mineral when given regimens that are not supplemented with trace minerals from additives. Clinical reports of TPN-induced deficiencies of copper, zinc, chromium, selenium, and molybdenum have appeared, and iron deficiency with or without anemia is a common consequence of the types of diseases for which parenteral alimentation is often indicated.

Additive solutions containing several minerals, alone and in combination, have recently been approved by the FDA for commercial production. Iron is the major exception, but recent experimental studies suggest that ferrous citrate may prove to be an acceptable, bioavailable, safe compound to use as an parenteral additive for iron.[18] The use of trace mineral additives requires judgment, prudence, and vigilance. Laboratory diagnosis of trace mineral status in humans is far from satisfactory, hampering the precise monitoring of patients for early detection of nutrient deficiency or toxic accumulation. The only compensatory strategy given the primitive state of our diagnostic acumen is the *careful* calculation of additive dosages, taking into account the intrinsic delivery of the nutrients by the TPN regimens and the particular features of the patient's disease and nutritional history. The physician should maintain a thorough, up-to-date familiarity with the biology of trace minerals and a keen awareness of the possibility that a trace mineral deficiency or imbalance may be at the root of a clinical problem that emerges prior to or during treatment with TPN. In the years ahead, improvements in our ability to determine whole-body trace mineral status should improve the precision with which long-term administration of complete TPN regimens can be prescribed and modified to provide optimal amounts of the essential trace minerals for both growing children and stable adults.

REFERENCES

1. Mertz, W.: The essential trace elements. Science, 18:1332–1338, 1981.
2. Riordan, J. F.: Biochemistry of zinc. Med. Clin. North Am., 60:661–674, 1976.
3. James, B. E., and MacMahon, R. A.: Trace elements in IV fluids. Med. J. Aust., 2:1161–1163, 1970.
4. Green, H. L., Hambidge, K. M., and Herman, R. F.: Trace elements and vitamins. Adv. Exp. Med. Biol., 46:131–144, 1974.
5. Bozian, R. C., and Shearer, C.: Copper, zinc, and manganese content of four amino acids and protein hydrolysate preparations. Am. J. Clin. Nutr., 29:1331–1332, 1976.
6. Freier, S., and Jungreis, E.: Zinc and acrodermatitis enteropathica. Lancet, 1:914, 1976.
7. Jacobson, S., and Wester, P. O.: Balance study of twenty trace elements during total parenteral nutrition. Br. J. Nutr., 37:107–126, 1977.
8. Jetton, M. M., Sullivan, J. F., and Burch, R. E.: Trace element contamination of intravenous volutions. Arch. Intern. Med., 136:782–784, 1976.
9. Okada, A., and Takagi, Y.: An importance of zinc in total parenteral nutrition. Jap. J. Surg., 6:189–191, 1976.
10. Solomons, N. W., Layden, T. J., Rosenberg, I. H., Vo-Khactu, K., and Sandstead, H. H.: Plasma trace metals during total parenteral alimentation. Gastroenterology, 70:1022–1023, 1976.
11. Hauer, E. C., and Kaminski, M. V.: Trace metal profile of parenteral nutrition solutions. Am. J. Clin. Nutr., 31:264–268, 1978.
12. Kerkhof, K. H.: Trace metal contamination in Travasol. Am. J. Clin. Nutr., 31:1717, 1978.
13. Ota, D. M., Macfadyen, B. V., Jr., Gunn, E. T., and Dudrick, S.: Zinc and copper deficiencies in man during intravenous hyperalimentation. *In* Hambidge, K. M., and Nichols, B. L., Jr. (eds.): Zinc and Copper in Clinical Medicine. New York, Spectrum, 1978, pp. 99–112.
14. Fell, G. S., Halls, D., and Shenkin, A.: Chromium requirements during intravenous nutrition. *In* Shapcott, D., and Herbert, J. (eds.): Chromium in Nutrition and Metabolism. Amsterdam, Elsevier/North Holland, 1979, pp. 105–111.
15. Seeling, W., Ahnefeld, F. W., Grunert, A., Kienle, K. H., and Swobodnik, M.: Chromium in parenteral nutrition. *In* Shapcott, D., and Herbert, J. (eds.): Chromium in Nutrition and Metabolism. Amsterdam, Elsevier/North Holland, 1979, pp. 95–104.
16. Van Rij, A. M., McKenzie, J. M., Robinson, M. F., and Thomson, C. D.: Selenium and total parenteral nutrition. J.P.E.N., 3:235–239, 1979.
17. Smith, J. L., and Goos, S. M.: Selenium nutriture in total parenteral nutrition: intake levels. J.P.E.N., 4:23–26, 1980.
18. Sayers, M. H., Johnson, D. K., Schumann, L. A., Ivey, M. F., Young, J. H., and Finch C. A.: Supplementation of total parenteral nutrition solution with ferrous citrate. J.P.E.N., 7:117–121, 1983.
19. Pollitt, E., Lewis, N. L., Leibel, R. L., and Greenfield, D. B.: Iron deficiency and play behavior in pre-school children. *In* Garry, P. H. (ed.): Human Nutrition: Clinical and Biochemical Aspects. Tennessee, Kingsport Press, 1981, pp. 290–301.
20. Tucker, D. M., Swenson, R. A., and Sandstead, H. H.: Neuropsychological effects of iron deficiency. *In* Dreosti, I. E., and Smith, R. M. (eds.): Neurobiology of the Trace Elements. Vol. 1: Trace Element Neurobiology and Deficiencies. Clifton, NJ, Humana Press, 1983, pp. 269–291.
21. Finch, C. A., Miller, L. R., Inamdar, A. R., Person, R., Seiler, K., and Mackler, B.: Iron deficiency in the rat. Physiological and biochemical studies of

muscle dysfunction. J. Clin. Invest., *58*:447–453, 1976.

22. Jacobs, A.: The non-haematological effects of iron deficiency. Clin. Sci. Mol. Med., *53*:105–109, 1972.

23. Munro, H. N.: Iron absorption and nutrition: Introduction. Fed. Proc., *36*:2015–2016, 1977.

24. Greene, R., Charlton, R., Seftel, H., Bothwell, T., Mayet, F., Adams, B., and Finch, C.: Body iron excretion in man: A collaborative study. Am. J. Med., *45*:336–353, 1968.

25. Cook, J., and Finch, C. A.: Assessing the iron status of a population. Am. J. Clin. Nutr., *32*:2115–2119, 1979.

26. Lipschitz, D. A., Cook, J. D., and Finch, C. A.: A clinical evaluation of serum ferritin as an index of iron stores. N. Engl. J. Med., *290*:1213–1216, 1974.

27. Fabri, P. J., Mirtello, J. M., and Ruberg, M. D.: Iron status before TPN—prospective evaluation and clinical correlates (abstract). Abstracts, 7th Clinical Congress of the American Society for Parenteral and Enteral Nutrition, Washington, D.C., January, 1983, p. 167.

28. Valberg, L. S., Sorbie, J., Corbett, W. E., and Ludwig, J.: Cobalt test for the detection of iron deficiency anemia. Ann. Intern. Med., *77*:181–187, 1972.

29. World Health Organization. Trace Elements in Human Nutrition. Geneva, WHO, 1973.

30. Mills, C. F.: Biochemical roles of trace elements. Prog. Clin. Biol. Res., *77*:179–188, 1981.

31. Fernandez-Madrid, F., Prasad, A. S., and Oberleas, D.: Effect of zinc deficiency on nucleic acids, collagen and non-collagen protein of connective tissue. J. Lab. Clin. Med., *82*:951–961, 1973.

32. Prasad, A. S., and Rabbani, P.: Nucleoside phosphorylase in zinc deficiency. Trans. Assoc. Am. Physicians, *94*:314–321, 1981.

33. Sandstead, H. H., Holloway, W. L., and Baum, V.: Zinc deficiency: Effect on polysomes. Fed. Proc., *30*:517, 1971.

34. Bettger, W. J., and O'Dell, B. L.: A critical physiological role of zinc in the structure and function of biomembranes. Life Sci., *28*:1425–1438, 1981.

35. Solomons, N. W.: On the assessment of zinc and copper nutriture in man. Am. J. Clin. Nutr., *32*:856–871, 1979.

36. Danks, D. M.: Diagnosis of trace metal deficiency—with emphasis on copper and zinc. Am. J. Clin. Nutr., *34*:278–280, 1981.

37. Juswigg, T., Batres, R., Solomons, N. W., Pineda, O., and Milne, D. B.: The effect of temporary occlusion on trace mineral concentrations in plasma. Am. J. Clin. Nutr., *35*:354–358, 1982.

38. Prasad, A. S., and Cossack, Z. T.: Neutrophil zinc: An index of zinc status in man. Trans. Assoc. Am. Physicians, *95*:165–176, 1982.

39. Jones, R. B., Keeling, P. W. N., Hilton, P. J., and Thompson, R. P. H.: The relationship between leucocyte and muscle zinc in health and disease. Clin. Sci., *60*:237–239, 1991.

40. Capel, I. D., Spencer, E. P., Daivies, A. E., and Levitt, H. N.: The assessment of zinc status by the zinc tolerance test in various groups of patients. Clin. Biochem., *15*:257–260, 1982.

41. Gordon, P. R., Woodruff, C. W., Anderson, H. L., and O'Dell, B. L.: Effect of acute zinc deprivation on plasma zinc and platelet aggregation in adult males. Am. J. Clin. Nutr., *35*:113–119, 1982.

42. Golden, M. H., Golden, B. E., Harland, P. S. E. G., and Jackson, A. A.: Zinc and immunocompetence in protein energy malnutrition. Lancet, *1*:1226–1227, 1978.

43. Ballester, O. F., and Prasad, A. S.: Anergy, zinc deficiency and decreased nucleoside phosphorylase activity in patients with sickle cell anemia. Ann. Intern. Med., *98*:180–182, 1983.

44. Kararskis, E. J., and Schuna, A.: Serum alkaline phosphatase after treatment of zinc deficiency in humans. Am. J. Clin. Nutr., *33*:2609–2612, 1980.

45. Sandstead, H. H.: Zinc deficiency in the United States. Am. J. Clin. Nutr., *26*:1251–1260, 1973.

46. Gordon, W., and White, P. J.: Zinc deficiency in total parenteral nutrition. S. Afr. Med. J., *54*:823–824, 1978.

47. Main, A. N., Hull, M. J., Russell, R. I., Fell, G. S., Mills, P. R., and Shenkin, A.: Clinical experience of zinc supplementation during intravenous nutrition in Crohn's disease: Value of serum and urine zinc measurement. Gut., *23*:984–991, 1982.

48. Fleming, C. R., Smith, L. M., and Hodges, R. E.: Essential fatty acid, copper, zinc and tocopheral deficiencies in total parenteral nutrition. Acta Chir. Scand. (Suppl.) *466*:20–21, 1976.

49. Tasman-Jones, C., Kay, R. G., and Lee, S. P.: Zinc and copper deficiency, with particular reference to parenteral nutrition. Surg. Ann., *10*:23–52, 1978.

50. Askari, A., Long, C. L., and Blakemore, W. S.: Zinc and copper and parenteral nutrition in cancer: A review. J.P.E.N., *4*:561–571, 1980.

51. McClain, C. J.: Trace metal abnormalities in adults during hyperalimentation. J.P.E.N., *5*:424–429, 1981.

52. MacMahon, R. A., LeMoine, P. M., and McKinnon, M. C.: Zinc treatment in malabsorption. Med. J. Aust., *2*:210–212, 1968.

53. Schlappner, O. L., Shelley, W. B., Ruberg, R. L., and Dudrick, J. J.: Acute papulo-pustular acne associated with prolonged intravenous hyperalimentation. J.A.M.A., *219*:877–880, 1972.

54. Kay, R. G., and Tasman-Jones, C.: Zinc deficiency and intravenous feeding. Lancet, *2*:605–606, 1975.

55. Kay, R. G., and Tasman-Jones, C.: Acute zinc deficiency in man during intravenous alimentation. Aust. N. Z. J. Surg., *45*:325–330, 1975.

56. Kay, R. G., Tasman-Jones, C., Pybus, J., Whiting, R., and Black, H.: A syndrome of acute zinc deficiency during total parenteral alimentation in man. Ann. Sur., *183*:331–340, 1976.

57. Solomons, N. W., Layden, T. J., Rosenberg, I. H., Vo-Khactu, K., and Sandstead, H. H.: Plasma trace metals during total parenteral alimentation. Gastroenterology, *70*:1022–1023, 1976.

58. Fleming, C. R., Hodges, R. E., and Hurley, L. S.: A prospective study of serum copper and zinc levels in patients receiving total parenteral nutrition. Am. J. Clin. Nutr., *29*:70–77, 1976.

59. Hankins, D. A., Riella, M. C., Scribner, B. H., and Babb, A. L.: Whole blood trace element concentrations during total parenteral nutrition. Surgery, *79*:674–477, 1976.

60. Lowry, S. F., Goodgame, J. T., Jr., Smith, J. C., Maher, M. M., Makuch, R. W., Henkin, R. I., and Brennan, M. F.: Abnormalities of zinc and copper during total parenteral alimentation. Ann. Surg., *189*:120–128, 1979.

61. Michie, D. D., and Wirth, F. H.: Plasma zinc levels

in premature infants receiving paenteral nutrition. J. Pediatr., 92:798–800, 1978.

62. Lockitch, G., Godolphin, W., Pendray, M. R., Tiddell, D., and Quigley, G.: Serum zinc, copper, retinol-binding protein, prealbumin and ceruloplasmin concentrations in infants receiving intravenous zinc and copper supplementation. J. Pediatr., 102:304–308, 1983.

63. Thorp, J. W., Boeck, R. L., Robbins, S., Horn, S., and Fletcher, A. B.: A prospective study of infant zinc nutrition during intensive care. Am. J. Clin. Nutr., 34:1056–1060, 1981.

64. Phillips, G. D., and Garnys, V. P.: Parenteral administration of trace elements to critically ill patients. Anesth. Intensive Care, 9:221–225, 1981.

65. Sivasubramanian, K. N., and Henkin, R. I.: Behavioral and dermatological changes and low serum zinc and copper concentrations in two premature infants after parenteral alimentation. J. Pediatr., 93:846–851, 1978.

66. Srouji, M. N., Balistreri, W. F., Caleb, M. H., South, M. A., and Starr, S.: Zinc deficiency during total parenteral nutrition: Skin manifestations and immune incompetence in a premature infant. J. Pediatr. Surg., 13:570–575, 1978.

67. Arlette, J. P., and Johnson, M. M.: Zinc deficiency dermatosis in premature infants receiving prolonged parenteral alimentation. J. Am. Acad. Dermatol., 5:37–42, 1981.

68. Herson, V. C., and Phillipps, A. F.: Acute zinc deficiency in a premature infant after bowel resection and intravenous alimentation. Am. J. Dis. Child., 135:968–969, 1981.

69. Vileisis, R. A., Deddish, R. B., Fitzsimmons, E., and Hunt, C. E.: Serial serum zinc levels in preterm infants during parenteral and enteral feedings. Am. J. Clin. Nutr., 34:2653–2657, 1981.

70. Schwarz, K., Peden, V. H., and Craddock, T.: Zinc deficiency in a premature infant with severe short bowel syndrome. Nutr. Rev., 40:81–83, 1982.

71. Arakawa, T., Tamura, T., Igarashi, Y., Suzuki, H., and Sandstead, H. H.: Zinc deficiency in two infants during total parenteral nutrition for intractable diarrhea. Acta Chir. Scand., (Suppl.) 466:16–17, 1976.

72. Arakawa, T., Tamura, T., Igarachi, Y., Suzuki, H., and Sandstead. H. H.: Zinc deficiency in two infants during total parenteral alimentation for diarrhea. Am. J. Clin. Nutr., 29:197–204, 1976.

73. Katoh, T., Iagarashi, M., Ohhashi, E., Ohi, R., Hebiguchi, T., and Seiji, M.: Acrodermatitis enteropathica eruption associated with parenteral nutrition. Dermatologica, 152:119–127, 1975.

74. Strobel, C. T., Byrne, W. J., Abramovitz, W., Newcomer, N. J., Bleich, R., and Ament, M. E.: A zinc-deficiency dermatitis in patients on total parenteral nutrition. Int. J. Dermatol., 17:575–581, 1978.

75. McCarthy, D. M., May, R. J., Maher, M., and Brennan, M. F.: Trace metal and essential fatty acid deficiencies during total parenteral nutrition. Am. J. Dig. Dis., 23:1009–1016, 1978.

76. Suita, S., Ikeda, K., Nagasaki, A., and Hagashida, Y.: Zinc deficiency during total parenteral nutrition in childhood. J. Pediatr. Surg., 13:5–9, 1978.

77. Oleske, J. M., Westphal, M. L., Shore, S., Gordon, D., Bogden, J. D., and Nahmias, A.: Zinc therapy of depressed cellular immunity in acrodermatitis enteropathica. Its correction. Am. J. Dis. Child., 133:915–918, 1979.

78. Pichanick, A. M., Thorn, J. C., and Hunter, J. C.: Zinc deficiency in total parenteral nutrition of neonates. S. Afr. Med. J., 56:246, 1979.

79. Stern, M., Gruttner, R., and Krumbach, J.: Protracted diarrhea, secondary monosaccharide malabsorption and zinc deficiency with cutaneous manifestation during total parenteral nutrition. Eur. J. Pediatr., 135:175–180, 1980.

80. Latimer, J. S., McClain, C. J., and Sharp, H. L.: Clinical zinc deficiency during supplemental parenteral nutrition. J. Pediatr., 97:434–437, 1981.

81. Palma, P. A., Conley, S. B., Crandell, S. S., and Densen, S. E.: Zinc deficiency following surgery in zinc supplemented infants. Pediatrics, 69:801–803, 1982.

82. Okada, A., and Takagi, Y.: An importance of zinc in total parenteral nutrition. Jap. J. Surg., 6:189–191, 1976.

83. Okada, A., and Takahi, Y., Itakura, T., Santoni, M., Manabe, H., and Iida, Y.: Zinc deficiency during intravenous hyperalimentation. Acta Chir. Scand., (Suppl.) 466:18–19, 1976.

84. Okada, A., Takagi, Y., Santoni, M., Manabe, H., Iida, Y., Taginaki, T., Iwasaki, M., and Kasahara, N.: Skin lesion during intravenous hyperalimentation: Zinc deficiency. Surgery, 80:629–635, 1976.

85. Tucker, S. B., Schroeder, A. L., Brown, P. W., and McCall, J. T.: Acquired zinc deficiency: Cutaneous manifestation typical of acrodermatitis enteropathica. J.A.M.A., 235:2399–2402, 1976.

86. Weismann, K., Hjorth, N., and Fischer, A.: Zinc depletion syndrome with acrodermatitis during long-term intravenous feeding. Clin. Exp. Dermatol., 1:237–242, 1976.

87. Bos, L. P., van Vloten, W. A., Smit, A. F., and Nube, M.: Zinc deficiency with skin lesions as seen in acrodermatitis enteropathica and intoxication with zinc during total parenteral nutrition. Neth. J. Med., 20:263–266, 1977.

88. Messing, B., Poitras, P., and Bernier, J. J.: Zinc deficiency in total parenteral nutrition. Lancet, 2:97–98, 1977.

89. Wexler, D., and Pace, W.: Acquired zinc deficiency disease of the skin. Br. J. Dermatol., 96:669–672, 1977.

90. de Leeuw, J., Peeters, R., and Croket, A.: Acquired trace element deficiency during total parenteral nutrition in a man with Crohn's disease. Acta Clin. Belg., 33:227–235, 1978.

91. Abou-Mourad, N. N., Farah, F. S., and Steel, D.: Dermatopathic changes in hypozincemia. Arch. Dermatol., 115:956–958, 1979.

92. Brazin, S. A., Johnson, W. T., and Abramson, L. J.: The acrodermatitis enteropathica–like syndrome. Arch. Dermatol., 115:597–599, 1979.

93. Chevrant-Breton, J., and Dreno, B.: Manifestations cutanées observées au cours des hyperalimentations veineuses prolongées. Annals Derm. Vener., 106:141–150, 1979.

94. Holbrook, I. B., Milewski, P. J., Clark, C., and Shipley, K.: Low serum zinc and long-term intravenous feeding. Am. J. Clin. Nutr., 33:1891–1892, 1979.

95. Hamit, H. F., David, H. E., and Stevens, J. C.: Dermatitis due to zinc deficiency associated with prolonged malnutrition and total parenteral nutrition. World J. Surg., 4:693–700, 1980.

96. McClain, C. J., Soutor, C., Steele, N., Levine, A. S., and Silvis, S. E.: Severe zinc deficiency presenting with acrodermatitis during hyperalimen-

tation: Diagnosis, pathogenesis, and treatment. J. Clin. Gastroenterol., 2:125–131, 1980.

97. Ferrandiz, C., Henkes, J., Peyri, J., and Sarmiento, J.: Acquired zinc-deficiency syndrome during total parenteral alimentation. Clinical and histopathological findings. Dermatologica, 163:255–266, 1981.

98. Goldwasser, B., Werbin, N., Stadler, J., and Wiznitzer, T.: Zinc deficiency during intravenous hyperalimentation. Isr. J. Med. Sci., 17:1155–1157, 1981.

99. Jarnum, S., and Ladefoged, K.: Long-term parenteral nutrition. I. Clinical experience in 70 patients from 1967 to 1980. Scand. J. Gastroenterol., 16:903–911, 1981.

100. Mozzillo, N., Ayala, F., and Federici, G.: Zinc deficiency syndrome in patient on long-term total parenteral nutrition. Lancet, 1:744, 1982.

101. Younoszai, H. D.: Clinical zinc deficiency in total parenteral nutrition. Zinc supplementation. J.P.E.N., 7:72–74, 1983.

102. Lowry, S. F., Smith, J. C., and Brennan, M. F.: Zinc and copper replacement during total parenteral nutrition. Am. J. Clin. Nutr., 34:1853–1860, 1981.

103. Freeman, J. B., Steglink, P. D., Meyer, P. D., Fry, L. K., and Denbesten, L.: Excessive urinary zinc losses during parenteral alimentation. J. Surg. Res., 18:463–469, 1975.

104. Steglink, L. D., Freeman, J. B., Denbesten, L., and Filer, L. J., Jr.: Maillard reaction products in parenteral nutrition. Prog. Food Nutr. Sci., 5:265–278, 1981.

105. Fry, L. K., and Steglink, L. D.: Formation of Maillard reaction products in parenteral alimentation solution. J. Nutr., 112:1631–1637, 1982.

106. Yancie, A. A., Kiez, R. W., Jr., and Kraikitpanitch, S.: Urinary zinc excretion following infusion of zinc sulfate, cysteine, histidine or glycine. Am. J. Physiol., 235:F40–F45, 1978.

107. Van Rij, A. M., McKenzie, J. M., and Dunckley, J. V.: Excessive urinary zinc losses and amino aciduria during intravenous alimentation. Proc. Univ. Otago Med. Sch., 53:77–78, 1975.

108. Godfrey, P. J., Van Rij, A. M., and McKenzie, J. M.: Differences in urinary zinc and amino acid excretion produced by the infusion of four amino acid preparations. Proc. Univ. Otago Med. Sch., 55:47–49, 1977.

109. Wolman, S. L., Anderson, G. H., Marliss, E. B., and Jeejeebhoy, K. V.: Zinc in total parenteral nutrition—requirements and metabolic effects. Gastroenterology, 76:458–467, 1979.

110. Ladefoged, K.: Intestinal and renal loss of infused minerals in patients with severe short bowel syndrome. Am. J. Clin. Nutr., 36:59–67, 1982.

111. Henzel, J. H., DeWeese, M. S., and Lichti, E. L.: Zinc concentration within healing wounds: Significance of post-operative zincuria on availability and requirements during tissue repair. Arch. Surg., 100:349–357, 1970.

112. Marceau, N., and Aspin, N.: The intracellular distribution of the radiocopper derived from ceruloplasmin and from albumin. Biochim. Biophys. Acta, 293:338–350, 1973.

113. O'Dell, B. L.: Biochemical basis of the clinical effects of copper deficiency. In Prasad, A. S. (ed.): Clinical, Biochemical and Nutritional Aspects of Trace Elements. New York, Alan R. Liss, 1982, pp. 301–314.

114. Holtzman, N.: Menkes' kinky hair syndrome: A genetic disease involving copper. Fed. Proc., 35:2276–2280, 1976.

115. Delves, H. T.: The microdetermination of copper in plasma protein fraction. Clin. Chim. Acta, 71:495–500, 1976.

116. Hambidge, K. M.: Increase in hair copper concentration with increasing distance from the scalp. Am. J. Clin. Nutr., 26:1212–1215, 1973.

117. Okahata, S., Mishi, Y., Hatano, S., Kobayashi, Y., and Usui, T.: Change in erythrocyte superoxide dismutase in a patient with copper deficiency. Eur. J. Pediatr., 134:121–124, 1980.

118. Castillo-Duran, C., Fisberg, M., Valenzuela, A., Egaña, J. I., and Uauy, R.: Controlled trial of copper supplementation during the recovery from marasmus. Am. J. Clin. Nutr., 37:898–903, 1983.

119. Blumenthal, I., Lealman, G. T., and Franklyn, P. P.: Fracture of the femur, fish odour, and copper deficiency in a preterm infant. Arch. Dis. Child., 55:229–231, 1980.

120. McGill, L. C., Boas, R. N., and Zerella, J. T.: Extremity swelling in an infant with copper and zinc deficiency. J. Pediatr. Surg., 15:746–747, 1980.

121. Klevay, L. M., and Viestenz, K. E.: Abnormal electrocardiograms in rats deficient in copper. Am. J. Clin. Nutr., 32:932, 1979.

122. Prohaska, J. R., and Heller, L. J.: Mechanical properties of the copper-deficient rat heart. J. Nutr., 112:2142–2150, 1982.

123. Tilson, M. D.: Decreased hepatic copper levels. A possible marker for the pathogenesis of aortic aneurysm in man. Arch. Surg., 117:1212–1213, 1982.

124. Karpel, J. T., and Peden, V. H.: Copper deficiency in long-term parenteral nutrition. J. Pediatr., 80:32–34, 1972.

125. Allen, T. M., Manoli, A., 2d, and LaMont, R. L.: Skeletal changes associated with copper deficiency. Clin. Orthop., 168:206–210, 1982.

126. Dunlap, W. M., James, J. C., and Hume, D. M.: Anemia and neutropenia caused by copper deficiency. Ann. Intern. Med., 80:470–476, 1974.

127. Heller, R. M., Kirchner, S. G., O'Neill, J. A., Jr., Hough, A. J., Jr., Howard, L., Kramer, S. S., and Green, H. L.: Skeletal changes of copper deficiency in infants receiving prolonged total parenteral nutrition. J. Pediatr., 92:947–949, 1978.

128. Bennani-Smires, C., Medina, J., and Young, I. W.: Infantile nutritional copper deficiency. Am. J. Dis. Child., 134:1155–1156, 1980.

129. Wiss, D. A., and Ledesma-Medina, J.: Skeletal changes in copper deficiency following prolonged total parenteral nutrition. Orthopedics, 3:969–973, 1980.

130. Joffe, G., Etzioni, A., Levy, J., and Benderly, A.: A patient with copper deficiency anemia while on prolonged intravenous feeding. Clin. Pediatr., 20:226–228, 1981.

131. Vilter, R. W., Bozian, R. C., Hess, E. V., Zellner, D. C., and Petering, H. C.: Manifestations of copper deficiency in a patient with systemic sclerosis on intravenous hyperalimentation. N. Engl. J. Med., 291:188–191, 1974.

132. Pulmissano, D. J.: Nutrient deficiencies after intensive parenteral alimentation. N. Engl. J. Med., 291:799, 1974.

133. Zidar, B. L., Shadduck, R. K., Zeigler, Z., and

Winkelstein, A.: Observation on the anemia and neutropenia of human copper deficiency. Am. J. Hematol., 3:177–185, 1977.

134. Askari A., Long, C. L., and Blakemore, W. S.: Net metabolic changes of zinc, copper, nitrogen and potassium balances in skeletal trauma patients. Metabolism, 31:1185–1193, 1982.

135. Shike, M., Roulet, M., Kurian, R., Whitewell, J., Stewart, S., and Jeejeebhoy, K. N.: Copper metabolism and requirements in total parenteral nutrition. Gastroenterology, 81:290–297, 1981.

136. Tyrala, E. E., Brodsky, N. L., and Auerbach, V. H.: Urinary copper losses in infants receiving free amino acid solutions. Am. J. Clin. Nutr., 35:542–545, 1982.

137. Hillman, L. S., Martin, L., and Fiore, B.: Effect of oral copper supplementation in premature infants. J. Pediatr., 98:311, 1981.

138. Sann, L., Rigal, D., Galy, G., Benvenu, F., and Bourgeois, J.: Serum copper and zinc concentration in premature and small-for-date infants. Pediatr. Res., 14:1041–1046, 1980.

139. Manser, J. L., Tran, N. N., Kotwal, M., and Hall, L.: Copper supplementation in premature infants. J. Pediatr., 100:511, 1982.

140. Shakespeare, P. G.: Studies on the serum levels of iron, copper and zinc and urinary excretion of zinc after burn injury. Burns Incl. Therm. Inj., 8:358–364, 1982.

141. Leach, R. M., Jr., and Lilburn, M. S.: Manganese metabolism and its function. World Rev. Nutr. Diet, 32:123–134, 1978.

142. Ash, D. E., and Schramm, V. L.: Determination of free and bound manganese (II) in hepatocytes from fed and fasted rats. J. Biol. Chem., 257:9261–9264, 1982.

143. Doisy, E. A.: Micronutrient controls on biosynthesis of clotting proteins and cholesterol. In Hemphill, D. D. (ed.): Trace Substances in Environmental Health—VI. Columbia, University of Missouri Press, 1972, pp. 193–199.

144. Versieck, J., Cornelius, R., Lemey, G., and De Rudder, J.: Determination of manganese in whole blood and serum. Clin. Chem., 26:531–532, 1980.

145. Versieck, J., Barbier, F., Speecke, A., and Hoste, J.: Manganese, copper, and zinc concentrations in serum and packed blood cells during acute hepatitis, chronic hepatitis and posthepatitic cirrhosis. Clin. Chem., 20:1141–1145, 1974.

146. Cotzias, G. C., Miller, S. T., and Edwards, J.: Neutron activation analysis: The stability of manganese concentrations in human blood and serum. J. Lab. Clin. Med., 67:836–849, 1966.

147. Pleban, P. A., and Pearson, K. H.: Determination of manganese in whole blood and serum. Clin. Chem., 25:1915–1916, 1979.

148. Mena, I., Horiuchi, K., Burke, K., and Cotzias, C. C.: Chronic manganese poisoning. Individual susceptibility and absorption of iron. Neurology, 19:1000–1006, 1969.

149. Paynter, D. I.: Changes in activity of the manganese superoxide dismutase enzyme in tissues of the rat with changes in dietary manganese. J. Nutr., 110:437–447, 1980.

150. de Rosa, G., Leach, R. M., and Hurley, L. S.: Influence of dietary Mn^{++} on the activity of mitochondrial superoxide dismutase. Fed. Proc., 37:594, 1978.

151. de Rosa, G., Keen, C. L., Leach, R. M., and Hurley, L. S.: Regulation of superoxide dismutase activity by dietary manganese. J. Nutr., 110:795–804, 1980.

152. Superoxide dismutase as an index of copper, zinc, and manganese status. Nutr. Rev., 38:326–327, 1980.

153. Hurley, L. S.: Teratogenic aspect of manganese, zinc and copper nutrition. Physiol. Rev., 61:249–295, 1981.

154. Lavin, J. P., Gimmon, Z., Miodovnik, M., Von Meyenfeldt, M., and Fischer, J. E.: Total parenteral nutrition in a pregnant, insulin-requiring diabetic. Surg. Obstet. Gynecol., 59:660–664, 1982.

155. Rotruck, J. T., Pope, A. L., Ganther, H. E., Swanson, A. B., Hafeman, D. G., and Hoekstra, W. G.: Selenium: Biochemical role as a component of glutathione peroxidase. Science, 179:588–590, 1973.

156. Awasthi, Y. C., Beutler, E., and Srivastava, S. K.: Purification and properties of human erythrocyte glutathione peroxidase. J. Biol. Chem., 250:5144–5149, 1975.

157. Hahn, H. K., Williams, R. V., Burch, R. F., Sullivan, J. F., and Novak, E. A.: Determination of serum selenium by means of solvent extraction combined with activation analyses. J. Lab. Clin. Med., 80:718–722, 1972.

158. Tappel, A. L., and Dillard, C. J.: In vivo lipid peroxidation measurement via exhaled pentane and protection by vitamin E. Fed. Proc., 40:174–178, 1981.

159. Van Rij, A. M., Thomson, C. D., McKenzie, J. M., and Robinson, M. F.: Selenium deficiency in total parenteral nutrition. Am. J. Clin. Nutr., 32:2076–2085, 1979.

160. Shils, M. E., Levander, O. A., and Alcock, N. W.: Selenium levels on long-term TPN patients. Am. J. Clin. Nutr., 35:838, 1982.

161. Lane, H. W., Dudrick, S., and Warren, D. C.: Blood selenium levels and glutathione peroxidase activities in university and chronic intravenous hyperalimentation subjects. Proc. Soc. Exp. Biol. Med., 167:383–390, 1981.

162. Robinson, M. F., Campbell, D. R., Stewart, R. D. H., Rea, H. M., Thomson, R. D., Snow, P. C., and Squires, J. A. W.: Effect of daily supplements of selenium on patients with muscular complaints in Otago and Canterbury, New Zealand. N. Z. Med. J., 93:289–292, 1981.

163. Kien, C., and Ganther, H. E.: Manifestations of chronic selenium deficiency in a child receiving total parenteral nutrition. Am. J. Clin. Nutr., 37:319–328, 1983.

164. King, W. W., Michel, L., Wood, W. C., Malt, R. A., Baker, S. S., and Cohen, H. J.: Reversal of selenium deficiency with oral selenium. N. Engl. J. Med., 304:1305, 1981.

165. Johnson, R. A., Baker, S. S., Fallon, J. T., Maynard, E. P., Ruskin, J. N., Wen, Z., Ge, K., and Cohen, H. J.: An occidental case of cardiomyopathy and selenium deficiency. N. Engl. J. Med., 304:1210–1212, 1981.

166. Fleming, C. R., Lie, J. T., McCall, J. T., O'Brien, J. F., Baillie, E. E., and Thistle, J. L.: Selenium deficiency and fatal cardiomyopathy in a patient on home parenteral nutrition. Gastroenterology, 83:689–693, 1982.

167. Shils, M. E., Jacobs, D. H., Cunningham-Rundles, S., Koziner, B., Levander, O. A., and Alcock, N.

W.: Selenium deficiency and immune functions in home TPN patients. Am. J. Clin. Nutr., 37:716, 1983.

168. Burk, R. F., Jr., Pearson, W. N., Wood, R. P., and Viteri, F.: Blood-selenium levels and in vitro red blood cell uptake of ^{75}Se in kwashiorkor. Am. J. Clin. Nutr., 20:723–733, 1967.

169. Levine, R. J., and Olson, R. E.: Blood selenium in Thai children with protein-calorie malnutrition. Proc. Soc. Exp. Biol. Med., 134:1030–1034, 1970.

170. Broghamer, W. L., Jr., McConnell, K. P., and Blotchy, A. L.: Relationship between serum selenium levels and patients with carcinoma. Cancer, 37:1384–1388, 1976.

171. Mertz, W.: Chromium occurrence and function in biological systems. Physiol. Rev., 49:185–239, 1969.

172. Mertz, W.: Chromium—an overview. In Shapcott, D., and Hubert, J. (eds.): Chromium in Nutrition and Metabolism. Amsterdam. Elsevier/North Holland, 1979, pp. 1–14.

173. Riales, R., and Albrink, M. J.: Effect of chromium chloride supplementation on glucose tolerance and serum lipids including high density lipoprotein in adult men. Am. J. Clin. Nutr., 34:2670–2678, 1981.

174. Offenbacher, E. G., and Pi-Sunyer, F. X.: Beneficial effects of chromium-rich yeast on glucose tolerance and blood lipids in elderly subjects. Diabetes, 29:919–925, 1980.

175. Hubert, J.: Techniques for measurement of chromium in biological materials. In Shapcott, D., and Hubert, J. (eds.): Chromium in Nutrition and Metabolism. Amsterdam, Elsevier/North Holland, 1979, pp. 15–30.

176. Guthrie, B., Wolf, W. R., and Veillon, C.: Background correction and related problems in the determination of chromium in urine by graphite furnace atomic aborption spectrophotometry. Anal. Chem., 50:1900–1902, 1978.

177. Liu, V. J. K., and Morris, J. S.: Relative chromium response as an indicator of chromium status. Am. J. Clin. Nutr., 31:972–976, 1978.

178. Rabinowitz, M. B., Levin, S. R., and Gonick, H. C.: Comparison of chromium status in diabetes and normal men. Metabolism, 29:355–364, 1980.

179. Gurson, C. T., and Saner, G.: The effect of glucose loading on urinary excretion of chromium in normal adults and individuals from diabetic families and in diabetes. Am. J. Clin. Nutr., 31:1158–1161, 1978.

180. Gurson, C. T., and Saner, G.: Urinary chromium excretion diurnal changes, and relationship to creatinine excretion in healthy and sick individuals of different ages. Am. J. Clin. Nutr., 34:1676–1979, 1981.

181. Saner, G.: Urinary chromium excretion during pregnancy and its relationship with intravenous glucose loading. Am. J. Clin. Nutr., 34:1676–1679, 1981.

182. Hopkins, L. L., Jr., Ransome-Kuti, O., and Majaj, A. S.: Improvement in impaired carbohydrate by chromium (III) in malnourished infants. Am. J. Clin. Nutr., 21:203–211, 1968.

183. Glinsmann, W. H., Feldman, F. J., and Mertz, W.: Plasma chromium after glucose administration. Science, 152:1243–1245, 1966.

184. Jeejeebhoy, K. N., Chu, R., Marliss, E. B., Greenberg, G. R., and Robertson, A. B.: Chromium deficiency, glucose intolerance and neuropathy

reserved by chromium supplementation in a patient receiving long-term total parenteral nutrition. Am. J. Clin. Nutr., 30:531–538, 1977.

185. Freund, H., Atamian, S., and Fischer, J. E.: Chromium deficiency during total parenteral nutrition. J.A.M.A., 241:496–498, 1979.

186. Shapcott, D.: The detection of chromium deficiency. In Shapcott, D., and Hubert, J. (eds.): Chromium in Nutrition and Metabolism. Amsterdam, Elsevier/North Holland, 1979, pp. 113–127.

187. Abumrad, N. N., Schneider, A. J., Steel, D., and Rogers, L. S.: Amino acid intolerance during prolonged total parenteral nutrition reversed by molybdate therapy. Am. J. Clin. Nutr., 34:2551–2559, 1981.

188. Versieck, J., Hoste, J., Barbier, F., Vanballenberge, L., DeRudder, J., and Cornelius, R.: Determination of molybdenum in human serum by neutron activation analysis. Clin. Chim. Acta, 87:135–140, 1978.

189. Kasperek, K., Iyengar, G. V., Kiem, J., Borberg, H., and Feinendegen, L. E.: Elemental composition of platelets. III. Determinations of Ag, Au, Cd, Co, Cr, Cs, Mo, Rb, Sb and Se in normal human platelets by neutron activation analysis. Clin. Chem., 25:711–719, 1979.

190. Versieck, J., Hoste, J., Vanballenberge, L., Barbier, F., Cornelius, R., and Waelput, I.: Serum molybdenum in diseases of the liver and biliary system. J. Lab. Clin. Med., 97:535–544, 1981.

191. Johnson, J. L., Waud, W. R., Rajagopalan, K. V., Duran, M., Beemer, F. A., and Wadman, S. K.: Inborn errors of molybdenum metabolism: Combined deficiencies of sulfite oxidase and xanthine dehydrogenase in a patient lacking the molybdenum cofactor. Proc. Natl. Acad. Sci. USA, 77:3715–3719, 1980.

192. Wretlind, A.: Complete intravenous nutrition: Theoretical and experimental background. Nutr. Metab., 14(Suppl.):1–57, 1972.

193. Shils, M. E.: Guidelines for total parenteral nutrition. J.A.M.A., 220:1721–1729, 1972.

194. American Medical Association. Guidelines for essential trace element preparation for parenteral use. J.A.M.A., 241:2051–2054, 1979.

195. Shenkin, A., Wretlind, A.: In Richards, J. R., and Kinney, J. H. (eds.): Nutritional Aspects of Care in the Critically Ill. Edinburgh, Churchill-Livingstone, 1977, pp. 345–365.

196. Steiger, E., Helbley, M., and Zlotkin, S. H.: Selenium in parenteral nutrition: Clinical experience in two medical centers (pamphlet). Chicago, Lyphomed, Inc., 1983.

197. Abumrad, N. N.: Molybdenum. Lyphomed Nutr. Nsltr., 2(4):1982.

198. Physician's Desk Reference. 37th ed. Oradell, NJ, Medical Economics Company, Inc., 1983, p. 1354.

199. Hamstra, R. D., Block, M. H., and Schocket, A. L.: Intravenous iron dextran in clinical medicine. J.A.M.A., 243:1726–1731, 1980.

200. Reed, M. D., Bertino, J. S., Jr., and Halpin, T. C., Jr.: Use of intravenous iron dextran injection in children receiving total parenteral nutrition. Am. J. Dis. Child., 135:829–831, 1981.

201. Halpin, T. C., Jr., Bertino, J. S., Rothstein, F. C., Kurczynski, E. M., and Reed, M. E.: Iron-deficiency anemia in childhood inflammatory bowel disease: Treatment with intravenous iron dextran. J.P.E.N., 6:9–11, 1982.

202. Kwong, K. W., and Tsallas, G.: Dilute iron dextran formulation for addition to parenteral nutrient solutions. Am. J. Hosp. Pharm., *37*:206–210, 1980.

203. Will, G., and Groden, B. M.: The treatment of iron deficiency anaemia by iron-dextran infusion: A radio-isotope study. Br. J. Haematol., *14*:61–64, 1968.

204. Thomson, A. B. R., Brust, R., Ali, M. A. M., and Valberg, L. S.: Iron deficiency in inflammatory bowel disease. Diagnostic efficacy of serum ferritin. Am. J. Dig. Dis., *23*:705–709, 1975.

205. Bothe, A., Jr., Benotti, P., Bistrian, B. R., and Blackburn, G. L.: The use of iron with total parenteral nutrition. N. Engl. J. Med., *293*:1153, 1975.

206. Barry, D. M., and Reeve, A. W.: Increased incidence of gram-negative neonatal sepsis with intramuscular iron administration. Pediatrics, *60*:908–912, 1977.

207. Becroft, D. M., Dix, M. R., and Farmer, K.: Intramuscular iron-dextran and susceptibility of neonates to bacterial infections. In vitro studies. Arch. Dis. Child., *52*:778–781, 1977.

208. Slødahl, S., Gutteberg, T. J., and Nordbø, S. A.: Septicaemia due to *Yersinia enterocolitica* after oral overdoses of iron. Br. Med. J., *285*:467–468, 1982.

209. Faintuch, J., Faintuch, J. J., Toledo, M., Nazario, G., Machado, M. C., and Raia, A. A.: Hyperamylasemia associated with zinc overdose during parenteral nutrition. J.P.E.N., *2*:640–645, 1978.

210. Brock, A., Reid, H., and Glazer, G.: Acute intravenous zinc poisoning. Br. Med. J., *1*:1390–1391, 1977.

211. McIntyre, N., Clink, H. M., Levi, A. J., Cumming, J. N., and Sherlock, S.: Hemolytic anemia in Wilson's disease. N. Engl. J. Med., *276*:439–444, 1967.

212. Deiss, A., Lee, C. R., and Cartwright, G. E.: Hemolytic anemia in Wilson's disease. Ann. Intern. Med., *73*:413–418, 1970.

213. Levander, O. A., Sutherland, B., Morris, V. C., and King, J. C.: Selenium balance in young men during selenium depletion and repletion. Am. J. Clin. Nutr., *34*:2662–2669, 1981.

214. Shils, M. E., and Levander, O. A.: Selenium stability in TPN Solutions. Am. J. Clin. Nutr., *35*:829, 1982.

CHAPTER 9

Nonglucose Carbohydrates in Parenteral Nutrition

J. van EYS

The primary carbohydrate in the bloodstream is glucose, which serves as the ubiquitous substrate under normal conditions. The glucose has an elaborate system for homeostasis, involving synthesis in the liver and elaboration in the bloodstream as well as uptake by peripheral tissues. Different tissues have a different preferential claim on circulating glucose, and the whole process is regulated by an intricate system of interdependent hormonal substances. Under stressful conditions, total parenteral alimentation can require large amounts of energy at a time when there are marked disturbances in glucose utilization. Historically, under such circumstances two approaches to carbohydrate administration have been taken: (1) the administration of glucose together with a high dose of insulin or (2) the combination of glucose with nonglucose carbohydrates. This chapter will summarize some of the background and rationale for the use of nonglucose carbohydrates in parenteral nutrition. Although the use of these substances is no longer generally advocated, some important observations were made during the period of their use. Furthermore, there are new concepts that might lead us to re-explore the use of such substances in special patients and under special disease conditions.

SCOPE OF SUGAR USE IN PARENTERAL NUTRITION

A significant number of carbohydrates and carbohydrate derivatives have been used, since the ideal carbohydrate for parenteral nutrition formulas has not yet been found. This chapter will concentrate on the sugar fructose and on the polyols sorbitol and xylitol. It should be noted, however, that other sugars have been used. Intravenous maltose has been evaluated.[1,2] Its use has been said to be effective in postoperative and diabetic patients.[3] Young and colleagues[4] have evaluated the metabolism of parenteral glucose oligosaccharides, using a glucose oligosaccharide mixture that contained only the α-D-1-4 anomeric linkage from hydrolyzed corn starch. This mixture contained maltose, maltotriose, maltotetrose, maltopentose, maltohexose, and maltoseptose. There was some free glucose in the material. Studies in healthy male volunteers showed that partial but significant quantities of these oligosaccharides could be metabolized after intravenous infusion, but it did require low infusion rates. Galactose has also been explored as an intravenous carbohydrate source in small infants.[5] However, so far all such sugars provide only an academic interest. Therefore, this discussion will concentrate on those sugars that have found relatively wide application for a period of time in parenteral nutrition.

Fructose, Sorbitol, and Xylitol

The structural formulas of sorbitol, xylitol, and fructose are shown in Figure 9–1. All substances are available in pure form and are natural products. Because of the widespread research in the utilization of these sugars and sugar substitutes in nutrition, dentistry, and

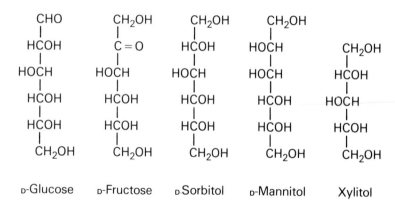

Figure 9–1. The structural formulas of D-glucose, D-fructose, D-sorbitol, D-mannitol, and xylitol. (*From* Wang, Y. M., and van Eys, J.: Nutritional significance of fructose and sugar alcohols. Ann. Rev. Nutr. 1:437, 1981, with permission. © 1981 by Annual Reviews, Inc.)

commercial application toward alternative sweeteners, the Life Science Research Office of the Federation of American Society for Experimental Biology has recently gathered the current information available on these substances under a contract with the Food and Drug Administration. They are available for fructose,[6] xylitol,[7] and sorbitol.[8]

Metabolism of Nonglucose Carbohydrates

Intermediate Metabolism

The three sugars and sugar derivatives—fructose, sorbitol, and xylitol—are all readily metabolized and interconverted to substrates and intermediates of glycolysis. Figure 9–2 summarizes the points at which sorbitol, fructose, and xylitol enter metabolism. Fructose is converted to fructose-1-phosphate through phosphorylation utilizing adenosine triphosphate (ATP). This is then split by aldolase into dihydroxyacetone phosphate and glyceraldehyde. Dihydroxyacetone phosphate is a direct intermediate of the glycolytic pathway. However, glyceraldehyde must be converted further to enter the pathway. This can happen in one of three ways: (1) through reduction to glycerol, (2) phosphorylation with ATP, or (3) conversion of the subsequent glycerol-3-phosphate to dihydroxyacetone phosphate. Alternatively, glyceraldehyde may be directly phosphorylated to glyceraldehyde phosphate, or glyceraldehyde can be oxidized to glyceric acid, which, in turn, gets phosphorylated to 3-phosphoglycerate. In humans, the direct phosphorylation of glyceraldehyde dominates.[9] Sorbitol and fructose are interconvertible. Fructose can be reduced to sorbitol and sorbitol can be reoxidized to fructose. Since

this oxidoreduction is nicotinamide adenine dinucleotide (NAD)–dependent, the metabolic thrust is toward oxidation of sorbitol to fructose. Conversely, sorbitol and glucose are interconvertible through an oxidoreduction process. This enzymatic step is dependent on nicotinamide adenine dinucleotide phosphate (NADP). In that interconversion, the thrust is toward reduction so that sorbitol is formed from glucose rather than the converse. Therefore, sorbitol tends to enter metabolism via fructose and the same subsequent pathways.

Sorbitol and fructose enter a main pathway of glycolysis. In contrast, xylitol is an intermediate in the so-called Touster cycle, through which glucose is converted to glucuronate via pentoses to xylulose phosphate, which then enters the hexose monophosphate shunt to be converted stepwise into intermediates of glycolysis. Xylitol, like sorbitol, can be oxidized by NAD to form D-xylulose—a direction that is preferred, as is the oxidation of sorbitol to fructose. Conversely, xylitol could be oxidized to L-xylulose, but this reaction requires NADP, which tends to favor the reduction of L-xylulose to xylitol. After xylitol is converted to D-xylulose it is phosphorylated to D-xylulose-5-phosphate, the intermediate of the hexose monophosphate shunt. The metabolism of the nonglucose carbohydrates has been summarized in many publications. A useful summary is published by Förster.[10]

Physiology and Whole-Animal Disposition

In contrast to the utilization of glucose, the utilization of fructose, sorbitol, and to a lesser degree xylitol is limited to special tissues. For instance, fructose turnover is pri-

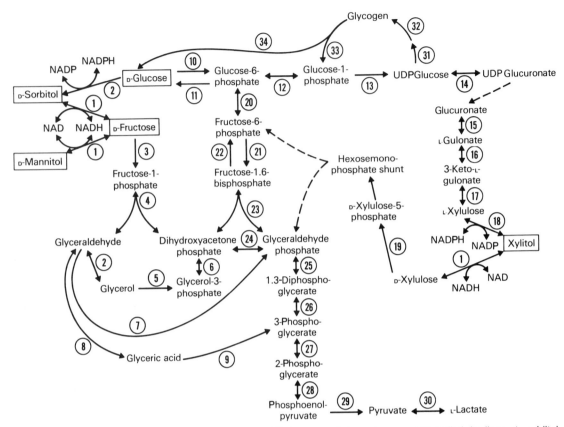

Figure 9–2. The metabolism of D-fructose, D-sorbitol, D-mannitol, D-glucose, and xylitol in liver. 1, L-Iditol dehydrogenase (E C 1.1.1.14), NAD-dependent polyol dehydrogenase (1.1.1.10); 2, aldose reductase (1.1.1.21); 3, ketohexokinase (2.7.1.3); 4, aldolase B (4.1.1.13); 5, glycerol kinase (2.7.1.30); 6, glycerol-3-phosphate dehydrogenase (1.1.1.94); 7, triosekinase (2.7.1.28); 8, aldehyde dehydrogenase (1.2.1.3); 9, glycerate kinase (2.7.1.31); 10, glucokinase (2.7.1.2); 11, glucose-6-phosphate (3.1.3.9); 12, phosphoglucomutase (2.7.5.1); 13, glucose-1-phosphate uridylyltransferase (2.7.7.9); 14, UDPG dehydrogenase (1.1.1.22); 15, glucuronate reductase (1.1.1.19); 16, L-gulonate dehydrogenase (1.1.1.45); 17, 3-keto-L-gulonate decarboxylase (4.1.1.34); 18, NADP-dependent xylitol dehydrogenase (1.1.1.9); 19, D-xylulokinase (2.7.1.17); 20, glucose phosphate isomerase (5.3.1.9); 21, phosphofructokinase (2.7.1.11); 22, fructose bisphosphatase (3.1.3.11); 23, fructose bisphosphate aldolase (4.1.2.13); 24, triose phosphate isomerase (5.3.1.1.); 25, glyceraldehyde-3-phosphate dehydrogenase (1.2.1.12); 26, phosphoglycerate kinase (2.7.2.3); 27, phosphoglycerate mutase (2.7.5.3); 28, enolase (94.2.1.11); 29, pyruvate kinase (2.7.1.40); 30, L-lactate dehydrogenase (1.1.1.27); 31, glycogen synthetase (2.4.1.11); 32, amylo-1-3,1-6 transglucosylase (2.4.1.18); 33, phosphorylase (2.4.1.1.); 34, oligo, 1-6-glucosidase (3.2.1.10). (*From* Wang, Y. M., and van Eys, J.: Nutritional significance of fructose and sugar alcohols. Ann. Rev. Nutr. *1*:437, 1981, with permission. © 1981 by Annual Reviews, Inc.)

marily limited to the liver and kidneys,[10,11] and there is some utilization of fructose by adipose tissue.[12] Sorbitol is primarily converted to fructose, and the enzyme responsible, L-iditol dehydrogenase, is present mainly in the liver, though it is also found in the kidneys and in several other tissues.[13] Fructose is not an adequate energy source for the isolated heart. However, it is a significant carbohydrate in supplying energy for spermatozoa motility.[14] Xylitol is also primarily metabolized by the liver. The enzyme responsible for the initial metabolism can be adapted, probably by adaptation of inducible hepatic xylitol dehydrogenases.[15] As much as

15 to 20 per cent of parenterally administered xylitol can be used extrahepatically in the kidney, lung, erythrocytes, fat storage, and myocardium.[16] Xylitol is handled by the kidney through simple glomerular filtration, and there is no reabsorptive mechanism.[17]

The usefulness of specific carbohydrates in parenteral alimentation is highly dependent on their rate of utilization. When one infuses the various sugars during a steady state in human volunteers, one can estimate a maximal utilization and the possible achievable cal/kg/hour. Zöllner[18] has summarized such data (Table 9–1). It can be seen from this table that at a rate advocated to be the

Table 9–1. COMPARISON OF MAXIMAL CARBOHYDRATE UTILIZATION DURING STEADY STATE

SUGAR	INFUSION RATE (gm/kg/h)	UTILIZATION (gm/kg/h)	CALORIES (cal/kg/h)
Glucose	1.5	1.390	5.5
Fructose	1.5	1.409	5.5
Xylitol	0.5	0.483	1.9
Sorbitol	0.5	0.436	1.7
Galactose	0.3	0.290	1.1
Maltose	0.5	0.350	0.15

maximal rate of infusion (to be explained later), xylitol and sorbitol can barely meet the caloric requirement of 1.6 cal/kg/hour.

Not everyone agrees with these figures. For instance, Baessler[19] reports the turnover constants of a variety of carbohydrates in healthy persons. The values for glucose, fructose, and xylitol are of the same order of magnitude. For instance, for glucose the reported ranges average 0.0349 kg (minute), with a half-life (T½) (minute) of 16.7. The figures for fructose are 0.0380 and 18.4, respectively, and for xylitol 0.300 and 23, respectively. Therefore, in the practice of parenteral nutrition one can hardly exceed the limit of their turnover capacity as long as the turnover is unimpaired.

It is clear that there is little effect of insulin on the metabolism of fructose, sorbitol, and xylitol. For instance, Baessler[19] summarized the turnover of these carbohydrates in rabbits, in healthy animals, and in alloxan-diabetic animals. These data, shown in Table 9–2, were obtained in long-term infusion at a constant rate, calculating the total clearance from the steady state blood level during equilibrium. Similar data are not clearly available in humans.

The disposition of xylitol is independent of insulin. In an eviscerated rat, the xylitol space is the same with or without insulin.[20] Fructose, sorbitol, and xylitol are not incorporated into glycogen in the isolated diaphragm in streptozotocin-treated rats.[21, 22] Fructose is slightly insulin-dependent for intake into adipose tissue in the absence of glucose.[23] In general, these sugars are considered to have less insulin dependence for their metabolism.

It is interesting to note that these sugars stimulate insulin secretion. Kosarka[24] was one of the earlier investigators to report the insulin secretion stimulation by xylitol. This stimulation actually exceeded that of the insulin response to glucose administration. Fructose was much less active, whereas mannitol showed no insulin secretory effect. The effect of xylitol insulin secretion is also seen in humans.[25] It is suppressed by the simultaneous administration of epinephrine.

Fructose, sorbitol, and xylitol are used as glucose precursors by the liver after oral or intravenous administration. Froesch and co-workers injected ^{14}C-labeled fructose, sorbitol, or xylitol in rats that were normal, fasted, or streptozotocin-treated, and again, with and without insulin.[21,22] All three sugars were rapidly converted to glucose by the liver, but no glycogen was formed from these substances in the absence of insulin.

The effects of glucose, fructose, sorbitol, and xylitol in healthy human volunteers, utilizing doses of 1.5 gm/kg of body weight in 20 per cent solutions over 20 minutes, showed no increase in glucose concentration in the blood except when glucose itself was infused. There was a significant rise in blood lactate levels, with the most marked effect being seen with fructose, followed by glucose and sorbitol. Xylitol had the least effect, with only a barely perceptible rise. Conversely, the lactate/pyruvate ratio, which would reflect the redox state in the liver, shows a marked increase when xylitol is used, with lesser increases seen from sorbitol, fructose, and glucose—in that order.[26-28] The effect of xylitol on cytoplasmic NAD reduction is not as marked as that seen following ethanol administration in humans when lactate pyruvate levels are also elevated. Förster[10] measured the conversion of uridine diphosphogalactose (UDP-galactose) to uridine diphosphoglucose (UDP-glucose) by hexose epimerase in the liver, which is the limiting factor in galactose metabolism. NAD must be kept in the oxidized state to be an effective coenzyme. Neither sorbitol nor xylitol inhib-

Table 9–2. ANIMALS WITH TURNOVER OF CARBOHYDRATES IN RABBITS DURING INTRAVENOUS INFUSION*

CARBOHYDRATES TOTAL CLEARANCE (ml/kg/h)	HEALTHY ANIMALS	ALLOXAN DIABETES
Fructose	32.0	29.2
Sorbitol	32.3	20.3
Xylitol	46.3	43.6

*The infusion rate was 0.50 gm/kg/h for all sugars.

ited galactose metabolism in healthy volunteers, in contrast to what is seen with ethanol administration.[29] There is an effect on lipid metabolism, with a reduction in unesterified fatty acids and a direct antiketogenic effect.[10]

RATIONALE FOR NONGLUCOSE CARBOHYDRATE UTILIZATION

In the normal state, it is clear that glucose is the preferred substrate and the most rapidly used carbohydrate. However, there are specific states in which there is a relative defect in glucose utilization. It is those states for which the utilization of nonglucose carbohydrates has been advocated. They include the premature newborn, extreme postsurgical, traumatic, or burn stress, and diabetes. Of these three conditions, the rationale for the use of nonglucose carbohydrates has been primarily advocated for severely traumatized patients. This section will briefly summarize this rationale for the utilization of nonglucose carbohydrates.

Neonatology

In term and older infants, glucose can be infused in parenteral hyperalimentation at a reasonable rate and usually can be increased to quantities of up to 12 to 14 mg/kg/hour without difficulty. However, there are a significant number of very low birth-weight infants who will develop serious hyperglycemia if the glucose infusion exceeds even 6 mg/kg/hour.[30] It is seen most often in the very immature infant. The hyperglycemia is not seen as frequently if amino acids are infused simultaneously.[31] Whether this effect is due to insulin stimulation is not known for certain. It is known that very low birth-weight infants do have an inadequate insulin response, especially when hyperglycemic infants are compared with normal glycemic ones.[32] Furthermore, infants are extremely sensitive to insulin.[33]

As already mentioned, an infusion of a mixture of glucose and galactose seemed to prevent hyperglycemia.[5] Glucose tolerance improves steadily after the first few days of life, because there is an increased amount of insulin secreted as well as an increased organ sensitivity to the insulin.[34]

Postoperative Catabolic States

Surgery, trauma, burns, and sepsis result in a complex series of metabolic responses in humans. A major component of this response is an increased catabolism of body protein, coupled with a significant insulin resistance, which results in hyperglycemia. These observations have been discussed many times and reviewed and extended in many publications. A recent review is that by Clowes and coworkers.[35] If one measures urea production in such patients, and infuses glucose, the response through a decreasing urea production is not as clear-cut with glucose alone as it is with glucose plus insulin.[36] Patients who are relatively glucose-resistant will not become hyperglycemic from the infusion of fructose or xylitol. For instance, Baessler and Schultis[37] have summarized experiments showing that xylitol has nitrogen-sparing and antiketogenic effects in the postoperative state (Table 9–3).

Table 9–3. METABOLIC PARAMETERS IN PREOPERATIVE AND POSTOPERATIVE STATES AND UNDER CONDITIONS OF INFUSION WITH RINGER'S SOLUTION, ALONE OR COMBINED WITH GLUCOSE OR XYLITOL

METABOLIC PARAMETERS	Preoperative State	POSTOPERATIVE STATE WITH INFUSION OF		
		Ringer's Solution	Ringer's and Glucose (100 gm/day)	Ringer's and Xylitol (100 mg/day)
N excretion in the urine (gm/day)*	—	7.8	5.2	2.9
Nonesterified fatty acids in the fasting serum (μEq/L)	699	742	778	670
Ketone bodies in the fasting blood (mg/100 ml)	0.753	4.754	5.006	0.805
Elimination constant for glucose (x/min)	1.92	1.02	1.02	1.47

*Mean values of 3 days each.

It is clear that even glucose utilization is improved by the infusion of xylitol.

Diabetes

Glucose resistance has made it attractive to use nonglucose carbohydrates as an energy source because it is better tolerated in diabetic patients. The literature on nonglucose carbohydrates and diabetes is extremely extensive. The nonglucose carbohydrates—fructose, xylitol, and sorbitol—do have an antiketogenic effect. However, that antiketogenic effect decreases with the severity of the diabetes. Nevertheless, it has been claimed that the infusion of xylitol during diabetic ketoacidosis improves blood ketone bodies and lowers blood sugar without concomitant administration of insulin.[38]

TOXICITY OF NONGLUCOSE CARBOHYDRATES

From the rationale of the utilization of nonglucose carbohydrates under certain physiologic and pathologic circumstances, one would expect that their use would be widespread. However, a number of toxicities have been reported, which has resulted in severe limitation of the use of these substances and even, on occasion, interdiction of their use by regulations within the country.[39-42] There are indeed significant toxicities associated with the nonglucose carbohydrates, which are to some degree common to all of them and in other instances are specific for a given substance.

General Toxic Effects

All three nonglucose carbohydrates generate, to a degree, excess NADH, resulting in lactic acidosis and lactate pyruvate elevations, as already discussed. The lactate increase in general remains within tolerable limits and is not necessarily a toxicity. However, there is a significant increase in serum bilirubin.[43,44] This effect is seen to a degree with high glucose and, in fact, with all carbohydrates.[45] Xylitol has the most marked effect on serum bilirubin, whereas glucose has the least. In model experiments in rabbits, the effect of xylitol on serum bilirubin and other metabolic parameters of liver tox-

icity is, in part, explained by the fact that many early experimenters and clinicians infused hypertonic solutions. Such hyperosmolar solutions clearly produce the hepatotoxicity indicated.[46]

A more common and clear side effect is an elevation of serum uric acid caused by an increased rate of serum uric acid production.[47-49] This coincides with a drop of adenine nucleotides in the liver. Sestoft and Gammeltoft[50] did biopsies in humans who were undergoing uncomplicated cholecystectomies. Xylitol was infused intravenously over a 30-minute period during the surgery, and the hepatic ATP concentration was measured. A 50-gm dose caused a decrease in the hepatic ATP concentration from 2.75 to 0.25 μm/liver with a concomitant drop in the concentration of inorganic phosphate. The overall concentration of adenine nucleotide was reduced to 30 per cent of the control value. This experiment demonstrated in human tissues what had been noted before in animal models—either in whole animals or perfused isolated livers. However, long-term infusions of fructose, in contrast to acute infusions, do not seem to change the levels of liver nucleotides significantly.[51]

All the side effects are, to a degree, dose- and infusion-rate-dependent. It must again be stressed that many arguments regarding side effects and their seriousness are strongly dependent on and aggravated by hyperosmolar effects, which are often found under circumstances of hyperalimentation.

Oxalate Production

In addition to the general side effects that have been mentioned, the most serious side effect that has been reported has been the deposit of oxalate crystals in the kidneys, as well as in the brain. This was observed in Australia[52, 53] and in Germany.[54, 55]

The Australians in particular attributed the death of the patients to oxalate deposits. Schröder has written a review about the oxalate deposits.[56] However, an analysis of data on 200 deceased intensive care unit patients showed that there was no statistical difference in the incidence in extent of oxalate deposits in patients who had received xylitol or no xylitol, or other carbohydrates.[57] Secondary oxalosis was seen in patients with renal insufficiency who were not receiving xylitol infusions.[58]

The Australian researchers have tried to link oxalate formation directly to xylitol. No such biochemical pathway has ever been demonstrated, but theoretic models have been proposed.[59] Rat experiments seemed to back up the contention that oxalate deposits from xylitol, especially in vitamin B_6-deficient rats.[60] However, in model experiments in the rabbit, Oshinsky and associates failed to show ^{14}C incorporation from xylitol into oxalate in a significant amount.[61] Treating the rabbits with vitamin B_1 or vitamin B_6 antagonists did not increase the amount of oxalate production from xylitol. Furthermore, in the same model, the amount of serum oxalate did not increase even with very high, near-toxic doses of xylitol.[62] Berg and colleagues[63] found no increase in serum oxalate in humans under steady state infusion of xylitol. Nevertheless, the oxalate scare gave the most pervasive argument for restricting the use of xylitol in parenteral alimentation in the United States. It is from such observations that the restriction by the German equivalent of the Food and Drug Administration suggested a maximal infusion rate of 0.25 gm/kg/body weight/hour.[41] Most observers agree that at such a rate the infusion is safe.

Genetic Considerations

On occasion, there are individuals incapable of metabolizing certain carbohydrates. For the purposes of this discussion, only hereditary fructose intolerance need be mentioned. In such patients there is an enzymatic deficiency of aldolase B in hepatic parenchymal cells and also in the cells of intestinal villi and renal cortex. Fructose-1-phosphate accumulates in the liver, kidneys, and intestines. This disease can occur in a relatively mild form that could be severely aggravated by the intravenous infusion of fructose. For a review, one can consult the monograph by Cornblath and Schwartz.[64]

APPLICATION OF NONGLUCOSE CARBOHYDRATES IN PARENTERAL HYPERALIMENTATION

There is no doubt that toxicity occurs from excessive quantities of nonglucose carbohydrates. At the same time, there were significant reasons to attempt to use nonglucose carbohydrates in hyperalimentation un-

der the circumstances previously elaborated upon. The literature on the use of nonglucose carbohydrates in parenteral alimentation is very voluminous, and many papers are repetitious. Furthermore, the initial enthusiasm that greets all new discoveries often is later tempered with better judgment. There is an upper limit of safe infusions. To summarize again briefly, the advantages of glucose in parenteral hyperalimentation solutions are obvious. It is the ubiquitous substrate under normal conditions. The disadvantages of glucose are that the sugar is poorly utilized after stress, and large amounts of insulin may be necessary. Sudden interruption can produce serious hypoglycemia. The advantages of nonglucose carbohydrates, the glucose substitutes, are that (1) there is no post-traumatic disturbance of utilization, (2) there is a slow formation of glucose from these substances so that there is no subsequent hyperglycemia, (3) the substances have good protein-sparing effects, and (4) there is a decline in the levels of unesterified fatty acids and ketones. The disadvantages of glucose substitutes are its low turnover rate (except for fructose) and the side effects of increased lactate and uric acid, and decreased liver adenine nucleotides. Finally, there is the rarely encountered genetically determined intolerance. It is no wonder then that a number of investigators have turned to combinations of sugars that would have the advantages of providing a given carbohydrate below a dose-limiting toxicity and yet increasing the caloric density while maintaining the advantages of all components. The most commonly used combinations are glucose-fructose mixtures and a mixture of glucose, fructose, and xylitol, which are most often used in the proportion of 1:2:1. The total dose is usually 0.5 gm/kg/hour of carbohydrate. A very large body of European experience has shown that this combination does, in fact, normalize fat metabolism and improves glucose tolerance without requiring exogenous insulin. The combinations have been continued for one to several weeks and, in general, no side effects have been noted. A concise and complete justification of the use of nonglucose carbohydrates in parenteral nutrition was given in a joint statement by its proponents.[65] Other ratios of sugars have been used. Georgieff and colleagues[66] used a glucose, fructose, and xylitol mixture in equal proportions. It was established that fructose was best used out of that combination. The only main side effect was a drop in inorganic phosphate in the blood. The individual sugars were administered at a rate of 0.25 gm/kg/hour for a total sugar load of 375 mg/kg/hour.

The mixture of glucose, fructose, and xylitol has been compared directly with glucose alone. For instance, in severely injured intensive care unit patients, it was thought that the glucose, fructose, and xylitol combination allowed easier control of blood sugar, though there was somewhat more xylitol loss.[67] Leutenegger and colleagues[68] published a detailed study of a comparison between glucose and the glucose, fructose, and xylitol combination for total parenteral nutrition in surgical intensive care patients. In these patients, the infusion ratio was 1:2:1 by weight, with a total dose of 600 gm/day in 2000 ml for glucose and 2500 ml for the mixture. Patients were given glucose or the mixture in alternating four-day blocks. A total of 12 patients were studied; 8 patients had two four-day cycles, 2 patients had three four-day cycles, and 2 patients had four such cycles. Patients were studied before and after the experimental infusions. The daily plasma insulin level was significantly lower in the patients on the mixture, whereas the insulin required for combatting hyperglycemia was significantly greater for patients who received glucose alone. The serum glucose concentration was significantly lower in patients on the mixture. However, there also was a greater spillage of calories, especially through xylitol loss. Although there was a difference between the lactate/pyruvate ratios, the drop in lactate and pyruvate seen after switching from the mixture to glucose disappeared after four days, at which time the value of the patients on glucose was the same as that seen with the mixture. Both groups of patients had a negative nitrogen balance, with no significant difference between groups. These authors concluded that from a clinical and biochemical point of view the infusion of glucose in combination with xylitol and fructose is justified in patients whose hyperglycemia during infusion of glucose alone is difficult to control, even with insulin.

A symposium on parenteral nutrition was held in which the experience and the superiority of the glucose, fructose, and xylitol mixture was documented by the experiences in post-traumatic patients, obstetric patients, and generally seriously ill patients.[69] As already mentioned, this enthusiasm is not generally shared, and several voices were raised that there are no recognizable indications that mixtures of hexoses and polyols have any advantages over the administration of hexoses alone.[18] Froesch and Jacob[70] stated "The use of sorbitol and xylitol for parenteral nutrition offers no advantage, but leaves the physician in the mistaken belief that he does not harm the patient because these polyols are easily 'utilized' without extra insulin." Conversely, Ahnefeld[65] went so far as to say that he and his colleagues consider "the use of these combinations to be suitable during the post-traumatic phase and that some, particularly surgeons, consider them to be indispensable."

Because of the reported side effects, the debate has settled down. Furthermore, because of the "watchdog" effect of the Food and Drug Administration, parenteral xylitol never had a general testing within the United States. However, it must be remembered that many of the arguments, such as the danger of fatty liver, are problems generally attributable to carbohydrate infusions, and are quite apart from the nature of the carbohydrate.[71] Triglyceride concentrations increase in the liver after the infusion of high carbohydrates; sorbitol is more prone to cause this increase than is xylitol, followed by fructose and glucose in that order. However, all solutions can cause it, including a 30 per cent glucose solution.

Fructose, either alone or in combination with glucose, has also been used. Very often invert sugar (an equal combination of glucose and fructose derived from sucrose hydrolysis) has been used.[72] There is a body of literature that shows that fructose infusion can decrease blood levels of and accelerate the elimination of ethyl alcohol in blood.[73] This is, in fact, an old observation.[74]

Potential Future Use of Nonglucose Carbohydrates in Parenteral Alimentation

In spite of the European proponents, nonglucose carbohydrates have never gotten a foothold in the United States. Recently, however, new interest has been shown in xylitol because of its remarkable effect in preventing dental caries. Most of those studies have been with oral xylitol. They have been recently reviewed by Raunhardt and Ritzel[75] and by Mäkinen and Scheinen.[76] For these reasons, there is some interest in re-examining the potential use of xylitol in parenteral alimentation for specific indications.

One application is the possible use of xylitol in the treatment and prevention of the effects of glucose-6-phosphate dehydrogenase. Glucose-6-phosphate dehydrogenase deficiency is found in 3 per cent of the world's population. Such individuals are very susceptible to drug or naturally induced hemolysis from peroxidative attacks. Any substance in the red cell that could generate NADPH, such as xylitol, might keep this peroxidative attack from destroying the red cell membrane. It was, therefore, proposed some years ago that xylitol could be used to treat glucose-6-phosphate dehydrogenase deficiency.[77,78] For that particular system the rabbit is an excellent model, especially when utilizing acetylphenylhydrazine-induced hemolysis. Quantitative experiments have shown that dosages of xylitol that are safe in the rabbit are effective in amelioration of such drug-induced hemolysis in those rabbits.[79] Again, the experiment has never been done in humans in the United States. Attempts have been made in Thailand and the Soviet Union to treat glucose-6-phosphate dehydrogenase deficiency in humans, with mixed results in the Soviet Union and some benefits in Thailand.

There are, however, more interesting possibilities. In rats bearing hepatocellular carcinomas, xylitol and glucose are not metabolized in the same proportion between the hepatoma and the normal liver.[80] The hepatocellular carcinoma is unable to convert xylitol to metabolites or glycogen and glycoproteins (Table 9–4). At the same time, it is clear that cancer, especially in its more extreme states, is an insulin-resistant state.[81] A high proportion of cancer patients have diabetic glucose tolerance curves, and this decreased glucose utilization becomes even more pronounced in the cachectic state.[82] There have been advocates for treating cancer cachexia with insulin, but that is not generally considered an acceptable treatment. However, the observation that tumor cells may not be capable of utilizing the xylitol quickly, together with a relative insulin resistance, might make a parenteral solution containing nonglucose carbohydrates an attractive possibility in patients with malignancy who require hyperalimentation. To date no systematic data on that use exist.

SUMMARY

The use of nonglucose carbohydrates in parenteral hyperalimentation as a preferred carbohydrate energy source in post-traumatic stress and similar insulin-resistant states has a body of physiologic observations that makes such use rational. Reports of toxicity precluded testing in the United States and made their use wane in Europe. New data

Table 9–4. COMPARATIVE METABOLISM OF GLUCOSE AND XYLITOL BETWEEN LIVER AND HEPATOMA*

EXPERIMENT	TISSUE	^{14}C-SUBSTRATE	% RECOVERED†		
			(^{14}C) XYLITOL	(^{14}C) GLUCOSE	OTHERS
1	Liver	Xylitol	8.4	60.9	30.7
2	Liver	Xylitol	6.6	54.0	39.4
3	AS-30D	Xylitol	81.4	5.3	13.3
4	AS-30D	Xylitol	93.4	0.0	6.6
5	Liver	Glucose		69.4	30.6
6	Liver	Glucose		65.7	34.3
7	AS-30D	Glucose		44.5	55.5
8	AS-30D	Glucose		43.7	46.3

*At the end of the elution in borate column chromatography (U-^{14}C xylitol or U-^{14}C) glucose was administered IV to rats bearing AS-30D hepatoma after 48 hours of fasting. The rats were sacrificed 45 minutes after infusion, and tissues were extracted with perchloric acid. The neutralized extracts were applied to a borate column; the eluates that contained more than 500 cpm/tube associating with the peaks of xylitol and glucose were pooled and recounted.

†Calculated as:

$$\frac{\text{cpm of xylitol or glucose recovered}}{\text{Total cpm of neutral sugar metabolites recovered}} \times 100$$
$$\text{after Amberlite MB-3 column chromatography}$$

(Adapted from Sato, J., Wang, Y. M., and van Eys, J.: Metabolism of xylitol and glucose in rats bearing hepatocellular carcinomas. Cancer Res., 41:3192, 1981.)

on xylitol and fructose and considerations of the disease states of drug-induced hemolysis in glucose-6-phosphate dehydrogenase deficiency and cancer cachexia suggest that the parenteral infusion of these substances be reinvestigated.

REFERENCES

1. Sprandel, U., Hueckenkamp, P-U, and Zöllner, N.: Utilization of intravenous maltose. Nutr. Metab., 19:96, 1975.
2. Finke, C., and Reinauer, H.: Ueber den Abbau von Infundierter Maltose beim Menschen. Z. Ernaehrungswiss, 15:231, 1976.
3. Yoshikawa, K., and Oda, T.: Metabolism of maltose during surgery in patients with diabetes mellitus under general anesthesia. Res. Exp. Med., 167:127, 1976.
4. Young, E. A., Fletcher, J. T., Cioletti, L. A., Hollrah, L. A., and Weser, E.: Metabolism of parenteral glucose oligosaccharides in man. J.P.E.N., 15:369, 1981.
5. Avery, J. B.: Galactose: its potential use in the glucose-intolerant immature infant. In Stein, L., Oh, W., and Friis-Hansen, B. (eds.): Intensive Care in the Newborn. II. New York, Masson, 1978, page 261.
6. Kimura, K. K., and Carr, C. J.: Dietary Sugars in Health and Disease. Bethesda, Maryland, Life Science Research Office, Federation American Society of Experimental Biology, 1976.
7. Fisher, K.: Dietary Sugars in Health and Disease. II. Xylitol. Bethesda, Maryland, Life Science Research Office, Federation American Society of Experimental Biology, 1978.
8. Allison, R. G.: Dietary Sugars in Health and Disease. III. Sorbitol. Bethesda, Maryland, Life Science Research Office, Federation American Society of Experimental Biology, 1979.
9. Heinz, F., Lampercht, W., and Kirsch, J.: Enzymes of fructose metabolism in human liver. J. Clin. Invest., 47:1826, 1968.
10. Förster, H.: Comparative metabolism of xylitol, sorbitol and fructose. In Sipple, H. L., and McNutt, K. W. (eds.): Sugars in Nutrition. New York, Academic Press, 1974, page 259.
11. Felber, J. P., Renold, A. E., and Zahnd, G. R.: The comparative metabolism of glucose, galactose and sorbitol in normal subjects and in disease states. Mod. Probl. Paediatr., 4:467, 1959.
12. Froesch, E. R., and Ginsberg, J. L.: Fructose metabolism of adipose tissue. I. Comparison of fructose and glucose metabolism in epididymal adipose tissue of normal rats. J. Biol. Chem., 237:3317, 1962.
13. Birnesser, H., Reinauer, H., and Hollman, S.: Comparative study of enzyme activities degrading sorbitol, ribitol, xylitol and gluconate in guinea pig tissues. Diabetologia, 9:30, 1973.
14. Chen, M., and Whistler, R. L.: Metabolism of D-fructose. Adv. Carbohydr. Chem. Biochem., 34:285, 1977.
15. Baessler, K. H.: Adaptive processes concerned with absorption and metabolism of xylitol. In Horecker, B. L., Lang, K., and Takagi, Y. (eds.): Metabolism,

16. Mueller, F., Strack, E., Kuhfahl, E., and Dettmer, D.: Der Stoffwechsel von Xylit bei normalen und alloxan diabetischen Kaninchen. Z. Gesamte. Exp. Med., 142:338, 1967.
17. Lang, K.: Utilization of xylitol in animals and man. In Horecker, B. L., Lang, K., and Takagi, Y. (eds.): Metabolism, Physiology and Clinical Uses of Pentoses and Pentitols. Berlin, Springer-Verlag, 1969, page 151.
18. Zöllner, N.: Evaluation of nonglucose carbohydrates in parenteral nutrition. In Johnston, J. D. A. (ed.): Advances in Parenteral Nutrition. Baltimore, University Park Press, 1978, page 61.
19. Baessler, K. H.: Physiological basis for the use of carbohydrates in parenteral nutrition. In Meng, H. C., and Law, D. H. (eds.): Parenteral Nutrition. Springfield, Illinois, Charles C Thomas, 1970, page 96.
20. Baessler, K. H., and Prellwitz, W.: Insulin und der Verteilungsraum von Xylit bei eviscerierten Ratten. Klin. Wochenschr., 42:94, 1964.
21. Froesch, E. R., Zapti, J., Keller, V., and Oelz, O.: Comparative study of the metabolism of U-14 C-fructose, U-14 C-sorbitol and U-14 C-xylitol in the normal and in the streptozotocin-diabetic rat. Eur. J. Clin. Invest., 2:8, 1971.
22. Keller, V., and Froesch, E. R.: Metabolism and oxidation of U-14 C-glucose, xylitol, fructose and sorbitol in the fasted and streptozotocin-diabetic rat. Diabetologia, 7:3492, 1971.
23. Froesch, E. R., and Jacob, A.: The metabolism of xylitol. In Sipple, H. L., and McNutt, K. W. (eds.): Sugars in Nutrition. New York, Academic Press, 1974, page 241.
24. Kosarka, K.: Stimulation of insulin secretion by xylitol administration. In Horecker, B. L., Lang, K., and Takagi, Y. (eds.): Metabolism, Physiology and Clinical Use of Pentoses and Pentitols. Berlin, Springer-Verlag, 1969, page 212.
25. Hirata, Y., Fujisawa, M., and Oguschi, T.: Effective intravenous injection of xylitol in plasma insulin. In Horecker, B. L., Lang, K., and Takagi, Y. (eds.): Metabolism, Physiology and Clinical Use of Pentoses and Pentitols. Berlin, Springer-Verlag, 1969, page 226.
26. Förster, H.: Grundlagen für die Verwendung der drei Zucker austauschstoffe Fructose, Sorbit, und Xylit. Med. Ernaehrung., 13:719, 1972.
27. Förster, H.: The effect of intravenous carbohydrates on various parameters in blood. Z. Ernaehrungswiss., 1:24, 1974.
28. Förster, H., Meyer, E., and Zige, M.: Erhöhung von Serumharnsäure und Serum-Bilirubin nacht Hochdosierten Infusionen von Sorbit, Fructose and Xylit. Klin. Wochenschr., 48:878, 1970.
29. Forsander, O. A.: The galactose tolerance test as a measurement of the redoxin potential of the liver. Scand. J. Clin. Lab. Invest., (Suppl.), 18:(92):143, 1966.
30. Dweck, H. S., and Cassady, G.: Glucose intolerance in infants of very low birth weight. I. Incidence of hyperglycemia in infants of birth weights of 1100 grams or less. Pediatrics, 53:189, 1974.
31. Chance, G. W.: Results in very low birth weight infants (less than 1300 grams birth weight). In Winters, R. W., and Hasselmeyer, E. G. (eds.): Intravenous Nutrition in the High Risk Infant. New York, John Wiley & Sons, 1975, page 39.

32. Cowett, R. M., Oh, W., Pollack, A., Schwartz, R., and Stonestreet, B. M.: Glucose disposal of low birth weight infants. Steady state hyperglycemia produced by constant intravenous glucose infusion. Pediatrics, 63(3):389, 1979.

33. Brans, Y. W.: Parenteral nutrition of the very low birth weight neonate: A critical review. Clin. Perinatol., 4:367, 1977.

34. Pollack, A., Cowett, R. M., Schwartz, R., and Oh, W.: Glucose disposal in low birth weight infants during steady state hyperglycemia: Effects of exogenous insulin administration. Pediatrics, 61:546, 1978.

35. Clowes, G. H. A., Jr., Randall, H. T., and Cha, C-J.: Amino acid and energy metabolism in septic and traumatized patients. J. P. E. N., 4:195, 1980.

36. Allison, S. P.: Effect of insulin metabolic response to injury. J.P.E.N., 4:175, 1980.

37. Baessler, K. H., and Schultis, K.: Metabolism of fructose, sorbitol, and xylitol and their use in parenteral alimentation. In Ghadimi, H. (ed.): Total Parenteral Nutrition Premises and Promises. New York, John Wiley & Sons, 1975, page 65.

38. Yamagata, S., Goto, Y., Ohneda, A., Anzi, N., Kawashima, S., Kikuchi, J., Chiba, M., Maruhama, Y., Yamaucha, Y., and Toyota, T.: Clinical application of xylitol in diabetes. In Horecker, B. ·L., Lang, K., and Takagi, Y. (eds.): Metabolism, Physiology and Clinical Use of Pentoses and Pentitols. Berlin, Springer-Verlag, 1969, page 316.

39. Berg, G., Matzkies, F., and Bickel, H.: Dosierungsgrenzen bei der Infusion von Glucose, Sorbit, Fructose, Xylit und Deren Mischungen. Dtsch. Med. Wochenschr., 99:633, 1974.

40. Huckenkamp, P. U.: Xylit in der Parenteralen Ernährung. Ernährungsumschau, 21:70, 1974.

41. Arzneimittelkommission der Deutschen Aerzteschaft: Achtung: Dosierungsgrenzen bei der Infusion von Zuckeraustauschstoffen Beachten. Dtsch. Aerztebl., 52:3399, 1972.

42. Interkantonale Kontrollstelle der Schweiz: Ersatzzucker für die Parenteralen Ernährung Monatsbericht. I.K.S., 10:589, 1975.

43. Donahoe, J. F., and Powers, R. J.: Biochemical abnormalities with xylitol. N. Engl. J. Med., 282:690, 1970.

44. Schumer, W.: Adverse effects of xylitol in parenteral nutrition. Metabolism, 20:345, 1971.

45. Förster, H.: Sind bei Infusion von Zuckeraustauschstoffen Echte Nebenwirkungen zu Erwarten? Dtsch. Med. Woschensschr, 98:839, 1973.

46. Wang, Y. M., King, S. M., Patterson, J. H., and van Eys, J.: Mechanism of xylitol toxicity in the rabbit. Metabolism, 22:885, 1973.

47. Förster, H., Boecker, S., and Ziege, M.: Anstieg der Konzentration der Serumharnsäure nacht Akuter und Chronischer Zufuhr von Saccharose, Fructose, Sorbit und Xylit. Med. Ernährr., 13:193, 1972.

48. Förster, H., Meyer, E., and Ziege, M.: Erhöhung von Serumharnsäure und Serum Bilirubin nacht Hochdosierten Infusionen von Sorbit, Xylit und Fructose. Klin. Wochenschr., 48:878, 1970.

49. Grunst, J., Dietz, E. G., Wicklmayr, M., Molz, S., Eisenburg, J., Mehnert, H., and Hepp, K. D.: Die Harnsäureproduktion der menschlichen Leber während Parenteraler Fructosezufuhr. Verhl. Dtsch. Ges. Inn. Med., 80:487, 1974.

50. Sestoft, L., and Gammeltoft, A.: The effect of intravenous xylitol on the concentration of adenine nucleotides in human liver. Biochem. Pharmacol., 25:2619, 1976.

51. Brinkrolf, H., and Bässler, K. H.: The adenine nucleotide content of rat liver during infusions of carbohydrates and polyols. Z. Ernährungswiss, 11:167, 1972.

52. Evans, G. W., Phillip, G., Mukherjee, T. M., Snow, M. R., and Lawrence, J. R.: Identification of crystals deposited in brain and kidney after xylitol administration by biochemical, histochemical and electron diffraction methods. J. Clin. Pathol., 26:32, 1973.

53. Thomas, D. W., Edwards, J. B., Gilligan, J. E., Lawrence, J. R., and Edwards, R. G.: Complications following intravenous administration of solutions containing xylitol. Med. J. Aust., 1:1238, 1972.

54. Beneke, G., and Paulini, K.: Morphologie und Mögliche Ursachen von Kristallablagerungen im Gebe Nach Infusions-Therapie. In: Beisbarth, H., Horatz, K., and Rittmeyer, P. (eds.): Die Bausteine der Parenteralen Ernährung. Stuttgardt, Enke Verlag, 1973, page 59.

55. Büngener, W.: Beobachtungen über Kristallablagerungen im Niere und Gehirn nach Infusionstherapie. In Beisbarth, H., Horatz, K., and Rittmeyer, P. (eds.): Die Bausteine der Parenteralen Ernährung. Stuttgardt, Enke Verlag, 1973, page 72.

56. Schröder R.: Störungen im Oxalsäurestoffwechsel bein parenteralen Ernährung mit Xylit. Dtsch Med Wochenschr., 105:997, 1980.

57. Pesch, H. J., Krampf, F. D., Menzel, H., Weiland, H., Eidam, Y-W, Prestele, H., and Heid, H.: Zur Wirkung von Kohlen Hydratinfusionen auf die Bildung von Calcium Oxalat-Niederschlägen in der Niere: Morphologische und Biochemische Befunde bei Verstorbenen und im Tierversuch. In Int. J. Vit. Nutr. Res. and Ritzel, G., and Brubacher, G. (eds.): Monosaccharides and Polyalcohols in Nutrition, Therapy and Dietetics. Verlag Bern, Hans Huber, 1970, page 193.

58. Balcke, P., Schmidt, P., Zazgornik, J., Kopsa, H., and Deutsch, E.: Secondary oxalosis in chronic renal insufficiency. N. Engl. J. Med., 303:944, 1980.

59. James, H. M., Bais, R., Edwards, J. B., Rofe, A. M., and Conyers, R. A. J.: Models for the metabolic production of oxalate from xylitol in humans: A role for fructokinase and aldolase. Aust. J. Exp. Biol. Med. Sci., 60:117, 1982.

60. Hannett, B., Thomas, D. W., Chalmers, A. H., Rofe, A. M., Edwards, J. B., and Edwards, R. G.: Formation of oxalate in pyridoxine or thiamine deficient rats during intravenous xylitol infusions. J. Nutr., 107:458, 1977.

61. Oshinsky, R. J., Wang, Y. M., and van Eys, J.: Xylitol infusion oxalate formation in rabbits. J. Nutr., 107:792, 1977.

62. Wang, Y. M., Oshinsky, R. J., Lantin, E., Ukab, W., and van Eys, J.: Zur Frage der Toxizität von Xylitinfusionen bei Kaninchen. Infusionstherapie, 4:251, 1977.

63. Berg, G., Matzkies, F., Heid, H., Fekl, W., and Conolly, M.: Wirkungen Einer Kohlenhydratkombinationslösung auf den Stoffwechsel bein Langzeitinfusion. Z. Ernährungswiss, 14:64, 1975.

64. Cornblath, M., and Schwartz, R.: Disorders of Carbohydrate Metabolism in Infancy. Philadelphia, W. B. Saunders Co., 1976, page 322.

65. Ahnefeld, F. W., Bässler, K. H., Bauer, B. L., Berg, G., Bergmann, H., Bessert, I., Dick, W., Dietze, G., Dölp, R., Dudziak, R., Förster, H., Geser, C. A., Grunst, J., Halmagyi, M., Heidland, A., Hel-

ler, L., Horatz, K., Kuhlmann, H., Kult, J., Lutz, H., Matzkies, F., Mehnert, H., Milewski, P., Paulini, K., Pesch, H. J., Peter, K., and Rittmeyer, P.: Suitability of nonglucose carbohydrates for parenteral nutrition. Eur. J. Intensive Care Med., *1*:105, 1975. (This paper has also been published in a German version in Infusionstherapie, *2*:227, 1975.)

66. Georgieff, M., Georgieff, E. M., Osswald, P., Schaub, P., and Lutz, H.: Das Verhalten Ciniger Wichtiger Stoffwechselparameter und-des Insulinspiegels bei 7 Tägiger totalen parenteralen Ernährung unter Prä- und Postoperative Bedingungen. Z. Ernaehrungswiss., *17*:93, 1978.

67. Lackner, F., Baumgartner, L., and Steinbereithner, K.: Thirty percent glucose versus a balanced mixture of levulose, glucose and xylitol (LGXL) in TPA of intensive care patients. Acta Chir. Scand. (Suppl.), *466*:48, 1976.

68. Leutenegger, A. F., Göschke, H., Stutz, K., Mannhart, H., Werdenberg, D., Wolff, G., and Allgöwer, M.: Comparison between glucose and a combination of glucose, fructose, and xylitol as carbohydrates for total parenteral nutrition of surgical intensive care patients. Am. J. Surg., *133*:199, 1977.

69. Ahnefeld, E. W., Burri, C., Dick, W., and Halmágyi, M. (eds.): Parenteral Nutrition. Berlin, Springer-Verlag, 1976.

70. Froesch, E. R., and Jacob, A.: The metabolism of xylitol. *In* Sipple, H. L., and McNutt, K. W. (eds.): Sugars In Nutrition. New York, Academic Press, 1974, page 241.

71. Machytka, B., Hoos, I., and Förster, H.: Fatty liver in rats following parenteral hyperalimentation with glucose or glucose substitutes. Nutr. Metab., *21*:(Suppl.1): 110, 1977.

72. Nube, M., Bos, L. P., and Winkelman, A.: Simultaneous and consecutive administration of nu-

trients in parenteral nutrition. Am. J. Clin. Nutr., *32*:1505, 1979.

73. Sprandel, U., Tröger H-D., Liebhardt, E. W., and Zöllner, N.: Acceleration of ethanol elimination with fructose in man. Nutr. Metab., *24*:324, 1980.

74. Carpenter, T. M., and Lee, R. C.: The effect of fructose on the metabolism of ethyl alcohol in man. J. Pharmacol. Exp. Ther., *6286*:295, 1937.

75. Raunhardt, O., and Ritzel, G.: Xylitol—Clinical Investigations in Humans. Bern, Hans Huber, 1982.

76. Mäkinen, K. K., and Scheinin A: Xylitol in dental caries. Ann. Rev. Nutr., *II*:133, 1982.

77. Wang, Y. M., Patterson, J. H., and van Eys, J.: The potential use of xylitol and glucose-6-phosphate dehydrogenase deficiency anemia. J. Clin. Invest., *50*:1421, 1971.

78. van Eys, J., Wang, Y. M., Chan, S., Tanphaichitr, V. S., and King, S. M.: Xylitol as a therapeutic agent in glucose-6-phosphate dehydrogenase deficiency. *In* Sipple, H. G., and McNutt, K. (eds.): Sugars In Nutrition. New York, Academic Press, 1974, page 613.

79. Ukab, W. A., Sato, J., Wang, Y. M., and van Eys, J.: Xylitol mediated amelioration of acetylphenylhydrazine-induced hemolysis in rabbits. Metabolism, *30*:1053, 1981.

80. Sato, J., Wang, Y. M., and van Eys, J.: Metabolism of xylitol and glucose in rats bearing hepatocellular carcinomas. Cancer Res., *41*:3192, 1981.

81. Lundholm, K., Holm, G., and Scherstén, T.: Insulin resistance in patients with cancer. Cancer Res., *38*:4665, 1978.

82. Jasani, B., Donaldson, L. J., Ratcliffe, J. G., and Sohhi, G. S.: Mechanism of impaired glucose tolerance in patients with neoplasia. Br. J. Cancer, *38*:287, 1978.

83. Wang, Y. M., and van Eys, J.: Nutritional significance of fructose and sugar alcohols. Ann. Rev. Nutr., *1*:437, 1981.

CHAPTER 10

Energy and Nitrogen Interactions

HARRY M. SHIZGAL

PROTEIN UTILIZATION IN THE BODY

Body protein is not a static component of body composition but is instead in a constant state of flux. The average young 70-kg adult man, with a total body protein of about 6 kg, ingests approximately 100 gm of dietary protein daily, whereas 70 gm are secreted into the lumen of the gastrointestinal tract. Only 10 gm of the 170 gm that appear daily within the GI tract are excreted, whereas the remaining 160 gm are absorbed. The daily urinary nitrogen loss is equivalent to 80 to 90 gm of protein.[1] Integumentary losses account for the difference between nitrogen intake and urinary excretion. These relatively large losses of nitrogen represent the oxidation of amino acids. Approximately 15 per cent of the resting energy expenditure results from the oxidation of amino acids.[2] Approximately 250 gm of protein are turned over daily. This large turnover results, in addition to the secretion of gut protein (70 gm), from the constant turnover of muscle (50 gm), plasma protein (20 gm), white cells (20 gm), and red cells (8 gm). In addition, there is large-scale recycling of the free amino acid pool. The size of the free amino acid pool has been estimated at approximately 70 gm. In the healthy adult, the synthesis rate is equal to the rate at which protein is being broken down, resulting in a constant total body protein.

Nitrogen Balance

Nitrogen intake equals nitrogen losses, resulting in nitrogen balance. Net positive nitrogen balance occurs when there is an increase in total body protein. This generally occurs with growth, with an increase in muscle mass as a result of exercise, or with the correction of protein malnutrition. Negative nitrogen balance indicates a net decrease in body protein and occurs when the protein catabolic rate exceeds the rate of protein synthesis. This is commonly seen when malnutrition is developing or with prolonged immobilization, resulting in a loss of muscle mass.

The healthy adult on a protein-free diet loses 54 mg of nitrogen/kg of body weight each day in the urine and stool and from the integument.[3] This represents 0.34 gm of body protein/kg of body weight. This protein loss must be replaced by the diet. To estimate the dietary protein required to replace this loss, corrections are required for both the efficiency of protein utilization and individual variation. The coefficient of variation of the mean daily loss is 15 per cent. To account for the efficiency of utilization, a further 30 per cent must be added. Thus, the daily requirement of dietary protein needed to achieve protein balance has been estimated at 0.59 gm of protein/kg of body weight. However, the average diet in the Western hemisphere consists of a protein that is only 75 per cent of the quality of egg protein. As a result, the protein requirement has been further increased to 0.8 gm/kg of body weight.[3] For a 70-kg individual this represents 56 gm of protein/day.

Injury and infection are associated with a rise in resting energy expenditure (REE) and an increased breakdown of body protein, with a resultant loss of body weight. These changes are all proportional to the magnitude and duration of the catabolic stress. Patients

210

undergoing elective surgical procedures of moderate severity will usually experience an increase in REE of about 10 to 15 per cent, with an increase in the daily nitrogen loss from the usual 12 gm/day to 15 to 18 gm/day.[4] An increase in the REE of 10 to 15 per cent with a daily nitrogen loss of 25 to 30 gm/day is commonly observed in the previously healthy patient who has sustained multiple fractures with a variable amount of soft tissue injury. A major infection such as peritonitis may result in an increase in the REE of 20 to 50 per cent above normal, with nitrogen losses of 30 to 35 gm/day. Major thermal burns are often associated with sustained increases in the REE of 50 to 100 per cent and nitrogen losses of as high as 40 gm/day. The REE and the magnitude of the protein breakdown tend to increase in a parallel fashion in proportion to the magnitude of the catabolic stress. The largest changes are seen in the well-nourished, muscular young adult male, whereas in the female, elderly, and the poorly nourished, the changes are much smaller.

In the healthy individual, nitrogen equilibrium is dependent not only on the quantity and quality of protein ingested but also on the adequacy of energy intake. Thus, when energy intake is less than required nitrogen balance becomes negative, in spite of adequate dietary protein. In a group of healthy men with an energy intake of 45 cal/kg, the mean requirement of egg protein for nitrogen equilibrium was 0.65 gm/kg of body weight.[5] When the energy intake was increased to 57 cal/kg, the mean requirement for nitrogen equilibrium fell to 0.46 gm/kg of body weight. Similarly, the requirements for nitrogen equilibrium with rice protein fell from 0.87 gm/kg to 0.58 gm/kg of body weight.

BODY COMPOSITION

Measurement of the Nutritional State

A variety of parameters have been monitored to assess the effects of nutritional support. The recording of morbidity and mortality has been widely employed. However, the variance of this measurement is, as a rule, large and therefore lacks sensitivity and specificity. The measurement of morbidity and mortality, as a measure of the response to nutritional therapy, can therefore be reliably applied only in experimental situations in which large differences are anticipated. The situation is similar with a battery of anthropometric, biochemical, and immunologic parameters, which have also been widely used to measure the nutritional state. With all of the commonly employed parameters, a statistically significant relationship has been demonstrated with the nutritional state. However, with the majority there are large 95 per cent confidence limits about the regression relating these parameters and the nutritional state.[6] As a result, these parameters are useful determinants of the mean nutritional state of a population, and as such are useful in epidemiologic studies, but are of little value in assessing an individual's nutritional state.

The determination of nitrogen balance is the technique most commonly employed to assess the results of nutritional therapy, because nitrogen balance is a measure of the net effect of protein synthesis and protein degradation, with the magnitude of positive and negative nitrogen balance directly proportional to anabolism and catabolism. There are, however, numerous problems associated with the measurement of nitrogen balance. They have been nicely summarized by Vinnars.[7] Accurate nitrogen balance measurements require the presence of a steady state. This is often difficult to achieve in the clinical environment. Furthermore, nitrogen intake tends to be overestimated, whereas output tends to be underestimated, resulting in a cumulative systematic error. A further limitation of nitrogen balance is that it is not a measure of the nutritional state, but rather measures only a change in the nutritional state. Nevertheless, the evaluation of nitrogen balance data requires an accurate knowledge of the pre-existing nutritional state. In the normally nourished individual, adequate nutritional support is indicated by the presence of nitrogen equilibrium, that is, balance. In the malnourished person, adequacy of nutritional support is indicated by positive nitrogen balance, whereas simple balance indicates an inadequate intake.

To overcome the difficulty associated with nitrogen balance measurements, a multiple isotope dilution technique was developed in our laboratory to evaluate body composition.[8-10] It involves the determination of total body water (TBW), total exchangeable potassium (K_e), and total exchangeable sodium (Na_e), which are measures of the lean body mass (LBM), the body cell mass (BCM), and the extracellular mass (ECM), respectively. The LBM is equivalent to the fat-free mass, whereas the BCM represents the total mass of living cells. The BCM is the component of the body that is metabolically active and is responsible for all of the oxygen consumption and carbon dioxide production. In contrast, the ECM is not metabolically active and does not consume oxygen, nor does it produce carbon dioxide. Its major function is transport and support. The measurement of body composition provides an accurate and precise measure of both the nutritional state and the response to nutritional support.

Malnutrition universally results in a contraction of the BCM accompanied by an expansion of the ECM, with a reversal of these changes as the nutritional state is corrected. As a result, the Na_e/K_e ratio is a sensitive index of the nutritional state. This ratio is a measure of the ECM expressed as a function of the BCM. In 25 normal volunteers, the BCM and ECM are approximately equal in size (Fig. 10–1). Thus, the mean Na_e/K_e in the normal volunteers was 0.98 ± 0.02, with an upper 95 per cent confidence limit of 1.22. With malnutrition this ratio increases.[9] The presence of a Na_e/K_e ratio in excess of 1.22 has been used to define a malnourished state.

PROTEIN SPARING

Starvation in a healthy, well-nourished adult results initially in the daily loss of 12 to 14 gm of nitrogen.[11] The normal fasting individual who is not subjected to catabolic stress adapts to this state with a reduction in the nitrogen loss to 8 gm/day by 10 days, with an eventual reduction in the daily nitrogen loss of 2 to 4 gm. Only a small amount of carbohydrate is available in the form of hepatic and muscle glycogen. This is rapidly depleted within the first 48 hours of total starvation. Gluconeogenic substrate from adipose tissue is limited to the glycerol component of triglycerides. Amino acid sources are thus the only significant gluconeogenic sources during periods of total starvation. Infusing glucose at a rate of 150 gm/day reduces nitrogen loss by about half.[12] Increasing the glucose infused further reduces protein breakdown, but cannot totally abolish it. Infusion of a lipid emulsion will also decrease the nitrogen loss of simple uncomplicated starvation. However, this effect has been attributed entirely to the carbohydrate precursor glycerol, which is present in the emul-

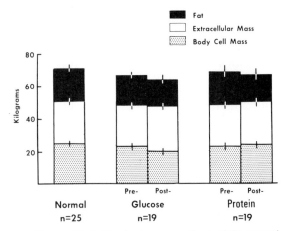

Figure 10–1. The body compositions of 25 normal volunteers, and the preoperative and postoperative body compositions of normally nourished patients undergoing elective surgery of moderate severity. Postoperatively, these patients received intravenous fluids containing either glucose or amino acids. (*From* Shizgal, H. M., Milne, C. A., and Spanier, A. H.: The effect of nitrogen-sparing intravenously administered fluids on postoperative body composition. Surgery, *85*:496, 1979, with permission.)

sion. A 10 per cent lipid emulsion provides 30 gm of glycerol for every 100 gm of available lipid. An amino acid infusion will also prevent the nitrogen loss associated with starvation. The addition of either glucose or lipid to the amino acid infusion improves the efficiency of amino acid utilization in proportion to the energy infused.[13]

The Postsurgical Patient

Elective surgery of moderate severity in the healthy normally nourished patient invariably results in a short period of intense catabolism, which is characterized by negative nitrogen and potassium balance with weight loss. The intensity and duration of this catabolic response is directly related to the magnitude of the surgical injury. Blackburn and associates[14,15] were the first to report a significant reduction in the postoperative nitrogen loss—that is, a sparing of body protein—when amino acids rather than the usual glucose-containing solutions were infused after operation. In the absence of an adequate caloric intake, the postoperative patient must rely on endogenous energy sources. They postulated that the infusion of glucose-containing intravenous solutions would elevate the plasma insulin concentration, which, in turn, would inhibit endogenous lipid mobilization. As a result, the patient receiving glucose-containing intravenous fluids must rely on the catabolic breakdown of body protein for energy. In support of this hypothesis, they reported the abolition of the usual postoperative nitrogen loss with the infusion of a 3 per cent amino acid solution. This was accompanied by a decrease in both the mean plasma glucose concentration and the serum immunoreactive insulin, whereas the plasma concentration of the free fatty acids and the ketone bodies was elevated when compared to the control patients receiving the usual glucose-containing solutions. Similar data have been reported by a number of investigators.[16-18] Protein-sparing was generally demonstrated by improved nitrogen balance in patients receiving intravenous amino acids. A reduction, rather than an abolition, in the postoperative negative nitrogen balance was reported. This may be related to the experimental error inherent in nitrogen balance measurements. To avoid the difficulties associated with nitrogen balance, Skillman and associates measured the albumin synthesis rate.[19] They reported an increased albumin synthesis rate following elective surgery in patients who received intravenous amino acids as compared with patients who received the usual glucose-containing solutions. These protein-sparing effects have been shown to be related to the infusion of amino acids and not to the absence of glucose in the infused solutions, as postulated by Blackburn and associates.[17,18]

Body composition measurements were performed in our laboratory to evaluate the postoperative protein-sparing effects of intravenous amino acid solutions.[8] Measurements were carried out in two groups of healthy, normally nourished patients who underwent an elective operation of moderate severity. The control group received the usual glucose-containing intravenous solutions, whereas in the experimental group intravenous glucose was excluded and they received instead a five per cent casein hydrolysate (Amigen—Baxter Laboratories, Canada). Body composition was determined, by multiple isotope dilution, prior to operation and again on the fifth postoperative day. The caloric intake of both groups was similar.

In both groups there was a statistically significant loss of body weight postoperatively. The patients who received glucose experienced a weight loss of 2.6 ± 0.6 kg, whereas the protein group lost 2.0 ± 0.5 kg,

a difference that was not significant (Fig. 10–1). However, the loss of weight in the glucose group resulted from a loss of both body fat (1.8 ± 0.9 kg) and BCM (3.2 ± 0.6 kg), whereas the ECM increased by 2.4 ± 0.5 kg. The body composition postoperatively in these patients was typical of mild malnutrition. The mean Na_e/K_e ratio increased significantly ($p < .05$) from 1.04 ± 0.08, which is within the normal range, to 1.29 ± 0.11, which is abnormally elevated. In contrast, the only change postoperatively in the patients who received amino acids was a loss of body fat (4.1 ± 0.8 kg), with the BCM and ECM remaining unchanged. Similarly, the Na_e/K_e ratio remained normal (1.00 ± 0.03). Thus, the administration of an intravenous amino acid solution effectively abolished the usual postoperative loss of BCM.

PROTEIN REQUIREMENTS

Protein-sparing involves simply the maintenance of the total body protein. This can be achieved by the provision of amino acids without a significant additional intake of nonprotein calories. However, the restoration of the depleted patient requires both the administration of an adequate supply of amino acids and of energy. The relationship between energy and protein has been nicely reviewed by Wilmore.[20] This relationship can be summarized as follows:

1. At any given energy intake, increasing the protein intake improves the efficiency of protein retention.

2. At any given protein intake, increasing the energy intake improves the efficiency of protein retention.

3. The efficiency of protein retention is greater in the malnourished patient.

4. The hypermetabolic response to trauma is associated with an increased protein breakdown, and there is less protein retention at any given protein and energy intake.

Total Parenteral Nutrition

To evaluate the relationship between energy and protein requirements, we evaluated the effect of total parenteral nutrition with two solutions containing different amino acid concentrations.[21] All patients requiring total parenteral nutrition (TPN) were randomized

Table 10–1. PROTEIN AND ENERGY INTER-RELATIONSHIP IN TPN PATIENTS

	NORMAL VOLUNTEERS	2.5% AMINO ACIDS		5% AMINO ACIDS	
		Pre-TPN	*Post-TPN*	*Pre-TPN*	*Post-TPN*
Weight (kg)	70.4 ± 2.5	56.1 ± 2.0	57.1 ± 2.0	54.4 ± 1.3	54.9 ± 1.4
Body fat (kg)	20.2 ± 1.4	10.4 ± 1.1	11.7 ± 1.1*	12.0 ± 1.1	12.2 ± 1.1
LBM (kg)	50.3 ± 1.9	45.7 ± 1.4	45.4 ± 1.2	42.4 ± 1.3	42.7 ± 1.3
BCM (kg)	24.7 ± 1.1	15.8 ± 0.6	16.6 ± 0.5*	14.3 ± 0.7	15.3 ± 0.7*
ECM (kg)	25.6 ± 0.9	29.9 ± 1.0	28.8 ± 1.1	28.1 ± 0.8	27.3 ± 0.9
K_e/TBW	80.0 ± 1.0	57.0 ± 1.3	61.1 ± 1.6*	55.0 ± 1.5	58.8 ± 1.7*
Na_e/TBW	77.5 ± 0.9	93.6 ± 1.3	90.1 ± 1.6*	91.1 ± 1.6	87.3 ± 1.6*
Na_e/K_e	0.98 ± 0.02	1.73 ± 0.08	1.57 ± 0.07*	1.73 ± 0.09	1.56 ± 0.07*
Patients	25	52		38	
TPN days		14.6 ± 0.2		13.8 ± 0.2*	
Nonprotein kcal/kg/day		48.8 ± 1.9		55.8 ± 1.7*	
Carbohydrate kcal/kg/day		43.9 ± 1.7		45.9 ± 1.4	
Protein gm/kg/day		1.23 ± 0.05		2.47 ± 0.08*	

*Significantly (p < 0.05) different from Pre-TPN by paired Student's t test.

to receive a solution containing either 2.5 per cent or 5 per cent crystalline amino acids (Travesol—Baxter Laboratories, Malton, Ontario, Canada). Both solutions contained 25 per cent dextrose. Five hundred milliliters of a 10 per cent lipid emulsion (Intralipid—Pharmacia Canada Ltd., Montreal, Quebec, Canada) was administered three times a week to prevent essential fatty acid deficiency. The efficacy of TPN with the two solutions was evaluated by measuring body composition at the onset of TPN, and at two-week intervals during the administration of TPN. The patients were divided into those who were normally nourished and those who were malnourished at the onset of each two-week period of TPN. The nutritional state was determined by the Na_e/K_e ratio. In the normally nourished patients, the body composition remained normal following two weeks of TPN. In the patients with pre-existing malnutrition, with both solutions there was a significant improvement in body composition, with a statistically significant increase in the BCM (Table 10–1). However, the change in BCM in both groups was similar. To further assess the effect of the protein intake on the rate at which a malnourished patient was restored, the data from the malnourished patients in both groups were combined, and a multiple linear regression was performed. The daily change in the BCM was correlated with the nonprotein and protein intake and the nutritional state, as determined by the Na_e/K_e ratio. The resultant multiple linear regression (see equation) was statistically significant (p<0.05), as were the regression coefficients associated with the nonprotein calories infused and the nutritional state as measured by the Na_e/K_e ratio.

$$BCM/day^* = -371.5 + 6.4 \text{ nonprotein kcal/kg/day} - 5.2 \text{ protein}^\dagger + 91.4 \text{ } Na_e/K_e$$

$$(p < 0.001) \qquad\qquad (ns) \qquad\qquad (p < 0.01)$$

According to this regression, the administration of TPN at a rate of 40 kcal/kg/day of nonprotein calories and 1.2 gm/kg/day of amino acids in the moderately malnourished patient (Na_e/K_e = 1.50), would increase the BCM at a rate of 28 gm/day. The mean amino acid intake for the patients receiving the 2.5 per cent solution was 1.2 gm/kg/day. If the nonprotein caloric intake was increased from 40 to 50 kcal/kg/day, the rate of change of the BCM would increase to 92 gm/day. Increasing the amino acid intake to 2.4 gm/day, which was the mean amino acid intake of the patients receiving the 2.5 per cent solution, would increase the BCM to only 98 gm/day. Thus, increasing the amino acid concentration from 2.5 to 5 per cent did not significantly alter the rate at which a malnourished individual was restored to normal. In the malnourished person, the rate of restoration of the BCM is therefore related to the nonprotein caloric intake and the nutritional state, and not to the protein infused in excess of 1.2 gm/kg/day.

*Daily change in BCM in gm/day
†Protein infused in gm/kg/day

The Malnourished Child

Traditionally, a high-protein diet was the recommended treatment for the child recovering from malnutrition. This arose because of the emphasis on protein deficiency as the main cause of malnutrition in less-developed countries and on the observation that kwashiorkor could be effectively treated with milk.[22] It was assumed that the beneficial effect of the milk diet was because of the protein content of milk. This led to the further assumption that a high-protein diet would be advantageous. However, with the traditional high-protein diets, malnourished children remained in the hospital for prolonged periods, often with an almost-stationary body weight. A number of recent reports have demonstrated that a high-protein diet is neither necessary nor desirable.[23-26] The protein requirement of the most rapidly growing infants is not greater than 7 to 8 per cent of the total caloric intake, which approximates the protein content of human milk.[26]

The protein content of cow's milk is more than twice this amount, whereas that of dried skim milk is four times greater. Recovery from malnutrition is not accelerated by providing protein in excess of this amount.

Ashworth and colleagues[23] determined the relationship between the protein content of the diet and the rate of recovery of malnourished children. One group of malnourished infants received a liquid diet containing 90 cal/L with a protein content of 2.2 gm/L, whereas the second group received a similar diet containing 135 cal/L and 3.1 gm/L of protein. A statistically significant relationship existed between the caloric intake and weight gain, which was not different for the two diets (Fig. 10–2). A multiple linear correlation was performed between weight gain (as the dependent variable) and the caloric and protein intakes (as the independent variables). In the resultant regression, the relationship between weight gain and calories was significant, whereas that between protein intake and weight gain was not.

$$\text{weight gain (gm/kg/day)} = 0.072 \text{ cal (kg/day)} + 0.283 \text{ protein (gm/kg/day)} - 3.57$$

$$(p > 0.01) \qquad\qquad (\text{ns})$$

These data demonstrate the relatively greater importance of calories as opposed to protein. This can be illustrated by the following example. According to the preceding regression, with an intake of 100 cal/kg/day and 3 gm/kg/day of protein, the weight gain would be 4.5 gm/kg/day. Increasing the caloric intake by 50 per cent to 150 cal/kg/day would increase the weight gain to 8.1 gm/kg/day, an 80 per cent increase. If instead, however, the protein intake was increased by 50 per cent, the weight gain would increase to 4.9 gm/kg/day, only a 9 per cent increase.

CALORIC REQUIREMENTS

Considerable controversy persists regarding both the magnitude and the nature of the nonprotein calories that are most appropriate for the malnourished patient. Moore has emphasized the importance of differentiating the energy needed for work from that required for protein synthesis.[27] During starvation, the energy required by the BCM to perform mechanical and chemical work is derived from the oxidation of endogenous fat. Although this endogenous source of energy can supply all of the energy required by the BCM to perform its various functions, it cannot support the requirements for protein synthesis. Thus, during periods of starvation there is a gradual wasting away of the BCM. In contrast, carbohydrates, even in relatively small amounts, will provide the energy required for protein synthesis, with a

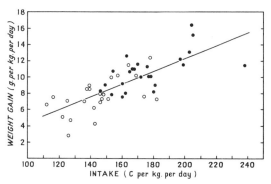

Figure 10–2. The relationship between caloric intake and weight gain. Open circles represent patients who received the low-protein diet, and the closed circles represent patients receiving the high-protein diet. The regression is given by the equation: weight gain (g/kg/day) = 0.078 caloric intake (cal/kg/day) − 3.30. (*From* Ashworth, A., Bell, R., James, W. P. T., and Waterlow, J. C.: Calorie requirements of children recovering from protein-calorie malnutrition. Lancet, 2:600, 1968, with permission.)

significant reduction in the net loss of body protein. The nitrogen-sparing effect of intravenous lipid emulsions in the normal starving subject can be accounted for by the glycerol content of the emulsion.[28] Moore has attributed this inability of fat oxidation to support protein synthesis to "an inborn error of metabolism."

Carbohydrate and Lipid Administration

A difference between the effect of carbohydrate and fat calories on protein metabolism has been reported for both the healthy subject and the patient subjected to a catabolic stress. In healthy young males, the substitution of fat, with an equal number of carbohydrate calories, resulted in a significantly improved nitrogen balance and dietary protein utilization.[29] Similarly, in a group of healthy male volunteers, the intravenous infusion of amino acids with glucose resulted in a more efficient amino acid utilization than with a similar isocaloric infusion of lipid emulsion with amino acids.[16] In patients who were clinically stable following injury or operation, the urinary urea excretion was inversely related to the carbohydrate intake and was directly related to the resting metabolic rate (Fig. 10–3).[30] Nitrogen excretion decreased as the carbohydrate dose increased, reaching a plateau as the carbohy-

drate caloric intake approached the resting metabolic rate. An additional improvement in amino acid utilization was achieved when exogenous insulin was administered. The additional intravenous infusion of a lipid emulsion did not alter the nitrogen excretion at any level of carbohydrate intake. Similarly, in patients with extensive burns who were receiving TPN, nitrogen balance decreased when infused lipid supplied more than 20 per cent of the total nonprotein caloric intake.[31] In contrast, Jeejeebhoy and associates[32] compared the effects of a TPN regimen containing 1 gm/kg amino acids and either hypertonic glucose or 83 per cent Intralipid with 17 per cent glucose. The two solutions were isonitrogenous and isocaloric and were administered for seven days in a cross-over manner to a group of patients with inflammatory bowel disease. The nitrogen balance was reported as positive to a comparable degree with both the lipid and glucose systems after the establishment of equilibrium (Fig. 10–4, Table 10–2). However, for the entire seven-day period, and for the first four days, the nitrogen balance with the glucose-containing solution was significantly more positive than when lipid supplied the majority of nonprotein calories. It was only during days five to seven that the differences were not statistically significant. However, the number of observations during this period was considerably less.

To evaluate the relative efficacy of car-

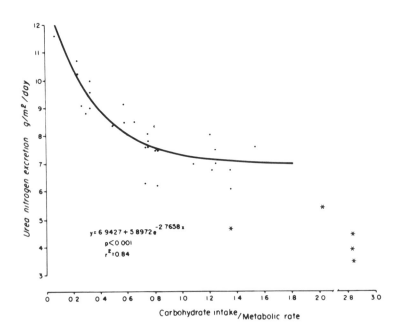

Figure 10–3. The relationship between urea excretion and caloric intake in clinically stable patients following injury or operation. Urea excretion decreased as the caloric intake increased until the caloric intake approximated the metabolic rate (i.e., when caloric intake:metabolic rate = 1). An additional improvement in amino acid utilization occurred with the administration of exogenous insulin (*). (*From* Long, J. M., Wilmore, D. W., Mason, A. D., and Pruitt, B. A.: Effect of carbohydrate and fat intake on nitrogen excretion during total intravenous feeding. Ann. Surg., *185*:417, 1977, with permission.)

Figure 10–4. Daily nitrogen balance in patients receiving TPN with either glucose or lipid as the major source of non-protein calories. The upper half of the figure shows results when the lipid system was administered first; the lower half of the figure shows results when the glucose system was administered first. (*From* Jeejeebhoy, K. N., Anderson, G. H., Nakhooda, A. F., Greenberg, G. R., Sanderson, I., and Marliss, E. B.: Metabolic studies in total parenteral nutrition with lipid in man. J. Clin. Invest., 57:125, 1976, with permission.)

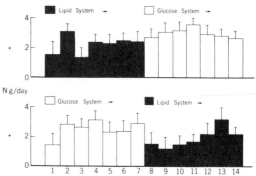

bohydrate and lipid calories in patients receiving TPN, patients were randomized to receive a solution containing 2.5 per cent crystalline amino acids (Travesol) with either 25 per cent glucose or a mixture containing 12.5 per cent dextrose and 5 per cent lipid (Intralipid). The efficacy of TPN with either solution was determined by measuring body composition at the onset of TPN and at two-week intervals.[33] In normally nourished patients, the body composition did not change significantly, except for a slight increase in body fat. The body composition was normal at the onset and, as expected, it remained so following a course of TPN. In the malnourished patients, TPN resulted in a significant increase in the BCM, which was similar in the two groups. However, the lipid group received significantly more calories than did the glucose patients.

The relationship between calories, the

type of calories, and the amino acids infused and the rate at which a depleted BCM is restored was determined by combining the data obtained in the malnourished patients who received the following TPN solutions:

1. 25 per cent glucose with 2.5 per cent amino acids (Table 10–3)
2. 25 per cent glucose with 5 per cent amino acids (Table 10–1)
3. 12.5 per cent glucose, 5 per cent lipid emulsion, 2.5 per cent amino acids (Table 10–3).

Two hundred and twelve TPN periods of approximately two weeks in duration were available for multiple linear regression. The mean daily change in BCM, as the dependent variable, was correlated with the carbohydrate, lipid, and protein intake and the nutritional state as evaluated by the Na_e/K_e ratio. The resultant regression was statistically significant ($p < 0.01$).

$$BCM^* = -348.5 + 4.9 \text{ CHO} + 3.2 \text{ lipid} + 4.7 \text{ protein} + 98.7 \text{ } Na_e/K_e$$

	(kcal/kg/body weight/day)	(kcal/kg body weight/day)	(kcal/kg body weight/day)	
	$p < 0.005$	$p < 0.05$	ns	$p < 0.001$

The preceding regression equation indicates that the rate at which a malnourished BCM is restored is dependent on the caloric intake and the nutritional state and is unaffected by increasing the amino acid concentration above 2.5 per cent. The regression coefficient associated with the carbohydrate intake is larger than that associated with lipid intake, indicating that carbohydrate calories are more efficient than lipid calories. This is demonstrated in Figure 10–5 in which the daily change in the BCM is plotted against the nonprotein caloric intake. An amino acid intake of 1.26 gm/kg/day and a Na_e/K_e ratio of 1.50, which is indicative of moderate malnutrition, is assumed. When all of the non-

protein calories are carbohydrate, the curve intercepts the abscissa at 36 cal/kg/day. This, therefore, is the caloric intake that will maintain the BCM. An intake in excess of this amount is required to achieve an increase in the BCM. Thus, with the infusion of 50 cal/kg/day, the BCM will increase at a rate of 69 gm/day. When lipid supplies all of the nonprotein calories, the intercept of the curve is 55 cal/kg/day, though with a mixture that supplies 50 per cent of the nonprotein calories as lipid and 50 per cent as carbohydrate, maintenance of the BCM is achieved with 44 cal/kg/day. Infusing this mixture at a rate of 50 cal/kg/day, will only increase the BCM at a rate of 16 gm/day.

The regression coefficient associated with the amino acid intake was not statistically significant. This does not mean that

---

*Change in BCM (gm/day)

Table 10–2. NITROGEN BALANCE IN GRAMS/DAY

BALANCE PERIOD	LIPID FOLLOWED BY GLUCOSE				GLUCOSE FOLLOWED BY LIPID			
	Lipid	*Glucose*	*n*	*p*	*Lipid*	*Glucose*	*n*	*p*
Days 1–7	2.27 ± 0.24	2.99 ± 0.20	86	< 0.005	2.49 ± 0.21	1.89 ± 0.21	95	< 0.001
Days 1–4	2.15 ± 0.34	3.14 ± 0.28	50	< 0.005	2.55 ± 0.28	1.46 ± 0.28	55	< 0.001
Days 5–7	2.41 ± 0.34	2.78 ± 0.30	36	ns	2.40 ± 0.33	2.52 ± 0.31	40	ns

(From Jeejeebhoy, K. N., Anderson, G. H., Nakhooda, A. F., Greenberg, G. R., Sanderson, I., and Marliss, E. B.: Metabolic studies in total parenteral nutrition with lipid in man. J. Clin. Invest., 57:125, 1976.)

Table 10–3. THE EFFECT OF TPN ON BODY COMPOSITION OF MALNOURISHED PATIENTS

	NORMAL VOLUNTEERS	2.5% AMINO ACIDS 25% DEXTROSE		5% AMINO ACIDS 12.5% DEXTROSE 5% LIPID	
		Pre-TPN	*Post-TPN*	*Pre-TPN*	*Post-TPN*
Weight (kg)	70.4 ± 2.5	57.5 ± 1.5*	58.6 ± 1.4*	57.4 ± 2.3	59.1 ± 2.4*
Body fat (kg)	20.2 ± 1.4	11.9 ± 0.9	12.4 ± 0.8	13.6 ± 1.6	15.5 ± 1.6*
LBM (kg)	50.3 ± 1.9	45.6 ± 1.1	46.2 ± 1.0	43.8 ± 1.5	43.6 ± 1.5
BCM (kg)	24.7 ± 1.1	15.5 ± 0.5	16.4 ± 0.4	14.6 ± 0.7	15.6 ± 0.8*
ECM (kg)	25.6 ± 0.9	30.1 ± 0.8	29.9 ± 0.9*	29.2 ± 1.1	28.0 ± 1.0
K_e/TBW	80.0 ± 1.0	56.1 ± 1.1	59.2 ± 1.3*	54.7 ± 1.4	58.2 ± 1.6*
Na_e/TBW	77.5 ± 0.9	94.6 ± 1.0	91.5 ± 1.2*	94.1 ± 1.3	91.3 ± 1.3
Na_e/K_e	0.98 ± 0.02	1.79 ± 0.07	1.66 ± 0.06*	1.85 ± 0.11	1.70 ± 0.11
Patients	25	55		29	
TPN periods		90		50	
TPN days		14.9 ± 0.3		14.0 ± 0.2	
Total kcal/kg/day		49.5 ± 1.4		57.1 ± 2.3	
Carbohydrate kcal/kg/day		43.6 ± 1.2		27.4 ± 1.1	
Lipid kcal/kg/day		0.8 ± 0.1		24.4 ± 1.2	
Protein kcal/kg/day		1.26 ± 0.04		1.36 ± 0.06	

*Significantly ($p < 0.05$) different by Student's t test.

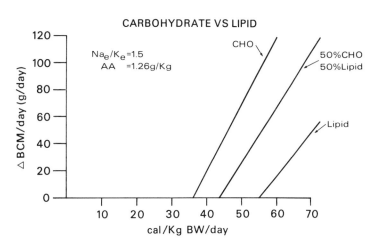

Figure 10–5. The relationship between the daily change in BCM and the nonprotein caloric intake with either glucose, lipid, or a mixture of half glucose and half lipid. The amino acid intake was set at 1.26 g/kg body weight/day and the Na_e/K_e at 1.50, indicative of mild malnutrition. The carbohydrate and lipid curves intercept the abscissa at 36 and 55 cal/kg/day, respectively. (*From* Shizgal, H. M., and Forse, R. A.: Protein and calorie requirements with total parenteral nutrition. Ann. Surg., *192*:562, 1980, with permission.)

amino acids do not influence the restoration rate of a depleted BCM. Rather, it indicates that the restoration rate of the BCM was not affected by the variation in amino acid intake within the range tested. The relationship between caloric intake and the daily change in the BCM, with amino acid intakes of 1.26 and 2.37 gm/kg/day, is depicted in Figure 10–6. These amino acid infusion rates are the mean rates for the patients who received the 2.5 per cent and 5 per cent amino acid solutions (see Table 10–1). A state of moderate

malnutrition is assumed, that is, the Na_e/K_e ratio was set at 1.50. Doubling the amino acid concentration of the infused solution shifted the curve to the left; therefore, at a similar caloric intake, there is a more rapid restoration of a depleted BCM with the higher amino acid intake. This apparent increased efficiency disappears when the calories associated with the additional amino acids are taken into account (the broken line in Fig. 10–6). The regression equation is consistent with the data in Table 10–1 in demonstrating that there was no advantage in increasing the amino acid concentration from 2.5 to 5 per cent.

The regression coefficient associated with the Na_e/K_e ratio was statistically significant, indicating that the rate at which a depleted BCM is restored is related to the nutritional state. This is demonstrated in Figure 10–7. As the Na_e/K_e ratio is increased, which is indicative of a more severe state of malnutrition, the intercept of the curve decreases, and hence less calories are required for maintenance of the BCM. At any given caloric intake above that required for maintenance, the restoration rate is greater in the more severely malnourished patient. Thus in the malnourished individual on a constant caloric and protein intake, the restoration rate of the BCM decreases continuously as the malnourished state is corrected. As the normally nourished state is approached, the rate of change of BCM approaches zero. Thus, in the normally nourished patient on TPN, the BCM does not change.

In a group of depleted patients, Elwyn and associates[34] infused a constant nitrogen intake (173 mg/kg of body weight) and varied

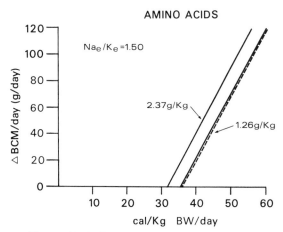

Figure 10–6. The relationship between the daily change in BCM and caloric intake with amino acid intakes of 1.26 and 2.37 g/kg body weight/day. The nonprotein caloric intake is all carbohydrate. A Na_e/K_e ratio of 1.50 is assumed. The broken line depicts the relationship associated with an amino acid infusion of 2.37 g/kg/day when the additional calories associated with the higher amino acid intake are taken into account. (*From* Shizgal, H. M., and Forse, R. A.: Protein and calorie requirements with total parenteral nutrition. Ann. Surg., *192*:562, 1980, with permission.)

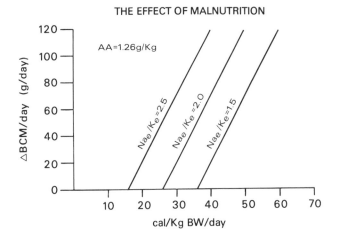

Figure 10–7. The relationship between caloric intake and the rate of change of BCM with varying degrees of malnutrition. All of the nonprotein calories are carbohydrate, and the amino acid intake is set at 1.26 g/kg body weight/day. (*From* Shizgal, H. M., and Forse, R. A.: Protein and calorie requirements with total parenteral nutrition. Ann. Surg., *192*:562, 1980, with permission.)

the energy intake, which was all carbohydrate. The following linear relationship existed between nitrogen balance and energy intake (Fig. 10–8).

Nitrogen balance (mg/kg body weight)
$$= -24.3 + 1.4 \text{ kcal/kg}$$

This relationship can be converted to the following by assuming that 1 gm of nitrogen is equivalent to 6.25 gm of protein and 25 gm of BCM:

BCM (gm/70 kg body weight)
$$= -42.4 + 2.4 \text{ kcal/kg}$$

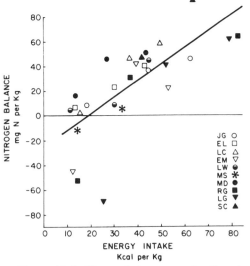

Figure 10–8. Nitrogen balance as a function of energy intake in ten depleted patients receiving TPN in whom the intake of amino acids was held constant, and the caloric intake in the form of glucose was varied. (*From* Elwyn, D. H., Gump, F. E., Munro, H. N., Iles, M., and Kinney, J. M.: Changes in nitrogen balance of depleted patients with increasing infusions of glucose. Am. J. Clin. Nutr., *32*:1597, 1979, with permission.)

Using both this equation and the preceding regression, the rate of change of the BCM was calculated for different caloric intakes (Table 10–4). Although the two equations predicted slightly different restoration rates, the magnitude of the predicted changes was similar. In a 70-kg individual receiving 50 kcal/kg, the Elwyn equation predicted a restoration rate of 77.6 gm/day, whereas the regression developed in our laboratory predicted a restoration rate of 68.2 and 117.6 gm/day with moderate ($Na_e/K_e = 1.5$) and severe ($Na_e/K_e = 2.0$) malnutrition, respectively. At this rate, almost two weeks are required to restore a 1-kg loss of BCM. A BCM loss of this magnitude develops in less than three days of uncomplicated starvation with a daily nitrogen loss of 15 gm/day.

The restoration of a malnourished state is therefore a slow process and requires a high energy intake. This is similar to the experience with malnourished children in less-developed countries,[24-26] in which a similar relationship between a high caloric intake and growth has been demonstrated (Fig. 10–9). This regression of weight gain on caloric intake indicates that at zero weight gain the caloric intake was 108 kcal/kg, and that 6.2 kcal was required for each gram of weight gained. Thus maintenance is approximately 100 kcal/kg/day, and for every 6 kcal above maintenance 1 gm of weight is gained. The use of high-caloric and low-protein feeding has resulted in growth rates in malnourished children that are 15 times normal. These high growth rates have resulted in much shorter stays in hospital, in contrast to the long hospitalizations that were the norm with the traditional high-protein diets.[22] Table 10–5 illustrates the relationship between weight

Table 10–4. RESTORATION OF A DEPLETED BCM IN GRAMS/DAY

CALORIC INTAKE (KCAL/KG)	ELWYN ET AL.[34]	SHIZGAL ET AL.[33]	
		$Na_e/K_e = 1.5$	$Na_e/K_e = 2.0$
30	29.6	−29.7	19.5
40	53.6	19.2	68.6
50	77.6	68.2	117.6

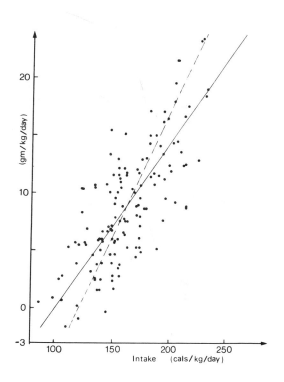

Figure 10–9. The relationship between caloric intake and weight gain in 50 children recovering from malnutrition. Each point represents the mean daily intake and weight increment calculated over a two-week period. The solid line indicates the least square fit of the equation: weight gain = −14.5 + 0.145 intake (r = 0.82, p < 0.01). The broken line represents the least square fit of: intake = 121.0 + 4.6 weight gain (r = 0.82, p < 0.01). (*From* Kerr, D., Ashworth, A., Picou, D., Poulter, N., Seakins, A., Spady, D., and Wheeler, E.: Accelerated recovery from infant malnutrition with high calorie feeding. *In* Gardner, L. I., and Amacher, P. (eds.): Endocrine Aspects of Malnutrition. The Kroc Foundation, Santa Ynez, Cal., 1973, p. 467, with permission.)

Table 10–5. GROWTH RATES*

CALORIC INTAKE (KCAL/DAY)	EXCESS CALORIES (KCAL/DAY)	WEIGHT GAIN (GM/DAY)	DAYS TO GAIN 3000 GM
700	0	0	
760	60	10	300
820	120	20	150
940	240	40	75
1180	480	80	38
1660	960	160	19

*A 7-kg child with a normal weight, according to height, of 10 kg.
Maintenance = 100 kcal/kg/day
Weight gain = excess kcal/6

gain and caloric intake for a 7-kg child whose expected weight for height is 10 kg. If this child consumed the normal intake for his weight, it would take a year to make up the deficit. To decrease this time, malnourished children were offered 240 kcal/kg/day.[26] Intakes in excess of 200 kcal/kg/day are frequently observed for limited periods and may even be as high as 300 kcal/kg/day without apparent complications.

The high energy requirements associated with normal growth and the repair of the malnourished state appear to be related to the energy cost associated with protein synthesis. The synthesis of a peptide bond has been estimated to require 29.2 kcal/mol.[35] However, only 5 kcal/mol of chemical energy is stored in the peptide bond, making a net cost for protein synthesis of 24.2 kcal/mol. In bacteria, 80 per cent of the metabolic energy expenditure has been attributed to protein synthesis. In humans, 15 to 20 per cent of the resting energy expenditure has been attributed to protein synthesis. Keys and colleagues estimated the caloric cost of weight change at approximately 6000 kcal/kg.[36] In malnourished subjects, the excess caloric requirements have been reported to vary from 6400 to 9800 kcal/kg.[37-39]

REFERENCES

1. Valgeirsdottir, K., and Munro, H. N.: Protein and amino acid metabolism. *In* Fischer, J. E. (ed.): Surgical Nutrition. Boston, Little Brown and Co., 1983, pages 129–164.
2. Wooflson, A. M. J.: Amino acids—their role as an energy source. Proc. Nutr. Soc., *42*:489, 1983.
3. Food and Agricultural Organization, World Health Organization Expert Committee Report: Energy and Protein Requirements. Technical report series No 522, WHO, Geneva, 1973.
4. Kinney, J. M., Long, C. L., Gump, F. E., and Duke, J. H.: Tissue composition of weight loss in surgical patients. I. Elective Operations. Ann. Surg., *168*:459, 1968.
5. Inoue, G., Fugita, Y., and Niiyama, Y.: Studies on protein requirements of young men fed egg protein and rice protein with excess and maintenance energy intakes. J. Nutr., *103*:1673, 1973.
6. Forse, R. A., and Shizgal, H. M.: The assessment of malnutrition. Surgery, *88*:17, 1980.
7. Vinnars, E.: Effects of intravenous amino acid administration on nitrogen retention. Scand. J. Clin. Lab. Invest. (Suppl.) 27(117):1, 1971.
8. Shizgal, H. M., Milne, C. A., and Spanier, A. H.: The effect of nitrogen-sparing, intravenously administered fluids on postoperative body composition. Surgery, *85*:498, 1979.
9. Shizgal, H. M.: The effect of malnutrition on body composition. Surg. Gynecol. Obstet., *152*:22, 1981.
10. Shizgal, H. M., Spanier, A. H., Humes, J., and Wood, C. D.: Indirect measurement of total exchangeable potassium. Am. J. Physiol., *233*(3):F253, 1977.
11. Cahill, G. J., Jr.: Starvation in man. N. Engl. J. Med., *282*:668, 1970.
12. Wolfe, B. M., Culebras, J. M., Sim, A. J. W., Ball, M. R., and Moore, E. D.: Substrate interaction in intravenous feeding. Ann. Surg., *186*:518, 1977.
13. Elwyn, D. H., Gump, F. E., Iles, M., Long, C. L., and Kinney, J. M.: Protein and energy sparing of glucose added in hypocaloric amounts to peripheral infusions of amino acids. Metabolism, 27:325, 1978.
14. Blackburn, G. L., Flatt, J. P., Clowes, G. H. A., Jr. et al.: Protein sparing therapy during periods of starvation with sepsis or trauma. Ann. Surg., *177*:588, 1973.
15. Blackburn, G. L., Flatt, J. P., Clowes, G. H. A., Jr. et al.: Peripheral intravenous feeding with isotonic amino acid solution. Am. J. Surg., *125*:447, 1973.
16. Freeman, J. B., Stegink, L. D., Wittine, M. F., and Thompson, R. G.: The current status of protein sparing. Surg. Gynecol. Obstet., *144*:843, 1977.
17. Greenberg, G. R., Marliss, E. B., Anderson, G. H. et al.: Protein sparing therapy in post-operative patients. N. Engl. J. Med., *294*:1411, 1976.
18. Hoover, H. C., Jr., Grant, J. P., Gorshboth, C. et al.: Nitrogen sparing intravenous fluids in postoperative patients. N. Engl. J. Med., *293*:172, 1975.
19. Skillman, J. J., Rosenor, V. M., Smith, P. C. et al.: Improved albumin synthesis in post-operative patients by amino acid infusion. N. Engl. J. Med., *295*:1037, 1976.
20. Wilmore, D. W.: Energy requirement for maximum nitrogen retention. *In* American Medical Association: Clinical Nutrition Update. Chicago, 1977, page 47.
21. Shizgal, H. M.: Protein requirements with total parenteral nutrition. Surg. Forum, *29*:60, 1978.
22. Waterlow, J. C.: The rate of recovery of malnourished infants in relation to the protein and calorie levels of the diet. J. Trop. Pediatr., *7*:16, 1961.
23. Ashworth, A., Bell, R., James, W. P. T., and Waterlow, J. C.: Calorie requirements of children recovering from protein-calorie malnutrition. Lancet, *2*:600, 1968.
24. Ashworth, A.: Growth rates of children recovering from protein-calorie malnutrition. Br. J. Nutr., *23*:835, 1969.
25. Graham, G. G., Cordano, A., and Baeril, J. M.: Studies in infantile malnutrition. II. Effect of protein and calorie intake on weight gain. J. Nutr., *81*:249, 1963.
26. Kerr, D., Ashworth, A., Picou, D., Poulter, N., Seakins, A., Spady, D., and Wheeler, E.: Accelerated recovery from infant malnutrition with high calorie feeding. *In* Gardner, L. I., and Amacher, P. (eds.): Endocrine Aspects of Malnutrition. Santa Ynez, California, The Kroc Foundation, 1973, page 467.
27. Moore, F. D.: Energy and the maintenance of the body cell mass. J. Parent. Ent. Nutr., *4*:288, 1980.
28. Brennan, M. F., Fitzpatrick, G. F., Cohen, K. H., and Moore, F. D.: Glycerol. Ann. Surg., *182*:386, 1975.
29. Richardson, D. P., Wayler, A. H., Scrimshaw, N. S., and Young, V. R.: Quantitative effect of isoenergetic exchange of fat for carbohydrate on dietary protein utilization in healthy young men. Am. J. Clin. Nutr., *32*:2217, 1979.

30. Long, J. M., Wilmore, D. W., Mason, A. D., and Pruitt, B. A.: Effect of carbohydrate and fat intake on nitrogen excretion during total intravenous feeding. Ann. Surg., *185*:417, 1977.

31. Long, J. M., Wilmore, D. W., Mason, A. D., and Pruitt, B. A.: Fat carbohydrate interaction: Nitrogen sparing effect of varying caloric sources for total intravenous feeding. Surg. Forum, *25*:61, 1974.

32. Jeejeebhoy, K. N., Anderson, G. H., Nakhooda, A. F., Greenberg, G. R., Sanderson, I., and Marliss, E. B.: Metabolic studies in total parenteral nutrition with lipid in man. J. Clin. Invest., *57*:125, 1976.

33. Shizgal, H. M., and Forse, R. A.: Protein and calorie requirements with total parenteral nutrition. Ann. Surg., *192*:562, 1980.

34. Elwyn, D. H., Gump, F. E., Munro, H. N., Iles, M., and Kinney, J. M.: Changes in nitrogen balance of depleted patients with increasing infusions of glucose. Am. J. Clin. Nutr., *32*:1597, 1979.

35. Lehninger, A. L.: Biochemistry. The Molecular Basis of Cell Structure. New York, Worth Pubs. Inc., 1975.

36. Keys, A., Brozek, J., Henschel, A., Mickelsen, O., and Taylor, H. L.: The biology of human starvation. Vol 2. Minneapolis, The University of Minnesota Press, 1950.

37. Passmore, R., Meiklejohn, A. D., Dewey, A. D., and Thow, R. K.: Energy utilization in overfed thin young men. Br. J. Nutr., *9*:20, 1955.

38. Walker, J., Roberts, S. L., Halmi, K. A., and Goldberg, S. C.: Caloric requirements for weight gain in anorexia nervosa. Am. J. Clin. Nutr., *32*:1396, 1979.

39. Dempsey, D. T., Crosby, L. O., Pertschuk, M. J., Feurer, I. D., Buzby, G. P., and Mullen, J. L.: Weight gain and nutritional efficacy in anorexia nervosa. Am. J. Clin. Nutr., *39*:236, 1984.

CHAPTER 11

Measurement of Energy Expenditure

IRENE D. FEURER
JAMES L. MULLEN

The recognition of the prevalence and severity of malnutrition in the clinical setting[1-7] has led to markedly improved efforts and methods of both identifying and supporting the malnourished patient. Enteral and parenteral nutritional therapy are essential components in caring for patients who are malnourished as well as for well-nourished patients who are at risk of developing malnutrition as a consequence of their disease process, injury, or treatment regimen (e.g., surgery necessitating a prolonged period without adequate oral nutrient intake). Of major concern when formulating a nutritional regimen is the determination of the patient's nonprotein energy requirement. When doing so, the clinician must consider: (1) the overall goal of therapy—nutritional repletion, maintenance, or weight reduction with preservation or repletion of visceral protein stores and skeletal musculature; (2) the patient's activity level (skeletal muscle activity not reflected while resting); (3) the patient's resting energy expenditure; and (4) the level of efficiency at which exogenous nutrients are converted to energy available at the cellular level.

The individual components of total daily energy expenditure are basal metabolism; resting energy expenditure; diet-induced thermogenesis; an increment for shivering and nonshivering thermogenesis; and the energy expended for physical activity. The contribution of each of these elements in normal persons is described in relation to resting energy expenditure in Figure 11–1. Basal metabolic rate is 90 per cent of resting energy expenditure. Diet-induced thermogenesis and the thermogenic effect of "coldness" add increments of 10 per cent and

periods of physical activity can increase metabolic rate to 200 per cent of true resting energy expenditure.

Indirect calorimetry provides a method whereby basal metabolic rate (BMR) or resting energy expenditure (REE) may be measured throughout the period of nutritional therapy, thus eliminating the necessity for estimating the combined effects of body composition, nutritional status, disease processes, trauma, or clinical events on metabolic rate. BMR is defined by Boothby and Sandiford to be "the minimal heat production of an organism, measured from twelve to eighteen hours after the ingestion of food and with the organism at complete muscular rest."[8] Measurements are performed early in the morning, in a thermoneutral environment, following greater than 30 minutes of skeletal muscle rest and a 12- to 18-hour fast and with the subject in the supine position.[8-11] It is our practice to measure BMR within the first 30 minutes of waking.

REE is measured in a thermoneutral environment after the subject has rested in a supine position in bed or in a comfortable recliner for greater than 30 minutes and has been without food for greater than 2 hours.[12, 13] Thus REE measured according to strict conditions includes the BMR, increases following awakening, and some thermic effect of food.[10, 12, 13] Accordingly, REE is 10 per cent higher than BMR.[10] The practical advantage of measuring energy expenditure under resting rather than basal conditions has made REE the optimal clinical procedure. Provided that the patient has rested appropriately and has been without dietary intake for greater than two hours, clinical determinations of REE may be performed throughout the day

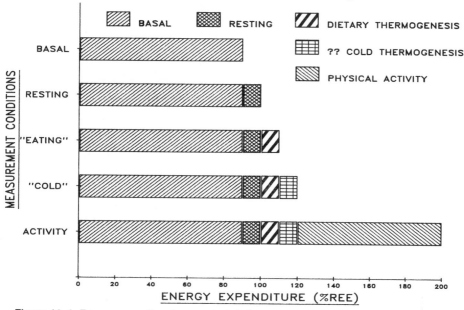

Figure 11–1. Energy expenditure in normals (relative to resting) during various nonresting conditions.

and require minimal advanced scheduling and patient preparation.

Although the principles of indirect calorimetry have been understood and employed for a variety of experimental and clinical purposes since the latter part of the 18th century, recent technologic advances and the rapid development of the field of clinical nutrition have enhanced the role of bedside measurements of REE as an integral part of nutritional care.

CALORIMETRY: HISTORICAL DEVELOPMENT AND TECHNICAL CONSIDERATIONS

Historical Development

Direct calorimetry is the process of measuring heat production as the temperature change of a medium. Bomb (*in vitro*) calorimetry, as described by Riche,[14] requires enclosing a weighed amount of a foodstuff in a steel cylinder. The foodstuff is rapidly ignited in an atmosphere of pure pressurized oxygen and the heat of combustion is measured from the temperature change of the water surrounding the cylinder. During the late 1700s, Lavoisier[15] measured the heat produced by a guinea pig by quantitating the amount of ice (surrounding the animal's chamber) that melted over a given period of time (1 kg melted ice = 80 kcal heat). His

observations relating gas exchange (oxygen consumption) to heat production led him and his coworkers to measure human oxygen consumption during a variety of circumstances using a metal facepiece apparatus.[16] Thus, direct calorimetry requires the measurement of heat production *per se*, and indirect calorimetry measures gas exchange: oxygen consumption ($\dot{V}O_2$) and carbon dioxide production ($\dot{V}CO_2$).

The pioneering investigators (Table 11–1) focused on developing the technology and establishing the agreement between direct and indirect calorimetric measurements.[15–18, 20, 22–24] During the middle to latter portion of the 19th century, closed- and open-circuit indirect calorimeters were used to study the effects of various diseases on human metabolism.[20–22, 26] However, the most fruitful clinical application of the technique proved to be in the diagnosis of thyroid dysfunction. Following Magnus-Levy's observations of an increased metabolic rate in patients with exophthalmic goiter (Graves' disease,)[26] several clinical investigators documented the effects of hypo- and hyperthyroidism on metabolic rate. Means and coworkers published several studies on the subject,[35, 36] and in 1935[36] they presented a description of the relationships among metabolic rate, symptomatology, and thyroid supplementation. It is important to note that it was then customary (and is frequently practiced today) to express a measured BMR relative to accepted normal stand-

Table 11–1. CALORIMETRY: EARLY DEVELOPMENT AND KEY HUMAN STUDIES

INVESTIGATORS	TIME PERIOD	COMMENTS
Black[17]	Late 1700s	Developed the distinction between latent heat and the temperature of a substance.
Lavoisier[15]	Late 1700s	Used an ice-jacketed calorimeter to relate oxygen consumption to heat production in animal studies.
Lavoisier[16]	1790	Documented experiments describing oxygen consumption in human subjects.
Regnault and Reiset[18]	1849	Used a closed-circuit calorimeter for animal studies.
Bidder and Schmidt[19]	Mid-1800s	Described the concept of interspecies similarities of BMR from gas exchange.
Pettenkofer and Voit[20]	Mid-1800s 1867	Built a respiration chamber for human studies. Reported observations on a diabetic patient.
Liebermeister[21]	1871	Measured carbon dioxide production patterns in two malaria patients.
Rubner[22, 23]	Latter 1800s	Performed direct and indirect calorimetric studies on dogs, which led to the establishment of the agreement between the two techniques. Noted interspecific similarities in heat production/unit body surface area in mammals. Observed and coined the term *specific dynamic action* of foodstuffs.
Zuntz and Geppert[22]	Late 1800s	Developed an open-circuit indirect calorimeter for human studies. Noted the importance of absolute skeletal muscle rest during measurements of REE.
Atwater, Rosa, and Benedict[22, 24]	Late 1800s	Developed a large respiration chamber for long-term human studies.
Magnus-Levy[25]	Circa 1894	Used the Zuntz-Geppert apparatus to study normal humans and observe the effects of food, age, gender, and pregnancy on metabolic rate.
Magnus-Levy[26]	1895	Demonstrated increased metabolic rate with Graves' disease.
Benedict[27]	Early 1900s	Continued extensive studies with humans using a variety of techniques while Director of the Nutrition Laboratory of the Carnegie Institute at Boston. Developed the first instrument suitable for clinical use.
Lusk[27]	Early 1900s	Directed experiments with respiration calorimeter at Bellevue Hospital—Russel Sage Institute of Pathology. Studied the effects of foods and intermediary metabolism.
Atwater and Benedict[28]	1903	Demonstrated the agreement between direct and indirect calorimetric measurements in humans.
Aub and DuBois[29]	1917	Published standards for normal REE.
Harris and Benedict[30]	1919	Published standards for normal REE frequently used in present-day practice.
Boothby and coworkers[31–33]	1920–1936	Published a detailed description of the measurement technique and standards for normal REE based upon *large* samples.
Benedict[34]	1930	Published a description of a "helmet" indirect calorimetric chamber to be employed with open- or closed-circuit systems that were mechanically ventilated by a blower. Principles of this system are applied today for long-term clinical studies.

ards. Means[36] expressed BMR in relation to the standards of Aub and DuBois.[29] For instance, a patient with hypothyroidism whose measured BMR was 70 per cent of standard was classified as having a BMR of −30.

The early 1900s saw the establishment of several major centers for the study of human metabolism. Three notable laboratories were the Nutrition Laboratory of the Carnegie Institute at Boston, Massachusetts, which was under the direction of F.G. Benedict; Graham Lusk's center at Bellevue Hospital in New York, New York, (Russel Sage Institute of Pathology); and Boothby's laboratory at the Mayo Clinic in Rochester, Minnesota. Comprehensive research projects conducted at these sites produced a wealth of information describing the nuances of the technique,[31] the influence of disease on metabolism,[32] and established standards for REE in large populations of normal subjects,[30, 32, 33] which continue to be referenced as the "gold standard" by current investigators.

Indirect Calorimetry: General Methodology and Calculations

Direct calorimetric measurements are still performed in research and clinical settings.[37–40] However, indirect calorimetry is much less cumbersome, costly, and time-consuming than the direct determination of heat production and is the most practical clinical method for measuring energy expenditure.

Gas exchange studies can be accomplished by either closed-circuit or open-circuit methods. Both systems require the ability to capture all expired gas and an accurate tool for the measurement of the volume of a gas expired. During a closed-circuit measurement, the subject breathes from a spirometer containing either oxygen or room air. Carbon dioxide is absorbed upon exhalation and the remaining expired air is directed back to the spirometer by means of a one-way valve. The decreased volume of gas in the spirometer represents the portion of oxygen that was assimilated over a precise time period.[41]

The open-circuit technique (most frequently employed in present-day studies) requires precise measurements of exhaled volume over time and accurate determinations of the composition of the mixed expired gas. The Douglas bag is an example of an open-circuit system. The subject breathes room air (or an enriched oxygen mixture) and exhales into the collection bag via a two-way valve. After a specific period of time, the volume and composition of the gas in the bag are determined and the volume of oxygen consumed ($\dot{V}O_2$) and the volume of carbon dioxide produced ($\dot{V}CO_2$) are calculated from the concentration differences between the inspired and expired gas mixtures, with volumes corrected for standard temperature, pressure, and dry gas concentrations (see below). Both techniques presuppose that there are no leaks of expired air at any point in the collection system and that the subject is in a steady state throughout the measurement.

Fowler and coworkers at the Mayo Clinic published a report in 1957 comparing results on 49 pairs of tests performed by closed- and open-circuit techniques.[42] They observed a strong correlation between the two techniques ($r = +0.84$), but noted that the results obtained by the closed-circuit method were less reproducible than those obtained on repeated open-circuit measurements. This led them to identify the increased magnitude of the error caused by leaks of expired air in the closed-circuit method as compared with the open-circuit technique. (An expiratory leak via the open-circuit method resulted in 1/25 the error in the final calculation of $\dot{V}O_2$ that would occur with the closed-circuit technique.) They concluded that open-circuit measurements were more reliable.

The concept of steady state is extremely critical to the accurate determination of REE or BMR. With the development of systems capable of performing continuous measurements of $\dot{V}O_2$ and $\dot{V}CO_2$,[43–51] it has become possible to identify a period of "equilibration" and to derive metabolic rate from documented steady state gas exchange values. This represents a major advantage over the Douglas bag technique.

Gas exchange is related to energy expenditure according to the following formulae:

(1) $EE = 4.83 \, (\dot{V}O_2)$[52]

(2) $EE = 3.9 \, (\dot{V}O_2) + 1.1 \, (\dot{V}CO_2)$[53]

(3) $EE = 3.941 \, (\dot{V}O_2) + 1.106 \, (\dot{V}CO_2) - 2.17 \, (UN)$[53]

---

(1) Inspired O_2 concentration (20.9 per cent if room air) − chamber O_2 concentration = Volume per cent O_2 extracted

(2) $\dfrac{\text{Volume gas expired}}{\text{Unit time}} \times \dfrac{\text{Volume per cent } O_2 \text{ extracted}}{1} = \dfrac{O_2 \text{ consumption}}{\text{Unit time}} = \dot{V}O_2$

(3) Inspired CO_2 concentration (0.04 per cent if room air) + chamber CO_2 concentration = Volume per cent CO_2 produced

(4) $\dfrac{\text{Volume gas expired}}{\text{Unit time}} \times \dfrac{\text{Volume per cent } CO_2 \text{ produced}}{1} = \dfrac{CO_2 \text{ production}}{\text{Unit time}} = \dot{V}CO_2$

EE   = energy expenditure (kcal/unit time)
$\dot{V}_{O_2}$ = oxygen consumption (L/unit time)
$\dot{V}_{CO_2}$ = carbon dioxide production (L/unit time)
UN   = urinary nitrogen excretion (gm/unit time).

Equation No. 1 requires only the measurement of $\dot{V}_{O_2}$ and is accurate to within ± eight per cent of the actual energy expenditure.[52] Equation No. 2 incorporates measurements of both oxygen consumption and carbon dioxide production and is accurate to within ± one to two per cent.[53] Equation No. 3 includes a factor to correct for incomplete protein metabolism in humans as reflected in urinary nitrogen excretion. Weir's factor[53] is based upon the assumption that 12.5 per cent of total caloric expenditure in humans arises from protein metabolism and that the individual has normal renal function. For routine clinical measurements, one may avoid the necessity of a 24-hour urine collection and use equation No. 2 in the following form to derive REE in kcal/day:

REE (kcal/day) =
    $[3.9\ (\dot{V}_{O_2}) + 1.1\ (\dot{V}_{CO_2})]$ 1440 minutes/day
$\dot{V}_{O_2}$ = oxygen consumption (L/minute)
$\dot{V}_{CO_2}$ = carbon dioxide production (L/minute)

The error generated by not measuring the energy reflected in urinary nitrogen excretion is usually less than two per cent.[53, 54]

Systems designed to measure both oxygen consumption and carbon dioxide production have the advantage of permitting the calculation of total respiratory quotient (RQ):

$$\text{Total RQ} = \frac{\dot{V}_{CO_2}}{\dot{V}_{O_2}}$$

If urinary nitrogen excretion is measured, the nonprotein RQ, which adjusts for the contribution of protein oxidation to gas exchange, may be calculated:

$$\text{Nonprotein RQ} = \frac{\dot{V}_{CO_2} - 4.754\ (UN)}{\dot{V}_{O_2} - 5.923\ (UN)}$$

The adjustment just described permits the calculation of the relative quantity of energy produced from carbohydrate, fat, and protein[55] oxidation and is based upon the fact that 1 gm of urinary nitrogen reflects the oxidation of a quantity of protein that would require 5.923 L of oxygen and would produce 4.754 L of carbon dioxide.[55] When a 24-hour urine collection is performed, one may calculate the nonprotein RQ and use the complete Weir formula (No. 3) to derive metabolic rate.

RQ reflects net substrate oxidation. A nonprotein RQ of 0.707 reflects net fat oxidation; a nonprotein RQ of 1.00 indicates net carbohydrate oxidation. Between these extremes, the relative proportions of energy produced from fat and carbohydrate oxidation change proportionally, with a nonprotein RQ of 0.85 being indicative of "mixed substrate oxidation" (50 per cent each from fat and carbohydrate) (Table 11–2).[57]

As is indicated in Table 11–2, the RQ can exceed 1.00 during periods of net lipogenesis. Although the stoichiometry indicates an RQ of 8.00 or greater,[56, 58] the whole-body RQ during synthesis of adipose tissue from carbohydrate is typically between 1.01 and 1.20. When performing indirect calorimetric studies, one must take special care to ascertain that an RQ that is observed to be greater than 1.00 is not reflecting a nonsteady state hyperventilation. Occasionally, the RQ may be observed to be less than 0.70 in subjects receiving ketogenic diets that are composed almost exclusively of protein,[59] during glu-

Table 11–2. ENERGY EQUIVALENTS AND RESPIRATORY QUOTIENT VALUES

SUBSTRATE	ENERGY (KCAL/GM) In Vitro Oxidation	ENERGY (KCAL/GM) Human Oxidation	STOICHIOMETRY	RESPIRATORY EQUIVALENT O_2 Kcal/L	RESPIRATORY EQUIVALENT CO_2 Kcal/L	RESPIRATORY EQUIVALENT RQ $\dot{V}_{CO_2}/\dot{V}_{O_2}$
Ethanol	7.1	7.1	1 ethanol + 6 $O_2 \rightarrow$ 4 CO_2 + H_2O	4.86	7.25	0.67
Fat	9.3	9.3	1 palmatate + 230 $O_2 \rightarrow$ 160 CO_2 + 16 H_2O	4.74	6.67	0.70
Protein	5.4	4.2	1 amino acid + 5.1 $O_2 \rightarrow$ 4.1 CO_2 + 2.8 H_2O + 0.7 urea	4.46	5.57	0.80
Carbohydrate	4.1	4.1	1 glucose + 6 $O_2 \rightarrow$ 6 CO_2 + 6 H_2O	5.05	5.05	1.00
Carbohydrate (lipogenesis)			13.5 glucose + 3 $O_2 \rightarrow$ $C_{55}H_{104}O_6$ + 26 CO_2 + 29 H_2O			8.67*

*Based upon the stoichiometry for equimolar synthesis of palmitic, stearic, and oleic acids from carbohydrate precursors (56). Net lipogenesis in humans is indicated by a steady state RQ >1.00 (1.01 − 1.20). (*Adapted from* Wilmore, D. W.: The Metabolic Management of the Critically Ill. New York, Plenum Publishing Corporation, 1977, p. 10.)

coneogenesis from fat,[58] or during the oxidation of ethanol. Typically, net RQ will range from 0.70 to 1.00, depending upon the amount of time that has elapsed between a subject's nutrient intake and the measurement. The subject's clinical condition is also a factor.

CURRENT CLINICAL TECHNIQUES

Systems

Present-day indirect calorimeters employ "state of the art" methods of gas analysis, volume or flow measurement, and data management and must be adapted for use with critically ill patients. One of the first such systems was developed by Kinney and co-workers.[44, 46, 60] It employs a transparent, rigid canopy in which the patient's head is enclosed by means of a neck seal. Air is delivered to the canopy at a fixed rate by a blower, and a spirometer measures tidal volume. Effluent gases are directed past a desiccant, pressure regulator, infrared carbon dioxide analyzer, and a paramagnetic oxygen analyzer. Data acquisition and the balance between input and output flow rates are controlled by a computer. Gas exchange is then calculated via material balance equations.[44, 46] This system affords the investigators the capability of making long-term measurements under tightly controlled conditions on critically ill patients who do not require supplemental oxygen. It is not a portable instrument, but rather is a computer-controlled system that enables simultaneous gas exchange monitoring on several patients located in the metabolic unit.

During the last decade a wide variety of systems have been developed for clinical use.[48–51, 60–64] Some are intended solely for use with patients who are being mechanically ventilated, whereas others are designed to measure gas exchange during mechanical ventilation with elevated inspired oxygen concentrations and on nonintubated patients breathing room air.[51, 60–64] At present, only one commercially available portable system offers the capability of measuring gas exchange on mechanically ventilated patients and on nonintubated patients breathing room air (during conditions of rest and exercise), is equipped with a canopy system, and incorporates fully automated calibration procedures and computerized data management (MMC Horizon, Sensor Medics Corp., Anaheim, California) (Fig. 11–2).[61]

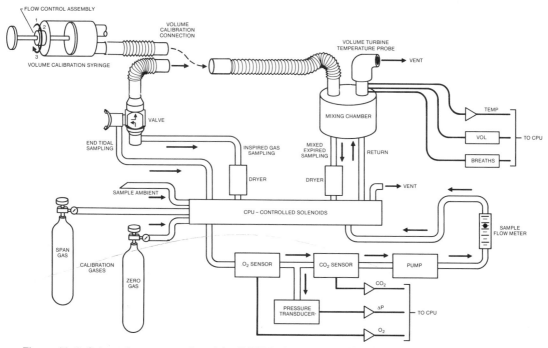

Figure 11–2. Schematic representation of the "MMC horizon system" (Sensor Medics Corp., Anaheim, CA).

Hardware Management

Regardless of the gas collection system employed (user-developed or commercial), standard precautions to prevent the transmission of infectious diseases must be taken. All equipment coming in contact with the patient's secretions or expired air must be sterilizable or disposable. Mouthpieces, valves, adapters, masks, and nose clips should be sterilized after each use. Depending upon the materials, these pieces may be gas sterilized (ethylene oxide) or soaked in a sterilizing and disinfecting solution (Cidex 7, Surgikos, Inc., Arlington, TX). Disposable tubing that directs expired air to the collection chamber should be replaced at regular intervals depending upon the circumstances of use, that is, daily with frequent use, after measuring a patient with a known respiratory infection, or prior to measuring a patient with compromised immune function. External surfaces of the instrument and the internal surface of the collecting chamber should be wiped down regularly with a disinfecting solution. The internal and external surfaces of the canopy chamber should be similarly disinfected after each use, or they may be sterilized with ethylene oxide.

Patient Preparation: REE and BMR

Routine monitoring of REE or BMR requires a portable system and a strict protocol for patient preparation, instrument calibration, and identification of steady state. Determinations of BMR are made early in the morning in a darkened room. We ask that subjects do not arise from bed prior to the measurement. REE is measured after the patient has rested in the supine position for greater than 30 minutes. Measurements of REE should not be performed on patients who are sitting in a chair. Although patients may appear to be comfortable and rested, the minimal skeletal muscle activity of sitting erect in a chair has been demonstrated to increase energy expenditure above the true resting conditions by eight per cent.[65] Patients should be returned to their beds and then tested after having completed at least 30 minutes of skeletal muscle rest.

The timing of a REE measurement relative to enteral nutrient intake (oral intake, bolus, or intermittent tube feedings) must also be strictly controlled, since it results in the thermogenesis first referred to by Rubner as "specific dynamic action."[22, 23] This increase in metabolic rate peaks within the first hour following a light meal and returns to within two per cent of baseline by the second and third hours.[66] For this reason, in the interest of clinical practicality, REE is measured longer than two hours following a light meal. Increases in resting metabolic rate are also associated with the infusion of hypercaloric parenteral nutrients.[67-69] Since parenteral nutrients are usually delivered continuously over the 24-hour period, one cannot avoid their thermic effect when measuring REE on patients receiving total parenteral nutrition. Under such circumstances, the operator should wait for at least two hours following a meal (if the patient is consuming an oral diet) and note the rate at which all parenteral nutrients (amino acids, carbohydrates, and lipid emulsions) are being infused at the time of measurement.

Calibration and Equilibration

The calibration procedures performed prior to a measurement of metabolic rate are dependent upon the system being used. In general, gas analyzers should be carefully calibrated to gas mixtures comparable in concentration to mixed expired air (16 per cent oxygen, 4 per cent carbon dioxide, and the balance nitrogen for patients inspiring room air). When measuring mixed expired gases during mechanical ventilation, calibration gas should simulate the elevated concentrations of oxygen present in the expired air. Similar considerations must be made during canopy measurements, for which calibration span gas must be 20 per cent oxygen, 0.75 per cent carbon dioxide, and the balance nitrogen. A general description of the span gas concentrations appropriate for various measurement conditions appears in Table 11-3. Volume-measuring devices should be calibrated to measure accurately at the appropriate rate of minute ventilation. Pressure transducers and temperature sensors should be calibrated as frequently as indicated by the instrument's stability.

Accurate measurements of BMR and REE are dependent upon meticulous attention to calibration procedures and rigid guidelines for identifying an equilibrated or steady state period during the measurement. Automated systems offer this capability.

Table 11–3. CALIBRATION GAS MIXTURES

COLLECTION MODE	INSPIRED O_2 CONCENTRATION (%)	SPAN GAS MIXTURE (%)		
		O_2	CO_2	N_2
Mask or Mouthpiece	20.93 (room air)	16.00	4.00	80.00
Ventilator	21.00–40.00	40.00	4.00	56.00
Ventilator	40.01–60.00	60.00	4.00	36.00
Canopy	20.00	20.00	0.75	79.25

Steady state requires that a defined number of consecutive determinations of oxygen consumption and carbon dioxide production do not vary by greater than a fixed amount. The specific criteria may be set by the individual, but the longer the duration of equilibration required and the narrower the range of variability accepted, the greater the assurance that one has accurately identified a period of gas exchange representative of either resting or basal metabolism. Our technique is to require five consecutive one-minute data periods having a standard deviation for $\dot{V}O_2$ and $\dot{V}CO_2$ that is less than or equal to five per cent of the mean for oxygen consumption and carbon dioxide production. The majority of patients will demonstrate such stability within 15 minutes or less. Only the mean values for $\dot{V}O_2$ and $\dot{V}CO_2$ from the equilibrated period are then used to derive BMR or REE via the abbreviated or complete Weir formula[53] and to calculate the RQ. Occasionally, patients do not demonstrate equilibration, in which case the data may not be used; the measurement should be repeated at a later time. Such patients may benefit from further familiarization with the collection system or the use of an alternate system (mask or canopy).

Gas Collection Set-ups

The most commonly used systems for routing expired air to the collection chamber when patients inspire room air are the mouthpiece and nonrebreathing valve with a nose clip or the nonrebreathing mask. Each system has its advantages and disadvantages. The mouthpiece, nonrebreathing valve, and nose clip system offers the best safeguard against leaks and is, in our experience, the system of choice for short-term measurements. Patients who find the mouthpiece or noseclip uncomfortable and do not equilibrate will usually achieve steady state with a facemask (plus or minus a nonre-

breathing valve, depending upon mask style). However, extreme care must be taken when using a mask. An airtight seal around the cuff must be present to prevent leaks of expired gases and the resultant erroneous measurements of metabolic rate. This can be accomplished by holding the mask in place by hand or by securing it firmly with a head strap. For short-term ($\leq$15 minutes) measurements we find the former system preferable. Special circumstances, such as altered facial configuration or the presence of a beard or tubing will dictate the use of one particular method (e.g., nasoenteric tubing causing leaks around the cuff of the mask, thus necessitating the use of the mouthpiece and nose clip), but most persons will tolerate either system.

Under specific conditions, one may obtain a complete collection of expired gases when the patient is breathing room air via a tracheostomy. This requires that the endotracheal cannula has an inflated cuff to prevent leaks through the mouth or nose. If no such leaks are present, a nonrebreathing valve may be placed directly onto the external portion of the tracheostomy cannula, directing expired air to the collecting chamber.

Measurements of gas exchange during mechanical ventilation require careful attention to detail. One must ensure that the patient is receiving a completely stable fraction of inspired oxygen (FiO_2) and that the concentration has been accurately measured at ambient pressure. Stability of FiO_2 is achieved by using an external blender and directing the preblended gas to both the oxygen and compressed air ports of the ventilator. This procedure effectively bypasses the ventilator's internal blending system, which in most cases delivers too variable an FiO_2 for the precision required during indirect calorimetric measurements.[70] An alternative to this approach is to deliver mixed gas to the ventilator and patient from a standing cylinder. If neither precaution is taken, erroneous values for $\dot{V}O_2$ may result, with the relative error in the $\dot{V}O_2$ calculation increasing in magnitude with FiO_2.[71] The end result of erroneous calculations of $\dot{V}O_2$ are inaccurate determinations of both energy expenditure and RQ.

Upon achieving FiO_2 stability, the concentrations of oxygen and carbon dioxide are typically measured by placing a sampling line into the inspired limb of the ventilator tubing and measuring unpressurized inspired gas. The sampling of unpressurized gas is accomplished by collecting an aliquot of inspired gas in an anesthesia bag and sampling from the bag. Alternatively, if one of the automated systems is being used, the measured pressure differential is mathematically accounted for by preprogrammed software adjustments.[61] The final step is to ensure that all expired gases are directed to the collecting chamber and that artifacts due to various ventilator modes are avoided by using the appropriate valving systems.

One commercially available instrument offers the capability of performing long-term metabolic measurements with a flow-through canopy system.[61] The description that follows pertains to the operation of that canopy system. The patient's head is enclosed in the canopy by means of a plastic collar and plastic ring–velcro strap seal. Ports are positioned on either side of the head, permitting the patient to touch his or her face. Smaller ports serve as exit sites for nasoenteric or intravenous tubing. An independent oxygen analyzer-alarm system samples canopy oxygen concentrations and emits an audible and visible signal if the oxygen concentration falls below a safe level.

After calibrating the instruments' oxygen and carbon dioxide analyzers with the appropriate gas mixture (Table 11–3), the blower that pulls room air through the canopy is set at a flow rate that will maintain the fraction of carbon dioxide in the range of 0.0065 to 0.0085. This setting (20–40 L/minute) is dependent upon the patient's minute ventila-

tion and is therefore related to body size. The final determinations of oxygen consumption and carbon dioxide production are calculated from the concentrations of oxygen and carbon dioxide in the mixed expired air and the measured rate at which air is pulled from the canopy. As with all other collection systems, one should watch for a period or periods of steady state and calculate REE and RQ from these equilibrated intervals. The advantages offered by the canopy system include the capability of performing metabolic measurements on patients who cannot tolerate a mouthpiece or mask system and the feasibility of long-term monitoring with maximal patient comfort.

CLINICAL EXPERIENCE AND IMPLICATIONS

Portable indirect calorimetry for bedside measurement of REE and RQ has been an integral component of the Nutrition Support Service at the Hospital of the University of Pennsylvania's assessment and monitoring procedures since 1979. To date we have performed more than 8000 measurements using commercially available instruments (Sensor Medics Corporation, Anaheim, California)[47, 51, 61, 72] and have experience with all collection systems.

Initial efforts were focused on the validation of the technique, that is, the reproduction of the known difference between BMR and REE and determining the repeatability of the measurement in both hospitalized patients and healthy control subjects using the mouthpiece and noseclip system. Data from these investigations are presented in Table 11–4. They demonstrate the typical 10 per cent increase in metabolic rate from basal to resting conditions, no statistically significant differences between repeated measurements of REE performed at midmorning and midafternoon on the same day

Table 11–4. MEASURED ENERGY EXPENDITURE (Kcal/day)*

STUDY SAMPLE	N	BASAL	RESTING (AM)	REPEAT RESTING (AM)	REPEAT RESTING (PM)	% CHANGE
Stable patients	10	1130 ± 242	1244 ± 263			10 ± 3
Stable patients	30		1287 ± 314		1289 ± 314	1 ± 9 (N.S.)
Healthy controls	26		1411 ± 289	1417 ± 269		0.2 ± 7.4 (N.S.)

*Values are expressed as mean ± SD. N.S. = differences not significant by paired students' t-test.

in stable patients, and excellent short-term reliability (two measurements within 1 hour) in control subjects. These findings established our current practice of measuring REE at any time of day provided that the strict conditions of premeasurement rest, greater than two hours without enteral (tube or orally-administered) nutrients, and equilibration are observed.

Reliability of RQ determinations must be assessed under extremely rigid circumstances. Not only must the patient be rested but he or she must also be in a steady state regarding net substrate oxidation. Nine stable patients who were receiving nothing by mouth and continuous infusions of total parenteral nutrition solutions (without fat emulsions on the day of study) had their RQ measured twice during the same day. Repeated RQ determinations under these circumstances were remarkably stable (0.90 ± 0.10 versus 0.91 ± 0.10), with no statistically significant difference existing according to paired Student's t-test. Under less rigid circumstances—for example, patients receiving an oral diet, cyclic parenteral nutrition, continuous parenteral nutrition with intermittent administration of lipids or supplemental amino acid solutions, or bolus tube feedings, and during periods of clinical instability—RQ will vary considerably because of natural shifts in nutrient oxidation or clinically related changes in whole-body substrate utilization patterns.

The major determinants of REE in hospitalized patients are body size, body composition, age, gender, disease, treatment modalities, clinical and nutritional status.[9, 10, 30, 65, 73, 74] When clinical measurements of REE are compared to standards such as the Harris-Benedict equations,[30] individual discrepancies between the measured REE and the standard occur at a frequency that is related to the patient's body composition, diagnosis and clinical condition.[75–78] It is important to note that although these standards are frequently referred to as predictors of BMR, the conditions of their development are those of REE. The Harris-Benedict multiple linear regression formulae were developed on the basis of normal individuals[30] and are a function of the relationships among height, weight, age, gender, and the size of the body cell mass or metabolically active compartment,[74] which is the prime determinant of REE in healthy persons with normal body composition.[73, 74] As such, these standards are appropriate for healthy populations with normal body composition and are not appropriate for hospitalized *individuals* with abnormal body composition, malnutrition, or disease.

Based upon the data of Harris, Benedict, and Boothby, the accepted normal range for measured REE is 90 to 110 per cent of their standard.[30, 32, 33] Boothby's data show 92 per cent of normal individuals to be within this range (± 10 per cent). When these criteria were applied to malnourished patients or patients who were thought to be at risk nutritionally, we observed the following: 40 per cent of 200 clinically stable patients (afebrile, >5 days postoperative, with no obvious clinical "stress") having a variety of primary diagnoses had REEs outside the normal range, with the majority of those being hypometabolic relative to the standard;[75] 59 per cent of 200 heterogenous cancer patients had abnormal REEs[76] as did 58 per cent of patients with gastrointestinal malignancies.[77] These data demonstrate that cancer patients are *not* uniformly hypermetabolic; rather, they document a wide range of individual variability in REE that appears to be related to duration of disease[76] and the site of the primary tumor.[77] The same analysis in patients with abnormal body composition (morbid obesity) showed the REE to be significantly over- or under-estimated via standards in 60 per cent of cases.[78] Persons with anorexia nervosa and substantial weight loss (averaging 52 per cent of ideal weight) demonstrated prerefeeding REEs that were, on the average, 30 per cent below standard using current weight.[79] This relative hypometabolism is in accordance with the effects of partial starvation on metabolic rate.[9, 65, 80, 81]

Clearly, applying standards that were developed on and for normal populations to hospitalized patients will result in a wide range of individual discrepancies, and there is at present no reliable method for identifying those individuals for whom a standard will or will not apply. At this time we can only characterize the frequency and magnitude of such occurrences within specific patient populations and describe the average effects of specific clinical conditions on REE.[10, 65, 75–79] We therefore *measure* the REE of all patients requiring specialized nutritional care.

A patient's total daily nonprotein caloric requirement is dependent upon several factors: the goal of therapy; total daily energy expenditure; and the level of efficiency at which various nutrients are utilized. The goal of therapy is a clinical decision based upon objective nutritional assessment parameters and clinical prognosis. The efficiency level for nutrient conversion to energy available at the cellular level is largely dependent upon the individual, disease or treatment factors and must be estimated to a major extent.

Total daily energy expenditure is composed of REE, BMR, SDA, shivering and nonshivering thermogenesis and the calories expended for activity. Since REE represents 75 to 100 per cent of total daily energy expenditure, depending upon the patient's voluntary activity and clinical status,[10, 82] measurements of REE eliminate the major portion of the guesswork involved in estimating total daily energy expenditure. It is then up to the clinician to devise a nonprotein caloric regimen that will create the desired energy balance (positive, negative, or equilibrium) based upon REE and an increment to adjust for the caloric cost of activity and any inefficiencies associated with nutrient absorption and utilization.

The optimal number of nonprotein calories in relation to REE for safe weight reduction (sustained negative energy balance) and maximal preservation of the protein compartment in well individuals has yet to be precisely defined. In the presence of adequate protein stores and intake, we recommend nonprotein calories in the range of 50 to 100 per cent of REE, after considering the magnitude of the energy deficit desired and the patient's physical activity and clinical status.

Provided that protein intake is optimal, our approach for minimally active hospitalized patients is to recommend (1) nonprotein calories at 1.3 × REE when the goals of nutritional therapy include maintenance of energy stores (energy equilibrium); and (2) 1.5 × REE in nonprotein calories when the nutritional goals include repletion of energy stores (positive energy balance). We then monitor nutritional and metabolic parameters, including REE and RQ, at regular intervals to assess the efficacy of the regimen and to assist in future clinical decisions.

REFERENCES

1. Butterworth, C.E., Jr.: Malnutrition in the hospital. J.A.M.A., 230:879, 1974.
2. Bistrian, B.R., Blackburn, G.L., Hallowell, E., and Handelle, R.: Protein status of general surgical patients. J.A.M.A., 230:858, 1974.
3. Butterworth, C.E., Jr.: The skeleton in the hospital closet. Nutr. Today, 9:4, 1974.
4. Bistrian, B.R., Blackburn, G.L., Vitale, J. et al: Prevalence of malnutrition in general medical patients. J.A.M.A., 235:1567, 1976.
5. Lundvick, J.L.: Evaluation of a nutritional screen when used on oncology patients. J.P.E.N., 3:521, 1979.
6. Mullen, J.L., Gertner, M.H., Buzby, G.P. et al: Implications of malnutrition in the surgical patient. Arch. Surg., 114:121, 1979.
7. Willcutts, H.D.: Nutritional assessment of 1,000 surgical patients in an affluent suburban community hospital. J.P.E.N., 1:25, 1977.
8. Boothby, W.M., and Sandiford, I.: Laboratory Manual of the Technique of Basal Metabolic Rate Determinations. Philadelphia, W.B. Saunders Co., 1920, page 11.
9. DuBois, E.F.: Basal Metabolism in Health and Disease, Edition 3. Philadelphia, Lea & Febiger, 1936, page 124.
10. Elwyn, D.H., Kinney, J.M., and Askanazi, J.: Energy expenditure in surgical patients. Surg. Clin. North Am., 61:545, 1981.
11. Wilmore, D.W.: The Metabolic Management of the Critically Ill. New York, Plenum Medical Book Co., 1977, page 18.
12. Kinney, J.M.: Energy Metabolism. In Fischer, J.E., (ed.): Surgical Nutrition. Boston, Little, Brown & Co., 1983, Pages 103 and 104.
13. Durnin, J.V.G.A., and Passmore, R.: Energy Work and Leisure. London, William Heinemann, Medical Books, Ltd., 1967, page 165.
14. Riche, J.A.: An improved type of calorimeter, to be used with any calorimetric bomb. Cornell Univ. Med. Bull., 4:Repr. 21, 1914.
15. Lavoisier, A.L., and DeLaPlace, P.S.: Memoire sur la chaleur (translated excerpts). In Benzinger, T.H. (ed.): Temperature, Part I. Arts and Concepts. Stroudsberg, Dowden, Hutchinson and Ross, 1977, page 145.
16. Kinney, J.M.: Energy Metabolism. In Fischer, J.E. (ed.): Surgical Nutrition. Boston, Little, Brown & Co., 1983, page 98.
17. Black, J.: Lectures on the elements of chemistry. In Benzinger, T.H. (ed.): Temperature, Part I. Arts and Concepts. Stroudsberg, Dowden, Hutchinson and Ross, 1977, page 116.
18. Regnault, and Reiset: Cited in DuBois, E.F.: Basal Metabolism in Health and Disease, Edition 3. Philadelphia, Lea & Febiger, 1936, page 10.
19. Bidder, and Schmidt: Quoted in DuBois, E.F.: Basal Metabolism in Health and Disease, Edition 3. Philadelphia, Lea & Febiger, 1936, page 11.
20. Pettenkofer, and Voit, C.: Cited in DuBois, E.F.: Basal Metabolism in Health and Disease, Edition 3. Philadelphia, Lea & Febiger, 1936, page 11.
21. Liebermeister: Cited in DuBois, E.F.: Basal Metabolism in Health and Disease, Edition 3. Philadelphia, Lea & Febiger, 1936, pages 11 and 12.
22. DuBois, E.F.: Basal Metabolism in Health and Disease, Edition 3. Philadelphia, Lea & Febiger, 1936, page 11.
23. Kinney, J.M.: Energy Metabolism. In Fischer, J.R. (ed.): Surgical Nutrition. Boston, Little, Brown & Co., 1983, page 99.
24. Atwater, W.O., and Rosa, E.B.: Quoted in Lusk, G.L.: The Elements and Science of Nutrition,

Edition 4. Philadelphia, W.B. Saunders Co., 1928, page 61.

25. DuBois, E.F.: Basal Metabolism in Health and Disease. Edition 3. Philadelphia, Lea & Febiger, 1936, page 12.

26. Magnus-Levy, A.: Ueber den respiratorischen gewechsel unter dem einfluss der thyroiden sowie unter verschiedenen pathologischen zustanden. Berl. Klin. Wochenschr., 32:650, 1895.

27. DuBois, E.F.: Basal Metabolism in Health and Disease, Edition 3. Philadelphia, Lea & Febiger, 1936, pages 11 and 12.

28. Atwater, W.O., and Benedict, F.G.: Experiments on the metabolism of matter and energy in the human body. USDA Office of Exp. Stations Bull. Pub. No. 136, 1903.

29. Aub, J.C., and DuBois, E.F.: Clinical Calorimetry XIX. Arch. Intern. Med., 19:823, 1917.

30. Harris, J.A., and Benedict, F.G.: Biometric studies of basal metabolism in man. Carnegie Institute of Washington Publ. No. 279, 1919.

31. Boothby, W.M., and Sandiford, I.: Laboratory Manual of the Technique of Basal Metabolic Rate Determinations. Philadelphia, W.B. Saunders Co., 1920.

32. Boothby, W.M., and Sandiford, I.S.: Summary of the basal metabolism of 8,614 subjects with especial reference to the normal standards for the estimation of the basal metabolic rate. J. Biol. Chem. 54:783, 1922.

33. Boothby, W.M., Berkson, J., and Dunn, H.L.: Studies on the energy metabolism of normal individuals: A standard for basal metabolism with a nomogram for clinical application. Am. J. Physiol., 116:468, 1936.

34. Benedict, F.G.: A helmet for use in clinical studies of gaseous metabolism. N. Engl. J. Med., 203:150, 1930.

35. Means, J.: Cited in DuBois, E.F.: Basal Metabolism in Health and Disease. Edition 3. Philadelphia, Lea & Febiger, 1936, pages 321 and 322.

36. Means, J., and Lehrman, J.: Symptomology of mixedema: its relation to metabolic levels, time intervals and rations of thyroid, Arch. Intern. Med. 55:1, 1935.

37. Webb, P., Annis, J.F., and Troutman, S.J., Jr.: Human calorimetry with a water cooled garment. J. Appl. Physiol., 32:413, 1972.

38. Jequier, E.: Studies with direct calorimetry in humans: thermal body insulation and thermoregulatory responses during excerise. In Kinney, J.M. (ed.): Assessment of Energy Metabolism in Health and Disease. Columbus, Ohio, Ross Laboratories, 1980, page 15.

39. Benzinger, T.H., and Kitzinger, C.: Gradient layer calorimetry-human calorimetry. In Herzfeld, C.M., and Hardy, J.D. (eds.): Temperature: Its Measurement and Control in Science and Industry. Vol. 3. New York, Reinhold, 1963, page 87.

40. McManus, C., Newhouse, H., Seitz, S. et al.: Human gradient-layer calorimeter: development of an accurate and practical instrument for clinical studies. J.P.E.N., 8:317, 1984.

41. Wilmore, D.W.: The Metabolic Management of the Critically Ill. New York, Plenum Publishing Corp., 1977, pages 11 and 14.

42. Fowler, W.S., Blackburn, C.M., and Helmholz, H.M., Jr.: Determination of basal rate of oxygen consumption by open and closed-circuit methods. J.C.E.M., 17:786, 1957.

43. Guyton, A.C., and Farish, A.C.: A rapidly responding continuous oxygen consumption recorder. J. Appl. Physiol., 14:143, 1959.

44. Kinney, J.M., Morgan, A.P., Domingues, F.J., and Gildner, K.J.: A method for continuous measurement of gas exchanges and expired radioactivity in acutely ill patients. Metabolism, 12:205, 1964.

45. Webb, P., and Troutman, S.J., Jr.: An instrument for continuous measurement of oxygen consumption. J. Appl. Physiol., 28:867, 1970.

46. Spencer, J.L., Zikria, B.A., Kinney, J.M. et al.: A system for continuous measurement of gas exchange and respiratory functions. J. Appl. Physiol., 34:523, 1972.

47. Jones, N. L.: Evaluation of a microprocessor-controlled exercise testing system. J. Appl. Physiol., 57:1312, 1984.

48. Bursztein, S., Saphar, P., Glaser, P. et al.: Determination of energy metabolism from respiratory functions alone. J. Appl. Physiol., 42:117, 1977.

49. Neuhof, N., and Wolf, H.: Method for continuously measured oxygen consumption and cardiac output for use in critically ill patients. Crit. Care Med., 6:155, 1978.

50. Bohrn, S.E., Hogman, B., Olsson, S.G. et al.: A new device for continuous measurement of gas exchange during artificial ventilation. Crit. Care Med., 8:705, 1980.

51. Norton, A.C.: Portable equipment for gas exchange. In Kinney, J.M. (ed.): Assessment of Energy Metabolism in Health and Disease. Columbus, Ohio, Ross Laboratories, 1980, pages 36–41.

52. Wilmore, D.W.: The Metabolic Management of the Critically Ill. New York, Plenum Publishing Corp., 1977, page 9.

53. Weir, J.B. de V.: New methods for calculating metabolic rate with special reference to protein metabolism. J. Physiol., 109:1, 1949.

54. Wilmore, D.W.: The Metabolic Management of the Critically Ill. New York, Plenum Medical Book Co., 1977, page 16.

55. Caldwell, F.T., Jr.: Measurement of oxygen consumption and CO_2 production in clinical nutritional assessment. In Kinney, J.M. (ed.): Nutritional Assessment—Present Status, Future Directions and Prospects. Columbus, Ohio, Ross Laboratories, 1981, pages 19–21.

56. Merrill, A.L., and Watt, B.K.: Energy Value of Foods. Agriculture Handbook No. 74. Washington, D.C., U.S. Government Printing Office, 1955.

57. Lusk, G.L.: The Elements of the Science of Nutrition, Edition 4. Philadelphia, W.B. Saunders Co., 1928, page 65.

58. Kleiber, M.: The Fire of Life: an Introduction to Animal Energetics. Huntington, Robert E. Krieger Publishing Co., 1975, page 89.

59. Schutz, Y., and Ravussin, E.: Respiratory quotients lower than 0.70 in ketogenic diets (letters to the editor). Am. J. Clin. Nutr., 33:1317, 1980.

60. Kinney, J.M.: The application of indirect calorimetry to clinical studies. In Kinney, J.M. (ed.): Assessment of Energy, Metabolism in Health and Disease, Columbus, Ohio, Ross Laboratories, 1980, pages 42–48.

61. Norton, A.C.: Development and testing of a microprocessor controlled system for measurement of gas exchange and related variables in man during rest and exercise. Beckman Reprint No. 025. Anaheim, California, Beckman Instruments Inc., 1982.

62. Dolcourt, J.L., and Cutler, C.A.: Automated measurement of oxygen consumption and respiratory quotient in critically ill newborn infants. J.P.E.N., 8:100, 1984.

63. Dechert, J.R., Wesley, J., Schafer, L. et al.: Measurement of resting energy expenditure in premature infants. J.P.E.N., 8:100, 1984.

64. Head, C.A., McManus, C.B., Seitz, S. et al.: A simple and accurate indirect calorimetry system for assessment of resting energy expenditure. J.P.E.N., 8:45, 1984.

65. Long, C.L., Schaffel, N., Geiger, J.W. et al.: Metabolic response to injury and illness: Estimation of energy and protein needs from indirect calorimetry and nitrogen balance. J.P.E.N., 3:452, 1979.

66. Boothby, W.M., and Sandiford, I.: Laboratory Manual of the Technique of Basal Metabolic Rate Determinations. Philadelphia, W.B. Saunders Co., 1920, page 24.

67. Elwyn, D.H., Kinney, J.M., Jeevanandum, M., Gump, F. E., and Broell, J. R.: Influence of increasing carbohydrate intake on glucose kinetics in injured patients. Ann. Surg., 190:117, 1979.

68. Askanazi, J., Carpentier, Y.A., Elwyn, D.H. et al.: Influence of total parenteral nutrition on fuel utilization in injury and sepsis. Ann. Surg., 191:40, 1980.

69. Shaw, S.N., Elwyn, D.H., Askanazi, J. et al.: Effects of increasing nitrogen intake on nitrogen balance and energy expenditure in nutritionally depleted adult patients receiving parenteral nutrition. Am. J. Clin. Nutr., 37:930, 1983.

70. Browning, J.A., Linberg, S.E., Turney, S., and Chodoff, P.: The effects of fluctuating FiO_2 on metabolic measurements in mechanically ventilated patients. Crit. Care Med., 10:82, 1982.

71. Ultman, J.S., and Bursztein, S.: Analysis of error in the determination of respiratory gas exchange at varying FiO_2. J. Appl. Physiol., 50:210, 1981.

72. Damask, M.C., Weissman, C., Askanazi, J. et al.: A systematic method for validation of gas exchange measurements. Anesthesiology, 57:213, 1982.

73. Kleiber, M.: The Fire of Life: an Introduction to Animal Energetics. Huntington, Robert E. Krieger Publishing Co., 1975, pages 210–214.

74. Moore, F.D., Olesen, K.H., McMurray, J.B., et al.: The Body Cell Mass and its Supporting Environment: Body Composition in Health and Disease. Philadelphia, W.B. Saunders Co., 1963.

75. Feurer, I.D., Crosby, L.O., and Mullen, J.L.: Measured and predicted resting energy expenditure in clinically stable patients. Clin. Nutr., 3:27, 1984.

76. Knox, L., Crosby, L., Feurer, I. et al.: Energy expenditure in malnourished cancer patients. Ann. Surg., 197:152, 1983.

77. Dempsey, D.T., Feurer, I.D., Knox, L. et al.: Energy expenditure in malnourished gastrointestinal cancer patients. Cancer, 53:1265, 1984.

78. Feurer, I.D., Crosby, L.O., Buzby, G.P., Rosato, E.F., and Mullen, J.L.: Resting energy expenditure in morbid obesity. Ann. Surg., 197:17, 1983.

79. Dempsey, D., Crosby, L., Pertschuk, M. et al.: Weight gain and nutritional efficacy in anorexia nervosa. Am. J. Clin. Nutr. 39:236, 1984.

80. Keys, A., Brozek, J., Henschel, A., Michelsen, O., and Taylor, H. L.: The Biology of Human Starvation. Minneapolis, University of Minnesota Press, 1950, page 303.

81. Kinney, J. M.: Energy metabolism. In Fischer, J.E. (ed.): Surgical Nutrition. Boston, Little, Brown & Co., 1983, pages 114–116.

82. Kinney, J.M.: Energy metabolism. In Fischer, J.E. (ed.): Surgical Nutrition. Boston, Little, Brown & Co., 1983, page 116.

CHAPTER 12

The Nutrition Support Team

ELIE HAMAOUI
JOHN L. ROMBEAU

In most settings, it is recognized that in order to provide nutritional support safely and effectively, a multidisciplinary team of health care professionals is desirable.[1–15] This chapter will discuss the following: (1) the rationale, goals, and organization of such a team; (2) the individual roles of its members; (3) the logistics of improving nutritional care in the hospital; and (4) an evaluation of the data concerning the efficacy of these teams. The terms *team* and *service* will both be used to refer to the group of health care professionals who provide nutritional support. The term *nutrition support team (NST)* will be used when the focus is on the inner workings of the team. *Nutrition support service (NSS)* will be used when this entity is discussed in the context of other hospital sections and its interactions with them.

RATIONALE AND GOALS OF THE NUTRITION SUPPORT TEAM

In order to properly define the goals of the NST, it is important to understand the circumstances in which a patient develops a need for nutritional support. To put it simply, a patient can be said to require nutritional support when his or her biologic machinery loses the capability to adequately resupply itself. This can occur in a wide spectrum of circumstances ranging from socioeconomic inability to obtain food, to loss of all gastrointestinal functions, to the metabolic impairments imposed by hepatic or renal disease or by various drug therapies. Regardless of the mechanism, the end result

is monotonously, if not ghastly, similar—malnutrition, that is, the lack of metabolic substrates and the consequent impairment of biologic functions that eventually leads to the arrest of life. In order to help such patients, one must first find them (before they become irreversibly depleted), diagnose precisely at what point their supply lines have been broken, and then proceed to reverse or bypass the particular nutritional block or blocks safely and effectively.

Clinical Goals

In view of this preface, the clinical goals of the nutritional support team are easily defined:

1. *Identification* of patients who are nutritionally impaired.

2. Performance of a *nutritional assessment that can adequately guide nutritional therapy*. (It is therapeutically more important to precisely define the patient's nutritional obstacles than to document the exact degree of the depletion through a multitude of overlapping parameters.)

3. Provision of nutritional support that is *safe and effective*.

In trying to achieve these three clinical goals, other goals become evident.

Didactic Goals

A number of studies have documented up to or even greater than a 50 per cent occurrence of malnutrition in hospitalized patients.[16–26] It is clearly impossible for most NSTs to be able to properly diagnose and treat such a large proportion of their hospital population. It becomes necessary therefore for the NST to educate the primary clinicians in the recognition of malnutrition and the therapy of at least its easily treatable forms. This allows the NST to concentrate on the more difficult cases.

Another didactic goal pertains to the NST's own education. The science and technology of clinical nutrition is rapidly developing. Unless the NST members keep abreast of these new developments, patients may get less than optimal therapy.

Research Goals

Because the field of clinical nutrition is so new, most nutritional regimens are at best approximations of physiologic patterns; at worst they may be life-threatening rather than life-saving. It therefore behooves clinical nutritionists to at least review their data periodically and systematically in search of improvements in the safety and efficacy of their nutritional care. Ideally, every effort should be made to participate in prospective randomized, controlled studies.

Nutrition Support Team Interactions

Team work in general can be categorized into one of two types. In the first type, the individual efforts are similar or identical, and the combination is required merely for the magnification of unit effect. In the other type of team effort, the contribution of each member is unique, and the combination is required for a complementary effect.

In the case of nutritional support, the team is needed because the required expertise traverses several disciplines. The specific contribution of each discipline will be reviewed. It should be pointed out, however, that as the collaborative and interactive experience of team members increases, the lines of demarcation distinguishing one member's functions from another's may almost vanish. In such a case, any one of the team members may be competent enough to discuss a given patient from the point of view of the physician, dietitian, nurse, or pharmacist. At that point, the complemen-

tary effect of the team effort becomes enhanced by a magnification effect.

It is particularly important for a newly developing NST to be aware of these two types of team-member interactions. Developing organizations in a new field tend to emulate those who have successfully established themselves. A problem of territoriality, however, may develop for the members of a new team if they blindly try to define the functions of a given member of their team in accordance with those of the corresponding member of some other team. Local pragmatic considerations may necessitate restricted or expanded individual roles in one team, but these considerations may not apply to another team. Thus, a direct translation from one team to another may be ill-advised. It is probably wiser for a new team to consider a complete set of functions that need to be performed and then to initially assign these functions to its members in accordance with previous training and experience. Subsequently, some changes may become necessary in job assignments.

Basic Nutrition Support Service Functions Required for Nutritional Support

The treatment of the malnourished patient involves four basic steps:

Diagnosis. As noted previously, malnutrition may be caused by a wide spectrum of factors. As for any other disease, a precise etiologic definition of the patient's problem is crucial in guiding therapy and in sparing the patient the unnecessary complications of unjustified interventions. For example, the therapeutic approach to anorexia must be guided by the knowledge of whether the cause is depression, drug toxicity, constipation, and so on. For the patient who merely lacks the ability to self-feed, parenteral nutrition can only offer unjustified risks. The patient's non-nutritional diseases also require a thorough evaluation to assess their severity and impact on the overall prognosis. This is crucial—not only for determining nutrient needs but also for appropriately matching the aggressiveness of nutritional support to the potential benefits that the given patient stands to gain. Thus it would be unreasonable to provide total parenteral nutrition (TPN) to a patient who is agonal, since death will occur long before any benefit could be derived from that intervention.

Planning Nutrient Delivery. After the patient's nutrient needs have been defined, a decision must be made as to which of the available modalities of nutritional support would be most suitable. This includes choosing the nutritional formulation as well as the route of administration.

Implementing Nutritional Support. As in many other types of therapy, one of the common causes of failure in nutritional therapy is incorrect implementation. Since most NSTs function as consulting services, it is important to make sure that their recommendations are properly carried out.

Monitoring Therapeutic and Adverse Effects of Nutritional Support. Again, as in many other therapies, nutritional support requires close monitoring, both clinical and biochemical, in order to ensure effectiveness and to avoid or treat complications.

Nutrition Support Team Composition and Individual Roles

It is generally agreed that the minimum composition of a NST consists of a physician, dietitian, pharmacist, and nurse.[1-14, 27] Each of these individuals contributes to the previously mentioned "basic functions," though ultimate responsibility for a given function should be assigned to a specific NST member.

The Physician's Role. The overall responsibility for any patient care rendered by the NST must, as in the rest of our medical system, be borne by the NST physician. In fairness to all involved, and especially to the patient, the treatment of malnutrition should have at least one thing in common with the treatment of any other deadly disease—it must be physician-directed and physician-supervised. Carrying such responsibility entails certain obligations. It is mandatory that the physician be knowledgeable about nutrient metabolism in health as well as in disease. The physician must be well versed in the pathophysiology and clinical manifestations of malnutrition in all its forms, as would be expected of any other specialist treating diseases encompassed by his or her area of competence. Also similar to any other specialist, the physician-nutritionist must possess at least a working knowledge of other diseases, particularly those that may

coexist with, mimic, exacerbate, or otherwise affect the therapeutic approach to the ailment for which a consultation is being requested. The physician must be fully knowledgeable about all forms of nutritional intervention and be well aware of their potential complications. When viewed from this perspective, there remains little doubt that an NST needs to be directed not merely by a physician but by a properly trained one. For such education the syllabus for the certifying examination of the American Board of Nutrition provides an appropriate basis.[28] This training is probably best obtained in a clinical nutrition fellowship program. A survey of such training programs was recently published by Howard and Bigaouette.[70]

If a physician director is mandatory, why is it that the NST in a number of centers is run by a nurse, dietitian, or pharmacist?[71] To answer this question, pragmatic considerations must be distinguished from fundamental ones. There are undoubtably centers in which no physician has been available to shoulder the responsibility of an NST, and a concerned nurse, dietitian, or pharmacist took it upon himself or herself to mobilize hospital resources and personnel to improve nutritional care. Such individuals deserve praise and admiration for their efforts to fill a medical gap and, in fact, have probably saved lives—but as Good Samaritans not as properly trained physicians. It is clear, however, that merely being a Good Samaritan is not an adequate credential for running an NST anymore than it is for running any other hospital service.

Heading a multidisciplinary team of professionals requires a clear understanding and a sincere appreciation of individual contributions, as well as an acknowledgement of the limitations of these individuals. In the case of the NST functions, it is important to realize that the dietitian, pharmacist, and nurse each have a unique role not only in the implementation of nutritional support but also in assessing and understanding the patient's condition and determining the nutritional prescription. Most physicians have no difficulty consulting with and learning from other physicians regarding a problem that lies outside their realm of expertise. The physician member of the NST must have at least a similar respect for the other members of the NST. There is much for the physician to learn from the daily interaction with a dietitian or pharmacist. This is especially true for new developments that have appeared in their respective professional literature and may be clinically helpful.

Coordinated nutritional support is a rather new and developing responsibility for most hospitals. The field is greatly indebted to many individuals from various disciplines who refused to accept a 50 per cent prevalence of hospital malnutrition as *status quo* and decided to do something about it—innovatively, resourcefully, and frequently single-handedly within their respective institutions. In their attempt to improve patient care, these individuals crossed the conventional bounds of their respective disciplines and performed duties that might have been done better by members of a different discipline, but that were in fact not being done at all. This innovative spirit should not be squelched; it should be nurtured—as long as patient care remains its highest priority. When faced with "out of discipline activities," the NST director can merely request that the appropriate member of the NST review the given activity, modify it as necessary, and continue to supervise it to ensure that it remains up to professional standards. In this way, individual initiative and creativity can be protected—though guided in the interest of patient welfare rather than choked in petty turf defense.

In addition to the responsibility in the orchestration of the clinical functions of the NST, the physician must personally perform or directly supervise those NST activities for which he or she is specifically trained. Such duties include obtaining a complete medical history, performing a physical examination, and requesting laboratory examinations or other professional consultations to properly assess the patient's overall medical condition and particularly the pathophysiology of the malnutrition. After appropriate consultation with the dietitian or pharmacist, or both, the physician must then recommend the optimal form of nutritional support. The insertion of central intravenous lines and most nasoenteral feeding tubes is also the physician's responsibility. Finally, he or she must recommend monitoring activities to ensure that the therapy is being properly implemented.

The Dietitian's Role. The dietitian's unique contribution* to NST functioning derives primarily from his or her expertise at the food-nutrient interphase.[33] This enables the dietitian to obtain an accurate dietary history and to interpret it for the other members of the NST into a meaningful nutrient profile. Without this information, one is often at a loss to prescribe appropriate supplemental nutritional support. Similarly, the implementation of a nutritional prescription that requires specific amounts of nutrients must await the dietitian's translation into a selection of foods that are acceptable to the patient. An exception to this procedure is when the route of nutrient administration is parenteral, in which case the pharmacist becomes the main translator of the nutritional prescription (see "The Pharmacist's Role"). Similarly, the NST dietitian should be the source of information regarding the dozens of formulas available for oral or enteral feeding, since they are in essence foods that are processed in ways that yield the various nutrient combinations that might be required in a nutritional prescription. It is certainly the dietitian's responsibility to choose the formulation that best fits the nutrient prescription for a given patient (except for parenteral nutrition) as well as to choose the formulations that the institution should regularly stock.

Many, if not most, dietitians can perform anthropometric measurements such as triceps skinfold thickness (TST) or midarm circumference (MAC). Should these measurements be considered specific functions of the dietitian? Strictly speaking they are part of the physical examination and one might assign them to the physician (along with other mechanically assisted procedures such as ophthalmoscopy or sigmoidoscopy), to the nurse (along with weight or blood pressure measurements), or to a medical technician (along with spirometry or sonography procedures). More importantly, the results of such measurements need to be interpreted and integrated with other results of patient assessment, such as the history of a nutritionally deficient diet or the presence of dehydration, myxedema, quadriplegia, or steroid therapy. The point is that the measurement of TST or MAC is an example

---

*Review of a number of reports[29-32] regarding the role definition of the dietitian leaves one with the sense of a certain identity crisis within the profession. Thus "Who and what are dietitians?" was a question posed by an ADA Study Commission on Dietetics in 1972.[30] Yet, 10 years later, role delineation was still of major concern.[31] The authors' purpose here is not to agree or disagree with any particular definition of a dietitian, but merely to point out those NST functions that are best performed by a trained dietitian and that require his or her presence on the team.

of a function that is not intrinsically a dietitian's responsibility, though it could be performed, and even taught by this member of the NST. Significantly, however, interpretation of that measurement is best done in light of a global multidisciplinary patient assessment, of which the dietitian's contribution is an integral part.

The Pharmacist's Role. There are two basic reasons for the need of a pharmacist on an NST.[34] The first, and usually more obvious one, pertains to his or her role in the preparation of TPN solutions. When given by the parenteral route, nutrients require the meticulous care with which the pharmacist normally handles drugs, especially the parenterally administered ones. This is because the parenteral route bypasses a number of defense mechanisms of the gut against various microbial and physico-chemical threats to the organism and against dangerous excesses of even nutrients. Of further help is the pharmacist's familiarity with the stability and physico-chemical compatibility of various compound preparations.

The other reason for having a pharmacist on an NST pertains to his or her knowledge of pharmacokinetics, drug metabolism, drug-drug interactions, and especially drug-nutrient interactions. This aspect of the pharmacist's contribution tends to be underutilized, though it could benefit a far greater number of patients than just those receiving TPN. Most patients who are on multiple, chronic drug therapies are likely to benefit from a thoughtful pharmacist's review of their drug regimens. For malnourished patients, however, this pharmacologic review should be as mandatory as any other part of the nutritional assessment, since drugs may affect nutrient flow from ingestion and digestion to metabolism and excretion.[34-36] Thus, the pharmacist's role is crucial not only for the implementation of parenteral nutrition but also for the metabolic assessment of all patients requiring nutritional support.

The Nurse's Role. The responsibility of the nurse member of the team is rather unique in that it derives not from a specialized understanding of the patient's pathophysiology, nutrient intake, or drug pharmacokinetics, but rather from the special knowledge she acquires from the individual patient as she observes his reactions to disease and to therapy.* Nurses correctly regard themselves as "vital links"[37] between the patient and the rest of the health care team.

Nurses are the ones who first observe whether the nutritional therapy is properly administered and if so whether it had the intended effect. In a manner similar to any other therapy, nutritional support—particularly when it involves enteral tube feeding or parenteral nutrition—is administered by the nurse directly to the patient. Hence, it is the nurse who is ideally suited to ensure that the right formula is given by the appropriate route at the recommended rate. Similarly, he or she is the first to notice the patient's clinical response to the nutritional prescription and may subsequently recommend modification or even complete change. Thus, the nurse's role is critical for implementation of nutritional support as well as for the ongoing assessment and understanding of the patient. Without the nurse's mediation, the patient might not derive any benefit from the efforts of the other team members.

Other Team Members and Their Functions. There are other professionals whose contributions to the NST effort are needed only in selected patients. Their inclusion as permanent members of the NST with the expectation that they should evaluate and follow every NST patient is therefore unnecessary and wasteful. Rather, their help should be requested selectively. Such professionals include the social worker, the physical therapist, and the dentist.

The Social Worker. Inasmuch as malnutrition sometimes develops because of socioeconomic factors, the therapeutic approach needs to include the social worker's input for the alleviation of such factors and the prevention of disease recurrence. In patients who receive TPN at home, the social worker plays a key role in emotional readjustment and financial securement.[38]

The Physical Therapist. Repletion of muscle mass may be impossible in an inactive individual, since the lack of activity—that is, muscle disuse—typically results in muscle atrophy. A severely cachectic but nonexercised patient may just accumulate fat rather than increase muscle mass, despite receiving an appropriately therapeutic diet. In such a case, the physical therapist may indeed

---

*Use of the feminine gender in reference to the nurse and masculine gender in reference to the patient is an arbitrary choice made for syntactic clarity in this sentence.

speed the patient's recovery by providing a graduated exercise program that enhances nutritional repletion.[4]

The Dentist. Food intake can be hampered by "mouth problems," such as the presence of tooth or gum pain or the loss of dentures. In such instances, a dental consultation may result in a much better nutritional intake than would trying to feed the patient a pureed diet, which is often unpalatable. Mouth care of tube-fed patients is another example in which consultation with a dentist may be helpful.

LOGISTICS OF IMPROVING NUTRITIONAL SUPPORT IN THE HOSPITAL

For most hospitals, nutrition support is either a newly established or, more frequently, a not yet established hospital service. What is often lacking, however, is not merely the staffing and equipment needed to run such a service, but even the notion that such a resource is needed. Thus, whereas the departure of a hospital's only cardiologist would elicit frantic attempts by the institution to fill the position, many hospitals (including some university affiliated and teaching hospitals) still have neither an NSS nor a "vacancy" for it—even though the number of patients in need of a nutritional consultation may be far greater than that of those in need of a cardiologic consultation.

It is very difficult to solve a problem whose presence is not recognized. Insofar as the malnourished hospitalized patient is concerned, it means that the physician does not even think of requesting a nutritional consultation and that the hospital administration has no reason to allocate resources for such a purpose. NSTs do not grow on such infertile grounds; their scientific and technical knowledge vanishes and, most sadly, their life-saving contribution to patient care is never realized. Thus, to establish an NSS, it is probably at least as important to learn how

to solve this public relations problem as it is to learn about catheter insertion or nutrient metabolism.

There are a number of publications on the various aspects of nutritional support logistics.[1, 3, 5, 15, 39-45] The purpose here is not to review all of them any more than it is to discuss general principles of hospital organization, business administration, or group psychology. Rather, the aim is to concentrate on those difficulties that one encounters when dealing with clinicians and administrators who are surrounded and enveloped by the manifestations of hospital malnutrition yet systematically fail to see the problem.

Although what follows is based primarily on the experience of one of us (E.H.) in organizing an NSS at the Brooklyn VA Medical Center, discussions with a number of colleagues at various other hospitals suggested that the obstacles that had to be surmounted were not unique to this hospital and that techniques that had succeeded here might well be effective elsewhere.

In an effort to assess the quality of nutritional care that had previously been provided, a chart audit was done at the outset. A list of all charts carrying a diagnosis of malnutrition (of any type) during the previous two-year period was obtained. The documented nutritional care in all available charts was then checked against a set of arbitrarily chosen minimum performance standards for a physician, nurse, and dietitian caring for a malnourished patient. It was expected that in dealing with such a patient the physician would write quantitative orders for nutritional repletion (e.g., "3000-calorie diet" or "high-protein diet," rather than "regular diet") and would order periodic weighing of the patient. The nurse was expected to chart an admission height and weight, follow-up weights, and at least one observation on food intake or apparent appetite. Finally, at least one chart entry by the ward dietitian was expected on every chart.

Table 12–1 shows that even if one assumed that the prevalence of malnutrition at

Table 12–1. DIAGNOSIS OF MALNUTRITION—BVAMC 1980–1981

	NUMBER OF ADMISSIONS	EXPECTED (25%)	DIAGNOSED	% OF EXPECTED
Medicine	11,903	2976	42	1.4
Surgery	5,756	1439	2	0.1
TOTAL	17,659	4415	44	1.0

this hospital were only half that reported for most others,[18, 21–25] the number of charts that in fact carried such a diagnosis was only one per cent of that expected. Table 12–2 further shows that only 14 per cent of that 1 per cent met all of the previously stated minimum standards for the management of malnutrition. It is interesting to note that although the lowest single function score was 43 per cent, the overall performance score was 14 per cent. This suggests that resource limitation (such as the lack of availability of bed scales) was not the limiting factor in the provision of nutritional care. Thus, rather than following the common medical practice of focusing limited resources on those patients that need them most, what appears to have happened is an uncoordinated and haphazard allocation of various nutritional care functions. Instead of evaluating, treating, and monitoring the sickest patient first, the patient who was evaluated tended not to be treated and the one who was treated was not likely to be monitored. In short, this audit showed that malnutrition was missed in 99 per cent of those who had it and mistreated in 86 per cent of the remaining patients.

In the face of such findings, it is clear that the first order of business must be to draw attention to the problem of malnutrition. Admittedly, once the disease is recognized complications of its therapy may then become the main concern of the NSS, especially in a teaching hospital. However, although misguided nutritional therapy may be as dangerous as malnutrition itself, it is an easier problem to come to grips with—the

clinician is likely to consult the NSS if the nutritional therapy appears to be producing adverse effects. This call for help, however, will not be sounded unless the clinician is aware of the problem. The question is how to reach the clinician.

Approach to the Clinician

Clinicians are generally well aware of the explosive rate of developments in modern medicine and of the vital need for continuing medical education. Information on new diseases, such as Legionnaires' disease or acquired immune deficiency syndrome (AIDS), is distributed and reaches clinicians either verbally (e.g., via lectures, conferences, symposia) or through the written word (e.g., articles, pamphlets, books, manuals). In this author's (E.H.) experience, both methods proved pitifully ineffective during the initial phases of introducing nutritional support in the hospital. Nutrition lectures, even when widely publicized and given by guest speakers of national repute, were uniformly very poorly attended. A manual of nutritional support distributed to all physicians and units within the hospital was either never read or never used, and in any case rapidly disappeared from sight, even though initially it was widely acclaimed within the institution and was eventually published.[46–48] The point is that conventional didactics do not work on those who are not aware of their ignorance.

Audits and surveys that document the prevalence of malnutrition and its neglect in a given medical center may be useful for generating some anxiety in a department chairman, but they do not usually result in improved nutritional care. When the results of the audit previously described were sent to all the service chiefs in the hospital, the chief of medicine sent copies of it to her entire staff and included a note concluding that "we are not even close to appreciating our patients' needs." It was subsequently gratifying to be told by colleagues that they had "seen the interesting audit"; however the nutrition consultation rate, which we used as a barometer of interest in clinical nutrition, did not rise.

Trying to raise the level of nutritional care in a training institution with a frequently rotating housestaff can be particularly frus-

Table 12–2. MANAGEMENT OF DIAGNOSED MALNUTRITION—BVAMC 1980–1981*

FUNCTION EXAMINED	% OF EXPECTED
Physician:	
Quantitative orders for repletion	70
Orders for weighing patient	50
Nurse:	
Admission height and weight	46
Follow-up weights	43
Qualitative chart notes on food intake	86
Dietitian:	
Dietitian's note in chart	57
All of above functions	14

*Based on all 28 complete charts available for review. (A total of 46 charts were identified as carrying a malnutrition diagnosis.)

trating. It is much like trying to keep a leaky tire inflated. By the time one has had a chance to instill some nutritional sophistication into the housestaff, they rotate, to be replaced by yet another set of physicians for whom the basics of clinical nutrition need to be rediscovered. This problem, however, is not unique to nutrition teaching; it is the daily fare of any teacher of clinical medicine. More importantly, it turns out that the system has some interesting advantages. During a physician's internship, most of the new information and much of the reflex responses to various clinical situations are obtained from the resident, with whom the intern spends most working hours and whose clinical advice he or she values more than the attending physician's. If one can somehow impress upon one intern the importance of nutritional care, particularly in the form of an unexpected clinical success, the benefit of that teaching may increase severalfold a year later when that intern becomes a resident and begins to "imprint" a new generation of interns.

Influencing nursing practice is no less of a challenge and requires still other factors to be considered. For instance, although providing proper nutritional care may seemingly mean little more for the physician than writing a few more orders on a patient's chart (such as weighing the patient periodically, feeding every three hours, and measuring and charting all intake and output), the amount of work that such orders generate for the nurse is very time-consuming and may be given low priority unless its importance to patient care has been adequately explained. More important, the nurse must see that the requested data is, in fact, reviewed and used rather than ordered and forgotten. Other nursing chores more specific to nutritional support, such as TPN catheter dressing change, require not only that the rationale be explained but also that the step-by-step procedure be demonstrated. Finally, any such training or education needs to be provided not to only one or two nurses but to every nurse of every shift on every ward.

How does one utilize all of this information about physicians and nurses to design a program that will indeed move the whole institution forward in nutritional care? For two years, one of us (E.H.) tried to answer this question, but to no avail. The problem was that the NST—then consisting of a part-time physician, a physician assistant, and a temporary research nurse—was so thinly spread out in this 900-bed hospital that its impact on the institution was diluted to extinction.

In an effort to define a more reasonably manageable task, the chief of medicine suggested that one of the medical wards be designated for a pilot project aimed at creating a unit in which nutritional care would be exemplary. The objectives were twofold. The first was to improve the nutritional state of malnourished patients. The second was to sensitize the housestaff physicians and the staff nurses of that ward to the patient's nutritional needs and to provide guidance in proper nutritional care.

The first hurdle, and probably the biggest for the entire project, was to get the ward's housestaff physicians together long enough to introduce to them the concept of the project. Housestaff physicians tend to feel, and in fact generally are, overworked. Second, in a teaching institution they also feel that they round and round daily to the point of vertigo. As a result, their scientific curiosity tends to be dulled by the fear of additional work or more rounding. When the resident of the designated ward was first approached and told that the project was being carried out at the request of the Service Chief, he grudgingly offered 10 minutes of time reserved for attending rounds to be introduced to the program. Luckily, the attending physician did not object.

In view of these limitations the following approach was taken. The allotted 10 minutes were used to make three points and one request, each accompanied by a pertinent handout. Table 12–3 was used to stress the high prevalence of malnutrition in a wide variety of hospitals. Figure 12–1 (which is a chart that appeared in a report by Heymsfield and associates[49]) was used to present the inexorable sequence of complications in untreated malnutrition. The third handout was a summary of a report by Lipschitz and Mitchell[50] that reported the reversal of a number of abnormalities in the elderly (such as anemia and confusion) by nutritional therapy. This particular study was chosen because of its clinical implications for that ever-growing group of patients who generate a major portion of house-staff frustration—the debilitated elderly patient with recurrent pneumonias, urinary tract infections, and persistent decubitus ulcers, all of which are complications that appear on the Heymsfield

Table 12–3. PREVALENCE OF MALNUTRITION IN HOSPITALIZED PATIENTS

	%	REFERENCE NO.*
Municipal hospital	32–88	4
	44–78	3
University hospital	12–45	1
	48	5
VA hospital (Philadelphia)	35–97	6
	25	7
Referral hospital (medical service)	17–45	1
General medical patients	17–45	1
	44–76	3
	48	5
General surgical patients	48–56	2
Rehabilitation patients	12–24	1

*References:
1. Bollet, A. J., et al.: Am. J. Clin. Nutr., 26:931–938, 1973.
2. Bistrian, B. R., et al.: J.A.M.A., 230:858–860, 1974.
3. Bistrian, B. R., et al.: J.A.M.A., 235:1567–1570, 1975.
4. Leevy, C. M., et al.: Am. J. Clin. Nutr., 17:259–271, 1965.
5. Weinsier, R. L., et al.: Am. J. Clin. Nutr., 32:418, 1979.
6. Mullen, J. L., et al.: Arch. Surg., 114:121–125, 1979.
7. V. A. Medical Service Newsletter: Dec. 26, 1979.

chart. Finally, the only request we made of the housestaff in return for the implied promises (the only "catch") was that they had to fill out a nutritional screening form (Fig. 12–2) that we would place on every chart and would require less than 60 seconds to complete. Based on the information that the physician entered and on simple criteria stated on the form itself, the physician could determine whether the patient needed referral to the NST. If so, a consult request form was to be filled out and placed in a folder that we taped to the wall in their office. The NST would then perform a complete nutritional assessment, place a formal nutritional consultation report on the chart, discuss the case with the responsible physician, continue to monitor the patient daily, and provide guidance as needed and *when it was convenient for the housestaff*.

Prior to initiating the project, contacts were made at several levels of the nursing service (including the chief of nursing, the associate chief for nursing education, and the ward head nurse) to stress the importance of the project and to solicit their assistance and suggestions. Several sessions were then held by the research nurse with the ward nurses to discuss ways of improving various monitoring aspects of nutritional state, the proper

usage of feeding tubes and feeding pumps, and so on. (At the nurses' request, she also demonstrated how to measure TST and MAC, procedures that appeared to have caught their fancy though were not required of them to perform.)

With this double-pronged preparation, the project was launched. The results were that over the next five weeks, the number of nutrition consultation requests made by that ward alone was greater than that produced by all the other five medical wards and intensive care unit together (13 versus 10). Interestingly, the screening form was not filled out for all or even most of the ward patients. Rather, it seemed to have been filled out mainly for those patients that the house-staff thought would need a nutritional consultation. Clearly, then, the recognition rate for

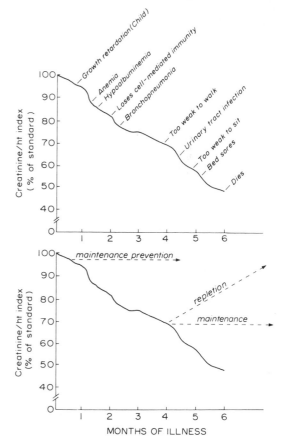

Figure 12–1. The natural history of protein-energy starvation *(top)* and prevention or correction by maintenance or repletion programs *(bottom)*. (*From* Heymsfield, S. B., Bethel, R. A., Ansley, J. D., Dixon, N. W., and Rudman, D.: Enteral hyperalimentation: An alternative to central venous hyperalimentation. Ann. Intern. Med. 90:63–71, 1979, with permission.)

Date: _____

Age: _____ Race: _____ Sex: _____ Date of admission: _____

Admitting Diagnosis:

Men Height			Medium Frame Ideal Weight	
Ft.	In.	cm	lb.	kg
5	2	157.5	124	56
5	3	160	127	57.6
5	4	162.6	130	59.1
5	5	165.1	133	60.3
5	6	167.6	137	62
5	7	170.2	141	63.8
5	8	172.7	145	65.8
5	9	175.3	149	67.6
5	10	177.8	153	69.4
5	11	180.3	158	71.4
6	0	182.9	162	73.5
6	1	185.4	167	75.6
6	2	188	171	77.6
6	3	190.5	176	79.6
6	4	193	181	82.2

Height: _____   Ideal weight: _____

Weight: _____   Usual weight: _____

Serum albumin: _____   gm/100 ml: _____

History of weight loss?   Yes _____ No _____

Tube feeding requirement?   Yes _____ No _____

TPN requirement?   Yes _____ No _____

Possible candidate for

Women Height			Medium Frame Ideal Weight	
Ft.	In.	cm	lb.	kg
4	10	147.3	101.5	46.1
4	11	149.9	104	47.3
5	0	152.4	107	48.6
5	1	154.9	110	50
5	2	157.5	113	51.4
5	3	160	116	52.7
5	4	162.6	119.5	54.3
5	5	165.1	123	55.9
5	6	167.6	127.5	58
5	7	170.2	131.5	59.8
5	8	172.7	135.5	61.6
5	9	175.3	139.5	63.4
5	10	177.8	143.5	65.2
5	11	180.3	147.5	67
6	0	182.9	151.5	68.9

  1. Major surgery?   Yes _____ No _____

  2. Antineoplastic therapy?   Yes _____ No _____

REQUEST NUTRITION SUPPORT TEAM CONSULTATION IF:

    1. Current weight 10% below usual weight or 15% below ideal body weight.

OR   2. Serum albumin less than 3.5 gm/100 ml.

OR   3. Answer was YES to any of above questions.

Figure 12–2. Screening nutritional assessment form. On the basis of measurements of height, weight, and serum albumin, one can identify the presence of marasmic and kwashiorkor-type malnutrition. The questions below these measurements are designed to identify those patients who may not be malnourished initially but are at risk of developing malnutrition subsequently.

malnutrition had been markedly enhanced, though it is not clear whether this was the result of the screening form, the daily presence of the NST on the ward, or, as we suspect, a combination of the two.

Nutritional monitoring by the nurses (specifically regarding the proper charting of weights and intake) became unquestionably superior on this ward when compared with that on the other medical wards. This was probably due to the constant, yet gentle and resourceful, prodding provided by the research nurse, since the advantage appeared to dwindle after she departed three weeks into the project.

A fair amount of *individual* housestaff teaching occurred during the daily NST visits to the ward, as a given patient would be discussed with his primary care physician. Some interest was expressed by the physicians in having a lecture in nutrition, which could have been scheduled and tailored to their convenience, but they apparently could not find time for it. It is of note, however, that when the interns on that ward rotated, the same ward resident was able to gather his new interns for 15 minutes one afternoon for a new orientation session—rather than expropriate time from attending rounds as he had done for the first orientation. The growth of that resident's interest in nutritional care appeared to stem in large measure from the fact that in a particular case, nutritional manipulations had cured the seemingly recalcitrant diarrhea of a tube-fed patient and, contrary to expectations, had allowed the patient to regain his strength, lose his confusion, and be discharged home in good health on an oral diet.

The impact of the "cure" was felt not only by that resident alone but also by all the physicians and nurses on that ward. In fact, the experience was electrifyingly new, even to the NST members. The nutritional recommendations made for this patient were similar to recommendations made previously for similar patients on other wards. Unlike before, however, this time there was collaboration by all involved. For a change, success was not foiled by misinterpretation or misimplementation of NST directions by physician or nurse.

The lessons gained from that pilot project were multiple. Limiting our scope of operation to one ward was not merely a fulfillment of the "divide and conquer" dictum. The achievement was not that we had done something better than we had done it before, but that we had accomplished that which we had never accomplished previously in patient care and especially in nutrition teaching. Interestingly, the key to success was success itself—the patient who improved. Attaining that first success was the most difficult. Fascinating lectures did not work—they were not attended. Shocking audit results on rampant malnutrition cured no one—they were at best politely acknowledged. Rather, the dramatic success was found at the end of a long, tedious, and most undramatic clinical journey in which the NST plodded along with this one patient's physicians and nurses until the patient recovered.

Gearing Up for a High Patient Load

In view of the high prevalence of malnutrition among hospitalized patients, it is very unlikely for any NSS to be able to supervise the day-to-day nutritional care of *every* malnourished patient at its institution. How then can one deal with such a high patient load?

To the extent that clinicians at a given center are trained to recognize and treat at least the mild or uncomplicated cases of malnutrition, the NSS is then able to focus its attention on a sicker but smaller—and hence more easily manageable—group of patients. The problem is that in the initial stages of setting up a nutrition effort within an institution little, if any, help can be expected from the clinicians.

For the identification of patients at risk, the previously noted nutritional screening form (Fig. 12–3) may be systematically incorporated into the data base of every patient's chart, though there is, of course, no guarantee that it will be filled out or that the NST will have time to collect and review these forms daily. In contrast, availability of a center computer may greatly facilitate the task of identifying patients who are nutritionally at risk. The routine admission procedure in many, if not most, hospitals includes a measurement of the patient's height and weight and of the serum albumin level. If the admitting nurse would enter the first two parameters on her ward terminal and the lab would enter the third parameter at its terminal, a list of patients with various degrees of marasmus or kwashiorkor, or both, could be generated daily by the computer with remarkably little effort, except for the initial period of training personnel in computer usage.

A center computer connecting wards, clinical laboratories, the pharmacy, and the dietetics department can greatly facilitate the teaching duties of the NSS. For instance, housestaff need to be taught to order TPN in terms of the patient's actual nutritional needs, in light of his latest laboratory data, and within the pharmaceutical, logistic, and cost constraints of TPN preparation. A center computer can remind the physician to add potassium if the last serum value was low or to suggest switching to a standard formulation if the tailor-made one that he ordered is very similar to it. Such a computer application was presented at the 1983 ASPEN Congress.[51] The same principles and mechanisms can be extended to the much-more-frequent ordering of formulas for enteral nutritional support.[52] Computer usage can also greatly facilitate nutritional assessment.[53–55]

What can one do in a hospital that is not yet computerized? In addition to the usage of simple screening forms such as that shown in Figure 12–3, one should pay particular attention to the design of standardized forms such as those used for ordering TPN. A TPN ordering form should not be a mere catalogue of available products. It must include some information on content and ordinary usage in order to facilitate rational utilization of this expensive and potentially dangerous form of therapy. A checklist format can help prevent important omissions. Such a form, however, should not be so overloaded with information as to be unwieldy.

Approach to the Hospital Administration

From the viewpoint of a hospital administrator, adding a new hospital service at a time when the country is in a budget-cutting mood and his hospital is frantically fighting to stay out of the red can only be pure folly. How then does one request funding to staff and equip an NSS? How does one rise at a clinical executive board meeting to demand $100,000 or $200,000 for TPN when across the table from him are the service chiefs who have just been told to drastically cut their staff and spending? To a nutritionist the weight of the evidence justifying such nutritional care expenditures may be overwhelm-

ing, but is the chairman of the board likely to have the patience to listen long enough to be swayed? How does one convince even a cooperative chief of nursing to assign a nurse to the NST when several of her nursing units are already understaffed and the hospital will not allow her an additional line?

It is clearly impossible to prescribe one approach for all administrators or for all institutions. In fact, just as each patient requires a diagnostic workup in order to institute appropriate therapy, so too does each institution need to be individually studied in order to effectively plan nutritional care within it.

There are several arguments to which hospital administrators may be particularly sensitive.

Cost Savings. The establishment of a knowledgeable NST with proper controls over the utilization of expensive enteral or parenteral nutritional formulations may reduce hospital spending. A comparison of TPN usage at the Brooklyn VA Medical Center showed a 32.8 per cent decrease in 1983 versus 1982 (despite a concomitant 27 per cent increase in the number of patients that the NSS had seen in consultation). This represented a saving of about $25,000 to the hospital.

Accreditation Requirements. Although the Joint Commission for the Accreditation of Hospitals (JCAH) does not yet have specific standards for nutritional support, the American Society for Parenteral and Enteral Nutrition (ASPEN) has recently published such standards[27] in the JCAH format. Once JCAH accepts these or similar standards, a hospital would have no choice but to comply or lose accreditation. For VA Medical Centers, there is a VA Central Office mandate[56, 57] to establish an NST consisting of a physician, nurse, pharmacist, and dietitian or stop providing TPN. Unfortunately the VA has not yet created new lines for such staffing. Nevertheless, it is still helpful to be able to tell the hospital administration that the hospital "is not in compliance with Central Office directives."

Avoiding Medicolegal Complications. With increasing public awareness of various sophisticated modalities of nutritional support as well as of the potentially adverse effects of such support, chances are that an increasing number of legal suits may be brought against hospitals for not providing nutritional support or for providing it inappropriately.[58, 59]

Reducing Morbidity and Mortality. A number of studies have demonstrated that nutritional support can reduce morbidity and mortality in a wide variety of diseases[60] and that the presence of a competent NST to monitor and guide nutritional support reduces the complication rate of that therapy.[7, 10, 11, 12, 61–66] (See section below for a critical review of this last point.)

In presenting the clinical benefits of nutritional support, there is a need to steer a middle course between two opposite tendencies. Nutritional support should not be presented as a panacea for all diseases. It is not. Nutritional therapy is treatment for malnutrition, not for Crohn's disease, cancer, or renal failure. Conversely, one should not sacrifice common sense on the scientific altar of "controlled double-blind studies." The absence of controlled double-blind studies showing that starvation is invariably fatal should not prevent anyone from emphatically stating that malnutrition kills.

Another helpful point to remember while arguing for nutritional support pertains to the form rather than the substance of the argument. It is well worthwhile to spend several hours searching for the one strongest point to make and for the specific sentence that will deliver it with the greatest punch to the administrators at an executive board meeting. "Journal club"–type presentations of scientific data will not touch them, and may in fact put them to sleep. This does not mean that one should not be prepared for a critical and detailed discussion of any aspect of the quoted study if someone should decide to raise a pointed question. It does mean that one should carefully distinguish between what is to be included in a short "banner headline" type of presentation and what needs to be kept in reserve for possible use after the first volley.

Finally, it is important to understand the data that might be used to argue against expenditures for nutritional support, such as the study showing no benefit from TPN in patients with small-cell lung carcinoma.[67] To a competent nutritionist such a study may mean that this particular form of nutritional support is not adequate for the type of malnutrition, or that this disease kills independently of malnutrition. The non-nutritionist, however, may incorrectly infer from such a report that one may completely ignore the nutritional needs of such a patient and allow him or her to starve to death, thus substituting a curable disease for an incurable one.

Death From Malnutrition is as Final as Death From Cardiac Standstill. The value of such a declaration lies not in the wisdom that it carries; it has none. Stating that "a pound of feathers is as heavy as a pound of lead" is just as silly. Rather its value pertains to its capacity to raise appropriate flags in the mind of clinicians and administrators alike, mobilizing them for action. In the minds of most clinicians, severe cardiac or pulmonary failure is clearly an entity requiring intensive care. For such a patient, the hospital is willing to assign staffing and resources galore. In contrast, the patient with severe nutritional depletion may be on the verge of total body failure and is therefore as much in need of intensive care, but frequently does not get it. Somehow, elevated ST segments across a patient's precordial leads make the doctor's heart skip a beat, whereas the report of a very low serum albumin level may elicit little reaction. Why is the response so different to these two patients in whom the potentially fatal outcome is identical? In one case it is recognized by the physician, in the other it is not. The solution to this problem follows Aristotelian didactics and consists simply of expressing the unfamiliar in terms that are familiar. Hence the value of equating pound to pound and death to death.

EVALUATION OF THE EFFICACY OF NUTRITIONAL SUPPORT TEAMS IN THE PREVENTION OF COMPLICATIONS OF NUTRITIONAL SUPPORT

Because of the increasing proliferation of NSTs and their potential for increasing personnel time and costs, it is important to examine the data regarding the overall effect of these teams on clinical care and the prevention of nutrition-related complications. The purpose of this section will be to review data on the current profile of NSTs in the United States and to examine the reports that have assessed the impact of NSTs on the administration of nutritional therapy.

The Ross Survey

In 1983, Ross Laboratories published an extensive survey on NST activities.[68] One thousand four hundred ninety-five hospitals were considered to be in need of an NST,

Table 12–4. DISTRIBUTION OF NST FUNCTIONS*

FUNCTION	AVERAGE PATIENTS/WEEK	PERCENTAGE
Total parenteral nutrition	7.8	19.1
Partial parenteral nutrition	4.7	11.9
Tube feeding and enteral supplements	14.3	36.2
Nutritional assessment only	12.7	32.1

*Survey of 180 teams.
(Modified from Sheridan and Calvert-Finn,[68] with permission.)

and these hospitals were surveyed. Five hundred twenty-one (34.8 per cent) indicated that they had an NST; this represented about 7 per cent of the 7000 hospitals in the United States or approximately 1 of every 14 hospitals having an NST. The average number of beds in the hospitals having NSTs was 489. The following discussion includes some of the summary data from the Ross Survey.

Table 12–4 lists the percentage distribution of team activities. Based on the current practices in hospitals that have NSTs, it is estimated that 1 of every 10 hospital admissions would require services from the NST. If one extrapolates to the hospitals that do not have teams, it is estimated that between 2500 and 2700 new NSTs would have to be formed to meet this demand. It is unrealistic to expect that this need will be met, especially in smaller hospitals. These data do emphasize the need for at least one person in every hospital who is qualified in clinical nutrition.

To identify proper allocation of NST personnel it is important to know the distribution of patients seen by the team. Table 12–5 shows the distribution as to referral specialties. The large percentage of surgical patients may be related to a high prevalence of perioperative nutritional problems in most hospitals or to insufficient recognition of malnutrition in nonsurgical patients. The finding

of similar rates of malnutrition among medical and surgical patients (see Table 12–3) would suggest that the latter interpretation is more correct.

Of great concern to hospital administrators is the ability of NSTs to become self-sufficient. Figure 12–3 lists the responses from 283 teams—58.6 per cent provided their services without charge, whereas 12.2 per cent operated strictly on a fee-for-service basis; 29.2 per cent charged for some services but not for others; and 25 per cent (68 of 269) indicated that they were financially self-supporting. These data will undoubtedly change with the onset of reimbursement by disease-related groupings (DRGs).

Of great importance are the qualifications of the team director. As noted previously, every effort should be made to select a *physician* director. The physician is the only person on the team who is responsible for the patient's total care. This is particularly important when complications are associated with nutritional care. Table 12–6 reveals the percentage distribution of team directors by profession.

Knowledge of the type and duration of feeding provides valuable information in estimating the cost of nutrition therapy. Table 12–7 lists the comparative duration of feeding for TPN and tube feeding for 253 teams. Of

Table 12–5. PERCENTAGE OF PATIENTS SERVED BY NUTRITION SUPPORT TEAMS BY REFERRAL SOURCE

	PERCENTAGE	NO. OF RESPONDENTS	PERCENTAGE	
			With Pediatrics	No Pediatrics
Surgery	42.0	265	45.3	45.9
Medicine	24.7	259	26.6	27.0
Oncology	17.6	227	19.0	19.2
Pediatrics	8.5	158	9.1	0.0
Other	7.2	61	0.0	7.9
	100.0	970	100.0	100.0

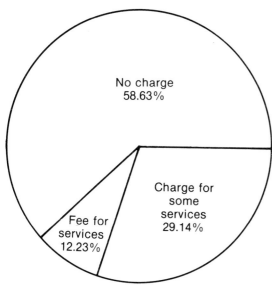

Figure 12–3. Nutrition support teams—basis for services.

Table 12–7. AVERAGE LENGTH OF FEEDING BY NUTRITION SUPPORT MODALITY

LENGTH OF TIME	PARENTERAL NUTRITION (PERCENTAGE)	ENTERAL TUBE FEEDING (PERCENTAGE)
Less than 2 days	0.4	0.4
2–5 days	3.2	4.6
6–10 days	21.3	26.4
11–15 days	37.9	33.2
16 days	37.2	35.4
(Rounded)	100.00	100.00

ies were excluded. Five reports met the selection criteria. They are summarized in Table 12–8 and are discussed individually in the following section.

The Ryan Study

As a component of their large prospective study of 200 patients, Ryan and colleagues[63] examined the effect of adherence to a standard protocol on the reduction of catheter sepsis. Adherence to the protocol was determined by the hyperalimentation nurse. Catheter sepsis was defined as an episode of sepsis for which no anatomic focus could be identified.

Eighty catheters were described as receiving improper care at the time of insertion or during maintenance of the catheter. There were 16 (20 per cent) episodes of sepsis in this group. Proper care was given to 275 catheters, and 9 of them (three per cent) became septic ($p < 0.01$). The authors concluded that TPN could be employed with an acceptable risk provided that catheter care was administered according to a protocol.

The Nehme Study

Nehme[10] examined the influence of an NST on the prevention of TPN-related complications in a prospective nonrandomized study of 375 patients for 24 months in a large city-county hospital. The NST had sole responsibility for 211 patients, whereas 164 patients were managed in a nonteam setting. Patients in both groups had reasonably comparable diagnoses.

The NST inserted 284 catheters, whereas 389 catheters were placed in the non-NST group. The non-NST patients had a 33 per

interest was the finding that 75 per cent of NSTs fed their patients for greater than 11 days. There were no significant differences in the duration of feeding between enteral and parenteral techniques. Less than 8 per cent of the teams provided TPN for 80 to 100 per cent of their patients, whereas more than three fourths of the teams provided TPN for 60 per cent or fewer patients.

The most important question relating to the presence of NSTs is whether they improve clinical outcome. Because of the many variables that influence clinical outcome and nutritional care, it is difficult to attribute the improvement in a patient's clinical course directly to the presence of an NST. Most reports that extoll the benefits of the NST are anecdotal and uncontrolled.[69]

A review of the literature was performed to identify and analyze controlled studies that related to the impact of the NST on clinical outcome and the prevention of complications. Abstracts and uncontrolled stud-

Table 12–6. PROFESSION OF NST DIRECTOR

	PERCENTAGE
Physician	80
Pharmacist	11.6
Dietitian	3.3
Nurse	1.8
Administrator or other	3.3

(From Sheridan and Calvert-Finn,[68] with permission)

Table 12–8. INFLUENCE OF NUTRITION SUPPORT TEAM ON NUTRITION-RELATED COMPLICATIONS

AUTHOR, YEAR, GROUP TYPE	NO. OF PATIENTS	NO. OF CATHETERS	COMPLICATIONS (NO. and %)			COMMENTS
			Metabolic	*Septic*	*Mechanical*	
Ryan, 1974	Total					Compared proper to improper care
Non-NST	Patients	80	—	16/80 20%	—	of catheters as determined by an
NST	200	275	—	9/275 0.3%	—	NST nurse
						p < 0.01
Nehme, 1980						
Non-NST	164	391	152	43/164 26.2%	33.5%	Catheter sepsis = defervescence
NST	211	284	24	5/211 1.3%	3.7%	upon catheter removal + blood
						and catheter tip cultures
Keohane, 1983	Total					
Non-NST	Patients	51	—	17/51 33%	9/51 18%	p < 0.001
NST	83	48	—	2/48 4%	3/48 6%	Catheter sepsis = + catheter tip
						culture or defervescence upon
						catheter removal
Dalton, 1983						
Non-NST	28	25	47.8%	1/28	7/20 35%	Compared loosely structured with
NST	29	20	26.3%	1/29	2/18 11%	more defined team approach
						p < 0.0005
						p < 0.1
Jacobs, 1984						
Non-NST	21	—	0.4%	5/21 24%	3/21 10%	Note: Transitional NST =
Transitional NST	35	—	0.9%	1/35 3%	2/35 6%	transitional period when one part
NST	22	—	0.1%	0/22 0%	0/22 0%	of the team was functioning.
						% abnormal hyperglycemia/patient/
						TPN day
						p < 0.05 vs. NST group

cent complication rate in catheter placement, whereas there was only a 3.7 per cent complication rate in the NST group. Patients in the non-NST group had a 26.2 per cent rate of catheter sepsis, whereas the incidence was reduced to 1.3 per cent in the NST group. Uncorrected electrolyte and pH changes that occurred for 48 hours were defined as metabolic complications. In the non-NST group, 40 per cent had metabolic complications, whereas the NST group had only an 11 per cent complication rate. The greatest difference between the two groups was in the frequency of electrolyte imbalance, which was attributed to inadequate monitoring in the non-NST group.

The study concluded that a protocol that is strictly adhered to by knowledgeable persons (preferably an NST) is necessary for the proper administration of TPN to the hospitalized patient.

The Dalton Study

In a prospective trial, Dalton and colleagues[64] examined the effects of a more defined approach to NST functions when compared with a loosely structured NST format. Their goal was to determine if the more defined approach reduced TPN-associated morbidity.

Twenty-eight consecutive patients were managed entirely by their primary physicians, with the role of the NST limited to consultative activities. The next 29 patients who received TPN were managed jointly by their primary physicians and the NST.

Mechanical complications were defined as technical complications of subclavian vein catheterization. Thirty-five per cent of the patients in the non-NST group had mechanical complications as compared with 11 per cent (p < 0.1) in the NST group.

Septic complications were defined as an episode of sepsis in which no focus for the infection could be identified other than the TPN catheter and which resolved upon its removal. Both groups had one episode of documented catheter sepsis. Nine catheters were removed for suspected sepsis in the non-NST group, whereas only two catheters were removed in the NST group.

Metabolic complications included abnormalities in electrolytes, pH, glucose, and vitamin K. Electrolyte, pH, and serum glucose abnormalities were defined as serum levels beyond the normal physiologic range that occurred during TPN therapy and were not corrected within 24 hours. An exception to the 24-hour correction period was inorganic phosphate, wherein a complication was defined as any level outside the normal range that occurred after the initiation of therapy. Complications of glucosuria were defined as urine sugar levels of 3+ or 4+, using a glucose oxidase method for one or more days. In addition, any abnormal prothrombin time that occurred during TPN was listed as a complication. In the non-NST group, 47.8 per cent of the patients had metabolic abnormalities, as compared with 26.3 per cent in the NST group. The imbalance rate was less for patients in the NST group in all measured metabolic abnormalities except serum bicarbonate.

It was concluded that modification of TPN to provide more control over its administration resulted in increased patient monitoring and adherence to infection control guidelines as well as decreased mechanical and metabolic complications.

The Keohane Study

In a prospective three-year study, Keohane and associates[65] examined the impact of an NST nurse on 83 patients who required 99 TPN catheters. The nursing care for the first 51 catheters was the responsibility of general and intensive care ward nurses, and a standard protocol was used. The subsequent 48 catheters were managed under the care of a specially trained NST nurse. The presence of an NST nurse led to a significant reduction of catheter sepsis from 33 to 4 per cent (p < 0.001).

It was concluded that rigorous aseptic NST nursing care was the most significant factor in the reduction of TPN catheter sepsis.

The Jacobs Study

Jacobs and colleagues[66] examined the impact of an NST on the reduction of complications in 78 consecutive patients who received TPN on the same VA surgical service. Patients were studied in three groups based on the evolution of the NST. The groups were as follows: Non-NST, 21 patients; transitional NST, 35 patients; and post-NST, 22 patients.

A mechanical complication was defined as being directly attributable to the insertion of the central venous catheter. There were no significant differences in mechanical complications among the three groups.

Catheter sepsis was defined as concurrent positive results of catheter and blood cultures of the same organism. In the absence of blood cultures, catheter sepsis was defined as defervescence within six hours of removing the catheter. The non-NST group had a significantly higher (p < 0.05) incidence of catheter sepsis than either the transitional NST or post-NST groups.

Metabolic abnormalities were reviewed in addition to the mean number of tests ordered/patient/TPN days. One-way analysis of variance revealed no significant differences among the three groups in (1) the mean number of tests/patient/TPN day, (2) the mean number of abnormal tests/patient/TPN day, and (3) the mean percentage of abnormal tests/patient/TPN day. Although the most common metabolic abnormality was hyperglycemia, the percentage of abnormal glucose tests/patient/TPN day was not significantly different among the groups.

Prior to the formation of the NST, the following inadequacies were identified: (1) lack of proper sterile technique in the insertion of central venous catheters; (2) lack of familiarity among the housestaff as to the calculation of specific nutrient requirements; (3) lack of a protocol for proper metabolic monitoring; (4) absence of nursing knowledge as to the appropriate methods of catheter care; and (5) routine administration of medications and measurement of central venous pressure via the TPN catheter. These inadequacies were corrected by the following changes: (1) insistence that all catheters for TPN be inserted with the aid of the NST nurse and with proper sterile technique; (2) "educational" consultations by the NST to indicate the methods for calculating nutrient requirements and making recommendations for nutritional therapy; (3) insistence that an overprint be provided on a standard order sheet to include routine metabolic monitoring for all patients who receive TPN; (4) nursing education as to proper catheter care; and (5) prohibition of the use of the TPN line for anything but TPN.

This study observed a significant reduction in catheter sepsis that was attributable to the establishment of an NST—specifically a nurse specialist and protocols for catheter insertion and care.

It is of note that of the three cited studies that looked at complications of catheter insertion and metabolic complications, this is the only one that failed to demonstrate a significant decrease in these types of complications. This may be the result of an already low complication rate at a hospital affiliate of the University of Pennsylvania, where central TPN originated and general clinicians are probably more familiar with this form of therapy than their counterparts elsewhere. Interestingly, however, all five studies demonstrated a significant reduction in the catheter sepsis rate that was related to the presence of a trained nurse enforcing a specific protocol for catheter care.

SUMMARY

The presence of an NST is recommended for the delivery of nutritional care to malnourished hospitalized patients. To fulfill its purpose, the team must collectively have a solid grounding in the science of clinical nutrition, as well as a thorough mastery of its techniques. Because the NST represents a new marriage of several disciplines, respective roles and chores should be innovatively rethought and perhaps redistributed in a new way, rather than recopied from the protocols of parent disciplines.

The challenge of establishing nutritional support at a medical center is in essence the attempt to make visible to others that which is obvious to nutritionists and to do so by inventing new modes of communication. Not surprisingly, success may require seemingly infinite patience and tact. However, perhaps no other field in medicine allows one to enjoy the science and art of medicine across so many worlds of nature, from the microcosm of nutrient interactions to the arenas of institutional dynamics.

REFERENCES

1. Blackburn, G.L., Bothe, A., and Lahey, M.A.: Organization and Administration of a Nutrition Support Service. Surg. Clin. North Am., 61:709–719, 1981.
2. Butterworth, C.E.: The advantages of a nutrition support team. Res. Staff Phys., 27(11):76–83, 1981.
3. Fisher, J.E.: The Organization of a parenteral nutrition unit. In Fisher, J.E. (ed.): Total Parenteral Nutrition, 127–131. Boston, Little, Brown & Co., 1976.
4. Grant, J.P.: A team approach. In Handbook of Total Parenteral Nutrition. Philadelphia, W.B. Saunders Co., 1980, pages 4–6.
5. Jensen, T.G., and Dudrick, S.J.: Implementation of a multidisciplinary nutritional assessment program. J. Am. Diet. Assoc., 79:258–266, 1981.
6. Shils, M.E.: Parenteral nutrition. In Goodhart, R.S., and Shils, M.E. (eds.): Modern Nutrition in Health and Disease. Philadelphia, Lea & Febiger, 1980, pages 1125–1152.
7. Skoutakis, V.A., Domingo, R.M., Miller, W.A., and Dobbie, R.P.: Team approach to total parenteral nutrition. Am. J. Hosp. Pharm., 32:693–697, 1975.
8. Seltzer, M.H., Slocum, B.A., Cataldi-Betcher, E.L. et al.: Nutrition support: team approach. Am. J. Intraven. Ther., 8:13–46, 1981.
9. Ferguson, D.G.: Total parenteral nutrition and the team. J.A.M.A., 243:1931, 1980.
10. Nehme, A.E.: Nutritional support of the hospitalized patient. The team concept. J.A.M.A., 243:1906–1908, 1980.
11. Carpentier, Y.A., Francois, N., Van Brandt, M., and Vanderveken, L. Total parenteral nutrition (TPN): The team concept. Acta Chir. Belg., 80:119–123, 1981.
12. Allen, J.R.: Prevention of infection in patients receiving total parenteral nutrition. Acta Chir. Scand. (Suppl.), 507:405–418, 1981.
13. MacDonald, H.L., Anderson, J.R., McLean Ross, A.H., Gove, L.F., Webb, A., Amos, A.A., and Walls, A.D.: Parenteral nutrition: the team approach. J.R. Coll. Surg. (Edinb.) 26:173–177, 1981.
14. Smith, E.M.: Total parenteral nutrition—a team concept. Nurs. Times, 77:1464–1465, 1981.
15. Pfeifer, E., Kaminsky, M.V., Jr., and Aquinas, M.: Metabolic support: how to form a service. Hospitals, 53:97–99, 1979.
16. Leevy, C.M., Cardi, L., Frank, O., et al.: Incidence and significance of hypovitaminemia in a randomly selected municipal hospital population. Am. J. Clin. Nutr., 17:259–271, 1965.
17. Bollet, A.J., and Owens, S.: Evaluation of nutritional status of selected hospitalized patients. Am. J. Clin. Nutr., 26:931–938, 1973.
18. Bistrian, B.R., Blackburn, G.L., Hallowell, E., and Heddle, R.: Protein status of general surgical patients. J.A.M.A., 230:858–860, 1974.
19. Hill, G.L., Blackett, R.L., Pickford, I., Burkinshaw, L., Young, G.A., Warren, J.V., Schorah, C.J., and Morgan, D.B.: Malnutrition in surgical patients: An unrecognized problem. Lancet, 1:689–692, 1977.
20. Butterworth, C.E., Jr.: Malnutrition in the hospital. J.A.M.A., 230:879, 1974.
21. Bistrian, B.R., Blackburn, G.L., Vitale, J., Cochran, D., and Nayloy, J.: Prevalence of malnutrition in general medical patients. J.A.M.A., 235:1567–1570, 1976.
22. Willard, M.D., Gilsdorf, R.B., and Price, R.A.: Protein-calorie malnutrition in a community hospital. J.A.M.A., 243:1720–1722, 1980.
23. Bushman, L., Russell, R., Warfield, L., Curry, G., and Iber, F.: Malnutrition among patients in an acute-care veterans facility. J. Am. Dietet. Assoc., 77:462–465, 1980.
24. Reinhardt, G.R., Mycofski, J.W., Wilkens, D.B. et al.: Incidence and mortality of hypoalbuminemic patients in hospitalized veterans. J.P.E.N., 4:357–359, 1980.
25. Mullen, J.L., Gertner, M.H., Buzby, G.P., Goodhart, G.L., and Rosato, E.F.: Implications of malnutrition in the surgical patient. Arch Surg., 114:121–125, 1979.

26. Tobias, A.L., and Van Itallie, T.B.: Nutritional problems of hospitalized patients. A preliminary survey. J. Am. Diet. Assoc., 71:253–257, 1977.

27. ASPEN Select Committee on Standards of Professional Practice: Standards for Nutrition Support—Hospitalized Patients. Washington, D.C., American Society for Parenteral and Enteral Nutrition, 1984.

28. Howard, L.: Certification of clinical nutrition specialists: the current role of the American Board of Nutrition. Am. J. Clin. Nutr., 38:811–812, 1983.

29. Schiller, M.R.: Profile of the dietitian. In Chernoff, R. (ed.): Interrelationships of Dietary and Pharmacy Services in Nutrition Support, Report of the Fourth Ross Roundtable on Medical Issues. Columbus, Ohio, Ross Laboratories, 1983, pages 7–12.

30. Study Commission on Dietetics: The Profession of Dietetics. Chicago, The American Dietetic Association, 1972.

31. The American Dietetic Association: Position paper on clinical dietetics. J. Am. Dietet. Assoc., 80:256, 1982.

32. Jensen, T.G., Brooks, B.J.: Marketing strategy: A key leverage point for dietitians. J. Am. Diet. Assoc., 79:267–273, 1981.

33. Johnson, D.: The dietitian—A translator of nutritional information. J. Am. Dietet. Assoc., 64:608–611, 1974.

34. Muller, R.J., Hoffman, D.M., and Mulligan, R.M.: Parenteral nutrition program in a major cancer center. Hosp. Pharm., 16:54–66, 1981.

35. Roe, D.A.: Interactions between drugs and nutrients. Med. Clin. North Am., 63:985–1007, 1979.

36. Maslakowski, C.J.: Drug-nutrient interactions/interrelationships. Nutr. Supp. Serv., 1:14–17, 1981.

37. Hoying, C.L.: Nutritional support nurses' role in nursing management. Nutr. Supp. Serv. 3(6):28–31, 1983.

38. Johnston, J.E.: Home parenteral nutrition: The "costs" of patient and family participation. Soc. Work. Health Care, 7:49–66, 1981.

39. Burke, W.A., Burkhart, VdP., Pierpaoli, P.G.: A Guide for a Nutritional Support Service. Deerfield, Illinois, Travenol Laboratories, Inc., 1980.

40. Blair, J., Burke, M., Chernoff, R., et al. (eds.): Establishing a Nutritional Support Service. Chicago, Abbott Laboratories, 1980.

41. Solassol, C., and Joyeux, H.: Logistic problems of artificial nutrition. Biomedicine, 28:85–88, 1978.

42. Shildt, R.A., Ross, M., Stollman, L., and Bell, B.: Organization of the nutritional support service at a medical center: one year's experience. Milit. Med., 147:55–58, 1982.

43. Tweedle, D.E.: Organizing nutritional support. Acta Chir. Scand. (Suppl.), 507:292–297, 1981.

44. Griffin, R.E., Lahey, M.A., and Blackburn, G.L.: Organization and management of a nutrition support service. Top. Hosp. Pharm. Manag., 2:51–60, 1982.

45. D'Eramo, D.: The hospital administrator's consideration of nutrition support teams. In Chernoff, R. (ed.): Interrelationships of Dietary and Pharmacy Services in Nutrition Support, Report of the Fourth Ross Roundtable on Medical Issues. Columbus, Ohio, Ross Laboratories, 1983, pages 15–17.

46. Hamaoui, E., Ahart, H.E., Eisen, R.F., Hinsdale, J.G., and Pollock, T.W.: Nutritional requirements

and considerations. Resid. Staff Phys., 29(1):40–56, 1983.

47. Hamaoui, E., Ahart, H.E., Eisen, R.F., Hinsdale, J.G., and Pollock, T.W.: Nutritional assessment and enteral nutrition. Resid. Staff Phys., 29(2):94–104, 1983.

48. Hamaoui, E., Ahart, H.E., Eisen, R.F., Hinsdale, J.G., and Pollock, T.W.: Total parenteral nutrition and peripheral alimentation. Resid. Staff Phys., 29(3):88–101, 1983.

49. Heymsfield, S.B., Bethel, R.A., Ansley, J.D., Nixon, D.W., and Rudman, D.: Enteral hyperalimentation: An alternative to central venous hyperalimentation. Ann. Intern. Med., 90:63–71, 1979.

50. Lipschitz, D.A., and Mitchell, C.O.: The correctability of the nutritional, immune, and hematopoietic manifestations of protein calorie malnutrition in the elderly. J. Am. Coll. Nutr., 1:17–25, 1982.

51. Larsen, K.: Application of the computer in TPN prescribing. Program of the Seventh Clinical Congress of the American Society for Parenteral and Enteral Nutrition. Washington, D.C., 1983, pages 63–65.

52. Geller, R.J., Blackburn, S.A., Glendon, D.H., et al.: Computer optimization of enteral hyperalimentation. J.P.E.N., 3:79–83, 1979.

53. Collins, C.D.: Microcomputers and nutritional assessment. NSS, 3(2):48–52, 1983.

54. McLaurin, N.K., Goodwin, C.W., Zitska, C.A., and Hander, E.W.: Computer generated graphic evaluation of nutritional status in critically injured patients. J. Am. Diet. Assoc., 82(1):49–52, 1983.

55. Schloerb, P.R.: Application of the computer in nutritional assessment. Symposium Session 8: Computer Applications in Clinical Nutrition. Program of the Seventh Clinical Congress. Washington, D.C., American Society of Parenteral and Enteral Nutrition, 1983.

56. Jacoby, W. J.: Requirement for Total Parenteral Nutrition (TPN). VA Circular 10(82):47, March 30, 1982.

57. Jacoby, W. J.: Requirement for Total Parenteral Nutrition (TPN). V.A. Circular, 10(83):52, March 23, 1983.

58. Martin, D.J., and Cerullo, T.C.: Medicolegal considerations in nutritional support. NSS, 1(4):21–22, 1981.

59. Cerrullo, T.C.: Legal considerations in implementing and maintaining a total parenteral nutrition program. U.S. Pharm., 4:21–31, 1979.

60. Grant, J.P.: Handbook of Total Parenteral Nutrition. Chapter 3. Philadelphia, W.B. Saunders Co., 1980, pages 7–46.

61. Weinsier, R.L., Bacon, J. and Butterworth, C.E., Jr.: Central venous alimentation: a prospective study of the frequency of metabolic abnormalities among medical and surgical patients. J.P.E.N., 6:421–425, 1982.

62. Sanders, R.A., and Sheldon, G.F.: Septic complications of total parenteral nutrition. A five year experience. Am. J. Surg., 132:214–220, 1976.

63. Ryan, J.A., Abel, R.A., Abbott, W.M., Hopkins, C., McChesney, T., Colley, R., Phillips, K., and Fischer, J.E.: Catheter complications in total parenteral nutrition. A prospective study of 20 consecutive patients. N. Engl. J. Med., 290:757–761, 1974.

64. Dalton, M.J., Schepers, G., Gee, J.P., Alberts, C.C.,

Eckhauser, F.E., and Korking, D.M.: Consultative total parenteral nutrition teams. The effect on the incidence of TPN related complications. J.P.E.N., 8:146–152, 1984.

65. Keohane, P.P., Attrill, H., Northover, J., Jones, B.J.M., Cribb, A., Frost, P., and Silk, D.B.A.: Effect of catheter tunneling and a nutrition nurse on catheter sepsis. A controlled trial. Lancet, 2:1388–1390, 1983.

66. Jacobs, D.O., Melnik, G., Forlaw, L. et al. Impact of a Nutritional Support Service on VA surgical patients. J. Am. Coll. Nutr., 3:311–315, 1984.

67. Shike, M.: Total parenteral nutrition in patients with lung cancer. Presented at the Seventh Clinical Congress of the American Society for Parenteral and Enteral Nutrition. Washington, D.C., 1983.

68. Sheridan, J.F., and Calvert-Finn, S.: The Nutrition Support Team—Results of a Comprehensive Hospital Survey. Columbus, Ohio, Ross Laboratories, 1983.

69. Koretz, R.: Nutritional Support and Clinical Outcome. Seventh Clinical Congress of the American Society for Parenteral and Enteral Nutrition, Washington, D.C., 1983.

70. Howard, L., and Bigaouette, J.: A survey of physician clinical nutrition training programs in the United States. Am. J. Clin. Nutr., 38:719–729, 1983.

71. NSS teams. NSS, 4(11):36–58, 1984.

CHAPTER 13

Parenteral Nutrition Equipment*

MURRAY H. SELTZER
BERNADETTE A. SLOCUM
EMMA L. CATALDI-BETCHER
DAVID J. GOLDBERGER
KENNETH W. JONES

A full discussion of the materials and devices related to parenteral nutrition is by definition too lengthy and immediately outdated to be included in any text when completed. In 1978, one of this chapter's authors (M.H.S.) was able to provide a cursory generic "state of the art" discussion composed of two pages that encompassed both parenteral and enteral equipment.[1] Such folly was rewarded with the privilege of coauthoring this more exhaustive chapter subsequent to a phenomenal proliferation of technology.

Review of the world's literature as well as available commercial product information and the authors' collective personal experience again dictate a discussion that is as generic as possible, in which important principles rather than important products are to be described in relation to parenteral nutrition equipment.

At times, the naming of a specific unique product or manufacturer may be unavoidable. Such mention is not intended to be an endorsement but rather an objective fact.

Equipment related to assessment, venous access, catheter dressings, pumps, ancillary intravenous equipment, pharmacy equipment, and home parenteral nutrition equipment will herein be described, as appropriate. Furthermore, for the reader's

continued self-education concerning new products Table 13–1 provides additional information concerning resource materials and their manufacturers.

NUTRITIONAL ASSESSMENT EQUIPMENT

In all the varied nutritional assessment techniques, the most readily available information relates to patient weight and height.

Height and Weight Measurements

Scales upon which the patient stands are, in general, either the spring type or the beam or lever balance type. Spring scales have the advantage of being portable and can easily be brought to the patient's bedside, whereas the beam or lever balance scale is usually in a fixed location to which the patient must be brought for weighing. Spring scales, however, have a tendency to loose accuracy when the spring stretches; thus, the beam or lever balance scales should be used when possible.

For patients who are unable to stand, there are two types of portable scales. The first consists of four weighing transducers (Aimex, Boston) that each fit permanently under a corner of the patient's bed and are connected to a control console. Accessory equipment (sheets, pillows) on the bed must be standardized for consistency, and the sys-

*The authors wish to acknowledge Donna Palardy for organizing many diversified materials and preparing the manuscript. Further acknowledgment goes to the Saint Barnabas Medical Center Librarians, A. Chris Connor, M.L.S., Louise Noll, B.A., and Sylvia Barrasso for their assistance in acquiring resource material.

Text continued on page 263

257

Table 13–1. EQUIPMENT

	ASSESSMENT	VENOUS ACCESS	DRESSING	PUMPS	ANCILLARY IV	PHARMACY	HOME TPN
Abbott Laboratories Hospital Products Division Abbott Park North Chicago, Illinois 60064 (312) 937-6100		X		X	X		
Acme United Corporation 100 Hicks Street Bridgeport, Connecticut 06609 (203) 384-1371			X				
Aimex Company 177 State Street Boston, Massachusetts 02109 (617) 227-7090	X						
American McGaw Division of American Hospital Supply 2525 McGaw Avenue · Irvine, California 92714 (714) 754-2000	X			X	X		X
American Pharmaseal P.O. Box 1300 Glendale, California 91209 (213) 240-8900		X					
Amtek Medical Specialties, Inc. 5656 Lincoln Drive Minneapolis, Minnesota 55436 (612) 933-1940				X	X		
American Scale Corporation P.O. Box 1776 Hartsdale, New York 10530 (914) 761-1745	X						
Anatros Corporation 1922 Junction Avenue San Jose, California 95031 (408) 298-3185				X			
Antek Instruments, Inc. 6005 N. Freeway Houston, Texas 77076 (713) 691-2265	X						
Antigen Supply House P.O. Box 2622 Canoga Park, California 91306 (800) 423-5783	X						
Argyle/Sherwood Medical 1831 Olive Street St. Louis, Missouri 63103 (314) 621-7788			X				
Argon Medical Corporation P.O. Box 1970 Athens, Texas 75751 (214) 675-9321 (800) 527-2983		X					
Arrow International, Inc. Hill and Georges Avenues Reading, Pennsylvania 19610 (215) 378-0131 (800) 523-8446		X					
Asimow Engineering Company 1818 Franklin Street Santa Monica, California 90404 (213) 828-7981	X						
Beckman Instruments, Inc. Physiological Measurements Operations 2500 Harbor Boulevard Fullerton, California 92636 (800) 526-3821	X						

Table 13–1. EQUIPMENT *Continued*

	ASSESSMENT	VENOUS ACCESS	DRESSING	PUMPS	ANCILLARY IV	PHARMACY	HOME TPN
Briarhills Medical 12077 Wilshire Boulevard Suite 718 Los Angeles, California 90025 (213) 390-4942 (800) 227-1617	X						
Burron Medical, Inc. 824 12th Avenue Bethlehem, Pennsylvania 18018 (215) 691-5400 (800) 523-9695					X		
Cambridge Scientific Industries Moose Lodge Road P.O. Box 265 Cambridge, Maryland 21613 (301) 228-5111 (800) 638-9566	X						
Clinipad Corporation P.O. Box 387 66 High Street Guilford, Connecticut 06437 (203) 453-6543 (800) 243-6548			X				
Concord Laboratories, Inc. Kit Street Keene, New Hampshire 03431 (603) 352-3812 (800) 258-5362			X				
Consolidated Medical Equipment, Inc. 10 Hopper Street Utica, New York 13501 (315) 797-8375		X					
Contamination Control Laboratories, Inc. 13324-T Farmington Road Livonia, Michigan 48150 (313) 427-8450						X	
Cormed, Inc. P.O. Box 470 591 Mahar Street Medina, New York 14103 (716) 798-4900		X		X	X		X
Critikon, Inc. P.O. Box 22800 Tampa, Florida 33622 (813) 876-5000		X	X		X		
Cutter Medical Division of Cutter Laboratories, Inc. 2200 Powell Street Emeryville, California 94608 (415) 420-4000				X	X		
Delmed, Inc. I.V. Catheter Division 27 Maple Avenue Holbrook, Massachusetts (800) 225-8634		X			X		
Deseret Medical Inc. 9450 State Street Sandy, Utah 84070 (800) 453-4538 (801) 255-6851		X	X		X		
Dow Corning Corporation P.O. Box 4767 Midland, Missouri 48640 (517) 496-4000 (517) 496-4067					X		
Drake Willock 13520 S.E. Pheasant Court Portland, Oregon 97222 (503) 659-3355				X			

Table 13–1. EQUIPMENT *Continued*

	ASSESSMENT	VENOUS ACCESS	DRESSING	PUMPS	ANCILLARY IV	PHARMACY	HOME TPN
Edcraft Industries, Inc. P.O. Box 609 Linden, New Jersey 07036 (201) 925-7760						X	
Eli Lilly and Company 307 East McCarty Street Indianapolis, Indiana 46285 (317) 261-2000	X						
Evermed P.O. Box 296 Medina, Washington 98039 (206) 827-1137		X					X
Extracorporeal Medical Specialties, Inc. Royal and Ross Roads King of Prussia, Pennsylvania 19406 (215) 337-2400				X			
Harvard Apparatus Company, Inc. 150 Dover Road Millis, Massachusetts 02054 (617) 376-2986				X			
Health Care Logistics, Inc. P.O. Box 25 Circleville, Ohio 43113 (800) 848-1633 (614) 477-1686					X		
Health Development Corporation 2551 Casey Avenue Mountainview, California 94043 (415) 961-9332		X			X		
Holtain Limited Bryberian, Crymmych Pembrokeshire, U.K.	X						
IMED Corporation 9925 Carroll Canyon Road San Diego, California 92131 (800) 854-2033 (714) 566-9000				X	X		
Invenex Laboratories 5885 Lakehurse Drive Orlando, Florida 32809 (305) 351-1400					X		
Inmed Corporation 2950 Pacific Drive Norcross, Georgia 30071 (800) 241-1926 (404) 449-6680		X					
IVAC Corporation 11353 Sorrento Valley Road San Diego, California 92121 (714) 453-4320				X			
Johnson & Johnson Products, Inc. Patient Care Division 501 George Street New Brunswick, New Jersey 08903 (800) 526-2459 (800) 352-4845			X				
LaBarge, Inc. Medical Product Division 500 Broadway Building St. Louis, Missouri 63102 (800) 325-3363				X			
Luther Medical Products, Inc. 3020 Enterprise Street Costa Mesa, California 92626 (714) 557-5963		X					

Table 13–1. EQUIPMENT *Continued*

	ASSESSMENT	VENOUS ACCESS	DRESSING	PUMPS	ANCILLARY IV	PHARMACY	HOME TPN
Lypho-Med, Inc. 4020 W. Division Street Chicago, Illinois, 60651 (800) 621-3334					X		
3-M Medical Products Division 225-5S 3-M Center St. Paul, Minnesota 55144 (612) 733-9033 (612) 733-8944			X				
Marion Scientific Corporation 9233 Ward Parkway Suite 350 Kansas City, Missouri 64114 (816) 363-4900			X				
Medical Packaging, Inc. 525 White Horse Pike Atco, New Jersey 08004 (609) 767-3604 (800) 257-5282					X		
Medlon, Inc. 3325 No. Glenoaks Boulevard Burbank, California 91502 (213) 954-9541					X		
Millipore Corporation Medical Products Division 80 Ashby Road Bedford, Massachusetts 02192 (800) 225-1380					X		
Norland Corporation Rt. 4, Norland Drive Fort Atkinson, Wisconsin 53538 (800) 558-0196 (414) 563-8456	X						
NuAire, Inc. 2100 Fernbrook Lane Plymouth, Minnesota 55441 (612) 553-1270						X	
Pall Biomedical Products Corporation 30 Sea Cliff Avenue Glen Cove, New York 11542 (516) 671-4000					X	X	
Paramedical, Inc. 570 Pleasant Street Watertown, Massachusetts 02172 (617) 926-8110					X		
Preston Company 60 Page Road Clifton, New Jersey 07035 (201) 777-2700	X						
Ross Laboratories 265 Cleveland Avenue Columbus, Ohio 43216 (614) 227-3333	X						
Scale-Tronix, Inc. 12 Baylor Circle White Plains, New York 10605 (914) 948-8117 P.O. Box 15 Wheaton, Illinois 60187 (312) 653-3377	X						
Scientific Industries, Inc. 70 Orville Drive Bohema, New York 11716 (516) 567-4700				X			

Table 13–1. EQUIPMENT *Continued*

	ASSESSMENT	VENOUS ACCESS	DRESSING	PUMPS	ANCILLARY IV	PHARMACY	HOME TPN
Shampaine/Wilson/AHP, Inc. Affiliated Hospital Products, Inc. 1920 South Jefferson Avenue St. Louis, Missouri 63104 (314) 772-7000					X		
Sigmamotor, Inc. 14 Elizabeth Street Middleport, New York 14105 (716) 735-3616				X	X		
Society of Actuaries 208 South LaSalle Street Chicago, Illinois 60604 (312) 236-3833	X						
Sorenson Research Company 4387 Atherton Drive P.O. Box 15588 Salt Lake City, Utah 84115 (801) 262-2688		X					
Squibb Pharmaceutical Company E. R. Squibb & Sons, Inc. P.O. Box 4000 Princeton, New Jersey 08540 (609) 921-4000			X				
Stewart-Riess Laboratories 18740 Oxnard Street Tarzana, California 91356 (213) 705-4300				X	X		
Stuart Pharmaceuticals P.O. Box 751 Wilmington, Delaware 19897 (800) 441-7758			X		X		
Superior Plastic Products Corporation Cumberland Industrial Park Cumberland, Rhode Island 02864 (401) 333-6061		X					
Travenol Laboratories, Inc. One Baxter Parkway Deerfield, Illinois 60015 (312) 948-2000		X	X	X	X		X
United Hospital Supply Corporation 1901 Route 130 P.O. Box 516 Burlington, New Jersey 08016 (609) 387-7580						X	
Valleylab, Inc. 5920 Longbow Drive P.O. Box 9015 Boulder, Colorado 80301 (303) 530-2300				X	X		
Wescor, Inc. 459 South Main Street Logan, Utah 84321 (801) 752-6011	X						
Wheaton Scientific (Wheaton Instruments) 1000 North Tenth Street Millville, New Jersey 08332 (609) 825-1400					X		

tem is limited in that it can be used by only one patient at a time. Such a system is advantageous for the patient who requires frequent weight measurement and is restricted to bed.

The second type of portable scale is one in which some type of stretcher or platform is placed under the patient and then a mechanized device lifts both the platform and the patient. A digital readout provides the patient's weight (Scale-Tronix, Wheaton, Illinois). The disadvantage of this system is that the patient must be moved, albeit only a small amount. The advantage of the system is that it can be transported rapidly from patient to patient. Disposable covers for the stretcher are available to avoid contamination.

Patient height is best determined by standing the patient against a truly vertical surface to which a measuring device has been permanently attached. The movable measuring rods attached to scales are less accurate. Further description of height and weight equipment has been provided by Murray.[2, 3] Information relative to average weights of men and women by height and age groups is available (Society of Actuaries, Chicago).

Other Measurements

Additional anthropometric information is obtained by using a caliper for a triceps skinfold determination and by using a tape measure for midarm circumference. Calipers range from the relatively inexpensive plastic (actually provided free) McGaw caliper and Ross adipometer to the more sophisticated spring-loaded metallic calipers such as the Lange or Holtain calipers. As would be expected, the more sophisticated calipers are more precise.[4] They are calibrated to a constant tension of 10 gm/mm^2 over a range of 2 to 40 mm of caliper openings on a contact area of 20 to 40 mm^2 and should read to $\pm$ 0.1 mm accuracy.[2] Tapes should be non-stretchable and should be manufactured from metal, paper, or fiberglass—but not from cloth.

Klidjian and associates[5] have measured grip strength as an assessment parameter, using a simple hand-grip dynamometer (Asimow, Santa Monica, California, or Preston, Clifton, New Jersey), and have found it useful in detecting malnutrition. Along a similar principle, the quantification of hair pluckability by a hand-held spring dynamometer (Trichotillometer), as designed by Krumdieck, has been described.[6]

Additional nutritional assessment parameters have been measured using metabolic carts, pulmonary function testing equipment, neutron activation analysis, total body isotope determination, and both direct and indirect calorimetry. The instrumentation required for such sophisticated determinations is not readily available in the average clinical setting and is beyond the scope of this chapter.

VENOUS ACCESS EQUIPMENT

Access to the venous system for the provision of fluids, electrolytes, minerals, nutrients, and medications has been the hallmark of medical progress over the past few centuries. The materials used for such access necessarily reflect "state of the art" technology at any given moment, and therefore they constantly change.

The materials used in this equipment have characteristics that require the closest attention. They include (1) the tensile strength related to breakage of the access device; (2) the thrombogenicity of the device and its propensity for bacterial or fungal colonization, and (3) its ease of use for the practitioner.

Catheter Materials and Their Complications

Rosenbauer and Herzer[7] studied seven different types of used and unused intravenous catheters and found them all to be of sufficient strength to preclude the possibility of spontaneous breakage secondary to the manufacturing process. Breakage or catheter embolization is probably most often related to improper usage. The authors further describe aberrations in the external and internal physical characteristics of needles and catheters with the use of the scanning electron microscope (SEM). They conclude that rough surfaces of the introducers or catheter walls may induce endothelial lesions and further enhance thrombus formation. Bair and Petersen,[8] in a similar study of four different types of used plastic (Teflon) catheters, demonstrated sufficient surface imperfections to account for possible thrombogenic complications.

Additional publications, including those by Nachnani and coworkers,[9] Hecker and coworkers,[10] Spanos and Hecker,[11] and Sawyer and coworkers[12] all support the concept that surface irregularities contribute to thrombosis or thrombophlebitis. In testing 14 different polymer surfaces, consisting of those commercially available as well as those considered experimental, Sawyer and associates[12] concluded that the ethylene acrylic acid (EAA) copolymer was the most satisfactory for decreasing thrombogenicity and phlebitis.

In evaluating five different catheter materials and catheters with SEMs, Locci and colleagues[13] found irregularities that were large enough to trap particles 0.5 to 1μ in size. In a subsequent work,[14] these same investigators found an amorphous material collected in the irregularities within the catheter lumina, favoring the growth of *Acinetobacter*, and *Pseudomonas* and particularly favoring coagulase-negative staphylococci. In the third part of their investigation,[15] these authors demonstrated that microbial adherence to the inner catheter surface is directly related to the presence and frequency of irregularities, particularly when such irregularities were located against the flow.

Turning to more clinically oriented studies, Valerio and colleagues,[16] using polyvinylchloride catheters, found a 27 per cent incidence of occult significant thrombus and a 4.5 per cent incidence of clinically evident thrombus. Animal studies[17, 18] have suggested that the incidence of catheter fibrin sleeve formation is decreased in silicone-coated or heparin-bonded catheters. In studying complications related to long-term central vein catheterization (median 4.5 months), Ladefoged and associates[19] noted a lower incidence of both sepsis and thrombosis in silicone rubber catheters when compared with those made of polyvinylchloride. By contrast, Brismar and coworkers in studying the occurrence of fibrin sleeve formation[20] and the effect of heparin on catheter thrombosis[21] noted no difference in the occurrence of these complications when either silastic or polyvinylchloride catheters were used. McDonald and coworkers,[22] in a study of peripherally inserted silicone catheters for total parenteral nutrition (TPN), concluded that the least satisfactory were short needles and long peripherally placed central venous

polyvinyl catheters. They noted further that polyvinyl and silastic subclavian catheters were equally efficacious. The most satisfactory catheter in their experience was a long silicone elastomer catheter inserted peripherally.

Flexible plastic catheters have been in use since 1945. New materials are constantly being developed to improve the efficacy of these catheters. Short-term access to the venous system has primarily been via the jugular, subclavian, extremity, or femoral vein routes, and most of the catheter materials used for these routes are those described in the preceding paragraphs. There are many variations among different products when either facilitating removal of a needle or actually introducing the catheter. Thus, breakaway needles, drum catheters, guidewires, introducers, peel-away sheaths, and split-sheath introducers are representative of the myriad products currently available, and they are destined to be improved upon.

A special discussion concerning long-term indwelling subclavian catheters is in order. As can be imagined, special problems related to catheter infection and displacement are encountered when catheters must stay in place for months and years. All such catheters are made of silicone rubber. They are much longer (approximately 90 cm) than short-term catheters so that they can reach the right atrium and can also be tunneled under the skin of the chest. They have Dacron cuffs to stimulate adherence of the catheter to the surrounding tissues. Broviac and colleagues[23] first described such a catheter for use with prolonged parenteral alimentation. Further experience with this catheter is described by Fleming and coworkers,[24] and Pollack and coworkers.[25]

A modification of the Broviac catheter by Hickman that resulted in a thicker-walled, larger-lumen catheter has been described.[26] Further experience with this catheter has been described in detail by Johnstone,[27] Merritt and colleagues,[28] and Ivey and colleagues.[29]

A double-lumen right atrial catheter has also been described by Sanders and associates.[30] The larger Hickman and smaller Broviac catheters are fused together to perform dual purposes. The smaller lumen is used for total parenteral nutrition, whereas the larger lumen is designed for additional functions.

In a detailed study by Begala and associates,[31] the infection rate was found to be five times higher in patients with Hickman catheters than in those with Broviac catheters. The cause for this disparity was not clear and was thought to be possibly related to the larger lumen size of the Hickman catheter. (Hickman and Broviac Catheters are trademarks of Evermed, Medina, Washington.) Virtually all of the short-term and long-term catheters are manufactured to be radiopaque.

There are a variety of commercially prepared kits containing all of the necessary components for the insertion of parenteral nutrition catheters.

DRESSINGS

The purpose of the dressing is twofold: first, it secures the catheter so that it will not become dislodged, and second, it minimizes the risks of infection. In the earlier days of nutrition support, dressing supplies, which were available at nursing stations, consisted of sterile gauze pads, sterile antibiotic ointment, an antiseptic, sterile gloves, and nonsterile tape. It was recognized that a kit containing appropriate materials should be available. Such kits were prepared upon request by the central supply sections of hospitals. Their preparation, being rather labor-intensive, resulted in significant costs. Thus, with the advent of the mass production of commercially prepared dressing kits, costs fell, whereas safety and efficiency increased.

Materials Used in Dressings

Many different materials have been evaluated for their appropriateness. Elastoplast,[32] Stomahesive,[33] and OpSite[34] (transparent, semipermeable polyurethane) have all been described as useful catheter dressing materials. Adhesive tape in some form is probably still the most widely used material to secure catheters and dressings.

Dressing changes have been greatly facilitated by the commercially prepared kits, which in general contain the following: acetone-alcohol preparation swabsticks, providone-iodine solution and ointment, sterile sponges, and sterile gloves. Masks, scissors, and specific dressing materials may either be in the prepackaged kit or may be provided separately.

INFUSION DEVICES

To avoid complications with intravenous nutrition support fluids, it is desirable to use some form of mechanical control for regulating intravenous administration. The topic of infusion device technology is both confusing and rapidly changing.

Pipp,[35] Vanderveen,[36] Kitrenos and associates,[37] and Turco[38] have addressed those factors leading to inaccuracies in intravenous flow rates and those features that are most desirable in infusion devices.

Gravity-Flow Systems

Turco[38] notes that in gravity-flow intravenous systems, the flow may be altered by volume, size of the drip chamber orifice, viscosity of the solution, plastic clamps, final filters, patient blood pressure and movements, extravasation, clots, kinks, height of the container, and temperature of the solutions. In studying factors influencing intravenous infusion drip rates, Flack and Whyte[39] found changes in the patient's venous pressure to be the most important factor.

Mechanical Infusion Devices

In addressing the preceding variables, we can define those features that are most desirable in infusion devices. The physical characteristics are important, and the device should be small, portable, quiet, lightweight, easy to use, and attachable to an intravenous pole. The flow rate should be independent of patient movement, viscosity of fluid, and tubing characteristics. The device should have electrical characteristics that provide appropriate safety with both alternating and direct currents. Control characteristics should include accuracy rates of ± five per cent and must have a flow range from keep vein open (KVO) to at least 300 ml/hour.

Alarms that monitor for occlusion, air in the line, empty solution container, infiltration, loss of electricity, broken or disconnected tubing, and rate variation are desirable. Such alarms should have both visual and audible features. Cost and servicing features must be appropriate for the institution in which the device is to be used.

Significant confusion exists in understanding the different types of infusion devices. Controllers, having no moving components, work by gravity and count drops electronically. They may extrude volumes of fluid electronically or mechanically, but they do not pump fluids and are therefore more simple mechanically. For most intravenous fluid administration, controllers are probably adequate.

Pumps are usually of either the piston (syringe) or peristaltic type. Piston-type pumps have a cylinder upon which, after filling, pressure is exerted to expel the fluid. Peristaltic-type pumps exert pressure externally on the fluid-filled chamber. This latter type of pump can have the peristalsis applied in either a linear or a rotary fashion.

With the advent of home hyperalimentation, a mobile infusion pump has also been developed (Cormed, Medina, New York).

A disposable flow controlling device that allows for the simultaneous administration of different sterilized parenteral nutrition solutions has been described by Engels and colleagues.[40] An excellent detailed description by Turco of pumps and controllers is available.[41] Rithalia and Tinker[42] also provide a comprehensive review of infusion devices.

ANCILLARY INTRAVENOUS EQUIPMENT

Filters

The use of filters during the administration of intravenous fluids also remains confusing to many. Filters are intended to remove particulate matter and air, reduce the incidence of phlebitis, and prevent sepsis. Thus, the ideal filter is one that will remove particulate matter and pathogens such as bacteria and fungi and exclude air. Jemison-Smith and Belman[43] have presented an in-depth description of the various types of in-line filters as well as a comprehensive discussion of their usage.

Essentially filters are either air-eliminating or nonair-eliminating, which refers to the filter's ability to vent air out of the intravenous system. Both 5- and 1-μ pore filters are nonair-eliminating filters. Filters that are 0.45 and 0.22 μ may be either air-eliminating or nonair-eliminating.

Although nonair-eliminating filters are usually less expensive, they are more likely to have their pores obstructed by larger air bubbles, necessitating more frequent filter changes.

Air-eliminating filters incorporate hydrophobic vents and effectively prevent air blockage so that even 0.22-μ filters of this type do not require a pressure infusion device to guarantee flow. This type of filter will not allow air to enter a patient if the intravenous line runs dry.

Integral in-line filters are those that are manufactured as an integral component within the administration set. Their advantage is that they decrease the likelihood of contamination, which is inherent to adding a filter. Their disadvantage is that they are located at a distance from the terminal end of the intravenous line and, therefore, are not available to filter more distally placed additives. The add-on filter, as the name implies, is added to the system and provides versatility in that the filter can be added at the desired location.

In 1979, the National Coordinating Committee on Large Volume Parenterals (NCCLVP)[44] recommended the use of particulate and microbe retentive filters for hyperalimentation. The committee further recommended the use of filters for immunocompromised patients, for patients receiving many heavily particulated additives, and when benefits appear to outweigh risks.

The NCCLVP further advises that filters should *not* be used for drugs administered in doses or concentrations of less than 5 μg/ml or when the total dose is less than 5 mg over a 24-hour period, or when both of these situations exist. The Committee advises that a 1-μ filter may be adequate for hyperalimentation needs. This recommendation must constantly be re-evaluated in light of newer information. Parent[45] recommends the use of a 0.22-μ filter to be changed at 24-hour intervals and to be used in conjunction with an infusion pump for patients receiving hyperalimentation.

Holmes and colleagues[46] give further support to the use of a 0.22-μ filter to be replaced every 24 hours. It should be noted that 0.22-μ filters will be obstructed by blood, blood fractions, emulsions, and suspensions. In studying the effect of filtration on trace metals, Boddapati and coworkers[47] noted no deleterious effect.

Although numerous studies[48–51] are available that suggest decreased complications when in-line filters are used, continued literature surveillance will be required to objectively evaluate the benefit to patients and the cost-benefit value of such practice if applied universally.

Lastly, Tortorici and associates[52] studied standards of practice in 90 hospitals in reference to in-line filtration and learned that 79 per cent of hospitals filtered TPN, and of these 84 per cent used a 0.22-μ filter. Filters were changed daily by 86 per cent of those using filters, and infusion pumps were used by 91 per cent. The reasons given for non-use of filters by the respondents were cost (66 per cent), clogging (66 per cent), rupture with infusion pumps (25 per cent), and impedance of flow (25 per cent).

Plastic Containers

Plastic containers for intravenous solutions have many advantages over glass containers.[53, 54] They include decreased storage space requirements, decreased weight, increased resistance to breakage, and the absence of air entering the container. Although such containers are more vulnerable to puncture, such a violation is easily recognized. The use of a 3-L bag has been described as improving preparation and delivery of fluids.[55]

Disadvantages include the possibility of chemicals being leached from the plastic into solution and the possibility of adsorption of intravenous drugs to the plastic. Compatability studies for commonly used additives with plastic containers are required by the Food and Drug Administration (Federal Regulation 43:58557, Dec. 15, 1978).

Intravenous Administration Sets

Drop size and flow rates can vary substantially.[56, 57] Merrick and Merrick[58] found that the number of drops the intravenous sets were calibrated to deliver and the number actually delivered ranged from 2.2 to 3.0 per cent of that predicted for minidrip sets and 1.3 to 17.4 per cent for regular sets. Ferenchak and colleagues[59] demonstrated as much as a 25 per cent increase in drop size for rapid infusion rates when compared to slower rates. This relationship was found to be linear. Microdrop tips were found to exhibit less variation.

Miscellaneous Devices

Geiss[60] has described a unique antiair-embolism device that firmly holds the intravenous tubing into the hub of the catheter.

PHARMACY EQUIPMENT

There are numerous equipment items that are of value in the pharmacy preparation of TPN. Most are devices to assist in the sterile transfer of liquid materials and include transfer sets, filling sets, additive sets, adapters, various needles, syringe caps, plugs, connectors, stopcocks, filters, bottle covers, caps, and adhesive foil covers.

Devices for Total Parenteral Nutrition

A rather unique formulating device for TPN has been described by McClendon,[61] in which three sterile fluids can be pumped simultaneously into one container. Such a device was shown to reduce mean per cent error in compounding from 5.3 to 1.8 per cent. It was further shown to save preparation time as well as cost while decreasing the possibility of contamination.

The one device that has produced the most dramatic change in the preparation of hyperalimentation fluids is the laminar flow hood, a device that propels filtered air across the intravenous fluid preparation site and thereby decreases contamination. Such devices are of either the horizontal or the vertical type. The ability to so effectively decrease contamination has enabled many more patients to be treated than would have otherwise been possible. Most hoods are similar in structure and range in size from three to six feet in width. They remove virtually all (99.99%) particulate matter 0.3 μ or larger via the use of a double filter system. The first filter used is a fiberglass prefilter and the second is a high efficiency particulate air filter (HEPA). It is this latter filter that is responsible for the removal of organisms and particles 0.3 μ in size. There are many features of importance in the construction of such hoods. Some of the more important ones clinically include lighting, blower speed control, degree of vibration, pressure gauges, electrical convenience outlet and shelving.

HOME TOTAL PARENTERAL NUTRITION EQUIPMENT

Since 1968, when Dudrick and associates[62] fed the first patient at home exclusively by intravenous hyperalimentation, others have attempted to facilitate the administration of such cumbersome care.

Systems for the Home Setting

Broviac and Scribner,[63] Solassol and associates,[64] and Jeejeebhoy and associates[65] were among the early investigators who attempted to develop workable systems, with the one described by Solassol being portable. MacNab described a portable peristaltic rotary infusion system for children.[66]

Although many of the previously described infusion devices are suitable for use in the home setting, they restrict the patient's geographic mobility. Dudrick and MacFadyen[66] described a hyperalimentation vest for ambulatory patients. Current vests are of lightweight materials and have two pockets that each house a 500-ml reservoir bag. The bags join each other via a Y-tubing connector on the patient's pump and catheter. The mobile infusion pump (Cormed, Medina, New York) has a rechargeable power pack that can operate for approximately 48 hours. The flow range is from 600 to 5000 ml/24 hours, depending upon the model.

The advantages of a vest system are self-evident in allowing the patient mobility; however, the disadvantage relates to the inconvenience and potential discomfort of being encumbered with such an appliance.

Goldfarb and Slater[68] describe the basic materials required for home intravenous nutritional support, which include a volumetric pump system, an intravenous administration set with an air-eliminating (0.22 µ) in-line filter, appropriate dressings, needles, syringes, heparin, latex injection ports, connector tubing, Keto-Diastix, a thermometer, a device for the destruction of needles, and alcohol wipes.

RESOURCE MATERIALS

Equipment for use with parenteral nutrition is constantly being developed and incorporates those materials that become available through advanced technology.

Thus, the remainder of this chapter is devoted to providing the reader with those resource materials that will most likely provide continuing sources of information pertinent to new developments.

This resource material will be presented in two forms: a list of publications most closely identified with intravenous nutrition support equipment and an alphabetized, categorized table of manufacturers (Table 13–1). Both have been prepared with great diligence; however, the authors apologize in advance for any omissions, all of which were unintentional.

PUBLICATIONS

Journals

American Journal of Clinical Nutrition
9650 Rockville Pike
Bethesda, Maryland 20814

American Journal of Hospital Pharmacy
4630 Montgomery Avenue
Bethesda, Maryland 20814

American Journal of Intravenous Therapy and Clinical Nutrition
83 Peaceable Street
Georgetown, Connecticut 06829

Hospital Pharmacy
Lippincott/Harper, Publishers
Subscriber Services Department
2350 Virginia Avenue
Hagerstown, Maryland 21740

Infusion
34 Ridge Street
Winchester, Massachusetts 01890

Journal of the American College of Nutrition
Alan R. Liss, Inc.
150 Fifth Avenue
New York, New York 10011

Journal of the National Intravenous Therapy Association
Lippincott/Harper, Publishers
Subscriber Service Department
P.O. Box 1600
Hagerstown, Maryland 21740

Journal of Parenteral and Enteral Nutrition
The Williams & Wilkins Co.
428 E. Preston Street
Baltimore, Maryland 21202

Nutritional Support Services: The Journal of Practical Application in Clinical Nutrition
12849 Magnolia Boulevard
North Hollywood, California 91607

Resource Manuals

A.S.P.E.N. Product Resource Manual
Edition 2, Revised
May, 1982
American Society for Parenteral and Enteral Nutrition (A.S.P.E.N.)
8605 Cameron Street
Suite 500
Silver Springs, MD 20910
(301) 587-6315

Emergency Care Research Institute (ECRI)
Health Devices Sourcebook
5200 Butler Pike
Plymouth Meeting, Pennsylvania 19462
(215) 825-6000

Nutrition Support Services: The Journal of Practical Application in Clinical Nutrition
2:11, November, 1982
12849 Magnolia Boulevard
North Hollywood, California 91607
(213) 980-4184

Texts

Deitel, M.: Nutrition in Clinical Surgery. Baltimore, The Williams & Wilkins Co., 1980.

Fischer, J.: Total Parenteral Nutrition. Philadelphia, W. B. Saunders Co., 1976.

Rhoads, J.: The general principles of nutrition. In Textbook of Surgery, Edition 5. Vol. 1. Philadelphia, J.B. Lippincott, 1977.

Schneider, H.: Nutritional Support of Medical Practice. New York, Harper & Row, 1976.

Shils, M.E.: Total parenteral nutrition. In Goodhart, R.S., and Shils, M.E. (eds.): Modern Nutrition in Health and Disease, Edition 5. Philadelphia, Lea & Febiger, 1973.

Silberman, H., and Eisenberg, D.: Parenteral and Enteral Nutrition for the Hospitalized Patient. Norwalk, Connecticut, Appleton-Century-Crofts, 1982.

REFERENCES

1. Seltzer, M.H.: How to—materials and devices. J.P.E.N., 2:572–573, 1978.
2. Murray, R.L.: Discussion and critique of current methods in anthropometry, Part I. Nutri. Support Serv., 1:31–36, 1981.
3. Murray, R.L.: Discussion of techniques in anthropometry, Part II. Nutri. Support Serv., 2:11–14, 1982.
4. Burgert, S.L., and Anderson, C.F.: A comparison of triceps skinfold values as measured by the plastic McGaw caliper and Lange caliper. Am. J. Clin. Nutr., 32:1531–1533, 1979.
5. Klidjian, A.M., Foster, K.J., Kammerling, R.M. et al.: Relation of anthropometric and dynamometric variables to serious postoperative complications. Br. Med. J. 281:899–901, 1980.
6. Chase, E.S., Weinsier, R.L., Laven, G.T., and Krumdieck, C.L.: Trichotillometry: The quantification of hair pluckability as a method of nutritional assessment. Am. J. Clin. Nutr., 34:2280–2286, 1981.
7. Rosenbauer, K.A., and Herzer, J.A.: Surface morphology and tensile force at breaking point of different kinds of intravenous catheters before and after usage. In Johari, O. et al.: Scanning Electron Microscopy. Part III. Chicago, SEM Inc., AMF O'Hare, 1981, pages 125–130.
8. Bair, J.N., and Petersen, R.V.: Surface characteristics of plastic intravenous catheters. Am. J. Hosp. Pharm., 36:1707–1711, 1979.
9. Nachnani, G.H., Lessin, L.S., Motomiya, T. et al.: Scanning electron microscopy of thrombogenesis on vascular catheter surfaces. N. Engl. J. Med., 286:139–140, 1972.
10. Hecker, J.F., Fish, G.C., and Farrell, P.C.: Measurement of thrombus formation on intravenous catheters. Anaesth. Intensive Care, 4:225–231, 1976.
11. Spanos, H.G., and Hecker, J.F.: Thrombus formation on indwelling venous cannulae in sheep: effects of time, size and materials. Anaesth. Intensive Care, 4:217–224, 1976.
12. Sawyer, P.N., Ramsey, W., Stanczewski, B. et al.: A comparative study of several polymers for use as intravenous catheters. Med. Instrum., 11:221–230, 1977.
13. Locci, R., Peters, G., and Pulverer, G.: Microbial colonization of prosthetic devices. I. Microtopographical characteristics of intravenous catheters as detected by scanning electron microscopy. Zentrabl. Bakteriol., 173:285–292, 1981.
14. Peters, G., Locci, R., and Pulverer, G.: Microbial colonization of prosthetic devices. II. Scanning electron microscopy of naturally infected intravenous catheters. Zentrabl. Bakteriol., 173:293–299, 1981.
15. Locci, R., Peters, G., and Pulverer, G.: Microbial colonization of prosthetic devices. III. Adhesion of staphylococci to lumina of intravenous catheters

perfused with bacterial suspensions. Zentrabl. Bakteriol., *173*:300–307, 1981.

16. Valerio, D., Hussey, J.K., and Smith, F.W.: Central vein thrombosis associated with intravenous feeding—A prospective study. J.P.E.N., *5*:240–241, 1981.

17. Welch, G.W., McKell, D.W., Silverstein, P. et al.: The role of catheter composition in the development of thrombophlebitis. Surg. Gynecol. Obstet., *138*:221–242, 1974.

18. Hoshal, V.L., Ause, R.G., and Hoskins, P.A.: Fibrin sleeve formation on indwelling subclavian venous catheters. Arch. Surg., *102*:353–358, 1971.

19. Ladefoged, K., Efsen, F., Krogh Christoffersen, J., and Jarnum, S.: Long-term parenteral nutrition. II. Catheter-related complications. Scand. J. Gastroenterol., *16*:913–919, 1981.

20. Brismar, B., Hardstedt, D., and Jacobson, S.: Diagnosis of thrombosis by catheter phlebography after prolonged central venous catheterization. Ann. Surg., *194*:779–983, 1981.

21. Brismar, B., Hardstedt, C., Jacobson, S. et al.: Reduction of catheter associated thrombosis in parenteral nutrition by intravenous heparin therapy. Arch. Surg., *117*:1196–1199, 1982.

22. MacDonald, A.S., Master, S.K.P., and Moffitt, E.A.: A comparative study of peripherally inserted silicone catheters for parenteral nutrition. Can. Anaesth. Soc. J. *24*:263–269, 1977.

23. Broviac, J.W., Cole, J.J., and Scribner, B.H.: A silicone rubber atrial catheter for prolonged parenteral alimentation. Surg. Gynecol. Obstet., *136*:602–606, 1973.

24. Fleming, C.R., Witzke, D.J., and Beart, R.W., Jr.: Catheter related complications in patients receiving home parenteral nutrition. Ann. Surg., *192*:593–599, 1980.

25. Pollack, P.F., Kadden, M., Byrne, W.J. et al.: 100 patient years' experience with the Broviac silastic catheter for central venous nutrition. J.P.E.N., *5*:32–36, 1981.

26. Hickman, R.O., Buckner, C.D., Clift, R.A. et al.: A modified right atrial catheter for access to the venous system in marrow transplant recipients. Surg. Gynecol. Obstet., *148*:871–875, 1979.

27. Johnstone, J.D.: Infrequent infections associated with Hickman catheters. Cancer Nurs., *5*:125–129, 1982.

28. Merritt, R.J., Ennis, C.E., Andrassy, R.J. et al.: Use of Hickman right atrial catheter in pediatric oncology patients. J.P.E.N., *5*:83–85, 1981.

29. Ivey, M.F., Adams, S.M., Hickman, R.O., and Gibson, D.L.: Right atrial indwelling catheters for patients requiring long term intravenous therapy. Am. J. Hosp. Pharm., *35*:1525–1527, 1978.

30. Sanders, J.E., Hickman, R.O., Aker, S. et al.: Experience with double lumen right atrial catheters. J.P.E.N., *6*:95–99, 1982.

31. Begala, J.E., Maher, K., and Cherry, J.D.: Risk of infection associated with the use of broviac and Hickman catheters. Am. J. Infect. Control., *10*:17–23, 1982.

32. Schwartz-Fulton, J., Colley, R., Valanis, B., and Fischer, J.E.: Hyperalimentation dressings and skin flora. J. Nat. Intraven. Ther. Assoc. (NITA), *4*:354–357, 1981.

33. McKenney, M.: Stomahesive dressing change procedure. Nutrit. Support Serv., *2*:53–54, 1982.

34. Palidar, P.J., Simonowitz, D.A., Oreskovich, M.R. et al.: Use of OpSite as an occlusive dressing for total parenteral nutrition catheters. J.P.E.N., *6*:150–151, 1982.

35. Pipp, T.L.: Intravenous infusion pumps—justification and selection and utilization. Infusion, *2*:45–57, 1978.

36. Vanderveen, T.W.: Consideration in infusion device usage. Am. J. Intraven. Ther., *5*:16–44, 1978.

37. Kitrenos, J.G., Jones, M., and McCleod, D.C.: Comparison of selected intravenous infusion pumps and rate regulators. Am. J. Hosp. Pharm., *35*:304–310, 1978.

38. Turco, S.J.: Inaccuracies in I.V. flow rates and the use of pumps and controllers. J. Parent. Drug Assoc., *32*:242–248, 1978.

39. Flack, F.C., and Whyte, T.D.: Behavior of standard gravity-fed administration sets used for intravenous infusion. Br. Med. J., *3*:439–443, 1974.

40. Engels, L.G.J., Bakker, J.H., Kapteyns, W.G., and van Tongeren, J.H.M.: An accurate flow controlling device to administer simultaneously different parenteral nutrition solutions. Am. J. Clin. Nutr., *35*:338–341, 1982.

41. Turco, S.: Mechanical and electronic equipment for parenteral and enteral use: An update. Am. J. Intraven. Ther., *9*:17–39, 1982.

42. Rithalia, S.V.S., and Tinker, J.: Recent developments in infusion devices. Br. J. Hosp. Med., *25*:69–75, 1981.

43. Jemison-Smith, P., and Belman, B.: Inline I.V. filters. Crit. Care Update, *8*:26–33, 1981.

44. National Coordinating Committee on Large Volume Parenterals: Problems and Benefits of Inline Filtration. Infusion, *4*:13–17, 1980.

45. Parent, B.: Filtration and TPN. Nutri. Support Serv., *2*:36–38, 1982.

46. Holmes, C.J., Kundsin, R.B., Ausman, R.K., and Walter, C.W.: Potential hazards associated with microbial contamination of in-line filters during intravenous therapy. J. Clin. Microbiol., *12*:725–731, 1980.

47. Boddapati, S., Yang, K., and Murty, R.: Intravenous solution compatibility and filter-retention characteristics of trace-element preparations. Am. J. Hosp. Pharm., *38*:1731–1736, 1981.

48. Biuins, B.A., Rapp, R.P., Deluca, P.P., McKean, H., and Griffen, W.O.: Final inline filtration: A means of decreasing the incidence of infusion phlebitis. Surgery, *85*:388–394, 1979.

49. Rusho, W.J., and Bair, J.N.: Effect of filtration on complications of postoperative intravenous therapy. Am. J. Hosp. Pharm., *36*:1355–1356, 1979.

50. Miller, R.C., and Grogan, J.B.: Efficacy of inline bacterial filters in reducing contamination of intravenous nutritional solutions. Am. J. Surg., *130*:585–589, 1975.

51. Ryan, P.B., Rapp, R.P., DeLuca, P.P. et al.: Inline final filtration—A method of minimizing contamination in intravenous therapy. Bull. Parent. Drug Assoc., *27*:1–14, 1973.

52. Tortorici, M., Nitschke, D., Heim, A. et al.: Survey of standards of practice for in-line filtration. Infusion, *5*:105–109, 1981.

53. Lamnin, M.: Advantages of plastic intravenous fluid containers. Am. J. Hosp. Pharm., *34*:1042, 1977.

54. Plastic containers for intravenous solutions. Med. Lett., *22*:43–44, 1980.

55. Fielding, L.P., Humfress, A., Mouchizadeh, J. et al.: Experience with three-litre bags. Pharmaceut. J., *226*:590–592, 1981.
56. Adelberg, H.: Intravenous administration sets. Arch. Intern. Med., *140*:133, 1980.
57. Kind, A.C., Williams, D.N., Persons, G., and Gibson, J.A.: Intravenous antibiotic therapy at home. Arch. Intern. Med., *139*:413–415, 1979.
58. Merrick, I.M., and Merrick, T.E.: Comparison of drop sizes of intravenous administration sets. Am. J. Hosp. Pharm., *37*:1346–1350, 1980.
59. Ferenchak, P., Collins, J.J., and Morgan, A.: Drop size and rate in parenteral infusion. Surgery, *70*:674–677, 1971.
60. Geiss, A.C.: Device to prevent complication of air embolism in parenteral nutrition and central venous catheterization. J.P.E.N., *3*:383–384, 1979.
61. McClendon, R.R.: Clinical evaluation of the I.V. 6500 formulator for fabricating TPN solutions. Am. J. Intraven. Ther. Clin. Nutr., *8*:17–20, 1981.
62. Dudrick, S.J., Englert, D.M., Van Buren, C.T., et al.: New concepts of ambulatory home hyperalimentation. J.P.E.N., *3*:72–76, 1979.
63. Broviac, J.W., and Scribner, B.H.: Prolonged parenteral nutrition in the home. Surg. Gynecol. Obstet., *139*:24–28, 1974.
64. Solassol, C., Joyeux, H., Mion, C., and Sausse, A.: A compact portable prosthesis for total parenteral nutrition (T.P.N.): Ambulatory parenteral feeding in the hospital and home. Trans. Am. Soc. Artific. Intern. Organs, *20A*:33–37, 1974.
65. Jeejeebhoy, K.N., Langer, B., Tsallas, G., et al.: Total parenteral nutrition at home: Studies in patients surviving 4 months to 5 years. Gastroenterology, *71*:943–953, 1976.
66. MacNab, A.J.: A portable infusion system for the ambulant child. J. Pediatr., *88*:654–658, 1976.
67. Dudrick, S.J., and MacFadyen, B.V., Jr.: A vest for ambulatory patients receiving hyperalimentation. Surg. Gynecol. Obstet., *148*:587–590, 1979.
68. Goldfarb, I.W., and Slater, H.: Techniques of administration. Am. J. Intraven. Ther. Clin. Nutr., *8*:25–34, 1981.

CHAPTER 14

Parenteral Nutrition Solutions

NANCY LOUIE
PAUL W. NIEMIEC

Several types of intravenous solutions are used in parenteral nutrition therapy. Energy balance and tissue synthesis require adequate protein, carbohydrate, fat, water, electrolyte, vitamin, and mineral components. Numerous parenteral nutrition products have been developed to provide these basic components. The number of products continues to increase as manufacturers meet the demands of clinical research and its advances toward individualization of parenteral nutrition formulas. Formulations may have general or specific indications. A thorough understanding of the indications along with that of product availability and formulation is essential to maximize the clinical application of parenteral nutrition theories.

Parenteral nutrition solutions, like other intravenous solutions, are available sterile, pyrogen-free, and free of particulate matter. Manufacturer precautions assure the delivery of a safe and effective single-component product. However, most parenteral nutrition components require admixture before they are administered. Organized admixture services can play an important role in the proper ordering, handling, and admixture of parenteral nutrition solutions.

Additional concerns arise with increasing interest in the use of parenteral nutrition solutions as drug delivery vehicles. Chemical stability and physical compatibility of both the parenteral nutrition components and the drug product should ideally be demonstrated before they are combined in the final solution.

This chapter describes and evaluates available parenteral nutrition solution products, solution admixture, scientific data regarding stability and compatibility of parenteral nutrition additives and components, and solution ordering procedures.

PARENTERAL NUTRITION PRODUCTS

Commercial products have been formulated to provide basic parenteral nutrition components. These components and their available substrates are listed in Table 14–1. Nutrition components are available as combined or single-substrate products. More recently, premixed solutions of combined nutrition components have become available. Although product availability will no doubt continue to change with advances in clinical research and product formulation, current commercially available nutrition components are described in the following section.

Energy Sources

Dextrose

Dextrose (glucose) is the most commonly used energy substrate for parenteral nutrition. It offers the advantages of being readily available, inexpensive, and efficiently metabolized in most patients. Dextrose may serve as the only nonprotein caloric source during parenteral nutrition. One gram of dextrose had been traditionally calculated as providing 3.75 kcal. However, commercially available dextrose is in the monohydrate form, which provides approximately 91 per cent of the caloric density of dextrose. Each gram of dextrose monohydrate provides 3.4 kcal, giving it a relatively low caloric density as an energy source. A liter of ten per cent dextrose

Table 14–1. BASIC NUTRIENT COMPONENTS
AND THEIR SUBSTRATES

COMPONENT	SUBSTRATES
Energy	Dextrose
	Fat
	Glycerol
	Fructose
	Invert sugar
	Alcohol
Protein	Crystalline amino acids
Essential fatty acids	Fat
Electrolytes	Salts of:
	Sodium
	Potassium
	Magnesium
	Calcium
	Chloride
	Phosphate
	Acetate
Vitamins	Fat-soluble:
	A
	D
	E
	K
	Water-soluble:
	Thiamine
	Riboflavin
	Pyridoxine
	Cyanocobalamin
	Ascorbic acid
	Folic acid
	Nicotinic acid
	Biotin
	Pantothenic acid
Trace minerals	Zinc
	Copper
	Manganese
	Chromium
	Iodine
	Selenium
	Molybdenum

provides only 340 kcal/liter. In order to increase caloric intake, dextrose solutions in parenteral nutrition are usually concentrated and thus hypertonic. The high osmolarity of concentrated dextrose solutions requires that precautions to minimize vein irritation be made upon administration. Normal serum osmolarity ranges from 275 to 295 mOsm/kg.[1] Dextrose solutions with osmolarities exceeding approximately 300 mOsm/L are defined as hypertonic. Hypertonicity and perhaps also the acidic pH of concentrated dextrose solutions warrant their administration via large veins such as the superior vena cava.[2] Peripheral vein tolerance to the hypertonic solution is highly patient-dependent, but administration is generally poorly tolerated as solution osmolarities approach 800 to 900 mOsm/L.

Admixed parenteral nutrition solutions rarely exceed 50 per cent final dextrose concentrations. Available concentrations of dextrose solutions are outlined in Table 14–2. Most adult standard formulas use a final dextrose concentration of 25 to 35 per cent, equivalent to a dextrose osmolarity of 1200 to 1700 mOsm/L. This high osmolarity precludes peripheral vein administration. A final dextrose concentration of 10 per cent is the maximum concentration generally administered via peripheral veins. Further administration considerations of the final dextrose/amino acid solution are discussed along with crystalline amino acids.

The acid pH of commercially available dextrose solutions is essential to ensure stability during autoclave sterilization and solution storage. Dextrose solution pH is approximately 3.5 to 5.5. Carmelization with discoloring of the solution may occur at higher pH ranges.[3] Dextrose solutions are made by several manufacturers and are available in filled glass bottles or plastic bags and also partially filled containers that simplify admixture. Like other large-volume solutions intended for intravenous use, dextrose solutions contain no bacteriostatic or antimicrobial agents. Strict aseptic admixture techniques must be exercised to maintain solution sterility. Aseptic admixture and antimicrobial growth potential of parenteral nutrition solutions are discussed further in a subsequent section of this chapter. Commercially avail-

Table 14–2. DEXTROSE SOLUTION DESCRIPTION

PREDILUTION CONCENTRATION	HYDROUS DEXTROSE (gm/100 ml)	KCAL/L	APPROXIMATE CALCULATED OSMOLARITY (mOsm/L)
10% dextrose	10	340	505
20% dextrose	20	680	1010
30% dextrose	30	1020	1515
40% dextrose	40	1360	2020
50% dextrose	50	1700	2525
60% dextrose	60	2040	3030
70% dextrose	70	2380	3535

able dextrose solutions may be stored at room temperature and should be protected from freezing and extreme heat.

Fat

Fat emulsions are utilized in parenteral nutrition as an energy source and as a source of essential fatty acids. Experimentation with intravenous fat emulsions occurred as early as the 1920s, when the Japanese experimented with fat emulsions consisting of butter fat and cod liver oil. Intravenous fat was used in the United States in the 1940s,[4] and a commercially available fat emulsion of cottonseed oil for parenteral administration was first marketed in the 1950s; this product was subsequently withdrawn from the market in the early 1960s owing to a high incidence of toxic reactions. A nontoxic intravenous soybean emulsion was developed in 1961.[5] Several intravenous fat emulsions are commercially available; they are compared in Table 14–3. Safflower oil contains a greater percentage of linoleic acid and very little linolenic acid compared with soybean oil. The clinical significance of this difference is not defined, as linolenic acid may be formed from the essential fatty acid linoleic acid. However, reformulations of commercially available fat emulsion products now provide low-dose linolenic acid from all major manufacturers. Thus, selection of a commercial fat emulsion product may be based on cost, availability, and, perhaps, compatibility.

All fat emulsion products contain significant amounts of the essential fatty acid linoleic acid. For an adult, it is generally recommended that four to ten per cent of the total weekly caloric intake be infused as fat emulsion.[6] This is equivalent to providing two to three bottles of 500 ml each of ten per cent fat emulsion per week to an adult patient.

Fat emulsions may also serve as useful energy sources, offering several advantages. Fat emulsions have a high caloric density (9 kcal/gm). Also, they are rendered isotonic by the addition of glycerin. Isotonicity allows administration by peripheral vein. This advantage is often utilized for short-term administration of parenteral nutrition solutions by peripheral veins. When infused continuously with the hypertonic dextrose/amino acid solution, the isotonic fat emulsion is used to reduce the overall osmolarity presented to the vein and, thus, to increase patient tolerance of peripheral vein

administration. Fat is also utilized as an energy source in parenteral nutrition administered by central vein in, for example, patients with poor glucose tolerance or fluid restriction, and patients on ventilators with large respiratory quotients from carbohydrate metabolism. In addition to appropriate clinical indications, adequate fat clearance, percentage of total calories as fat, and cost of therapy should be considered when fat is used as a caloric source. The maximum recommended daily intake of fat calories is 60 per cent of the total infused calories, with the remaining 40 per cent supplied as carbohydrate and protein. A 500-ml bottle of 10 or 20 per cent fat emulsion provides 550 kcal or 1000 kcal, equivalent to 1.1 or 2.0 kcal/ml, respectively.

Fat emulsions have not traditionally been admixed with other components of the parenteral nutrition solution because of reported physical instability of the emulsions and the likelihood that divalent cations such as calcium and magnesium may further interfere.[7–10] Fat emulsions may be "piggybacked" to the dextrose/amino solution using a distal intravenous tubing injection site or "Y" set. If a final in-line filter is being used for parenteral nutrition solution administration, the fat emulsion must be piggybacked below the filter, because the emulsion particle size exceeds the filter pore size. A phthalate-free administration set is advisable for patients receiving frequent fat emulsion administration.[7–10] Otherwise, during infusion, fat may extract diethyl hexyl phthalate, a plasticizer in conventional administration sets. Special admixture equipment and techniques commonly utilized in Europe[11] and Canada allow all parenteral nutrition components, including fat, to be admixed and administered in one bag. The compatibility, stability, and growth potential considerations for this combined formulation are discussed in the solution admixture section of this chapter.

A test dose of fat emulsion is recommended prior to the full infusion. In adults, 10 per cent fat emulsion should be infused at a rate of 1 ml/min for the first 15 to 30 minutes, or 20 per cent fat emulsion at a rate of 0.5 ml/min for the first 15 to 30 minutes. The remainder of a 500-ml bottle of 10 per cent fat emulsion should be infused over at least four hours. In pediatric patients, a test dose of 10 per cent fat emulsion should be infused at a rate of 0.1 ml/min for 15 to 20 minutes, or a 20 per cent fat emulsion at a rate of 0.05 ml/min. The maximum fat infu-

Table 14-3. COMMERCIAL FAT EMULSION PRODUCTS

	INTRALIPID 10% (KABI VITRUM)	LIPOSYN II 10% (ABBOTT)	SOYACAL 10% (ALPHA THERAPEUTIC)	TRAVAMULSION 10% (TRAVENOL)	INTRALIPID 20% (KABI VITRUM)	LIPOSYN II 20% (ABBOTT)	SOYACAL 20% (ALPHA THERAPEUTIC)
Oil	*Soybean*	*Safflower and Soybean*	*Soybean*	*Soybean*	*Soybean*	*Safflower and Soybean*	*Soybean*
Fatty Acid Content (%)							
Linoleic	54.0	65.8	49.0–60.0	56.0	50.0	65.8	49.0–60.0
Oleic	26.0	17.7	21.0–26.0	23.0	26.0	17.7	21.0–26.0
Palmitic	9.0	8.8	9.0–13.0	11.0	10.0	8.8	9.0–13.0
Linolenic	8.0	4.2	6.0–9.0	6.0	9.0	4.2	6.0–9.0
Stearic	0	3.4	3.0–5.0	0.0	0	3.4	3.0–5.0
Egg Yolk Phospholipids (%)	1.2	1.2	1.2	1.22	1.2	1.2	1.2
Glycerin (%)	2.25	2.5	2.21	2.25	2.25	2.5	2.21
Calories/ml	1.1	1.1	1.1	1.1	2.0	2.0	2.0
Osmolarity (mOsm/L)	280	320	280	270	330	340	315
How Supplied (ml)	50, 100, 500	25, 50, 100, 200, 500	250, 500	500	50, 100, 250, 500	25, 50, 200, 500	250

sion load in pediatrics is 1 gm/kg over four hours; the total daily dose should not exceed 4 gm/kg body weight. As in adults, a maximum of 60 per cent of the total calories received should be infused as fat.[7] Fat emulsions may be stored at room temperature but should be protected from freezing and extreme heat.

Glycerol

Glycerol (glycerin) is a naturally occurring sugar alcohol. Small amounts (2.21 to 2.50 per cent) of glycerin are contained in fat emulsions, but glycerol has not commonly been utilized as an energy source. Numerous investigators have studied glycerol metabolism and utilization. It has a caloric density of 4.32 kcal/gm and appears to have the same metabolic effect on protein breakdown as assessed by urinary nitrogen loss that fat emulsion does.[12] However, its introduction as a single energy source in parenteral nutrition is relatively recent. Glycerol is now marketed as the sole energy source (three per cent glycerol) in a premixed solution combined with three per cent amino acids and electrolytes. The product is intended for nutritional maintenance in postoperative protein sparing therapy.[13] Toxicities from intravenous administration of low-dose glycerol (three per cent) are much less common than those associated with high or low dose of glycerol administered subcutaneously.[14] However, the use of this product should be preceded by assessment of individual patient nutritional requirements and further cost-benefit considerations.

Fructose

Fructose, a ketohexose, is a naturally occurring monosaccharide that may be used as a source of carbohydrate calories in parenteral nutrition. Fructose has been widely used in combination with glucose and xylitol in Europe,[15] but its use in the United States has not yet gained popularity. A ten per cent fructose (levulose) in water solution and five and ten per cent fructose in water solutions with electrolytes are available for intravenous administration. The ten per cent solution without electrolytes is hypertonic at 555 mOsm/L and provides 375 to 400 kcal/L, or 3.75 to 4.00 kcal/gm of fructose.[16] Fructose offers several advantages over dextrose as a calorie source: It does not require insulin for phosphorylation and conversion to glucose

and thus may be more efficiently metabolized even by patients with insulin deficiency; it is more readily converted to glycogen; and it produces lower serum glucose levels and less glycosuria than similar doses of dextrose.[13, 17] Its use as a single energy source is limited by total dose and infusion rate. Fructose is contraindicated in patients with fructose intolerance and also should not be used in the therapy of acute hypoglycemia.[16] Side effects of fructose administration, including uricemia, lactic acidosis, and hypophosphatemia, are related to total dose and rate of infusion.[15] A dose of 0.25 gm/kg/hr is recommended.[15] A maximum delivery of 1 gm/kg/hr should not be exceeded in either infants or adults.[16]

Invert Sugar

Invert sugar is composed of equal parts of dextrose (glucose) and fructose (levulose). Although infrequently associated with parenteral nutrition therapy, invert sugar may be used as a carbohydrate energy source. The combination of sugars results in better carbohydrate utilization. Invert sugar is available in 5 and 10 per cent solutions with electrolytes and a 5 per cent solution without electrolytes.[18] The 5 and 10 per cent solutions with electrolytes are hypertonic at approximately 400 mOsm/L and 800 mOsm/L, respectively.[18] The 5 per cent invert sugar in water solution is isotonic at 278 mOsm/L. Invert sugar has a caloric density of approximately 4 kcal/gm.[18]

Alcohol

Administration of alcohol may increase caloric intake, but alcohol is not recommended as a caloric source in parenteral nutrition. It has a relatively high caloric density, 7.0 kcal/gm, but it may be associated with adverse effects if infused too rapidly, may interact significantly with drug therapy, and may aggravate or worsen a patient's disease state.

Other Energy Substrates

Sorbitol and xylitol may also serve as alternative fuel sources; however, their use in parenteral nutrition remains limited.

Sorbitol (D-glucitol) is a naturally occurring hexitol or sugar alcohol. Its metabolic fate is similar to that of fructose.[19] Like fructose, it does not cause increased insulin production or hyperglycemia upon administration. However, its use is not favored in parenteral nutrition because it does not offer any advantage over fructose.[20]

Xylitol is a nonglucose carbohydrate that has long been investigated as a potential calorie source in parenteral nutrition. It offers several of the same metabolic advantages as fructose; the initial step has little or no insulin dependence, glycogen formation occurs independent of plasma glucose levels, and it has an antiketogenic effect.[20] *In vitro* investigations demonstrate that xylitol may selectively feed the normal cell over the cancer cell in the hepatoma model.[20] However, the toxicity of xylitol in hyperosmolar solutions or at high infusion rates has limited its use in humans.[21]

Protein Sources

Crystalline Amino Acids

Amino acids are currently the most commonly utilized source of nitrogen in parenteral nutrition. Nitrogen for protein synthesis was originally provided by hydrolysates of naturally occurring proteins (fibrin, casein). Protein hydrolysates require further breakdown by the liver prior to their utilization in protein synthesis. Incomplete hydrolysis (85 per cent utilizable nitrogen), resulting in a large concentration of dipeptides and tripeptides, poor utilization of the nitrogen, and a high incidence of elevated blood ammonia levels, has put protein hydrolysates in disfavor. They are infrequently utilized in parenteral nutrition today. Crystalline or synthetic amino acids, which are 100 per cent utilizable and may be used directly to build protein, have replaced the earlier-used hydrolysates.

Commercially available crystalline amino acid solutions provide, in a concentrated form, a physiologic ratio of biologically utilizable substrates for protein synthesis. Solutions contain a combination of essential (40 to 50 per cent) and nonessential (50 to 60 per cent) amino acids. Commercially available amino acid concentrations are listed in Table 14–4. Representative solutions available from three manufacturers are compared in Table 14–5. The products differ in their available concentrations, individual amino acid profiles, and electrolyte profiles. In addition, several products are available that contain premixed maintenance electrolytes. The

Table 14–4. COMMERCIALLY AVAILABLE AMINO ACID CONCENTRATIONS

MANUFACTURER	CONCENTRATIONS AVAILABLE (%)
Abbott Laboratories (Aminosyn)	3.5, 5, 7*, 8.5*, 10
Cutter Biological (Novamine)	8.5, 11.4
McGaw Laboratories (FreAmine)	3*, 8.5, 10
Travenol Laboratories, Inc. (Travasol)	5.5*, 8.5*, 10

*Available with electrolytes.

maintenance electrolyte contents of two representative solutions are shown in Table 14–6.

The availability of a wide range of amino acid concentrations facilitates compounding of parenteral nutrition solutions to meet individual patient needs. Significant differences in amino acid profile between the commercially available general amino acid products are few. Products differ slightly in the amounts of essential and nonessential amino acids, but the clinical significance of these differences has not been demonstrated for the general amino acids. The presence of small amounts of glutamic and aspartic acids, two nonessential amino acids that are metabolically very reactive, may be desirable; however, superiority of solutions containing them has not yet been demonstrated.[22, 23] The presence of cysteine may be preferable in neonates who lack the enzyme necessary to form cysteine from methionine. Cysteine is unstable over time, however, and eventually is converted to insoluble cystine.[24] Thus, any advantage of commercial general amino acid solutions that include cysteine upon manufacture may be diminished upon storage.

A more significant difference in amino acid products in the past was electrolyte content. This was of greater concern with products containing chloride salt forms of amino acid. The high chloride load frequently led to complications of hyperchloremic acidosis. These products have been reformulated to provide amino acids in their free-base forms. Clinical comparison of two different commercial amino acid products found no significant difference in nitrogen balance, measurements of renal function, liver function, or acid-base balance.[25] However, considerable differences between amino acid products lie in the area of drug and nutrient stability and compatibility; this topic is discussed in detail later in this chapter.

Table 14–5. COMPOSITION OF FOUR COMMERCIAL AMINO ACID SOLUTIONS
(8.5 PER CENT CONCENTRATIONS)

	AMINOSYN 8.5% (ABBOTT)	FREAMINE III 8.5% (McGAW)	NOVAMINE 8.5% (CUTTER)	TRAVASOL 8.5% (TRAVENOL)
L-Amino acids (gm/100 ml)	8.5	8.5	8.5	8.5
Total nitrogen (gm/100 ml)	1.3	1.3	1.35	1.4
Osmolarity (mOsm/L)(calculated)	850	810	785	860
Approximate pH	5.3	6.5	5.6	6.0
Essential amino acids (mg/100 ml)				
L-Leucine	810	770	590	526
L-Isoleucine	620	590	420	406
L-Valine	680	560	550	590
L-Phenylalanine	380	480	590	526
L-Tryptophan	150	130	140	152
L-Methionine	340	450	420	492
L-Threonine	460	340	420	356
L-Lysine	624	620	673	492
Nonessential amino acids (mg/100 ml)				
L-Alanine	1100	600	1200	1760
L-Arginine	850	810	840	880
L-Histidine	260	240	500	372
L-Proline	750	950	500	356
L-Serine	370	500	340	—
L-Tyrosine	44	—	20	34
L-Glutamic acid	—	—	420	—
L-Aspartic acid	—	—	250	—
Glycine (AAA, USP)	1100	1190	590	1760
Cysteine	—	20	40	—
Electrolytes				
Sodium (mEq/500 ml)	—	5	—	—
Potassium (mEq/500 ml)	2.7	—	—	—
Magnesium (mEq/500 ml)	—	—	—	—
Chloride (mEq/500 ml)	17.5	1.5	—	17
Acetate (mEq/500 ml)	45	36	—	26
Phosphate (mM/L)	—	5	—	—

General amino acid solutions are available as single, usually 500-ml or 1000-ml volume units, in glass or plastic containers. They are also available in "TPN kits," which contain 500 ml of dextrose in a partially filled one-liter container, 500 ml of amino acid solution, and a transfer set to facilitate admixture of the two base components into the one-liter bottle. Amino acid solutions may be stored at room temperature but should be protected from freezing or extreme heat. In addition, all amino acid solutions that contain tryptophan, which is photolabile, should be protected from light in order to increase its stability. Amino acid products generally have a shelf life of one to two years when stored properly unopened.

Protein Sparing. Lower-concentration (3.0 to 5.5 per cent) general amino acid solutions with maintenance electrolytes have

Table 14–6. MAINTENANCE ELECTROLYTE CONTENT OF TWO COMMERCIAL AMINO ACID
SOLUTIONS
(8.5 PER CENT CONCENTRATION)

	AMINOSYN 8.5% WITH ELECTROLYTES (ABBOTT)	TRAVASOL 8.5% WITH ELECTROLYTES (TRAVENOL)
Electyrolytes		
Sodium (mEq/500 ml)	35	35
Potassium (mEq/500 ml)	33	30
Magnesium (mEq/500 ml)	5	5
Chloride (mEq/500 ml)	49	35
Acetate (mEq/500 ml)	71	67.5
Phosphate (mM/500 ml)	15	15
Osmolarity (mOsm/L)	1160	1160

been formulated for "protein-sparing therapy." Like the glycerol-containing product discussed earlier, these products rely on a patient's body fat as the major energy source. They are usually infused without dextrose and provide only an amino acid substrate for protein synthesis. Thus, these solutions are indicated specifically in patients who may not be protein-depleted and who have adequate fat stores. Low-concentration amino acid solutions with electrolytes indicated for protein-sparing therapy (Aminosyn M 3.5%, Travasol M 3.5%, FreAmine III 3%) are nearly isotonic, with osmolarities of 400 to 450 mOsm/L. The solutions are available in 1000-ml units.

Formulas for Specific Disorders

Renal Failure. Amino acid formulas high in essential amino acids (EAA) have been formulated with specific indications for patients with renal failure. Three EAA products are described in Table 14–7. In addition to supplying concentrated EAA, the formulations also contain L-histidine, which appears to enhance amino acid utilization in uremia and L-arginine; one product also includes some nonessential amino acids, which may enhance nitrogen balance and weight gain.[26] Significant clinical advantages of high EAA products over low-dose standard amino acid solutions in renal failure patients remain controversial.[27-31] This consideration is important in the utilization of the most cost-effective and clinically effective parenteral nutrition therapies.

One unit of high–essential amino acid solution (equivalent to 300 ml of Aminosyn RF 5.2%, 250 ml Nephramine 5.4%, or 250 or 500 ml of RenAmin) is intended for admixture with 500 ml of 50 or 70 per cent dextrose solution prior to administration. This dilution provides the appropriate calorie/nitrogen ratios indicated for renal failure therapy.

Formulas for Hepatic Disease. Two types of solutions high in branched-chain amino acid (BCAA) are currently commercially available (Table 14–8). The first was formulated for use in the treatment of hepatic encephalopathy in patients with cirrhosis or hepatitis. This product provides a concentrated amino acid source high in BCAA (leucine, isoleucine, and valine) for patients who require parenteral nutrition and are intoler-

Table 14–7. COMPOSITION OF HIGH–ESSENTIAL AMINO ACID FORMULAS

CONTENT	AMINOSYN RF, 5.2% (ABBOTT)	NEPHRAMINE, 5.4% (McGAW)	RENAMIN (TRAVENOL)
Essential amino acids (mg/100 ml)			
L-Leucine	726	880	600
L-Isoleucine	462	560	500
L-Phenylalanine	726	880	490
L-Methionine	726	880	500
L-Threonine	330	400	380
L-Valine	528	640	820
L-Lysine	535	640	450
L-Tryptophan	165	200	160
Nonessential amino acids (mg/100 ml)			
L-Arginine	600	—	630
L-Histidine	429	250	420
L-Cysteine	—	20	—
L-Alanine	—	—	560
L-Proline	—	—	350
L-Serine	—	—	300
L-Tyrosine	—	—	40
Glycine (AAA, USP)	—	—	300
Electrolytes (mEq/100 ml)			
Acetate	10.5	4.4	6.0
Chloride	—	—	3.1
Sodium	—	0.6	—
Potassium	0.54	—	—
L-Amino acid content (gm/100 ml)	5.2	5.4	6.5
Total nitrogen (gm/100 ml)	0.79	0.65	1.0
Approximate pH	5.2	6.5	6.0
Approximate osmolarity (mOsm/L)	475	440	600
How supplied (ml)	300	250	250, 500

Table 14–8. COMPOSITION OF HIGH-BCAA PRODUCTS

	HEPATAMINE 8% (MCGAW)	FREAMINE HBC 6.9% (MCGAW)
Essential amino acids (mg/100 ml)		
L-Isoleucine	900	760
L-Leucine	1100	1370
L-Valine	840	880
L-Lysine	610	410
L-Methionine	100	250
L-Phenylalanine	100	320
L-Threonine	450	200
L-Tryptophan	66	90
Nonessential amino acids (mg/100 ml)		
L-Alanine	770	400
L-Arginine	600	580
L-Histidine	240	160
L-Proline	800	630
L-Serine	800	330
Glycine (AAA, USP)	900	330
L-Cysteine	20	20
Electrolytes		
Sodium (mEq/L)	10	10
Acetate (mEq/L)	62	57
Chloride (mEq/L)	3	3
Phosphate (mM/L)	10	—
L-*Amino acid content (gm/100 ml)*	8.0	6.9
Approximate pH	6.5	6.5
Osmolarity (mOsm/L) (calc.)	785	625
How supplied (ml)	500	750

ant of general amino acid formulations. The use of these products for this indication remains controversial and is further discussed in Chapter 35. A 500-ml volume of Hepatamine 8% is intended for admixture with 500 ml of 50 or 70 per cent dextrose prior to administration.[32]

Formulas for Stress or Trauma. The second high-BCAA product (see Table 14–8) was formulated specifically for high-risk, hypercatabolic trauma or stress patients. Like the solution for hepatic encephalopathy, this product has been formulated to balance abnormalities in serum amino acid levels associated with the disease states. Investigation concerning the role of each BCAA on nitrogen balance and the clinical impact of altered serum amino acid levels continues. Further studies and analysis to define amino acid needs during the course of specific disease states as well as patient-specific cost:benefit ratios should precede widespread clinical use of this product. Before administration, the 750-ml, partially filled bottle of FreAmine HBC 6.9% should be admixed with 250 ml of 70 per cent dextrose.[33]

Neonatal Amino Acid Formulas. Trophamine 6% is an amino acid solution for-

mulated to normalize plasma amino acid concentrations and promote growth in neonatal and pediatric patients. The formulation differs from adult general amino acid formulations in that it has a higher concentration of histidine and tyrosine, which are considered essential for infants, as well as other amino acid pattern adjustments that are associated with normalization of the plasma amino acid profile.[34] Investigations are currently ongoing to evaluate the clinical significance of normalized plasma amino acid profiles, effects on correcting elevated liver function tests, and infant morbidity and mortality.

Single-Component Amino Acid Formulations. L-Cysteine HCl, an amino acid generally considered to be essential in infants,[35] is available in a single-use, prefilled 10-ml syringe. The concentration of cysteine is 50 mg/ml. This product is intended for admixture with neonatal parenteral nutrition solutions. Owing to the conversion of cysteine to insoluble cystine, parenteral solutions with added cysteine should be refrigerated immediately and used within 24 hours of mixing.[35]

Administration Considerations. The osmolarity of dextrose and amino acid solutions with final concentrations of 25 to 35 per cent dextrose and 3.5 to 5 per cent amino acids is calculated at approximately 1200 to 1500 mOsm/L. This hypertonicity precludes their administration by peripheral vein. Although clinical indications for peripheral vein administration of parenteral nutrition may be limited, dextrose and amino acid solutions that do not exceed final concentrations of 10 per cent dextrose and 4.25 per cent amino acids may be tolerated for short periods by peripheral veins, even though they are moderately hyperosmolar. The addition of heparin sodium, 1000 U/L, to a parenteral nutrition solution may reduce the thrombophlebitis of the peripheral veins.[36] Co-administration of isotonic fat emulsion via a "Y" connection site may further diminish the osmolarity presented to peripheral veins. The incidence of venous irritation may also be lessened by using larger peripheral veins, slowing the rate of infusion, or using an in-line filter on the dextrose and amino acid solution to reduce particulates.[37] A liter of 10 per cent dextrose and 4.25 per cent amino acid supplies only 510 total calories. Thus, adequate peripheral vein nutrition can often be given only to patients who can tolerate large fluid volumes.

Electrolytes

Intracellular and extracellular electrolytes required for maintenance and correction of deficiency must be provided to patients receiving parenteral nutrition. Electrolyte solutions are available as single- or multiple-electrolyte products that provide salts of sodium, potassium, chloride, acetate, phosphate, magnesium, and calcium. Commercially available electrolyte salt forms are listed in Table 14–9.

All electrolyte salts except bicarbonate may be added to the parenteral nutrition solution after determination of compatibility. The basic pH of the bicarbonate ion precludes its addition directly to the acidic parenteral nutrition solution. Readily metabolized bicarbonate precursor salts such as acetate or lactate are compatible with parenteral nutrition components and may be added.

Multiple-electrolyte formulations intended for maintenance administration in parenteral nutrition patients are also available. These formulations simplify parenteral nutrition solution admixture but are not routinely indicated in patients with renal, hepatic, cardiac, or pulmonary disease, for whom individualized electrolyte administration may be preferred. Commercially available multiple-electrolyte formulations vary in electrolyte composition. For compatibility reasons, most formulations are deficient in calcium or phosphate salts. These two electrolytes are important in cellular function and should be added if a multiple-electrolyte formulation is used. The contents of a commercial multiple electrolyte formulation are shown in Table 14–10.[38] In addition to containing no phosphate, this formulation has a lower potassium content than could usually meet potassium requirements in parenteral nutrition patients. It is important to note that

Table 14–10. A COMMERCIAL MULTIPLE-ELECTROLYTE FORMULATION[38]

ELECTROLYTE	CONCENTRATION (mEq/20 ml)
Sodium	35
Potassium	20
Calcium	4.5
Magnesium	5
Chloride	35
Acetate	29.5

additional phosphate as the potassium salt is intended for addition to make up the deficiency of phosphate. Attention must be given to the completeness of multiple electrolyte formulations when they are selected for use in maintenance. Amino acid solutions with maintenance electrolytes are also available (see Table 14–6); these solutions can further simplify admixture and reduce costs when indicated, but like some multiple electrolyte formulations, they require addition of a maintenance calcium source. The fact that the inherent electrolyte content of amino acid solutions varies with each manufacturer (see Table 14–5) may need to be considered in determining additive compatibility.

Vitamins

Vitamins are well-established essential components in metabolism and maintenance of cellular function and integrity. General guidelines for maintenance vitamin supplementation for adult and pediatric patients on parenteral nutrition have been established by the American Medical Association Nutrition Advisory Group (AMA/NAG).[39] Several products have been formulated to specifically follow the adult or pediatric AMA/NAG guidelines (Table 14–11). The vitamins are separated to minimize the degradation of folic acid, B_{12}, and biotin that may occur when they are stored with other vitamins.

Adult multiple-vitamin products do not contain vitamin K. Vitamin K should be administered intramuscularly for repletion or treatment of vitamin K deficiency. From clinical experience, maintenance requirements for vitamin K have been adequately met when the vitamin is admixed with other nutrient components in the parenteral nutrition solution.

It is important to emphasize that malnutrition, specific disease states, and drug

Table 14–9. ELECTROLYTE SALT FORMS

Sodium chloride
Sodium acetate
Sodium bicarbonate
Sodium lactate
Sodium phosphate
Potassium chloride
Potassium acetate
Potassium phosphate
Magnesium sulfate
Calcium chloride
Calcium gluconate
Calcium gluceptate

Table 14–11. MULTIPLE-VITAMIN PRODUCTS FORMULATED TO MEET ADULT AND PEDIATRIC GUIDELINES OF THE AMA/NAG

	VITAMIN CONTENT													HOW SUPPLIED
	A (IU)	D (IU)	E (IU)	Thiamine (mg)	Riboflavin (mg)	Niacin (mg)	Pantothenic Acid (mg)	Pyridoxine (mg)	C (mg)	Folic Acid (mg)	B_{12} (μg)	Biotin (μg)	K (μg)	
Daily AMA/NAG guidelines for adults	3300	200	10	3.0	3.6	40	15	4	100	400	5	60	—	—
Adult Products														
Berocca Parenteral Nutrition (Roche)	3300	200	10	3.0	3.6	40	15	4	100	400	5	60	—	2 solutions; 2 single-dose ampules (1-ml) or 2 multi-dose vials (10-ml)
Multivitamin Additive (Abbott)	3300	200	10	3.35*	4.93*	40	15	4.86*	100	400	5	60	—	2 solutions; 2 single-dose Abbojet vials (5-ml)
MCV-Plus (Ascot)	3300	200	10	3.0	3.6	40	15	4	100	400	5	60	—	2 solutions, 1 single-dose duo-vial (10-ml)
MCV 9 + 3 (Lyphomed)	3300	200	10	3.0	3.6	40	15	4	100	400	5	60	—	2 solutions; 1 single-dose mix-o-vial (10-ml) or 2 single-dose vials (5-ml)
MVI-12 (Armour)	3300	200	10	3.0	3.6	40	15	4	100	400	5	60	—	2 solutions; 2 single-dose vials (5-ml) or lyophilized sterile powder for reconstitution in single-dose vials
Daily AMA/NAG guidelines for children up to 11 years old	2300	400	7	1.2	1.4	17	5	1	80	140	1	20	200	—
Pediatric Product MVI Pediatric (Armour)	2300	400	7	1.2	1.4	17	5	1	80	140	1	20	200	Single-dose lyophilized sterile powder for reconstitution (10-ml vials)

*Provided in appropriate salt form equivalent to AMA recommendations.

therapy may often predispose some patients to vitamin deficiencies, for which additional vitamin supplementation is indicated. Parenteral multivitamin products and individual vitamins are available to provide additional fat and water-soluble vitamins. Single-entity products for vitamins A, D, E, K, B_1 (thiamine), B_2 (riboflavin), B_3 (niacin), B_6 (pyridoxine), B_{12} (cyanocobalamin), folic acid, and C are commercially available.[40] Single-entity products and recommended routes of administration are listed in Table 14–12.

Trace Minerals

Commercially available trace mineral solutions have eliminated the necessity to compound trace mineral formulations within the pharmacy. Zinc, copper, chromium, and manganese contaminants are present in commercially available parenteral nutrition solutions. Concentrations of each element vary with the manufacturer, solution concentration, and lot number. Additional trace mineral supplementation has been recommended for adult and pediatric parenteral nutrition patients.[41] The AMA/NAG guidelines for adult and pediatric trace mineral supplementation in parenteral nutrition and several multiple-element products that provide adult and pediatric maintenance dosages are listed in Table 14–13. In addition, single-entity solutions are also commercially available. Recommendations have been made for zinc, copper, manganese, and chromium. Single-entity products are available for iodide (as sodium iodide) and trace minerals such as selenium (as selenious acid) and molybdenum (as ammonium molybdate tetrahydrate), for which requirements are not well defined but appear significant in long-term total parenteral nutrition.

SOLUTION ADMIXTURE

Maintenance of solution sterility during admixture and handling is critical to reducing the incidence and complications of sepsis in parenteral nutrition patients. Evaluations of solution growth potential have described organisms most likely to proliferate in parenteral nutrition solutions and methods to minimize rapid proliferation. An understanding of the microorganism growth potential in

Table 14–12. SINGLE-ENTITY PARENTERAL VITAMINS[40]

VITAMIN	PRODUCT* (MANUFACTURER)	VITAMIN CONTENT	ROUTE(S) OF ADMINISTRATION
A	Aquasol A (Armour)	50,000 IU/ml, vitamin A	IM only
D	Calciferol (Kremers-Urban)	5,000,000 IU/ml, vitamin D_2	IM only
E	Vitamin E (various)	200 IU/ml	IM only
K	Aqua Mephyton (MSD)	2 mg/ml or 10 mg/ml phytonadione	SC, IM, or slow IV
	Konakion (Roche)	2 mg/ml or 10 mg/ml phytonadione	IM only
Folic acid	Folvite (Lederle)	5 mg/ml	SC, IM, or IV
	Folic acid (Pasadena Research)	10 mg/ml	SC, IM, or IV
B_1	Thiamine HCl (various)	100 mg/ml	IM, IV†
B_2	Riobin-50 (Pasadena Research)	50 mg/ml, riboflavin	
B_3	Nicotinic Acid (Consolidated Midland)	50 mg/ml	SC, IM, or slow IV
	Nicotinic Acid (various)	100 mg/ml	SC, IM, or slow IV
	Nicotinamide (various)	100 mg/ml	SC, IM, or slow IV
B_6	Pyridoxine HCl (various)	100 mg/ml	IV, IM
B_{12}	Cyanocobalamin, crystalline (various)	1000 μg/ml	SC, IM, or IV‡
	Hydroxocobalamin, crystalline (various)	1000 μg/ml	IM only
C	Ascorbic acid (various)	100 mg/ml	SC, IM, or slow IV
	Ascorbic acid (Pasadena Research)	200 mg/ml	SC, IM, or slow IV
	Ascorbic acid (various)	250 mg/ml	SC, IM, or slow IV
	Cevalin (Lilly)	500 mg/ml, ascorbic acid	SC, IM, or slow IV
	Sodium ascorbate (various)	250 mg/ml	SC, IM, or slow IV
	Cenolate (Abbott)	562.5 mg/ml sodium ascorbate (equivalent to 500 mg/ml ascorbic acid)	SC, IM, or slow IV
	Calsorbate (O'Neal, Jones & Feldman)	100 mg/ml, calcium ascorbate	SC, IM, or slow IV

*Use in neonates should include consideration of preservative content per dose administered.
†Deaths have resulted from IV use.
‡Avoid IV for pernicious anemia.
Data extrapolated from reference 40.

Table 14–13. MULTIPLE-ELEMENT TRACE MINERAL PRODUCTS FORMULATED TO MEET ADULT AND PEDIATRIC GUIDELINES OF THE AMA/NAG[41]

	ZINC CONTENT (AS SULFATE)	COPPER CONTENT (AS SULFATE)	MANGANESE CONTENT (AS SULFATE)	CHROMIUM CONTENT (AS CHLORIDE)	SELENIUM CONTENT (AS SELENIOUS ACID)
Daily AMA/NAG Guidelines for Adults (dose per ml)	2.5–4.0 mg	0.5–1.5 mg	0.15–0.8 mg	10–15 µg	—
Adult Products (dose per ml)					
Multiple Trace Element Additives (Abbott)	4.0 mg	1.0 mg	0.8 mg	10.0 µg	—
Multiple Trace Element Solution (American Quinine)	1.0 or 5.0 mg	0.4 or 1.0 mg	0.1 or 0.5 mg	4.0 or 10.0 µg	—
Multiple Trace Metal Additive (IMS)	4.0 mg	1.0 mg	0.5 mg	10.0 µg	—
MTE-4 (Lyphomed)	1.0 mg	0.4 mg	0.1 mg	4.0 µg	—
MulTE-Pak-4 (Solo Pak)	1.0 or 5.0 mg	0.4 or 1.0 mg	0.1 or 0.5 mg	4.0 or 10.0 µg	—
MTE-5 (Lyphomed)	1.0 mg	0.4 mg	0.1 mg	4.0 µg	20.0 µg
MulTE-Pak-5 (Solo Pak)	1.0 mg	0.4 mg	0.1 mg	4.0 µg	20.0 µg
Daily AMA/NAG Guidelines for Children (dose per kg)	100–300 µg	20 µg	2–10 µg	0.14–0.2 µg	—
Pediatric Products (dose per ml)					
Trace Element Solution (American Quinine)	0.5 mg	0.1 mg	30 µg	1.0 µg	—
Pak-4 (Solo Pak)	1.0 mg	0.1 mg	25 µg	1.0 µg	—

parenteral nutrition solutions and the corresponding risk of infection reinforces the importance of aseptic technique and handling in parenteral nutrition solution admixture.

Microorganism Growth Potential

As nutrient sources, parenteral nutrition solutions can be a natural growth medium for microorganisms. If contamination occurs during admixture or handling, the risk of sepsis is increased if the contaminating organisms can proliferate in the parenteral nutrition solution. Numerous studies have investigated microbial growth potential of parenteral nutrition solutions in order to better define the organisms and conditions that may favor rapid microbial proliferation.[42–50]

Rapid proliferation of both bacteria and fungi was evident in dextrose and the older protein hydrolysate solutions.[42] Appreciable multiplication and survival of organisms appears to have been reduced in dextrose and crystalline amino acid solutions after 24 hours for all species except for *Candida albicans*.[42–44] The reduced growth potential is apparently due to the lack of large proteins, which can provide peptides necessary for the growth of organisms. Although hypertonicity and acidity of commercially available parenteral nutrition solutions do not present ideal conditions for microbial growth, some pathogens may proliferate very rapidly at room temperature. A reduction in the growth of *C. albicans* and incidence of fungal septicemia occurs

when the solutions are cooled to 4°C.[42, 47] If parenteral solutions must be stored after admixture, it is recommended that they be refrigerated immediately.[42, 45, 51] It is further recommended that parenteral solutions be used within 24 hours after final admixture.[51] Addition of albumin to crystalline amino acid parenteral solutions increases bacterial and fungal growth potential.[46] Substantial growth of microorganisms may also occur in intravenous fat emulsions[48–50] and is especially significant if fat emulsions are admixed with dextrose–amino acid solutions in large volumes with expiration times exceeding 12 hours. The incidence of parenteral nutrition–associated infection may be reduced by strict adherence to carefully designed aseptic admixture and infection control protocols.

Aseptic Admixture

Aseptic admixture, along with aseptic handling during all phases of administration, is needed to ensure that a sterile parenteral nutrition solution is delivered to the patient. Parenteral nutrition therapy is often used in seriously ill patients with a high potential for the development of sepsis. Nosocomial infections traced to pharmaceutical preparations emphasize the need for quality control in the preparation of parenteral nutrition solutions.[52–54]

Microbial growth potential and the numerous additive steps in parenteral nutrition solution admixture render admixture techniques that are less than aseptic unacceptable.

Parenteral nutrition solutions should be prepared in the clean air environment provided by a laminar flow hood. The hood should be located in a separate IV admixture room or in an area away from contamination sources and the normal flow of traffic and air currents. Admixture should be performed by specially trained personnel using strict aseptic techniques. A hospital pharmacist familiar with solutions and additive handling, storage, stability, and compatibility is also essential.

The incidence of sepsis may be as high as 27 per cent without uniform protocols for parenteral nutrition admixture.[55] A pharmacy-based admixture program allows an efficient and uniform program of quality control in parenteral nutrition preparation. Many IV admixture pharmacies have developed guidelines for admixture of parenteral nutrition solutions. Specific guidelines will vary from institution to institution, but should generally address the following issues: (1) solution and additive handling and storage; (2) aseptic admixture training; (3) admixture preparation procedures; (4) personnel dress code; (5) admixture personnel and product quality assurance; (6) environmental maintenance procedures; (7) environmental quality assurance; (8) solution and additive stability, compatibility, and expiration; (9) solution labeling; (10) recording of solution prescription and preparation; (11) visual inspection of solutions; and (12) corrective procedures.

SOLUTION STABILITY AND COMPATIBILITY

Stability and compatibility considerations are essential in providing a safe and effective parenteral nutrition solution. Guidelines used in practice for base solutions and additive admixture should reflect the most recent scientific literature. The literature concerning base solution and nutrient and drug additive stability and compatibility are reviewed in the following sections.

Base Solution

Base solution refers to the combined dextrose and amino acid components of a parenteral nutrition solution. The National Coordinating Committee on Large Volume Parenterals (NCCLVP)[51] has made the general recommendation that large-volume parenterals, including parenteral nutrition solutions, should be administered immediately after compounding. If they are not started immediately, they should be refrigerated within one hour; if refrigerated, they should be used in 24 hours.[51] The goal of the NCCLVP was to insure that patients receive a parenteral as prescribed, free of microbial or particulate contamination and unaltered by incompatibility of interacting additives.[51] Less stable TPN additive components (i.e., vitamins) should be utilized immediately after compounding. However, growing interest in the use of parenteral nutrition as outpatient as well as inpatient therapy has created interest in bulk parenteral nutrition compounding and base solution storage for periods longer than 24 hours.

Microbial growth is a major limiting factor in both short- and long-term storage of parenteral nutrition base solutions.[42-50] Laegeler and associates[56] demonstrated that strict aseptic admixture techniques can eliminate yeast and bacterial growth in dextrose and amino acid solutions stored at 4°C, 25°C, and 37°C for up to three months. However, although no microbiologic growth appeared, significant amino acid deterioration, color formation, and pH depression occurred in solutions stored at 25°C and 37°C. Higher temperatures and increased length of solution storage favors entrance of dextrose into the complex Maillard (carmelization) reaction. The most obvious characteristic of this reaction is color formation and darkening from yellow to dark brown.[57, 58] However, the first step in this reaction is the formation of colorless glycosamines from the reaction of amino groups with free aldehyde groups of sugars.[57-59] Thus, the rate of color formation alone is not an accurate assessment of solution stability.

Amino acid analysis in the investigation by Laegeler and associates[56] did not include tryptophan. Jurgens and colleagues[60] studied long-term stability of tryptophan, the most labile of the amino acids, and other amino acids, in an 8.5 per cent amino acid and 50 per cent dextrose base solution. Except for tryptophan, amino acid concentrations, pH, and particulate analysis parameters remained unchanged within the range of normal experimental variation after two weeks when the solution was either stored at room temperature (approximately 25°C) or refrigerated (maintained at 4°C). Refrigeration was better for tryptophan stability, with a reported reduction to 94.1 per cent remaining of original tryptophan concentration during storage for two weeks at room temperature and 97.5 per cent under refrigeration.[60] Two-week stability has also been demonstrated with base solutions of dextrose and protein hydrolysates.[43] However, the demonstration of bacterial growth, which is more favored in protein hydrolysate base solutions,[42, 44] leads us to re-emphasize that microbial growth is the rate-limiting factor in base solution stability.

Freezing of base solutions with electrolytes and subsequent thawing at room temperature or by microwave was investigated by Ausman and co-workers.[61] Changes in amino acid and electrolyte concentrations were small. The greatest amino acid change occurred in tryptophan. Amino acid concentrations were assessed after 60 days of refrigerated storage, after 60 days of freezing followed by an overnight room temperature thaw, and after 60 days of freezing followed by a 30-minute microwave thaw; tryptophan concentration was 92, 93, and 95 per cent of original concentration, respectively. Additional descriptions of freeze-thaw effects on parenteral nutrition containers is needed before this method of practice is initiated.

Equipment and techniques commonly used in Europe and Canada, which allow admixture of fat emulsions with dextrose–amino acid base solutions, have recently been accepted in the United States. Concerns regarding this admixture were for fat emulsion instability (i.e., flocculation, oiling out) resulting from admixture with hypertonic glucose and varying doses of calcium, magnesium, sodium, and potassium.[62–66] However, amino acids may exert a "butterfly" effect upon overall solution pH and improve fat emulsion stability following admixture. Consequently, admixture of amino acids with fat or carbohydrate prior to combining the fat emulsion with dextrose or electrolytes may minimize admixture pH changes and enhance fat emulsion stability.[67] In vitro compatibility[67–70] and stability[71–73] as well as in vivo metabolic effects in animals and humans[67, 74] have been investigated for combined admixture and administration. Guidelines for admixture of specifically outlined parenteral nutrition components are currently available for a commercially available fat emulsion product.[75] Stability of this system may vary with various crystalline amino acid products, electrolyte content, and other additives. Because the potential for microbial growth may be enhanced with this combination, strict aseptic technique, restricted expiration dating, and cost considerations should be observed before this technique is used clinically. An in-line filter should not be used on admixtures that contain fat emulsions.

Suppliers of commercially available amino acid solutions recommend that they be protected from light, freezing, and excessive heat during storage. Various expiration dates have been assigned to completely admixed parenteral nutrition solutions.[76] However, the storage guidelines of a 24-hour expiration outlined by the NCCLVP[51] are the most widely followed. Storage practices for noncomplete parenteral nutrition base solutions vary widely. Electrolytes and trace minerals are frequently admixed with the base solution for long-term storage, although further investigations with these components are needed. The results of investigations of stability and microbial growth suggest that recommendations for long-term storage (greater than 24 hours) of base solutions include the following:

1. Solutions should be admixed using crystalline amino acid–dextrose combinations rather than solutions of protein hydrolysate–dextrose.

2. Solutions should be admixed with strict aseptic technique by trained personnel.

3. Solutions should be refrigerated and stored with protection from light, freezing, and excessive heat.

4. Base solution can be stored up to two weeks until further investigations document otherwise.

Nutrient and Drug Additives

The complex composition of parenteral nutrition solutions renders them highly susceptible to compatibility and stability problems. Since parenteral nutrition formulations differ in many respects from dextrose-saline solutions, determination of nutrient and drug compatibility in these formulations has proved to be a unique and formidable challenge.[77] Numerous parenteral nutrition compatibility studies have been published in the last six years.[78] The increasing sophistication of life-support systems has rekindled interest in this subject and has placed a renewed emphasis upon obtaining compatibility information that is based on sound, scientific methodology.

Varying study methodologies of published reports preclude the simple and sole use of tables or charts to designate compatibility. Review of the extensive literature on calcium and phosphate interrelationships alone demonstrates how differing study conditions have resulted in a wide range of "compatible" salt concentrations. Some compatibility data have been generated from direct syringe admixture of concentrated ingredients, and these findings should not be confused with compatibility studies reflecting admixture in large-volume parenterals or in association with auxiliary medication infusion units. Furthermore, compatibility studies may have serious flaws or limitations in study design that subsequently limit their realistic application.[78] Critical evaluation of the primary literature report is encouraged, whenever possible, to aid the practitioner in assessing the valid application of study results to a given clinical situation.

Parenteral nutrition solutions possess titratable acidity as a result of their amino acid and electrolyte (i.e., acetate) content,[79] whereas dextrose-saline intravenous fluids have minimal buffering capacity.[80] Consequently, parenteral nutrition solutions are more resistant to pH change, with additives generally having minimal effect upon overall solution pH. Depending upon the optimal pH range for an additive's stability and the exposure time, additive compatibility in parenteral nutrition solutions may differ from that in standard intravenous fluids. Compatibility designations may also differ among crystalline amino acid products, because titratable acidity is highly dependent upon amino acid concentration and product used.[79]

Historically, compatibility designations have been based on visual criteria or pH change. Visual assessment is subject to interpretation and, depending upon method, may fail to detect particles less than 50 microns in size.[81] Recent studies employing microbiologic assays, high-pressure liquid chromatography, and atomic absorption spectroscopy have attempted to provide more meaningful data by simulating actual conditions of use as closely as is feasible. Athanikar and colleagues,[82] Kobayashi and King,[83] and Schuetz and King[84] evaluated the complexity of calcium-phosphate salt relationships and the visual compatibility of numerous medications. Importantly, these reports emphasized the limitations of visual compatibility assessment and the need for chemical verification of stability. Dextrose, amino acid, and electrolyte components, including magnesium sulfate, potassium acetate, potassium chloride, sodium acetate, and sodium chloride, are generally considered compatible when admixed in commonly used dosages. The following paragraphs critically address the compatibility of select nutrient and drug additives with, and their stability in, parenteral nutrition formulas.

Nutrient Admixture

INSULIN

Insulin is considered to be chemically stable in parenteral nutrition solutions and clinically effective upon admixture in controlling serum glucose concentrations when dosage is titrated to patient response. Insulin admixture in parenteral nutrition formulations provides a continuous exogenous supply of the hormone during glucose delivery with minimal risk of hypoglycemia if the parenteral nutrition infusion is interrupted.

Decreased availability of insulin from parenteral nutrition delivery systems occurs because of adsorptive losses to the solution container, administration set, and in-line filter.[85-95] Numerous studies since the 1950s have documented nonspecific insulin adsorption to glass and polyvinyl chloride (PVC) surfaces, thus decreasing availability of insulin from intravenous delivery systems.[89] Adsorptive losses of insulin have varied from three to 80 per cent, depending upon study methodology. Adsorption can significantly decrease initial insulin availability from continuous low-dose infusions[88-93] and parenteral nutrition solutions,[85, 86] with the extent of adsorption determined by insulin concentration,[88] type of intravenous solution,[89] temperature,[93] previous insulin tubing flush,[90] and the presence of albumin, polygeline,[94] whole blood,[95] and electrolytes.[91] Additions of albumin (0.25 to 2 per cent) have been used to decrease insulin adsorption to intravenous delivery systems during continuous insulin infusion,[90, 96-100] but insulin infusion without the addition of albumin has been successfully employed in the management of diabetic ketoacidosis.[98, 99, 102]

Weber and associates[85] examined factors contributing to insulin loss from a parenteral nutrition delivery system. Because solution components may influence kinetics of insulin adsorption,[86] it is noteworthy that these authors used crystalline amino acid and protein hydrolysate–dextrose solutions with typical electrolyte and vitamin additives. They compared the effects of glass and PVC solution containers, administration tubing with extension set, in-line filters, and the addition of albumin upon insulin loss during a simulated infusion over six hours. Insulin loss was increased 17 per cent by use of an in-line filter and seven per cent with PVC bag and was reduced by seven per cent with the addition of 0.37 per cent albumin. The authors concluded from their model that insulin loss to a parenteral nutrition infusion system may be as high as 47 per cent and that the minimal reduction in adsorption resulting from albumin addition did not justify its costly admixture in parenteral nutrition solutions for this purpose.[85]

It is apparent that numerous variables may affect insulin adsorption kinetics, confounding the interpretation of study findings and accurate prediction of insulin loss from a given delivery system. The potential benefit of simultaneous glucose-insulin infusion during parenteral nutrition supports the admixture of insulin to parenteral nutrition formulations with the realization that as much as 50 per cent adsorptive loss of insulin may occur.

CALCIUM AND PHOSPHATE SALTS

Compatibility concerns in parenteral nutrition solutions have traditionally involved admixture of calcium (Ca) and phosphate (P) salts. The compatibility of these salts in parenteral nutrition solutions depends on a complex set of interrelationships among factors that affect Ca-P solubility.[82, 103]

The chemical interaction between Ca and P salts in an aqueous solution depends on concentration[82, 84, 103–106] and pH[82, 103, 104] and appears to depend also on temperature,[103, 105–107] amino acid concentration,[103–108] calcium salt form,[105] infusion time,[109, 110] and order of salt admixture.[82, 84] Factors favoring precipitate formation include: (1) high molar Ca-P salt concentrations;[82] (2) increases in solution pH;[103, 104] (3) low amino acid concentrations, especially less than 2.5 per cent;[103, 108, 111] (4) increases in environmental temperature;[103, 107, 109] (5) Ca admixture prior to P admixture or to maximal formula dilution;[82, 84] (6) increases in standing time or slow infusion rates;[82, 103, 109] and (7) use of Ca as the chloride salt.[105] Precipitation may occur immediately in the solution container, hours later in the administration tubing/filter, or in the paren-

teral nutrition catheter, causing occlusion.[82, 109, 111]

Ca-P precipitation primarily occurs in the form of dibasic Ca-P, which is less soluble than the monobasic form in an aqueous medium and is highly pH-dependent.[103, 113] Increases in solution pH predispose to Ca-P precipitation, because more dibasic phosphate is available to bind with Ca.[103] Commercially available crystalline amino acid products vary greatly with respect to solution pH and titratable acidity,[80] with these factors directly influencing the resultant pH of a given formulation after admixture completion and solution tolerance of Ca and P addition. Dilution of amino acids to varying concentrations with dextrose and water decreases the mixed solution's overall titratable acidity in a linear fashion (Fig. 14–1).[108] Because buffering capacity decreases as a direct function of amino acid dilution, parenteral nutrition formulas containing lower concentrations of protein (i.e., less than 2.5 per cent) are less tolerant of Ca and P addition before precipitation occurs. Addition of potassium phosphate injection (pH approximately 6.9) to parenteral nutrition solutions containing low amino acid concentrations results in a dramatic dose-related increase in pH (Fig. 14–2).[108] In addition, amino acids in solution at mid-range pH form soluble complexes with Ca and P, thus decreasing free salt concentrations available for interaction.[106]

Increasing the solution temperature decreases Ca-P solubility by increasing Ca and P salt dissociation to their free forms, which are then available for interaction.[107, 109] Temperature is a crucial variable influencing Ca-P precipitation and catheter occlusion in preterm infants placed in incubators and in patients with Hickman catheters. Ca chloride

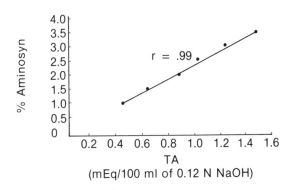

r = .99

*endpoint pH ≤ 6.5

Figure 14–1. Titratable acidity* (TA) as a function of per cent Aminosyn in 20 per cent dextrose.

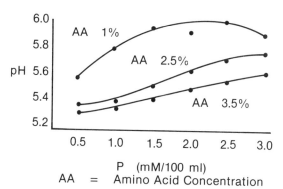

Figure 14–2. Initial solution pH after addition of KPO_4 to Aminosyn in 20 per cent dextrose.

reportedly dissociates in solution to a greater extent than Ca gluconate, so use of the chloride salt may result in Ca-P precipitation at lower molar Ca-P salt concentrations.[105] The presence of magnesium in solution may further influence the reaction between Ca and P;[112, 113] thus, any study of Ca-P precipitation in a parenteral nutrition model should include pharmacologic amounts of magnesium. Ca-P precipitation may occur in stages as a function of salt concentration and pH.[114] Precipitation may progress through a time-related "induction period," with gradual formation of well-defined crystals. Consequently, Ca-P solubility may decrease over 24 hours, as evidenced by substantial decreases in solution pH accompanying gradual precipitate formation.[109, 115] Scheutz and King[84] have previously noted the delayed onset of precipitation over 12 to 24 hours in parenteral nutrition solutions bordering on compatibility. Precipitation during parenteral nutrition infusion may not be observed until 12 or more hours after solution preparation unless conditions favor an immediate flocculent precipitation.

Although numerous studies have addressed Ca-P compatibility relationships in an attempt to establish maximal salt concentrations that can be mixed,[82, 84, 103–106, 112, 116, 117] conflicting findings have been presented owing to varying experimental conditions and methodology and to lack of appreciation of amino acid concentration as an important variable. A recent review article addresses some of the methodologic differences among these studies.[117] Eggert and co-workers[103] examined various factors affecting Ca-P solubility, including solution pH, temperature, time, amino acid and dextrose concentrations, and mixing with lipid emulsion. Precipitation curves were presented for Amino-

syn 1% and 2% and FreAmine III 1%, 2% and 4% with varying concentrations of dextrose. Curves incorporated variables such as amino acid concentration, temperature, and time. Despite limitations in this report, their precipitation model was stressed by higher temperatures, thus providing a reasonable assessment of Ca-P solubility under differing conditions of use.

Any study of Ca-P salt compatibility in parenteral nutrition solutions is specific for the amino acid product, the tested amino acid concentration, and the testing limitations of the model (i.e., time, temperature, salt form). Solutions of borderline compatibility should be regarded as potentially disastrous with regard to possible catheter occlusion due to minor environmental changes such as warming, decreases in amino acid concentration, or co-infusion with lipids[103] or alkaline medications.[118] Because of the numerous variables influencing Ca-P precipitation and the role of "induction time" in solutions bordering on compatibility, parenteral nutrition solutions should be observed carefully for Ca-P incompatibility during administration as well as during preparation. Ca-P incompatibility must be included in a differential assessment of administration problems involving suspected occlusion of catheters or in-line filters. It is prudent to avoid "borderline" compatibilities whenever possible, because they are most susceptible to factors influencing solution stability. A reasonable approach is to use the Ca-P precipitation curves generated by Eggert and co-workers,[103] with the conditions and limitations of their study kept in mind.

SODIUM BICARBONATE

The availability of acetate and lactate salts to serve as bicarbonate precursors generally precludes the need for admixture of sodium bicarbonate to parenteral nutrition solutions. Admixture with acidic parenteral nutrition solutions results in carbon dioxide formation with loss of the bicarbonate ion, as well as potential formation of insoluble calcium and magnesium carbonates.[118]

ALBUMIN

Albumin appears to be physically compatible in parenteral nutrition solutions for 24 hours. Parenteral nutrition admixture of 12.53 to 37.5 gm/L is employed in some centers to increase serum albumin levels and oncotic pressure. Occlusion of in-line filters has been noted with additions of albumin exceeding 25 gm/L. Prior to routine albumin admixture, due consideration must be given to the cost of albumin,[119] the appropriateness of its use,[120, 121] and the reported enhanced potential for parenteral nutrition solutions containing albumin to support bacterial and fungal growth.[46] Albumin admixture is generally not recommended for the purpose of decreasing insulin adsorption to parenteral nutrition delivery systems, because overall adsorption may be decreased by less than 10 per cent.[85, 89]

VITAMINS

Specific vitamin stability information has not been readily available in commonly used references. Numerous factors may affect vitamin stability in parenteral nutrition solutions, including solution pH, presence of electrolytes, other vitamins, and environmental conditions of storage time, temperature, and light exposure. The topic of vitamin stability in parenteral nutrition fluids has been subject to speculation of vitamin-vitamin interactions and vitamin degradation secondary to light exposure. Frequently, concerns for vitamin instability have been based upon uncontrolled observations using massive vitamin dosages tested over weeks under varying conditions. These results have been perpetuated through various compatibility charts, with consideration seldom given to establishing whether losses observed were clinically significant with normal parenteral nutrition solution expiration dating.

Parenteral multivitamin manufacturers claim greater than 95 per cent potency of labeled constituent vitamins for 24 hours upon admixture with parenteral nutrition solutions under reasonably normal temperature and lighting conditions. In addition to stability considerations, vitamin availability from parenteral nutrition delivery systems must also be considered. Recent reports of selected vitamin losses observed during parenteral nutrition, as well as the establishment of new guidelines for parenteral vitamin usage,[39] support the need for careful evaluation of parenteral nutrition vitamin delivery.

Folic Acid. The effects of the B-complex vitamins on decomposition of folic acid were first quantified in 1947 by Foss and colleagues.[122] Riboflavin was found to have the greatest and most injurious effect on folic acid decomposition, followed in descending order by thiamine, ascorbic acid, nicotinamide, pantothenic acid, and pyridoxine. Scheindlin and associates[123] were able to describe the reactions that take place in the chemical decomposition of folic acid by riboflavin. Under combined effects of light and riboflavin, a dehydrogenation of folic acid occurs, with subsequent oxidative cleavage to form para-amino-benzoyl-glutamic acid and a carbonyl compound, presumed to be 2-amino, 4-hydroxy, 6-pteridine carboxaldehyde.[123] The newly formed compounds do not possess folic acid activity. Polyvitamin mixtures have also been shown to exert a destructive effect on folic acid in oral liquid preparations.[124, 125] Storage at room temperature and the presence of other vitamins appear to provide favorable conditions for folic acid degradation.[124]

Physical stability of folic acid has been demonstrated in parenteral nutrition solutions.[84] However, chemical degradation of folic acid does not result in the formation of a precipitate.[126, 127] On the basis of early investigations of folic acid instability in oral solutions, folic acid is reported to be unstable with riboflavin, thiamine, light,[128–129] reducing agents, oxidizing agents, and heavy metal ions.[128]

Louie and Stennett[130] assessed the chemical stability of folic acid in a parenteral nutrition model including added multivitamins under varying conditions of light, temperature, and folic acid concentration. Folic acid was found to be stable for 48 hours in a dextrose amino acid solution. Stability was retained under refrigeration (4°C) or at room temperature (25°C) under both light and dark storage conditions (Fig. 14–3).[130] Manufacturers' overages may prevent total loss of vitamin potency as a result of short-term instability. Folic acid stability in parenteral nutrition solutions without multivitamins has been determined over a two-week period. Stability was retained in these solutions, providing that the acidity of the solution remained above pH 5.0[131] Folic acid has also been found to pass through an in-line filter with negligible loss.[132]

Vitamin K. There is a lack of published documentation concerning the stability of phytonadione in parenteral nutrition solutions and in the presence of ascorbic acid. Although concern has been expressed about the light sensitivity of phytonadione,[133] the vitamin is reported to be physically and chemically stable over 24 hours in parenteral nutrition solutions containing typical addi-

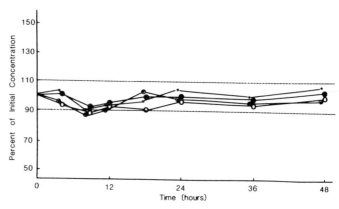

Figure 14–3. Time as a function of per cent of initial folic acid concentration.[131] (——●——) = 0.25 ng/L, (——○——) = 0.5 ng/L, (——•——) = 0.75 ng/L, (——⊙——) = 1.0 ng/L. (From Louie, N., and Stennett, D. J.: Stability of folic acid in 25% dextrose, 3.5% amino acids, and multivitamin solution: J.P.E.N., 8:424, 1984.)

tives.[82, 84, 134] A lyophilized pediatric multivitamin preparation containing phytonadione is commercially available, with vitamin stability demonstrated over 24 hours following reconstitution and admixture. Addition of vitamin K to parenteral nutrition solutions containing other vitamin additives has resulted in maintenance of prothrombin time. Prophylactic administration of vitamin K has received increasing attention in the malnourished patient receiving broad-spectrum antibiotics, especially certain cephalosporins.[135–137]

Vitamin A. A basic assumption has been that vitamin A admixture in a parenteral nutrition solution results in effective delivery of the dose to the patient.[138–140] Poor delivery of vitamin A has been demonstrated from parenteral nutrition delivery systems, with losses of 40 to 75 per cent reported, depending upon storage conditions and duration.[141–146] The chemical properties of this vitamin may favor absorption from a parenteral nutrition solution into the plastic matrix of intravenous administration sets, resulting in a strong physiochemical bond.[147] Increases in exposure time and temperature favor enhanced diffusion and decreased availability of vitamin A from a parenteral nutrition system.[147] Moorhatch and Chion[147] demonstrated a sustained decrease in unbound retinol acetate over 24 hours with light protection, using PVC intravenous bags, with losses approaching 75 per cent. The majority of vitamin A availability studies have not supported significant vitamin sensitivity to room lighting as opposed to net delivery losses, although significant vitamin A losses have been attributed to exposure to sunlight.[148]

Howard and associates[143] reported on a home parenteral nutrition patient who experienced repeated episodes of night blindness despite having 3000 units of retinol in the daily formula. The patient presented with decreased serum concentrations and hepatic stores of vitamin A accompanied by normal levels of retinol-binding protein and plasma zinc. *In vitro* analysis demonstrated that one week of storage at 4°C of the mixed parenteral nutrition solution in a PVC bag resulted in a 50 per cent loss of vitamin A due to oxidation and absorption. A portion of the "missing" vitamin was successfully extracted from the plastic bag with an ether-ethanol solvent.

It becomes apparent that significant losses of vitamin A may be occurring during parenteral nutrition solution delivery, with the magnitude of loss related to solution storage time, temperature, infusion time, and type of administration equipment used.[148] Further vitamin destruction may occur if solutions are exposed to strong lighting. These studies suggest that the availability of vitamin A from parenteral nutrition systems may be as low as 25 per cent. The potential magnitude of this loss has important implications for neonatal and chronic nutritional support, wound healing, and the establishment of parenteral vitamin requirements in disease and stress. Because the availability of vitamin A from parenteral nutrition systems cannot be assumed, it may be preferable at present to supplement severely vitamin A–depleted patients by the intramuscular or oral route as feasible. These concerns are further highlighted by recent formulation changes in parenteral multivitamin products, including substantial decreases in vitamin A content, to conform to recently recommended dietary allowances.[39]

Thiamine. Despite claims of thiamine stability in various crystalline amino acid products, a recent report has raised concern over potential thiamine degradation in bisulfite-containing parenteral nutrition solutions.[149] The influence of solution pH, temperature, time, and the inactivating effect of sulfite upon the thiamine molecule have been of pharmaceutical interest for decades.[150] Hydrolytic cleavage of thiamine to inactive products may occur rapidly in solutions containing greater than 160 mg/L of bisulfite at a pH of greater than or equal to 6.[150–152]

Scheiner and colleagues[149] recently compared the degree of thiamine degradation in two crystalline amino acid injections (without added dextrose) under varying study conditions. They observed 33 to 97 per cent losses of thiamine over 24 hours, with the magnitude of loss depending on pH of solution, amino acid product, storage time, and temperature; lighting had a negligible effect. The authors concluded that the loss of thiamine in bisulfite-containing solutions is substantial under refrigeration or normal conditions of administration and that these solutions are unsuitable vehicles for administration of parenteral vitamins containing thiamine. Unfortunately, their model did not realistically simulate the amino acid–dextrose mixtures employed clinically. Chen and co-workers[152] attributed a 26 per cent thiamine loss in a parenteral nutrition model over eight hours to the effect of direct sunlight (minimal losses with fluorescent light or indirect sunlight) without addressing the role of bisulfite. In contradiction to the findings of Scheiner and colleagues,[149] Bowman and Nguyen[153] recently reported that thiamine was stable for 24 hours in Travasol that was further diluted with dextrose, providing final sulfite concentrations of less than 0.05 per cent.

Determination of parenteral nutrition thiamine stability must account for differences in pH and bisulfite content among commercially available crystalline amino acid products. Until thiamine stability in parenteral nutrition formulations is absolutely confirmed, predisposed patients should be monitored for signs of thiamine deficiency during nutrition support, and alternative approaches to thiamine supplementation should be anticipated. Aggressive provision of carbohydrate calories may enhance thiamine utilization and precipitate thiamine deficiency.[154] Owing to the importance of thiamine in the biochemical pathways of carbohydrate metabolism and the dangers of thiamine deficiency in chronic malnutrition, in alcoholism, and with prolonged intravenous feeding,[154–156] the availability of thiamine during parenteral nutrition therapy must be clearly established by well-designed studies employing baseline and concentration versus time assays. Concern for this issue is further supported by the recent reduction in AMA/NAG[39] guidelines for thiamine content of parenteral multivitamin products.

Medication Admixture with Parenteral Nutrition Solutions

Whereas numerous studies have assessed medication stability in dextrose-saline fluids, parenteral nutrition solutions have traditionally been reserved for nutrients only. Limited compatibility information, caution regarding admixture with proteinaceous substances, and concern for bacterial contamination associated with additional admixtures has precluded the use of parenteral nutrition solutions as "drug-delivery vehicles." Admixture of drugs with parenteral nutrition solutions may facilitate management of patients who have severe fluid restriction, limited peripheral venous access, or are receiving home nutrition support. Correlation of drug dosage and nutrient requirements with parenteral nutrition infusion rate necessitates a cautious and responsible approach, especially if the medication has a narrow therapeutic range. This subject requires cautious development, with attention given to stability of additives and nutrients, as well as documented pharmacologic effectiveness following admixture. Studies should differentiate between drug stability in the large-volume parenteral nutrition solution versus stability after co-infusion or administration by auxiliary medication unit. Consideration must be given to the therapeutic appropriateness of continuous drug administration via large-volume parenteral nutrition admixture, with admixture being less desirable for drugs requiring careful titration of dosage based upon clinical response (i.e., dopamine, antiarrhythmics). Consideration must also be given to alternative means of drug administration, hospital policy governing medication administration during parenteral nutrition, and container labeling.

HEPARIN

Heparin is physically compatible in parenteral nutrition solutions in concentrations up to 20,000 U/L.[82, 83, 157] Admixture of low-dose heparin with parenteral nutrition solutions (1 to 3 U/ml) has been advocated to decrease the incidence of subclavian vein thrombosis without altering clotting time,[158–161] although a recent report[162] utilizing 1 U/ml does not support this claim. Conflicting data suggest that a certain critical concentration of heparin may be needed to be effective in hypercoagulable states. Another recent report cites the effectiveness of 20,000 U/day in reducing the risk of central vein thrombosis with silicone and PVC catheters, but hemorrhagic complications were noted.[163] It is unknown whether the routine addition of heparin to parenteral nutrition solutions can significantly deplete lipoprotein lipase stores or represents an added risk for the hemodialysis patient receiving lipid infusion.[164–167]

CIMETIDINE

The chemical stability of 300 mg/L of cimetidine hydrochloride injection in various parenteral nutrition solutions over 24 hours has been clearly demonstrated.[168, 169] Tsallas and Allen[168] employed high-pressure liquid chromatography to demonstrate 96 to 100 per cent recovery of 300 mg/L over 24 hours in a parenteral nutrition model containing typical additives. Other investigators are currently attempting to determine the stability of larger cimetidine dosages. The preliminary results appear favorable at concentrations of up to 1200 mg/L. Continuous intravenous infusion of parenteral nutrition solutions providing 900 to 1300 mg/day of cimetidine resulted in steady-state serum concentrations of 0.6 to 1.0 μ/ml in four patients over seven to 16 days.[170] Cimetidine is a routine addition in some centers for the prevention of stress ulceration and to combat metabolic alkalosis secondary to nasogastric suctioning or use of high acetate–containing crystalline amino acid solutions.[171–173] Cimetidine may be incompatible in solution with iron, aminophylline, various antibiotics, and hydrochloric acid.[169, 174]

AMINOPHYLLINE

Dilute aminophylline concentrations found in intravenous infusions appear to be stable over a wide pH range.[175, 176] Athanikar and colleagues[82] found negligible changes in pH in particulate matter levels in association with the addition of 500 mg/L to a parenteral nutrition solution. Niemiec and co-workers[177] recently reported on the chemical stability of aminophylline injection in concentrations of up to 1500 mg/L over 24 hours in three

parenteral nutrition models containing typical additives. High-pressure liquid chromatographic analysis revealed mean recovery rates in all models of 100 per cent after 24 hours and more than 94 per cent after 48 hours. Aminophylline stability was not affected by refrigeration or decreases in amino acid concentration. Addition of aminophylline to parenteral nutrition solutions containing low amino acid concentrations (i.e., 1.0 to 2.5 per cent) and maximal amounts of calcium and phosphate may result in calcium phosphate precipitation.[177] With admixture, aminophylline dosage must be carefully correlated to the parenteral nutrition infusion rate.

AMPHOTERICIN B

Addition of 100 mg/L of amphotericin B to a parenteral nutrition solution resulted in visual turbidity and unacceptable particulate matter counts.[82] Disruption of the colloidal drug dispersion is enhanced in solutions containing crystalline amino acids and electrolytes, and in solutions possessing pH values less than 6.06.[82, 178]

IRON DEXTRAN

Iron dextran has been added to parenteral nutrition solutions to provide 1 to 100 mg/L of iron, thus serving to avoid painful and inconvenient intramuscular injections. Despite the predicted negative iron balance in chronically ill patients receiving prolonged parenteral nutrition,[179] iron is not routinely added to parenteral nutrition formulations. Parenteral nutrition admixture of 1 to 8 mg/L of iron as dextran is practiced in some centers for inpatients and outpatients following administration of a test dose.[179, 180] Skepticism concerning iron dextran admixture has focused on issues of compatibility,[182] availability,[183] and concern for increasing patient susceptibility to infection in conjunction with hypotransferrinemia or periods of hyperferremia.[184–186] Since iron dextran injection is not approved for mixture with any vehicle, the need exists to evaluate the safety and efficacy of iron administration by parenteral nutrition admixture to facilitate care of patients receiving prolonged parenteral nutrition.

Wan and associates[186] assessed the chemical stability of iron dextran (100 mg/L) in a parenteral nutrition solution containing typical additives and found greater than 86 per cent recovery of total iron content after

18 hours without observing physical incompatibility. The findings of this report are difficult to interpret owing to limitations in the study design. The effect of iron dextran–parenteral nutrition admixture for longer than 18 hours, under differing conditions of temperature and pH and upon vitamin stability, remains to be clarified before routine admixture can be recommended.

Methods of iron replacement currently used include: "total dose" replacement over a few days using the parenteral nutrition solution as a vehicle, "total dose" replacement using dextrose-saline infusions with temporary interruption of parenteral nutrition therapy,[187, 188] and blood transfusions.[189] Sayers and colleagues[182] have reported on the potential benefits of parenteral nutrition admixture using ferrous citrate. A prospective study recently evaluated the restoration of serum iron levels during iron dextran–parenteral nutrition admixture, in which optimal rises in serum iron correlated with dosages of 12.5 mg/day.[179] Adverse reactions to intravenous iron administration were not observed, and the incidence of sepsis was not increased according to study criteria. Serum ferritin levels were not measured to assess iron body stores. It has been suggested that the use of iron dextran complex may confuse the interpretations of serum iron measurements, because some iron may continue to circulate as the dextran complex in addition to transferrin-bound iron.[182]

The chemical stability and availability of intravenous iron salts from parenteral nutrition formulations remains to be clearly demonstrated, with testing performed over a minimum of 24 hours under simulated conditions of use, prior to their routine admixture. Vitamin stability with iron admixture should also be assessed. Further study of patient response to parenteral nutrition–delivered iron is indicated; serum ferritin level should be assessed because it appears to be a more appropriate indicator of marrow iron stores during visceral protein malnutrition.[182, 190–192]

ANTIBIOTICS

Use of a parenteral nutrition solution as a vehicle for antibiotic administration is clinically attractive in patients with fluid restriction or limited venous access. Potential benefits of co-administration include decreases in intravenous sites or amount of infusion equipment used and improved use of fluid volumes for nutritional purposes. The relative risks of catheter contamination and central vein thrombosis associated with intermittent antibiotic administration and frequent line manipulation for medication delivery are largely unknown. Clinicians have generally hesitated to add antibiotics directly to parenteral nutrition formulas because of the lack of stability data. Simultaneous delivery of specific antibiotics and parenteral nutrition (by large-volume admixture or intermittent co-infusion) has been employed in pediatric and oncology patients and is generally performed on the basis of negative visual evidence of incompatibility.

Antibiotic stability studies traditionally involve dextrose-saline intravenous solutions. Because these solutions possess negligible titratable acidity in comparison with parenteral nutrition formulations,[79, 80] stability data generated in routine IV fluids that undergo pH change upon antibiotic admixture do not apply to parenteral nutrition solutions that are relatively resistant to pH change. Studies evaluating the visual compatibility[82, 84] of various antibiotics with parenteral nutrition solutions as well as assessing stability by microbiologic assay[82, 193–195] have been published. The majority of studies employed insensitive tests of stability, found no correlation between physical incompatibility and decreased antibiotic activity, and did not address the stability and feasibility of antibiotic-parenteral nutrition co-infusion for periods less than 24 hours. Another consideration concerns equivalent antibiotic efficacy in comparisons of administration by continuous infusion with intermittent administration by auxiliary medication unit (providing higher peak serum levels).[196–201] The feasibility of continuous antibiotic infusion may depend upon the pathogen involved, site of infection, and minimum inhibitory concentration of bacteria. Several studies by Bodey and co-workers[196–198] have successfully employed continuous aminoglycoside infusions in immunocompromised adult patients but have noted a poor response rate for Klebsiella infections during continuous infusion. Colding and associates[199] have reported on the achievement of therapeutic serum levels of gentamicin and ampicillin and positive clinical response following parenteral nutrition admixture and continuous infusion in neonates. Reed and colleagues[202] cite the advantages of cyclic parenteral nutrition therapy in facilitating the administration of chemotherapy, amphotericin B, and trimethoprim-sulfamethoxazole during parenteral nutrition infusion-free periods.

As suggested by preliminary microbiologic assay reports, it is probable that many antibiotics are reasonably stable with parenteral nutrition fluids, especially upon co-infusion. On the basis of available information, it is difficult to define conditions under which numerous antibiotics retain or lose significant activity. Further study is indicated to clearly delineate the stability and feasibility in the administration of select antimicrobials by co-infusion or as additives to parenteral nutrition formulas. Sensitive and specific assays should be employed (i.e., high-pressure liquid chromatography), with stability testing at short enough intervals to clarify the feasibility of "piggybacking" antibiotics with parenteral nutrition solutions. Optimal confirmation of compatibility should include molecular stability study by quantitative assay in conjunction with anti-infective activity determination by microbiologic assay. Until such data are accumulated, it would seem prudent to limit antibiotic admixture via parenteral nutrition delivery systems. Stability of a single antibiotic in a parenteral nutrition solution does not confer compatibility with other antibiotics in solution.[194]

HYDROCHLORIC ACID

Hydrochloric acid (100 mEq/L) availability from a parenteral nutrition model has been demonstrated with minimal alteration of amino acid content.[203] Admixtures may be useful for short-term treatment of severe, refractory metabolic alkalosis.

CORTICOSTEROIDS

There is a general lack of published compatibility data pertaining to corticosteroid admixture with parenteral nutrition solutions. One report did cite the admixture of hydrocortisone sodium succinate (5 mg/L) to a parenteral nutrition solution without noting incompatibility, but B vitamins were not added to this solution owing to a speculated interaction.[204] Solu-Cortef is believed to be physically compatible in a concentration of 500 mg/L in a dextrose–FreAmine II model containing electrolytes, vitamins, insulin, and heparin.[205] Solu-Medrol, 250 mg/L, has been reported to be physically compatible in a dextrose–FreAmine II solution without additives.[82] Various centers have admixed up to 250 mg/L of Solu-Cortef or Solu-Medrol

with parenteral nutrition formulas without noting visual incompatibility. At present, however, most clinicians prefer to administer corticosteroids by IV push or co-infusion.

METOCLOPRAMIDE

Metoclopramide is reported to be chemically stable for 72 hours at room temperature in concentrations of 5 and 20 mg/L in a Travasol 2.75 per cent–dextrose 25 per cent model including electrolytes. Metoclopramide reportedly facilitates an increase in gastric emptying time and pyloric sphincter relaxation[206–209] and may be helpful in gastroparesis associated with tumor burden, diabetes, and postoperative gastric atony.[209–213] Controlled observations are required to establish the drug's efficacy in facilitating enteral feeding tube placement and enteral nutrition in association with parenteral nutrition or postoperative ileus.[206, 213]

NARCOTICS

Narcotic analgesics have not generally been added to or co-infused with parenteral nutrition formulations because of the lack of stability data. Because venous access may be quite limited in cancer patients receiving nutrition support, co-infusion or admixture of morphine, meperidine, hydromorphone, and levorphanol with parenteral nutrition solutions has been used in hospitalized and ambulatory patients. Visual incompatibility has not been observed with typical daily dosages, and pain relief has been successfully maintained. Chemical stability studies are currently in progress. Hydromorphone hydorchloride has been reported to be compatible with various amino acid products in concentrations up to 80 mg/L, but tested solutions did not simulate actual parenteral nutrition formulations being used clinically.[215] Should current stability studies document compatibility of select narcotics, use of a parenteral nutrition solution to deliver narcotic analgesia will require consideration of the potential risks of continuous infusion.[216–218]

DIGOXIN

Because a major portion of digoxin is absorbed in the upper small bowel[219] and because its intramuscular administration is unpleasant and incomplete, patients with significant small-bowel resection requiring chronic digoxin therapy and parenteral nutrition would benefit from data supporting the stability and availability of digoxin from parenteral nutrition solutions. The intravenous preparation is carefully formulated in a nonaqueous propylene glycol solvent; therefore, concern has been raised that this poorly water-soluble drug may preferentially partition into plastic intravenous delivery systems when placed in an aqueous environment and infused over time.[220] Thus, stability studies should carefully assess both stability and availability of digoxin in a parenteral nutrition delivery system.

Digoxin reportedly does not undergo substantial hydrolytic cleavage in solution at a pH of 5 to 8 over 24 hours at 37°C.[220] It is reported to be chemically stable in concentrations of 0.25 mg/99 ml in dextrose–saline IV fluids upon storage at 4 and 23°C for 48 hours in glass.[221] Blackstone and colleagues[222] have reported physicochemical stability of 0.25 to 1.0 mg/L digoxin in parenteral nutrition fluid by radioimmunoassay for up to 96 hours when the solution is stored in plastic IV bags at 4°C. Success in maintaining adequate serum digoxin concentrations and therapeutic response following admixture has been reported in limited numbers of patients.[222, 223] Previous reports have demonstrated that the potency of specific drugs administered in small dosages may be reduced during in-line filtration,[224, 225] although digoxin has been reported not to bind significantly to cellulose or polycarbonate membrane filters.[219, 220]

INOTROPIC AGENTS AND VASODILATORS

Assessment of dopamine-parenteral nutrition compatibility has not been conducted owing to the need for continuous titration of dopamine infusions to hemodynamic response. Direct parenteral nutrition admixture (as a large-volume parenteral) of dopamine, dobutamine, nitroprusside, nitroglycerin, isoproterenol, and norepinephrine would be unlikely, would require numerous stability and dosage considerations, and would be therapeutically unsuitable. However, the feasibility of co-infusing these medications with parenteral nutrition formulas may deserve exploration. Factors to consider in such a study should include the influence of solution pH and electrolyte and trace mineral content upon drug stability and the attainment of pharmacologic response associated with co-infusion.

5-FLUOROURACIL

Speculation exists in the medical literature concerning the relative toxicity and efficacy of 5-FU when administered as an intravenous bolus and when diluted with prolonged infusion.[226, 227] It has been suggested that dilutions of 5-FU may not provide adequate therapeutic effects and that administration by prolonged infusion may be less myelotoxic and less effective than bolus injection with comparable dosages.[226] Athanikar and colleagues[82] found 500 mg/L to be physically compatible in a parenteral nutrition model over 24 hours at 4°C. The chemical stability of 1 mg/ml has been reported in a parenteral nutrition model.[228, 229]

Trace Minerals

Boddapati and co-workers[230] reported stability of combined trace minerals (zinc, copper, manganese, chromium) in a representative parenteral nutrition formulation over 24 hours at elevated temperatures and under refrigeration. Differences in mineral recovery were not demonstrated between glass and plastic intravenous containers, and in-line filtration did not alter recovery during a three-hour infusion.

Conclusion

Tables 14–14 to 14–16 have been compiled to serve as supplements to the preceding monographs, with the realization that compatibility designations expressed in tabular form represent many sources and may not adequately identify the limitations of the original report or compatibility.

There remains a continuing need for practical, applied research dealing with parenteral nutrition compatibility that is based upon sound, scientific technique. Suggestions for conducting and reporting stability studies have been offered in a recent editorial by Trissel.[78] Adequate description of methods and materials and the use of specific baseline and replicate sample assays in future studies will help to provide meaningful information and minimize contradictory findings. It is optimal to evaluate the primary literature report and evaluate the validity of the study design, limiting conditions, and appropriateness of extrapolating the findings. Consideration must be given to availability of nutrients and drugs from, as well as their stability in, parenteral nutrition delivery systems.

Table 14–14. ADDITIVES COMPATIBLE WITH AMINO ACID–DEXTROSE SOLUTION*

ADDITIVE	VISUAL COMPATIBILITY (AMOUNT/L)	CHEMICAL STABILITY (AMOUNT/L)	COMMENTS
Albumin	12.5–37.5 gm		Anecdotal experience; high concentrations may occlude in-line filters
Insulin	100 U		Variable adsorptive losses less than 60%
Vitamins, Multiple	10 ml		Manufacturer claims 24-hour stability of constituent vitamins under normal environmental conditions
Folic Acid	5 mg	1 mg	Avoid direct sunlight
Vitamin K	10 mg		Maintains prothrombin time following admixture
Aminophylline	500 mg	1500 mg	May alter solution tolerance of calcium phosphate
Cimetidine		300 mg	Pharmacologic serum concentrations attained
Hydrochloric Acid		100 mEq	
Heparin	20,000		

*Refer to text for further elaboration.

Table 14–15. ADDITIVES INCOMPATIBLE OR CONDITIONALLY COMPATIBLE WITH AMINO ACID–DEXTROSE SOLUTIONS*

ADDITIVE	AMOUNT/L	COMMENTS
Incompatible		
Sodium bicarbonate	—	Acid-base reaction, interaction with calcium and magnesium salts
Amphotericin B	100 mg	Visual turbidity
Ampicillin	1 g	Further stability study required for short intervals
Conditionally Compatible		
Calcium-phosphate salts	—	Dependent upon numerous factors
Thiamine	—	Further stability study required
Antibiotics (numerous)	—	See Table 14–17
Digoxin	0.25–1.0 mg	Further stability and availability studies required
Hydrocortisone sodium succinate	500 mg	Further stability study required
Methylprednisolone sodium succinate	250 mg	Further stability study required
Narcotic analgesics	—	Physical compatibility noted with selected agents; stability studies pending
Iron dextran	100 mg	Further stability study required
Vitamin A	—	Variable availability from delivery systems; further study required

*Refer to text for further elaboration.

Table 14–16. ANTIBIOTIC COMPATIBILITY STUDIES IN PARENTERAL NUTRITION SOLUTIONS*

AUTHOR		ATHANIKAR[82]		SCHUETZ[84]		FEIGIN[193]				REED[194]		COLDING[195]	
TYPE STUDY		VISUAL (PARTICULATE)		MICRO (DISK DIFFUSION) VISUAL		MICRO (DISK DIFFUSION)				MICRO (TUBE DILUTION) VISUAL		MICRO (DISK DIFFUSION) VISUAL	
SOLUTION		CAA/D, NO ADDITIVES		CAA/D + ADDITIVES		CAA/D + ADDITIVES				PH/D + ADDITIVES		CAA/F + ADDITIVES	
TEMPERATURE (TIME)		4°C (22 HR) ROOM (2 HR)		22°C (24 HR)		24 HR 4°C	25°C	37°C		4°C, ROOM (24 HR)		29°C (24 HR)	
		Amount/L	Result	Amount	Result	Amount				Amount	Result	Amount	Result
Antibiotic													
Ampicillin, Na	(G)	1.0	X	0.5, 1.0	Visual C / Micro C (12 hr)	1.0 C	C (6 hr) X (24 hr)	X				1.5	Visual C / Micro X
Carbenicillin, diNa	(G)	8.0	C			1.0 C	C	C		1.5	Visual C / Micro C	6.0	Visual C / Micro X
Cephalothin, Na	(G)	2.0	C	2.0	Visual C / Micro C (12 hr)	1.0 C	C	X		0.6	Visual C / Micro C		
Cefazolin, Na	(G)	1.0	C								Visual C / Micro C		
Chloramphenicol, Na Succ	(G)									0.7	Visual C / Micro C		
Clindamycin phosphate	(G)	0.6	C			0.25 C	C	C		0.1	Visual C / Micro C		
Erythromycin gluceptate	(G)	1.0	C										
Gentamicin SO₄	(mg)	80	C	80	Visual C / Micro C (12 hr)					50	Visual C / Micro C	50	Visual C / Micro C
Kanamycin SO₄	(G)	0.5	C	0.5	Visual C / Micro C (12 hr)	0.25 C	—	X (6 hr)		1.5	Visual C / Micro C		
Methicillin, Na	(G)	1.0	C			1.0 C	C	X		1.5	Visual C / Micro C		
Oxacillin, Na	(G)	0.5	C										
Penicillin G	(m.u.)	1.0	C			5.0 C	C	C		0.4	Visual C / Micro C		
Polymyxin B SO₄	(mg)											40	Visual C / Micro C
Tetracycline HCl†	(G)	0.5	C										
Tobramycin SO₄	(mg)	80	C							50	Visual C / Micro C		

*CAA = crystalline amino acid; PH = protein hydrolysate; D = dextrose; F = fructose; C = compatible; X = incompatible.
†May chelate with Ca, Mg in solution.

SOLUTION ORDERING

The multicomponent nature of parenteral nutrition solutions has generated the development of ordering forms that simplify, standardize, or prompt completeness in ordering of parenteral nutrition solutions. Forms for parenteral nutrition solution ordering should meet the needs of each nutrition support team or institution. Some forms are limited to the ordering of the parenteral nutrition solutions, whereas more comprehensive standardized forms include the options to order placement of central venous catheters, baseline metabolic monitoring parameters, and other multidisciplinary services to maximize support of total parenteral nutrition patients. An example of a comprehensive standardized form is illustrated in Figure 14–4.

It is important to emphasize that the use of standardized forms should not be abused, especially in light of the need for cost containment in clinical practice. Preprinted standardized forms should serve to prompt ordering of comprehensive services in an efficient and simplified manner. However, inefficient utilization of standard services in all parenteral nutrition patients should be discouraged. Requiring individual indications for each service or test ordered rather than a signature on several pages of preprinted orders may facilitate the continued therapeutic and cost-effective thought process needed in the care of parenteral nutrition patients.

PARENTERAL NUTRITION ORDERS

1. X-ray for central line catheter placement.
2. Central line IV: DIOW at 20 ml/hr until parenteral nutrition solution started.
3. Start parenteral nutrition solution as ordered below after catheter placement confirmed.
4. Parenteral nutrition solution (check A for standard formula, or specify modified formula B)

☐A. Standard Formula (vol: 1000 ml)   ☐B. Modified Formula (vol: _____ ml)

Dextrose	25%		Dextrose	_____
Amino acids	4.25%		Amino acids	_____
NaCl	50mEq		NaCl	_____
KCl	10mEq		NaAcetate	_____
KPhos	20mEq		KCl	_____
MgSO$_4$	8mEq		KPhos	_____
CaGluconate	4.7mEq		MgSO$_4$	_____
MVI-12	10ml/day		CaGluconate	_____
Trace minerals	1ml/day		MVI-12	_____
Other_____			MVI concentrate	_____
_____			Trace minerals	_____
			Other _____	

Rate_____ ml/hr   Rate_____ ml/hr

5. Lipids: ☐20% or ☐10%, _____ml at _____ml/hr.
6. ☐Parenteral nutrition monitoring protocol
   includes: Baseline electrolytes, Mg, Phos, glucose, Cr, chemical profile
   Electrolytes daily for 3 days, then 3 × /wk
   Urine glucose every shift, call MD if ≥3 +
   Chemical profile 2 × /wk
   ABC 2 × /wk
7. ☐Social Services _____
   ☐Physical Therapy_____

_____ M.D.

Date:_____   Time:_____

U.C._____   R.N._____

Figure 14–4. Standardized solution ordering form.

PHARMACIST'S ROLE

The role of the nutrition support pharmacist will vary with individual interest, expertise, and availability of expertise of other professionals involved in nutrition support at their respective institutions. The nutrition support pharmacist is uniquely qualified in several aspects of nutrition support practice, including cost-effective formulary product solution, solution admixture and quality control, solution stability and compatibility, and cost-effective formulation ordering. Practicing nutrition support pharmacists often integrate this background into providing clinical services in daily patient care, conducting clinical and laboratory research, and teaching.

REFERENCES

1. Garb, S.: Laboratory Tests in Common Use, 6th ed. New York, Springer Verlag, 1976, p. 91.
2. Vere, D.W.: Venous thrombosis during dextrose infusion. Lancet, 1:627, 1960.
3. Dextrose Monograph. In The United States Pharmacopeia, 20th ed. Easton, PA, Mack, 1980, p. 218.
4. McKibbin, J.M., Pope, A., and Thayer, B.A.: Parenteral nutrition: Studies on fat emulsions for intravenous alimentation. J. Lab. Clin. Med., 30:488, 1945.
5. Schuberth, O., and Wretlind, A.: Intravenous infusion of fat emulsions, phosphatides, and emulsifying agents. Acta Chim. Scand., 278 (Suppl.):1021, 1961.
6. Elwyn, D.H.: Nutritional requirements of adult surgical patients. Crit. Care Med., 8:9, 1980.
7. Prescribing Information for Intralipid Intravenous Fat Emulsion. Berkeley, CA, Cutter Laboratories, Inc., 1981.
8. Prescribing Information for Liposyn Intravenous Fat Emulsion. Chicago, Abbott Laboratories, Inc., 1981.
9. Prescribing Information for Soyacal Intravenous Fat Emulsion. Los Angeles, Alpha Therapeutic Corp., 1982.
10. Prescribing Information for Travamulsion Intravenous Fat Emulsion. Deerfield, IL, Travenol Laboratories, Inc., 1981.
11. Pennington, C.R., and Richards, J.M.: Three-liter bags containing Intralipid for parenteral nutrition (letter). J.P.E.N., 7:304, 1983.
12. Brennan, M.F., et al.: Glycerol: major contributor to the short-term protein-sparing effect of fat emulsions in normal man. Ann. Surg., 182:386, 1975.
13. Prescribing Information for Procalamine, 3% Amino Acid and 3% Glycerin Injection with Electrolytes. Irvine, CA, American McGaw, 1982.
14. Tao, R.C., et al.: Glycerol: its metabolism and use as an intravenous energy source. J.P.E.N., 7:479, 1983.
15. Singh, V.N.: Non-glucose carbohydrate as an alternate energy source (abstract). 7th Clinical Congress, American Society of Parenteral and Enteral Nutrition, Washington, D.C., 1983.
16. Trissel, L.A.: Handbook of Injectable Drugs, 2nd ed. Bethesda, MD, American Society of Hospital Pharmacists, 1980, p. 583.
17. Friedman, G.J.: Diet in the treatment of diabetes mellitus. In Goodhart, R.S., and Shils, M.E. (eds.): Modern Nutrition in Health and Disease. Philadelphia, Lea & Febiger, 1980, p. 984.
18. Facts and Comparisons. J.B. Lippincott Company. St. Louis, Missouri. 1980, p. 39.
19. Ahnefeld, F.W., Bassler, K.H., Bauer, B.L., et al.: Suitability of non-glucose carbohydrates for parenteral nutrition. Eur. J. Intensive Care Med., 1:105, 1975.
20. van Eys, J.: Alternate fuel sources (abstract). 7th Clinical Congress, American Society of Parenteral and Enteral Nutrition, Washington, D.C., 1983.
21. Thomas, D.W., et al.: Complications following intravenous administration of solutions containing xylitol. Med. J. Aust., 1:1238, 1972.
22. Prescribing Information for Novamine Amino Acid Injection. Berkeley, CA, Cutter Laboratories, 1983.
23. Winters, R.W.: Aminosyn, FreAmine III, Travasol and Novamine: What are the differences? In The Supplement. Fairfield, NJ, HNS, 1983.
24. Stegink, L.D., and Baker, G.L.: Infusion of protein hydrolysates in the newborn infant: Plasma amino acid concentrations. J. Pediatr., 78:595, 1971.
25. Mirtallo, J.M., et al.: Clinical comparison of two 8.5% amino acid injection products. Am. J. Hosp. Pharm., 38:83, 1981.
26. Prescribing Information for RenAmin Amino Acid Injection Renal Formula. Deerfield, IL, Travenol Laboratories, Inc., 1982.
27. Montgomerie, J.Z., Kalmanson, G.M., and Guze, L.B.: Renal failure and infection. Medicine, 47:132, 1968.
28. Mirtallo, J.M., et al.: A comparison of essential and general amino acid infusions in the nutritional support of patients with compromised renal function. J.P.E.N., 6:109, 1982.
29. Freund, H., et al.: Comparative study of parenteral nutrition in renal failure using essential and nonessential amino acid–containing solutions. Surg. Gynecol. Obstet., 151:652, 1980.
30. Blumenkrantz, M.S., et al.: Total parenteral nutrition in the management of acute renal failure. Am. J. Clin. Nutr., 31:1831, 1978.
31. Blackburn, G.L., Etter, G., and Mackenzie, T.: Criteria for choosing amino acid therapy in acute renal failure. Am. J. Clin. Nutr., 31:1841, 1978.
32. Prescribing Information for Hepatamine Amino Acid Injection. Irvine, CA, American McGaw, 1982.
33. Prescribing Information for FreAmine HBC Amino Acid Injection. Irvine, CA, American McGaw, 1982.
34. Prescribing Information for Trophamine 6% Amino Acid Injection. Irvine, CA, American McGaw, 1983.
35. Prescribing Information for L-Cysteine. Chicago, Abbott Laboratories, Inc., 1982.
36. Fong, W.L., and Grimley, G.W.: Peripheral intravenous infusion of amino acids. Am. J. Hosp. Pharm., 38:652, 1981.
37. Akers, M.J., Schrank, G.D., and Russell, S.: Partic-

ulate evaluation of parenteral nutrition solutions by electronic particle counting and scanning electron microscopy. Am. J. Hosp. Pharm., 38:1304, 1981.

38. Prescribing Information for TPN Electrolytes Multiple Electrolyte Additive. Chicago, Abbott Laboratories, Inc., 1978.

39. American Medical Association, Department of Foods and Nutrition: Multivitamin preparations for parenteral use. A statement by the Nutrition Advisory Group. J.P.E.N., 3:253, 1979.

40. Facts and Comparisons. St Louis, J.B. Lippincott Company, 1984, p. 18–34.

41. American Medical Association, Department of Foods and Nutrition: Guidelines for essential trace element preparations for parenteral use. A statement by the nutrition advisory group. J.P.E.N., 3:263, 1979.

42. Goldmann, D.A., Martin, W.R., and Worthington, J.W.: Growth of bacteria and fungi in total parenteral nutrition solutions. Am. J. Surg. 126:314, 1973.

43. Rowlando, D.A., Wilkinson, W.R., and Yoshimura, N.: Storage stability of mixed hyperalimentation solutions. Am. J. Hosp. Pharm., 30:436, 1973.

44. Gelbert, S.M., Reinhardt, G.F., and Greenlee, H.B.: Multiplication of nosocomial pathogens in intravenous feeding solutions. Appl. Microbiol., 26:874, 1973.

45. Brennan, M.F., et al.: The growth of Candida albicans in nutritive solutions given parenterally. Arch. Surg., 103:705, 1971.

46. Mirtallo, J.M., et al.: Growth of bacteria and fungi in parenteral nutrition solutions containing albumin. Am. J. Hosp. Pharm., 38:1907, 1981.

47. Wilkinson, W.R., Floreo, L.L., and Pagoves, J.N.: Growth of microorganisms in parenteral nutritional fluids. Drug Intell. Clin. Pharm., 7:226, 1973.

48. Keammerer, D., et al.: Microbial growth patterns in intravenous fat emulsions. Am. J. Hosp. Pharm., 40:1650, 1983.

49. Deitel, M., Fuksa, M., Kaminski, M.V., et al.: Growth of microorganisms in soybean oil emulsion: Clinical implication. Int. Surg., 64:27, 1971.

50. Crocker, K.S., et al.: Microbial growth comparisons of five commercial parenteral lipid emulsions. J.P.E.N., 8:391, 1984.

51. National Coordinating Committee on Large Volume Parenterals: Recommendations to pharmacists for solving problems with large volume parenterals. Am. J. Hosp. Pharm., 33:231, 1976.

52. Sanders, L.H., Mabadeje, S.A., Avis, K.E., et al.: Evaluation of compounding accuracy and aseptic techniques for intravenous admixtures. Am. J. Hosp. Pharm., 35:531, 1978.

53. Sarubbi, F.A., Wilson, M.B., Lee, M., et al.: Nosocomial meningitis and bacteremia due to contaminated amphotericin B. J.A.M.A., 239:416, 1978.

54. Plouffe, J.F., Brown, D.G., Silva, J., et al.: Nosocomial outbreak of Candida parapsilosis fungemia related to intravenous infusions. Arch. Intern. Med., 137:1686, 1977.

55. Goldmann, D.A., and Maki, D.G.: Infection control in total parenteral nutrition. J.A.MA., 223:1360, 1973.

56. Laegeler, W.L., Tio, J.M., and Blake, M.I.: Stability of certain amino acids in a parenteral nutrition solution. Am. J. Hosp. Pharm., 31:776, 1974.

57. Schroeder, L.J., Iacobellis, M., and Smith, A.H.: The influence of water and pH on the reaction between amino compounds and carbohydrates. J. Biol. Chem., 212:973, 1955.

58. Foster, A.B., and Horton, D.: Aspects of the chemistry of the amino sugars. Adv. Carbohydr. Chem., 14:213, 1959.

59. Ellis, G.P.: The Maillard reaction. Adv. Carbohydr. Chem., 14:63, 1959.

60. Jurgens, R.W., Henry, R.S., and Welco, A.: Amino acid stability in a mixed parenteral nutrition solution. Am. J. Hosp. Pharm., 38:1358, 1981.

61. Ausman, R.K., Kerkhof, K., Holmes, C.J., et al.: Frozen storage and microwave thawing of parenteral nutrition solutions in plastic containers. Drug Intell. Clin. Pharm., 15:440, 1981.

62. Koida, Y., Matsuda, S., and Miura, H.: Preparation of infusion for total parenteral nutrition. Acta Chir. Scand., 466(Suppl.):116, 1976.

63. LeVeen, H., Giordano, P., and Johnson, A.: Flocculation of intravenous fat emulsions. Am. J. Clin. Nutr., 16:129, 1965.

64. Black, C., and Popovich, N.: Stability in intravenous fat emulsions. Arch. Surg., 115:891, 1980.

65. Davis, S.: The stability of fat emulsions for intravenous administration. In Johnston I. (ed.): Advances in Clinical Nutrition: Selected Proceedings of the Second International Symposium. Lancaster, MTP Press, Limited, 1983, p. 213.

66. Hardy, G., Cotter, R., and Dawe, R.: The stability and comparative clearance of TPN mixtures with lipid. In Johnston, I. (ed.): Advances in Clinical Nutrition: Selected Proceedings of the Second International Symposium. Lancaster, MTP Press, Limited, 1983, p. 241.

67. Ang, S., et al.: Clinical use of an admixture of amino acids, dextrose, and fat emulsion: Compatibility and stability (Abstract). 7th Clinical Congress, American Society of Parenteral and Enteral Nutrition, Washington, D.C., 1983.

68. Kirkland, W.D., et al.: Compatibility of Intralipid IV fat emulsion in total parenteral nutrition admixtures (Abstract). 7th Clinical Congress, American Society of Parenteral and Enteral Nutrition, Washington, D.C., 1983.

69. Black, C.D., and Popovich, N.G.: A study of intravenous emulsion compatibility: Effects of dextrose, amino acids, and selected electrolytes. Drug Intell. Clin. Pharm., 15:184, 1981.

70. Cotter, R., et al.: Comparison of the physical stability and metabolism of lipid emulsions administered in varying total parenteral nutrition regimens (abstract). 7th Clinical Congress, American Society of Parenteral and Enteral Nutrition, Washington, D.C., 1983.

71. Burnham, W.R., et al.: Stability of a fat emulsion based intravenous feeding mixture. Int. J. Pharm., 13:9, 1983.

72. Pamperl, H., and Kleinberger, G.: Stability of intravenous fat emulsions. Arch. Surg., 117:859, 1982.

73. O'Neill, M., et al.: Comparison of two methods of fat emulsion infusion in total parenteral nutrition (TPN) (abstract). 7th Clinical Congress, American Society of Parenteral and Enteral Nutrition, Washington, D.C., 1983.

74. Epps, D.R.: Clinical results with total nutrient admixture for intravenous infusion. Clin. Pharmacol., 2:268, 1983.

75. Prescribing Information for Intralipid Admixture. Berkeley, Cutter Laboratories, 1983.

76. Malky, M.J., and Haspela, N.A.: The national survey of neonatal intravenous alimentation services. Am. J. Intrav. Ther. Clin. Nutr., 2:43, 1980.

77. Cluxton, R.: Some complexities of making compatibility studies in hyperalimentation solutions. Drug Intell. Clin. Pharm., 5:177, 1971.

78. Trissel, L.: Avoiding common flaws in stability and compatibility studies of injectable drugs. Am. J. Hosp. Pharm., 40:1159, 1983.

79. Sturgeon, R., Athanikar, N., Henry, R., et al.: Titratable acidities of crystalline amino acid admixtures. Am. J. Hosp. Pharm., 37:388, 1980.

80. Chan, J., Malekzadeh, M., and Hurley, J.: pH and titratable acidity of amino acid mixtures used in hyperalimentation. J.A.M.A., 220:1119, 1972.

81. Athanikar, N., Boyer, B., Deamer, R., et al.: Visual compatibility of 30 additives with a parenteral nutrient solution. Am. J. Hosp. Pharm., 36:511, 1979.

82. Schuetz, D., and King, J.: Compatibility and stability of electrolytes, vitamins and antibiotics in combination with 8% amino acid solution. Am. J. Hosp. Pharm., 35:33, 1978.

83. Kobayashi, N., and King, J.: Compatibility of common additives in protein hydrolysate/dextrose solutions. Am. J. Hosp. Pharm., 34:589, 1977.

84. Turco, S., and King, R.: Sterile Dosage Forms. Philadelphia, Lea & Febiger, 1979, p. 276.

85. Weber, S., Wood, W., and Jackson, E.: Availability of insulin from parenteral nutrient solutions. Am. J. Hosp. Pharm., 34:353, 1977.

86. Tate, J., and Cowan, G.: Insulin kinetics in hyperalimentation solution and routine intravenous therapy. Am. J. Surg., 43:811, 1977.

87. Goldberg, N., and Levin, S.: Insulin adsorption to an in-line membrane filter (letter) N. Engl. J. Med., 298:1480, 1978.

88. Whalen, F., LeCain, W., and Latiolais, C.: Availability of insulin from continuous low-dose insulin infusions. Am. J. Hosp. Pharm., 36:330, 1979.

89. Petty, C., and Cunningham, N.: Insulin adsorption by glass infusion bottles, polyvinyl chloride infusion containers, and intravenous tubing. Anesthesiology, 40:400, 1974.

90. Peterson, L., Caldwell, J., and Hoffman, J.: Insulin adsorbance to polyvinyl chloride surfaces with implications for constant-infusion therapy. Diabetes, 25:72, 1976.

91. Hirsch, J., Fratkin, M., Wood, J., et al.: Clinical significance of insulin adsorption by polyvinyl chloride infusion systems. Am. J. Hosp. Pharm., 34:583, 1977.

92. Twardowski, Z., Nolph, K., McGary, T., et al.: Insulin binding to plastic bags: A methodologic study. Am. J. Hosp. Pharm., 40:575, 1983.

93. Twardowski, Z., Nolph, K., McGary, T., et al.: Influence of temperature and time on insulin adsorption to plastic bags. Am. J. Hosp. Pharm., 40:583, 1983.

94. Kraegen, E., Lazarus, L., Meler, H., et al.: Carrier solutions for low-level intravenous insulin infusion. Br. Med. J., 3:464, 1975.

95. Kerchner, J., Colaluca, D., and Juhl, R.: Effect of whole blood on insulin adsorption onto intravenous infusion systems. Am. J. Hosp. Pharm., 37:1323, 1980.

96. Genuth, S.: Constant intravenous insulin infusion in diabetic ketoacidosis. J.A.M.A., 223:1348, 1973.

97. Kidson, W., Casey, J., Kraegen, E., et al.: Treatment of severe diabetes mellitus by insulin infusion. Br. Med. J., 2:691, 1974.

98. Page, M., Alberti, K., Greenwood, R., et al.: Treatment of diabetic coma with continuous low-dose infusion of insulin. Br. Med. J., 2:687, 1974.

99. Semple, P., White, C., and Manderson, W.: Continuous intravenous infusion of small doses of insulin in treatment of diabetic ketoacidosis. Br. Med. J. 2:694, 1974.

100. Weisenfeld, S., Podolsky, S., Goldsmith, L., et al.: Adsorption of insulin to infusion bottles and tubing. Diabetes, 17:766, 1968.

101. Felig, P.: Insulin: Rates and routes of delivery. N. Engl. J. Med., 291:1031 (editorial), 1974.

102. Sacks, H., Shahshahani, M., Kitabchi, A., et al.: Similar responsiveness of diabetic ketoacidosis to low-dose insulin by intramuscular injection and albumin-free infusion. Ann. Intern. Med., 90:36, 1979.

103. Eggert, L., Rusho, W., MacKay, M., et al.: Calcium and phosphorus compatibility in parenteral nutrition solutions for neonates. Am. J. Hosp. Pharm., 39:49, 1982.

104. Johnston, I.: Advances in Parenteral Nutrition. Lancaster, MTP Press, Limited, 1978, pp. 267, 418.

105. Henry, R., Jurgens, R., Sturgeon, R., et al.: Compatibility of calcium chloride and calcium gluconate with sodium phosphate in a mixed TPN solution. Am. J. Hosp. Pharm., 37:673, 1980.

106. Kaminski, M., Harris, D., Collins, C., et al.: Electrolyte compatibility in a synthetic amino acid hyperalimentation solution. Am. J. Hosp. Pharm., 31:244, 1974.

107. Henry, R., Jurgens, R., Harbison, H., et al.: Temperature effects on calcium phosphate precipitation in a mixed parenteral nutrition solution (abstract). 15th Annual ASHP Midyear Clinical Meeting, San Francisco, 1980.

108. Niemiec, P., Fochtman, F., Giudici, R., et al.: Compatibility guidelines pertaining to calcium and phosphate addition to a parenteral nutrient solution. Thesis, Duquesne University, 1981.

109. Robinson, L., and Wright, B.: Central venous catheter occlusion caused by body-heat–mediated calcium phosphate precipitation. Am. J. Hosp. Pharm., 39:120, 1982.

110. Pomerance, H., and Rader, R.: Crystal formation: A new complication of total parenteral nutrition. Pediatrics, 52:864, 1973.

111. Knight, P., Buchanan, S., and Clatworthy, W.: Calcium and phosphate requirements of preterm infants who require prolonged hyperalimentation. J.A.M.A., 243:1244, 1980.

112. Boulet, M., Marier, J., and Rose, D.: Effect of magnesium on formation of calcium phosphate precipitates. Arch. Biochem. Biophys., 96:629, 1962.

113. VanDenBerg, L., and Soliman, F.: Composition and pH changes during freezing of solutions containing calcium and magnesium phosphate. Cryobiology 6:10, 1969.

114. Boulet, M., and Marier, J.: Precipitation of calcium phosphates from solutions at near physiological concentrations. Arch. Biochem. Biophys., 93:157, 1961.

115. Poole, R., Rupp, C., and Kerner, J.: Calcium and phosphorus in neonatal parenteral nutrition solutions. J.P.E.N., 7:358, 1983.

116. Knight, P., Heer, D., and Abdenour, G.: Ca × P

and Ca/P in the parenteral feeding of preterm infants. J.P.E.N., 7:110, 1983.

117. Niemiec, P., and Vanderveen, T.: Compatibility considerations in parenteral nutrient solutions. Am. J. Hosp. Pharm., 41:893, 1984.

118. Trissel, L.: Handbook on Injectable Drugs, 2nd ed. Washington, D.C., American Society of Hospital Pharmacists, 1980, p. 485.

119. Mirtallo, J., Schneider, P., and Ruberg, R.: Albumin in TPN solutions: Potential savings from a prospective review. J.P.E.N., 4:300, 1980.

120. Tullis, J.: Albumin. I: Background and use. J.A.M.A., 237:355, 1977.

121. Tullis, J.: Albumin. II: Guidelines for clinical use. J.A.M.A., 237:460, 1977.

122. Foss, N.E., Scheller, G.H., and Sullivan, C.F.: Folic acid. Calco Tech. Bull., 721:9, 1947.

123. Scheindlin, S., Lee, A., and Griffith, I.: The action of riboflavin on folic acid. J. Am. Pharm. A, Sci. Ed., 41:420, 1952.

124. Scheindlin, S., and Griffith, I.: The action of ascorbic acid on folic acid. Am. J. Pharm., 123:78, 1951.

125. Bergy, G.: Folic acid incompatibilities. Am. Prof. Pharm., 16:523, 1950.

126. Lewis, G.P., and Rowe, P.B.: Oxidative and reductive cleavage of folates: A critical appraisal. Anal. Biochem., 93:91, 1979.

127. Trissel, L.A.: Handbook on Injectable Drugs, 2nd ed. Bethesda, Maryland, American Society of Hospital Pharmacists, 1980, p. 225.

128. Wade, A. (ed.): Martindale: The Extra Pharmacopoeia, 27th ed. London, The Pharmaceutical Press, 1977, pp. 1683.

129. American Hospital Formulary Service. Maryland, American Society of Hospital Pharmacists, 1982, p. 1683.

130. Louie, N., and Stennett, D.: Stability of folic acid in 25% dextrose, 3.5% amino acids and multivitamin solution. J.P.E.N., 8:424, 1984.

131. Barker, A., Hebron, B., Beck, P., et al.: Folic acid and total parenteral nutrition. J.P.E.N., 8:3, 1984.

132. Butler, L., Munson, J., and DeLuca, P.P.: Effect of in-line filtration on the potency of low-dose drugs. Am. J. Hosp. Pharm., 37:935, 1980.

133. Longe, R.: Stability of phytonadione in hyperalimentation fluids (letter). Am. J. Hosp. Pharm., 31:759, 1974.

134. Frear, R., and Patel, J.: Stability of phytonadione in parenteral nutrition solutions (abstract). 16th Annual American Society of Hospital Pharmacists Midyear Clinical Meeting, New Orleans, 1981.

135. Rymer, W., and Greenlaw, C.: Hypoprothrombinemia associated with cefamandole. Drug Intell. Clin. Pharm., 14:780, 1980.

136. Fainstein, V., Bodey, G., McCredie, K., et al.: Coagulation abnormalities induced by beta-lactam antibiotics in cancer patients. J. Infect. Dis., 148:745, 1983.

137. Hooper, C., Haney, B., and Stone, H.: Gastrointestinal bleeding due to vitamin K deficiency in patients on parenteral cefamandole. Lancet 1:39, 1980.

138. Stromberg, P., Shenkin, A., Campbell, R., et al.: Vitamin status during total parenteral nutrition. J.P.E.N., 5:295, 1981.

139. Nichoalds, G., Meng, H., and Caldwell, M.: Vitamin requirements in patients receiving total parenteral nutrition. Arch. Surg., 112:1061, 1977.

140. Lowry, S., Goodgame, J., Maher, M., et al.: Parenteral vitamin requirements during intravenous feeding. Am. J. Clin. Nutr., 31:2149, 1978.

141. Hartline, J., and Zachman, R.: Vitamin A delivery in total parenteral nutrition solution. Pediatrics, 58:448, 1976.

142. Shenai, J., Stahlman, M., and Chytil, F.: Vitamin A delivery from parenteral alimentation solution. J. Pediatrics, 99:661, 1981.

143. Howard, L., Chu, R., Feman, S., et al.: Vitamin A deficiency from long term parenteral nutrition. Ann. Intern. Med., 93:576, 1980.

144. Gillis, J., Jones, G., and Pencharz, P.: Delivery of vitamins A, D and E in total parenteral nutrition solutions. J.P.E.N., 7:11, 1983.

145. Kishi, H., Yamaji, A., Kataoka, K., et al.: Vitamin A and E requirements during total parenteral nutrition. J.P.E.N., 5:420, 1981.

146. McKenna, M., and Bieri, J.: Loss of vitamin A from total parenteral nutrition (TPN) solutions (abstract 1561). Fed. Proc., 39:561, 1980.

147. Moorhatch, P., and Chiou, W.: Interactions between drugs and plastic intravenous fluid bags. Am. J. Hosp. Pharm., 31:72, 1974.

148. Niemiec, P., and Walker, J.: Vitamin A availability from parenteral nutrition delivery systems. Nutr. Supp. Serv., 3:53, 1983.

149. Scheiner, J., Araujo, M., and DeRitter, E.: Thiamine destruction by sodium bisulfite in infusion solutions. Am. J. Hosp. Pharm., 38:1911, 1981.

150. Trissel, L.: Handbook on Injectable Drugs, 2nd ed. Washington, D.C., American Society of Hospital Pharmacists, 1980, p. 515.

151. Sokoloski, T., and Visconti, J.: IV admixtures: An approach to avoid problems. In Therapeutics Monograph. Smith Kline and French Laboratories, 1980.

152. Chen, M., Boyce, W., and Triplett, L.: Stability of the B vitamins in mixed parenteral nutrition solution. J.P.E.N., 7:462, 1983.

153. Bowman, B., and Nguyen, P.: Stability of thiamin in parenteral nutrition solutions. J.P.E.N., 7:567, 1983.

154. Davidson, S., Passmore, R., Brock, J., et al.: Human Nutrition and Dietetics, 7th ed. Edinburgh, Churchill Livingstone, 1979, p. 129.

155. Harper, C.: Sudden, unexpected death and Wernicke's encephalopathy: A complication of prolonged intravenous feeding. Aust. N.Z. J. Med., 10:230, 1980.

156. Harper, C.: Thiamine deficiency. Med. J. Aust., 2:280, 1980.

157. Trissel, L.: Handbook on Injectable Drugs, 2nd ed. Washington, D.C., American Society of Hospital Pharmacists, 1980, p. 247.

158. Fabri, P., Mirtallo, J., Ruberg, R., et al.: Incidence and prevention of thrombosis of the subclavian vein during total parenteral nutrition. Surg. Gynecol. Obstet., 155:238, 1982.

159. Blackburn, G.: Hyperalimentation in the critically ill patient. Heart Lung, 8:67, 1979.

160. Valerio, D., Hussey, J., and Smith F.: Central vein thrombosis associated with intravenous feeding: A prospective study. J.P.E.N., 5:240, 1981.

161. Bailey, M.: Reduction of catheter-associated sepsis in parenteral nutrition using low-dose intravenous heparin. Br. Med. J., 1:1671, 1979.

162. Ruggiero, R., and Aisenstein, T.: Central catheter fibrin sleeve—heparin effect. J.P.E.N., 7:270, 1983.

163. Brismar, B., Hardstedt, C., Jacobson, S., et al.: Reduction of catheter-associated thrombosis in parenteral nutrition by intravenous heparin therapy. Arch. Surg., *117*:1196, 1982.

164. Pelham, L.: Rational use of intravenous fat emulsions. Am. J. Hosp. Pharm., *38*:198, 1981.

165. Bergrem, H.: Dialysis death and increased free fatty acids. Lancet, *2*:1160, 1978.

166. Huttunmen, J., Pasternack, A., Vanthinen, I., et al.: Lipoprotein metabolism in patients with chronic uremia. Acta Med. Scand., *204*:211, 1978.

167. Rugegni, M.: Heparin-induced lipolysis in the elderly. Lancet, *2*:903, 1974.

168. Tsallas, G., and Allen, L.: Stability of cimetidine hydrochloride in parenteral nutrition solutions. Am. J. Hosp. Pharm., *39*:484, 1982.

169. Rosenberg, H., Dougherty, J., Mayron, D., et al.: Cimetidine hydrochloride compatibility. I. Chemical aspects and room temperature stability in intravenous infusion fluids. Am. J. Hosp. Pharm., *37*:390, 1980.

170. Moore, R., Feldman, S., Treuting, J., et al.: Cimetidine and parenteral nutrition. J.P.E.N., *5*:61, 1981.

171. Rowlands, B., Tindall, S., and Elliott, D.: The use of dilute hydrochloric acid and cimetidine to reverse severe metabolic alkalosis. Postgrad. Med. J., *54*:118, 1978.

172. Doherty, N., Shekeeb, S., Palvides, C., et al.: Cimetidine in the treatment of severe metabolic alkalosis secondary to short bowel syndrome. Int. Surg., *63*:140, 1978.

173. Barton, C., Vaziri, N., Ness, R., et al.: Cimetidine in the management of metabolic alkalosis induced by nasogastric drainage. Arch. Surg., *114*:70, 1979.

174. Yuhas, E., Lofton, F., Rosenberg, H., et al.: Cimetidine hydrochloride compatibility. III: Room temperature stability in drug admixtures. Am. J. Hosp. Pharm., *38*:1919, 1981.

175. Trissel, L.: Handbook on Injectable Drugs, 2nd ed. Washington, D.C., American Society of Hospital Pharmacists, 1980, p. 26.

176. King, J.: Guide to Parenteral Admixtures. Berkeley, CA, Cutter Laboratories, 1982.

177. Niemiec, P., Vanderveen, T., Hohenwarter, M., et al.: Stability of aminophylline injection in three parenteral nutrition solutions. Am. J. Hosp. Pharm., *40*:428, 1983.

178. Jurgens, R., DeLuca, P., and Papadimitriou, D.: Compatibility of amphotericin B with certain large-volume parenterals. Am. J. Hosp. Pharm. *38*:377, 1981.

179. Norton, J., Peters, M., Wesley, R., et al.: Iron supplementation of total parenteral nutrition: A prospective study. J.P.E.N., *7*:457, 1983.

180. Gilbert, L., Dean, R., and Karaganis, A.: Iron-dextran administration via TPN solution in malnourished patients with low transferrin levels. J.P.E.N., *3*:494, 1979.

181. Swenson, J., Edwards, D., Chamberlain, M., et al.: A total parenteral nutrition protocol. Drug Intell. Clin. Pharm., *11*:714, 1977.

182. Sayers, M., Johnson, D., Schumann, L., et al.: Supplementation of total parenteral nutrition solutions with ferrous citrate. J.P.E.N., *7*:117, 1983.

183. Bothe, A., Benotti, P., Bistrian, B., et al.: Use of iron with total parenteral nutrition. N. Engl. J. Med., *293*:1153, 1975.

184. Weinberg, E.: Infection and iron metabolism. Am. J. Clin. Nutr., *30*:1485, 1977.

185. McFarlene, H., Reddy, S., Adcock, K., et al.: Immunity, transferrin, and survival in kwashiorkor. Br. Med. J., *4*:268, 1970.

186. Wan, K., and Tsallas, G.: Dilute iron-dextran formulation for addition to parenteral nutrient solutions. Am. J. Hosp. Pharm., *37*:206, 1980.

187. Halpin, T.: Use of intravenous iron-dextran in sick patients receiving TPN. Nutr. Supp. Serv., *2*:19, 1982.

188. Halpin, T., Bertino, J., Rothstein, F., et al.: Iron-deficiency anemia in childhood inflammatory bowel disease: Treatment with intravenous iron-dextran. J.P.E.N., *6*:9, 1982.

189. Askari, A., Long, C., and Blakemore, W.: Zinc, copper, iron and manganese in blood and blood products. Nutr. Supp. Serv., *3*:28, 1983.

190. Lipschitz, D., Cook, J., and Finch, C.: A clinical evaluation of serum ferritin. N. Engl. J. Med., *290*:1213, 1974.

191. Thomson, A., Brust, R., Ali, M., et al.: Iron deficiency in inflammatory bowel disease: Diagnostic efficacy of serum ferritin. Am. J. Dig. Dis., *23*:705, 1975.

192. Stead, N., Curtis, M., and Grant, J.: Changes in ferrokinetics during parenteral nutrition. J.P.E.N., *4*:585, 1980.

193. Feigin, R., Moss, K., and Shackelford, P.: Antibiotic stability in solutions used for intravenous nutrition and fluid therapy. Pediatrics, *51*:1016, 1973.

194. Reed, M., Perry, E., Fennell, S., et al.: Antibiotic compatibility and stability in a parenteral nutrition solution. Chemotherapy, *25*:336, 1979.

195. Colding, H., and Anderson, G.: Stability of antibiotics and amino acids in two synthetic L-amino acid solutions commonly used for total parenteral nutrition in children. Antimicrob. Agents Chemother., *13*:555, 1978.

196. Bodey, G., Chang, H., Rodriguez, V., et al.: Feasibility of administering aminoglycoside antibiotics by continuous intravenous infusion. Antimicrob. Agents Chemother., *8*:328, 1975.

197. Keating, M., Bodey, G., Valdivieso, M., et al.: A randomized comparative trial of three aminoglycosides: Comparison of continuous infusions of gentamicin, amikacin and sisomicin combined with carbenicillin in the treatment of infections in neutropenic patients with malignancies. Medicine, *58*:159, 1979.

198. Valdivieso, M., Feld, R., Rodriguez, V., et al.: Amikacin therapy of infections in neutropenic patients. Am. J. Med. Sci., *270*:453, 1975.

199. Colding, H., Moller, S., and Andersen, G.: Continuous intravenous infusion of ampicillin and gentamicin during parenteral nutrition in 88 newborn infants. Arch. Dis. Child., *57*:602, 1982.

200. Van Etta, L., Kravitz, G., Russ, T., et al.: Effect of method of administration on extravascular penetration of four antibiotics. Antimicrob. Agents Chemother., *21*:873, 1982.

201. Thys, J., Klastersky, J., and Mombelli, G.: Peak or sustained antibiotic serum levels for optimal tissue penetration. J. Antimicrob. Chemother., *8*(Suppl. C):29, 1981.

202. Reed, M., Lazarus, H., Herzig, R., et al.: Cyclic parenteral nutrition during bone marrow transplantation in children. Cancer *51*:1563, 1983.

203. Mirtallo, J., Rogers, K., Johnson, J., et al.: Stability of amino acids and the availability of acid in total parenteral nutrition solutions containing hydrochloric acid. Am. J. Hosp. Pharm., *38*:1729, 1981.

204. Isaacs, J., Millikan, W., Stackhouse, J., et al.: Par-

enteral nutrition of adults with a 900 milliosmolar solution via peripheral veins. Am. J. Clin. Nutr., *30*:552, 1977.

205. King, J.: Guide to Parenteral Admixtures. Berkeley, CA, Cutter Laboratories, 1982.

206. Albibi, R., and McCallum, R.: Metoclopramide: Pharmacology and clinical application. Ann. Intern. Med., *98*:86, 1983.

207. Pinder, R., Brogden, R., Sawyer, P., et al.: Metoclopramide: A review of its pharmacological properties and clinical use. Drugs, *12*:81, 1976.

208. Ponte, C., and Nappi, J.: Review of a new gastrointestinal drug: Metoclopramide. Am. J. Hosp. Pharm., *38*:829, 1981.

209. Shivshanker, K., Bennett, R., and Haynie, T.: Tumor-associated gastroparesis: Correction with metoclopramide. Am. J. Surg., *145*:221, 1983.

210. McClelland, R., and Horton, J.: Relief of acute, persistent postvagotomy atony by metoclopramide. Ann. Surg., *188*:439, 1978.

211. James, W., and Hume, R.: Action of metoclopramide on gastric emptying and small bowel transit time. Gut, *9*:203, 1968.

212. Arvanitakis, C., Gonzalez, G., and Rhodes, J.: The role of metoclopramide in peroral jejunal biopsy. Am. J. Digest. Dis., *21*:880, 1976.

213. Davidson, E., Hersh, T., Brunner, R., et al.: The effects of metoclopramide on postoperative ileus. Ann. Surg., *190*:27, 1979.

214. Cutie, M., and Waranis, R.: Compatibility of hydromorphone hydrochloride in large-volume parenterals. Am. J. Hosp. Pharm., *39*:307, 1982.

215. Church, J.: Continuous narcotic infusions for relief of postoperative pain. Br. Med. J., *1*:977, 1979.

216. Orr, I., Keenan, D., and Dundee, J.: Improved pain relief after thoracotomy: Use of cryoprobe and morphine infusion. Br. Med. J., *283*:945, 1981.

217. Rutter, P., Murphy, F., and Dudley, H.: Morphine: Controlled trial of different methods of administration for postoperative pain relief. Br. Med. J., *1*:12, 1980.

218. Batenhorst, R., and Graves, D.: Risks of continuous narcotic infusions (letter). Am. J. Hosp. Pharm., *39*:2084, 1982.

219. Keys, P.: Digoxin. *In* Evans, W., Schentag, J., and Jusko, W. (eds.): Applied Pharmacokinetics. San Francisco, Applied Therapeutics, 1980, p. 319.

220. Sternson, L., and Shaffer, R.: Kinetics of digoxin stability in aqueous solution. J. Pharm. Sci., *67*:327, 1978.

221. Shank, W., and Coupal, J.: Stability of digoxin in common large-volume injections. Am. J. Hosp. Pharm., *39*:844, 1982.

222. Blackstone, M., Lee, P., and Reynolds, E.: Use of digoxin in total parenteral nutrition fluids. Poster presented at the 15th Annual ASHP Midyear Clinical Meeting, San Francisco, CA, 1980.

223. Fagerman, K., and Dean, R.: Daily digoxin administration in parenteral nutrition solution. Am. J. Hosp. Pharm., *38*:1955, 1981.

224. Rusmin, S., Welton, S., DeLuca, P., et al.: Effect of in-line filtration on the potency of drugs administered intravenously. Am. J. Hosp. Pharm., *34*:1071, 1977.

225. DeLuca, P.P.: Binding of drugs to in-line filters (letter). Am. J. Hosp. Pharm., *36*:151, 1979.

226. Siefert, P., Baker, L., Reed, M., et al.: Comparison of continuously infused 5-fluorouracil with bolus injection in treatment of patients with colorectal adenocarcinoma. Cancer, *36*:123, 1975.

227. Lane, M.: Chemotherapy of cancer. *In* DelRegato, J., and Spjut, H. (eds.): Cancer: Diagnosis, Treatment and Prognosis, 5th ed. St. Louis, C. V. Mosby, 1977, p. 119.

228. Hardin, T., Clibon, U., Page, C., et al.: Compatibility of 5-fluorouracil and total parenteral nutrition solutions. J.P.E.N., *6*:163, 1982.

229. Hardin, T., and Clibon, U.: The stability of 5-fluorouracil in a crystalline amino acid solution. Am. J. I.V. Ther. Clin. Nutr., January 1982, p. 39.

230. Boddapati, S., Yang, K., and Murty, R.: Intravenous solution compatibility and filter-retention characteristics of trace-element preparations. Am. J. Hosp. Pharm., *38*:1731, 1981.

CHAPTER 15

Catheter Access

JOHN P. GRANT

Solutions that are used in total parenteral nutrition—and that provide all nutrients, including carbohydrate, protein, electrolytes, minerals, and vitamins—are by necessity very hypertonic, being three to eight times normal serum osmolality. Infusion of such solutions into small vessels or into vessels with low blood flow results in severe burning and rapid thrombosis of the vein. Hemolysis has also been observed. The development of total parenteral nutrition has therefore required techniques to gain access to veins with high blood flow, such as the superior vena cava, the right atrium, the inferior vena cava, or a surgically created arteriovenous fistula. In addition to the requirement of rapid dilution by high blood flow, vascular access for total parenteral nutrition should be easily established, well tolerated by the patient, and capable of remaining in place for long periods of time, and it should not restrict joint mobility or otherwise interfere with physical activity.

HISTORY

The most common vascular access used for total parenteral nutrition is a percutaneously placed subclavian vein catheter. This technique was first introduced in 1952 by Aubaniac, who found that the technique provided rapid access to the central venous system with minimal complications in patients suffering from military injuries.[1] Use of the technique was first reported in the United States by Wilson and associates in 1962.[2] Over the next five years, experience with the subclavian catheter was gained primarily from its use for central venous pressure mon-

itoring. The catheters were seldom left in place for more than 14 days and usually for only 3 to 4 days. When prolonged central venous pressure measurements were required, it was suggested that the catheter be changed every two to five days to avoid subclavian vein thrombosis and infection.[3, 4] The use of the subclavian catheter for intravenous nutritional support was first proposed by Dr. Stanley Dudrick in his early work at the University of Pennsylvania in 1969.[5] Since then, the percutaneous subclavian vein catheterization technique has gained widespread use for total parenteral nutrition because of the ease of placement and dressing management and the low infection complication rate.

In 1965, Yoffa described a supraclavicular approach to the subclavian vein, claiming it was a safer technique with a higher percentage of successful catheterizations.[6] Since 1969, others have found occasion to utilize the internal jugular vein, the external jugular vein, the basilic vein, and even the right atrial appendage. Although first described in 1949 by Duffy, the use of an inferior vena caval catheter via the femoral vein has found little clinical application because of the high risk of infection and thrombosis.[7] This chapter will discuss placement of the more commonly used central venous catheters, with some comments on particular clinical situations requiring specialized catheter placement.

BASIC PRINCIPLES

There are four basic principles that must be observed to ensure optimal safety and success in the placement of central venous catheters: (1) proper patient preparation, (2) proper timing of catheterization, (3) proper skin preparation, and the (4) availability of proper equipment and supplies.

Proper Patient Preparation

Prior to the placement of a central venous catheter, the nurse and physician should thoroughly explain to the patient the reason for the catheter placement and the technique to be used to allay any fears or misconceptions the patient might have of the procedure. When properly informed, the patient will rarely require sedation, though on occasion a sedative will be helpful. The patient should be cautioned to expect some discomfort, even though a local anesthetic will be used. For cannulation of the antecubital fossa or femoral vein, the patient should lie flat in bed. For catheterization of vessels in the head and neck area, the patient should be placed in the Trendelenburg position. Visible engorgement of the external jugular vein will assure the presence of positive pressure and minimize the possibility of air embolization during catheterization (up to 100 ml of air/second can pass through a 14-gauge needle). For cannulation of the subclavian vein, a small rolled towel should be placed longitudinally between the scapula from the 7th cervical vertebra to the 10th or 12th thoracic vertebra to allow the shoulders to fall back onto the bed. This will permit easy access to the subclavian vein and will avoid cannulation of the subclavian artery. It is also helpful to instruct the patient to "reach for the toes" to bring the clavicle into a horizontal position and to establish the normal curve of the subclavian and axillary vein from the thoracic outlet into the arm. If the shoulders are in a shrugged position, the vein will be at a variable distance below the lower edge of the clavicle and may take a tortuous course. If the bed is particularly soft, it may be necessary to place a wooden board under the patient to allow proper positioning.

It has been proposed that proper head positioning is important when attempting to pass a catheter from the subclavian vein into the superior vena cava. Some claim that if the head is turned away from the cannulation site, there will be a higher incidence of successful cannulation of the superior vena cava rather than of the internal jugular vein. Others have suggested that turning the head toward the cannulation site is of value. There has, however, been no documentation of any significant change in the angle between the internal jugular vein and the subclavian vein the head turning. The patient's head should be positioned in the most comfortable angle for cannulation.

Proper Timing of Catheterization

Placement of a central venous catheter for total parenteral nutrition should always be done on an elective basis when proper patient preparation can best be established. Proper time should be taken in patient preparation, skin preparation, definition of landmarks, and catheter insertion. Placement of catheters in emergency situations has been shown to be associated with a significantly increased complication rate due to suboptimal conditions.[8]

Proper Skin Preparation

The area of proposed cannulation is first shaved carefully because the removal of any hair assists in the sterile preparation and subsequent placement of tape when applying the bandage. Since it is desirable for these catheters to remain in place for extended periods of time, strict attention must be paid to aseptic technique during catheter placement. A thorough cleansing of a wide area around the proposed cannulation site should be performed using an antiseptic soap; the skin should then be defatted with ether, acetone, or trichlorotrifloroethane; a povidone-iodine solution should be applied; and sterile draping should follow (Fig. 15–1). The physician should cleanse the hands with antiseptic soap and should wear a mask and gown. Earlier practice was to perform the procedure in the operating room only. This has been found not to be necessary, and most cannulations are performed in the patient's room. The number of people in the room should be limited to avoid airborne contamination, and all those present should wear masks.

Availability of Proper Equipment and Supplies

The placement of central venous catheters is facilitated by having the help of a trained assistant, such as a hyperalimenta-

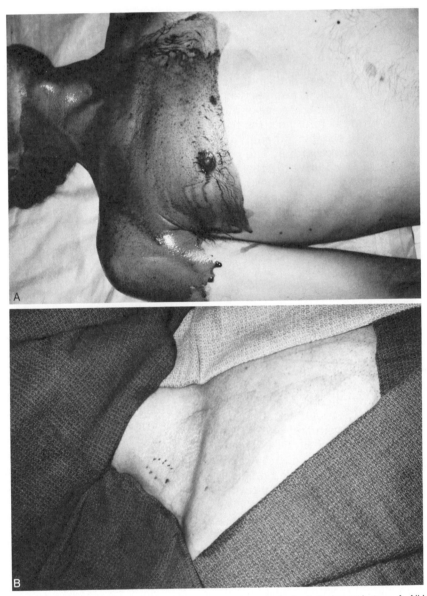

Figure 15–1. Preparation of skin of chest for percutaneous placement of subclavian catheters. *A,* All hair is removed by shaving, and the skin is prepared with an antiseptic soap, followed by a defatting agent and then a povidone-iodine solution. *B,* The area is draped with sterile towels.

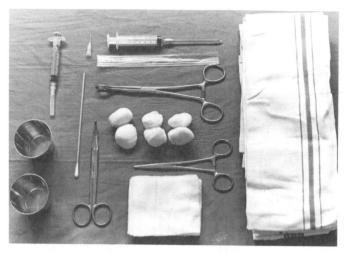

Figure 15–2. Materials included on a tray for percutaneous placement of subclavian catheters. (*From* Grant, J. P.: Handbook of Total Parenteral Nutrition. Philadelphia, W. B. Saunders Company, 1980, p. 49, with permission.)

tion nurse, and appropriate instruments. Most institutions have found it cost-effective to develop a catheter insertion tray, which consists of basins, clamps, syringes, and sponges (Fig. 15–2). This author has found the use of reusuable material preferable to the use of disposable kits; however, others have been quite satisfied with the disposable kits. In addition to the tray materials, a cart containing the various preparation solutions, gowns, gloves, masks, and catheters will greatly assist in catheterization (Fig. 15–3). A wide number of catheters are available for use in central venous catheterization. Selection of a catheter depends upon personal preference and familiarity. New materials are continuously being investigated in hopes of discovering a material with significantly lower thrombogenicity. Currently available materials include the standard polyvinylchloride, Silastic, Teflon, polyurethane, and heparin-coated catheters. To date no significant decrease in the incidence of thrombosis has been found with any of these catheters, though the investigations continue.[9, 10]

CENTRAL VENOUS CANNULATION

Percutaneous Infraclavicular Subclavian Vein Cannulation

Landmarks used in subclavian vein catheterization by the infraclavicular route should be based on anatomic relationships (Fig. 15–4). The axillary vein passes obliquely across the axilla toward the middle third of the clavicle at which point it becomes the subclavian vein at the lateral border of the first rib. The subclavian vein arches behind the clavicle over the first rib anterior to the insertion of the anterior scalene muscle. At this point just medial to the midpoint of the clavicle, the vein reaches its most cephalad portion in its arch over the rib, and it is at this point that the safest cannulation can be achieved. At the medial border of the anterior scalene muscle, the subclavian vein joins the internal jugular vein to form the brachiocephalic vein. It is therefore suggested that the appropriate landmark for subclavian vein cannulation is the insertion of the anterior scalene muscle on the tubercle of the first

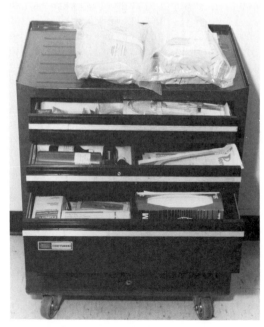

Figure 15–3. Catheter insertion cart containing prep solutions, gowns, gloves, masks, and catheters.

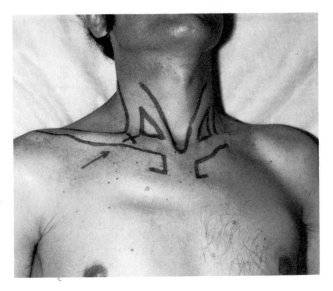

Figure 15–4. Landmarks used in the placement of a percutaneous subclavian catheter by the infraclavicular route. A postage-stamp–sized area is defined by the superior and inferior margins of the clavicle, a line extended from the lateral head of the sternocleidomastoid muscle inferiorly across the clavicle, and the completion of the square medially. The posterior border is marked by the insertion of the anterior scalene muscle on the tubercle of the first rib, and the anterior border is marked by the posterior surface of the clavicle. (*From* Grant, J. P.: Handbook of Total Parenteral Nutrition. Philadelphia, W. B. Saunders Company, 1980, p. 52, with permission.)

rib, which lies just posterior to the clavicle. This postage-stamp-sized area contains no other major structures, and cannulation at this point should be entirely safe. Advancement of the needle more medially can result in pneumothorax, advancement more posteriorly can result in arterial puncture, and advancement more superiorly and posteriorly can result in brachial plexus injury.

After adequate patient preparation, a small wheal of local anesthetic should be placed at the proposed puncture site, which should be approximately 2 cm below the clavicle at a point that allows access to the target area. Usually this will allow placement of the barrel of the syringe and needle in the deltopectoral groove, further reducing the difficulties if a patient cannot extend the shoulders fully back onto the bed, such as might occur in uncooperative patients or those with marked arthritis. The needle is then advanced through the anesthetized skin toward the target area, maintaining the barrel of the syringe horizontal to the floor, which assures no penetration into the area of the artery or lung. As the needle is advanced, intermittent aspiration on the syringe will confirm passage into the subclavian vein by a rapid rush of blood into the barrel of the syringe. Depending on the kind of system being used, once the needle has been advanced into the subclavian vein, the catheter is advanced either through the needle or over a wire spring that is advanced through the needle, with the subsequent removal of the needle. Care must be taken in all procedures to avoid air aspiration or shearing of the

catheter. Failure of the catheter or spring to advance easily usually means that the needle is no longer within the vein or that it is against the wall at the junction of the internal jugular vein and the subclavian vein (Fig. 15–5). In the latter case, withdrawing the needle a short distance will often allow passage of the catheter or wire further into the venous system. Once the catheter is in place, documentation of its placement in a large-bore vein can be done by free aspiration of blood. Easy and rapid confirmation that the catheter has not been passed into the internal jugular vein can be accomplished by gently aspirating blood from the catheter while

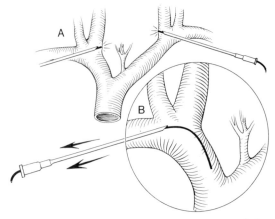

Figure 15–5. *A,* Difficulty in advancement of the catheter into the subclavian vein may be due to its abutment against the wall of the internal jugular vein. The *inset (B)* shows the technique of slightly withdrawing the needle from the vein to allow the catheter to curve and go distally into the superior vena cava.

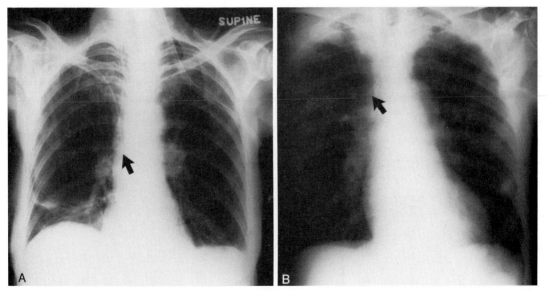

Figure 15–6. Following placement of a subclavian catheter, a chest x-ray is necessary to confirm its proper position in the superior vena cava and to rule out the presence of a pneumothorax. *A*, Proper placement of a catheter inserted from the right subclavian vein. *B*, Proper placement of a catheter inserted from the left subclavian vein.

firmly pressing along the course of the internal jugular vein with the tip of the finger. If the tip of the catheter lies within the internal jugular vein, occlusion of the vein by pressure of the finger will result in a sudden stoppage of blood flow into the syringe during aspiration. If this is encountered, the catheter should be partially withdrawn, rotated, and reinserted, and this procedure should be repeated until one is certain that the catheter does not lie in the internal jugular vein. Experience from thousands of subclavian vein catheterizations and antecubital placement of central venous catheters has demonstrated that approximately 10 per cent of these catheters will pass into the internal jugular vein; some testing of the catheter's position, therefore, is mandatory prior to performing a chest x-ray to avoid the cost of an unnecessary film.[11] Following the presumed proper placement of the subclavian catheter, a chest x-ray film is necessary to document the position of the catheter as well as to rule out the presence of pneumothorax (Fig. 15–6). This x-ray should be performed prior to connecting the catheter to any hypertonic solution. A five per cent dextrose solution, with or without electrolytes, should be connected to the catheter to maintain its patency until an x-ray is taken. Following proper catheter placement, a sterile dressing should be applied using either gauze or plastic.

Supraclavicular Percutaneous Approach to the Subclavian Vein

The landmarks used in the supraclavicular cannulation of the subclavian vein are identical to those used for the infraclavicular approach, except that the skin puncture site is located in the angle between the lateral head of the sternocleidomastoid muscle and the clavicle (Fig. 15–7). At this point, a small wheal of local anesthetic is placed in the skin. The catheterization needle is inserted through this wheal of anesthetized skin, with the tip directed just behind the clavicle at a 45-degree angle to the sagittal plane and pointed 15 degrees forward of the coronal plane. Thus, as the needle is advanced it is safely moving away from the structures of the subclavian artery and cupula of the lung. Gentle aspiration is intermittently applied to the syringe as the needle is advanced until the vein is entered just anterior to the tubercle of the first rib. Once within the vein, the syringe is lowered toward the shoulder to align the needle with the vein. The catheter or wire stylet is inserted, and the cannulation procedure is performed as for the infraclavicular approach. With the supraclavicular approach, retrograde cannulation of the internal jugular vein is rarely encountered. However, the catheter can still go out the subclavian vein on the same or opposite side or pass into the mammary veins or other

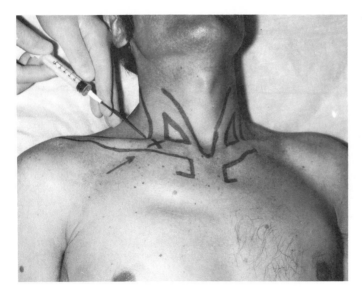

Figure 15–7. Landmarks used in the percutaneous placement of a subclavian catheter via the supraclavicular approach. Skin puncture site is located in the angle formed by the lateral head of the sternocleidomastoid muscle and the superior border of the clavicle. (*From* Grant, J. P.: Handbook of Total Parenteral Nutrition. Philadelphia, W. B. Saunders Company, 1980, p. 57, with permission.)

small tributaries. It is therefore important to check for ease of blood flow by aspirating on the syringe and also to check for proper catheter positioning with a postplacement chest x-ray film. A sterile dressing should be applied, as discussed in a later section. Occasionally, it has been useful to tunnel the catheter over the anterior surface of the clavicle down to a point on the anterior chest wall to make application of a sterile dressing easier and more comfortable for the patient rather than placing the dressing in the more mobile, hairbearing area of the neck.

Internal and External Jugular Vein Catheterization

Utilization of the internal and external jugular veins for central venous access has found less use in long-term total parenteral nutrition than in short-term central venous pressure monitoring in the intensive care unit. Because of the higher positioning of the puncture site on the neck, difficulties of maintaining a sterile dressing limit their long-term use. In addition, the small size of the external jugular vein can result in thrombosis of this system, with tender thrombophlebitis extending distally from the puncture site and presenting a clinical problem for the patient. The use of these two access sites is not recommended for total parenteral nutrition, but in extenuating circumstances they can be used temporarily until more permanent access can be achieved.

Basilic Vein in the Antecubital Fossa

Experience with using polyvinylchloride catheters through the basilic vein in the antecubital fossa has demonstrated a high incidence of thrombophlebitis that occurs within 4 to 10 days of catheter placement. This has seriously limited the use of the basilic vein for long-term total parenteral nutrition. Recently, the development and use of silicone elastomer catheters has improved the experience, with catheters being left in place for 20 to 40 days with few complications.[12] Catheterization is performed as per routine, but instead of placement of a polyvinylchloride catheter, the Teflon-coated catheter is passed into the superior vena cava. To avoid any contamination of the catheter with talc, special gloves must be worn during the insertion. Skin preparation and dressing care is the same as that used in subclavian vein catheterization. Dressings should be changed routinely (as outlined later), and the system should be isolated for total parenteral nutrition. The catheters do limit the mobility of the arm and are somewhat less comfortable than the subclavian catheters for long-term use.

Other Vascular Access Sites Useful in Extenuating Circumstances

As mentioned earlier, Duffy described using the femoral vein for cannulation of the inferior vena cava in 1949.[7] When no upper veins are available, for example, following thrombosis of both subclavian veins, the femoral approach has been used with variable success. The vein can be cannulated percutaneously and a catheter inserted until the tip is within the right atrium as observed under fluoroscopy. This vein can subsequently be used for total parenteral nutrition. Great care must be exercised in maintaining the exit site of the catheter to avoid skin-borne contamination. These patients must be monitored carefully for the development of phlebitis and particularly for intermittent pulmonary embolism because the foreign body in the inferior vena cava carries a high risk of these complications. This author has acquired some recent experience with the use of Silastic catheters placed via the femoral system and advanced into the right atrium in patients receiving home intravenous support. With limited clinical experience, these patients have been maintained on low dose anticoagulation with sodium warfarin (Coumadin) to avoid complications of thrombosis.

On rare occasions when superior vena caval thrombosis is present and the risks of using the inferior vena cava are too high, catheters have been placed via a small anterior thoracotomy through the right atrial appendage into the right atrium. Experience with these catheters in thoracic surgery for monitoring pulmonary artery pressure has shown them to be quite safe in short-term use. Whether the catheters can be maintained for long-term intravenous feeding has yet to be demonstrated.

A few authors have suggested using an arteriovenous (AV) fistula or shunt for long-term vascular access in total parenteral nutrition.[13-15] When a shunt is employed, a small T is placed in the shunt, and access is achieved through the T, infusing the solution through the catheter while blood flow is maintained. When an AV fistula is used, a small-bore needle is percutaneously placed into the access, much as is done when performing dialysis. The feeding solutions are infused either continuously or cyclicly. Use of an AV fistula or shunt is associated with an increased risk of thrombosis of the vascular access. Fear of separation of the AV shunt and exsanguination limits its use to patients who are alert and cooperative.

The percutaneously placed subclavian catheters used in hemodialysis have also been used to supply hypertonic total parenteral nutrition solutions. Typically, one lumen of these two-lumen catheters is used during the time when dialysis is not being performed. The solution is interrupted for the two to six hours of dialysis. Since these catheters are typically placed for short-term use only, their use is somewhat limited for total parenteral nutrition. A more permanent access must be established once the dialysis catheter is removed.

Finally, one of the portals of a Swan-Ganz catheter or a triple-lumen subclavian catheter has been used for total parenteral nutrition. The use of these catheters is likely associated with an increased risk of infection and is therefore limited to short-term use during acute illness.

Long-Term Vascular Access

Specially designed catheters are now available for long-term access to the central venous system. These catheters are particularly useful for patients receiving nutritional support at home, but they have also been used in the hospital for extended periods of care. Several designs are available, but in general they consist of a single- or dual-lumen tubing with Luer-Lok caps on the end and a Dacron cuff positioned to be placed in the subcutaneous tissues to anchor the catheter in place. Most of these catheters are composed of Silastic and come presterilized. Catheters made of erythrothane, which claims a lower thrombogenicity index, are under investigation.

Initially these catheters were all placed in the operating room by a small cutdown to the cephalic vein or external jugular vein and then advanced under fluoroscopic control into the right atrium.[16] The catheters were then advanced through a subcutaneous tunnel to exit at or just slightly below the nipple line. Subsequently, techniques have been modified so that these catheters are placed percutaneously.[17] Experience with these catheters has shown them to be very safe, with a low infectious complication rate.[18, 19] There is a certain incidence of subclavian vein thrombosis that may range as high as three to five per cent. The catheters are of significant bore to allow easy passage of the total parenteral nutrition solutions, including fat emulsions. They come in sizes for use in infants, adolescents, and adults.

SPECIAL CLINICAL CONSIDERATIONS IN VASCULAR ACCESS

Following head and neck surgery or placement of a tracheostomy, patients have a higher incidence of subclavian vein catheter infection. This is likely caused by contamination of the area and the subsequent migration of bacteria along the course of the catheter in the subcutaneous tissues. To decrease the incidence of catheter-related sepsis in these patients, it has been recommended that following placement of the catheter in the superior vena cava the end of the catheter be tunneled subcutaneously away from the catheterization site for a distance of approximately 8 to 10 cm (Fig. 15–8). The original puncture site is then closed with a single suture, and the dressing is moved laterally to the new catheter exit site.

Patients who have suffered extensive burns of the shoulders, upper extremities, and head and neck area can be given intravenous nutritional support through the central veins of the neck if no other access is available. In general, if an adequate dressing cannot be maintained because of the burned area, it is suggested that the catheter be sutured in place and left uncovered by gauze. The skin around the catheter should be cleansed every two to four hours and povidone-iodine ointment applied to cover the exit site. The catheter should be removed and placed at another site approximately every 48 to 72 hours.

Patients with clotting abnormalities or very low platelet counts present special risks for central vein cannulation. Little difficulty will be encountered if the catherization technique is uncomplicated. However, puncture of a major artery or arterial tributary can result in significant bleeding, which leads to hemothorax and hemomediastinum and possibly cardiac tamponade and shock. If possible, it is suggested that prior to any cannulation, the clotting difficulty be corrected by the administration of fresh-frozen plasma, platelets, or specific clotting factors. If heparin is being administered, it is suggested that it be interrupted and that the bleeding time or partial thromboplastin time be allowed to

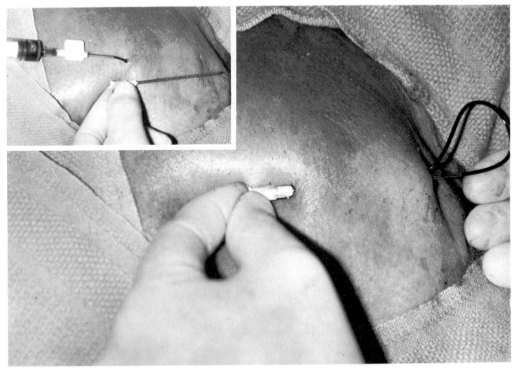

Figure 15–8. Technique of tunnelling the catheter away from the puncture site. This procedure is particularly useful if there is contamination in the area of the head and neck. The needle used in placing the catheter in the subclavian vein is introduced more laterally, tunnelled subcutaneously, and made to exit through the initial puncture hole for subclavian vein cannulation. The end of the catheter is then fed through the needle while the needle is drawn out through the skin, thus transplanting the exit site more laterally. The proximal catheterization site is closed with a simple suture. (*From* Grant, J. P.: Handbook of Total Parenteral Nutrition. Philadelphia, W. B. Saunders Company, 1980, p. 54, with permission.)

return to normal prior to cannulation. Following uncomplicated placement of the catheter, heparin therapy can be resumed immediately.

Patients who are allergic to povidone-iodine solutions should undergo vigorous skin preparation with an antiseptic soap such as Hibiclens or pHisoHex and undergo subsequent defatting with acetone, ether, or trichlorotrifluoroethane. Catheterization should then be accomplished with subsequent catheter dressing using a non-povidone-iodine ointment such as Bacitracin or Neosporin. Note should be made that many patients claiming a sensitivity to povidone-iodine solutions will tolerate the placement of a povidone-iodine ointment and often a povidone-iodine solution when applied to the small area of the catheter exit site and dressing. A trial application should be undertaken before the catheter care is compromised by not applying the povidone-iodine solution.

REFERENCES

1. Aubaniac, R.: Une nouvelle voie d'injection ou de ponction veineuse: La voie sous-claviculaire. Semin. Hop. Paris, 28:3445–3447, 1952.
2. Wilson, J.N., Grow, J.B., Demong, C.V., Prevedel, A.E., and Owens, J.C.: Central venous pressure in optimal blood volume maintenance. Arch. Surg., 85:55–70, 1962.
3. Ashbaugh, D., and Thomson, J.W.W.: Subclavian-vein infusion. Lancet, 2:1138–1139, 1963.
4. Estridge, C.E., Hughes, F.A., Prather, J.R., and Clemmons, E.E.: Use of central venous pressure in the management of circulatory failure. Review of indications and technique. Am. Surg., 32:121–125, 1966.
5. Dudrick, S.J., Wilmore, D.W., Vars, H.M., and Rhoads, J.E.: Can intravenous feeding as the sole means of nutrition support growth in the child and restore weight loss in an adult? An affirmative answer. Ann. Surg., 169:974–984, 1969.
6. Yoffa, D.: Supraclavicular subclavian venipuncture and catheterization. Lancet, 2:614–617, 1965.
7. Duffy, B.J., Jr.: The clinical use of polyethylene tubing for intravenous therapy: A report on seventy-two cases. Ann. Surg., 130:929–936, 1949.
8. Bernard, R.W., and Stahl, W.M.: Subclavian vein catheterizations, a prospective study. Ann. Surg., 173:184–190, 1971.
9. Hoshal, V.L., Jr., Ause, R.G., and Hoskins, P.A.: Fibrin sleeve formation on indwelling subclavian central venous catheters. Arch. Surg., 102:353–358, 1971.
10. Welch, G.W., McKeel, D.W., Silverstein, P., and Walker, H.L.: The role of catheter composition in the development of thrombophlebitis. Surg. Gynecol. Obstet., 183:421–424, 1974.
11. Grant, J.P.: Handbook of Total Parenteral Nutrition. Philadelphia, W.B. Saunders Co., 1980, pages 61–62.
12. Hoshal, V.L., Jr.: Total intravenous nutrition with peripherally inserted silicone elastomer central venous catheters. Arch. Surg., 110:644–648, 1975.
13. Scribner, B.H., Cole, J.J., Christopher, T.G., Vizzo, J.E., Atkins, R.C., and Blagg, C.R.: Long-term total parenteral nutrition. J.A.M.A., 212:457–463, 1970.
14. Shils, M.E.: Guidelines for total parenteral nutrition. J.A.M.A., 220:1721–1729, 1972.
15. Heizer, W.D., and Orringer, E.P.: Parenteral nutrition at home for 5 years via arteriovenous fistulae. Gastroenterology, 72:527–532, 1977.
16. Heimbach, D.M., and Ivey, T.D.: Technique for placement of a permanent home hyperalimentation catheter. Surg. Gynecol. Obstet., 143:634–636, 1976.
17. Vander Salm, T.J., and Fitzpatrick, G.F.: New technique for placement of long-term venous catheters. J.P.E.N., 5:326–327, 1981.
18. Pollack, P.F., Kadden, B.A., Byrne, W.J., Fonkalsrude, E.W., and Ament, M.E.: 100 patient years' experience with the Broviac silastic catheter for central venous nutrition. J.P.E.N., 5:32–36, 1981.
19. Hickman, R.O., Buckner, C.D., Clift, R.A., Sanders, J.E., Stewart, P., and Thomas, D.: A modified right atrial catheter for access to the venous system in marrow transplant recipients. Surg. Gynecol. Obstet., 148:871–875, 1979.

CHAPTER 16

Central Venous Catheter Care

*LORETTA FORLAW**
MICHAEL H. TOROSIAN

SEPSIS

Catheter-Care Protocols

Meticulous catheter care has dramatically decreased the incidence of septic and mechanical complications associated with the use of central venous catheters.[2, 37, 43] The development of strict protocols regarding insertion and maintenance techniques of total parenteral nutrition (TPN) catheters is primarily responsible for this reduction in catheter-related complications. During the initial years of TPN administration (1969–1972), the incidence of catheter-related sepsis ranged from 14 to 27 per cent.[21, 26, 30, 52] In one study, in fact, infectious complications occurred in 93 per cent of infants and children receiving parenteral nutrition.[10] The morbidity associated with septic complications in patients receiving TPN was soon recognized, necessitating the institution of catheter care protocols specifically designed to eliminate such complications. Numerous clinical investigations have subsequently demonstrated that aseptic placement and proper maintenance of the TPN catheter are essential in preventing catheter-related complications.[31, 37, 71, 79, 87]

In 1969, Wilmore and Dudrick[86] managed all central venous catheters with strict

aseptic technique and changed catheters only as clinically indicated. After 700 patient-days of TPN, no instances of bacterial or fungal sepsis were observed. The excellent results of this early study contrast with contemporary reports and demonstrate the efficacy of aseptic catheter care. In 1972, Freeman and colleagues[37] observed an incidence of septic complications of only 1.3 per cent in patients who had catheters inserted and managed according to strict protocol. In this study, a TPN team was organized to assume the implementation of catheter maintenance according to a strict, aseptic protocol.

Prior to the institution of this coordinated approach to catheter care, a sepsis rate of 21 per cent was observed in a comparable group of patients. In 1976, Sanders and Sheldon[76] reported a similar reduction in the incidence of sepsis following the development of a TPN team. In a sequential series of patients, the sepsis rate decreased from 29 to 8 per cent after the TPN team was established.

Subsequent reports have confirmed these observations and indicate that septic complications of central venous catheters are largely preventable with meticulous catheter care. Deviation from such protocol is associated with a significant increase in bacterial and fungal infection rates. Ryan and colleagues[74] observed a 7.5-fold increase in septic complications in patients whose catheter care deviated from a previously established protocol. Additional complications ob-

*The opinions or assertions contained herein are the private views of the authors and are not to be construed as official or as reflecting the views of the Department of the Army or the Department of Defense.

served in patients receiving TPN include subclavian vein thrombosis, catheter malposition, and catheter dysfunction.[2, 43] These catheter-related events are potentially serious and require early recognition and appropriate therapy. Strict aseptic technique and proper catheter care are mandatory so that TPN can be provided to patients with minimal morbidity and mortality.

Handwashing

Numerous studies[2, 74, 86] have demonstrated the efficacy of scrupulous central venous catheter care. Techniques and protocols vary significantly from institution to institution with apparent success in minimizing catheter-related sepsis. The only absolute agreement in methods of care is that strict adherence to aseptic principles is essential.

Handwashing is the single most effective measure for the prevention of nosocomial disease. A recent study has documented that hospital personnel in the intensive care units of a university and private hospital setting complied with recommended handwashing procedures less than 50 per cent of the time.[1] The results of this study stress the need to continually re-educate hospital personnel about the importance of handwashing. Two appropriate methods for handwashing follow:

1. Between patient contacts, between performing more than one procedure for a specific patient, and after handling equipment, wash hands vigorously with soap for 15 to 30 seconds under a stream of warm water.

2. Before performing surgical or invasive procedures,[1, 20] wash hands vigorously with an antiseptic for three to five minutes under a stream of warm water.

When sinks with knee or foot pedals are not available, the paper towel used to dry the hands should also be used to touch the faucet when turning off the water. The filter or trap in the faucet should be cleaned or changed regularly to avoid the trapping of bacteria, which can contaminate the hands of personnel. Rings and nail polish make it more difficult to wash the hands properly.

Skin Asepsis

The skin is the body's first line of defense against infection. The initial routine preparation of the skin must be meticulous to minimize catheter-related sepsis. Any disruption of the skin's integrity provides an opportunity for bacterial or fungal invasion of the body.

Shaving the skin at the catheter insertion site should be avoided. Hamilton and colleagues[44] have shown, with the use of a scanning electron microscope, that a safety razor produces gross cuts and electric clippers tend to injure the skin at creases, but depilatory preparations do not injure the skin. Thus, trimming excessive hair or using depilatory preparations is preferable to shaving.

Numerous antiseptics are available for cleansing the skin. These same antiseptics are also sufficient for cleansing hair. The characteristics of those most commonly used appear in Table 16–1.[11, 28, 29]

The use of antibiotic or antiseptic ointments has been questioned, particularly since their effectiveness is generally diminished within 12 hours of application, and dressings are changed every 24 to 72 hours.[2, 50, 55] Currently, there is also much debate regarding defatting of the skin. Although the theoretic advantages and disadvantages of skin lipids are known, there are no definitive studies to prove or disprove these theories in the clinical setting.[2, 59] The protocols that were introduced to reduce infection associated with the care of the central venous catheter site in parenteral nutrition frequently recommended the use of acetone, and later acetone-alcohol solutions. Patients have received site care with acetone-alcohol solutions for months to years without skin disruption or other apparent skin-related difficulties.[34, 86] Thus, many practitioners are hesitant to discontinue the use of defatting agents until appropriate clinical studies provide optimal guidelines. Unfortunately, studies to date remain conflicting, without adequate data for strong support of either option.

Catheter Placement and Dressing Changes

The initiation of TPN therapy in adults is always an elective procedure and thus allows time for careful aseptic placement of the central venous catheter. Insertion of the catheter is a minor surgical procedure. Caps, masks, gowns, and sterile gloves should be worn by all personnel participating in the procedure (Fig. 16–1).[2, 4, 43, 86]

Aseptic catheter dressing changes need to be performed for the duration of the

Table 16–1. CHARACTERISTICS OF ANTISEPTICS COMMONLY USED FOR SKIN CLEANSING

ANTISEPTIC	RECOM-MENDED DILUTION	MODE OF ACTION	Residue	Inactivated by Organic Matter	Skin Irritant	Eye Irritant	Respiratory Irritant	Toxic
					CHARACTERISTICS*			
Isopropyl Alcohol	70%	Denaturation of proteins; high level of disinfectant activity.	−	−	−	+	−	+
Hydrogen peroxide	3%	Destruction of membrane lipids, DNA and other components of the cell; high level of disinfectant activity.	−	−	+	+	−	+
Iodophors	1–2% Free iodine	Penetration of the cell wall of the microorganism, with disruption of protein and nucleic acid structure and synthesis; intermittent level of disinfectant activity.	+	+	+	+	−	+
Acetone	10–100%	Loosening of the horny layer of the epidermis; intermittent level of disinfectant activity.	−	+†	−	+	−	+
Chlorohexidine	0.5%	Disruption of the plasma membrane of the cell; high level of disinfectant activity.	−	−	−	+	−	+

*+ = yes, − = no.
†Acetone 10% and isopropyl alcohol 70% are frequently used for skin cleansing and do not produce irritation.

patient's TPN therapy. The frequency of dressing changes varies from daily to weekly (with transparent polyurethane dressings).[2, 21-23, 26, 34, 73, 86] The lowest infection rates have been reported with daily dressing changes.[34, 51] Infection rates have been kept as low as two to five per cent with the most commonly reported dressing change frequency of three times per week. An infection rate of less than one per cent was maintained for four years using the catheter dressing procedure outlined in Figure 16–2.[34]

A modified dressing procedure for the patient with a Broviac-Hickman catheter, who has a closed catheter-cutaneous junction, is shown in Figure 16–3. Dressing care techniques for central venous catheters will continue to be diverse until definitive, prospective, patient-matched, controlled studies are conducted. Until these studies become available, strict protocols using the scientific information available should be followed to minimize catheter-related sepsis.

Central venous catheter infections are also related to the improper use of delivery systems and associated biomedical devices (Fig. 16–4). Measures for minimizing infec-

tion are outlined in Table 16–2.[2, 7, 54, 63, 72] There is a greater risk of septicemia developing when careful technique is not used with central lines for TPN or when the patient has more than one central line.

Management of Catheter-Related Sepsis

Signs, Symptoms, and Diagnosis

Regardless of the etiology, sepsis presents with a set of characteristic signs and symptoms. Clinical evidence of sepsis includes fever, chills, hypotension, and a deteriorating clinical or mental status. Systemic arterial infection, confirmed by positive blood cultures, leukocytosis, and unexplained glycosuria, provides laboratory support for the diagnosis of sepsis. In patients receiving TPN, the central venous catheter must always be suspected as a primary source of sepsis and this type of sepsis must be distinguished from sepsis originating at distant sites (see later discussion) (Fig. 16–5).[3, 13-15, 25, 56] Appropriate therapy for the septic state demands that the source for sepsis and the

EQUIPMENT

Caps
Masks
Clean gown for assistant
Sterile gowns for physicians inserting catheter
Sterile gloves
Sterile drapes
Appropriate parenteral fluid and tubing
Paper or plastic bag
Central venous catheter insertion tray containing:
    Three acetone-10% isopropyl
      alcohol-70% swabsticks
    Three povidone-iodine scrub
      swabsticks
    Three isopropyl alcohol 70%
      swabsticks
    Three povidone-iodine solution
      swabsticks

Telfa pad
Povidone-iodine ointment
Scissors
Elastoplast
Tincture of benzoin, Skin Prep or Cliniguard
Needle carrier
4″ × 4″ gauze sponges
2″ × 2″ gauze sponges
4-0 silk on a cutting needle
One alcohol swab
1% Lidocaine
Two 10 ml syringes
One 22-gauge needle
One 20-gauge needle
Tape

(If swabsticks are not available, tray will need five medicine glasses, a hemostat, additional 4″ × 4″ and 2″ × 2″ gauze sponges. The solutions listed will also be needed.)

PROCEDURE	RATIONALE
Explain procedure to patient.	Promotes patient's understanding and minimizes anxiety.
Organize supplies at bedside.	
Assistant dons gown, cap, mask.	Avoids contamination of site.
Wash hands—turn faucet off with paper towel.	Mechanical removal of bacteria decreases contamination of area if tear in glove occurs while touching catheter site.
Open and prepare insertion tray.	Minimizes time patient is in Trendelenburg position.
Place patient supine and in Trendelenburg position with towel between scapulae and with head turned away from site of insertion. Drape patient.	Promotes maximum filling and distention of the subclavian vein to the angle between the clavicle and the first rib.
Wash hands, again turning faucet off with paper towel.	
Don sterile gloves and cleanse area thoroughly with sterile acetone-alcohol swabsticks or saturated gauze pads. Cleanse with friction, using a circular motion from center to periphery. Acetone may be necessary if patient has had adhesive tape on site previously.	Removal of skin fats and oils, which may harbor pathogens.
Cleanse area with povidone-iodine scrub swabsticks or saturated gauze pads. Cleanse with friction, using a circular motion from center to periphery.	Removal of bacteria and fungi from skin.
Remove povidone-iodine scrub with sterile isopropyl alcohol swabstick or saturated gauze pad. Use a circular motion from center to periphery.	Povidone-iodine scrub is contaminated with skin organisms.
Blot skin dry.	
Paint area from center to periphery with povidone-iodine solution swabsticks or saturated gauze pad. Blot any pooled solution.	Provides a protective barrier against skin organisms. Pooled solution may cause iodine burns.
Apply sterile drapes.	Provides sterile field.
Physician wearing sterile gown, mask, cap, and sterile gloves will insert catheter.	
Connect fluid to central venous line; use extension tubing. Solutions containing more than 10% dextrose should not be infused prior to confirmation of catheter placement in superior vena cava.	Minimizes risk of thrombosis of subclavian or internal jugular vein.
Catheter should be secured to skin.	Minimizes movement of catheter and prevents accidental dislodgement.
Remove any blood from area with isopropyl alcohol. Blot area dry.	Blood left on skin may provide media for bacterial growth.
Apply povidone-iodine solution. Blot dry.	Pooled solution may cause iodine burns.
Apply povidone-iodine ointment to catheter insertion site.	May decrease bacterial and fungal growth at catheter site.
Cover catheter insertion site with a 2″ × 2″ gauze pad.	
Cover 2″ × 2″ gauze pad and catheter sheath with Telfa pad.	Prevents dislodging of catheter and pulling on sutures when removing Elastoplast.
Paint skin with tincture of benzoin, Skin Prep pad, or Cliniguard swabstick. Do not include catheter-cutaneous junction.	Enhances "sticking" of Elastoplast and tape and decreases damage to skin during removal of tape.
Apply Elastoplast to include junction of catheter and extension tubing; apply in a manner that does not interfere with joint movement.	Semiocclusive dressing to prevent air contamination of catheter site.
Tape extension tubing to Elastoplast with "butterfly" or "chevron" crossing of tape. Loop and secure extension on tubing to dressing. Tape all connections.	Prevents dislodgement of tubing. Decreases possibility of air embolism with accidental disconnection of tubing.
Label dressing. Include date of change and initials of person performing dressing change.	Provides unit personnel with date of last change.
Remove supplies and clean work area.	
Chart dressing change, patient tolerance, and any problems encountered.	Provides information for unit personnel and maintenance of medical records.
Ensure that chest x-ray film to check correct placement is obtained.	Documents proper placement of catheter.

Figure 16–1. Procedure for central venous catheter placement.

EQUIPMENT

Cap
Two masks
Clean gown
Tape
Central venous pressure or TPN tray containing:
  One pair gloves
  Three acetone-alcohol swabsticks
  One triple-pack povidone-iodine scrub swabsticks
  One triple-pack 70% isopropyl alcohol swabsticks
  Two 2″ × 2″ cotton gauze sponges
  One fenestrated drape

One triple-pack povidone-iodine solution swabsticks
Two cotton-tipped applicators
One protective dressing pad or swabstick
One povidone-iodine ointment
One 2″ × 2″ nonwoven split sponge
Two 2″ × 2″ cotton gauze sponges
One 2″ × 2″ nonadhering pad
One 1″ × 4″ nonadhering pad
One 3/4″ × 2″ nonadhering pad
One 3″ × 6″ elastic bandage
One pair scissors
One dressing change label

PROCEDURE	RATIONALE
Explain procedure to patient. Check for povidone-iodine or tape allergy.	Promotes patient understanding of care. Decreases anxiety.
Organize supplies at bedside.	
Wash hands. Turn off faucet with paper towel.	Mechanical removal of bacteria. Decreases contamination of area if tear in glove occurs while touching catheter site.
Don gown, cap, and mask.	Avoids contamination of catheter site.
Instruct patient to put on mask or to turn head away from the catheter and drape.	Avoids contamination of catheter site.
Open central venous pressure–dressing tray.	Avoids contamination of catheter site.
Remove old dressing carefully and place in paper bag.	
Inspect catheter site and surrounding skin for signs of irritation, leakage, edema, erythema, kinking, or altered position of catheter.	Detects complications such as infection, deterioration of catheter, or skin irritation.
Don sterile gloves and cleanse a 3″ × 6″ area thoroughly with sterile acetone-alcohol swabstick. Cleanse with friction, using a circular motion from center to periphery. Include protective plastic sheath. Repeat three times.	Acetone-alcohol removes skin fats and oils that may harbor pathogens.
Cleanse 3″ × 6″ area with sterile povidone-iodine scrub swabsticks. Cleanse with friction, using a circular motion from center to periphery. Include protective plastic sheath. Repeat three times.	Removes bacteria and fungi from skin.
Remove povidone-iodine scrub with sterile 70% isopropyl-alcohol swabsticks.	Povidone-iodine scrub is contaminated with skin pathogens.
Clamp existing extension tubing. Fill new extension tubing with fluid. Have patient take a breath and hold it during connection of extension tubing to catheter.	Prevents fibrin sleeve formation from "bleeding back" into catheter. Prevents air embolism.
Remove first pair of sterile gloves.	First pair of sterile gloves became contaminated with removal of extension tubing.
Don second pair of sterile gloves.	
Drape area with fenestrated drape.	Maintains a sterile field during final preparation of skin.
Prepare 3″ × 6″ area from center to periphery with sterile povidone-iodine solution swabsticks. Blot any pooled solution and allow to dry.	Provides a protective barrier against skin pathogens. Pooled solution may cause iodine burns.
Apply povidone-iodine ointment to catheter insertion site.	May decrease bacterial and fungal growth at catheter site.
Cover catheter insertion site with a 2″ × 2″ gauze pad.	
Cover 2″ × 2″ gauze pad and catheter sheath with Telfa pad.	Prevents dislodging of catheter and pulling on sutures when removing Elastoplast.
Paint skin with tincture of benzoin, Skin Prep pad or Cliniguard swabstick. Do not include catheter-cutaneous junction.	Enhances "sticking" of Elastoplast and tape and decreases damage to skin during removal of tape.
Apply Elastoplast to include junction of catheter and extension tubing; apply in a manner that does not interfere with joint movement.	Semiocclusive dressing to prevent air contamination of catheter site.
Tape extension tubing to Elastoplast with "butterfly" or "chevron" crossing of tape. Loop and secure extension tubing to dressing; tape all connections.	Prevents dislodgement of tubing. Decreases possibility of air embolism with accidental disconnection of tubing.
Label dressing. Include date of change and initials of person performing dressing change.	Provides unit personnel with date of last change.
Remove supplies and clean work area.	
Chart dressing change, appearance of catheter site, and any problems encountered.	Provides information for unit personnel and maintenance of medical records.

Figure 16–2. Dressing change procedure for central venous catheters.
(Modified from Forlaw, L.: Parenteral nutrition in the critically ill child. Crit. Care Quart., 3:7, 1981.)

EQUIPMENT

Four 2″ × 2″ gauze pads
Sterile scissors
One 10% acetone-70% isopropyl alcohol
  swabstick (single swabstick)
Povidone-iodine solution swabstick (three per package)

Sterile gloves
Small bottle povidone-iodine scrub or Hibiclens
Two masks
Tape

PROCEDURE	RATIONALE
Put on mask (patient must also mask when in the hospital.)	Avoids contamination of catheter site.
Wash hands with povidone-iodine scrub or Hibiclens. Use paper towel to turn off faucet.	Mechanical removal of bacteria.
Open 2″ × 2″ gauze pads—make a slit in two of them.	Allows easy placement around catheter.
Remove old dressing—check area for any redness, swelling, drainage, or irritation. Call staff nurse, or physician or clinical nurse specialist before cleaning the site when in hospital.	Detects any signs of irritation or infection.
Clean catheter exit site with 10% acetone-70% isopropyl alcohol swabstick. Work in a circular fashion from point of catheter exit. Blot skin dry with a folded 2″ × 2″ gauze pad.	Defats skin, leading to a decrease in bacteria.
Apply povidone-iodine solution. Work in circular fashion from point of catheter exit.	Provides a protective barrier against skin pathogens.
Blot skin dry with a folded 2″ × 2″ gauze pad—check under catheter for any pooling of povidone-iodine solution.	Pooled solution may cause iodine burns.
Put on sterile gloves.	Avoids contamination of gauze pads.
Apply 2″ × 2″ gauze pad with slit under and over catheter, then place a 2″ × 2″ gauze pad on top of catheter exit site.	Completely covers wound and decreases potential for infection. Supports catheter.
Tape dressing in place.	Secures catheter in place and decreases chance of dislodgement.
Anchor catheter to dressing.	Secures catheter in place and decreases chance of dislodgement.
Chart procedure in nursing or doctor's progress notes.	Provides information for unit personnel and maintenance of medical records.

For Children: The child's head should be turned away from the dressing. Child may wear mask or be draped appropriately. *Do not* cover face or tracheostomy *completely*. Be sure child can breathe.

Figure 16–3. Modified dressing change procedure for Broviac-Hickman catheter exit site used after closure of catheter-cutaneous junction.

infecting organism or organisms be accurately identified.

Evaluation of the septic patient begins with a systematic and thorough search for the locus of infection. After reviewing the history, a careful clinical examination of the nose, throat, ears, chest, abdomen, surgical wound, and intravenous access sites should be performed. Gram stains of the urine and sputum, urine and sputum cultures, a sensitivity chest roentgenogram, and additional radiologic and laboratory tests are performed as clinically indicated. An essential aspect of the initial evaluation is obtaining multiple blood cultures for aerobic and anaerobic bacteria and fungi cultures. Sensitivity testing of all organisms cultured from the bloodstream is necessary to ensure the selection of appropriate antibiotic therapy. Blood cultures may be drawn either through the central line or at a peripheral site. In either case, a positive blood culture merely indicates the presence of bacteria or fungi in the bloodstream. Blood samples obtained through a central venous catheter do not reflect the status of the catheter itself.[9, 42]

Fungal sepsis is frequently more difficult to diagnose than is bacterial sepsis.[81] *Candida* is an opportunistic organism that commonly causes catheter-related sepsis in patients receiving broad-spectrum antibiotics.[8, 18-20, 73] Although venous blood cultures often remain negative despite the presence of systemic candidemia, positive fungal cultures may be obtained from arterial blood samples.[70] Persistent isolation of *Candida* from the urine, fungal endophthalmitis, or the presence of intraleukocytic fungal forms on blood smear may confirm the diagnosis of fungal septicemia.[36, 57]

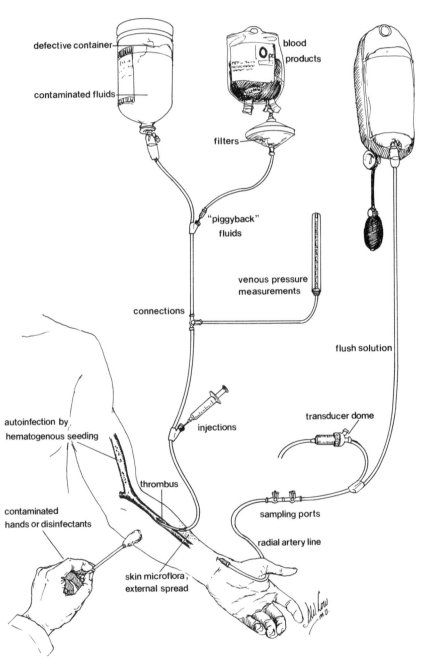

Figure 16–4. Potential sources of contamination of venous and arterial access catheters.

Table 16–2. METHODS FOR MINIMIZING COMPLICATIONS FROM CENTRAL VENOUS CATHETERS

GENERAL USE	RATIONALE	PARENTERAL NUTRITION	RATIONALE
Avoid stopcocks		Stopcocks are not used	Closed system is maintained
Stopcocks should be covered at all times	Open stopcocks provide entry for bacteria from sheets, patient's skin, dressings, wounds, personnel's hands		Open stopcocks provide entry for bacteria from sheets, patient's skin, dressings, wounds, personnel's hands
Stopcocks should be changed at least daily or when blood collects within them	Blood within stopcocks may provide media for bacterial growth		Blood within stopcocks may provide media for bacterial growth
Avoid injecting medicines and "piggybacks" through central venous lines, avoid use of multidose vials	Decreases possibility of bacterial contamination	Medications are not injected or piggybacked	Decreases possibility of bacterial contamination
Needles used for piggybacking must be securely taped	Bacteria may be pistoned into system from latex	Fat emulsions may be given via a Y-connector if no peripheral access	Peripheral route is always preferred
Use Y-connectors, multilumen connectors or solusets for administering medications			Fat emulsions support bacterial growth
		The fat emulsion and parenteral nutrition are added to the infusion via the Y-connector and are discontinued simultaneously	Avoids excessive opening of the system
Clamp extension tubing when adding or clamping intravenous fluid container	To avoid bleeding back into catheter and promotion of an internal fibrin sheath, decreases catheter occlusion	Clamp extension tubing when adding or changing parenteral nutrition or fat emulsion solution container	To avoid bleeding back into the catheter and promoting an internal fibrin sheath, decreases catheter occlusion
Blood transfusions may be given through catheter when necessary	Catheters are generally for short-term use, platelets may adhere to the catheter and form an internal fibrin sheath	Blood transfusions are not given through catheters used for parenteral nutrition	Catheters are generally for longer use, platelets may adhere to the catheter and form an internal fibrin sheath
Blood should not be drawn through catheter	Possible formation of internal fibrin sheath Risk of air embolism Increases potential for clotting of catheter, Hickman or similar catheters are an exception	Blood should not be drawn through catheter	Possible formation of internal fibrin sheath Risk of air embolism Increases potential for clotting in catheter
Catheter is used for monitoring central venous pressure, use of transducer is preferable to manometer	Generally for short-term use May be changed over a Selinger wire if necessary for long-term use	Catheter is not used for monitoring central venous pressure	Possible increased formation of internal fibrin sheath Risk of hypoglycemia Risk of glucose intolerance Avoids bleeding back into the catheter with possible formation of internal fibrin sheath
Transducers should be changed at once if retrograde blood flows into dome or disruption of the integrity of any attached connectors, stopcocks occurs	May be necessary for adequate monitoring, may become contaminated by retrograde blood flow into dome, by contaminated cleansing solution or flush, leaks from dome, intraflow or connecting stopcocks	Are not used with parenteral nutrition catheter	May decrease possibility of bacterial contamination
Tape all connections securely, Luer-Lok connections may be helpful if standardized and attached appropriately	To avoid accidental disconnection of catheter and connecting tubing, thus decreasing risk of bleeding back into or clotting in catheter, decreases risk of air embolism	Tape all connections securely, Luer-Lok connections may be helpful if standardized and attached appropriately	To avoid accidental disconnection of catheter and connecting tubing, thus decreasing risk of bleeding back into or clotting in catheter, decreases risk of air embolism
Patients with tracheostomy, nasotracheal tubes, nasogastric tubes, neck wounds should have dressing covered with an absorbent abdominal dressing pad that can be changed frequently if necessary	To prevent contamination of site, plastic covering may promote moisture retention	Patients with tracheostomy, nasotracheal tubes, nasogastric tubes, neck wounds should have dressing covered with an absorbent abdominal dressing pad that can be changed frequently if necessary	To prevent contamination of site, plastic covering may promote moisture retention

(Modified from Forlaw, L., and Mullen, J. L.: Care of central venous catheters. Crit. Care Monitor, March 1981.)

EQUIPMENT

Two pair sterile gloves
One 10 ml syringe
Two sterile suture removal sets
Two packages 10% acetone-70% isopropyl alcohol
  swabstick
One each mask, gown, cap, plastic bag
One package povidone-iodine swabsticks

One culturette
One sterile drape
Two 2" × 2" gauze pads
Tape
Two sterile culture tubes
Three microbiology request slips

PROCEDURE

Explain procedure to patient and gather equipment.
Put on cap, mask, and gown.
Wash hands—turn off faucet with paper towel.
Remove dressing, place in plastic bag, inspect site—if drainage is present, culture with culturette.
Cleanse skin around catheter, sutures, catheter hub, and extension tubing with acetone-alcohol swabstick. Allow skin to dry. Carefully remove all crusts and ointment. Repeat with povidone-iodine swabstick.
Open suture removal tray, cut and remove sutures with scissors and forceps.
Turn off IV fluid. Don sterile gloves.
Grasp hub of catheter. Ask patient to take deep breath and hold. Remove IV tubing, swab inside of hub with culturette. Attach syringe to catheter.
If patient is septic—temperature of 101° F—draw blood for culture.
Have patient take deep breath and hold. Withdraw catheter. Handle catheter only by hub and pull catheter upward away from skin.

Allow blood to drain from catheter onto sterile drape.
With sterile scissors from second suture set, cut two 5- to 7-cm segments: (1) proximal segment beginning inside the former skin-catheter interface; (2) the tip. Place each segment in a separate dry sterile culture tube.
If any purulent material is expressed from the catheter site, culture it using a culturette. Place 2" × 2" gauze pad over site. Tape in place.
If the patient has signs of sepsis and a temperature of 101° F, draw a blood culture from a peripheral site before removing catheter or one hour after removing catheter.
Label samples with patient's name.
Fill out microbiology slips completely.
Chart procedure and patient's tolerance in doctor's progress or nursing notes.
Take cultures to laboratory immediately to prevent drying of the specimen and loss of the organisms.

Figure 16–5. Procedure for culturing central venous catheters 20- to 30-cm (8- to 12-inch) long.

Catheter Removal

If an obvious source of sepsis is discovered distant to the TPN catheter, treatment of the primary site of infection is immediately indicated. Although hematogenous seeding of the fibrin sheath surrounding the catheter may occur, this complication is unlikely with appropriate treatment of the primary infection.[19, 54] If the patient remains clinically stable and becomes afebrile with initial therapy, most studies indicate that the central venous catheter may remain in place. In a prospective study of 200 consecutive patients receiving TPN, Ryan and colleagues[74] reported that 75 per cent of the TPN catheters discontinued during septic episodes were, in retrospect, not causing infection and did not require removal. Thus, excellent clinical judgment is required to determine which catheters may be left in place during the initial evaluation of the septic patient.

Persistence of fever or positive blood cultures without a known source of infection, cardiovascular instability, or continued deterioration of clinical or mental status dictate immediate catheter removal. All TPN catheters removed for suspected catheter sepsis must be cultured. The semiquantitative method of culturing the catheter tip as described by Maki and associates in 1977 is preferable to culturing in broth (Fig. 16–5).[58, 78] because the high-density colonization (fifteen colonies per plate) obtained in semiquantitative culture is more specific for diagnosing catheter-related sepsis. Low-density colonization (fifteen colonies per plate) on semiquantitative culture indicates catheter contamination, but essentially eliminates the central venous catheter as the primary site of infection. Catheter-related sepsis is strictly defined as a clinical episode of systemic infection that resolves with catheter removal and for which no distant locus is identified.[2, 43] Growth of the same organism on high-density semiquantitative culture of the catheter tip and in the blood confirms this diagnosis.[2, 54, 58]

In patients who have Hickman catheters for long-term intravenous access, several modifications of the previously described protocol exist (Fig. 16–5).[43, 66] The initial evaluation of febrile episodes in these patients is identical to that outlined for patients with percutaneous subclavian catheters. However, because of the difficulty in obtaining alternate sites of central venous access in these patients, a more persistent attempt is made to preserve the indwelling catheter. If the patient remains clinically stable, most investigators recommend waiting 48 to 72 hours for microbial culture results and catheter removal is considered only with positive blood cultures in the absence of another identifiable locus of infection.[17, 66, 73] Despite the persistence of fever, Hickman catheters may be left *in situ* for several days unless hypotension or clinical instability necessitates earlier removal. Identification of a distant site of infection can be managed appropriately without catheter removal. If fever persists and no other source of infection is apparent, the catheter is removed. Complete resolution of sepsis may require surgical excision of the subcutaneous Dacron cuff.

In 1980, Glynn and coworkers reported successfully treating patients with infected Hickman catheters with urokinase and systemic antibiotic therapy. It was postulated that the urokinase-induced thrombolysis at the tip of the Hickman catheter rendered the organisms in this vicinity susceptible to subsequent antibiotic therapy. In this study, fever resolved and blood cultures became negative in 7 of 20 patients treated with this technique. Although further study is required for thorough evaluation, this technique represents another attempt to avert surgical intervention in this difficult patient population.

Antibiotics and Antibacterial Agents

In fact, the majority of patients with catheter-related sepsis can be treated with catheter removal alone—regardless of whether a bacterial or a fungal organism is implicated as the etiologic agent.[5, 40, 74, 75] Although resolution of catheter-related sepsis occurs promptly with catheter removal in most cases, some investigators recommend that antibiotics be administered routinely in all patients with presumed catheter sepsis.[32] The presence of hypotension, continued deterioration of clinical status, or the persistence of fever necessitates immediate institution of broad-spectrum antibiotics. Evidence of tissue invasion by fungi or the development of additional septic foci similarly require the use of systemic fungal or antibacterial agents.[4, 41] When any doubt exists regarding the etiology of a febrile episode, the central venous catheter must be suspected and should be removed immediately and cultured. The severity of the patient's clinical condition dictates the urgency with which systemic antibiotics and additional supportive measures are instituted.

Guide Wire Technique for Changing the Central Venous Catheter

An alternative approach exists for managing the febrile patient with a central venous catheter who remains clinically stable. If the patient maintains normal cardiovascular, neurologic, and renal function throughout the febrile episode, the indwelling central venous catheter may be replaced with another catheter by changing over a sterile guide wire.[42] This technique permits evaluation of the catheter tip upon removal, but avoids the complications associated with obtaining central venous access at another site. Changing a central venous catheter over a guide wire, however, must be regarded as a diagnostic, not a therapeutic, technique. Thus, any catheter inserted through an infected or colonized subcutaneous tract must be removed as soon as positive culture results are obtained.[42] Although controversy exists over whether catheter infection originates at the cutaneous puncture site or intravascularly, numerous studies have demonstrated that the subcutaneous tunnel and adjacent segment of catheter are colonized with the same organism as the intravascular fibrin sheath.[27, 36, 37, 58] It must be emphasized that the persistence of fever, hypotension, or deteriorating clinical status is a contraindication to using this guide wire technique, and any one of these events dictates immediate catheter removal.

CENTRAL VENOUS THROMBOSIS

Central venous thrombosis following subclavian vein catheterization was first recognized by McDonough and Altemeier in 1971.[60] Since this initial observation, the reported incidence of subclavian vein thrombosis with polyvinylchloride catheters has ranged from 3 to 71 per cent.[2, 13, 14, 27, 67] Several factors are responsible for this obvious discrepancy among studies reporting the incidence of catheter-related thrombosis. First, multiple methods of diagnosing central venous thrombosis exist and include clinical examination, radiographic studies (dye contrast and radionuclide), and autopsy studies.[13, 65] By monitoring symptoms and clinical signs alone, patients with clinically silent central venous thrombosis will be overlooked.[13, 27] Fifty to 58 per cent of patients with subclavian vein thrombosis may be asymptomatic and lack obvious clinical evidence of central venous occlusion. These clinically occult cases of thrombosis will be detected only by radiography or autopsy examination.[2] Second, the definition of catheter-related thrombosis is often extended to include radiographic findings other than subclavian vein occlusion. For instance, the presence of a fibrin sleeve or thrombus of the catheter tip are frequently observed venographic findings that are defined by some investigators to represent catheter-related thrombosis. Associating these relatively minor venographic changes with central venous occlusion will certainly increase the observed incidence of subclavian vein thrombosis. Third, the risk of thrombogenicity in any patient is multifactorial and may significantly influence results among different study populations. Differences in catheter size and composition, pH of infusate, duration of infusion, presence of bacteria, and venous flow characteristics are several factors known to alter the thrombogenic potential of intravenous catheters.[33, 48, 49, 83, 85]

In a recent review, Grant proposed an incidence of approximately three per cent for symptomatic subclavian vein thrombosis associated with plastic catheters.[43] In 1981, Padberg and colleagues reported a 4.8 per cent incidence of clinically apparent central venous thrombosis in 104 patients receiving TPN.[67] Clinically occult thrombosis of the central venous system was subsequently demonstrated in 4 of 19 patients after autopsy examination. In 1980, Valeri and associates studied 18 patients with central venous polyvinylchloride catheters in a prospective manner.[84] Although only one instance (4.4 per cent) of symptomatic subclavian vein thrombosis was observed, venographic abnormalities of the central venous system were demonstrated in six patients (33 per cent). Thus, radiographic evidence of central venous thrombosis is common despite the relatively infrequent occurrence of clinically evident thrombosis.

The significance of central venous thrombosis is shown by an infrequent but serious complication of this entity—pulmonary embolism. Frior in 1972, Ryan and coworkers in 1974, and Singh and coworkers in 1979 have all reported thromboembolic events that are presumed to have arisen from catheter-related thrombosis.[32, 74, 80] The embolic potential of central venous thrombi demands that definitive diagnosis be pursued and appropriate therapy instituted. Thorough physical examination and selected radiographic studies are required to detect thrombosis in high-risk patients.

Management

In patients with clinically evident or presumed central venous thrombosis, venography should be performed to confirm the diagnosis.[2, 61] Venography is most readily performed through the indwelling central venous catheter, which is immediately removed after confirmation of the diagnosis. Since embolic complications are potential sequelae of central venous thrombi, systemic heparin should be administered to attain therapeutic anticoagulation. Heparin therapy should be continued until symptoms resolve (if present) or until initial venographic abnormalities improve.[2, 12, 54, 61, 80]

If only the TPN catheter is occluded, without thrombosis of the surrounding intravascular system, recent studies have reported restoring catheter patency with the local instillation of fibrinolytic solutions into the occluded line.[39, 49]

Both streptokinase-streptodornase and urokinase have been used for this purpose with no evidence of systemic fibrinolysis. Occlusion of percutaneous subclavian and indwelling Hickman catheters has been successfully treated with this technique.

Catheter Composition and Thrombogenicity

Numerous methods have been investigated in an attempt to decrease the incidence of catheter-related thrombosis. Catheter composition, an important determinant of thrombogenicity, has been extensively studied in recent years.[64, 85] In a canine model, Welch and associates demonstrated a dramatic reduction in the gross and histologic inflammatory reaction observed in veins cannulated with silicone catheters when compared to those catheterized with polyethylene catheters.[85] Clinical studies have similarly demonstrated an improvement in thrombosis associated with the use of silicone central venous catheters.[69] In 1982, McLean-Ross and coworkers reported a series of 118 consecutive silicone elastomer subclavian catheter insertions with an average catheter life of 19.4 days.[61] An incidence of symptomatic and asymptomatic central venous thrombosis approximated 4 per cent; one episode of major pulmonary embolism occurred in this study. In 1982, Dolcourt and Bose studied a series of newborn infants with percutaneous silicone catheters placed for TPN delivery and reported no instances of clinically evident central venous thrombosis.[24] Other studies have reported similar results, and they indicate an apparent reduction in the incidence of central venous thrombosis associated with silicone catheters.[47, 53] The influence of catheter composition on the occurrence of major pulmonary embolism originating from central venous thrombi, however, remains to be determined.

Heparin coating of the central venous catheter has also been tried, but it significantly increased the stiffness of the catheter material.[46, 68] No reduction in thrombogenicity has been observed with heparin-coated catheters, perhaps because of mechanical damage to the vessel wall caused by the rigidity of these catheters.[12, 46, 68] Several studies have demonstrated a slight reduction in thrombophlebitis and catheter-related sepsis with the addition of heparin (1 to 3 IU/ml) to the TPN solution.[6, 82] However, additional reports demonstrate no efficacy from this prophylactic measure.[62] Finally, intermittent heparin administration through the central venous catheter has recently been studied, with one report indicating a reduction in venographically proven thrombosis.[12] However, the efficacy of continuous or intermittent heparin therapy in preventing major thromboembolic complications of central venous catheterization remains controversial.

CATHETER MALPOSITION

Catheter malposition is a common complication of percutaneous subclavian vein cannulation. Misdirection of the catheter tip into the ipsilateral internal jugular vein occurs most frequently. The contralateral innominate and subclavian vein, small venous tributaries, or anomalous veins represent relatively uncommon sites of inadvertent cannulation.[66] In 1978, Bradley and associates reported malposition of the catheter tip in 5.6 per cent of 178 central venous catheterizations.[9] In 1978, Herbst reported only one instance of internal jugular vein cannulation in 117 subclavian catheter attempts.[45] In a recent retrospective review of 524 consecutive infraclavicular subclavian vein catheterizations, Gatti and Mullen reported a 5.9 per cent incidence of catheter misdirection involving the internal jugular vein.[38]

Complications

Delivery of TPN through an intravenous catheter with its tip outside the superior vena cava or right atrium is inadvisable. Previous studies have clearly demonstrated an increased risk of phlebitis and thrombosis with infusion of hypertonic fluid through an improperly positioned catheter.[43] Only by placing the catheter tip in the superior vena cava or right atrium is the venous flow rate sufficient to reduce these complications to an acceptable level.

Thrombosis of the internal jugular vein may be associated with significant morbidity and may present with the symptoms of pseudotumor cerebi.[77] This syndrome consists of diplopia, headache, bilateral papilledema, and sixth cranial nerve injury.

To avoid complications of catheter malposition, chest roentgenograms are required to confirm proper catheter placement prior to TPN administration. If the catheter is improperly located, correct positioning of the catheter tip is mandatory and may be accomplished by several techniques. Repeated percutaneous attempts to cannulate the superior vena cava are occasionally necessary. However, with each attempt at percutaneous catheter insertion, the patient is exposed to a multitude of mechanical complications associated with central line placement. In an effort to avoid this source of potential morbidity, alternative techniques for repositioning the catheter tip without catheter removal have been devised. Grant reported successful positioning of misdirected catheter tips by partially withdrawing the catheter, rotating it, and reinserting it in 32 of 50 cases.[43] A guide wire may similarly be used to place the catheter tip in the superior vena cava after partially withdrawing the previously inserted catheter.[38] A repeat roentgenogram of the chest is required to document proper repositioning of the catheter tip in the superior vena cava. Finally, the use of fluoroscopy may be a helpful adjunct in expediting correct catheter placement. The safety and efficacy of each of these techniques has been previously documented.

FUTURE TRENDS: IMPLANTABLE VASCULAR DEVICES

Implantable vascular access devices may provide an alternate delivery system for patients who are unable to comply with the care requirements related to permanent indwelling catheters such as the Broviac or Hickman.[88]

Huber needles are used to access the device to avoid damage to the septum. Careful attention to adequate preparation of the skin is essential to minimize infectious complications related to puncture of the skin or to the device for delivery of intravenous fluids or heparinization.

SUMMARY

Catheter-related complications during TPN administration are largely preventable. Aseptic placement and maintenance of central venous catheters according to rigorous protocol have dramatically reduced the incidence of catheter-related complications. Sepsis, thrombosis, and catheter malposition are potentially serious complications that require early recognition and prompt therapy. The diagnosis and treatment of catheter-related complications, as well as guidelines for catheter care, are presented so that TPN may be administered to patients with minimal morbidity and mortality.

REFERENCES AND SELECTED READINGS

1. Albert, R.K., and Condie, F.: Hand-washing patterns in medical intensive-care units. N. Engl. J. Med., *304*:1465, 1981.
2. Allen, J.R.: The incidence of nosocomial infection in patients receiving total parenteral nutrition. *In* Johnston, I.D.A. (ed.): Advances in Parenteral Nutrition. Lancaster, England, MTP Press Ltd., 1978.
3. Attman, R.P., and Randolph, J.C.: Application and hazards of total parenteral nutrition in infants. Am. Surg., *174*:84, 1971.
4. Anderson, A.O., and Yardley, J.H.: Demonstration of *Candida* in blood smears. N. Engl. J. Med., *286*:108, 1972.
5. Ashcraft, K.W., and Keape, L.L.: *Candida* sepsis complicating parenteral feeding. J.A.M.A., *212*:454, 1970.
6. Bailey, M.J.: Reduction of catheter-associated sepsis in parenteral nutrition using low-dose intravenous heparin. Br. Med. J., *1*:1671, 1979.
7. Band, J.D., and Maki, D.G.: Safety of changing intravenous delivery systems at longer than 24-hour intervals. Ann. Intern. Med., *91*:173, 1979.
8. Bentley, D.W., and Lepper, M.H.: Septicemia related to indwelling venous catheter. J.A.M.A., *206*:1749, 1968.
9. Bradley, J.A., Halsall A., Hill, G.L., and McMahon, M.J.: A prospective study of subclavian catheters used exclusively for the purpose of intravenous feeding. Br. J. Surg., *65*:393, 1978.
10. Boeckman, C.R., and Krill, C.E.: Bacterial and fungal infections complicating parenteral alimentation in infants and children. J. Pediatr. Surg., *5*:117, 1970.
11. Boyd, J.R. (ed.): Drug Facts and Comparisons. Philadelphia, J.B. Lippincott Co., 1982, pages 1700, 1701, and 1705.
12. Brismar, B., Hardstedt, C., Jacobson, S., Kager, L., and Malmborg, A.: Reduction of catheter-associated thrombosis in parenteral nutrition by intravenous heparin therapy. Arch. Surg., *117*:1196, 1982.
13. Brismar, B., Hardstedt, C., and Jacobson, S.: Diagnosis of thrombosis by catheter phlebography after prolonged central venous catheterization. Ann. Surg., *194*:779, 1981.
14. Brismar, B., Hardstedt, C., and Malmborg, A.S.: Bacteriology and phlebography in catheterization for parenteral nutrition: a prospective study. Acta Chir. Scand., *146*:115, 1980.
15. Buxton, A.E., Highsmith, A.K., Garner, J.S., Stamm, W.E., Dixon, R.E., and McGowan, J.E.: Contamination of intravenous infusion fluid: effects of changing administration sets. Ann. Intern. Med., *90*:764, 1979.
16. Cleri, D.J., Corrado, M.L., and Seligman, S.J.: Quantitative culture of intravenous catheters and other intravenous inserts. J. Infect. Dis., *141*:781, 1980.
17. Colley, R., Wilson, J., et al.: Fever and catheter-related sepsis in total parenteral nutrition. J.P.E.N., *3*:32, 1979.
18. Copeland, E.M., MacFayden, B.V., and Dudrick, S.J.: Prevention of microbial catheter contamination in patients receiving parenteral hyperalimentation. South. Med. J., *67*:303, 1974.
19. Copeland, E.M., MacFayden, B.V., McGown, C., and Duduck, S.J.: The use of hyperalimentation in patients with potential sepsis. Surg. Gynecol. Obstet., *137*:377, 1974.
20. Crow, S.: Understanding asepsis practices. Supervis. Nurse, Vol. 11, Nov: 28, 1980.
21. Curry, C.R., and Quie, P.G.: Fungal septicemia in patients receiving parenteral hyperalimentation. N. Engl. J. Med., *285*:1221, 1971.
22. Curtas, S., and Grant, J.: Evaluation of Op-site as a

total parenteral nutrition dressing. N.I.T.A., 4:414, 1981.

23. Dillon, J.D., Jr., Schaffner, W., Van Way, C.W., and Meng, H.C.: Septicaemia and total parenteral nutrition. J.A.M.A., 223:1341, 1973.

24. Dolcourt, J.L., and Bose, C.L.: Percutaneous insertion of Silastic central venous catheters in newborn infants. Pediatrics, 70:484, 1982.

25. Driscoll, J.M., Jr., Heird, W.C., Schullinger, J.N., Gongaware, R.D., and Winters, R.W.: Total intravenous alimentation in low-birth-weight infants: a preliminary report. J. Pediatr., 81:145, 1972.

26. Dudrick, S.J., Graff, D.B., and Wilmore, D.W.: Long-term venous catheterization in infants. Surg. Gynecol. Obstet., 129:805, 1969.

27. Fabri, P.J., Mirtallo, J.M., Ruberg, R.L., Kudsk, K.A., Denning, D.A., Ellison, E.C., and Schaffer, P.: Incidence and prevention of thrombosis of the subclavian vein during total parenteral nutrition. Surg. Gynecol. Obstet., 155:238, 1982.

28. Falconer, M.W., Sheridan, E., Patterson, H.R., and Gustafson, E.A.: The Drug, The Nurse, The Patient. Philadelphia, W. B. Saunders Co., 1978.

29. Favero, M.S.: Iodine—champagne in a tin cup. Infect. Control, 3:30, 1982.

30. Filler, R.M., and Eraklis, A.J.: Care of the critically ill child: intravenous alimentation. Pediatrics, 46:456, 1970.

31. Filler, R.M., Eraklis, A.J., and Das, J.B.: Total parenteral nutrition in pediatrics, rationale and clinical experience. *In* Gadini, H. (ed.): Total Parenteral Nutrition. New York, John Wiley and Sons, 1975.

32. Firor, H.V.: Pulmonary embolization complicating total intravenous alimentation. J. Pediatr. Surg., 7:81, 1972.

33. Fonkalsrud, E.W.: The effect of pH in glucose infusions on development of thrombophlebitis. J. Surg. Res., 8:539, 1968.

34. Forlaw, L.: Parenteral nutrition in the critically ill child. Crit. Care Quart., 3:7, 1981.

35. Forlaw, L., and Mullen, J.L.: Care of central venous catheters. Crit. Care Monitor, March 1981.

36. Freeman, J.B., Davis, P.L., and MacLean, L.: *Candida* endophthalmitis associated with intravenous hyperalimentation. Arch. Surg., 108:237, 1974.

37. Freeman, J.B., Lemire, A., and MacLean, L.: Intravenous alimentation and septicemia. Surg. Gynecol. Obstet., 135:708, 1972.

38. Gatti, J.E., and Mullen, J.L.: The malpositioned subclavian catheter. Surg. Gynecol. Obstet., 153:91, 1981.

39. Glynn, M.F.X., Langer, B., and Jeejeebhoy, K.N.: Therapy for thrombotic occlusion long-term intravenous alimentation catheters. J.P.E.N., 4:387, 1980.

40. Goldmann, D.A., and Maki, D.G.: Infection control in total parenteral nutrition. J.A.M.A., 223:1360, 1973.

41. Goldstein, E., and Hoesprich, P.D.: Problems in the diagnosis and treatment of systemic candidiasis. J. Infect. Dis., 125:190, 1972.

42. Graeve, A.H., Carpenter, C.M., and Schiller, W.R.: Management of central venous catheters using a wire introducer. Am. J. Surg., 142:752, 1981.

43. Grant, J.P.: Handbook of Total Parenteral Nutrition. Philadelphia, W. B. Saunders Co., 1980.

44. Hamilton, H.W., Hamilton, K.R., and Lone, F.J.: Preoperative hair removal. Can. J. Surg., 20:269, 1977.

45. Herbst, C.A.: Indications, management, and complications of percutaneous subclavian catheters. Arch. Surg., 113:1421, 1978.

46. Hoar, P.F., Stone, J.G., Wicks, A.E., et al.: Thrombogenesis associated with Swan-Ganz catheters. Anesthesiology, 48:445, 1978.

47. Hoshal, V.L.: Total intravenous nutrition with peripherally inserted silicone elastomer central venous catheters. Arch. Surg., 110:644, 1975.

48. Hoshal, V.L., Ause, R.G., and Hoskins, P.A.: Fibrin sleeve formation on indwelling subclavian central venous catheters. Arch. Surg., 102:353, 1971.

49. Hurtubise, M.R., Bottino, J.E., et al. Restoring patency of occluded central venous catheters. Arch. Surg., 115:212, 1980.

50. Jarrard, M., and Freeman, J.: The effects of antibiotic ointments and antiseptics on the skin flora beneath subclavian catheter dressings during intravenous hyperalimentation. J. Surg. Research, 22:521, 1977.

51. Jarrard, M.M., Olson, C.M., and Freeman, J.B.: Daily dressing change effects on skin flora beneath subclavian catheter dressing during total parenteral nutrition. J.P.E.N., 4:391, 1980.

52. Johnson, J.D., Abritton, W.L., and Sunshine, P.: Hyperammonemia accompanying parenteral nutrition in newborn infants. J. Pediatr., 81:154, 1972.

53. MacDonald, A.S., Master, S.K.P., and Moffitt, E.A.: A comparative study of peripherally inserted silicone catheters for parenteral nutrition. Can. Anaesth. Soc. J., 24:263, 1977.

54. Maki, D.G.: Sepsis arising from extrinsic contamination of the infusion and measures for control. *In* Phillips, I., Meers, P.D., and D'Arcy, P.F. (eds.): Microbiological Hazards of Infusion Therapy, Lancaster, England, MTP Press, Ltd., 1976.

55. Maki, D.G., and Band, J.D.: Study of polyantibiotic idophor ointments in prevention of vascular catheter related infection. Am. J. Med., 70:739, 1981.

56. Maki, D.G., Goldmann, D.A., and Rhame, F.S.: Infection control in intravenous therapy. Ann. Intern. Med., 79:867, 1973.

57. Maki, D.G., Jarrett, F., and Sarafin, H.W.: A semiquantitative culture method for identification of catheter-related infection in the burn patient. J. Surg. Res., 22:513, 1977.

58. Maki, D.G., Weise, C.E., and Sarafin, H.W.: A semiquantitative culture method for identifying intravenous catheter-related infection. N. Engl. J. Med., 296:1306, 1977.

59. Maki, D.G., and McCormick, K.N.: Acetone defatting in cutaneous antisepsis Crit. Care Med., 9:202, 1981.

60. McDonough, J.J., and Altemeier, W.A.: Subclavian venous thrombosis secondary to indwelling catheters. Surg. Gynecol. Obstet., 133:397, 1971.

61. McLean-Ross, A.H., Griffith, D.M., Anderson, J.R., and Grieve, D.C.: Thromboembolic complications with silicone elastomer subclavian catheters. J.P.E.N., 6:61, 1982.

62. McNair, T.J., and Dudley, H.A.F.: The local complications of intravenous therapy. Lancet, 2:365, 1959.

63. Millan, D.A.: Final inline filters. A.J.N., 79:1272, 1979.

64. Nejad, M.S.: Clotting on the outer surface of vascular catheters. Radiology, 91:248, 1968.

65. Nordlund, S., and Thoren, L.: Catheter in the superior vena cava for parenteral feeding. Acta Chir. Scand., 127:39, 1964.

66. O'Reilly, R.J.: Aberrant venous catheter position within the left chest. Contemp. Surg., 12:29, 1978.

67. Padberg, F.T., Ruggiero, J., Blackburn, G.L., et al.: Central venous catheterization for parenteral nutrition. Ann. Surg., 193:264, 1981.

68. Peters, W.R., Bush, W.H., Jr., McIntyre, R.D., et al.: The development of fibrin sheath on indwelling venous catheters. Surg. Gynecol. Obstet., 137:43, 1973.

69. Pollack, P.F., Kadden, M., Byrne, W.J., Fonkalsrud, E.W., and Ament, M.E.: 100 patient years' experience with the Broviac silastic catheter for central venous nutrition. J.P.E.N., 5:32, 1981.

70. Portnoy, J., Wolf, P.L., Webb, M., et al.: *Candida* blastospores and pseudohyphae in blood smears. N. Engl. J. Med., 285:1010, 1971.

71. Powell-Tuck, J., Lennard-Jones, J.E., Lowes, J.A., Danso, K. T., and Shaw, E. J.: Intravenous feeding in a gastroenterological unit: a prospective study of infective complications. J. Clin. Pathol., 32:549, 1979.

72. Rhoades, C., Adcock, M., and Jovanovich, J.F.: Prevention of nosocomial infection in critical care units. *In* Anking, L.M., and McArthur, B.J. (eds.): Infection Control. Nurs. Clin. North Am., 15:803, 1980.

73. Ryan, J.A., Jr.: Complications of total parenteral nutrition. *In* Fischer, J.E. (ed.): Total Parenteral Nutrition. Boston, Little, Brown & Co., 1976.

74. Ryan, J.A., Abel, R.M., Abbott, W.M., et al.: Catheter complications in total parenteral nutrition: a prospective study of 200 consecutive patients. N. Engl. J. Med., 290:757, 1974.

75. Sanderson, I., and Deitel, M.: Intravenous hyperalimentation without sepsis. Surg. Gynecol. Obstet., 136:577, 1973.

76. Sanders, R.A., and Sheldon, G.F.: Septic complications of total parenteral nutrition. Am. J. Surg., 132:214, 1976.

77. Sazena, V.K., Heilpern, R.J., and Murphy, S.F.: Pseudotumor cerebri. A complication of parenteral hyperalimentation. J.A.M.A., 235:2124, 1976.

78. Shafer, K., and Forlaw, L.: WRAMC Protocol, Walter Reed Army Medical Center Dept. of Nursing, Washington, D.C., 1983.

79. Simmons, B.P.: CDC guidelines for the prevention and control of nosocomial infections—guideline for prevention of intravascular infections. Am. J. Infect. Control, 11:183, 1983.

80. Singh, A.K., Dykvizan, D.L., and Vargas, L.L.: Acute superior vena cava obstruction with intravenous thrombosis: a complication of central venous catheterization. Cardiovasc. Dis., 6:308, 1979.

81. Stone, H.H., Kolb, L.D., Currie, C.A., Geheber, C.E., and Cuzzell, J.Z.: *Candida* sepsis; pathogenesis and principles of treatment. Ann. Surg., 179:697, 1974.

82. Tanner, W.A., Delaney, P.V., and Hennessy, T.P.: The influence of heparin on intravenous infusions: a prospective study. Br. J. Surg., 67:311, 1980.

83. Tse, R.L., and Lee, M.W.: pH of infusion fluids; a predisposing factor in thrombophlebitis. J.A.M.A., 215:642, 1971.

84. Valerie, D., Hussey, J.K., and Smith, F.W.: Central vein thrombosis associated with subclavian catheterization for intravenous feeding. Proceedings of the 2nd European Congress of Parenteral and Enteral Nutrition. PJ4:72, 1980.

85. Welch, G.W., McKeel, D.W., Silverstein, P., et al.: The role of catheter composition in the development of thrombophlebitis. Surg. Gynecol. Obstet., 138:421, 1974.

86. Wilmore, D.W., and Dudrick, S.J.: Safe long-term venous catheterization. Arch. Surg., 98:256, 1969.

87. Wilmore, D.W., Groff, D.B., Bishop, H.C., et al.: Total parenteral nutrition in infants with catastrophic gastrointestinal anomalies. J. Pediatr. Surg., 4:181, 1969.

88. Winters, V.: Implantable vascular access devices. Oncology Nursing Forum 11:25 1984.

CHAPTER 17

Potential Complications and Monitoring of Patients Receiving Total Parenteral Nutrition

SAMUEL D. ANG
JOHN M. DALY

COMPLICATIONS AND MONITORING

The use of total parenteral nutrition (TPN) to replenish malnourished individuals and support hospitalized patients who are unable to eat has gained widespread acceptance since its development in 1967. Advances in technology, standardized methods of catheter placement, increased understanding of substrate metabolism, and improved patient monitoring have reduced morbidity associated with parenteral nutritional support. Complications of TPN may occur, however, and may be divided into three areas: mechanical, metabolic, and infectious. In this chapter, potential mechanical and metabolic complications are outlined; infectious complications are discussed in the chapter on catheter care.

Mechanical Complications

The incidence of complications accompanying percutaneous insertion of subclavian vein catheters has ranged from 4.2 to 12.5 per cent.[1-3] In a review of the English language literature, Grant[1] noted 430 complications in 10,130 subclavian vein catheterizations. Increased operator experience and improved catheterization techniques play an important role in diminishing the number of complications associated with percutaneous catheter placement.[4, 5] Other factors related to morbidity include the indications for and circumstances requiring central vein catheterization. In a prospective series evaluating central venous catheter insertion, Bernard and Stahle found that emergency percutaneous subclavian vein catheterization was performed in 2.5 per cent of all patients with central venous catheters, but it resulted in 44 per cent of the technical complications.[4] Cannulation complications are minimized by meticulous attention to neurovascular, clavicular, and chest wall anatomic relationships. Common complications include pneumothorax; hemothorax; pneumohemothorax; hemomediastinum; subclavian artery, brachial plexus, and thoracic duct injuries; air embolism; catheter embolization; cardiac arrhythmias; subclavian vein thrombosis; and improper catheter tip placement. Early recognition is the key to successful management of any complication.

Pneumothorax

Pneumothorax, the most frequent complication associated with subclavian vein catheterization, occurs when the needle tip penetrates or lacerates the pleura or the apex of the lung.[1] Pneumothorax occurs most frequently in emergency situations; in thin, malnourished patients; and in situations in which an inadequate Trendelenburg position does not allow the subclavian vein to fill maximally. Following this complication, the

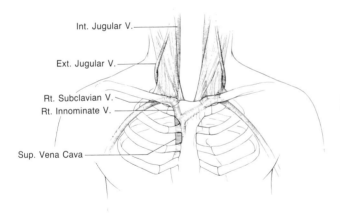

Figure 17–1. The subclavian vein courses medially, joining the internal juglar vein to form the innominate vein. It is usually located at the medial one-half or one-third mark on the clavicle.

patient usually complains of the sudden onset of sharp, lancinating pain around the area in which the needle was inserted. Coughing occurs secondary to pleural irritation. In most cases the air leak is self-limiting, and the patient's symptoms improve. However, if the patient complains of progressive dyspnea or severe chest pains, develops cyanosis, or becomes hypotensive, the diagnosis of tension pneumothorax should be suspected and confirmed clinically. Catheterization attempts should be abandoned, and an ipsilateral tube thoracostomy should be performed without delay. If symptoms occur but do not progress, the catherization procedure should be halted temporarily, and a chest roentgenogram should be obtained to confirm the diagnosis. Most asymptomatic, small (<20 per cent) pneumothoraces resolve spontaneously over several days without further treatment. However, chest tube insertion and underwater seal drainage is indicated for prophylaxis in the preoperative patient who requires endotracheal intubation and positive pressure ventilation. If serial chest roentgenograms reveal a progressive increase in the size of the pneumothorax or if clinical symptoms develop, chest tube thoracostomy should be performed. The chest tube is connected to underwater seal drainage for several days until the air leak ceases, and then the tube is withdrawn. A chest roentgenogram should be obtained to confirm the absence of residual pleural air. A thorough understanding of the anatomy of the subclavian vein and costoclavicular space is essential in preventing this complication. The subclavian vein is situated in the costoclavicular-scalene triangle (Fig. 17–1). It overlies the dome of the pleura as it courses medially to join the internal jugular vein behind the sternoclavicular joint to form the innominate

vein. The subclavian vein overlies the apex of the lung (Fig. 17–2). Placing the patient in the Trendelenburg position before subclavian vein cannulation results in maximal distention of the vein. The needle should be advanced in a horizontal direction, with the tip of the needle as close to the clavicle as possible to minimize the occurrence of a pneumothorax.

Subclavian Artery Injury

Subclavian artery injury occurs when the advancing needle is directed lateral to the subclavian vein. Penetration of the subclavian artery is recognized by the return of pulsatile bright red blood into the syringe. As in pneumothorax, this complication is avoided by a thorough knowledge of the anatomic relationship between the subclavian artery and vein. The subclavian artery

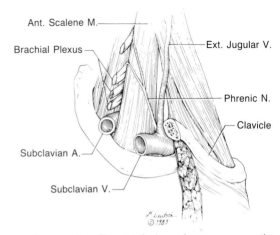

Figure 17–2. The subclavian vein courses over the first rib and overlies the dome of the pleura. It is separated from the subclavian artery by the anterior scalene muscle. The subclavian artery lies lateral and dorsal to the vein.

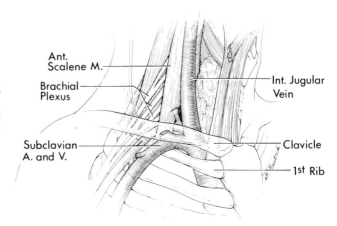

Figure 17–3. The brachial plexus, subclavian artery, and subclavian vein are intimately related. Knowledge of the anatomy of the subclavicular area is essential to avoid any technical complications during percutaneous central venous catheterization.

is dorsal and lateral to the vein and is separated from the subclavian vein medially by the anterior scalene muscle (Fig. 17–3). Once subclavian artery penetration is recognized, the needle should be withdrawn immediately, and local pressure should be applied for 10 minutes, both anteriorly and posteriorly to the clavicle at the point of arterial penetration. The patient should have frequent monitoring of vital signs and distal ipsilateral pulses for at least six hours. A chest roentgenogram should be obtained for evaluation of a widened mediastinum, which is an indication of arterial hemorrhage into the mediastinum.

Air Embolism

Air embolism occurs when the intrathoracic pressure becomes negative compared with the atmospheric pressure at the open needle during the subclavian catheter insertion,[6] while changing the intravenous tubing,[7] or during accidental separation of the tubing.[8] As much as 100 cc of air can enter a 14-gauge needle in one second.[9] Entry of 100 to 200 cc of air intravenously in a rapid fashion is fatal.[8-10] Aspiration of a small amount of air usually is asymptomatic. However, intravenous aspiration of a larger amount of air will cause sharp pain, dyspnea, cyanosis, tachycardia, elevated venous pressure manifested by distended neck veins, and hypotension. When the air embolus is located at the pulmonary outlet, a characteristic churning murmur may be heard over the precordium. Cardiac arrest may result from blockage of blood flow by the air embolus. Immediate recognition is crucial, since treatment requires immediate placement of the patient in a Trendelenburg and left lateral

decubitus position to limit intracardiac air to the right atrium. This also prevents intracardiac air from blocking the pulmonary outlet.[11, 12] The air embolus may then be aspirated through a central vein catheter that is inserted into the right atrium. Shires and O'Banion reported successful resuscitation of a patient with an air embolus using emergency thoracotomy and direct aspiration of the right ventricle.[13]

Intravenous air embolism is avoided by placing the patient in a Trendelenburg position and having the patient perform a Valsalva maneuver while disconnecting the needle and syringe and inserting the catheter through the needle and into the subclavian vein. All intravenous connections should be tightly taped to avoid accidental disconnection. Patients should be instructed about the dangers of intravenous line disconnection. In the event of an accidental disconnection, the patient should be instructed to put a finger on the open needle or catheter. Application of a bactericidal ointment and an occlusive dressing over the skin insertion site after the catheter has been removed can prevent intravenous air aspiration, since air embolism through a patent catheter-sinus tract has been reported.[14]

Catheter Embolization

When the catheter is pulled back through the needle during unsuccessful subclavian vein cannulation, a portion of the catheter inside the vein may be sheared off and embolized intravascularly.[2] The catheter tip can lodge any place from the subclavian vein to the pulmonary arterial system. Congenital heart anomalies may allow embolization of the catheter into the arterial system.[15]

Catheter embolization may cause cardiac arrhythmias. Burri and Krischak noted a 39.5 per cent mortality rate when the embolized catheter was left in either the heart or the lung.[2] The embolized catheter can be retrieved transvenously under fluoroscopy with a guide wire snare as described by Block.[16] To avoid this complication, the catheter should never be withdrawn through the needle during a difficult cannulation; both the needle and the catheter should be withdrawn simultaneously.

Venous Thrombosis

The reported incidence of great vein thrombosis varies. Burri and Krischak found 15 cases of clinical thrombosis in 1098 catheterizations, an incidence of 1.3 per cent.[2] Ryan and colleagues noted eight cases of clinically apparent venous thrombosis in 200 patients, an incidence of four per cent.[3] Padberg and associates found an incidence of 8.7 per cent.[17] However, a recent review by Grant noted only 36 cases of clinically diagnosed venous thrombosis in 10,130 catheterizations, an incidence of 0.3 per cent.[1] Great vein thrombosis probably occurs more frequently than is clinically recognized by ipsilateral arm and neck swelling.[6, 18] A fibrin sheath caused by irritation to the intima often originates at the point of catheter penetration. This fibrin sheath, which forms around the catheter, usually precedes the formation of thrombus.[19] Catheter composition influences thrombus formation. Silastic catheters are less thrombogenic than are polyethylene or polyvinylchloride catheters.[20, 21] The patient's clinical disease or general condition influences the likelihood of great vein thrombosis. Hypercoagulable states, sepsis, prolonged bed rest, venous stasis, dehydration, and the presence of certain malignancies predispose to this complication.

Great vein thrombosis is usually asymptomatic when the thrombi are small and there is minimal venous occlusion.[22] The first sign of subclavian vein thrombosis may be the inability to recannulate the affected vein. When thrombosis extends to the internal jugular vein, the patient may exhibit the symptoms of pseudotumor cerebri, such as persistent headaches, diplopia, papilledema, and sixth nerve palsy.[23] Other clinical signs include distention of neck veins and swelling of the ipsilateral arm and face. In burn patients, subclavian vein thrombosis may pro-

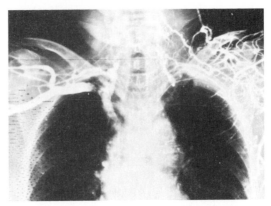

Figure 17–4. Thrombosis of the left subclavian vein with resultant opening of collateral venous channels.

gress to septic thrombophlebitis.[24] If unrecognized, this complication is often fatal.[25]

Definitive diagnosis of venous thrombosis is made with venous flow studies using radioisotopes or contrast materials (Fig. 17–4). Treatment of clinically apparent subclavian vein thrombosis includes immediate removal of the catheter and institution of intravenous heparin therapy. Heparin is continued for 7 to 10 days until the arm or neck swelling subsides. In cases of suspected septic thrombophlebitis, an appropriate antibiotic should be started after the catheter is removed, and the catheter tip should be cultured and blood drawn for culture and sensitivity testing. Great vein thrombosis can be minimized by using less-thrombogenic silicone catheters[20, 21] or by adding heparin to the nutrient solutions.[17, 22] In a prospective, randomized study using radionuclide venography, Fabri and coworkers found an 8 per cent incidence of subclavian vein thrombosis in a group of patients receiving 3000 U of heparin/L of solution, compared with an incidence of 32 per cent in the control group of patients who did not receive heparin.[22] Administration of heparin did not result in a change of the coagulation parameters. Padberg and colleagues[17] routinely add 6000 U of heparin/day to their TPN solutions and found a reduced incidence of central vein thrombosis.

Catheter Tip Misplacement

The catheter tip should normally be situated in the midportion of the superior vena cava. However, catheter tip misdirection is a fairly common complication that is recognized radiographically. One report cited an incidence of 11.5 per cent.[7] The tip of the catheter may enter the internal jugular vein, the opposite subclavian vein, or any abnormal venous channel.[26] This complication can be prevented by directing the bevel of the needle caudally while inserting the catheter through it. The catheter should be redirected into the superior vena cava using a guide wire. Frequently, fluoroscopy may be required for successful repositioning. Aberrant catheter tips in the atrium or ventricle can cause heart perforation and tamponade.[27-30] Cardiac arrhythmias can be triggered when the catheter tip is located near an irritable locus in the atrium.[31]

Perforation of the great veins is an infrequent complication.[32] It occurs by direct penetration during catheter insertion or through gradual erosion of the vessel wall.[32] It usually results in hemothorax and hemomediastinum[33] or hydrothorax.[34-36] Perforation during catheterization is diagnosed when a free flow of blood cannot be obtained. The needle and catheter should be removed immediately, and the patient should be monitored closely for signs of respiratory distress. Delayed perforation through vessel erosion is more difficult to diagnose. Patients often complain of chest pain or difficulty in breathing. Chest roentgenograms may reveal hydrothorax or an abnormally widened mediastinum. Treatment consists of removing the catheter and close observation of the patient.

Technical complications associated with central venous catheterization can be minimized by adhering to established cannulation techniques and thoroughly understanding the anatomy of the costoclavicular-subclavian area. With careful methodology, complication rates in severely malnourished and immunologically compromised patients can be minimized.[37]

Metabolic Complications

During the early years of TPN administration, many metabolic complications were related to the infusion of inadequate or excessive amounts of substrates, vitamins, and minerals.[38] During the last decade, increased knowledge of the metabolism of substrates, electrolytes, vitamins, and trace minerals have defined requirements for patients with various disease states, and improved patient monitoring has reduced the occurrence

of metabolic complications. Consequently, these complications are now reported with less frequency.

Glucose Metabolism

Blood glucose concentration depends upon glucose supply, utilization, and excretion. A healthy 70-kg man utilizes 0.4 to 1.2 gm/kg/hour of glucose, depending on his age and metabolic state. Utilization of glucose is maximal in infants and decreases with advancing age. Disease states such as diabetes mellitus, sepsis, shock, elective operations, or major trauma usually decrease glucose utilization, which is mediated principally by insulin and glucagon in the presence of glucocorticoids and catecholamines. A healthy adult responds to a carbohydrate intake of up to 500 gm a day by increasing endogenous insulin production to four to six times the basal level within six hours.[39, 40] By slowly increasing the amount of infused glucose, up to 1500 gm of glucose can be infused/day without abnormalities in blood or urine glucose levels. Thus, normal pancreatic beta cells have a large capacity to increase insulin production.[41]

Hyperglycemic, Hyperosmolar, Nonketotic Coma. The syndrome of hyperglycemic, hyperosmolar, nonketotic coma (HHNC) was a commonly reported complication during the development of TPN support.[38, 42-44] Mortality rates of up to 50 per cent were reported.[44, 45] With improved understanding and closer monitoring of glucose metabolism in patients receiving TPN, this problem has become less frequent. HHNC coma develops because of dehydration resulting from osmotic diuresis. Abnormal neurologic symptoms include disorientation, lethargy, stupor, and convulsions, which lead to coma and death.[46] Blood glucose levels greater than 1000 mg per dl are common with serum osmolarities greater than 350 MOsm/L.

Careful monitoring of blood and urinary glucose levels in patients receiving TPN will prevent this complication. In the event a patient develops HHNC, the TPN solution should be discontinued immediately. Hypoosmolar solutions in the form of 0.45 per cent normal saline should be administered initially at 250 ml/hour. Regular insulin is added to the intravenous fluid and is given at a rate of 10 to 20 U/hour, depending upon the severity of hyperglycemia and clinical symptomatology. Metabolic acidosis is corrected with intravenous infusion of sodium bicarbonate according to the following formula:

$$\text{mEq HCO}_3^- = \text{Body weight (kg)} \times (24 - \text{plasma HCO}_3^-) \times 0.6$$

One half of the calculated requirement for $NaHCO_3$ is given rapidly, and the remainder is infused over the following six hours. Arterial blood pH, Po_2, and Pco_2 are monitored every six hours until the pH normalizes. Similarly, serum osmolarity is monitored closely either by direct measurement or by calculation from the following formula:

$$\text{Serum osmolarity} = (Na^+ + K^+) + \text{blood sugar}/18 + \text{BUN}/2.8$$

The patient's clinical sensorium, vital signs, urine output, serum glucose and electrolyte levels, and arterial blood pH, Po_2 and Pco_2 are monitored hourly until the condition stabilizes. Care should be taken to lower the blood sugar level slowly to avoid the danger of cerebral edema resulting from rapid influx of water from the relatively hypotonic plasma into the hypertonic cerebrospinal fluid.

Hypoglycemia. Sudden cessation of the infusion of hypertonic dextrose–amino acid solutions in patients unable to ingest food is sometimes followed by a rapid drop in serum glucose levels to below normal within 30 minutes.[38, 39, 47] Patients may experience headaches, sweating, thirst, disorientation, paresthesias, convulsions, and eventual coma. As in other medical emergencies, rapid recognition and immediate treatment are crucial. Treatment consists of the bolus infusion of a 50 per cent dextrose solution intravenously until the abnormal symptoms or signs disappear. Hypertonic dextrose TPN solutions should be tapered slowly before discontinuation. The infusion rate is initially decreased to one half the usual rate for 12 hours. The solution is then switched to five per cent dextrose in water at 50 to 100 ml/hour for the next 12 hours before complete cessation and removal of the subclavian catheter. When the TPN solution has to be discontinued abruptly because of an emergency, 10 per cent dextrose in water should be administered to maintain normoglycemia. More rapid infusion tapering methods done over several hours have been used for patients who received cyclic hyperalimentation and usually result in no adverse sequelae.

Carbon Dioxide Retention. Infusion of calories in excess of energy requirements may be harmful. Recently, Askanazi and colleagues reported the development of respiratory distress due to increased CO_2 production during infusion with glucose-based TPN in a septic patient.[48] They noted that CO_2 production increased by 20 per cent, and minute ventilation rose an average of 26 per cent in patients who received only glucose as nonprotein calories compared with patients who received calories as a combined glucose-lipid mixture.[49] Subsequent reports confirmed the association of excessive glucose infusion rates with increased basal energy expenditure, O_2 consumption, CO_2 production, alveolar ventilation, minute ventilation, and respiratory quotient.[50-52] The degree of elevation of those determinants, however, was dependent on the patient's metabolic state. Askanazi found that the respiratory quotient was elevated in malnourished patients receiving excess glucose calories to greater than 1. This increase in respiratory quotient was not seen in hypermetabolic patients because increased CO_2 production from excess glucose was accompanied by increased energy expenditure and O_2 consumption. Hypermetabolic patients continued to mobilize and oxidize endogenous fat even when all their calories were supplied as glucose, suggesting obligatory fat oxidation.[53, 54] The increased CO_2 production in malnourished hypermetabolic groups stimulated a compensatory increase in minute ventilation. Consequently, the risk of developing CO_2 production is very high in patients with impaired pulmonary function.[51] This problem may first become manifest when attempting to wean patients with chronic obstructive pulmonary disease.[48]

Treatment of CO_2 retention should include tapering the glucose-based TPN and replacing a portion (40 to 50 per cent) of the glucose with an isocaloric fat infusion. In patients with significant obstructive or restrictive lung disease, TPN should be administered using isocaloric amounts of dextrose and fat emulsions given simultaneously.

Protein Metabolism

Abnormalities of protein metabolism, such as azotemia, hyperammonemia, and hyperchloremic metabolic acidosis, occurred more frequently during the early development and clinical use of TPN. Prerenal azotemia results when excessive amounts of protein hydrolysates or amino acids are infused,[38, 55] and is aggravated by underlying dehydration. Providing insufficient nonprotein calories results in the infused amino acids being used to meet immediate energy needs rather than for protein synthesis.[56] Patients usually present with laboratory signs of dehydration and an elevation of serum blood urea nitrogen. If the condition is not corrected, the patient may develop progressive lethargy and perhaps coma.[38] Close monitoring of bodyweight, fluid balance, and serum blood urea nitrogen prevents this complication.

A closely related problem is hyperammonemia, which occurs when casein or fibrin hydrolysates are infused, since these solutions contain up to 40,000 μg of free ammonia/dl.[57, 58, 75] With the advent of crystalline amino acid solutions, in which free ammonia is absent, this problem has become much less prevalent. Although Heird and colleagues reported hyperammonemia in pediatric patients receiving crystalline amino acids, this complication was probably related to deficiency of arginine, which is an important substrate in the Krebs-urea cycle, in which ammonia is converted to urea.[59] Clinical manifestations of hyperammonemia include progressive lethargy and malaise, coma, and grand mal seizures. Treatment is again preventive. In infants receiving TPN, serum ammonia levels should be closely monitored. Heird treated hyperammonemia in pediatric patients by administering 2 to 3 mol/kg/day of arginine; he reported successful prevention of this complication with daily administration of 0.5 to 1.0 mol/kg/day of arginine.[59]

Acid-base disturbances are potentially dangerous in patients receiving TPN. Earlier protein hydrolysates often resulted in metabolic acidosis because of the acidic nature of these solutions.[60] Hyperchloremic metabolic acidosis also occurred with infusion of the first-generation crystalline amino acid solutions because chloride ions were released as the amino acids were utilized.[59] Excess chloride ions are reabsorbed with sodium in the renal tubules, and fewer hydrogen ions are secreted in exchange for sodium, thus producing metabolic acidosis. Infusion of large amounts of acidic amino acids such as arginine, histidine and lysine may cause acidosis because they release hydrogen ions when metabolized.[61] Hyperchloremic metabolic acidosis may be prevented by administering sodium and potassium as acetate, lactate, or phosphate salts.[62]

Fat Metabolism

Patients maintained on hypertonic glucose and amino acids without supplemental fat for three to six weeks will eventually develop essential fatty acid deficiency (EFAD).[63-65] Goodgame and colleagues found that patients receiving TPN without fat supplementation developed serum biochemical evidence of EFAD in four weeks.[66] Similar findings were reported by Wine and coworkers.[67] The three polyunsaturated fatty acids (linoleic, arachidonic, linolenic) cannot be synthesized by humans and thus are classified as essential fatty acids. However, it has been found that arachidonic acid can be synthesized in vivo when sufficient linoleic acid is present.[68-70] Essential fatty acids are important in maintaining membrane structure and transport processes in the cell because they make up the majority of cholesterol esters and phospholipids in the body.[71, 72] The metabolic consequences of EFAD include a decrease in high-energy phosphate bonds and a diminished efficiency of caloric utilization.[73, 74] Clinically, patients manifest scaliness and dryness of the skin, coarsening and loss of hair, impaired wound healing, hepatomegaly, and bone changes.[75-79] Freund and colleagues reported increased intraocular pressure as a result of prostaglandin deficiency.[80] EFAD is diagnosed by its characteristic serum biochemical changes. Low serum levels of linoleic and arachidonic acids occur with elevated serum levels of 5,8,11,14-eicosatetraenoic acid, and an increase in the serum triene/tetraene ratio, which is normally 0.4.[68-70] Other abnormal laboratory findings include elevated serum liver function tests, increased red blood cell fragility, anemia, thrombocytopenia, and decreased levels of serum prostaglandin.[65] EFAD is prevented by administering fat emulsions (500 ml of a 10 per cent solution) to patients on TPN at least twice weekly.[66] Intravenous requirements of linolenic acid are estimated at 25 to 100 mg/kg/day in an adult.[75-77]

Hypophosphatemia

Phosphate is used intracellularly for the synthesis of adenosine triphosphate (ATP), DNA, and membrane phospholipids. The need for phosphate increases in a malnourished patient receiving TPN because of the heightened utilization of phosphate for glucose metabolism and protein synthesis.[81, 82] The intracellular transfer of glucose and phosphorus is mediated by insulin, and the predominant sites of phosphate incorporation are the liver and skeletal muscles. About 1 to 2 mol of phosphate are incorporated/gram of nitrogen synthesized. Hill and colleagues studied phosphorus utilization in starved rats using radiolabeled phosphorus and found that there was a rapid incorporation of phosphorus into muscle tissues after a period of catabolism.[82]

Hypophosphatemia may be caused by alkalosis.[83] Alkalosis stimulates glycolysis and phosphorylation of carbohydrates intracellularly, which may increase intracellular transport of phosphate. Gram-negative septicemia may result in hypophosphatemia due to hyperventilation and respiratory alkalosis.[84, 85] Persistent vomiting and malabsorption alcoholism and liver failure may result in hypophosphatemia, either by increased loss or decreased intake of phosphate.[86-89] Medical conditions such as vitamin D deficiency, hyperparathyroidism, and Fanconi's syndrome may cause phosphorus depletion by increasing renal phosphate clearance. Iatrogenic causes of hypophosphatemia include administration of phosphate-binding antacids such as magnesium or aluminum hydroxide and administration of phosphate-poor TPN solutions to malnourished patients.[90, 91]

Clinical signs and symptoms of hypophosphatemia usually appear when serum inorganic phosphate concentrations fall below 1 mg/dl.[38, 91, 93] Patients may become progressively lethargic and develop anorexia, muscle weakness, paresthesias, and long bone pain. If hypophosphatemia is not corrected, the patient's mental status will deteriorate, resulting in coma.[89, 91, 93, 94] The metabolic consequences of hypophosphatemia are severe and include a shift of the oxyhemoglobin dissociation curve, with increased affinity of oxygen to hemoglobin; depletion of red blood cell and platelet ATP, with resultant shortened survival of red blood cells and platelets; impaired white blood cell chemotaxis and phagocytosis, leading to increased susceptibility to infection, and finally, depression of myocardial function.[92, 95-101] Hypophosphatemia is generally an iatrogenic condition. Phosphate requirements are

dictated by the degree of malnutrition before TPN is initiated, the presence of predisposing medical conditions, and the amount of glucose calories in the solutions being administered. In general, 20 mEq PO_4 is required for each 1000 calories of TPN solution administered.[102-104]

Abnormalities of Liver Function

Patients who are maintained on TPN from one to three weeks often develop abnormalities in serum liver function tests.[105-110] Serum glutamic-oxaloacetic transaminase (SGOT), serum glutamic-pyruvate transaminase (SGPT), serum alkaline phosphatase, and rarely, serum bilirubin levels become elevated during the course of TPN administration and usually return to normal spontaneously when the infusion is stopped. In a long-term clinical study by Wagman and associates, 143 patients receiving glucose-based TPN were followed for up to seven weeks. Serum transaminase levels became elevated during the first one to two weeks and then plateaued. Serum alkaline phosphatase levels generally rose progressively, whereas total bilirubin, direct bilirubin, and serum lactate dehydrogenase (LDH) levels did not rise significantly.[111] MacFadyen and colleagues reported persistent elevations of serum bilirubin and alkaline phosphatase levels in 15 patients who had initially abnormal levels of serum bilirubin, SGPT, SGOT, and alkaline phosphatase and who received TPN.[112] The etiology of changes in serum liver function tests remains obscure. Almost all components of the nutrient solution have been implicated as the cause of hepatic dysfunction. The rate of glucose infusion is most frequently cited as causing hepatic fatty infiltration.[107, 108, 110, 113-117] Lowry and Brennan noted that patients receiving glucose calories in excess of their basal energy requirement invariably developed abnormal serum liver function tests.[117] Similar findings were reported in pediatric patients.[118-123] It has been suggested that infusion of an imbalanced amino acid solution or a solution lacking in all essential amino acids causes abnormal bile salt formation and flow and the development of hepatic dysfunction.[105, 107, 124] Grant and colleagues postulated that tryptophan degradation products in nutrient solutions were responsible for the hepatic dysfunction.[105] EFAD has been reported as a possible cause of hepatic dysfunction, since the infusion of fat emulsions corrected the serum abnormalities.[125-127] Conversely, the administration of fat calories in excess of glucose calories has also been reported to cause abnormalities in serum liver enzyme levels.[128] Liver dysfunction is therefore probably influenced by a variety of factors. Histologic findings include fatty infiltration of the hepatic parenchyma, glycogen deposition, intrahepatic cholestasis, bile duct proliferation, and bile plugs.[107] The clinical course of patients receiving TPN with elevated serum liver enzymes is usually benign. Serum transaminases may rise after one week of TPN administration, whereas serum bilirubin and LDH levels generally remain within the normal range. Any elevation of serum bilirubin and LDH should alert the clinician to look for another cause. In summary, almost all components of the nutrient solutions have been implicated in liver dysfunction in patients receiving TPN. Patients should be administered balanced TPN solutions according to their caloric requirements. Serum liver enzyme levels should be monitored at least once a week during TPN administration.

Magnesium Abnormalities

Magnesium plays an important role in cellular metabolism and oxidative phosphorylation.[129, 130] It is the metalloenzyme of ATP and is active in the transfer of phosphate radicals to and from ATP. Magnesium reduces cardiac irritability and is involved in the maintenance of structural integrity of DNA and RNA.[131] Of the approximately 2000 mEq of magnesium in the body, 60 per cent is situated in the bone, and the remainder is in the soft tissues, primarily the liver and muscles.[132] Normal plasma magnesium concentration ranges from 1.4 to 2.2 mEq/L. It is absorbed primarily in the small intestine with dietary excesses being excreted in the urine and feces.

Hypomagnesemia occurs in a variety of gastrointestinal disorders, especially the malabsorption syndrome,[133] massive small bowel resection,[134] intestinal fistulae[135] and acute pancreatitis.[136] It is also noted in patients on prolonged nasogastric suction.[137] Renal diseases such as glomerulonephritis, renal tubular necrosis, nephrosclerosis, pyelonephritis, and hydronephrosis may cause hypomagnesemia because of renal loss of magnesium.[138] In patients receiving TPN, the requirements for magnesium are increased because of new tissue synthesis. About 0.5 mEq of magnesium is required for 1 gm of nitrogen utilized for protein synthesis.[1] Clinical symptoms due to hypomagnesemia develop when the serum concentration falls below 1 mEq/L.[130] Patients may manifest muscle weakness, depression, apathy, nausea, vomiting, and irritability bordering on psychosis.[139] Clinical signs include a positive Trousseau's sign, muscle tremors and fasciculations, hyporeflexia, ataxia, and vertigo.[139] In severe cases, convulsions may occur. The clinical signs and symptoms of hypomagnesemia are similar to those of hypocalcemia; thus, serum levels of both ions should be measured to distinguish between the two conditions. In the presence of convulsions, treatment consists of slowly infusing 10 per cent magnesium sulfate intravenously or intramuscularly.[140] Magnesium deficiency is prevented by supplying at least 0.35 to 0.45 mEq/kg/day in patients receiving TPN.[139] In the patient with impaired renal function, as suggested by a creatinine clearance of less than 30 ml/minute, hypermagnesemia should be avoided.[141] Hypermagnesemia is manifested by increasing drowsiness, weakness, nausea, vomiting, cardiac arrhythmias, and if severe, hypotension, coma, and cardiac arrest. Serum levels of greater than 3 mEq/L result in adverse clinical symptoms. A level of 25 mEq/L is fatal.[141] Treatment of hypermagnesemia includes peritoneal dialysis or hemodialysis. Intravenous infusion of calcium gluconate may temporarily relieve the adverse effects. This condition is best prevented by monitoring serum magnesium levels once weekly. In patients with impaired renal function, serum magnesium levels should be monitored at least twice weekly.

Monitoring

Monitoring of patients on TPN should include accurate measurement of the patient's temperature, pulse rate, respiratory rate, and blood pressure every eight hours; urine sugar and acetone levels every six hours; fluid balance every eight hours; and daily bodyweights. Serum electrolytes, blood urea nitrogen, and glucose levels are determined daily until the serum levels stabilize within normal ranges, and then every two to three days thereafter. Weekly measurements of serum calcium, phosphorus, magnesium, albumin, total bilirubin, direct bilirubin,

SGOT, SGPT, and alkaline phosphatase should be done to ensure adequate mineral replacement and monitoring of liver function.

Blood and urine glucose levels should be measured regularly to avoid osmotic diuresis and the potential for development of non-ketotic hyperglycemic coma. The nutrient solution should be maintained at a rate that will not allow the blood glucose level to exceed 200 mg/dl or the urinary glucose level to exceed 2 gm/dl (equivalent to 3+ nitroprusside reaction). Insulin can be administered in the same container if indicated. Occasionally, the rate of TPN infusion will have to be decreased for several days to allow better control of blood sugar. The persistence of hyperglycemia despite these precautions may indicate impending or underlying sepsis. This should be vigorously searched for and treated.

SUMMARY

A knowledge of potential complications associated with the administration of TPN can reduce their frequency. The development of multidisciplinary nutritional support teams—qualified individuals who follow established techniques, remain alert to potential complications, and intervene quickly to minimize the morbidity associated with complications—has made TPN a safe and effective adjunct in clinical management. These potential complications are largely avoided by adhering to basic metabolic principles of nutrient administration and anatomic details of catheter insertion as well as precise monitoring of the patient's response to TPN infusions.

REFERENCES

1. Grant, J.P.: Subclavian catheter insertion and complications. In Grant, J.P.: Handbook of Total Parenteral Nutrition. Chapter 4. Philadelphia, W.B. Saunders Co., 1980.
2. Burri, C., and Krischak, G.: Techniques and complications of administration of total parenteral nutrition. In Manni, C., Magalini, S.I., and Sorascia, E. (eds.): Total Parenteral Nutrition. New York, American Elsevier Scientific Publishing Co., 1976, pages 306–315.
3. Ryan, J.A., Jr., Abel, R.M., Abbott, W.H., Hopkins, C.C., Chesney, T. McC., Colley, R., Phillips, K., and Fischer, J.E.: Catheter complications in total parenteral nutrition. A prospective study of 200 consecutive patients. N. Engl. J. Med., 290:757, 1974.
4. Bernard, R.W., and Stahle, W.M.: Subclavian vein catheterization: A prospective study. Ann. Surg., 173:184, 1971.
5. Wilson, J.N., Grow, J.B., Demong, C.V., Prevedel, A.E., and Owens, J.C.: Central venous pressure in optimal blood volume replacement. Arch. Surg., 85:55, 1962.
6. Johnson, C.L., Lazarchick, J., and Lynn, H.B.: Subclavian venipuncture: Preventable complications; reports of 2 cases. Mayo Clin. Proc., 45:712, 1970.
7. Green, H.L., and Nemir, P., Jr.: Air embolism as a complication during parenteral alimentation. Am. J. Surg., 121:614, 1971.
8. Ordway, C.B.: Air embolus via CVP catheter without positive pressure: Presentation of case and review. Ann. Surg., 179:479, 1974.
9. Flanagan, J.P., Gradisar, I.A., Gross, R.J., and Kelly, T.R.: Air embolus—a lethal complication of subclavian venipuncture. N. Engl. J. Med., 281:488, 1969.
10. Yeakel, A.E.: Lethal air embolism from plastic blood storage container. J.A.M.A., 204:267, 1969.
11. Oppenheimer, M.J., Durant, T.M., and Lymes, P.: Body position in relation to venous air embolism and the associated cardiovascular respiratory changes. Am. J. Med. Sci., 225:362, 1953.
12. Durant, I.M., Long, J., and Oppenheimer, M.J.: Pulmonary (venous) air embolism. Am. Heart J., 33:269, 1947.
13. Shires, T., and O'Banion, J.: Successful treatment of massive air embolism producing cardiac arrest. J.A.M.A., 167:1483, 1958.
14. Paskin, D.L., Hoffman, W.S., and Tuddenham, W.J.: A new complication of subclavian vein catheterization. Ann. Surg., 179:266, 1974.
15. Nash, G., and Moylan, J.S.: Paradoxical catheter embolism. Arch. Surg., 102:213, 1971.
16. Block, P.C.: Transvenous retrieval of foreign bodies in the cardiac circulation. J.A.M.A., 224:241, 1973.
17. Padberg, F.T., Ruggiero, J., Blackburn, G.L., et al.: Central venous catheterization for parenteral nutrition. Ann. Surg., 193:264, 1981.
18. McDonough, J.J., and Altemeier, W.A.: Subclavian venous thrombosis secondary to indwelling catheters. Surg. Gynecol. Obstet., 136:71, 1973.
19. Hashal, V.L., Jr., Ause, RG., and Hoskins, P.A.: Fibrin sleeve formation on indwelling subclavian central venous catheters. Arch. Surg., 102:353, 1971.
20. Welch, G.W., McKell, D.W., Silverstein, P., and Walker, H.L.: The role of catheter composition in the development of thrombophlebitis. Surg. Gynecol. Obstet., 138:426, 1974.
21. McLean, A.H., Griffith, C.D.M., Anderson, J.R., and Grieve, D.C.: Thromboembolic complications with silicone elastomer subclavian catheters. J.P.E.N., 6(1):61, 1982.
22. Fabri, P.J., Mirtallo, J.M., Ruberg, R.L., Dudsk, K.A., Denning, D.A., Ellison, E.C., and Schaffer, P.S.: Incidence and prevention of thrombosis of the subclavian vein during total parenteral nutrition. Surg. Gynecol. Obstet. 115:238, 1982.
23. Saxena, V.K., Halpern, R.J., and Murphy, S.F.: Pseudotumor cerebri; a complication of parenteral hyperalimentation. J.A.M.A., 235:2124, 1976.
24. Pruitt, B.A., Stein, J.M., Foley, F.D., Moncrief, J.A., and O'Neill, J.A.: Intravenous therapy in burn patients—suppurative thrombophlebitis

and other life threatening complications. Arch. Surg., *100*:399, 1970.

25. Stein, J.M., and Pruitt, B.A.: Suppurative thrombophlebitis: A lethal iatrogenic disease. N. Engl. J. Med., *282*:1452, 1970.

26. O'Reilly, R.J.: Aberrant venous catheter position within the left chest. Contemp. Surg., *12*:29, 1978.

27. Brown, C.A., and Kent, A.: Perforation of right ventricle by polyethylene catheter. South. Med. J., *49*:466, 1956.

28. Friedman, B.A., and Jurgeleit, H.C.: Perforation of atrium by polyethylene CV catheter. J.A.M.A., *203*:1141, 1968.

29. Defalque, R.J., and Campbell, C.: Cardiac tamponade from central venous catheters. Anesthesiology, *50*:249, 1979.

30. Johnson, C.E.: Perforation of right atrium by a polyethylene catheter. J.A.M.A., *195*:584, 1966.

31. Brody, R.E., and Weinberg, P.M.: Atrioventricular conduction disturbance during total parenteral nutrition. J. Pediatr., *88*:113, 1976.

32. Jekson, P.J., and Rempe, L.E.: Perforation of intrathoracic great veins by parenteral nutrition catheters. J.P.E.N., *6*:528, 1982.

33. Bernard, R.W., and Stahl, W.M.: Mediastinal hematoma. N.Y. State J. Med., *1*:83, 1974.

34. Spriggs, D.W., and Brantley, R.E.: Thoracic and abdominal extravasation: A complication of hyperalimentation in infants. Am. J. Roentgenol., *128*:419, 1977.

35. Carvell, J.E., and Pearce, D.J.: Bilateral hydrothorax following internal jugular catheterization. Br. J. Surg., *63*:381, 1976.

36. Reilly, J.J., Cosimi, A.B., and Russell, P.S.: Delayed perforation of the innominate vein during hyperalimentation. Arch. Surg., *112*:96, 1977.

37. Daly, J.M., Lawson, M., Speir, A., and Raaf, J.H.: Angioaccess in cancer patients. Curr. Probl. Cancer, *5*:1, 1981.

38. Dudrick, S.J., MacFadjen, B.V., VanBuren, C.T., Ruberg, R.L., and Maynard, A.T.: Parenteral hyperalimentation, metabolic problems and solutions. Ann. Surg., *176*:259, 1972.

39. Sanderson, I., and Deitel, M.: Insulin response in patients receiving concentrated infusions of glucose and casein hydrolysate for complete parenteral nutrition. Ann. Surg., *179*:387, 1974.

40. Genuth, S.: Insulin responses to intravenous alimentation. N. Engl. J. Med., *289*:107, 1973.

41. Porte, D., and Bagdale, J.D.: Human insulin secretion: An integrated approach. Ann. Rev. Med., *21*:219, 1970.

42. Sament, S., and Schwartz, S.: Severe diabetic stupor without ketosis. S. Afr. Med. J., *31*:893, 1957.

43. Rea, W.S., Wynick, W.J., McClelland, R.V., and Webb, W.R.: Intravenous hyperosmolar alimentation. Arch. Surg., *100*:393, 1970.

44. Wyrick, W.J., Rea, W.J., and McClelland, R.N.: Complications of hyperosmotic IV fluids. J.A.M.A., *211*:1697, 1970.

45. Flanigan, W.J., Thompson, B.W., Casali, R.E., and Caldwell, F.T.: The significance of hyperosmolar coma. Am. J. Surg., *120*:652, 1970.

46. Doromal, N.M., and Cauter, J.W.: Hyperosmolar hyperglycemia nonketotic coma complicating intravenous hyperalimentation. Surg. Gynecol. Obstet., *136*:729, 1973.

47. Kaplan, M.S., Mares, A., Quintana, P., Strauss, J., Huxtable, R.F., Brennan, P., and Hays, D.M.: High calories glucose-nitrogen infusions. Post-operative management of neonatal infants. Arch. Surg., *77*:567, 1969.

48. Askanazi, J., Elwyn, D.H., Silverberg, P.A., Rosenbaum, S.A., and Kinney, J.M.: Respiratory distress secondary to a high carbohydrate load: A case report. Surgery, *88*:596, 1980.

49. Askanazi, J., Nordenstrom, J., Rosenbaum, S.H., Elwyn, D.H., Hyman, A.I., Carpenter, Y.A., and Kinney, J.M.: Nutrition for patients with respiratory failure. Anesthesiology, *54*:373, 1981.

50. Covelli, H.D., Black, J.W., Olsen, M.S., and Beekman, J.F.: Respiratory failure precipitation by high carbohydrate loads. Ann. Intern. Med., *95*:579, 1981.

51. Askanazi, J., Rosenbaum, S.H., Hyman, A.I., Silverberg, P.A., Milic-Emili, J., and Kinney, J.M.: Respiratory changes induced by the large glucose loads of total parenteral nutrition. J.A.M.A., *243*(14):1444, 1980.

52. Askanazi, J., Carpentier, Y.A., Elwyn, D.H., Nordenstrom, J., Jeevanandam, M., Rosenbaum, S.H., Gump, F.E., and Kinney, J.M.: Influence of total parenteral nutrition on full utilization in injury and sepsis. Ann. Surg., *191*:40, 1980.

53. Carpentier, Y.A., Askanazi, J., Elwyn, D.H., Jeevanandam, M., Gump, F.E., Hyman, A. I., Burr, R., and Kinney, J.M.: Effects of hypercaloric glucose infusion on lipid metabolism in surgery and sepsis. J. Trauma, *19*:649, 1979.

54. Burke, J.F., Wolfe, R.R., Mullany, C.J., Mathews, D.E., and Beer, D.M.: Glucose requirements following burn injury. Parameters of optimal glucose infusion and possible hepatic and respiratory abnormalities following excessive glucose intake. Ann. Surg., *190*:274, 1979.

55. Ausman, R.K., Aust, J.B., and Friend, J.E.: Parenteral nutrition with a new amino acid solution. Acta Surg. Scand.(Suppl.), *466*:32, 1976.

56. Ausman, R.K., and Meng, H.C.: The effect on nitrogen balance and other parameters of varying doses of intravenous protein and calories. Acta Surg. Scand.(Suppl.), *466*:26, 1976.

57. Ghadimi, H., and Kumar, S.: High ammonia content of protein hydrolysates. Biochem. Med., *5*:548, 1971.

58. Walker, F.A.: Ammonia in fibrin hydrolysates. N. Engl. J. Med., *285*:1324, 1971.

59. Heird, W.C., Nicholson, J.F., Driscoll, J.R., Jr., Schullinger, J.N., and Winters, R.W.: Hyperammonia resulting from intravenous alimentation using a mixture of synthetic L-amino acids: A preliminary report. J. Pediatr., *81*:162, 1972.

60. Chan, J.C.M., Asch, M.J., Lin, S., and Hays, D.M.: Hyperalimentation with amino acid and casein hydrolysate solutions. Mechanism of acidosis. J.A.M.A., *220*:1700, 1972.

61. Heird, W.C., Dell, R.B., Driscoll, J.R., Jr., Grebin, B., and Winters, R.W.: Metabolic acidosis resulting from intravenous alimentation mixtures containing synthetic amino acids. N. Engl. J. Med., *287*:943, 1972.

62. Pitts, R.F.: Physiology of the Kidney and Body Fluids, Edition 2. Chicago, Year Book Medical Publishers, Inc., 1972, page 188.

63. Fleming, C.R., Smith, L.M., and Hodges, R.E.: Essential fatty acid deficiency in adults receiving total parenteral nutrition. Am. J. Clin. Nutr., *29*:976, 1976.

64. O'Neill, J.A., Caldwell, M.D., and Meng, H.C.: Essential fatty acid deficiency in surgical patients. Ann. Surg., *185*:535, 1977.

65. Paulsrud, J.R., Pensler, L., Whitten, C.F., Stewart, S., and Holman, R.T.: Essential fatty acid deficiency in infants induced by fat free intravenous feeding. Am. J. Clin. Nutr., 25:897, 1972.

66. Goodgame, J.T., Lowry, S.T., and Brennan, M.F.: Essential fatty acid deficiency in total parenteral nutrition: Time course of development and suggestions for therapy. Surgery, 84(2):271, 1978.

67. Wine, J.D., Connor, W.E., and denBesten, L.: The development of essential fatty acid deficiency in healthy men fed fat-free diets intravenously and orally. J. Clin. Invest., 56:127, 1975.

68. Richardson, T.J., and Sgoutas, O.: Essential fatty acid deficiency in four adult patients during total parenteral nutrition. Am. J. Clin. Nutr., 28:258, 1975.

69. Tashiro, T., Ogata, H., Yokoyama, H., Mashima, Y., and Iwasaki, I.: The effects of fat emulsions on essential fatty acid deficiency during intravenous hyperalimentation in pediatric patients. J. Pediatr. Surg., 10:203, 1975.

70. Riela, M.D., Broviac, J.W., Wells, M., and Scribner, B.H.: Essential fatty acid deficiency in human adults during total parenteral nutrition. Ann. Intern. Med., 83:786, 1975.

71. Sinclair, H.M.: Effects of deficiency of essential fatty acid deficiency in lower animals. In Sinclair, H.M. (ed.): Essential Fatty Acids. Fourth International Conference on Biochemical Problems of Lipids. Chapter 36. London, Butterworth & Co., 1958.

72. Lehninger, A.L.: The enzymatic and morphologic organization of the mitochondria. Pediatrics, 26:466, 1960.

73. Klein, P.D., and Johnson, R.M.: Phosphorus metabolism in unsaturated fatty acid deficient rats. J. Biol. Chem., 211:103, 1954.

74. Soderhjeem, L., Wiese, H.F., and Holman, R.T.: The role of polyunsaturated acids in human nutrition and metabolism. Prog. Chem. Fats Other Lipids, 9:555, 1970.

75. Holman, R.T.: The ratio of trienoic:tetraenoic acids in tissue lipids as a measure of essential fatty acid requirements. J. Nutr., 70:405,1960.

76. Hansen, A.Z., Haggard, M.E., Boelsche, A.N., Adams, D.J.D., and Wiese, H.F.: Essential fatty acids in infant nutrition III. Clinical manifestations of linoleic acid deficiency. J. Nutr., 66:565, 1958.

77. Caldwell, M.D., Jonsson, H.T., and Othersen, H.B., Jr.: Essential fatty acid deficiency in an infant receiving prolonged parenteral alimentation. J. Pediatr., 81:894, 1972.

78. Collins, F.D., Sinclair, A.J., Royle, J.P., Coats, D.A., Maynard, A.T., and Leonard, R.F.: Plasma lipids in human linoleic acid deficiency. Nutr. Metab., 13:150, 1971.

79. Heird, W.C., and Winters, R.W.: Total parenteral nutrition: The state of the art. J. Pediatr., 86:2, 1975.

80. Freund, H., Floman, N., Schwartz, B., and Fischer, J.E.: Essential fatty acid deficiency in total parenteral nutrition: Detection by changes in intraocular pressure. Ann. Surg., 190:139, 1979.

81. Groeir, J., Willebrands, A.F., Kamminga, C.E., et al.: Effects of glucose administration on the potassium and inorganic phosphate content of blood serum and the ECG in normal individuals and non-diabetic patients. Acta Med. Scand., 141:352, 1952.

82. Hill, G.L., Gunn, E.J., and Dudrick, S.J.: Phosphorus distribution in hyperalimentation induced hypophosphatemia. J. Surg. Res., 20:527, 1976.

83. Mastellar, M.E., and Tuttle, E.P.: The effects of alkalosis on plasma concentration and urinary excretion of inorganic phosphate in man. J. Clin. Invest., 43:138, 1964.

84. Okel, B.B., and Hurst, J.W.: Prolonged hyperventilation in man: Associated electrolyte changes and subjective symptoms. Arch. Intern. Med., 108:757, 1961.

85. Riedler, G.F., and Schertlin, W.A.: Hypophosphatemia in septicemia: Higher incidence in GN than GP infections. Br. Med. J., 1:753, 1969.

86. Betro, M.G., and Pain, R.W.: Hypophosphatemia and hyperphosphatemia in hospitalized population. Br. Med. J., 1:273, 1972.

87. Stein, J.H., Smith, W.O., and Ginn, H.E.: Hypophosphatemia in acute alcoholism. Am. J. Med. Sci., 252:78, 1966.

88. Roberts, K.E., Vanamee, P., Poppell, J.W., Rubin, A., Braverman, W., and Randall, H.T.: Electrolyte alteration in liver disease and hepatic coma. Med. Clin. North Am., 40:901, 1956.

89. Frank, B.W., and Kern, F., Jr.: Serum inorganic phosphorous during hepatic coma. Arch. Intern. Med., 110:865, 1962.

90. Bloom, W.L., and Flinchum, D.: Osteomalaria with pseudofractures caused by the ingestion of albumin hydroxide. J.A.M.A., 174:1327, 1960.

91. Bollens, P.A., Norwood, W., Kjellstrand, C., and Brown, D.M.: Hypophosphatemia with muscle weakness due to antacids and hemodialysis. Am. J. Dis. Child., 120:350, 1970.

92. Travis, S.F., Sugerman, J.H., Ruberg, R.L., Dudrick, S.J., Delivaria-Papadopoulous, M., Miller, L.D., and Oski, F.A.: Alterations of red cell glycolytic intermediates and oxygen transport as a consequence of hypophatemia in patients receiving intravenous hyperalimentation. N. Engl. J. Med., 285:763, 1971.

93. Silvis, S.E., and Paragas, P.D., Jr.: Paresthesias, weakness, seizures, and hypophosphatemia in patients receiving hyperalimentation. Gastroenterology, 62:513, 1972.

94. Lotz, M., Zisman, E., and Bartter, F.C.: Evidence for a phosphorus depletion syndrome in man. N. Engl. J. Med., 278:409, 1968.

95. Harken, A.H., and Woods, M.: The influence of oxyhemoglobin affinity on tissue oxygen consumption. Ann. Surg., 183:130, 1976.

96. Lichtman, M.A., Miller, D.R., Cohen, J., and Waterhouse, C.: Reduced red cell glycolysis. 2,3-diphosphoglycerate and adenosine triphosphate concentration, and increased hemoglobin-oxygen affinity caused by hypophosphatemia. Ann. Intern. Med., 74:562, 1971.

97. Chanutin, A., and Crunish, R.R.: Effect of organic and inorganic phosphates on the oxygen equilibration of human erythrocytes. Arch. Biochem., 121:96, 1967.

98. Jacob, H.S., and Amaden, T.: Acute hemolytic anemia with rigid red cells in hypophosphatemia. N. Engl. J. Med., 285:1446, 1971.

99. Nakao, K., Wada, T., Kamiyama, T., Nakao, M., and Nogano, K.: A direct relationship between adenosine triphosphate level and in vivo viability of erythrocytes. Nature (London), 194:877, 1962.

100. Craddock, P.R., Yawata, Y., VanSanten, L., Gilberstadt, S., Silvis, S., and Jacob, H.S.: Acquired

phagocyte dysfunction. A complication of the hypophosphatemia of hyperalimentation. N. Engl. J. Med., 290:1043, 1974.

101. O'Conner, L.R., Wheeler, W.S., and Bethune, J.E.: Effect of hypophosphatemia on myocardial performance in man. N. Engl. J. Med., 297:901, 1977.

102. Sheldon, G.F., and Grzyb, S.: Phosphate depletion and repletion: Relation to parenteral nutrition and oxygen transport. Ann. Surg., 182:683, 1975.

103. Sheldon, G.F.: Defective hemoglobin function: A complication of hyperalimentation. J. Trauma, 13:971, 1973.

104. Sedgwick, C.E., and Viglotti, J.: Hyperalimentation. Surg. Clin. North Am., 51:681, 1971.

105. Grant, J.P., Cox, L.E., Kleinman, L.M., Maher, M.M., Pittman, M.A., Tangrea, J.A., Brown, J.H., Gross, E., Beazley, R.M., and Jones, R.S.: Serum hepatic enzyme and bilirubin elevations during parenteral nutrition. Surg. Gynecol. Obstet., 145:573, 1977.

106. Host, W.R., Serlur, O., and Rush, B.F., Jr.: Hyperalimentation in cirrhotic patients. Am. J. Surg., 123:57, 1972.

107. Sheldon, G.F., Peterson, S.R., and Sanders, R.: Hepatic dysfunction during hyperalimentation. Arch. Surg., 113:504, 1978.

108. Parsa, M.H., Ferrer, J.M., and Habif, D.V.: Safe Central Venous Nutrition. Springfield, Illinois, Charles C Thomas, 1974, page 232.

109. Rutten, P., Blackburn, G.L., Flah, J.P., Hallowell, E., and Cochran, D.: Determination of optimal hyperalimentation infusion rate. J. Surg. Res., 18:477, 1975.

110. Maini, B., Blackburn, G.L., Bistrian, B.L., Flatt, J.P., Pasa, J.G., Bothe, A., Benotti, P., and Rienhoff, H.Y.: Cyclic hyperalimentation: An optimal technique for preservation of visceral protein. J. Surg. Res., 20:515–525, 1976.

111. Wagman, L.D., Burt, M.E., and Brennan, M.F.: The impact of total parenteral nutrition on liver function tests in patients with cancer. Cancer, 49:1249, 1982.

112. MacFadyen, B.V., Dudrick, S.J., Baquero, G., and Gunn, E.T.: Clinical and biological changes in liver function during intravenous hyperalimentation. J.P.E.N., 3:438, 1979.

113. Ikeda, Y., Yoshikawa, K., Soda, S., Okada, A., and Kawashima, Y.: Are hepatomegaly and jaundice attributable to glucose overload? J.P.E.N., (Abstr.) 2:39, 1978.

114. Mashima, Y., Ohno, K., and Suwandi, K.: The effect of caloric overload on puppy livers during parenteral nutrition. J.P.E.N., 3:139, 1980.

115. Skidmore, F.D., Tweedle, D.E.F., Gleave, E.N., Gowland, E., and Knoss, D.A.: Abnormal liver function during nutritional support in post-operative cancer patients. Ann. Roy. Coll. Surg. Engl., 61:183, 1979.

116. Hirai, V., Sanada, Y., Fujiwara, T., Hasegawa, S., and Kuwabara, N.: High caloric infusion-induced hepatic impairments in infants. J.P.E.N., 3:146, 1979.

117. Lowry, S.F., and Brennan, M.F.: Abnormal liver function during parenteral nutrition: Relation to infusion excess. J. Surg. Res., 26:300, 1979.

118. Touloukian, R.J., and Downing, S.E.: Cholestasis associated with long term parenteral hyperalimentation. Arch. Surg., 106:56, 1973.

119. Peden, V.H., Witzleben, C.L., and Skelton, M.A.: Total parenteral nutrition. J. Pediatr., 78:180, 1977.

120. Ghadimi, H., Abaci, F., Kumar, S., and Rathi, M.: Biochemical aspects of intravenous alimentation. Pediatrics, 48:955, 1971.

121. Wigger, J.H.: Hepatic changes in premature infants receiving intravenous alimentation. Toronto, Pediatric Pathology Club (Abstr.), 1971.

122. Postuma, R., and Trevenen, C.L.: Liver disease in infants receiving total parenteral nutrition. Pediatrics, 63:110, 1979.

123. Cohen, I.T., Dahms, B., and Hays, D.M.: Peripheral total parenteral nutrition employing a lipid emulsion (Intralipid): Complications encountered in pediatric patients. J. Pediatr. Surg., 12:837, 1977.

124. Popper, H.: Cholestasis. Ann. Rev. Med., 19:39, 1968.

125. Barr, L.H., Dunn, G.D., and Brennan, M.F.: Essential fatty acid deficiency during total parenteral nutrition. Ann. Surg., 193:304, 1981.

126. Langer, B., McHattie, J.D., and Zbhrab, W.J.: Prolonged survival after complete bowel resection using intravenous alimentation at home. J. Surg. Res., 15:226, 1973.

127. McDonald, A.T.J., Philips, M.J., and Jeejeebhoy, K.N.: Reversal of fatty liver by intralipid in patients on total parenteral alimentation. Gastroenterology, 64:885, 1973.

128. Salvian, A.J., and Allardyce, D.B.: Impaired bilirubin secretion during total parenteral nutrition. J. Surg. Res., 28:547, 1980.

129. Vitale, J.J., Nakamura, M., and Hegsted, D.M.: The effect of magnesium deficiency on oxidative phosphorylation. J. Biol. Chem., 228:573, 1957.

130. Walker, W.E.C., and Parisi, A.F.: Magnesium metabolism. N. Engl. J. Med., 278:658–662, 712, 772, 1968.

131. Rodgers, A.: Magnesium ions and the structure of *Escherichia coli* ribosomal ribonucleic acid. Biochem. J., 100:102, 1966.

132. Jones, J.E., Manalo, R., and Flink, E.B.: Magnesium requirements in adults. Am. J. Clin. Nutr., 20:632, 1967.

133. Balint, J.A., and Hirschowitz, B.I.: Hypomagnesium with tetany in nontropical sprue. N. Engl. J. Med., 265:631, 1961.

134. Opie, L.H., Hunt, B.G., and Finlay, J.M.: Massive small bowel resection with malabsorption and negative magnesium balance. Gastroenterology, 47:415, 1964.

135. Fishman, R.A.: Neurological aspects of magnesium metabolism. Arch. Neurol., 12:562, 1965.

136. Edmondson, H.A., Berne, C.J., Hamann, R.E., Jr., and Westman, M.: Calcium, potassium, magnesium, amylase disturbances in acute pancreatitis. Am. J. Med., 12:34, 1952.

137. Kellaway, G., and Ewen, K.: Magnesium deficiency complicating prolonged gastric suction. N.Z. Med. J., 61:137, 1962.

138. Wacker, W.E.C., and Vallec, B.L.: Magnesium metabolism. N. Engl. J. Med., 259:431, 475, 1958.

139. Shils, M.E.: Experimental human magnesium depletion. Medicine, 48:61, 1969.

140. Flink, E.B.: Therapy of magnesium deficiency. Ann. N.Y. Acad. Sci., 162:901, 1969.

141. Randall, R.E., Jr., Cohen, M.D., Spray, C.C., Jr., and Rossmeisl, E.C.: Hypermagnesium in renal failure. Etiology and toxic manifestations. Ann. Intern. Med., 61:73, 1964.

CHAPTER 18

Computer Applications in Clinical Nutrition

TERRY P. CLEMMER
KEITH G. LARSEN
JAMES F. ORME

Computers have become an integral part of modern medical care. The care team's ability to collect, correlate, and evaluate data has been markedly enhanced by computer use. For example, computerization of x-ray and laboratory instruments routinely aids the physician in patient diagnosis and treatment. Computers are able to monitor patients in real time, allowing physicians to continually assess their changing physiologic status and the efficacy of therapy.[1] They process large quantities of data, increasing our knowledge of epidemiology, changing patterns of disease, and environmental influences on humans.

Eliminating many routine tasks, computers have improved the efficiency of the delivery of health care. Computer technology helps physicians to observe the anatomic, physiologic, and biochemical changes occurring in their patients. This permits the basic and clinical sciences to interweave as never before. Special techniques, which 10 to 20 years ago were performed only in very specialized research laboratories, are now performed routinely at the bedside. This has allowed clinical research to develop rapidly, improving our understanding of the pathophysiology of disease states.

Nutrition and metabolism are particularly suited to computer application. Computers are quickly being applied to increase our understanding of the patient, to improve the delivery of care, and to allow research to develop in areas previously too complex to understand. This chapter will look at the current art of computer application in nutrition.

TYPES OF HARDWARE SYSTEMS

There are a variety of hardware systems available for use in nutritional support. The most common are the small hand-held calculators used for simple calculations. They are carried by most dietitians and nurses who regularly deal with clinical nutrition. Although they are extremely inexpensive and very reliable, they have limited capacities and memories. The more sophisticated programmable pocket calculators can be programmed with magnetic cards to perform preset tasks. Their expanded memories and storage allow for more sophisticated data processing at a relatively low cost, yet they can be used at the bedside. These systems save time and reduce computation errors. Although these calculators have expanded memory, their storage capacity remains limited, and they lack long-term storage and recall of patient data. The programmable calculator is task-oriented. Each program is rigid, allowing few options to the user except in the ability to change the program with another magnetic card. Good examples of the use of a pocket programmable calculator are described by Rich,[2] who uses this system to analyze nutritional intake of patients, and by el-Lozy,[3] who uses it in nutritional assessment.

Larger desktop programmable calculators have expanded capacities and memories. They are frequently connected to printers to allow more complex programs to be written and displayed. Although moderately expensive, they are used for more complex dietary nutrient analysis and assessment programs.[4]

Microcomputers with expanded data storage and long-term recall are capable of handling more elaborate programs. They can simultaneously perform several tasks, such as assessment, dietary analysis, and formulation of solutions, and they have some long-term data storage. The long-term memory and more sophisticated programming permits formulation of solutions[5, 6] and user interactive programs with increased versatility.[7, 8]

Larger, stationary, multiple-use computers have the added advantages of a greatly expanded long-term storage capacity; multiple ports for input and output of data, allowing for the simultaneous interaction of users at several terminals; extended computing power, permitting the development of much more elaborate programs; and the integration of several hospital services. They are used, often simultaneously, for nutrient analysis, patient assessment, formulation of parenteral and enteral solutions,[9, 10] monitoring of patient care,[11] menu planning,[12, 13] billing and inventory, and research. Some have developed integrative programs between various departments such as the laboratory, pharmacy, nursing units, nutritional support services, and administration. Such systems can routinely screen for high-risk, nutritionally depleted patients[14] and can provide decision-making capabilities that alert personnel to problems, help physicians formulate solutions, and aid in pharmacy preparation.

The type of system depends on the patient volume requiring nutritional support, the needs of the nutritional support and dietary services, the research interests of the institution, the availability of personnel to develop the programs, and costs.

Broad areas in which computers can be used by the nutritional support services include (1) nutrient analysis; (2) patient assessment; (3) prescription and formulation of menus and enteral and parenteral solutions; (4) monitoring; (5) inventory, supply ordering, and billing; (6) education; and (7) research.

puter, which referenced 1692 selected items. Using punch cards containing the food items and the weighted amounts, the computer prints out the nutrients in each item and the total daily nutrients received by the patient, comparing them to recommended daily dietary allowances according to the patient's sex and age. The stored data generated nutrient equivalent lists for specific nutrients such as potassium, sodium, and fats. This aided in formulating specific menus for metabolic studies and clinical purposes.

The computer has also analyzed food table inconsistencies. By pinpointing discrepancies among food tables and by using more recent data that identify up to 100 specific nutrients, more precise nutrient values are being developed.

Many of these early programs, however, were very expensive, requiring large computers and consuming much of the user's time to enter and retrieve data. Therefore, they were not generally accepted for routine use. More recently, programs have been developed for the smaller, more affordable microcomputers. These programs have been refined for easier use.[8, 19] They lack the depth of the large storage-capacity computers but allow the user to analyze, at least, the common hospital food. Many such programs are now commercially available for common desktop computers.[4, 20, 21] Other telephone-linked systems are accessible, allowing several hospitals to share a single large computer system that has greater depth at reasonable costs.[22] In many of these newer programs, foods can be entered by their common names and standard amounts without converting to code numbers in tables and changing units to the metric system.[22]

The computer's major contribution in this area is to improve our data on food nutrients, to reduce the workload of dietary personnel in analyzing patient diets, and to assist them in menu planning for specific dietary restrictions. They also aid the metabolic researcher in achieving more precise studies.

NUTRIENT ANALYSIS

Digital computers have assisted dieticians and researchers in analyzing nutrients in foods since the early 1960s.[15, 16] In 1973, De St. Jeor and coworkers[17] coded Table 1 of Agriculture Handbook No. 8 into the com-

PATIENT ASSESSMENT

Several data-processing methods assist in patient assessment. In 1976, Slack and colleagues[23] described a computer program that essentially interviews the patient to obtain dietary history and behavior. They demonstrated that the computer interview reduced the time that the nutritionist spent with the patient and made the patients more aware of their dietary habits. Compared to the nutritionist, however, the computer program was not very good at generating meal plans.

In 1978, el-Lozy[24] described the use of a small, programmable pocket calculator to assist in the analysis of anthropometric measurements in children, allowing the bedside calculation of nutritional status index.[25]

More sophisticated patient analysis programs have been described using larger desktop computers.[5, 26] They incorporate anthropometric measurements and laboratory data comparing the assessed results to stored ideal standards. The prognostic nutritional indices, along with a complete nutritional analysis of the patient's status, is then computed.

In noncritically ill patients, computers have also made possible a quick and accurate bedside evaluation of oxygen consumption, carbon dioxide production, and respiratory quotient. If nitrogen excretion is known, the computer can calculate the protein, fat, and carbohydrate utilization.[27] Small microprocessors also lend themselves to more sophisticated body composition and metabolic measurements, such as high-energy neutron bombing for nitrogen activation[28, 29] and continuous expired gas analysis in the critically ill.[30] Thus, with the aid of computers, more exact patient nutritional assessment becomes possible, allowing development of better metabolic studies and research techniques.

PRESCRIPTION AND FORMULATION OF MENUS AND ENTERAL AND PARENTERAL SOLUTIONS

As early as 1976, Hoover described the use of the computer in menu planning.[31, 32] In the hospital, it enhanced the ability to plan modified diets that coordinate with the general menu, thus reducing costs. Recently, more sophisticated systems for menu planning and an integrated management system of food service permit on-line, real time menu management, overcoming some limitations of the batch system menu planning. These sophisticated systems require a large computer with a large master menu file, menu transaction file, and production file and provide for direct user interaction.[24]

Recently, the computer has been used to optimize enteral hyperalimentation solutions for individual patient needs.[33] Following the input of standard patient data—which includes sex, age, height, and weight—the computer compares the patient to standard tables stored in the computer and calculates the energy and protein needs. The computer then selects the best-suited, standard, prepackaged tube feeding from a list. When the user interacts with the computer, it can specifically tailor the formulation, set fluid and electrolyte limitations, and clarify the needs for elemental formulations. With a daily print-out, the user can review the patient's past feedings and current pertinent data.

Programs for pediatric patients have been developed that reduce the time required to calculate the appropriate nutrients in parenteral solutions,[7, 34, 35] reducing the time required by the pharmacist in preparing the solutions.[6]

With larger computers that interface directly with all nursing units, the laboratory, the pharmacy, the dietary unit, and the nutritional support team, much more sophisticated systems have been developed.

Larsen and associates[36] describe a parenteral solution–prescribing program developed on a large central computer using an integrated hospital information system. The prescribing program is designed so that the patient's physician can prescribe either a pediatric or an adult formulation. It is characterized by the presentation of a series of computer screens that teach and guide the physician through the ordering procedure. Pertinent patient information, including the sex, age, height, weight, Basal Energy Expenditure (BEE), previous parenteral order, past 24-hour nutritional summary, and laboratory results, are recalled automatically from the computer's memory and presented during ordering. The computer asks the physician to make clinical judgments about the patient's nutritional needs for the next 24 hours and translates those needs into an ingredient order for the pharmacist's convenience. The ordering presentation begins with the previous day's order and an analysis of it based on current patient status (Fig. 18–1). If satisfactory, the order can simply be reordered. If unsatisfactory, the electrolytes can be separately modified if that is the only change, or if necessary, the entire order can be rewritten. The computer terminal screens that are presented when a new formulation is ordered depend on whether the patient is a child or an adult. A physician ordering a pediatric solution is asked to prescribe calo-

```
* THE PREVIOUS ORDER FOR THIS PATIENT SUPPLIED THE FOLLOWING:
     2420 ML TOTAL THERAPY
     1920 ML OF TPN SOLUTION
      500 ML OF LIPID 20% EMULSION  (0.83 GM/KG/DAY)
      848 NON-PROTEIN CALORIES / GM NITROGEN
     3689 TOTAL NON-PROTEIN CALORIES ( 1.55 TIMES PATIENT'S BEE)
            2689 DEXTROSE CALORIES
            1000 LIPID CALORIES
     3836 TOTAL CALORIES ( 1.61 TIMES PATIENT'S BEE)
       37 GM  PROTEIN (  0.3 GM / KG / DAY)


 *   NEPHRAMINE 5.4%      354 CC      ( 19.1 GM PROTEIN)     *
 *   DEXTROSE  41.2%                  ( 1400.5 CAL DEXTROSE)*
 *   SODIUM        25.0 mEq    *  ACETATE     75.0 mEq      *
 *   POTASSIUM     58.0 mEq    *  PHOSPHATE   10.9 mEq      *
 *   CALCIUM        4.6 mEq    *  SULFATE      4.0 mEq      *
 *   MAGNESIUM      4.0 mEq    *  GLUCONATE    4.6 mEq      *
 *   ZINC           3.0 ms     *                           *
 *   COPPER         0.6 ms     *  MVI-12       5.1 cc       *
 *   MANGANESE      0.3 ms     *  INSULIN     15.0 units    *
 *   IODINE        84.0 mcs    *                           *


 OPTIONS: (1) RE-ORDER,(2) MODIFY ELECTROLYTES ONLY,(3) WRITE NEW ORDER:B
```

Figure 18–1. Computer screen image that recalls previous TPN order, with yesterday's nutritional summary at the top and individual ingredients below. The option to reorder the same solution, modify only the electrolyte composition, or rewrite the entire order is given.

```
* ELECTROLYTE ORDERING *
CURRENT LAB RESULTS:
    DATE          NA+    K+    CL-    CO2   CA++   PO4   MG++   CREAT   BUN
    1/ 3/83  3:30  130   5.1   104    22    0.0    0.0          0.0     0
    1/ 2/83  3:25  127   5.3   107    20    0.0    0.0          0.0     0

ELECTROLYTES IN THE TPN SOLUTION:

   1.   4.0 MEQ/KG   NACL            8.   10.0 ML    MVI-12
   2.   0.0 MEQ/KG   KCL             9.  200.0 MCG   VITAMIN K
   3.   0.0 MEQ/KG   NA ACETATE     10.    0.1 ML    TRACE ELEMT/100ML TPN
   4.   3.0 MEQ/KG   K ACETATE      11.    1.0 UNIT  HEPARIN/ML TPN
   5.   0.3 MEQ/KG   MG SULFATE
   6.   2.0 MEQ/KG   CALCIUM GLUCONATE
   7.   1.0 MM/KG    PHOSPHATE



MODIFICATIONS MARKED WITH AN *

 ENTER NUMBER TO CHANGE OR PRESS RETURN IF DONE:
   (ENTER CHOICES SEPARATED BY COMMAS) 6,7
 ENTER NEW CALCIUM GLUCONATE DOSE (mEq/kg): 3
 ENTER NEW PHOSPHATE DOSE (mM/kg): 2                                    A
─────────────────────────────────────────────────────────────────────────
ELECTROLYTES IN THE TPN SOLUTION:

   1.   4.0 MEQ/KG   NACL            8.   10.0 ML    MVI-12
   2.   0.0 MEQ/KG   KCL             9.  200.0 MCG   VITAMIN K
   3.   0.0 MEQ/KG   NA ACETATE     10.    0.1 ML    TRACE ELEMT/100ML TPN
   4.   3.0 MEQ/KG   K ACETATE      11.    1.0 UNIT  HEPARIN/ML TPN
   5.   0.3 MEQ/KG   MG SULFATE
   6.   3.0 MEQ/KG   CALCIUM GLUCONATE *
   7.   2.0 MM/KG    PHOSPHATE *



MODIFICATIONS MARKED WITH AN *

 ENTER NUMBER TO CHANGE OR PRESS RETURN IF DONE:
   (ENTER CHOICES SEPARATED BY COMMAS)                                  B
```

Figure 18–2. These computer screen images show the standard pediatric electrolyte formula *(A)* and how they are modified by the user *(B)*. In this case, the calcium and phosphate (nos. 6 and 7) are increased. *B*, The new formulation for the user to review.

ries, lipid, protein, daily fluid intake, and electrolytes on a per weight basis. Standard per weight amounts of each of these factors based on the patient's age are presented as a beginning point for ordering. Each factor can be modified by the prescribing physician. During the formulation, the latest laboratory results from the patient's data files are presented to assist in ordering electrolytes (Fig. 18–2).

The screens that appear for the adult solutions depend on whether the patient is to be alimented peripherally or centrally. Standard formulations are presented along with an analysis of how they meet the patient's nutritional needs. One of the standard formulas (regular, fluid-restricted, or renal failure) may be chosen, or a modified solution may be selected in which the calories, stress factor, quantity of lipid, protein, nitrogen, or caloric nitrogen ratio can be manipulated individually for a custom solution (Fig. 18–3). Calories are prescribed on the basis of the patient's basal energy expenditure, which the computer calculates from its data base information. Both carbohydrate and lipid calories are given in appropriate amounts in

order to avoid side effects and to reduce waste of standard packaged nutrients. The protein and nitrogen are prescribed on a per weight basis starting from a standard amount. The calories and the protein can also be manipulated by specifying the desired caloric nitrogen ratio. The standard electrolyte packages are presented to the physician along with the patient's current laboratory data. The physician either accepts one of the standard packages or modifies the electrolyte quantities as necessary (Fig. 18–4).

As it is formulated by the physician, the program automatically tests for problems in the order. These tests include checks for excess glucose and lipids, insufficient or excess protein, excess volume, and ingredient incompatability. The program points out problems and directs the user to possible solutions by calculating the presenting alternative ways to order. For example, the computer resolves a calcium and phosphate incompatability by presenting either the option to lower the calcium or phosphate, or both, from the prescribed levels to specific calculated levels or the option of giving the phosphate through a separate line (Fig. 18–5). The

```
CENTRAL PARENTERAL NUTRITION PRESCRIBING FACTORS:

1-    3689 TOTAL NP-CALORIES / DAY          6- 151.42 GM PROTEIN / DAY
2-    1.55 TIMES BEE REQUIREMENT            7-  24.00 GM NITROGEN / DAY
3-     770 LIPID CALORIES / DAY             8- FREAMINE III
4-    0.58 GM LIPID / KG / DAY              9-     154 NP-CALORIES / GM NITROGEN
5-    1.26 GM PROTEIN / KG / DAY           10-    4264 ML TOTAL VOLUME / DAY

ENTER INDEX OF ITEM TO CHANGE OR RETURN TO CONTINUE: 9
ENTER NEW VALUE FOR CALORIC-NITROGEN BALANCE: 600

THE NEW CALORIC-NITROGEN RATIO (      600 ) IS GREATER THAN PREVIOUS RATIO
OF      154 CHOOSE ONE OF THE FOLLOWING MODIFICATIONS:
    1- INCREASE CALORIES
    2- DECREASE PROTEIN (E.G. FOR RENAL IMPAIRMENT)
    3- RETURN TO OLD VALUE FOR RATIO

ENTER INDEX OF CHOICE: 2                                                   A
```

```
CENTRAL PARENTERAL NUTRITION PRESCRIBING FACTORS:

1-    3689 TOTAL NP-CALORIES / DAY          6-  38.80 GM PROTEIN / DAY
2-    1.55 TIMES BEE REQUIREMENT            7-   6.15 GM NITROGEN / DAY
3-     770 LIPID CALORIES / DAY             8- FREAMINE III
4-    0.58 GM LIPID / KG / DAY              9-     600 NP-CALORIES / GM NITROGEN
5-    0.32 GM PROTEIN / KG / DAY           10-    2890 ML TOTAL VOLUME / DAY

ENTER INDEX OF ITEM TO CHANGE OR RETURN TO CONTINUE:
    CURRENT LAB DATA BEING RETRIEVED                                      B
```

Figure 18–3. These computer screen images demonstrate how the computer-selected formula can be easily modified. From the patient's sex, age, height, weight, and BEE, the computer formulated the solution in A. Any or all of the prescribing factors can be selected for modification. In this case no. 9, the calorie-nitrogen ratio, was selected for modification and increased from 154:1 to 600:1. The computer presented the option of increasing the nonprotein calories or reducing the protein. B, The new formula for user review. Other modifications could be made if desired.

```
* ELECTROLYTE ORDERING *
CURRENT LAB RESULTS:
DATE            NA+   K+    CL-   CO2   CA++  PO4   MG++  CREAT  BUN   GLUC
 1/ 3/83 10: 0                                      2.2
 1/ 3/83  5:20                                      2.1
 1/ 3/83  5:20  146   2.5   116   19    0.0   0.0          4.7   79     0
 1/ 2/83  8:56  149   3.0   113   20    0.0   0.0          4.6   71     0
ELECTROLYTE PACKAGES:
     ELECTROLYTES GIVEN PER LITER TPN BOTTLE *(2.2 BTLE WILL BE GIVEN TODAY)*.
     CHOOSING ONE OF THESE PACKAGES REDUCES THE COST TO THE PATIENT.
ELECTROLYTE        PACK#1      PACK#2

   SODIUM          41.0 mEq    41.0 mEq
   POTASSIUM       20.0 mEq    40.5 mEq
   CALCIUM          5.0 mEq     5.0 mEq
   MAGNESIUM        5.0 mEq     8.0 mEq
   CHLORIDE        30.0 mEq    33.5 mEq
   ACETATE         25.0 mEq    40.6 mEq
   GLUCONATE        0.0 mEq     5.0 mEq
   PHOSPHATE       24.0 mEq    24.0 mEq

1- PACK#1    3- PACK#1 MODIFIED
2- PACK#2    4- PACK#2 MODIFIED

ENTER OPTION NUMBER: 3                                                     A
```

```
ELECTROLYTE PACKAGE FOR MODIFICATION
 1- 20.0 mEq  NaCl             SODIUM     41.0 mEq
 2-  5.0 mEq  Na ACETATE       POTASSIUM  20.0 mEq
 3-  0.0 mEq  KCl              CHLORIDE   30.0 mEq
 4- 20.0 mEq  K ACETATE        ACETATE    25.0 mEq
 5-  5.0 mEq  MAGNESIUM        MAGNESIUM   5.0 mEq
 6-  5.0 mEq  CALCIUM          CALCIUM     5.0 mEq
 7- 16.0 mEq  Na PHOSPHATE     PHOSPHATE  24.0 mEq
 8-  0.0 mEq  K PHOSPHATE      GLUCONATE   0.0 mEq
                              SULFATE     0.0 mEq


 ENTER INDEX OF ELECTROLYTE INGREDIENT TO CHANGE OR RETURN TO CONTINUE:
    (ENTER CHOICES SEPARATED BY COMMAS) 1,2,3,4,7,
ENTER NEW VALUE FOR NaCl (PER TPN BOTTLE): 0
ENTER NEW VALUE FOR Na ACETATE (PER TPN BOTTLE): 20
ENTER NEW VALUE FOR KCl (PER TPN BOTTLE): 20
ENTER NEW VALUE FOR K ACETATE (PER TPN BOTTLE): 60
ENTER NEW VALUE FOR Na PHOSPHATE (PER TPN BOTTLE): 0                       B
```

```
ELECTROLYTE PACKAGE FOR MODIFICATION
 1-  0.0 mEq  NaCl             SODIUM     20.0 mEq
 2- 20.0 mEq  Na ACETATE       POTASSIUM  80.0 mEq
 3- 20.0 mEq  KCl              CHLORIDE   20.0 mEq
 4- 60.0 mEq  K ACETATE        ACETATE    80.0 mEq
 5-  5.0 mEq  MAGNESIUM        MAGNESIUM   5.0 mEq
 6-  5.0 mEq  CALCIUM          CALCIUM     5.0 mEq
 7-  0.0 mEq  Na PHOSPHATE     PHOSPHATE   0.0 mEq
 8-  0.0 mEq  K PHOSPHATE      GLUCONATE   5.0 mEq
                              SULFATE     5.0 mEq


 ENTER INDEX OF ELECTROLYTE INGREDIENT TO CHANGE OR RETURN TO CONTINUE:
    (ENTER CHOICES SEPARATED BY COMMAS)                                    C
```

Figure 18–4. Three computer screen images demonstrate the ordering of electrolytes. *A,* The patient's latest electrolytes are given first, followed by two prepackaged electrolyte additives. If neither packet is acceptable, it can be modified by choosing number 3 or 4. *B,* The modification ingredients are listed, and the user can modify any number as demonstrated at the bottom of the screen. *C,* The new formulation is presented for review. The total quantity of each electrolyte is shown on the right.

```
PRESENT CONCENTRATIONS OF CALCIUM AND PHOSPHATE ( 21.4 MEQ/L AND 14.3
   MM/L ) IN  1.9% PROTEIN MAY PRECIPITATE OUT. (G 3,  238.69)
   CHOOSE ONE OF THE FOLLOWING SOLUTIONS:

     1- DECREASE CALCIUM FROM   3.0 MEQ/KG TO   0.6 MEQ/KG

     2- DECREASE PHOSPHATE FROM   2.0 MM/KG TO   0.5 MM/KG

     3- DECREASE CALCIUM FROM   3.0 MEQ/KG TO   1.2 MEQ/KG AND
        DECREASE PHOSPHATE FROM   2.0 MM/KG TO   0.9 MM/KG

     4- TRY YOUR OWN MODIFICATIONS OF CALCIUM AND PHOSPHATE

     5- GIVE THE PHOSPHATE IN A SEPARATE LINE

     6- GIVE THE LIPID IN A SEPARATE LINE
        (MAY NOT COMPLETELY SOLVE THE PROBLEM)
```

Figure 18–5. This screen image demonstrates a computer check to prevent calcium-phosphate precipitation. It presents to the user several options to prevent the problem.

physician indicates the desired action, and the program makes the necessary changes automatically.

The computer automatically adds appropriate daily amounts of vitamins and trace elements. In addition to prescribing the parenteral solution, the program allows the physician to order laboratory monitoring tests. The monitoring tests, recommended by the nutritional support service, are presented along with the protocol-recommended frequency and the last performed test (Fig. 18–6). The physician indicates which of the tests will be done that day.

With the prescribing completed, the program uses the prescribing factors to calculate the ingredients needed to satisfy the patient's needs. The resulting order consists of four parts: (1) pharmacy orders, (2) nursing orders, (3) laboratory orders, and (4) nutritional analysis. The pharmacy order is the recipe of ingredients in the volume needed to fulfill the physician's requirements (Fig. 18–7). If more than a 1-L volume is necessary for nutritional requirements, the pharmacy orders are listed in ingredients per 1000-ml bottle and the number of bottles used in 24 hours. The nursing orders supply the nurse with the infusion rate of the solutions, or in the case of peripheral alimentation, the infusion rate of the lipid-parenteral solution mixture through the Y-connector. The nurse is also instructed on the bedside tests to perform and their frequency. The laboratory order section lists the day's tests that were ordered by the physician. The nutritional analysis section indicates the amount of calories (separating out the dextrose, lipid, nonprotein, and total calories), the relationship of the calories to the patient's basal energy expenditure as a stress factor, the amount of protein, the caloric/nitrogen ratio

```
**************
* LABORATORY TEST ORDERING *

    LAB TEST              TPN PROTOCOL RECOMMENDATIONS              LAST DONE
                      (INITIAL)    (INTERMEDIATE)    (STABLE)

1 - SMA-7          TU,W,TH,SAT,SUN        W         W AND F      1/ 3/83   5:20
2 - SMAC-20        M AND F           M AND F         M           1/ 2/83   5:10
3 - SERUM MG       M AND F           M AND F         M           1/ 3/83  10: 0
4 - URINE UREA     M,W, AND F        M AND F         M           1/ 3/83   7:50
5 - UR. CREATIN.   M,W, AND F        M AND F         M           1/ 3/83   7:50
6 - TIBC           Q 2 WKS           Q 2 WKS         Q 2 WKS     12/29/82 10: 0
7 - CBC WITH       Q 2 WKS           Q 2 WKS         Q 2 WKS      1/ 3/83   5:20
    DIFF.

ENTER INDEX OR INDICES OF TESTS TO DO TODAY:
   (ENTER CHOICES SEPARATED BY COMMAS) 2,3,4,5
```

Figure 18–6. The recommended schedule for monitoring of unstable, intermediate, and stable TPN patients. The user has the option of selecting those laboratory tests he or she wishes to have done today.

```
************************     ****  CENTRAL   SOLUTION ****
                                    4S30      3005725              1/ 3/83

1-   41 YEARS OLD          4- 188.00 cm  HEIGHT
2-      M                  5- 120.00 kg  WEIGHT
3- 2380.0 BEE              6- NOT FLUID RESTRICTED
*************************************************************
* PHARMACY ORDERS *                                         *
*                                                           *
*    201.0 ML   FREAMINE III 8.5%                           *
*    731.0 ML   DEXTROSE 50%                                *
*     10.0 ML   SODIUM ACETATE ( 2.0 mEq/ml )               *
*     10.0 ML   POTASSIUM CHLORIDE ( 2.0 mEq/ml )           *
*     30.0 ML   POTASSIUM ACETATE ( 2.0 mEq/ml )            *
*      1.2 ML   MAGNESIUM SULFATE 50%                       *
*     10.0 ML   CALCIUM GLUCONATE 10%                       *
*      4.6 ML   MVI                                         *
*      1.4 ML   TRACE ELEMENTS                              *
*     20.0 UN   REGULAR INSULIN                             *
*   1000.0 ML   * TOTAL VOLUME *                            *
*                                                           *
*          MAKE 3 BOTTLES                                   *
*          SEND  700 ML OF LIPID EMULSION 10%               *
*          SEND VITAMIN K  5 MG, IM, TODAY                  *
*************************************************************
PRESS RETURN TO CONTINUE:
*************************************************************
* NURSING ORDERS *                                          *
*            - RUN TPN BOTTLES AT  98 ML PER HOUR           *
*            - RUN LIPID 10% EMULSION AT 125 ML PER HOUR    *
*               UNTIL  700 ML OF LIPID HAVE BEEN INFUSED    *
*************************************************************
*************************************************************
* LAB ORDERS *                                              *
*    - ROUTINE MONITORING (WT., I&O, AND UR GLUC Q6H)       *
*    - SERUM MG++                                           :
*    - 24 HR URINE WITH UREA NITROGEN                       *
*    - 24 URINE WITH CREATININE                             *
*************************************************************
PRESS RETURN TO CONTINUE:
```

Figure 18–7. The order and label that will be printed out in the pharmacy. The patient's name, age, sex, height, weight, and BEE are on the top. The pharmacy orders are given in milliliters rather than grams or milliequivalents. The quantity to mix and the infusion rates are calculated, and the nursing and laboratory orders are given.

of the solutions, and the electrolytes the patient will receive during the next 24 hours. The physician can confirm the accuracy of the entry by reviewing the factors displayed in the final nutritional analysis section (Fig. 18–8).

Three copies of the order are printed at the nursing division for the physician's signature. One copy is also automatically printed in the pharmacy. It includes the order's billing information, along with labels for the solution bottles.

MONITORING

In nutritionally supported patients, calculators and computers are useful as monitoring tools. Recently, calculator programs have been described that facilitate the monitoring of fluids, electrolytes, and nutrients received by neonatal[37] and adult patients.[2] If the composition and quantity of the solutions are entered, or the solution or a combination of solutions from a menu of enteral and parenteral items is selected, the calculators will compute and display the calories; grams of carbohydrate, fat, and protein; nitrogen intake; the caloric/nitrogen ratio; percentages of calories from each food substrate; and electrolyte intakes.

Larger computers, which integrate many hospital services and have large storage capacities, can greatly reduce the work of the nutritional support services. When personnel resources are limited, such programs can be used to support the daily monitoring of all nutritional therapy patients. Such a system has been developed[38] and is characterized by a central patient data file in which multiple

```
EACH BOTTLE OF TPN (TOTAL VOLUME 1000 ML) SUPPLIES THE FOLLOWING:

 *     FREAMINE III 8.5%    201 cc    ( 16.5 GM PROTEIN)       *
 *     DEXTROSE   36.5%                ( 1242.1 CAL DEXTROSE)*
 *     SODIUM       20.0 mEQ   *  CHLORIDE    20.0 mEQ       *
 *     POTASSIUM    80.0 mEQ   *  ACETATE     80.0 mEQ       *
 *     CALCIUM       4.6 mEQ   *  SULFATE      5.0 mEQ       *
 *     MAGNESIUM     5.0 mEQ   *  GLUCONATE    4.6 mEQ       *
 *     ZINC          2.8 ms    *                             *
 *     COPPER        0.6 ms    *  MVI-12       4.6 cc        *
 *     MANGANESE     0.3 ms    *  INSULIN     20.0 units     *
 *     IODINE       78.4 mcs   *                             *

 * NUTRITIONAL SUMMARY FOR 24 HOURS:
      3050 ML TOTAL THERAPY
      2350 ML OF TPN GIVEN
       700 ML OF LIPID 10% EMULSION   (0.58 GM/KG/DAY)
       600 NON-PROTEIN CALORIES / GM NITROGEN
      3689 TOTAL NON-PROTEIN CALORIES ( 1.55 TIMES PATIENT'S BEE)
             2919 DEXTROSE CALORIES
              770 LIPID CALORIES
      3844 TOTAL CALORIES ( 1.62 TIMES PATIENT'S BEE)
        39 GM  PROTEIN  (  0.3 GM / KG / DAY)

PLACE ORDER WITH PHARMACY (Y OR N OR C): N
```

Figure 18–8. The final formulation with the electrolytes given in mEq. The vitamins and trace elements are given in appropriate quantities to deliver the daily requirements. A nutritional summary is given for review. The user then either places the order with the pharmacy or, by answering "No," rewrites the order as appropriate.

hospital service areas are able to store and review patient data. These service areas include the pharmacy, the hematology and chemistry laboratories, the x-ray department, the blood gas laboratory, intensive care units (ICUs), the electrocardiograph (ECG) department, and the admitting and medical records departments.

The computerized laboratory, blood gas, and ICU summary reports are used daily by the nutritional support services in monitoring patients.[39] A report of laboratory results (Fig. 18–9) for each patient is printed daily before rounds. This report includes the most current laboratory data that is available as soon as the test is completed, along with the past data for following trends. The blood gas report (Fig. 18–10) displays the most current blood gas test results along with a data analysis. The availability of this data facilitates rounds, allowing for timely review of infectious and metabolic problems.

In the ICUs, in which even more data on the patients is entered, the shift reports (Fig. 18–11) display the vital signs, intake and output, all drugs, weights, and hemodynamic and blood gas data.[39] On the daily generated weekly summary reports, the nutritional data for each 24-hour period is also displayed (Fig. 18–12). All of this data can also be displayed on any hospital terminal.

Ready access to such data not only improves efficiency but also helps provide better care, since the required data for proper decisions is available when needed.

In addition to patient monitoring, the computer, with two computerized questionnaires, can audit the service and care. One questionnaire is used by the nutritional support services nurse and dietician, and the other is used by the infectious disease control nurse. The questionnaires consist of computer-prompted, multiple choice, and numeric entry questions, in which the answer to certain questions will determine the next question. For example, if total parenteral nutrition (TPN) has been discontinued, the reasons for therapy discontinuation are listed. If a complication caused discontinuation, the type of complications are listed. The team members go through the questionnaire daily, spending about three minutes per patient. The infectious disease questionnaire is similar. The criteria for answering both questionnaires has been standardized to ensure consistent meaning to the entered data. The computer generates regular reports for audits, allowing the nutritional support service to identify specific problems, to modify the emphasis to solve such problems, and to evaluate the effectiveness of such efforts by subsequent audits.

3024387   3W05

LAB DATA - CBC

DATE	TIME	WBC	RBC	HGB	HCT	MCV	MCH	MCHC
27DEC	05:20	8.9	3.75	12.0	34.8	92.8	32.0	34.5
26DEC	05:30	9.5	3.65	11.4	33.8	92.6	31.3	33.8
25DEC	21:00	13.0	4.11	13.4	37.8	91.9	32.6	35.4
25DEC	05:35	11.7	3.72	11.8	34.6	92.8	31.6	34.0
24DEC	05:20	13.3	3.77	12.0	35.0	92.8	31.7	34.2

LAB DATA - PROTIME

DATE	TIME	CONTROL	PATIENT
25DEC	05:35	12.0	11.5
20DEC	05:30	12.0	11.5
17DEC	05:15	12.0	11.0
13DEC	05:20	12.0	11.1
12DEC	14:50	12.0	10.4

LAB DATA - SMA-7

DATE	TIME	NA+	K+	CL-	CO2	BUN	GLUC	CREAT
26DEC	05:30	132	3.6	100	24	12	131	0.8
25DEC	21:00	128	4.5	96	24	10	99	0.5
25DEC	05:35	132	3.8	99	23	8	139	0.7
24DEC	18:00	0	3.4	0	0	0	0	0.0
24DEC	11:35	121	3.5	0	0	0	0	0.0

LAB DATA - LACTIC ACID

DATE	TIME	VALUE
14DEC	05:25	1.2
13DEC	05:20	2.0
12DEC	18:54	2.3

LAB DATA - URINE UREA NITROGEN

DATE	TIME	MG/DL	GM/SPEC	VOL	TIME
25DEC	11:30	380	13.4	3520	24
		COMMENT 24 HOUR URINE SPECIMEN			
20DEC	07:58	1060	13.3	1250	24
		COMMENT 24 HOUR URINE SPECIMEN			
19DEC	09:30	1020	12.2	1200	24
		COMMENT 24 HOUR URINE SPECIMEN			
18DEC	07:50	720	10.8	1500	24
		COMMENT 24 HOUR URINE SPECIMEN			
17DEC	08:05	820	18.0	2200	24
		COMMENT 24 HOUR URINE SPECIMEN			

Figure 18–9. Computer printout of laboratory data. The latest data are at the top of each section and are immediately available at any hospital terminal as soon as they are obtained and entered in the laboratory.

```
JAN 05 83    PH   PCO2 HCO3   BE  HB  CO/MT PO2 SO2  O2CT %O2  PK/ PL/PP MR/SR
NORMAL HI  7.45  40.0 25.0   2.5 19.0  2/ 1  85  95  25.4
NORMAL LOW 7.35  34.0 19.0  -2.5 15.0  0/ 1  68  93  19.6

05 08:21 V 7.48  28.4 21.1  -0.5 12.3  2/ 1  36  63  10.9  50  22/ 17/ 0 10/ 0
05 08:20 A 7.51  24.7 19.7  -0.9 12.2  1/ 3  69  89  15.3  50  22/ 17/ 0 10/ 0
           SAMPLE #  14, TEMP 37.8, BREATHING STATUS : ASSIST/CONTROL
           MODERATE ACUTE RESPIRATORY ALKALOSIS
           HYPERVENTILATION NOT IMPROVED
           LESS THAN NORMAL ANION GAP ( 7.5 MEQ/L)
           AV O2 CONTENT DIFF  4.53
           R-TO-L SHUNT  30%
           A-A GRADIENT 203, A/A  25% (EST ALV PO2 272)
           MILD HYPOXEMIA
05 03:56 V 7.47  30.4 22.0   0.0 11.4  2/ 8  34  60   9.6  50   0/  0/ 0 15/ 0
05 03:55 A 7.50  25.3 19.7  -1.3 11.5  2/ 1  68  93  15.0  50   0/  0/ 0 15/ 0
05 01:00 A 7.49  27.0 20.5  -0.7 12.5  1/ 1  69  93  16.4  50   0/  0/ 0 15/ 0
05 00:01 V 7.46  30.0 21.2  -0.8 12.6  2/ 1  40  69  12.2  60  26/ 15/ 0 16/ 0
05 00:00 A 7.50  25.3 19.7  -1.1 12.6  2/ 1  91  96  17.1  60  26/ 15/ 0 16/ 0
ENTER T TO ENTER TIME, P TO PRINT, P* TO PRINT ALL, B FOR MORE DATA -->
: SNAPSHOT
```

Figure 18–10. Computer printout of blood gas report, including a computer interpretation.

By giving timely feedback to the nursing units about nursing care—such as accurate intake and output, daily weights, breaks in dressing techniques, the head nurse can compare her staff to other nursing units and emphasize specific areas. Infection control personnel can also use this information to help analyze and prevent infectious complications related to nutritional support.

made available technology in metabolic monitoring, body composition analysis, and data processing, which allow more precise metabolic studies and make possible large epidemiologic and population research projects. As computer technology advances, the sophisticated animal research models will be feasible at the bedside, allowing for even faster advances in metabolism and nutrition.

EDUCATIONAL AND RESEARCH APPLICATIONS

Large computers can be adapted for educational purposes. When formulation of solutions is done with the computer, prompting questions can be asked to guide the physician. Questions about fluid restriction, overfeeding with lipids or glucose, caloric/nitrogen ratio in patients with elevated blood urea nitrogen levels, and vitamin K when the protime is prolonged force the physician to think about new, possibly unfamiliar areas. The audits can lead the team to new concepts and previously unrecognized questions. Routine presentation of patient nutritional data teaches the nurse and the physician to routinely think about this aspect of care and to modify their behavior.

Many research areas have been opened up by computers. Microcomputers have

ADMINISTRATIVE USES

The computer can save time for the nutritional support service, pharmacy, nursing personnel, billing, and central services. Inventories can be kept; ordering of supplies facilitated; labels printed; units converted from milliequivalents to milliliters; intake and outputs recorded; nutrients delivered, calculated, and stored; and billing automated, with the computer reducing lost charges. In addition to saving time, the accuracy is improved, and more precise data is available to the clinician for decision-making.

The computer streamlines monitoring so that the team can work more efficiently in real time. Patient data may be accessed anywhere in the hospital for review when consulting on nutritional problems. This helps to provide a more efficient service and improves care.

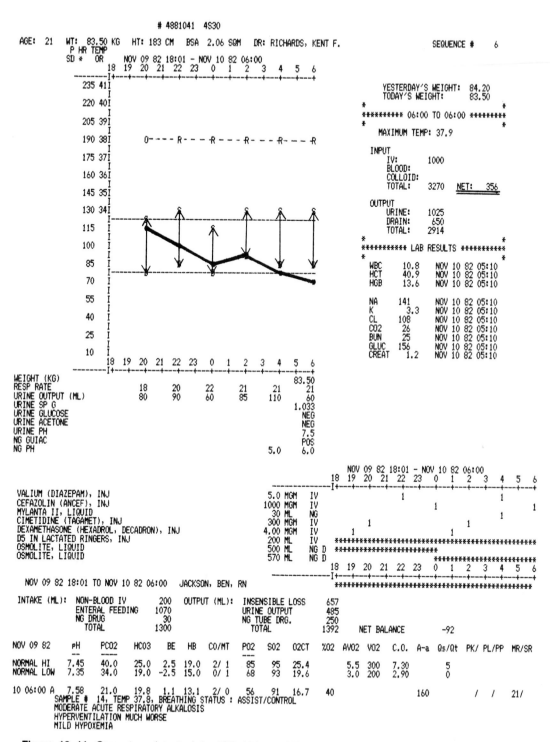

Figure 18–11. Computer printout of the ICU 12-hour shift report. All measures of vital signs, hemodynamics, intakes, outputs, and medications are available on the report, along with the latest blood gas report, CBC, and SMA-7. A new printout is posted at the bedside at 0600 and 1800 hours.

```
I C U    N U T R I T I O N A L    S U M M A R Y
```

```
                    4877130 4S30    AGE 21   HT 182 CM   BEE 1858

DATE:              NOV 04 82   NOV 05 82   NOV 06 82   NOV 07 82   NOV 08 82

WEIGHT          KG
TOTAL INTAKE    ML      12126       2867        8665        7373        5967
TOTAL OUTPUT    ML       5454       8946        9280        7739        7958
NET BALANCE     ML       6672      -6079        -615        -366       -1991

NP ENERGY       KCAL     2741        991        2513        2302        2652
TOTAL ENERGY    KCAL     3039       1131        2786        2570        3043
PROTEIN         GM         75         35          68          67          98
FAT             GM         50          0          50          50          40
CHO             GM        644        291         577         515         662
NP ENERGY/N2    KCAL/GM   249        165         228         230         176

N2 IN           GM         11          6          11          10          15
URINE UREA N    GM                    22                      18          19
N2 BALANCE      GM                   -20                     -12          -8

URINE NA+       MEQ
URINE K+        MEQ
```

Figure 18–12. Computer printout of the nutritional summary of the past five days. Such a printout is posted daily on the patient's bedside chart at the bottom of a 24-hour summary sheet that also summarizes the past five days of patient care.

REFERENCES

1. Clemmer, T.P., Gardner, R.M., Orme, J.F., Jr.: Computer support in critical care medicine. Washington, D.C., Proceedings of the Fourth Annual Symposium on Computer Applications in Medical Care, November, 1980, page 1557.

2. Rich, A.J.: A programmable calculation system for the estimation of nutritional intake of hospital patients. Am. J. Clin. Nutr., 34:2276–2279, 1981.

3. el-Lozy, M.: Programmable calculators in the field assessment of nutritional status. Am. J. Clin. Nutr., 31:1718–1719, 1978.

4. Kee, B.L., and Kilby, M.E.: Use of a programmable calculator for nutrient analysis. J. Am. Diet. Assoc., 72:629–630, 1978.

5. Edwards, F.H.: Computer-assisted planning of parenteral hyperalimentation therapy. Crit. Care Med., 10:539–543, 1982.

6. Rich, D.S., Karnack, C.M., and Jeffrey, L.P.: An evaluation of a microcomputer in reducing the preparation time of parenteral nutrition solutions. J.P.E.N., 6:71–75, 1982.

7. Klotz, R., Smith, A.E., and Isakson, C.: Using a microcomputer to support clinical nutrition services in a pediatric hospital. Nutr. Support Serv., 2:25–32, 1982.

8. Witschi, J., Kowaloff, H., Bloom, S., and Slack, W.: Analysis of dietary data: An interactive computer method of storage and retrieval. J. Am. Diet. Assoc., 78:606–613, 1981.

9. May, F., and Robbins, G.: A computer program for parenteral nutrition solution preparation. J.P.E.N., 2:646–651, 1978.

10. Shearing, G.: Parenteral and enteral nutrition: Computers and prescribing. Acta Chir. Scand. (Suppl.), 507:356–363, 1981.

11. Wright, P.D., Shearing, G., Rich, A.J., and Johnston, I.D.A.: The role of a computer in the management of clinical parenteral nutrition. J.P.E.N., 2:652–657, 1978.

12. Hoover, L.W., Waller, A.L., Rastkar, A., and Johnson, V.A.: Development of on-line, real-time menu management system. J. Am. Diet. Assoc., 80:46, 1982.

13. Hoover, L.W., and Leonard, M.S.: Automated hospital information system function for dietetics. J. Am. Diet. Assoc., 80:46–52, 1982.

14. Fisher, M.M., and Munro, I.: A computer programme for nutritional surveillance. Aust. N.Z. J. Surg., 50:512–516, 1980.

15. Brisbane, H.M.: Computing menu nutrients by data processing. J. Am. Diet. Assoc., 44:453, 1964.

16. Hjortland, M.C., Duddleson, W.G., Porter, C., and French, A.B.: Using the computer to calculate nutrients in metabolic diets. J. Am. Diet. Assoc., 49:316, 1966.

17. De St. Joer, S.T., Millar, R., and Tyler, F.H.: The digital computer in research dietetics. J. Am. Diet. Assoc., 56:404, 1970.

18. Hertzler, A.A., and Hoover, L.W.: Review of nutrient data-bases: development of food tables and use with computers. J. Am. Diet. Assoc., 70:20–31, 1977.

19. Williamson, M., Azen, C., and Acosta, P.: A computerized procedure for estimating nutrient intake. J. Toxicol. Environ. Health, 2:481–487, 1976.

20. Dorea, J.G., Horner, M.R., and Johnson, N.E.: Dietary analysis with programmable calculator: a simplified method. J. Am. Diet. Assoc., 78:161–162, 1981.

21. McConnell, F.G., and Wilson, A.: Computerized nutritional analysis in the dietetic department of a teaching hospital. J. Hum. Nutr., 76:405–413, 1976.

22. Danford, D.F.: Computer applications to medical nutrition problems. J.P.E.N., 5:441–446, 1981.

23. Slack, W., Porter, D., Witshi, J., et al.: Dietary interviewing by computer: An experimental approach to counseling. J. Am. Diet. Assoc., 69:514–517, 1976.

24. el-Lozy, M.: The assessment of nutritional state by

composite anthropometric measurement. J. Trop. Pediatr., *18*:3, 1972.

25. el-Lozy, M.: Computers, multivariate analysis, and the assessment of nutritional state. *In* McLaren, D.S., and Daghir, N.J. (eds.): Proceedings of the Sixth Symposium on Nutrition and Health in the Near East. Beirut; American University, 1971, page 305.

26. Nazari, S., Dionigi, R., Dionigi, P., and Bonoldi, A.: A multivariable pattern for nutritional assessment. J.P.E.N., *4*:499–500, 1980.

27. Norton, A.C.: Development and testing of a microprocessor-controlled system for measurement of gas exchange related variables in man during rest and exercise. Beckman Reprint No. 25.

28. Hill, G.L., McCarthy, I.D., Collins, J.P., et al.: A new method for the rapid measurement of body composition in critically ill surgical patients. Br. J. Surg., *65*:732–735, 1978.

29. Oxby, C.B., McCarthy, I., Burkinshaw, L., Ellis, R.E., and Hill, G.L.: A technique for measuring total body nitrogen in clinical investigations using the ^{14}N (n, 2n) ^{13}N reaction. Int. J. Appl. Radiat. Isot., *29*:205–211, 1978.

30. Kinney, J.M., Morgan, A.P., Domingues, F.J., and Gildner, K.T.: A method for continuous measurement of gas exchange and expired radioactivity in acutely ill patients. Metabolism, *13*:205, 1964.

31. Hoover, L.W., and Meylor, D.J.: Clinical dieticians use computer-generated worksheet. J. Am. Diet. Assoc., *76*:404–406, 1976.

32. Hoover, L.W.: Computers in dietetics: State-of-the-art. J. Am. Diet. Assoc., *76*:39–42, 1976.

33. Geller, R.J., Blackburn, S.A., Glendon, D.H., Henneman, W.H., and Steffee, W.P.: Computer optimization of enteral hyperalimentation. J.P.E.N., *3*:79–83, 1979.

34. Giacoia, G.P., Warden, L.K., and Canfield, B.G.: Computerized total parenteral nutrition formulas for newborn infants. Am. J. Hosp. Pharm., *37*:22–24, 1980.

35. Giacoia, G.P., and Chopa, R.: The use of a computer in parenteral alimentation of low birth weight infants. J.P.E.N., *5*:328–331, 1981.

36. Larsen, K.G., Clemmer, T.P., Nicholson, L., Conti, M.J., and Petersen, H.: Computer support in monitoring of nutritional therapy. Nutritional Support Services, *3*:7–16, 1983.

37. Neu, J., Crim, W., Kien, C.L., and Kelly, K.: Calculation-assisted monitoring of nutrition, fluids, and electrolytes. Crit. Care Med., *10*:461, 1982.

38. Larsen, K.G., and Clemmer, T.P.: Application of computers by TPN prescribing. Washington, D.C., A.S.P.E.N.'s Seventh Clinical Congress, January, 1983.

39. Gardner, R.M., West, B.J., Pryor, A., Larsen, K.G., Warner, H.R., Clemmer, T.P., and Orme, J.F., Jr.: Computer-based ICU data acquisition as an aid to clinical decision-making. Crit. Care Med., *10*:823, 1982.

CHAPTER 19

Cost-Effectiveness of Nutritional Support*

PATRICK L. TWOMEY
STEVEN C. PATCHING

LIMITED RESOURCES IN NUTRITIONAL SUPPORT

Special nutritional support, especially intravenous support, is expensive—no one denies that. The money flowing through the intravenous nutrition industry is being reckoned in hundreds of millions of dollars a year,[1] and Wall Street analysts are describing these high-technology health care industries as "attractive growth opportunities." However, for the individual health professional, the guiding principle continues to be to seek the best possible care for the individual patient. In addition, few patients ask that their case be the one on which greater economizing is begun.

Nevertheless, the specter of rationing is upon us, even in the wealthiest countries of the West. (Poorer countries have always had it.) In England nearly 20 years ago, Mr. Enoch Powell pointed to the inevitability of health care rationing because demand is potentially unlimited, whereas resources are limited.[2] In the United States, dissemination of certain procedures (heart transplantation) and equipment (computerized tomography [CT] scanners) has been curtailed, chiefly or solely on the basis of cost.[3-5] In nutrition, we know of hospitals that are on fixed budgets and in which a ceiling has been set on the number of patients who are allowed to receive total parenteral nutrition (TPN) on any given day. Administrators pointed out that exceeding this quota would mean running out of money before the year's end, with nothing for the next patient, no matter how great the need.[6]

Clearly, decisions regarding allocation of resources must be made. Tradition, emotion, and politics all feed into the decision-making process in these difficult areas. The need for a systematic framework within which to present data bearing on these decisions has brought techniques of cost-benefit analysis and cost-effectiveness analysis into health care planning.[7-11] Broadly speaking, these techniques are exercises in speculative accounting that tote up the pluses and minuses associated with a given strategy. The literature on these analyses has been increasing even faster than the medical-care costs themselves.[12] Nonetheless, the application of formal cost-benefit and cost-effectiveness analysis to hospital nutritional support is still in its infancy.[13, 14]

DEFINITION OF TERMS

Four distinct but related forms of analysis are now popular in medical circles:

Risk-Benefit Analysis compares the morbidity and mortality of the proposed strategy to the reductions in morbidity and mortality and the improved quality of life that will result. Cost is not a direct consideration. For example, a recent study analyzed a strategy of routine cerebral angiography to detect asymptomatic berry aneurysms in a high-risk group (patients with polycystic kidney disease) and found that only under the most optimistic assumptions could this approach produce more good than harm.[15] In nutrition, a randomized trial of adjuvant hyperalimentation during chemotherapy for lymphoma found that TPN had no impact on survival or drug toxicity but was associated with an 11 per cent rate of subclavian

*Reprinted from J.P.E.N., 9(1):3–10, 1985, with permission.

vein thrombosis in the treated group.[16] If this observation is correct, the judgment that this population should not be given TPN under these conditions is an example of a simple risk-benefit calculation.

Cost-Benefit Analysis (CBA) relates the monetary cost of a presumably beneficial therapy or strategy to the benefits produced. A major component of the analysis is the attempt to put all the costs and benefits into the same unit, for example, dollars. In medicine, this quickly runs afoul of the difficulty of quantitating the value of pain avoided, function restored, or a life saved. A few intrepid souls have attempted to provide an acceptable formula for valuing years of human life based on future production potential or the willingness of people to pay to reduce risks to their lives.[17] Such exercises may be useful in the context of public policy, such as planning programs for auto safety or pollution control. They have less appeal to the health professional dealing here and now with an individual patient.

Cost-Effectiveness Analysis (CEA) attempts to avoid these dilemmas by selecting the benefit or good to be achieved and comparing the monetary costs of various ways of achieving it. Thus, competing strategies to prevent death might be compared on the basis of "dollars spent to save one life," or equivalently "number saved per million dollars expended." Such analysis is particularly suited to preventive care programs, such as immunization and mass screening. For example, it has been used to highlight the populations to whom the first supplies of hepatitis B vaccine might best be given[18] and to guide the use of guaiac testing of stool as a screen for gastrointestinal cancer.[19]

Sensitivity Analysis assesses the impact of varying the starting assumptions in the CBA or the CEA previously described. Since the data are often incomplete, and the true costs and benefits are hard to quantify, this additional juggling of the numbers provides a feel for the stability of the conclusions.

In summary, risk-benefit analysis answers the question "Is more harm than good being done?" CBA addresses "What can we afford to do?" CEA asks "Which way costs less?" Sensitivity analysis looks at "How sure is the conclusion?" None of these approaches in itself answers the jackpot question "Is it worth it?" This requires a value judgment beyond the scope of the analysis.[20, 21] The value of CBA and CEA is not their ability to render a decision that is acceptable to all.

Rather, these approaches offer a chance to elevate the level of debate over resource allocation to a higher plane by displaying gaps in the data and replacing statements of opinion with testable hypotheses.

COSTS OF SPECIALIZED NUTRITIONAL SUPPORT

The first step in CBA or CEA is the determination of costs. However, finding the "true costs" of individual hospital services is difficult if not impossible. One quickly runs into the fact that economic cost (value of resources consumed) and charges (what the patient or third party was asked to pay) are very different things. Finkler, who is an accountant, lucidly explains the fundamental importance of this distinction to meaningful analysis of health care costs.[22] He also points out several cases in which ignoring this distinction has led to uninterpretable analyses. For a scientific approach to CBA-CEA, the most useful data would be economic cost. However, as Finkler points out, many forces act to make that difficult to determine in practice.

Consider, for example, a 1-liter bottle of amino acid–dextrose solution to be used for TPN. The price paid by the pharmacy to the vendor for the needed amino acids and dextrose varied from $7 to $15 in five metropolitan California hospitals we surveyed in 1983. Additives and equipment for mixing cost the hospital a similar amount. However, the pharmacy charge to the patient for this liter ranged from $60 to $120, with a median increase in price ("markup") of about 400 per cent (Fig. 19–1). A small amount of the increase can be attributed to labor costs for the pharmacist or technician mixing, labeling, storing, and delivering the solutions.[23] At a salary of $16/hour for one-half hour this amounts to no more than an additional $8/liter. To ferret out the source of the remaining charge one needs first to delve into the hospital's method of cost accounting and price setting (Table 19–1).

Each hospital department that generates charges must also bill for numerous items of overhead, such as depreciation on the space and equipment it uses, administrative costs, building maintenance, utilities, and so on. Provision for future expansion must be made, and certain money-losing departments within the hospital must be subsidized. Bad debts and underreimbursed patients must be

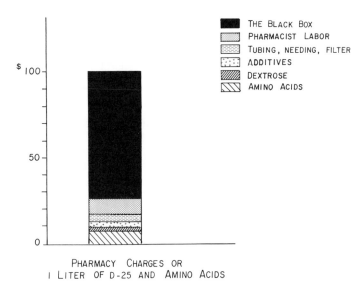

THE BLACK BOX
PHARMACIST LABOR
TUBING, NEEDING, FILTER
ADDITIVES
DEXTROSE
AMINO ACIDS

PHARMACY CHARGES OR
I LITER OF D-25 AND AMINO ACIDS

Figure 19–1. Pharmacy charges for one liter of 25 per cent dextrose and 4 per cent amino acids. Summarized here is the result of an informal survey of five California hospitals in 1983. The largest part of the amount charged to the patient is "markup," a "black box" whose specific contents were very difficult to ascertain.

covered, since the hospital's first financial imperative is to stay solvent. Finally, and most unpredictably, the hospital administration often adjusts charges further based on what competing institutions charge, and, above all, on what third-party payers will pay.[24] There may even be two different rates for the same service, depending on who's picking up the bill.

Of course, overhead, cross subsidization, consensus pricing, and other "black box" charges are not limited to the pharmacy. The clinical laboratory, radiology, and other departments are also among those asked to help keep the hospital in the black. Since many of these departments also provide important services to the TPN patient, the "eco-nomic cost" of a course of TPN (in terms of resources consumed or opportunities foregone) becomes ever more elusive. Thus, for the purposes of the subsequent discussion, we will confine ourselves to *charges*, namely, what the patient sees as costs to him or her, since that data is both more available and of greater concern to the ultimate payer.

Table 19–2 shows representative charges taken from patient bills in five California hospitals in 1983. This summary estimate is based on a 10-day course of TPN such as might be given preoperatively to a surgical patient. One-time costs, such as insertion fees, are prorated over the 10-day course. We noted that laboratory charges for standard tests, such as a complete blood count or serum electrolyte levels, varied over a wide range. The total patient charge fluctuated even more because of great institutional variability in "standard" monitoring for the TPN patient. Some institutions have standing orders that suggest frequent determinations of not only routine blood chemistries but also trace element levels, lipid panels, urine collections for nitrogen balances, and the like. Thus, for the patient who has a metabolic abnormality to begin with, or in situations where the physician simply wishes to "cover all the bases," charges for laboratory work can approach those for TPN solutions.

Professional fees for monitoring nutritional support are even less standardized. Some institutions have independent nutritional support teams who visit the patients daily, providing consultation, serial nutritional assessment, and other services. This

Table 19–1. CONTRIBUTORS TO MARKUP

Overhead
  Depreciation of building space, equipment and so on
  Housekeeping and maintenance
  Employee services (laundry, cafeteria, parking)
  Administration
  Future expansion
Allowance for Bad Debts
  Nonpaying patients and staff
  Partial reimbursement by third parties
Cross-Subsidization of Money-Losing Departments
Profit (Proprietary hospitals)
Adjustment for Concensus Pricing
  Rates set to resemble similar nearby institutions
  Rates set under pressure from Blue Cross, Medicare,
    or the like

"Black box" charges for hospital services such as pharmacy, laboratory, and radiology often greatly exceed the direct cost of materials and labor consumed. This table indicates some of the other sources of final patient charges.

CATEGORY	MEDIAN (DOLLARS)	RANGE (DOLLARS)
Pharmacy and Supplies		
solutions (3 L of D-25/AA)	280	240–380
lipid 2 × per week (prorated)	20	10–30
tubing, filters, pump	28	0–50
dressings, antibiotic ointment	10	0–25
Insertion Costs (Prorated)		
gowns, gloves, tray, catheters 100		
physician's fee 80		
x-rays and readings 120		
300/10 days	30	20–40
Lab monitoring (averaged to daily)	92	25–210
Professional Fees (Nutrition Support Service)	40	0–140
Treatment of Complications (Prorated)	13	0–100
Subtotal—Daily Cost of TPN Given Incidental to Hospitalization	503	
Cost of hospital bed—semiprivate	300	200–400
Total Daily Cost of Hospitalization Extended for TPN Only	800	

Representative daily charges for TPN in five California hospitals informally surveyed in 1983. The wide variation in charges reflects both differences in hospital pricing and different patterns of medical practice and patient populations. Items such as professional fees are estimates subject to considerable uncertainty.

attention may result in direct charges over and above those of the primary physician or physicians, or they may be submerged in pharmacy, laboratory, or hospital bed charges.

The cost of complications of TPN and their treatment can only be estimated. Pneumothorax, the most common mechanical complication of subclavian catheter insertion, has been reported in about four per cent of several large series. Catheter sepsis that is serious enough to require removal and reinsertion of the catheter can regularly be kept to less than 1/100 patient days of TPN. Together, the estimated prorated cost of these complications constitutes less than 10 per cent of the total daily cost of nutritional support (Table 19–3), even if additional hos-

pital days are allocated to their treatment. Metabolic complications such as hyperglycemia seldom generate major additional cost, and in this table are subsumed under laboratory charges. Other reported complications, such as catheter migration or arterial injury, contribute little to the daily cost of TPN in the average patient because of their relative rarity or the absence of need for expensive or prolonged treatment. The even-rarer fatal complications, such as massive air embolus, sudden overwhelming sepsis, and the like, are difficult to associate with a dollar cost. They can perhaps be dealt with better in a *risk*-benefit than in a *cost*-benefit calculation. Any measurable improvement in survival or prolongation of life in a given patient group should offset these small risks.

The total of the patient charges for TPN in Table 19–2 is greater than that mentioned in passing in several other reports, even after adjustment for inflation.[1, 13, 25, 26] However, these earlier reports have generally used the solution cost to the pharmacy or the hospital as the main basis for "cost" determination. As already noted, this "economic cost" (the value of resources consumed) is not only harder to completely detect but is also less relevant to the payers than the final patient charges. Moreover, adding monitoring costs, professional fees, and, when appropriate, hospital bed charges to the earlier reported solution costs brings their totals closer to those given here.

Enteral Feeding

In comparison with amounts charged for parenteral nutrition, enteral feeding charges seem quite modest. Material costs for standard isotonic, complete lactose-free commercial mixtures are often less than for meals prepared in the kitchen, and markup charges are less, with final charges often less than $10/day.[13, 26] Nasoenteric tubes, bags, and connecting tubing contribute less than $2/day, and laboratory monitoring, x-ray fees, and rental for simple controllers totals less than $10 daily in many institutions. Although there are no good data published on the cost of complications of feeding by this route, the major serious complication (aspiration pneumonia) in the alert patient who can protect the airway should be rare enough to add only a few dollars more to the average patient's costs. We can find no representative data on professional fees for tube-feeding

Table 19–3. ESTIMATED COSTS OF SOME COMPLICATIONS OF TPN/1000 PATIENT-DAYS
(100 PATIENTS EACH RECEIVING 10-DAY COURSE)

	COST/EPISODE (DOLLARS)		COST/1000 PATIENT-DAYS (DOLLARS)
Systemic Sepsis			
Blood and catheter cultures, 10 at $20	200		
IV antibiotics	300		
Catheter replacement	300		
Additional hospitalization—2 days	600		
	1400		
Frequency: 5/1000 patient-days	× 5	=	7000
Pneumothorax requiring chest tube			
Tube thoracostomy tray	80		
Three-bottle suction and tubes	120		
Surgeon's fee	150		
Chest x-rays and readings 4 × 120	480		
	830		
Frequency: 4/100 insertions	× 4	=	3320
Subclavian Vein Thrombosis—Symptomatic			
Venogram and professional fees	200		
IV heparin and laboratory monitoring—10 days	500		
Extra hospitalization—5 days	1500		
	2200		
Frequency: 1/1000 patient-days	× 1	=	2200
Total for 1000 Patient-Days			$12,520.00
Prorated Cost for One Patient-Day			$ 12.50

Charges for some common complications of TPN. Cost estimates were made using published incidence figures for the complications. Even using "worst case" assumptions, such as sepsis persisting after catheter removal, the prorated contribution of these charges to the daily TPN cost is small.

monitoring but believe this is unlikely to push the total cost above $30/day, exclusive of hospital room charges.

On the other side of the ledger there is some evidence from animal[27] and human[28] studies suggesting that in subjects with normal gut function, enteral feeding is more efficacious than parenteral feeding in raising resistance to septic challenge and in prolonging survival. Hence, in patients with functioning gastrointestinal tracts the adage, "If the gut works, use it!" reflects both good physiology and good economics.

Intangible Costs

Complete CBA-CEA requires not only tallying dollar charges for goods and services but also attempting to value the other "costs" to the patient, such as discomfort, immobility, psychologic feeling of dependency, and lost time from other activity as a result of special nutritional support or its complications.[29] Conversely, the intangible benefits of the therapy should also be recognized. In virtually every trial of TPN or other specialized support, patients gain weight—though not always lean body mass. Many improve their functional status and subjective well-being, though this is not yet well quantitated. Patients generally respond positively to these changes and appreciate the feeling that "something is being done."

These intangible costs and benefits may not always be in balance, since they are weighted differently by different people. Furthermore, placing a monetary value on the net balance of these feelings is very difficult. However, viewed in the context of any measurable reduction in mortality or major morbidity, we believe the contribution of these intangibles to the balance among costs, risks, and benefits is small for the typical patient, and thus have not included them in the analyses that follow. Also excluded is the vexing issue of the legal costs of giving or withholding such therapy. We do know of instances in which legal penalties have been imposed after complications ensued that were thought to be due in some cases to giving and in other cases to not giving special nutritional support. However, their imposition has been so capricious and uncertain as to defy systematic analysis. Fortunately, such cases are still rare.

BENEFITS OF NUTRITIONAL SUPPORT—TPN

Benefits must be demonstrable in order to justify risks or costs in this analysis. Theoretic advantages do not suffice. In the case of therapy such as TPN, such demonstration usually requires analysis of controlled clinical trials. Fortunately, several have now been completed. Unfortunately, they often do not rule in or out the presence of clinically important benefits because of problems in experimental design—above all small sample size.[30] This topic has recently been reviewed by Koretz, who found 25 trials possibly qualifying as prospective and randomized.[31] Only three of these trials demonstrated important improvements in morbidity or mortality. However, we have calculated the 95 per cent confidence limits within which the "true differences" are likely to lie.[31] For most trials these limits are wide and often still include clinically important benefits as being "possible" (Fig. 19–2).[32] Furthermore, in retrospect it seems that some of these trials can be criticized on the grounds that inappropriate patient populations were studied or that inadequate nutritional support was given. Hence, for many clinical situations of interest the question remains open.

One exception to the need for controlled clinical trials is the situation in which the course of the disease is so well known and predictable and the effects of therapy so dramatic that no one familiar with the disease can deny the efficacy of therapy. The use of penicillin in pneumococcal pneumonia is often cited. For TPN, the existence of short gut syndrome, for example, less than 40 cm of small bowel, satisfies this requirement. In these cases the benefit is clear—life would not continue without TPN. The costs can be added up, and the analytic part of the CBA-CEA exercise is complete.

A second category of use, providing TPN in various advanced malignancies, has generally failed to show clinically important benefit. Although weight gain has sometimes been demonstrated, serum protein levels have seldom risen, and no important outcome variable has improved convincingly.[1, 31] However, confidence intervals in these trials, too, are wide (Fig. 19–2). Many patient subgroups remain to be studied, and the proper selection of the combination of antineoplastic agents and nutritional support is still unknown. In fact, many workers in this field believe it is only the absence of effective specifically antineoplastic agents that prevents the repletion of the malnourished patient with advanced cancer. For the present, the lack of demonstrated and quantifiable clinical benefits in available controlled trials makes comparison with costs moot.

A third category that has been studied is the preoperative use of TPN in an attempt to reduce postoperative morbidity and mortality. There have been reports of six trials using this approach that had at least some degree of prospective randomization.[33-38] Only two trials met the twin criteria of providing sufficient TPN so that a clinical effect would be anticipated and including enough patients so that important differences might be detected. Both trials did show some benefit from TPN and warrant further analysis.

The first trial was conducted by Heatley and colleagues in Wales[35] who randomized 7 to 10 days of preoperative TPN against regular diet in 74 patients with gastric or esophageal cancer. The TPN group had a lower rate of wound infection, anastomotic leak, other infections, and death, though only the the first of these groups achieved conventional statistical significance. Interestingly, in a kind of informal cost-benefit analysis Heatley concluded: "This small benefit has to be set against the morbidity associated with intravenous nutrition and the costly and time-consuming nature of the therapy. It is doubtful that the limited benefit achieved justifies the routine use of this type of regime, even in patients whose nutritional status has been impaired by upper gastrointestinal malignancy."

The second trial randomized 10 days of preoperative parenteral feeding in 125 patients with gastrointestinal carcinoma and was conducted by Müller and associates in Cologne, West Germany.[34] They also found reductions in wound infections, pneumonia, other major complications, and mortality in the TPN group (Table 19–4). The latter two categories reached conventional statistical significance, and the authors concluded that the routine use of TPN in such patients could be recommended.

QUANTITATION OF BENEFITS IN SURGICAL TPN TRIALS

Surgical TPN trials reported benefits in three areas: better wound healing, reduction

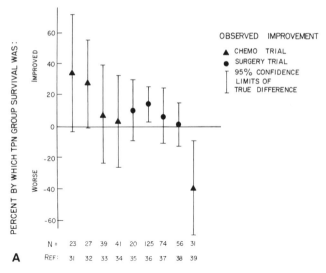

CHANGE IN SURVIVAL WITH TPN
RANDOMIZED, CONTROLLED TRIALS

PERCENT BY WHICH TPN GROUP SURVIVAL WAS: IMPROVED / WORSE

OBSERVED IMPROVEMENT
▲ CHEMO TRIAL
● SURGERY TRIAL
┬ 95% CONFIDENCE
│ LIMITS OF
┴ TRUE DIFFERENCE

N = 23 27 39 41 20 125 74 56 31
REF: 31 32 33 34 35 36   37 38 39

A

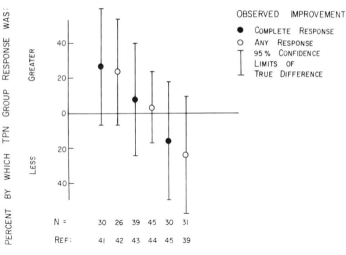

CHANGE IN RATE OF RESPONSE TO CHEMOTHERAPY
WITH TPN IN RANDOMIZED, CONTROLLED TRIALS

PERCENT BY WHICH TPN GROUP RESPONSE WAS: GREATER / LESS

OBSERVED IMPROVEMENT
● COMPLETE RESPONSE
○ ANY RESPONSE
┬ 95% CONFIDENCE
│ LIMITS OF
┴ TRUE DIFFERENCE

N = 30 26 39 45 30 31
REF: 41 42 43 44 45 39

B

Figure 19–2. The 95 per cent confidence intervals for differences between treated and control groups in randomized trials of TPN. By definition, brackets excluding zero indicate a "statistically significant difference" with p < .05. Conversely, differences within the brackets have not been ruled at this p value. For most trials, "no difference" remains possible. However, the sample sizes in many of the trials are to small to exclude clinically important differences. For example, six of the eight "negative" trials in *A* lack the power to rule out an improvement in survival of 20 per cent with TPN (e.g., 30 per cent control survival increasing to 50 per cent in the TPN group). Similarly, four of the six trials reporting chemotherapy response *(B)* and six of the seven trials reporting postoperative complication rates *(C)* do not rule out a 20 per cent improvement at the p < .05 level. Other negative trials have been reported but were either quite small or included insufficient data for calculation of confidence intervals.[30, 44]

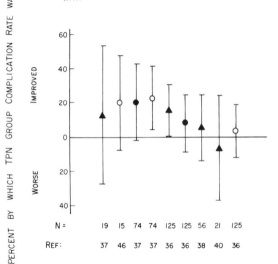

CHANGE IN SURGICAL COMPLICATION RATE
WITH TPN IN RANDOMIZED, CONTROLLED TRIALS

PERCENT BY WHICH TPN GROUP COMPLICATION RATE WAS: IMPROVED / WORSE

OBSERVED IMPROVEMENT
○ WOUND INFECTIONS
● OTHER INFECTIONS
▲ MAJOR COMPLICATIONS

┬ 95% CONFIDENCE
│ LIMITS OF
┴ TRUE DIFFERENCE

N = 19 15 74 74 125 125 56 21 125
REF: 37 46 37 37 36   36   38 40 36

C

Table 19–4. PREOPERATIVE TPN IN GASTROINTESTINAL CANCER. (BENEFITS IN TWO LARGEST RANDOMIZED TRIALS)

	TPN	CONTROL
Wound Infection		
Cologne	14/66	15/59
Wales	3/38	11/36
Total	17/104	26/95
	(16.3%)	(27.4%)
Major Complications		
Cologne	11/66	19/59
Wales	11/38	19/36
Total	22/104	38/95
	(21.1%)	(40.0%)
Death		
Cologne	3/66	11/59
Wales	6/38	8/36
Total	9/104	19/95
	(8.7%)	(20.0%)

Benefits associated with preoperative TPN in randomized trials. Data from the two largest published trials[34, 35] were pooled in an attempt to estimate the reduction in morbidity and mortality that may be expected from TPN. Note that the inclusion of data that did not achieve statistical significance (e.g., "deaths" in the study from Wales) results in a more conservative estimate of benefit than including only the results more favorable to TPN.

magnitude. In using published cost data from different years, allowance must also be made for the effects of inflation. Here we have adjusted all monetary amounts to 1982 dollars using the index of medical care prices.[39]

The cost of a postoperative wound infection has been estimated in published trials of antibiotic prophylaxis in surgery. One report from Atlanta gave an additional cost (adjusted to 1982 dollars) of $1921.[40] A similar study from Boston gives an adjusted cost of about $2100 for postoperative infectious complications, including wound infections.[41] Hence we have assigned a value of $2000 for each wound infection avoided.

Much larger dollar benefits accrue from avoiding a major complication such as anastomotic leak, renal failure, or intra-abdominal abscess. Here the data are less secure, since costs, patient management practice, and hospital populations vary. One carefully done study from Boston reported an additional cost to the patient of the equivalent of $54,000 (in 1982 dollars) for postsurgical complications of this magnitude.[42] A similar inflation-adjusted figure of $57,600/major complication emerges from an earlier study of misadventures after colon surgery by the same group.[43] These large amounts reflect the enormous cost of additional hospitalization, intensive care unit charges, reoperations, dialysis, drugs, diagnostic studies, and so on. Nor was money "saved" when the patient died. Charges for treatment of those who ultimately succumbed were double those of the survivors. Furthermore, since these reports included only hospital charges (professional fees being billed separately), they actually

in other, often septic, complications, and decreased mortality. Neither these authors nor any other performing similar trials have published data on the costs of avoided unfavorable outcomes. Hence we must rely on other sources, acknowledging the dangers of pooling data from different institutions (not to mention different countries). If we assume that similar reductions in morbidity occur elsewhere, we can hope that such extrapolation is correct at least to within an order of

Table 19–5. COSTS AND BENEFITS BALANCE SHEET (10 DAYS' PREOPERATIVE TPN IN 100 PATIENTS WITH GASTROINTESTINAL CANCER)

BENEFITS					
Wound infections avoided	11 ×				
Cost/infection	$2000	=	$ 22,000		
Major complications avoided	19 ×				
Cost/complication	$50,000	=	$950,000		
				TOTAL:	$972,000
COSTS					
Direct TPN costs:					
$500/day × 10 days × 100 patients	$500,000				
Room costs at $300/day	$300,000				
				TOTAL:	$800,000
				NET SAVINGS:	$172,000
				or	$1720/patient

Example of a cost-effectiveness calculation for TPN. Under the assumptions put forward in Tables 19–2 to 19–4 and in the text, a net dollar savings results from complications avoided using preoperative TPN in this patient group. In addition, on the average 11 lives/100 patients may be saved. Note again that these results are no more reliable than the data used to generate them, which at present contain many uncertainties.

represent an underestimate. Since the complications reported in the randomized trials of TPN (see Table 19–3) were generally similar to the ones in these latter trials, we have used the figure of $50,000/major complication in the following cost-effectiveness analysis.

Analysis

Using the amounts already derived, the calculation of the net patient costs of a course of preoperative TPN is straightforward. Employing a weighted average of the benefits shown in the two largest trials (see Table 19–4), the value of the complications avoided, and the median charges for a 10-day course of TPN (see Table 19–2), we can subtract the charges from the savings for a bottom-line figure (Table 19–5). *Under these assumptions*, a calculated savings of $1720/patient results from the use of preoperative TPN in this population, even when the patient is kept in the hospital solely for nutritional support. In addition, there is an average saving of the lives of 11 patients out of each 100 patients operated on. However, these numbers are subject to considerable uncertainty because of the inadequacies of the data base from which they are derived.

Sensitivity Analysis. Since reduction in major complications is the major source of savings in this calculation, we should investigate the effect of varying this reduction over its likely range. The cost assigned to a wound infection is low enough that no plausible change in its rate will influence the conclusions of the analysis. In addition, the charges

for nutritional support can be varied, for example, by attributing the hospital room charges to the patient's underlying illness rather than to the TPN ("incidental TPN"). Even bigger changes result if the costs of tube feeding are used in place of those for TPN. The result of such a sensitivity analysis is shown in Figure 19–3.

Limitations. One major weakness of this sample CEA is the large influence of one reported trial[34] on establishing the presence and magnitude of benefit of TPN in the preoperative patient. Although as reported, this study shows good design and adequate patient numbers with a clear-cut improvement in morbidity, some concern has been raised in a recent presentation by its first author that a third patient group, not yet reported, was also given a special regimen of parenteral nutritional support without improvement.[44] While awaiting clarification of this point, all can agree that a confirmatory trial is in order.

If the reductions in morbidity and mortality are actually much more modest than those presented in Tables 19–3 and 19–4, the proper pricing of a course of TPN becomes another critical ingredient in the calculation. Third-party payers are showing considerable interest in opening the "black box" of Figure 19–1 in order to produce more equitable and economical reimbursement.[45] Hopefully, results of these inquiries will be made public so that future analyses can narrow the gap between "economic cost" and patient charges.

Improving Cost-Effectiveness of Nutritional Support. The preceding exercise helps

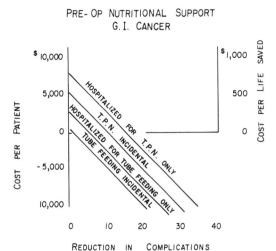

PRE-OP NUTRITIONAL SUPPORT
G.I. CANCER

Figure 19–3. Sensitivity analysis of the cost-effectiveness calculation in Table 19–5. Under the conditions put forth in the text, the reduction in complications is the major variable affecting cost-effectiveness. Other important contributors are (1) the need to extend hospitalization solely for nutritional support as opposed to giving it "incidentally" and (2) the route chosen for administration.

The right-hand axis shows the cost of support per life saved under the constant assumption of an 11 per cent reduction in postoperative mortality, as in Table 19–4. Note that in the region below the horizontal axis, preoperative nutritional support not only reduces morbidity and mortality but also saves money (given the assumptions made at the outset).

highlight the areas in which costs can best be controlled. Figure 19–1 illustrates that major improvements in the cost-effectiveness of hospital nutritional support are not likely to come from shaving a few cents/liter from the amino acid stock solution contract in the pharmacy. A glance at Figure 19–3 restates the obvious fact that use of TPN in patients whose complication rate is not demonstrably reduced can be very expensive. If money is to be saved, one place to start may be the advance identification of those patients unlikely to benefit from TPN, thereby avoiding the expenses, discomforts, and risks of useless intervention. The concept that the use of special nutritional assessment techniques will identify those most likely to benefit from special nutritional support has not yet been subjected to the scrutiny of a prospective randomized trial. Although there is little doubt that these techniques can identify patients at high risk, it is less clear that the benefit of nutritional support is concentrated in the patients so identified. The authors of the largest trial showing benefit from TPN concluded that standard nutritional assessment techniques were not useful in patient selection,[34] an opinion shared by others.[26] The rigorous demonstration of a means of identifying the patients that are most able to benefit from parenteral nutritional support, for example, would be a major scientific as well as economic step forward.

Another way to increase cost-effectiveness includes the use of the enteral route when feasible, since this not only saves money but also may be better physiologically.[27, 28] Timing nutritional intervention so that it is incidental to hospitalization (during testing or therapy of concomitant conditions) can reduce the room-rent portion of costs. Also, since in many places laboratory expenses are "big ticket" items, consideration could be given to streamlining and pruning the standing orders for laboratory tests when patients are stable and risks of rare deficiencies are low. A list (in descending order of impact) of some of the possible ways to improve cost-effectiveness follows:

1. Patient selection—use only in patients who will demonstrably benefit.

2. Incidental nutritional support—avoid hospitalization for nutritional support only.

3. Reduce noncontributory laboratory work.

4. Reduce direct professional charges.

5. Reduce complications below rates reported in the literature.

6. Use standardized solutions.

7. Reduce vendor charges for ingredients and supplies.

CONCLUSION—THE MISSING DATA

It should be clear that our ability to manipulate exceeds the strength of the data and that the exercise of CEA presented here cannot be used to "prove" that a given patient should or should not be given special support. As we noted at the outset, its value is in highlighting the areas for future investigation and pointing out gaps in the data. The major gap, we believe, is the lack of controlled trials of adequate size to rule in or out clinically important benefits from special support, especially TPN. Since such trials may require 200 or more patients with similar diagnoses to reach a firm conclusion, multi-institutional cooperative studies will be needed. In addition, more accurate data on costs are needed, both "economic" costs of resources consumed and final patient charges and their genesis. Both hospitals and insurance companies show a paradoxic reluctance to provide such information, even anonymously. Free discussion of this important issue is overdue, and all could benefit from a broader data base on which to base the discussion.

There is virtual unanimity on one point: costs must be controlled. We submit that organized analysis along the lines illustrated here will help ensure that the difficult choices ahead are made in the least painful way. It may also help identify ways in which nutritional support not only improves outcome but also reduces costs.

REFERENCES AND SELECTED READINGS

1. Brennan, M.F.: Total parenteral nutrition in the cancer patient. N. Engl. J. Med., 305(7):375, 1981.
2. Lister: Medical intelligence. N. Engl. J. Med., 293(13):651, 1975.
3. Moloney, T.W., and Rogers, D.E.: Medical technology—a different view of the contentious debate over costs. N. Engl. J. Med., 301(26):1413, 1979.
4. Knox, R.A.: Heart transplants: to pay or not to pay. Science, 209:570, 1980.
5. Centerwall, B.S.: Cost-benefit analysis and heart transplantation. N. Engl. J. Med., 304(15):901, 1981.
6. Hiatt, H.H.: Protecting the medical commons: who is responsible? N. Engl. J. Med., 293(5):235, 1975.

7. Shepard, D.S., and Thompson, M.S.: First principles of cost-effectiveness in health. Public Health Rep., 94(6):535, 1979.
8. Weinstein, M.C., and Statson, W.B.: Foundations of cost-effectiveness analysis for health and medical practices. N. Engl. J. Med., 296(13):716, 1977.
9. Pauker, S.G., and Kassirer, J.P:.: Therapeutic decision making: a cost-benefit analysis. N. Engl. J. Med., 293(5):229, 1975.
10. Barnes, B.A.: Cost-benefit and cost-effective analysis in surgery. Surg. Clin. North Am., 62(4):737, 1982.
11. Bunker, J.P., Barnes, B.A., and Mosteller, F.: Costs, Risks, and Benefits of Surgery. New York, Oxford University Press, 1977.
12. Warner, J.E., and Hutton, R.C.: Cost-benefit and cost-effectiveness analysis in health care: growth and composition of the literature. Med. Care, 28(11):1069, 1980.
13. Roberts, D., Thelen, D., and Weinstein, S.: Parenteral and enteral nutrition: a cost-benefit audit. Minn. Med., 65:707, 1982.
14. Koretz, R.L.: Preoperative total parenteral nutrition in upper gastrointestinal cancer: how much for how much. Abstract. Gastroenterology, 84:1214, 1983.
15. Levey, A.S., Paker, S.G., and Kassirer, J.P.: Occult intracranial aneurysms in polycystic kidney disease: when is cerebral arteriography indicated? N. Engl. J. Med., 308(17):986, 1983.
16. Popp, M.B., Fisher, R.I., Wesley, R., et al.: A prospective randomized study of adjuvant parenteral nutrition in the treatment of advanced diffuse lymphoma: influence on survival. Surgery, 90(2):195, 1981.
17. Landefeld, J.S., and Seskin, E.P.: The economic value of life: linking theory to practice. Am. J. Public Health, 72(6):555, 1982.
18. Mulley, A.G., Silverstein, M.D., and Dienstag, J.L.: Indications for use of hepatitis B vaccine, based on cost-effectiveness analysis. N. Engl. J. Med., 307(11):644, 1982.
19. Neuhauser, D., and Lewicki, A.M.: What do we gain from the sixth stool guaiac? N. Engl. J. Med., 293(5):226, 1975.
20. Fuchs, V.R.: What is CBA/CEA, and why are they doing this to us? N. Engl. J. Med., 303(16):937, 1981.
21. Berwick, D.M., and Komaroff, A.L.: Cost-effectiveness of lead screening. N. Engl. J. Med., 307(20):1270, 1982.
22. Finkler, S.A.: The distinction between costs and charges. Ann. Intern. Med., 96(1):102, 1982.
23. Vanderveen, T.W., and Robinson, L.A.: Total parenteral nutrition solution preparation utilizing amino acid sources with and without pre-added electrolytes: a time and cost comparison. J.P.E.N., 3(2):84, 1979.
24. Marty, A.T., Matar, A.F., Danielson, R., et al.: The variation in hospital charges: a problem in determining cost/benefit for cardiac surgery. Ann. Thorac. Surg., 24(5):409, 1977.
25. Wateska, L.P., Sattler, L.L., and Steigher, E.R.: Cost of a home parenteral nutrition program. J.A.M.A., 244(20):2303, 1980.
26. Michel, L., Serrano, A., and Malt, R.A.: Nutritional support of hospitalized patients. N. Engl. J. Med., 304(19):1147, 1981.
27. Kudsk, K.A., Carpenter, G., Petersen, S., et al.: Effect of enteral and parenteral feeding in malnourished rats with E. coli-hemoglobin adjuvant peritonitis. J. Surg. Res., 31(2):105, 1981.
28. Sako, K., Loré, J.M., Kaufman, S., et al.: Parenteral hyperalimentation in surgical patients with head and neck cancer: a randomized trial. J. Surg. Oncol., 16:391, 1981.
29. Brett, A.S.: Hidden ethical issues in clinical decision analysis. N. Engl. J. Med., 305(19):1150, 1981.
30. Freiman, J.A., Chalmers, J.C., Smith, H., Jr., et al.: The importance of beta, the type II error and sample size in the design and interpretation of the randomized control trial: survey of 71 "negative" trials. N. Engl. J. Med., 299(13):690, 1978.
31. Koretz, R.L.: What supports nutritional support? Dig. Dis. Sci., 29(6):577, 1984.
32. Remington, R.D., and Schorla, M.A.: Statistics with Applications to the Biological and Health Sciences. Englewood Cliffs, New Jersey, Prentice-Hall, 1970.
33. Simms, J.M., Oliver, E., and Smith, J.A.R.: A study of total parenteral nutrition in major gastric and esophageal resection for neoplasia. Abstract. J.P.E.N., 4(4):422, 1980.
34. Müller, J.M., Brenner, U., Dienst, C., et al.: Preoperative parenteral feeding in patients with gastrointestinal carcinoma. Lancet, 1:68, 1982.
35. Heatley, R.V., Williams, R.H.P., and Lewis, M.H.: Preoperative intravenous feeding—a controlled trial. Postgrad. Med. J., 55(646):541, 1979.
36. Holter, A.R., and Fischer, J.E.: The effects of perioperative hyperalimentation on complications in patients with carcinoma and weight loss. J. Surg. Res., 23(1):31, 1977.
37. Jordan, W.M., Valdivieso, M., Frankmann, C., et al.: Treatment of advanced adenocarcinoma of the lung with ftorafur, doxorubicin, cyclophosphamide, and cisplatin and intensive IV hyperalimentation. Cancer Treat. Rep., 65:197, 1981.
38. Thompson, B.R., Julian, T.B., and Stremple, J.F.: Perioperative total parenteral nutrition in patients with gastrointestinal cancer. J. Surg. Res., 30(5):497, 1981.
39. Statistical Abstract of the United States: Washington, D.C., U.S. Government Printing Office, Table 157, 1982–1983.
40. Stone, H.H., Hooper, C.A., Kolb, L.D., et al.: Antibiotic prophylaxis in gastric, biliary and colonic surgery. Ann. Surg., 184(4):443, 1976.
41. Shapiro, M., et al.: Benefit-cost analysis of antimicrobial prophylaxis in abdominal and vaginal hysterectomy. J.A.M.A., 249(10):1290, 1983.
42. Couch, N.P., Tilney, N.L., Rayner, A.A., et al.: The high cost of low-frequency events: the anatomy and economics of surgical mishaps. N. Engl. J. Med., 304(11):634, 1981.
43. Couch, N.P., Tilney, N.L., and Moore, F.D.: The cost of misadventures in colonic surgery: a model for the analysis of adverse outcomes in standard procedures. Am. J. Surg., 135:641, 1978.
44. Müller, J.: Presentation at 1983 Clinical Congress of American Society for Parenteral and Enteral Nutrition. Washington, D.C., 1983.
45. Williams, S.V., Finkler, S.A., Murphy, C.M., et al.: Improved cost allocation in case-mix accounting. Med. Care, 20(5):450, 1982.
46. Coquin, J.Y., et al.: Influence of parenteral nutrition on chemotherapy and survival of acute leukaemias; preliminary results of a randomized trial. J.P.E.N., 4:437, 1980.
47. Shamberger, R.C., Pizzo, P.A., Goodgame, J.T., Jr., et al.: The effect of total parenteral nutrition on chemotherapy-induced myelosuppression: a randomized study. Am. J. Med., 74:40, 1983.

48. Serrou, B., Cupissol, D., Plagne, R., et al.: Parenteral intravenous nutrition (PIVN) as an adjunct to chemotherapy in small cell anaplastic lung carcinoma. Cancer Treat. Rep. (Suppl.) 65(5):151, 1981.

49. Valdivieso, M., Bodey, G.D., Benjamin, R.S., et al.: Role of intravenous hyperalimentation as an adjunct to intensive chemotherapy for small cell bronchogenic carcinoma. Cancer Treat. Rep. (Suppl.) 65(5):145, 1981.

50. Issel, B.F., et al.: Protection against chemotherapy toxicity by IV hyperalimentation. Cancer Treat. Rep., 62:1139, 1978.

51. Serrou, B., Cupissol, D., Plagne, R., et al.: Follow-up of a randomized trial for oat cell carcinoma evaluating the efficacy of peripheral intravenous nutrition (PIVN) as adjunct treatment. Rec. Res. Cancer Res., 40:246, 1982.

52. Nixon, D.W., Moffitt, S., Lawson, D.H., et al.: Total parenteral nutrition as an adjunct to chemotherapy of metastatic colorectal cancer. Cancer Treat. Rep.(Suppl.), 65(5):121, 1981.

53. Samuels, M.L., Selig, D.E., Ogden, S., et al.: IV hyperalimentation and chemotherapy for stage III testicular cancer: a randomized study. Cancer Treat. Rep., 65:615, 1981.

54. Moghissi, K., Hornshaw, J., Teasdale, P.R., et al.: Parenteral nutrition in carcinoma of the esophagus treated by surgery: nitrogen balance and clinical studies. Br. J. Surg., 64:125, 1977.

CHAPTER 20

Perioperative Total Parenteral Nutrition

JORGE E. ALBINA
MARK J. KORUDA
JOHN L. ROMBEAU

The presence of protein-calorie malnutrition in hospitalized patients has been documented extensively[1, 2] and has been reported to occur in nearly 50 per cent of surgical patients in a major urban hospital.[3] Protein-calorie malnutrition is characterized by decreases in visceral protein, skeletal muscle, and fat stores. These decreases are associated with an adverse postoperative outcome.[4] There is an observed increase in postoperative morbidity and mortality in malnourished patients,[5] and with weight loss,[6] hypoalbuminemia,[7, 8] decreased total lymphocyte counts,[9] and low serum transferrin levels.[10]

Efforts have been made to improve the perioperative nutritional status of malnourished patients with the use of total parenteral nutrition (TPN) in an attempt to improve their postoperative courses. The rationale for the use of perioperative TPN involves several assumptions: (1) protein-calorie malnutrition can be adequately defined; (2) protein-calorie malnutrition leads to increased morbidity and mortality; (3) adequate nutritional support can reverse protein-calorie malnutrition; and (4) the reversal of protein-calorie malnutrition results in a decrease in morbidity and mortality.[5]

There is substantial evidence to support the validity of the first three assumptions. The premise for the use of perioperative TPN is based, however, on the final assumption that reversal of protein-calorie malnutrition results in improvement in postoperative morbidity and mortality. Can this assumption be substantiated? Total parenteral nutrition is not without complications and it is also expensive. Therefore, close scrutiny is currently being applied to identify the most efficacious use of TPN in the perioperative setting.

IDEAL CRITERIA FOR PERIOPERATIVE TPN

Ideally, the use of perioperative TPN should

1. *Improve the clinical outcome.* Improvement can be measured as decreased morbidity rate, prolonged survival, improved response to other treatment modalities, decreased hospital stay, or reduced total hospital costs.

2. *Be relatively inexpensive.* The daily cost of TPN has been estimated at $150 to $300 per day.[11] The cost-benefit ratio should not encumber its use.

3. *Not unduly delay the need for surgery.* The amount of time needed to replete the patient nutritionally should be realistic and should not unduly delay needed surgery.

4. *Be restricted to patients who cannot be fed enterally,* either orally or via a feeding tube. TPN should not be used if the gastrointestinal tract can be used safely.

5. *Be safe.* The complication rate of TPN should be acceptably low and the risk-benefit ratio should be low.

6. *Be provided in amounts that meet nutritional needs.* The nutrients supplied should fulfill requirements for protein, calorie, vitamin, and mineral maintenance or repletion.

7. *Cause improvement in nutritional status.* Supplying "adequate" nutrition is expected to improve nutritional assessment indices, as noted previously.

In this chapter, the current literature on

the use of TPN in the perioperative period is reviewed and how well the perioperative TPN studies fulfill the proposed criteria, as outlined in this chapter, is determined.

PERIOPERATIVE TPN STUDY DESIGN

There are numerous reports of the use of perioperative TPN.[12-31] The designs of such studies are often fraught with shortcomings, and the ideal protocol is often not followed. Elements of the ideal protocol for evaluation of the efficacy of perioperative TPN are: (1) proper patient selection and definition of *malnutrition;* (2) "adequate" nutritional repletion; (3) adequate population size; (4) prospective and randomized design; (5) matching of control group for multiple variables; and (6) precise definition of complications.

First, there is the problem of identifying those patients at increased postoperative risk from malnutrition. Apart from specific macronutrient or micronutrient deficiency syndromes (Vitamin C, zinc, iron), malnutrition appears to be a multifactorial problem. A further problem is the inability to *precisely* measure the degree of malnutrition in individual patients.[32, 33] Therefore, care must be taken to determine how malnutrition is defined when critically evaluating and comparing reported studies.

Second, the definition of "adequate" nutrition is not easily determined. Total parenteral nutrition in the perioperative setting implies supplying nutrients via the intravenous route in excess of maintenance requirements in order to replete the malnourished patient. Nutrient requirements can only be estimated for stressed surgical patients. Also, the appropriate duration of preoperative repletion has not been confirmed. Mullen and associates[15] and Williams and colleagues[34] suggest that at least seven days of preoperative TPN constitutes "adequate" repletion. Lehr and co-workers[35] state that the preoperative correction of total body potassium deficiency is the end-point for repletion of Crohn's disease patients. To date, there are no objective measures to indicate when a surgical patient has undergone "adequate" nutritional repletion to significantly reduce postoperative risks.

A third problem encountered when evaluating the effects of TPN is the selection of a proper control population. To perform an adequate analysis of the impact of nutritional support on surgical outcome, it is necessary to isolate this form of therapy from other concurrent treatments that may also influence clinical outcome. Most malnourished surgical patients suffer from major illnesses such as cancer, burns, sepsis, and trauma, all of which severely affect outcome. Other factors that enter into the control group selection include age, sex, extent of disease, severity and type of nutritional problem, and type of operative procedure. It may be impossible to isolate the effect of malnutrition or repletion from other forms of therapy or from the consequences of the patient's disease. It is therefore necessary to gather a large cohort population in order to avoid type II statistical errors.

Finally, complications should be precisely defined. Each should be categorized as to its likelihood of its being related to malnutrition and whether it would be expected to be prevented by nutritional treatment. For example, it is questionable that perioperative nutritional support could reduce the prevalence of wound hematomas or urinary tract infections.

PREOPERATIVE TPN

The administration of preoperative TPN to malnourished surgical patients has been evaluated in many studies. These include abstracts[14, 36] retrospective or uncontrolled trials,[15-22, 29] and studies that compare diverse routes of nutritional delivery.[23] The beneficial effects of preoperative nutritional repletion has been advanced by several authors; however, this review will discuss five prospective and two retrospective studies.

Prospective Studies

Only five reports to date partly fulfill the criteria for a definitive prospective, randomized study (Table 20–1).

The Moghissi Study.[24] This 1977 report clearly illustrates the difficulties in performing a clinical trial. Patients with carcinoma of the esophagus were admitted to the study if they had complete or almost complete dysphagia and their tumors proved to be resectable. They were alternately allocated to receive TPN (Group A) or not to receive TPN (Group B). Group A consisted of ten patients who received TPN for five to seven days before operation and for six to seven days

Table 20–1. PROSPECTIVE CONTROLLED TRIALS OF PREOPERATIVE TOTAL PARENTERAL NUTRITION*

STUDY	DIAGNOSIS	PREOPERATIVE NUTRITIONAL ASSESSMENT INDICES	NO. DAYS PREOPERATIVE TPN	NO. PATIENTS		NO. PATIENTS WITH COMPLICATIONS§ (%)				TPN-Related	NO. DEATHS (%)		COMMENTS
						Major		Minor					
				S†	C‡	S†	C‡	S†	C‡		S†	C‡	
Moghissi et al.[24]	Esophageal cancer	Dysphagia	5–7	10	5	See text‖	See text‖	See text‖		NR	0	0	Postoperative course was termed "smoother and more satisfactory" in the TPN group.
Holter and Fischer[25]	GI cancer	>10-lb. weight loss	3	30	26M 28W	4/30 (20)	5/26M (19) 2/28W (7)	7/30 (23)	6/26M (23) 6/21W (21)	NR	2/30 (7)	2/26M (8) 0W	Only 3 days of preoperative TPN.
Heatley et al.[26]	Esophageal and gastric cancer	NR	7–10	38	36	2/10 (20)	4/11 (36)	3/38** (8)	11/36** (31)	See text	6 (16)	8 (22)	Patients not randomized according to preoperative nutritional status. 5 patients in control group received postoperative TPN.
Thompson et al.[27]	GI cancer	>10-lb. weight loss	5–14	12	9M 20C	2/12 (17)	1/9M (11) 2/20C (10)	3/12 (25)	2/9M (22) 4/20C (20)	1	0	0M 2/10C (20)	
Müller et al.[28]	GI cancer	>5-kg weight loss; albumin <3.5 g/dl; anergy	10	66	59	19/66** (29)	11/59** (19)	NS	NS	4	11** (5)	3** (18)	Nutritional status not considered in randomization. 59% of TPN group and 62% of control group malnourished.

*NR = not reported; NS = not significant.
†S = TPN.
‡C = no TPN; M = malnourished controls; W = well-fed controls.
§Major complications intra-abdominal abscess, peritonitis, anastomotic leak, and wound dehiscence. Minor complications included wound infections, pulmonary complications, etc.
‖Hospital course was subjectively evaluated.
**p < 0.05.

after operation. The regimen included 34 to 36 kcal/kg/day and nitrogen at 0.18 to 0.20 gm/kg/day. The caloric source was a mixture of dextrose, fructose, ethanol, and 20 per cent fat emulsion. Patients in Group B received 6 kcal/kg/day intravenously and no nitrogen. Patients' sex, age, degree and duration of dysphagia, weight loss, and general condition were reported. Nitrogen balance studies were conducted over the duration of hospital stay. The postoperative courses were evaluated for adequacy of wound healing, presence of wound sepsis, weight changes, and general progress. Unfortunately, wound healing and general progress could only be gauged by subjective judgment and were as good, fair, poor, or bad. The only objective findings of this study were the presence of weight gain and positive nitrogen balance in the TPN patients and of weight loss and negative nitrogen balance in the non-TPN patients. On the basis of clinical judgment, the postoperative course was considered to have been "smoother and more satisfactory" in the patients on TPN.

The Holter and Fischer Study.[25] These authors reported a study in which they provided TPN for 72 hours before operation to a group of patients with gastrointestinal malignancies who had lost ten pounds of body weight over the preceding two or three months. A group of patients with similar diagnoses and weight loss was randomized not to receive preoperative total parenteral nutrition. A third group of patients without weight loss was used as controls. Age, sex, and extent of disease were not reported. Patients in the TPN group received approximately 2000 calories and 80 gm of protein hydrolysate or amino acids per day. No other components of the solutions were reported. Patients in the TPN group were fed intravenously after surgery for ten days or until 1500 kcal/day were taken orally. Patients in the TPN group had increases in serum albumin level and body weight. No difference was detected in the incidences of either major or minor complications among the groups. The authors concluded that the duration of the course of TPN might have been too short to provide nutritional repletion. We would concur that it is doubtful that nutritional deficiencies that have developed over many months could be corrected with only 72 hours of preoperative nutritional support.

The Heatley Study.[26] A prospective randomized trial of preoperative total parenteral nutrition was conducted in 1979 in Cardiff, South Wales. Patients with cancer of the esophagus and stomach were randomized by year of birth to one of two groups. Group 1 included 36 patients who were encouraged to eat and drink as much as possible of either a standard hospital diet or a liquid diet that contained 3000 calories and 15 gm of nitrogen and vitamins. The amount of diet actually consumed was not reported. In Group 2, 39 patients were provided with the same diet as Group 1 and also received intravenous nutrition in the form of Aminoplex 5. This product contained synthetic L-amino acids, with ethanol and sorbitol as the energy substrates. Patients in the TPN group received 40 kcal/kg of body weight per day. Solutions were infused by gravity drip through a catheter inserted into an antecubital vein. TPN was given for seven to ten days immediately before operation. The two groups were comparable as to mean age, male-to-female ratio, and diagnoses.

Nutritional status at admission and concomitant disease(s) were not reported. Two patients in the control group who underwent esophageal anastomoses received postoperative intravenous nutrition for five days. The remaining patients did not receive intravenous nutrition after surgery.

A rather high incidence of catheter complications was encountered. Intravenous catheters were replaced 25 times in 17 patients owing to swelling of the arm, occlusion of the catheter, or infection. This occurrence may have been related to placement of the catheters via the antecubital vein. Two patients had documented thrombosis of the subclavian vein. In both cases, catheter tips were located in the subclavian vein and not in the superior vena cava. There was one episode of catheter sepsis.

Postoperative follow-up and assessment included measurements of body weight, duration of hospital stay, tests of immune function, and serum chemistry evaluation. Wound infection was diagnosed according to the presence of purulent discharge or erythema and induration of the incision.

The findings of this study included a reduction of mortality and of three measurements of morbidity (anastomotic leakage, wound infection, and other infections) in the TPN group. Only in the case of wound infection did this difference reach statistical significance. Of those patients who underwent total gastrectomies, five developed anastomotic leakage (two of the ten TPN patients, three of the nine controls). One of the two patients in the control group who underwent an esophagectomy developed an anastomotic leak that closed spontaneously after 15 days of intravenous nutrition. There was no significant difference between incidences of anastomotic disruption in the groups.

Nine patients in the TPN group had infection in sites other than the wound in the TPN group, and 16 in the control group. This difference was not significant. Wound infection was significantly lower in the TPN group (three of 39) than in the control group (11 of 36). Patients with serum albumin levels below 3.5 gm/dl at the time of admission had an even greater reduction in the incidence of wound infections: none of eight in the TPN group, and five of nine in the control group. No differences were found in the results of immunologic tests in the two groups.

Several questions arose from this study. First, patients on TPN showed a large urinary urea excretion; however, no data were reported as to the actual nitrogen and calorie intakes. If one assumes full consumption of oral feedings, patients seemed to have been in negative to marginally positive nitrogen balance. The authors stated that most of the amino acids provided were converted to urea and excreted. The caloric sources, ethanol and sorbitol, may have accounted for the apparently low nitrogen retention values. The authors also reported that patients complained frequently of feeling unwell when the solution was infused faster than the recommended rate; these complaints may have been related to the ethanol content of the solutions. No mention was made of energy expenditure of the patients, either measured or estimated, or whether nutritional support was tailored to meet estimated requirements. The authors stated that the three major complications in the study were problems with the intravenous cannula, folate deficiency, and deep vein thrombosis. The use of a long catheter from the antecubital fossa and the malpositioning of the catheters that resulted in subclavian vein thrombosis presumably led to some of the complications. The exact incidence of folate deficiency was not reported.

The authors concluded that the small benefit of a reduced wound infection rate had to be evaluated against the morbidity, cost, and time required by TPN.

The Thompson Study.[27] All patients with gastrointestinal cancers who were admitted to the surgical service of the Pittsburgh VA Medical Center during a certain interval were eligible for this study. Twenty patients without history of weight loss were used as well-fed controls. Twenty-one patients with a weight loss of more than ten pounds within the preceding three to six months were randomized to receive either TPN for a mean of eight days prior to surgery and during the postoperative course (12 patients) or no TPN (nine patients). Patients were not matched for sex, age, or extent of disease. Patients in the TPN group received 40 to 50 kcal/kg/day as glucose-based TPN. Protein, mineral, and vitamin contents of the TPN were not reported. Intake for the other groups was not reported. Serum albumin levels and delayed cutaneous hypersensitivity were measured before and at the end of the study. Serum albumin levels in the control group were higher preoperatively; however, there were no differences in these levels among the groups at the end of the study. Postoperative complications were equally distributed among the three groups. One abscess and one colocutaneous fistula occurred in the well-nourished control group. In the malnourished control group, one patient had an intra-abdominal abscess. In the TPN group, one patient developed an empyema and one a pelvic abscess. Minor complications did not differ among groups. Only two deaths occurred, both in the well-nourished control group. There was one complication of TPN, a pneumothorax at the time of catheter insertion. The authors concluded that no difference in complication rates could be detected among the three groups and that a larger number of patients would be required to make definitive conclusions.

The Müller Study.[28] Müller and associates, in Cologne, West Germany, studied 125 surgical patients with cancer of the gastrointestinal tract. Malnutrition was defined as: the presence of a weight loss greater than five kilograms over the preceding three months, serum albumin levels below 3.5 gm/dl, and/or a negative response to delayed hypersensity skin testing. Surprisingly, nutritional status was not considered as a criterion for randomization or admission into the study. Patients were allocated in a random fashion either to receive or not to receive TPN before surgery. The control· group received a regular hospital diet; however, no mention was made of the amount of food actually consumed. The TPN group received a solution composed of amino acids at 1.5 gm/kg/day and glucose at 11 gm/kg/day. Electrolytes, trace elements, and vitamins were added to the nutrient solution. Patients received TPN for ten days before surgery and again postoperatively until they resumed oral intake. The nutritional intake after operation in the control group was not given.

Sixty-six patients were entered into the TPN group, although only 41 per cent were considered to be malnourished at the time of admission. The control group included 59 patients, 62 per cent of whom were classified as malnourished on admission. The groups were comparable as to age, sex, tumor localization and stage, preoperative risk factors, and type and duration of surgical procedure. Several biochemical and immunologic parameters were monitored. Postoperative morbidity and mortality rates were calculated. Major complications were defined as the occurrence of intra-abdominal abscesses, peritonitis, anastomotic leakage, and ileus. Wound infections and pneumonia were reported separately.

Complication rates in both groups and mortality in the control group were high. The incidence of wound infections was above 20 per cent in both groups, and pneumonia occurred in 40 per cent of the control group and 30 per cent of the TPN group. The overall major complication rate was 30 per cent in the control group and nearly 20 per cent in the TPN group. The mortality rate was 18.6 per cent in the control group and 4.5 per cent in the TPN group.

As noted, the group that received TPN had significantly fewer major complications and postoperative deaths. Necropsies were performed in 13 of the 14 patients that died, and in 11 of these, the cause of death was a complication at the site of operation. Two patients succumbed from pneumonia, but the final cause of death was complication of an anastomotic leak. Complications of TPN included a subclavian artery puncture, one pneumothorax, and two episodes of catheter sepsis.

This study has been justifiably criticized for including well-nourished patients in the TPN group. It is logical to question why TPN should reduce surgical complications in the absence of malnutrition. If it does so, could the effects of TPN be independent of total nutritional repletion? Could the same results be obtained more economically by infusing only some of these components (e.g., amino acids, vitamins, or minerals)? Despite these very valid criticisms, the Müller study is the most confirmatory report in favor of preoperative TPN.

Retrospective Studies

The Mullen Study.[15] Mullen and associates reviewed the clinical course of patients who received at least a seven-day course of preoperative TPN. Nutritional status was retrospectively determined by a prognostic nutritional index (PNI).[37] The hospital course of the TPN group was compared with that of a similar population that did not receive TPN before surgery. The two groups showed no apparent differences in nutritional status or other important variables. Analysis of the malnourished group of patients revealed that preoperative TPN reduced postoperative complications 2.5-fold, postoperative major sepsis six-fold, and mortality five-fold.

The Daly Study.[16] The effect of preoperative TPN was retrospectively assessed in malnourished patients with esophageal cancer. The outcomes for patients who received a five-day course of preoperative TPN was compared with those for a similar group of patients with esophageal cancer who did not receive TPN preoperatively during the same period. A historical control group treated before the use of TPN was also analyzed. The groups were similar in age, sex, tumor stage, and treatment modality. The TPN group, however, had more complications on admission and appeared to have a poorer preoperative nutritional status. Postoperatively, there was no difference in major organ failure or mortality rates among the groups. There was a significant reduction in rates of major wound infection and anastomotic complications in the TPN group.

Conclusion. These retrospective reports only imply the association of preoperative TPN with improved clinical outcome and are subject to the criticism of pretreatment bias.

POSTOPERATIVE TPN

The use of TPN solely in the postoperative period constitutes a separate issue. The theoretic advantage of repleting the malnourished patient prior to the operative procedure is lost when TPN is administered only postoperatively. TPN initiated early in the postoperative period, before the patient is able to receive complete enteral nutrition, improves nitrogen balance and restores the plasma levels of transferrin and prealbumin.[12, 13] As with the use of preoperative TPN, the question remains whether the observed improvement in nutritional indices correlates with an improved postoperative course.

Two prospective, randomized studies have been reported that evaluated the clinical outcome of patients receiving solely postoperative TPN.

The Abel Study.[30] Abel and associates reported a 1976 randomized controlled study that investigated the effect of poor nutrition on the results of cardiac surgery. Immediate postoperative nutrient repletion via TPN was given in an attempt to favorably influence the postoperative course. Candidates for this study included all patients over 18 years of age who were to undergo open heart procedures. Malnourished patients were identified as those with a history of recent weight loss (greater than 4.5 kg in the preceding 12 months), a body weight less than 15 per cent below ideal, or the clinical impression of malnutrition. A control group of nonmalnourished patients (22 patients) who were to undergo similar procedures was also selected. The malnourished group (44 patients) was then randomized for two treatment protocols. One group (24 patients) received total parenteral nutrition following completion of heart surgery. TPN was continued for five to six days, with an average daily calorie and nitrogen delivery of 1000 kcal and 5 gm, respectively. Oral intake was allowed as soon as the endotracheal tube was removed. The remaining 20 patients were included as malnourished controls. Both the malnourished and nonmalnourished control groups received normal maintenance intravenous fluids with gradual liberalization of their diets, which were unrestricted by the end of the first postoperative week.

The findings of this study revealed that those patients judged to be malnourished had less satisfactory results after cardiac procedures than the well-nourished patients. Complications were more common in the malnourished patients than in the well-nourished controls. The malnourished TPN group developed more postoperative complications than the malnourished non-TPN group.

Although this study identified the adverse effects of preoperative malnutrition on the results of cardiac surgery, it failed to demonstrate benefit from the early postoperative administration of TPN at an intake level of 1000 kcal/day and 5 gm/day nitrogen. No significant differences were detected in nitrogen balance between the TPN group and the malnourished non-TPN control population. This lack of significant difference may reflect inadequate calorie/nitrogen supplementation of the TPN group. The nutrition supplied to the TPN patients was insufficient to improve nitrogen balance and, therefore, may have been of inconsequential nutritional benefit. No other nutritional indices were reported to further confirm this hypothesis. Inasmuch as no nutritional benefit was observed in the TPN group, the lack of clinical improvement was not surprising.

The Hill Study.[12, 13, 31] The second postoperative TPN study was reported by Collins and associates from Leeds in 1978. They studied patients who underwent abdominoperineal resections for benign or malignant diseases. By closely matching for age, weight, previous weight loss, and diagnosis, these researchers divided 30 patients into three groups. Group I did not receive nutritional therapy except for routine maintenance intravenous fluids. Group II received only 4.25 per cent amino acids by central venous catheter, equivalent to 0.23 ± 0.02 gm/kg/day of nitrogen. Group III received a full course of TPN that consisted of amino acids equivalent to 0.23 ± 0.02 g/kg/day of nitrogen and 25 per cent glucose equivalent to 36.5 ± 3.5 kcal/kg/day. Amino acid or TPN infusions were begun on the second or third postoperative day and were continued for approximately 13 days. The nutritional indices, which were matched preoperatively and followed postoperatively, included plasma protein levels (transferrin, prealbumin, retinol-binding protein, albumin), body composition, and plasma amino acid levels.

This study revealed no significant differences in septic morbidity or mortality among the three groups. Compared with the amino acid and control groups, the TPN group showed a significantly shorter healing time for perineal wounds and also a significant decrease in the length of hospital stay. Weight loss was observed in the control and amino acid groups. Positive nitrogen balances were obtained in the amino acid and TPN groups. Plasma protein levels, which were decreased in all three groups postoperatively, were restored to normal in only the TPN group. Similarly, TPN spared more body protein and fat and restored plasma amino acids to normal levels. This study elegantly presented the beneficial effect of administering adequate postoperative TPN, which not only improved abnormal nutritional parameters but also enhanced clinical outcome.

SUMMARY AND CONCLUSIONS

It is obvious from the preceding analysis that a conclusion cannot be reached as to the efficacy of perioperative total parenteral nutrition. Most of the studies that we reviewed had design deficits. Study variables, especially TPN formulations and amount of nutrients consumed by control patients, were not always available or well defined. Despite these criticisms, most studies of preoperative TPN showed a trend toward better results in the TPN-treated patients, and the Müller study[28] "sanctified" this trend with statistical significance. Similarly, the Collins study[31] demonstrated a significant improvement in outcome in patients who were treated solely with postoperative TPN. The inability of the other studies to achieve statistically significant results may have been due to the rather small groups of patients that were studied in the presence of many unmatched variables.

On the basis of the aforementioned trends in the literature, we believe that there is probably a clinically beneficial but small effect from the use of perioperative TPN in selected patients. This effect is probably more evident in the very severely malnourished patient. A definitive conclusion and cost-benefit analysis will be possible only when large-scale, well-controlled, multicenter studies are performed. At this time, a multicenter, randomized clinical trial of preoperative total parenteral nutrition in malnourished surgical patients is underway at ten VA Medical Centers.

In view of the limited number of controlled trials, the question of when to prescribe total parenteral nutrition in the perioperative period remains unanswered. One option is to withhold its use until conclusive reports from clinical trials confirm its efficacy. This approach will certainly save money, but it might deny potential benefits to needy patients. Furthermore, it may be impossible to unequivocally prove or disprove the value of perioperative TPN. Our approach is to prescribe TPN selectively in the perioperative period for the indications shown in Table 20–2.

TPN has undeniably improved the survival of those patients with short-bowel syndrome (see Chapter 25); the use of TPN in the treatment of enterocutaneous fistulas is not as well defined as initially expected (see Chapter 24). However, if high fistula output precludes the use of the enteral route, TPN is indicated. In our opinion, patients who

Table 20–2. INDICATIONS AND CONTRAINDICATIONS FOR PERIOPERATIVE TOTAL PARENTERAL NUTRITION

Indications	Short-bowel syndrome
	High-output enterocutaneous fistula
	Prolonged postoperative ileus
	NPO status for more than 1 week during medical management or preoperative workup
	Severe malnutrition (80% of usual body weight or serum albumin levels <3.0 gm/dl)
Relative indications	Low-output enterocutaneous fistula
	Moderate malnutrition (80–90% of usual body weight or serum albumin level 3.0–3.5 gm/dl)
Contraindications	Ability to be fed enterally
	Terminal disease with poor prognosis
	Adequate nutritional status

develop postoperative ileus for longer than seven days should be started on TPN. Preoperative evaluations, such as endoscopies, radiographic procedures, and bowel preparations, frequently impair adequate nutrient intake. TPN is advised if the period of impaired intake is expected to exceed one week in a patient who is to undergo major surgery. Similarly, malnourished patients who are potential surgical candidates and whose medical treatment involves receiving nothing by mouth for longer than one week should be given TPN. Examples of these circumstances include management of gastric outlet obstruction secondary to ulcer disease, treatment of inflammatory bowel disease, and the conservative management of bowel obstruction. Finally, preoperative TPN should be provided to those patients in need of major surgery who are severely malnourished, as defined by a 20 per cent loss of body weight or a serum albumin level less than 3.0 gm/dl.

It is suggested that perioperative TPN for the moderately malnourished patient (as defined by a recent weight loss of ten to 20 per cent of usual body weight and/or a serum albumin level of 3.0 to 3.5 gm/dl) should be used selectively. Variables such as magnitude of proposed surgery, age of patient, rate of occurrence of malnutrition, and associated illnesses should be considered. We suggest that these patients may benefit from nutritional repletion. TPN should be administered to these patients only after the potential risks, costs, and benefits are assessed.

Total parenteral nutrition is contraindicated in several conditions. When the gastrointestinal tract is functioning normally, enteral nutrition, as provided orally or via a feeding tube, is the preferred route. Patients who are adequately nourished and have normal fat and protein stores would receive no potential benefit from TPN under most circumstances. The administration of TPN to patients with terminal malignancies or with very poor prognoses is, in most instances, unjustifiable. We do not recommend that TPN be given to such patients if other therapies (antineoplastic, surgical, antibiotic, etc.) are not being considered. In general, TPN is not indicated for those patients whose diseases preclude extraordinary treatment modalities.

We conclude that despite the many unanswered questions concerning the use of total parenteral nutrition in the perioperative period, evidence is supportive of its safe and efficacious prescription to a select group of patients.

REFERENCES

1. Butterworth, E.E., and Blackburn, G.L.: Hospital malnutrition and how to assess the nutritional status of a patient. Nutrition Today (Mar.-Apr.) Teaching Aid #18, 1976.
2. Hill, G.L., Pickford, I., Young, G.A., Schorah, C.J., Blackett, R.L., Burkinshaw, L., Warren, J.U., and Morgan, D.B.: Malnutrition in surgical patients. An unrecognized problem. Lancet, 1:689, 1972.
3. Bistrian, B.R., Blackburn, G.L., Hallowell, E., and Heddle, R.: Protein status of general surgical patients. J.A.M.A., 230:858, 1974.
4. Rombeau, J.L., Goldman, S.L., Apelgren, K.N., et al.: Protein-calorie malnutrition in patients with colorectal cancer. Dis. Colon Rectum, 21:587, 1978.
5. Mullen, J.L., Gertner, M.H., Buzby, G.P., Goodhart, G.L., and Rosato, E.F.: Implications of malnutrition in the surgical patient. Arch. Surg., 114:121, 1978.
6. Studley, H.O.: Percentages of weight loss: A basic indicator of surgical risk in patients with chronic peptic ulcer. J.A.M.A., 106:458, 1936.
7. Rhoads, J.E., and Alexander, C.E.: Nutritional problems of surgical patients. Ann. N.Y. Acad. Sci., 63:268, 1955.
8. Hickmann, D.M., Miller, R.A., Rombeau, J.L., Twomey, P.L., and Frey, C.F.: Serum albumin and body weight as predictors of postoperative course in colorectal cancer patients. J.P.E.N., 4:314–317, 1980.
9. Lewis, R.T., and Klein, H.: Risk factors in postoperative sepsis: significance of preoperative lymphopenia. J. Surg. Res., 26:365, 1979.
10. Harvey, K.B., Ruggiero, J.A., Regan, C.S., et al.: Hospital morbidity-mortality risk factors using nutritional assessment. J. Clin. Nutr., 26:581, 1978.
11. Goodgame, J.T.: A critical evaluation of the results of total parenteral nutrition in various disease states: Cost and benefit. In Fischer, J.E. (ed.): Surgical Nutrition. Boston, Little, Brown, 1983, p. 179.
12. Young, G.A., Collins, J.P., and Hill, G.L.: Plasma proteins in patients receiving intravenous amino acids or intravenous hyperalimentation after major surgery. Am. J. Clin. Nutr., 32:1192, 1979.
13. Young, G.A., and Hill, G.L.: A controlled study of protein-sparing therapy after excision of the rectum. Ann. Surg., 192:183, 1980.
14. Sims, J.M., Oliver, E., and Smith, J.A.R.: A study of total parenteral nutrition in major gastric and esophageal resection for neoplasia (abstract). J.P.E.N., 4:422, 1980.
15. Mullen, J.L., Buzby, G.P., Mathews, D.G., et al.: Reduction of operative morbidity and mortality by combined pre-operative and postoperative nutritional support. Ann. Surg., 192:604–613, 1980.
16. Daly, J. M., Massar, E., Giacco, G., et al.: Parenteral nutrition in esophageal cancer patients. Ann. Surg., 196:203–208, 1982.
17. Gibbons, G.W., Blackburn, G.L., Harken, D.E., et al.: Pre- and postoperative hyperalimentation in the treatment of cardiac cachexia. J. Surg. Res., 20:439–444, 1976.
18. Eisenberg, H.W., Turnbull, R.B., and Weakley, F.L.: Hyperalimentation as preparation for surgery in transmural colitis (Crohn's disease). Dis. Colon Rectum, 17:469–475, 1974.
19. Allardyce, D.B.: Pre-operative parenteral feeding in Crohn's disease: Pre-operatively, to induce remission and at home. Am. Surg., 44:510–516, 1978.
20. Frazier, T.G., Copeland, E.M., Khalil, K.G., Dudrick, S.J., and Mountain, C.F.: Intravenous hyperalimentation as an adjunct to colon interposition for carcinoma of the esophagus. Cancer, 39:410–412, 1977.
21. Balzola, F., Bianco, L., Boggio-Bertinent, A., and Domeniconi, D.: La Renutrizione preoperatoria nei pazienti affetti da stenosi dell'esofago. Minerva Med., 69:3435–3444, 1978.
22. Dietel, M., Alexander, M., and Hew, L.R.: Hyperalimentation and cancer. Can. J. Surg., 23:11–13, 1980.
23. Lim, S.T.K., Choa, R.G., Lam, K.H., Wong, J., and Ong, G.B.: TPN versus gastrostomy in the preoperative preparation of patients with carcinoma of the esophagus. Br. J. Surg., 68:69–72, 1981.
24. Moghissi, K., Hornshaw, J., Teasdale, P.R., and Dawes, E.A.: Parenteral nutrition in carcinoma of the esophagus treated by surgery: Nitrogen balance and clinical studies. Br. J. Surg., 64:125–128, 1977.
25. Holter, A.R., and Fischer, J.E.: The effects of hyperalimentation on complications in patients with carcinoma and weight loss. J. Surg. Res., 23:31–34, 1977.
26. Heatley, R.V., Lewis, M.H., and Williams, R.H.P.: Pre-operative intravenous feeding—a controlled trial. Postgrad. Med. J., 55:541–545, 1979.
27. Thompson, B.R., Julian, T.B., and Stremple, J.T.: Peri-operative total parenteral nutrition in patients with gastrointestinal cancer. J. Surg. Res., 30:497–500, 1981.
28. Müller, J.M., Dienst, C., Brenner, U., and Pichlmaier, H.: Preoperative parenteral feeding in patients with gastrointestinal carcinoma. Lancet, 1:68–71, 1982.
29. Rombeau, J.L., Barot, L.R., Williamson, C.E., and Mullen, J.L.: Preoperative total parenteral nutri-

tion and surgical outcome in patients with inflammatory bowel disease. Am. J. Surg., *143*:139, 1982.

30. Abel, R.M., Rischer, J.E., Mortimer, J.B., et al.: Malnutrition in cardiac surgical patients: Results of a prospective randomized evaluation of early postoperative parenteral nutrition. Ann. Surg., *111*:45, 1976.

31. Collins, J.P., Oxby, C.B., and Hill, G.L.: Intravenous amino acids and intravenous hyperalimentation as protein-sparing therapy after major surgery. A controlled clinical trial. Lancet, *1*:788, 1978.

32. Twomey, P., Ziegler, D., and Rombeau, J.: Utility of skin testing in nutritional assessment: a critical review. J.P.E.N., *6*:50, 1982.

33. MacBurney, M., and Wilmore, D.W.: Rational decision making in nutritional care. Surg. Clin. North Am., *61*:571, 1981.

34. Williams, R.A., Heatley, R.V., Lewis, M.H., et al.: A randomized controlled trial of preoperative intravenous nutrition in patients with stomach cancer. Br. J. Surg., *63*:667, 1976.

35. Lehr, L., Schober, O., Hundeshagen, H., et al.: Total body potassium depletion and the need for preoperative nutritional support in Crohn's disease. Ann. Surg., *196*:709, 1982.

36. Mueller, J.M., Brenner, M., Roecki-Mueller, C., and Pichlmaier, H.: Preoperative parenteral nutrition in surgery for carcinoma of the upper GI tract—a prospective randomized trial. J.P.E.N., *5*:570, 1981.

37. Buzby, G.P., Mullen, J.L., Matthews, D.C., et al.: Prognostic nutritional index in gastrointestinal surgery. Am. J. Surg., *139*:150, 1980.

CHAPTER 21

Malnutrition and Inflammatory Bowel Disease: Indications for and Complications of Parenteral Nutritional Support

DANNY O. JACOBS
ROLANDO ROLANDELLI
ROBERT FRIED
JOHN L. ROMBEAU

Inflammatory bowel disease (IBD) refers to a group of chronic disorders that, in addition to affecting the bowel and other organ systems, commonly affect nutrient intake and absorption. Disease activity is often directly influenced by the patient's nutritional status. Thus, maintenance of adequate nutrition is an important consideration in the management of patients with inflammatory bowel disease. Because many patients with IBD are unable to eat, they need to be fed parenterally. In this chapter, we discuss the prevalence and etiology of malnutrition and review the nutrient needs of, as well as the therapeutic role of parenteral nutritional support in, patients with inflammatory bowel disease.

PREVALENCE OF MALNUTRITION IN IBD

One of the problems of documenting malnutrition in any group of patients is the manner in which the term *malnutrition* is defined. This has been the subject of many recent reviews.[1-5] The most useful and perhaps most accurate assessments are those that address the relationship of malnutrition to clinical outcome. Clinical outcome is markedly affected by protein and calorie deficits in patients with IBD. Body weight and serum albumin levels, two indices that are thought to be measures of protein calorie malnutrition, are easily determined in most hospitals.

The relationship of weight loss to disease activity in IBD has been studied extensively. Crohn and Yarnis[6] noted a 70 per cent incidence of weight loss in patients with regional ileitis. Weight loss is also fairly common in patients with ulcerative colitis. Incidences of 18 to 62 per cent have been reported.[7] More recently, efforts have been directed to defining the amount and rate of weight loss that is clinically significant. Dudrick and colleagues[8] and Mullen and associates[9] introduced the concept of *significant weight loss* as measured weight loss over time and identified losses of 0.2 per cent of the usual weight per day over seven days as an important index of malnutrition.

Hypoalbuminemia is frequently observed in patients with IBD. Driscoll and Rosenberg[10] estimated the incidence of hypoalbuminemia to be 25 to 80 per cent in patients with Crohn's disease and 25 to 50 per cent in patients with ulcerative colitis. Mullen and co-workers,[11] in a ten-year review of 74 patients with IBD, found a mean serum albumin level of 2.9 ± .13 gm/dl. Similarly, deDombal[12] studied 46 ulcerative colitis patients with "severe" attacks and found a mean serum albumin level of 3.34 gm/dl.

ETIOLOGY OF MALNUTRITION IN IBD

Many factors may be responsible for malnutrition in patients with IBD, including decreased nutrient intake, greater nutrient needs, increased nutrient losses (e.g., protein-losing enteropathy), malabsorption, and surgical complications.

Decreased Intake and Greater Nutrient Need

Anorexia commonly accompanies the active phase of IBD; however, its etiology is uncertain.[11] Nevertheless, as would be expected, the oral intake of patients with active IBD is often decreased. As in other disease states, multiple factors, including malaise, weakness, and mineral deficiencies (zinc, copper, nickel, and niacin), may alter taste and smell. Some or all of these factors may be active in patients with IBD.[13-16] Nutrient intake may also be influenced by disease activity. Nitrogen balance studies have shown strong correlations between disease activity and decreased nitrogen uptake and increased urinary nitrogen excretion.[17] Catabolic stress secondary to intra-abdominal sepsis may increase nutrient requirements in patients with IBD.[11] Peritonitis increases the metabolism of endogenous protein and elevates resting energy expenditures to 40 per cent above normal.[18] Bistrian and colleagues[19] suggested that serum albumin concentrations would decrease to less than 3.5 gm/dl as a result of the "response to catabolic stress" and hypocaloric infusions of carbohydrate. Hill and associates[3] studied 74 IBD patients in an effort to identify those patients at risk for malnutrition. The authors divided the study patients into six groups on the basis of disease activity: group 1, patients with ileostomies for more than one year's duration;

group 2, patients whose disease had been in remission for seven to eight years; group 3, patients admitted for elective surgery with chronic continuous disease; group 4, patients with acute attacks (moderate to severe disease); group 5, patients requiring urgent surgery (severe colitis); and group 6, patients who developed post-operative complications (e.g., sepsis, fistulas). Weight loss was demonstrated in all groups except group 1. Mean serum albumin and transferrin levels were significantly lower in groups 4, 5, and 6 than in controls.

Although the studies just cited could not control for the numerous other causes of malnutrition in IBD, they do reinforce the theory that malnutrition is related to catabolic stress and is reflected in disease activity. Patients with malnutrition and active IBD have a diminished ability to convert from the catabolic phase of stress to the anabolic phase of convalescence. Moore and Brennan[20] described that phenomenon as "late nutritional failure" and noted that it was commonly accompanied by failure of fistulas to close, poor wound healing in general, and immunoincompetence.

Protein-Losing Enteropathy

The mechanisms of hypoproteinemia in IBD have been examined extensively. An early study by Steinfeld and co-workers,[21] conducted at the National Institute of Health, documented exudative protein loss in patients with IBD. Using ^{131}I-labeled albumin and polyvinylpyrrolidine (PVP), a water-soluble and nonmetabolizable macromolecule, the authors were able to demonstrate logarithmic relationships between albumin turnover and total exchangeable albumin over time. In this prospective trial, low serum albumin, circulating albumin, and total exchangeable albumin concentrations were found in patients with IBD. The authors also found an overall increase in albumin degradation (8.6 per cent in patients vs. 4.8 per cent in controls, expressed as percentage of total body albumin per day), unimpaired albumin synthesis, and higher fecal excretion of labeled parenteral albumin in patients than in controls. On the basis of their data, an absorptive defect could not be absolutely excluded; however, the exudative loss of protein into the gut was strongly implicated as the primary mechanism of hypoproteinemia. Because there was also a higher fecal loss of

PVP, the loss of protein into the gut lumen was believed to be nonspecific.

Jarnum and associates[22] further characterized the protein loss in IBD using ^{59}Fe-labeled dextran. Fecal losses of this macromolecule were higher in ten patients with Crohn's disease. Albumin "catabolism" was positively correlated with the excretion of ^{59}Fe in the feces. In addition, an inverse relationship between albumin catabolism and serum albumin levels was demonstrated.

Studies conducted by Beeken and colleagues[23] and Nygaard and Rootwelt[24] confirmed these early findings. Their studies cited mucosal ulceration or lymphatic obstruction as causes of protein-losing enteropathy in IBD. It was suggested that sites of protein leak could occur in either small or large bowel.[25]

More recently, it has been suggested that gastrointestinal protein loss in IBD may be similar to renal protein loss in the nephrotic syndrome.[25,26] There is also evidence that alpha$_1$-antitrypsin could serve as an inexpensive marker of protein-losing enteropathy in patients with IBD.[27]

Malabsorption

Primary malabsorption of essential nutrients has been proposed as yet another mechanism of malnutrition in IBD.[11,28] Small bowel mucosal abnormalities have been noted in patients with IBD, and there have been attempts to link these abnormalities with deficiencies of intestinal absorption, digestion, and enzymatic function.[29,30]

Initial investigations into structural and enzymatic changes of the bowel mucosa in patients with IBD were reported by Salem and Truelove.[31,32] These authors studied a group of 63 ulcerative colitis patients and a control group consisting of 27 patients with irritable bowel syndrome, 14 patients with psoriasis, and 14 patients with anemia. Mucosal changes as noted via light microscopy were graded 1 through 4, with grade 1 changes rated as normal. The normal mucosa had villi with "slender finger-like projections" on microscopic examination. Grade 4, or subtotal villous atrophy, was described as a mucosal surface devoid of villi. Variations from the normal villous architecture were graded according to villous height. Their findings were as follows: Three of 52 controls had abnormal villous architecture of a mild (grade 1 to 2) degree. Fourteen of 60 (23 per

cent) ulcerative colitis patients had pronounced (grade 3 to 4) villous abnormalities. Although these studies were not controlled for age or sex, were not analyzed statistically, and did not review the histologic slides in a blinded fashion, several important questions regarding mucosal function were raised: Are there mucosal changes in the radiologically normal areas? Is ulcerative colitis indeed a diffuse lesion of the GI tract? Are these mucosal changes related to disease activity? Are these mucosal changes associated with abnormalities of small bowel absorption or digestion?

Later studies confirmed the presence of mucosal abnormalities in both ulcerative colitis and Crohn's disease in areas that did not appear to be affected on radiologic or histologic study.[30,33-36] Researchers have found villous abnormalities of the intestinal mucosa in areas of the bowel that appeared to be grossly unaffected by IBD.[29-32,34] Collectively, these works suggest that IBD is a diffuse lesion of the gastrointestinal tract.

There are conflicting findings from at least two well-controlled studies concerning the mucosal changes seen in IBD and their relationship to disease activity.[30,34] The study by Dunne,[30] published in 1977, suggests that there is no association between mucosal changes and disease activity as measured by serum albumin, hemoglobin, or serum mucoid level.

Abnormalities of small bowel digestive function, as measured by disaccharidase activity, have been associated with mucosal atrophy in several disease states, including adult celiac disease, tropical sprue, and kwashiorkor.[37-42] It has been suggested that disaccharidase deficiencies may contribute to malnutrition by provoking nausea, vomiting, and diarrhea.[43,44] These deficiencies appear to be related to abnormalities of mucosal microvilli. Disaccharidase deficiency in IBD has also be studied.[30,32,45,46] Lactase deficiency occurs in patients with IBD but probably with no greater frequency than in normal populations.[45,46] Moreover, it has been suggested that a factor other than lactose may contribute to milk intolerance in these patients.[46] Deficiencies of other disaccharidases have been reported.[30,33] In addition to the direct effects of IBD on intestinal absorption, malabsorption may occur secondary to indirect effects of disease, such as the blind loop syndrome and surgical resection. In Crohn's disease, overgrowth of the normal small bowel flora occurs secondary to partial obstruction due to fistulas or bypassing of loops of bowel. Bacterial overgrowth has generally not been considered a problem in ulcerative colitis, although there have been reports of bacterial contamination of the small bowel after a Koch pouch ileostomy.[47]

Clinical features of the blind loop syndrome that produce protein calorie malnutrition include steatorrhea, carbohydrate malabsorption, and reduced serum protein concentrations. Steatorrhea generally occurs in the blind loop syndrome if the stagnant loop involves the duodenum or jejunum. The etiology of steatorrhea in the blind loop syndrome is thought to be related to alterations in bile salt metabolism induced by the contaminating bacteria. Certain bacterial species, especially *Bacteroides*, are able to deconjugate bile salts and form free bile acids that are poorly soluble at the low pH of the upper intestine. The resulting precipitated bile acids may form crystals that readily enlarge to form enteroliths. If the rate of deconjugation is sufficiently great to reduce the concentration of conjugated bile acid below that necessary for micelle formation, steatorrhea results. Furthermore, anaerobic bacteria may aggravate steatorrhea by dehydroxylating triglycerides into free fatty acids that have a greater water solubility and are therefore lost more easily in liquid stools. Carbohydrate malabsorption is fairly common with blind loop syndromes and may be identified by detection of impaired D-xylose absorption.[48-51]

Finally, patients with blind loop syndrome may develop hypoproteinemia.[51,52] Serum protein concentrations may fall as low as those seen in protein-calorie malnutrition.[53,54] The precise mechanism by which this protein deficit occurs is unknown.

Surgical Complications

Protein-calorie malnutrition occurs in patients with Crohn's ileitis who have undergone ileal resection. The clinical abnormalities that result include vitamin B_{12} deficiency, diarrhea, steatorrhea, an increased incidence of cholelithiasis, renal calculi, and dyslipoproteinemia.[28,55-58]

Steatorrhea, diarrhea, cholelithiasis, and renal calculi in these patients are all manifestation of "broken" enterohepatic circulation and the resultant bile salt wastage. It is well known that bile salts allow water-insoluble fatty acids to exist in diffusible form.[59] It was also observed quite early that bile salts are absorbed poorly from the jejunum but rapidly from the ileum.[28] The observation that distal small bowel resection (i.e., ilectomy) resulted in fat malabsorption was first proposed in several animal studies.[58,60] These findings were later confirmed in humans with bile salt malabsorption and steatorrhea after ileal resection.[58]

The size of the bile salt pool and the turnover rate have been estimated by isotope-labeled bile salt dilution techniques. After labeled salts are given orally or parenterally, enteral samplings are performed and bile salt activity is measured over time. By this method, the size of the normal bile acid pool has been estimated at 3 to 4 gm with a half-life of 3.9 days. Normally, more than 90 per cent of bile salts are reabsorbed in the enterohepatic cycle. When bile salt reabsorption is interrupted (e.g., by ilectomy), bile salts are lost in the ascending colon. These losses are normally compensated for by hepatic synthesis. The normal liver can increase bile salt synthesis by ten- to 20-fold when the bile salt pool size is decreased. Using the isotope dilution technique, researchers have been able to quantify the degree of bile salt malabsorption after ilectomy and have correlated the extent of resection and the length of disease in the excised segment with the degree of bile salt wastage. Hofmann[61] could not demonstrate a significant increase in fecal bile salts with resections of less than ten centimeters of distal ileum. However, he was able to demonstrate a greater than 50 per cent increase in the concentration of fecal bile salts with a 30-cm distal ileal resection and an 80 per cent increase with a distal ileal resection of more than 90 cm. A poor correlation exists between fecal bile salt concentration and the length of disease in the ileal segment.

Experimentally, when approximately 100 cm of distal ileum is resected or diseased, hepatic synthesis can no longer compensate for fecal bile salt wastage, the bile salt pool contracts, and steatorrhea results.[58,61] This condition is manifested by ineffective bile salt micelle formation, and malabsorption of fat and the fat-soluble vitamins, A, D, E, and K. In addition, diarrhea occurs once the enterohepatic circulation is disrupted by the transformation by bacteria of bile salts to conjugated dihydroxy bile salt forms. These conjugated bile salts are very similar in structure to the active cathartic agent in castor oil, ricinoleic acid, and are known to decrease colonic fluid and electrolyte absorption and to stimulate colonic secretion and motility (see later discussion).[62-64]

Ileal resection in Crohn's disease patients may also affect serum lipoprotein concentrations. Bile salt malabsorption decreases serum cholesterol, presumably by increasing hepatic bile salt synthesis from serum cholesterol. The small intestine also secretes fatty acids into the serum in the form of very-low-density lipoproteins (VLDL). Johansson[65] found a negative correlation between the length of resected intestine and total serum cholesterol (low-density and high-density lipoproteins).[65] Total serum triglyceride concentrations were maintained in all patients despite limited fat intake and ileal resection. Johansson suggested that lipolysis might be increased in these patients in order to supply free fatty acids to the liver to be used for triglyceride synthesis, as generally occurs with catabolism and stress.

Anemia

Anemia occurs in both ulcerative colitis and Crohn's disease and is thought to be closely related to the patient's nutritional status. Twenty-five to 85 per cent of patients with Crohn's disease have anemia.[66-69]

The pathogenesis of anemia in patients with Crohn's disease is most likely multifactorial, whereas the anemia of patients with ulcerative colitis is thought to occur primarily from a single cause. Causes of anemia in Crohn's disease include deficiencies of iron, folate, and B_{12} or a combination of these factors.[66-70]

A number of indices, such as the peripheral smear, serum transferrin saturation, bone marrow iron stores, and serum ferritin and iron concentrations, and TIBC, have been used to determine the incidence of iron deficiency. These indices are unreliable, however, in establishing a diagnosis of iron deficiency anemia in IBD patients, because of the difficulty in differentiating the anemia of iron deficiency from the anemia of chronic disease. Serum iron studies may overestimate the incidence of iron deficiency in IBD patients. The serum iron level has been shown to be decreased in up to 65 per cent of patients with Crohn's disease; however, bone marrow iron stores were low in only 39 per cent of the same patients.[66-68] Examination of bone marrow iron stores is the most sensitive determinant of iron deficiency anemia.

It is however, a subjective, semiquantitative, and invasive measure.

The overall incidence of iron deficiency in ulcerative colitis patients has been estimated to be 36 per cent on the basis of bone marrow studies and is the primary cause of anemia in these patients. Iron deficiency in ulcerative colitis patients has long been believed to be secondary to intestinal ulceration and fecal blood loss, although blood has not always been demonstrable in the feces.

Iron deficiency anemia frequently occurs in Crohn's disease patients. Bone marrow examinations confirm the presence of iron deficiency anemia in 22 to 44 per cent of all cases.[66-69] Numerous pathophysiologic mechanisms have been proposed, including decreased intake, excessive losses, and malabsorption of iron compounds.

Megaloblastic anemia occurs primarily in patients with Crohn's disease, with an incidence of approximately 79 per cent.[28,66] Low serum folate concentrations are found in 62 to 80 per cent of Crohn's disease patients with megaloblastic anemia.[70]

Several reports have suggested that malabsorption is the primary cause of megaloblastic anemia in patients with IBD. Although the proximal small bowel is known to be the primary site of folate absorption, there has been no study effectively linking disease in this area with folate malabsorption.

Theoretically, chronic inflammation, and thereby increased inflammatory cell production, could lead to higher utilization of folate and megaloblastic anemia when intake is insufficient. Evidence to support this theory comes from Dyer and Dawson,[28] who found hypercellular marrows with increased numbers of leukocytes and their precursors as well as low serum folate levels in patients with active Crohn's disease. Finally, Gerson and colleagues[71] suggested that reduced dietary intake of folate is responsible for megaloblastic anemia in Crohn's disease patients in whom vitamin B_{12} levels are normal. In all probability, the etiology of folate deficiency in Crohn's disease is multifactorial.

The incidence of B_{12} deficiency in unoperated Crohn's disease patients is estimated to be 16 to 39 per cent.[71] Dyer and Dawson[28] noted significantly lower serum B_{12} levels in unoperated patients with Crohn's disease than in controls. Some patients had severe vitamin B_{12} deficiencies.

Both bacterial overgrowth and Crohn's disease of the stomach contribute to vitamin

B_{12} malabsorption in patients with Crohn's disease. The severity of vitamin B_{12} malabsorption varies with the amount and severity of distal ileal disease. Megaloblastosis and megalocytosis of small intestinal crypts and villous cells have been noted and are associated with abnormalities of B_{12} absorption.[68,69] Certainly, malabsorption of fat and B_{12} occurs before and after intestinal resection in patients with Crohn's disease.[66-68] Bacterial overgrowth, especially of obligate anaerobes like *Bacteroides*, can result in fat and vitamin B_{12} malabsorption.[54,72] Impaired intestinal motility is thought to be an important predisposing factor to bacterial overgrowth and B_{12} deficiency.

NUTRITION AND GROWTH RETARDATION IN CHILDREN WITH IBD

Failure to grow and gain weight is a prominent feature of IBD in some prepubertal patients. Growth retardation has been noted to affect 16 to 58 per cent of young people with Crohn's disease and from two to 20 per cent of young people with ulcerative colitis.[73,74]

The growth retardation of IBD in adolescent patients is characterized by short stature. Height and weight are proportional, but skeletal maturation is retarded. Puberty is delayed, as is the development of secondary sexual characteristics. Occasionally, these abnormalities may become manifest years before the colitis is clinically evident.

When examining affected children, it is important to differentiate the pathologic growth retardation of patients with IBD from genetic short stature. Pathologic growth retardation is characterized by deceleration of height and weight on growth curves such as the Tanner growth standards. Radiologic bone age is also a useful diagnostic tool. Patients with pathologic growth retardation generally manifest a bone age one or two years behind their chronologic age.

Several mechanisms have been proposed to explain the growth retardation seen in IBD patients, including the use of steroid therapy, nutritional abnormalities, and hormone deficiencies.[75] However, protein-calorie malnutrition is now recognized as a major cause of growth retardation in youngsters.[76]

Chronic caloric deprivation can cause a characteristic form of growth retardation known as nutritional dwarfing.[75-78] This disorder is characterized by a depressed linear growth. In this syndrome, weight is proportional to height. Growth retardation in IBD is similar in character to that in nutritional dwarfing.[79] Numerous reports cite reversal of growth retardation with intensive protein calorie repletion or with the supplementation of dietary intake with trace metals.[73,79-81]

Normal skeletal growth and maturation depend on the proper interaction of hormones secreted from the thyroid and adrenal glands. Several investigators have examined these hormones in growth-retarded children with IBD. McCaffery and colleagues[82] examined several hormones in a group of 130 youngsters with ulcerative colitis and Crohn's disease. The indices examined included urinary gonadotrophins, 17-ketosteroids, 17-hydroxycorticosteroids, protein-bound iodine, basal metabolic rate, T_3 resin uptake, pre-thyroxine, 24-hour radioactive iodine uptake, and the response of serum growth hormone to insulin-induced hypoglycemia. These researchers also reported low urinary gonadotrophins in four patients, equivocally low thyroid function tests in four other patients, and a depressed growth hormone response to insulin-induced hypoglycemia in 11 of 13 patients tested. On the basis of their data, the authors suggested that some patients with IBD have an acquired secondary hypopituitarism. Other investigators who examined thyroid and adrenal function in children with IBD have found no evidence of hypopituitarism.[81,83,84]

McCaffery and colleagues,[85] in a second study, administered growth hormone over six months to three children with Crohn's disease and growth retardation. They could not detect accelerated growth in these youngsters.

The response of growth hormone to a number of different provocative tests, including arginine, propranolol, and L-dopa tests as well as sleep induction, have been found to be normal.[81,83,84] The response of growth hormone to insulin-induced hypoglycemia, has been varied, but most authors have observed decreased responsiveness. Gotlin and Dubois,[84] in a study of three children, noted that high blood insulin levels were accompanied by comparative decreases in serum glucose. These authors suggested that a decreased tissue response to insulin exists in growth-retarded children with IBD; such a decrease could also explain the reduced response of serum growth hormone to insulin-induced hypoglycemia.

Growth hormone is thought to act through intermediary small polypeptide hormones called somatomedins. These hormones are thought to be secreted by the liver and to exert a positive effect on linear growth through their action upon cartilage. Tenore and associates[83] and others have hypothesized that there is a nutritionally related deficit of somatomedin levels that causes growth retardation in youngsters with IBD. Although this hypothesis is quite attractive, depressed somatomedin levels have not yet been demonstrated in subsequent studies of growth-retarded children with IBD.

NUTRIENT REQUIREMENTS AND DEFICIENCIES IN INFLAMMATORY BOWEL DISEASE

Severe inflammatory bowel disease predisposes patients to fluid and electrolyte imbalances. Patients with Crohn's disease, especially those with colonic involvement, may develop sodium and potassium deficiencies secondary to chronic diarrhea and an inadequate electrolyte intake. Diarrheal losses in patients with severe ulcerative colitis can cause significant dehydration and electrolyte depletion. Children are especially prone to develop these electrolyte abnormalities. Excessive losses of some cations, especially magnesium and zinc, and their respective deficiency syndromes are described in patients with inflammatory bowel disease.[13,86] Therefore, cation losses in inflammatory bowel disease are clinically important.

Small Intestine and IBD

The normal small intestine has a great capacity to absorb nutrients and a tremendous functional reserve. Normally, carbohydrate, fat, most vitamins, and trace minerals are absorbed in the proximal small intestine. A large amount of the intestine may be diseased, bypassed, or resected before nutrient absorption is impaired. In addition, the small bowel has the ability to adapt. Undiseased or unresected normal small bowel can increase its absorptive capacity to compensate for the loss of normal activity in diseased areas. Diarrhea, steatorrhea, and nutrient malabsorption can be expected to occur only when the reserve capacity of the small bowel

is exceeded. In patients with inflammatory bowel disease, especially Crohn's disease, varying amounts of bowel are affected, and thus their absorptive capacities are impaired to different degrees.

The intestinal absorption of fluids and electrolytes in diseased segments and grossly normal segments of bowel has been studied in patients with Crohn's disease. The absorption of water and electrolytes from diseased bowel roughly correlates with disease severity.[87] Studies suggest that the intestinal mucosa in Crohn's disease may not function normally with respect to electrolyte transport. This holds true for both involved and grossly uninvolved tissue from the small intestine. Abnormal fluid and electrolyte transport can be further aggravated by osmotic and secretory effects of malabsorbed nutrients (e.g., carbohydrates and fatty acids).

Effects of Ileal Resection

It is clear that extensive disease of the small bowel, particularly the ileum, or extensive small bowel resection can impair the absorption of bile acids and induce fat malabsorption. Bile acids and fatty acids reduce colonic absorption and can cause a net secretion of fluid into the colonic lumen. Ricinoleic acid, which is the major active ingredient of castor oil and is used to simulate endogenous overload of the colon by fatty acids, inhibits the net absorption of water and electrolytes by the colon.[58,88] This substance at higher doses can also induce fluid secretion, as mentioned previously.[58,88] The mechanism by which bile acids and fatty acids induce secretion is uncertain at present, but it may be secondary to the effects of these agents on adenylate cyclase activity.[89] Increased adenylate cyclase activity elevates mucosal cyclic AMP levels, which in turn increase chloride secretion. Other possible mechanisms of action for bile and fatty acids include direct mucosal damage[90] and a bile acid–induced increase in colonic motility and transit time.[91] The effects of resection of the ileum and colon on diarrhea are directly related to the amount of bowel removed. In this instance, the mechanism appears to involve the loss of colonic surface area for absorption and a decrease in production of short-chain fatty acids, which diminish sodium absorption.[92] Diarrhea due to ileal resection appears to vary directly with the amount of colon resected or the extent of disease in the colon. When the amount of fatty acids and/or bile acids reaching the colon is increased as a result of disease or surgery and the absorptive capacity of the colon is exceeded, diarrhea results.

Pathologic Changes in the Colon

Disturbances of fluids and acid-base balance typically occur as a result of colonic disease only when the disease is severe and acute. Losses of fluids and electrolytes from the inflamed colon are in the ranges of 100 to 1500 ml of fluid, 10 to 70 mM of sodium, and 20 to 50 mM of potassium daily.[93] A metabolic or mixed alkalosis may occur in patients with severe ulcerative colitis, in contrast to the metabolic acidosis that commonly occurs in other diarrheal states. Excess chloride is lost in the stools, suggesting defective chloride and bicarbonate exchange.[93,94] The mechanism of sodium loss in patients with severe colitis is thought to be due to a decreased flux of sodium from mucosa to serosa in the face of relatively normal sodium secretion.[95] Alternatively, back-diffusion of sodium may occur, so that absorbed sodium leaks back into the lumen because of enhanced mucosal permeability.[96] In vivo studies have demonstrated impaired absorption of sodium, water, chloride, and potassium in patients with ulcerative colitis and Crohn's colitis.[97,98]

Recent studies have investigated the role of prostaglandins in electrolyte and fluid transport.[99-101] Much of this work is preliminary in nature. In vivo dialysis studies of inflammatory bowel disease patients have demonstrated decreased sodium and water absorption and increased potassium secretion in association with an increased flux of prostaglandin E_2.[99] However, infusions of prostaglandin E_2, which did increase ileal flow, did not affect colonic absorption.[100] Campieri and associates[101] did not detect any beneficial effects of the use of prostaglandin inhibitors in patients with ulcerative colitis. Increased prostaglandin release in patients with colitis may merely reflect changes induced by colonic inflammation as a general phenomenon.

Energy Requirements

Barot and colleagues[102,103] have determined the energy requirements of nonseptic patients with inflammatory bowel disease using indirect calorimetry. They also found that patients with weight losses of greater than 10 per cent of their ideal body weight have higher energy expenditures than would be estimated using the Harris-Benedict formula.[102,103] This difference between measured energy expenditure and calculated basal energy expenditure is thought to be secondary to elevated disease activity. For example, it appears that patients with a Crohn's disease activity index (CDAI) greater than 225 have an increase in Na^+, K^+-ATPase activity measured as the number of ouabain binding sites per erythrocyte.[104] Under normal conditions, the human organism may expend 30 to 40 per cent of its energy in sodium-potassium pump exchange activity. An increase in activity of 30 per cent above the normal level could account for the ten per cent difference in energy expenditure noted by Barot and colleagues.[102,103]

These investigators suggest that in the absence of significant weight loss or sepsis, inflammatory bowel disease does not significantly alter basal metabolism, and that calculations of the basal energy expenditure (BEE) based on the Harris-Benedict formula are statistically equivalent to the resting energy expenditure obtained with indirect calorimetry. In general, calorie requirements for nonseptic, fairly weight-stable patients are 1.75 times the BEE. The level of caloric intake should provide sufficient calories to promote anabolism and/or to minimize weight loss where appropriate. It should be remembered that the energy requirements of patients with IBD may be extremely variable. In situations where multiple stress factors are combined with acute changes in nutritional status, techniques such as indirect calorimetry that measure the actual energy expenditure may be preferable.

Carbohydrate and Fat Requirements

Little research has been done to determine which energy substrates are optimal, if any, in patients with inflammatory bowel disease. For the patient without complications, energy needs can be met with typical concentrated dextrose sources. In patients in need of parenteral feeding, an intravenous lipid source is added twice weekly to meet the requirements for essential fatty acids. As yet, there is no evidence that patients with IBD need to be treated any differently, in terms of energy substrates, from any other critically ill patient requiring parenteral nutrition. Parenteral formulas should be administered carefully in order to avoid overfeeding of carbohydrate, which may aggravate or induce hepatic dysfunction in patients with IBD.

Protein Requirements

As noted, patients with Crohn's disease may have reduced pancreatic enzymatic output, so the rate of proteolytic digestion may be impaired by as much as 30 per cent.[105] In addition, mucosal disease may interfere with peptide and amino acid absorption, and bacterial overgrowth can interfere with protein homeostasis.[72,106] Rutgeerts and co-workers[72] noted that the activation of proteolytic enzymes was impaired and brush border peptidase activity reduced in patients with bacterial overgrowth. Furthermore, severe protein malnutrition may result from small bowel overgrowth.[54] Bacteria that catabolize tryptophan and tyrosine to produce indicans and phenols may cause a deficiency of these amino acids and impair host synthesis.[107] Free amino acid transport may also be impaired.[108] These changes, coupled with the loss of endogenous plasma proteins from inflamed mucosa, can accelerate the rate of protein loss in patients with IBD. For these reasons, patients may present with severe protein deficiency, and their protein requirements may be greater than anticipated— especially when diarrhea, steatorrhea, hematochezia, or melena continues.

Vitamins

Vitamin balance is altered only when the small intestine, which is the primary site of vitamin absorption, is affected by significant disease. Recent evidence suggests that the transport of vitamins, especially those that are water soluble, across the small bowel is mediated by membrane-bound carriers. The absorption of vitamin C, thiamine, riboflavin, nicotinic acid, biotin, folic acid, inositol, and choline appears to be dependent on mucosa-serosa sodium gradients, suggesting a sodium-coupled transport system.[109,110] Theoretically, anorexia in the presence of reduced vitamin intake and malabsorption could lead to deficiency states.

Defective fat digestion and absorption may cause the fat-soluble vitamins, D, A, K, and E, to be malabsorbed as well. Vitamin D deficiency occurs in patients with Crohn's disease and probably reflects reduced dietary intake and malabsorption.[111]

Trace Minerals

Mineral deficiencies are now being characterized in patients with inflammatory bowel disease. Iron deficiency is commonly found in patients with Crohn's disease, as discussed earlier. Dietary intake may be inadequate and requirements may be increased because of acute or chronic blood loss. Cox and O'Donnell[112] have suggested that there are high-affinity iron binding sites in the intestine that mediate absorption across the microvilli. It is not known whether the number of binding sites is decreased in Crohn's disease or whether the number of these sites fails to increase in the presence of iron deficiency.

Symptomatic magnesium deficiency has also been reported in patients with inflammatory bowel disease.[13,113,114,115] The clinical importance of magnesium deficiency relates not only to skeletal muscle function but also to cardiac muscle function. Levine and associates[115] reported a case of ventricular tachycardia secondary to magnesium deficiency in a patient with ulcerative colitis who was receiving TPN. Main and co-workers[113] surveyed serum magnesium levels in patients with IBD during intravenous alimentation and noted hypomagnesemia in 36 per cent of all IVH periods in eight patients with severe IBD. Fifty per cent of the patients followed as outpatients continued to have low magnesium levels in association with severe diarrhea and steatorrhea. Two-thirds of these patients were symptomatic. Main and co-workers[113] concluded that because magnesium deficiency may be a long-term problem in IBD patients with severe diarrhea, magnesium supplementation is warranted. They recommended that at least 5 mM of magnesium per day are needed to maintain or replete patients with IBD. In normal adults, only about one-third of all ingested magnesium is absorbed; less may be absorbed in malabsorptive states and after surgical resections.[113] In another study, Main and co-workers[114] measured serum and 24-hour urine magnesium concentrations and noted magnesium depletion in 15 of 17 (88 per cent) patients with severe Crohn's disease. Serum magnesium levels were lower in patients with Crohn's disease than in a group of matched hospitalized controls. Urine levels were also decreased in most patients and appeared to be more sensitive indicators of magnesium depletion than serum levels alone.

Other researchers have not found significant hypomagnesemia in patients with IBD who receive total parenteral nutrition.[116] The appearance of symptomatic magnesium deficiency varies both with the intracellular magnesium concentration and with the amount of magnesium bound to protein.[116] Magnesium is a true intracellular cation. Thus, serum and urine magnesium levels may not reflect the body's true magnesium status, and there may be no correlation between serum magnesium levels and total body magnesium stores. Nevertheless, patients with IBD, especially Crohn's disease, would appear to be at risk for magnesium deficiency. Severe uncontrolled diarrhea would appear to be a major predisposing factor.[13] A significant amount of magnesium may be bound to lipid and lost in steatorrhea.[117] Magnesium deficiency is also seen in patients with diarrheal disorders other than IBD.[118]

Patients with inflammatory bowel disease, especially Crohn's disease, may also develop zinc deficiencies.[86,117,119] Zinc is important for nucleic acid and protein synthesis and is therefore very important for normal growth and healing. The gut is the main excretory route for zinc,[120] but the contribution of intestinal secretions and epithelial desquamation to fecal zinc levels is unknown. Solomons and associates[86] noted that plasma zinc levels correlate well with plasma albumin concentrations. Possible causes of zinc deficiency include: anorexia and hypogeusia, decreased absorption by disease bowel secondary to disease or surgery, internal redistribution secondary to the production of leukocyte endogenous mediator, serum hypoalbuminemia, as mentioned previously, and excessive losses from inflamed mucosa. McClain and colleagues[121] proposed that zinc malabsorption plays a primary role in the etiology of zinc deficiency in patients with Crohn's disease, because when these patients were given an oral dose of zinc, their serum zinc levels are much lower than those of controls. Very low serum zinc levels have been noted in growth-retarded adolescents with Crohn's disease.[86]

In most instances, it is not clear whether zinc deficiency results from a deficient dietary intake or from increased losses secondary to diarrhea. In many patients, both mechanisms may be active. As with magnesium, it is difficult to determine the body's zinc status precisely, because serum and urine zinc levels are indirect guides to intracellular zinc concentrations. Main and associates[122] surveyed serum and urine zinc levels in ten patients with IBD before and during 59 patient weeks of intravenous nutrition. The authors found these levels to be significantly less than in control patients. However, no patients with IBD developed signs of zinc deficiency before or during therapy. Furthermore, there was no significant change in serum zinc concentrations despite improvements in anthropometric characteristics, the achievement of positive nitrogen balance, and improvements in serum albumin and transferrin concentrations. IBD serum zinc levels remained significantly lower than control levels despite the provision of intravenous zinc supplements. Urine zinc levels increased by a mean of 11-fold during IVH, and a positive relationship was noted between zinc uptake and urine zinc excretion. The authors proposed that zinc supplied by the intravenous route could be inefficiently transported to the tissues. Zinc administered intravenously chelates with amino acids and sugars to form low-molecular-weight complexes, which can be filtered into the urine. Main and associates[122] stated that decreased zinc levels in Crohn's disease are not simply secondary to decreased albumin concentrations, because serum zinc levels do not necessarily increase in IBD patients in whom serum albumin levels rise. In the opinion of these researchers, anabolism in the face of an inadequate supply of zinc is responsible for the clinical syndromes of zinc deficiency when they occur.

Mills and Fell[123] confirmed these findings when they studied total plasma and 24-hour urinary zinc levels in 40 patients with IBD who were not being treated with steroids. They found no significant disturbance of serum zinc levels in patients with active Crohn's disease or inactive ulcerative colitis. However, significantly high urinary zinc excretion was noted in patients with ulcerative colitis, and the level of zincuria was related to the severity of the ulcerative disease. Mills and Fell[123] hypothesized that urinary zinc excretion was closely related to muscle protein catabolism. Amino acid–zinc complexes released by muscle catabolism can be ultra-filtered by the kidneys. Crohn's patients would have the additional factor of zinc malabsorption. Fecal excretion of zinc could be higher in Crohn's patients than in patients with ulcerative colitis, thereby modifying their urinary response. In summary, in this study by Mills and Fell,[123] no biochemical evidence for acute zinc deficiency could be found in patients with IBD, but tissue zinc depletion could not be ruled out. Other researchers have commented on the role of leukocyte endogenous mediator (LEM) in stimulating the uptake of amino acids by the liver and thereby lowering the ultrafilterable amino acid–bound zinc fraction.[122] Plasma zinc levels and the amount of zinc available for excretion would be lowered as a consequence of the action of LEM.[122] Differences in disease activity and therefore in LEM release may account for the different incidences of hypozincemia reported in patients with IBD.[123,124]

Solomons and Rosenberg[124] have summarized the current concepts of zinc metabolism in inflammatory bowel disease. Hypoalbuminemia can be associated with reduced serum zinc levels. Malabsorption, exudative losses, and hyperzincuria can all contribute to zinc deficiency in patients with IBD and may be responsible for the varying incidences of hypozincemia noted by different researchers. Finally, patients with severe zinc losses who required intravenous repletion typically are in a negative nitrogen balance. On the basis of current knowledge, Solomons and Rosenberg[124] note that one can expect to find a substantial number of patients with active IBD in whom serum zinc levels are decreased. However, a decrease in serum zinc concentrations does not necessarily imply low or abnormal total body zinc stores, because a reduced albumin binding capacity or LEM-mediated redistribution could account for decreased serum levels without significantly altering body zinc stores. Patients with severe disease and significant diarrhea may need zinc supplementation, because they are at increased risk for zinc deficiency. Along with other trace elements, zinc should be added to the parenteral alimentation formulas of patients with IBD.[125,126] Solomons and Rosenberg[124] raise one final important issue—controlled therapeutic trials have yet to answer the question of whether zinc supplementation in zinc-depleted patients with IBD improves healing of inflammatory lesions or reverses growth retardation.

TOTAL PARENTERAL NUTRITION AND INFLAMMATORY BOWEL DISEASE

TPN may be used as adjunctive, supportive, or primary therapy. Typically, TPN is used in patients who are being prepared for surgery, who develop postoperative complications with transitory gut failure, or who undergo massive intestinal resections and have permanent gut failure. In these instances, the goal of TPN is to replete or maintain the nutritional status.

Patients with inflammatory bowel disease may require TPN in all of the aforementioned circumstances. More frequently, TPN may be indicated for patients whose IBD is refractory to medical treatment. When classic medical treatment fails to control an exacerbation of inflammatory bowel disease, the patient is usually started on "bowel rest." Although he or she may improve symptomatically with this regimen, nutritional depletion will progress if only standard intravenous solutions of five per cent dextrose are provided. Until the introduction of TPN, adequate nutrition with bowel rest was an impossibility in patients with severe inflammatory bowel disease.[127-129] The advent of TPN has made the use of bowel rest nutritionally feasible and has prompted consideration of TPN, bowel rest, and anti-inflammatory medications as primary therapy in IBD.

Although Crohn's disease and ulcerative colitis share several pathologic features, the overall prognosis, success of surgical therapy, and long-term sequelae are different for each condition. Therefore, it is essential that the two diseases be analyzed separately in consideration of TPN as primary therapy. On the other hand, the benefits of perioperative TPN, as either adjunctive or supportive therapy, are more likely due to improvements in nutritional status than to effects on disease activity. For this reason, the results of perioperative TPN in Crohn's disease and ulcerative colitis may be analyzed inclusively.

In this section we review the published trials of TPN and IBD that have addressed the following issues: (1) TPN as primary therapy in Crohn's disease; (2) TPN as primary therapy in ulcerative colitis; (3) Preoperative treatment of IBD with TPN; and (4) Complications of TPN in IBD.

TPN as Primary Therapy in Crohn's Disease

TPN is considered primary therapy for Crohn's disease when it is indicated after failure of standard medical treatment but surgical treatment is not performed. Medical treatment may or may not be continued during TPN. In 1973, Anderson and Boyce[130] studied six patients with advanced Crohn's disease who were treated with TPN as primary therapy. The effectiveness of TPN was assessed on the basis of changes in weight and serum albumin levels, the presence or absence of abdominal pain and diarrhea, and radiographic findings. Clinical improvement was achieved in five patients, although none had radiographic improvement. In all cases, symptoms returned within three months after TPN was discontinued. One patient received two courses of TPN. Although the first course was successful in controlling clinical symptoms, the second course was not and the patient developed catheter sepsis.

In 1973, Fischer and associates[131] reported a series of IBD patients treated with TPN at the Massachusetts General Hospital; this experience was updated in 1976 by Reilly and colleagues.[132] In these studies, a total of 23 patients received TPN for either enteritis or enterocolitis. Fourteen of 23 patients experienced clinical remissions, whereas in the remaining nine patients, TPN failed to induce remission, and surgery was required. One of the patients who required surgery for Crohn's enterocolitis died in the postoperative period owing to systemic candidiasis.

Vogel and co-workers[133] reported their experience with TPN as primary therapy in eight patients with Crohn's disease. Clinical remission was achieved in seven patients, allowing steroid requirements to be reduced in five patients and withdrawn in two. Unfortunately, at follow-up periods of four months to three years, only four patients remained symptom free. Eisenberg and associates[134] reported nine patients who were treated with TPN as primary therapy for Crohn's disease. Three were patients with short-bowel syndrome, three had intestinal fistulas, and the remaining three severe malnutrition. Remission was obtained in five patients. One of the patients with fistulas healed spontaneously. One patient on TPN improved considerably. Therapy failed in two patients, including one with short-bowel syndrome who died.

Greenberg and colleagues[135] conducted a prospective study of 43 patients, who were then treated with TPN for an average of 25 days after they had failed to respond to other forms of therapy. There were four indications for treatment: enteric fistulas (14 patients), obstruction (4), inflammatory masses (14), and unremitting disease (11). There was evidence of clinical improvement in 33 of the 43 patients. Of 32 patients available for follow-up at two years, 29 remained in remission.

Fazio and co-workers[136] reported a five-year experience with 18 patients who received TPN as primary therapy for Crohn's disease. The indications were short-bowel syndrome, intestinal fistulas, inadequate response to conventional therapy, and malnutrition. TPN was successful in 11 patients, but the other seven patients had to undergo surgical treatment. Long-term follow-up of these patients was reported by Harford and Fazio,[137] who found that only four patients had not had some surgical treatment within 27 months of the original remission.[137]

In Mullen's group of 33 patients with Crohn's disease who were treated with TPN as primary therapy, 19 patients responded well and did not require surgery during their index hospitalizations, but nine had recurrence of the disease at six months to ten years.[138] In a series of patients discussed by Driscoll and then reported by Elson and colleagues,[139] 20 patients with Crohn's disease were treated with TPN. Thirteen patients improved clinically during the original hospitalization, but during follow-up periods of two to four years, only three remained symptom free. In eight of the ten patients reported by Holm,[140] TPN was used for primary treatment. Clinical improvement was obtained in seven patients, but three of these had recurrence within 18 to 72 months. Shiloni and Freund[141] reported that six of nine patients with Crohn's disease responded to TPN as primary treatment.

Recently, Müller and associates[142] published a prospective study on the effects of TPN as the sole therapy in Crohn's disease. TPN was administered through a permanent Silastic catheter to 30 patients with Crohn's disease for three weeks in the hospital and then nine weeks at home. In five patients disease was not controlled by this therapy and they underwent surgery. Seventeen of the 25 patients who experienced remission had recurrences within 48 months.

The results of all of the studies cited are summarized in Table 21–1. This table includes only those patients who reportedly

Table 21–1. RESULTS OF TPN GIVEN AS PRIMARY THERAPY FOR CROHN'S DISEASE

STUDIES	NO. PATIENTS	NO. DAYS OF TPN	NO. REMISSIONS	NO. IMPROVEMENTS	NO. FAILURES	FOLLOW-UP† (MONTHS)	NO. RECURRENCES
Anderson et al.[130]	6	30	—	5	—	14	5
Fischer et al.[131] and Reilly et al.[132]	23	32	14	—	9	—	—
Vogel et al.[133]	8	32	5	2	1	4–36	3
Eisenberg et al.[134]	9	32	5	2	2	4	1
Greenberg et al.[135]	43	25	33	—	10	24	14
Fazio et al.[136] and Harford and Fazio[137]	18	20	11	—	7	20–45	5
Mullen et al.[138]	33	26	19	—	14	6–120	8
Elson et al.[139]	20	36	8	5	7	20–45	5
Holm[140]	8	71	4	3	1	18–72	3
Müller et al.[142]	30	84	25	—	5	12–48	17
Shiloni and Freund[141]	9	45	6	—	3	—	—
Totals	207	—*	130	17	60		63
Rates	—	—	62.8%	8.2%	28.9%		54.78%
			147	71.0%			

*Average no. TPN days for whole group: 39.36 ± 19.17.
†Follow-up was reported in nine studies accounting for 175 of the 207 patients, 115 of whom initially had remission.

received TPN as primary treatment and not those who received TPN as perioperative support. For this reason, the number of patients listed for each study may differ from the total number discussed in the report of the study. When one considers these 207 patients as one group, the overall success rate for TPN is 71 per cent. In 62.8 per cent (130 patients), "remission" was achieved, and in 8.2 per cent (17 patients), condition improved. A large variety of TPN formulas were administered for a mean of 39.9 ± 19.1 days. The calculated overall success rate is in agreement with the remission rates reported in each study individually. One hundred seventy-five of the 207 patients were followed for periods ranging from four months to ten years, during which more than half of the patients whose disease originally remitted had recurrences; when these patients are excluded from the success category, the overall success rate is reduced to 36.5 per cent.

Müller and associates[142] surveyed recurrence rates over three separate periods. Whereas the overall remission rate was 83 per cent at six weeks, it was reduced to 56.6 per cent by the first year and to 23.3 per cent at four years. When these patients were compared with historic controls who underwent surgical resections, the recurrence rate was four times higher in patients who received only TPN. The use of historic controls is of questionable validity, however. Furthermore, the comparison is less than ideal, because the goal of TPN as primary therapy is to avoid a surgical resection, rather than to achieve better perioperative results. Nevertheless, this study does underscore the over-all failure of TPN as primary therapy in patients with Crohn's disease.

Recently, Lochs and co-workers[143] reported a prospective study in which patients were randomized to receive TPN with and without bowel rest. Patients were entered into the study when they weighed less than 80 per cent of ideal body weight and/or the Crohn's disease activity index (CDAI) was above 150. Medications were discontinued in all but three patients. Subjects randomized to the study group were maintained NPO, and they received TPN and bowel rest. Patients in the control group were allowed to have a low-residue liquid diet *ad libitum* in addition to TPN. TPN was discontinued when the patients reached at least 80 per cent of ideal body weight and their CDAIs were reduced by 40 per cent. Patients in both groups gained weight and CDAIs fell; however, there were no significant differences between the two groups with respect to these two variables. The authors concluded that if TPN has any beneficial effect in the treatment of IBD, it is not related to bowel rest.

It is clear that, with the exception of biopsy techniques, which obviously cannot be used routinely, there is no reliable method to assess disease activity. The indices evaluated in most clinical studies, such as general well-being, body weight, and nutritional status, reflect nutritional status rather than disease activity. It is not necessarily surprising that these indices improve. Unfortunately, none of the improvements has been proven to correlate with remission of the pathologic features of Crohn's disease. The relative inefficacy of using these nutritional indices to assess disease activity is demonstrated by the high incidence of recurrences found after remissions.

TPN as Primary Therapy in Ulcerative Colitis

There are two main differences between ulcerative colitis and Crohn's disease that must be considered in an analysis of the effects of TPN on disease activity in IBD. First, in ulcerative colitis, disease is restricted to the colon, with minimal or no small bowel involvement. Second, patients with ulcerative colitis may be cured by surgical treatment, i.e., total colectomy. Patients with small bowel involvement tend to have more severe nutritional deficits and may have more favorable responses to bowel rest. One must consider that curative surgical therapy of patients with inflammatory bowel disease may be delayed by efforts to use TPN as primary therapy.

Truelove and colleagues[144] developed an intravenous regimen, which included nutrients, corticosteroids, and antibiotics, for patients with severe attacks of ulcerative colitis. This regimen, the exact composition of which was not described, was administered centrally over four days while the patients were kept NPO. In 100 courses of this intravenous regimen, a temporary remission was obtained in 75 per cent of cases of severe colitis. Fifty-two per cent of the patients were in remission at six weeks, and 33 per cent at 31 months. Dickinson and associates[145] reported the results of a prospective study in which patients with acute colitis were randomized to receive either TPN or a regular hospital diet. Most of these patients (27 of 36) had ulcerative colitis, and those with Crohn's disease had only large bowel in-

volvement. All patients followed a strict steroid-weaning schedule and were evaluated as to whether or not TPN accelerated steroid withdrawal or enabled avoidance or delay of surgery. The initial remission rates were the same in the two groups, as were the recurrence rates over four months to three years. An interesting observation in this study was the discordance between total body nitrogen content and body weight. Although patients in both groups gained weight, those who did not receive TPN lost a mean of 108 gm of total body nitrogen as measured by neutron activation, whereas those who did receive TPN preserved total body nitrogen.

Table 21–2 summarizes the results of these studies, in which TPN was used as primary therapy in ulcerative colitis. When these 60 patients are regarded as a group, the overall success rate of TPN is approximately 48 per cent. Eighteen patients (30 per cent) had remissions, and 11 (18 per cent) improved. Forty-nine patients were followed for between four months and ten years. In sixteen of seventeen patients with initial remission, disease recurred within the follow-up period; when these patients are excluded from the success category, the overall success rate for TPN in ulcerative colitis is then reduced to 24 per cent.

Preoperative TPN in IBD

Some of the aforementioned studies also included patients who received TPN as preoperative treatment. The data for 139 patients are available for analysis (Table 21–3). These patients received TPN for a mean of 24.9 days before operation; 26.6 per cent of them had postoperative morbidity, half of which could be classified as septic complications.

Reilly and associates[132] reported a 20 per

Table 21–2. RESULTS OF TPN GIVEN AS PRIMARY THERAPY FOR ULCERATIVE COLITIS

STUDIES	NO. PATIENTS	NO. DAYS OF TPN	NO. REMISSIONS	NO. IMPROVEMENTS	NO. FAILURES	FOLLOW-UP† (MONTHS)	NO. RECURRENCES
Fischer et al.[131] and Reilly et al.[132]	11	29	1	—	10	—	—
Fazio et al.[136] and Harford and Fazio[137]	5	20	4	—	1	27.3	4
Mullen et al.[138]	17	9	9	—	8	6–120	3
Elson et al.[139]	10	36	1	3	6	44	1
Dickinson et al.[145]	17	21	3	8	6	4–36	8
Totals	60	*	18	11	31		
Rates	—	—	30% 29	18.3% 48.3%	51.6%	—	57.14%

*Average no. TPN days for whole groups: 23 ± 9.0.
†Follow-up was reported for 17 of the 18 patients.

Table 21–3. EFFECTS OF PREOPERATIVE TPN IN INFLAMMATORY BOWEL DISEASE*

STUDIES	NO. PATIENTS	NO. DAYS OF PREOP TPN	NO. OF COMPLICATIONS			LENGTH POSTOP HOSPITAL STAY (DAYS)
			Total	Sepsis	Other	
Fischer et al.[131] and Reilly et al.[132]	19	32	5	NR	NR	27
U.C. TPN	10	23	2	2	—	24
Cont.	16†	—	8	4	4	27.4
Vogel et al.[133]	6	14	1	NR	NR	NR
Eisenberg et al.[135]	25	21	2	—	2	NR
Mullen et al.[138]	24	26	5	—	5	NR
Elson et al.[139]	17	36	6	—	2	NR
Bos[149]	26	37	2	2	—	NR
Rombeau et al.[146]						
TPN	22	11.5	1	1	—	37.7
Cont.	11†	—	5	4	1	31
Totals	139	—†	37	18	7	—
Rates	—	—	26.6%	72%	28%	—

*NR = not reported.
†Average no. days preop TPN for whole group: 24.9.
‡Excluded from the total of patients.

cent incidence of postoperative complications in 10 patients who received TPN for ulcerative colitis preoperatively. When they compared these ten patients with 16 control patients with ulcerative colitis who did not receive preoperative TPN, a slightly higher incidence of complications was observed in the patients who received TPN, but this difference was not statistically significant. The authors suggested that more aggressive procedures were performed in the patients who received TPN. Their theory was indirectly supported by the significantly lower remission rate identified in patients who received preoperative TPN than in those who did not.

Fazio and co-workers[136] published the results of a study of 58 patients with IBD who were also given TPN preoperatively. In 36 patients, surgery proceeded as planned. Surgery was avoided in 13 patients who improved during parenteral alimentation. In nine patients, the surgical plan was modified after the course of TPN was completed. These patients underwent more radical operations than originally planned because their overall physical condition and nutritional status had improved.

Mullen and colleagues[138] reported that 87 per cent of the surgical procedures performed in their patients treated with TPN were resections. They also observed that patients with ulcerative colitis had fewer complications when they received corticosteroids in addition to TPN in the preoperative period.

Rombeau[146] analyzed a group of patients IBD who received or did not receive preoperative TPN. The two groups had similar age and sex distributions, underwent the same types of surgical procedures, and had similar histologic diagnoses. Patients who received preoperative TPN, for a mean of 11.5 days, had significantly fewer postoperative complications (one of 22) than those who did not (five of 11). Hospital stay for the patients who received TPN was slightly longer but not significantly different on statistical analysis.

Complications of TPN in IBD

In general, complications of TPN can be divided into three major categories: (1) mechanical (e.g., pneumothorax, thrombosis, catheter dislodgment, catheter fracture with embolism of catheter fragments); (2) infectious (e.g., catheter sepsis, local infection); and (3) metabolic (e.g., abnormal liver function parameters, mineral deficiencies, electrolyte imbalances, hyperglycemia). Patients with IBD may have higher risks for any of these complications because they may receive multiple courses of TPN over extended periods. For example, the frequency of mechanical complications appears to be higher in patients with IBD owing to repeated subclavian vein catheterizations. Often, alternative routes of intravenous access are needed because of subclavian vein thrombosis.

A case study of a patient who developed a superior vena cava thrombosis after 12 subclavian catheter insertions was reported by Apelgren and co-workers.[147] This patient with Crohn's disease needed direct right atrial catheterization for TPN. Three weeks later, the atrial catheter migrated to the pleural space and induced a pleural effusion and pneumothorax.

The incidence of infectious complications in patients with inflammatory bowel disease who receive TPN varies from 2.1 to 26 per cent (Table 21–4). Although patients with IBD are thought to be predisposed to catheter sepsis, the mean incidence calculated from all reported series is only 7.9 per cent, a figure within the range of incidences reported in surveys encompassing patients with all types of disease.

Abnormal liver function is strikingly frequent in patients with IBD during total parenteral nutritional therapy. Anderson and Boyce[130] reported that SGOT and alkaline phosphatase concentrations were elevated in five of eight patients with IBD. Liver biopsies were performed in three of these five patients but did not reveal any consistent histologic pattern. Hepatic enzymes returned to normal once TPN was discontinued. The TPN formula given to these patients was based solely on carbohydrates for the energy source and provided approximately 67 kcal/kg body weight.

Vogel and associates[133] noted a patient in their series who developed cholestatic jaundice with elevated alkaline phosphatase and SGOT levels. These blood chemistry parameters returned to normal once TPN was discontinued, only to rise again when TPN was restarted. This patient received a TPN formula that provided 72 kcal/kg body weight and used carbohydrate as the only energy source.

In a study by Elson and co-workers,[139] 21 of 30 patients with IBD who received TPN had elevated serum transaminase levels. Eight of these patients also had hepatomegaly and right upper quadrant tenderness. The authors compared the patients with normal and abnormal liver function values. There was no correlation between the presence of abnormal liver function values and age, sex, weight loss before TPN, weight gain with TPN, duration of TPN, or caloric dose. However, patients with hepatic dysfunction had significantly higher rates of weight gain—1.9 ± 0.66 kg/week (2.9 ± 1.4 kg in the week before symptoms), compared with 1.2 ± 0.48 for patients with normal hepatic function (p = 0.01). On the basis of this observation, and in hopes of avoiding hepatic dysfunction, the authors recommended that parenteral prescriptions be adjusted so that weight gain does not exceed one kg/week.

In the prospective study by Müller and associates,[142] all 30 patients with IBD who were treated with TPN had elevated SGOT, SGPT, and alkaline phosphatase concentrations.[142] Four patients had liver biopsies because of intrahepatic cholestasis; histologic examination of the specimens showed fatty infiltration of the peripheral type and pericholangitis. In this study, TPN was given at 30 to 45 kcal/kg body weight. Twenty-five per cent of the total caloric prescription was administered as intravenous lipid. Transient decreases of serum liver function parameters occurred as calorie/nitrogen ratios or relative

Table 21–4. COMPLICATIONS OF TOTAL PARENTERAL NUTRITION IN INFLAMMATORY BOWEL DISEASE*

STUDIES	NO. PATIENTS	MECHANICAL COMPLICATIONS			INFECTIOUS COMPLICATIONS		METABOLIC COMPLICATIONS	
		Pneumothorax	*Thrombosis*	*Other*	*Probable*	*Sepsis*	*Liver Dysfunction*	*Other*
Anderson et al.[130]	8	—	—	—	—	1 (12.5)	5	—
Fischer et al.[131] and Reilly et al.[132]	34	2	—	—	—	6 (17)	—	—
Vogel et al.[133]	15	—	—	—	—	4 (26)	1	2
Eisenberg et al.[134]	46	—	—	2	—	1 (2.1)	(?)	6
Fazio et al.[136]	71	2	1	1	—	—	—	—
Dean et al.[128]	16	—	—	—	—	1 (6.25)	—	—
Mullen et al.[138]	74	3	—	—	—	3 (4)	—	2
Elson et al.[139]	30	—	—	1	4	—	21	20
Bos[149]	115	7	5	3	9	19 (16.5)	7	5
Milewski and Irving[129]	50	—	—	—	—	2 (4)	—	—
Holm[140]	10	—	—	—	—	—	1	—
Shiloni and Freund[141]	19	2	2	—	—	1 (5.2)	—	—
Müller et al.[142]	30	—	—	2	—	3 (10)	—	—
Totals (%)	518	16 (3)	8 (1.5)	9 (1.7)	13 (2.5) 87 (16.8)†	41 (7.9)	35 (6.8)	35 (6.8)

*Numbers in parentheses indicate percentages.
†Excluding metabolic complications.

percentages of fat and dextrose changed, but liver function parameters returned to normal and remained normal only when the patients resumed oral alimentation. Müller and associates[142] proposed that hepatic dysfunction occurs in patients with IBD who receive TPN as a result of overloading the liver with nutrients after it has adapted to malnutrition.

Other clinical studies on the pathogenesis and prevention of hepatic dysfunction during TPN have been performed in patients with IBD. Conclusions from these studies are not necessarily limited to patients with IBD. Fouin-Fortunet and colleagues[148] analyzed bile acids, via duodenal aspiration, from patients with IBD before and after TPN. Whereas lithocholic acid was undetectable or represented less than one per cent of the total bile acid concentration before TPN, it constituted seven to 15 per cent of the total pool in patients who had elevated transaminases and alkaline phosphatase concentrations during TPN. Recently, Capron and co-workers[150] provided more data on the pathogenesis and prevention of hepatic dysfunction during TPN in IBD patients. Sixteen patients with Crohn's disease were randomized to receive TPN with or without the addition of metronidazole (500 mg twice a day). The group who did not receive metronidazole had significantly higher serum alkaline phosphatase, gammaglutamyltransferase, and alanine-aminotransferase concentrations after 30 days of TPN than the group that did receive metronidazole. The authors concluded that metronidazole prevented hepatic dysfunction during TPN by reducing the number of anaerobic bacteria in the intestine. Overgrowth of the intestine with organisms during bowel rest could lead to the production of hepatotoxic substances, e.g., bacterial endotoxins or bile acid metabolites, which may be responsible for the hepatic dysfunction observed in patients with IBD.

CONCLUSIONS

Some conclusions can be formulated concerning the use of TPN in patients with IBD. First, nutritional indices, such as body weight, serum proteins, and nitrogen balance, can be improved in almost all patients, provided that sufficient calories and protein are given. However, nutritional improvement does not necessarily correlate with a reduction of disease activity. Second, a temporary remission can be expected in 70 per cent of patients with Crohn's disease and 50 per cent of those with ulcerative colitis. Approximately half of these patients will still be in remission on follow-up after extended periods. Third, the use of preoperative TPN not only may allow more aggressive and often more curative surgical procedures to be performed. but also may reduce postoperative complications. Finally, in patients with IBD there appears to be a high incidence of hepatic dysfunction associated with TPN; this dysfunction may be secondary to the primary disease.

At present, one would consider TPN to be indicated in the following patients with IBD: (1) nutritionally depleted patients, in order to prepare them for surgery and to maintain them during the postoperative period if complications develop such that enteral feeding is impossible; (2) patients with Crohn's disease who fail to respond to medical treatment and in whom surgery is to be avoided, if possible (e.g., patients with previous resections of small bowel, who are at risk to develop short-bowel syndrome); (3) selected patients with growth retardation who do not respond to oral and/or enteral therapy; and (4) patients with permanent or transitory gut failure.

REFERENCES

1. Blackburn, G.L., Bistrian, B.R., Maini, B.S., et al.: Nutritional and metabolic assessment of the hospitalized patient. J.P.E.N., 1:11–22, 1977.
2. Rosenberg, I.H.: Nutritional support in inflammatory bowel disease. Gastroenterology, 77:393–395, 1979.
3. Hill, G.L., Blackett, R.L., Pickford, M.D., et al.: A survey of protein nutrition in patients with inflammatory bowel disease—a rational basis for nutritional therapy. Br. J. Surg., 64:894–896, 1977.
4. Dudrick, S.J., Jensen, T.G., and Rowlands, B.J.: Nutritional support: Assessment and indications. In Dietel, M. (ed.): Nutrition in Clinical Surgery. Baltimore, Williams & Wilkins, 1980, pp. 19–28.
5. Guthrie, H.A., and Guthrie, G.M.: Factor analysis of nutritional status from ten state nutritional surveys. Am. J. Clin. Nutr., 29:1238–1241, 1976.
6. Crohn, B.B., and Yarnis, H.: The diagnosis of regional ileitis. In Regional Ileitis. New York, Grune & Stratton, 1958, p. 108.
7. Wall, A.J., and Kirsner, J.B.: Ulcerative colitis and Crohn's disease of the colon: Symptoms, signs, and laboratory aspects. In Kirsner, J.B., and Shorter, R.G. (eds.): Inflammatory Bowel Disease. Philadelphia, Lea & Febiger, 1975, pp. 101–108.
8. Dudrick, S.J., Wilmore, D.W., Vars, H.M., et al.: Long-term parenteral nutrition with growth, development, and positive nitrogen balance. Surgery, 64:134–142, 1968.

9. Mullen, J.L., Gertner, M.H., Buzby, G.P., Goodhart, G.L., and Rosato, E.F.: Implications of malnutrition in the surgical patient. Arch. Surg., 114:121–125, 1979.

10. Driscoll, R.H., and Rosenberg, I.H.: Total parenteral nutrition in inflammatory bowel disease. Med. Clin. North Am., 62:185–201, 1978.

11. Mullen, J.L., Hargrove, W.C., Dudrick, S.J., Fitts, W.T., and Rosato, E.F.: Ten years experience with intravenous hyperalimentation and inflammatory bowel disease. Ann. Surg., 187:523–529, 1978.

12. deDombal, F.T.: Prognostic value of the serum protein during severe attacks of ulcerative colitis. Gut, 9:144–149, 1968.

13. Gerlach, K., Morowitz, D.A., and Kirsner, J.B.: Symptomatic hypomagnesemia during severe attacks of ulcerative colitis. Gastroenterology, 59:567–574, 1970.

14. Henkin, R.I., Schechter, P.J., Hoyer, R., and Mattern, C.F.: Idiopathic hypogeusia with disgeusia, hyposmia and dysosmia. J.A.M.A., 217:434–440, 1971.

15. Henkin, R.I.: Disorders of taste and smell. J.A.M.A., 218:1946, 1971.

16. Cohen, I.K., Schechter, P.J., and Henkin, R.I.: Hypogeusia, anorexia and altered zinc metabolism following thermal burn. J.A.M.A., 223:914–916, 1973.

17. Clark, R.G., Lauder, N.M.: Undernutrition and surgery in regional ileitis. Br. J. Surg., 56:736–738, 1969.

18. Kinney, J.M.: A consideration of energy exchange in human trauma. Bull. N.Y. Acad. Med., 36:617–631, 1960.

19. Bistrian, B.R., Blackburn, G.L., Hallowell, E., et al.: Protein status of general surgical patients. J.A.M.A., 230:858–860, 1974.

20. Moore, F.D., and Brennan, M.F.: Surgical injury: Body composition, protein metabolism and neuroendocrinology. In American College of Surgeons (eds.): Manual of Surgical Nutrition. Philadelphia, W.B. Saunders, 1975, p. 212.

21. Steinfeld, J.L., Davidson, J.D., Gordon, R.S., and Greene, F.E.: The mechanism of hypoproteinemia in patients with regional enteritis and ulcerative colitis. Am. J. Med., 29:405–415, 1960.

22. Jarnum, S., Westergaard, H., Yssing, M., et al.: Quantitation of gastrointestinal protein loss by means of Fe59 labeled dextran. Gastroenterology, 55:229–241, 1968.

23. Beeken, W.L., Busch, H.J., and Sylvester, D.L.: Intestinal protein loss in Crohn's disease. Gastroenterology, 62:207–215, 1972.

24. Nygaard, K., and Rootwelt, K.: Intestinal protein loss in rats with blind segments of the small bowel. Gastroenterology, 54:52–55, 1969.

25. Bendixen, G., Jarnum, S., Soltoft, J., et al.: IgG and albumin turnover in Crohn's disease. Scand. J. Gastroenterol., 3:481–489, 1968.

26. Kingham, J.G.C., and Loehry, C.A.: Selectivity of small intestinal exudate in celiac disease and Crohn's disease. Am. J. Dig. Dis., 23:33–38, 1978.

27. Bernier, J.J., Florent, C., Desmazures, C., Aymes C., and L'Hirondel, C.: Diagnosis of protein-losing enteropathy by gastrointestinal clearance of alpha$_1$-anti-trypsin. Lancet, 2:763–764, 1978.

28. Dyer, N.H., and Dawson, A.M.: Malnutrition and malabsorption in Crohn's disease with reference to the effect of surgery. Br. J. Surg. 60:134–140, 1973.

29. Shiner, M., and Drury, R.A.: Abnormalities of the small bowel mucosa in Crohn's disease (regional enteritis). Am. J. Dig. Dis., 7:744–759, 1962.

30. Dunne, W.T., Cooke, W.T., and Allan, R.N.: Enzymatic and morphometric evidence for Crohn's disease as a diffuse lesion of the gastrointestinal tract. Gut, 18:290–294, 1977.

31. Salem, S.N., Truelove, S.C., and Richards, W.C.D.: Small-intestinal and gastric changes in ulcerative colitis: A biopsy study. Br. Med. J., 5380:394–398, 1964.

32. Salem, S.N., and Truelove, S.C.: Small-intestinal and gastric abnormalities in ulcerative colitis. Br. Med. J., 5438:827–831, 1965.

33. Jankev N., and Price, L.A.: Small-intestinal histochemical and histological changes in ulcerative colitis. Gut, 10:267–269, 1969.

34. Cooper, B.T., Lucas, M.L., and Lei, F.M.: Abnormal jejunal surface pH in Crohn's disease. New evidence that Crohn's disease is a diffuse lesion of the gastrointestinal tract. Gut, 18:423, 1977.

35. Ferguson, R., Allan, R.N., and Cooke, W.T.: A study of the cellular infiltrate of the proximal jejunal mucosa in ulcerative colitis and Crohn's disease. Gut, 16:205–208, 1975.

36. Goodman, M.J., Skinner, J.M., and Truelove, S.C.: Abnormalities in the apparently normal bowel mucosa in Crohn's disease: Lancet, 1:275–278, 1976.

37. Plotkin, G.R., and Isselbacher, K.J.: Secondary disaccharidase deficiency in adult celiac disease, (nontropical sprue) and other malabsorption states. N. Engl. J. Med., 271:1033–1037, 1964.

38. Weser, E., and Sleisenger, M.H.: Lactosuria and lactase deficiency in adult celiac disease. Gastroenterology, 48:571–578, 1965.

39. Jeejeebhoy, K.N., Desai, H.G., and Verghese, R.V.: Milk intolerance in tropical malabsorption syndrome. Role of lactose malabsorption. Lancet, 2:666–667, 1964.

40. Bowie, M.D., Brinkman, G.L., and Hanson, J.D.L.: Acquired disaccharide intolerance in malnutrition. J. Pediatr., 66:1083–1091, 1965.

41. James, W.P.T.: Intestinal absorption in protein-calorie malnutrition. Lancet, 1:333–335, 1965.

42. Viteri, F.E., Flores, J.M., Alvarado, J., and Behar, M.I.: Intestinal malabsorption in malnourished children before and during recovery. Relation between severity of protein deficiency and the malabsorption process. Am. J. Dig. Dis., 18: 201–211, 1973.

43. Owen, G.M.: Metabolic alkalosis with diarrhea and chloride-free urine. J. Pediatr., 65:849–857, 1964.

44. Clark, J.T.: Chronic diarrhea and failure to thrive due to intestinal disaccharidase insufficiency. Pediatrics, 34:807, 1964.

45. Chalfin, D., and Holt, P.R.: Lactase deficiency in ulcerative colitis, regional enteritis and viral hepatitis. Am. J. Dig. Dis., 12:81–87, 1967.

46. Goodman-Hoyer, E., and Varnum, S.: Incidence and clinical significance of lactose malabsorption in ulcerative colitis and Crohn's disease. Gut, 11:338–343, 1970.

47. Gelernt, I.M.: Experience and late results with the continent ileostomy. In Korelitz, B.I. (ed.): Inflammatory Bowel Disease—Experience and Controversy. Littleton, MA, John Wright-PSG, Inc., 1982, pp. 207–219.

48. Benson, J.A., Culver, P.J., Ragland, S., et al.: The D-xylose absorption test in malabsorption syndromes. N. Engl. J. Med., 256:335–339, 1957.

49. Fordtran, J.S., Soergel, K.N., and Ingelfinger, F.J.: Intestinal absorption of D-xylose in man. N. Engl. J. Med., 267:274–279, 1962.

50. Goldstein, F., Karacadag, S., Wirts, C.W., and Kowlessar, O.D.: Intraluminal small intestinal utilization of D-xylose by bacteria: A limitation of the D-xylose absorption test. Gastroenterology, 59:380–386, 1970.

51. Neale, G., Gompertz, D., Schonsby, H., Tabaqchali, S., and Booth, C.C.: The metabolic and nutritional consequences of bacterial overgrowth in the small intestine. Am. J. Clin. Nutr., 25:1409–1417, 1972.

52. Jones, E.A., Cragie, A., Tavill, A.S., et al.: Protein metabolism in the intestinal stagnant loop syndrome. Gut, 9:466–469, 1968.

53. Yap, S.H., Hafikensheid, J.L.M., Van Tongeren, J.H., et al.: Rate of synthesis of albumin in relation to serum levels of essential amino acids in patients with bacterial overgrowth of the small bowel. Eur. J. Clin. Invest., 4:279–284, 1974.

54. King, C.E., and Toskes, P.P.: Small intestine bacterial overgrowth. Gastroenterology, 76:1035–1055, 1979.

55. Cohen, S., Kaplan, M., Gottlieb, L., and Patterson, J.: Liver disease and gallstones in regional enteritis. Gastroenterology, 60:237–245, 1971.

56. Smith, L.H., Fromm, H., and Hofmann, A.F.: Acquired hyperoxaluria, nephrolithiasis and intestinal disease: Description of a syndrome. N. Engl. J. Med., 286:1371–1375, 1972.

57. Hylander, E., Jarnum, S., Jensen, H., and Thale, M.: Enteric hyperoxaluria: Dependence on small intestine resection, colectomy and steatorrhea in chronic inflammatory bowel disease. Scand. J. Gastroenterol., 13:577–588, 1978.

58. Hofmann, A.F., and Poley, J.R.: Role of bile acid malabsorption in pathogenesis of diarrhea and steatorrhea in patients with ileal resection. Gastroenterology, 62:918–934, 1972.

59. Wilson, F.A., Sallee, V.C., and Dietschy, J.M.: Unstirred water layers in the intestine: Rate determination of fatty acid absorption from micellar solutions. Science, 174:1031–1033, 1971.

60. Corcino, J.J., Waxman, S., and Herbert, V.: Absorption of malabsorption of vitamin B_{12}. Am. J. Med., 48:562–569, 1970.

61. Hofmann, A.F.: The syndrome of ileal disease and the broken enterohepatic circulation: Choleretic enteropathy. Gastroenterology, 52:752–757, 1965.

62. Ammon, H.V., and Phillips, S.F.: Inhibition of colonic water and electrolyte absorption by fatty acids in man. Gastroenterology, 65:744–749, 1973.

63. Bright-Asare, P., and Binder, H.J.: Stimulation of colonic secretion of water and electrolytes by hydroxy fatty acids. Gastroenterology, 64:81–88, 1973.

64. Binder, H.J., and Rawlins, C.L.: Effect of conjugated dihydroxy bile salts on electrolyte transport in rat colon. J. Clin. Invest., 52:1460–1466, 1973.

65. Johansson, C.: Studies of gastrointestinal interactions. VIII: Characteristics of the absorption pattern of sugar, fat, and protein from composite meals in man. A quantitative study. Scand. J. Gastroenterol., 10:33–42, 1975.

66. Dyer, N.H., Child, J.A., Mollin, D.L., et al.: Anemia in Crohn's disease. Q. J. Med., 164:419–436, 1972.

67. Cox, E.V., Meyhill, M.J., Cooke, W.T., and God-die, R.: The folic acid excretion test in the steatorrhea syndrome. Gastroenterology, 35:390–397, 1958.

68. Hoffbrand, A.V., Stewart, V.S., Booth, C.C., and Mollin, A.L.: Folate deficiency in Crohn's disease: Incidence, pathogenesis and treatment. Br. Med. J., 2:71–75, 1968.

69. Thompson, A.B.R., Burst, R., Mam, Ali, Mant, M.J., and Valverg, L.S.: Iron deficiency in inflammatory bowel disease: Diagnostic efficacy of serum ferritin. Am. J. Dig. Dis., 23:705–709, 1978.

70. Klipstein, F.A.: The urinary excretion of orally administered tritium labelled folic acid as a test of folic acid absorption. Blood, 21:626–639, 1963.

71. Gerson, L.D., Cohen, N., and Janowitz, H.J.: Small intestine absorptive function in regional enteritis. Gastroenterology 64:907–912, 1973.

72. Rutgeerts, P., Ghoos, Y., Vantrappen, G., and Eyssen, H.: Ileal dysfunction and bacterial overgrowth in patients with Crohn's disease. Eur. J. Clin. Invest., 11:199–206, 1981.

73. Booth, I.W., and Harries, J.T.: Inflammatory bowel disease in childhood. Gut, 25:188–202, 1984.

74. Nutritional supplementation and growth restoration in juvenile Crohn's disease: A new approach. Nutr. Rev., 40:199–201, 1982.

75. Hansen, J.D.L., Freeseman, C., Moodie, A.D., et al.: What does nutritional growth retardation imply? Pediatrics, 47:299–313, 1971.

76. Toch, M.B., and Symthe, P.M.: Does undernutrition during infancy inhibit brain growth and subsequent intellectual development? Arch. Dis. Child., 38:546–552, 1963.

77. Waterloo, J.L.: Classification and determination of protein-calorie malnutrition. Br. Med. J., 2:566–569, 1972.

78. Hansen, J.D.L., Brinkman, G.L., and Bowie, M.D.: Body composition and protein-calorie malnutrition. S. Afr. Med. J., 39:491–495, 1965.

79. Kelts, D.G., Grand, R.J., Shen, G., Watkins, J.B., Werlin, S.L., and Boehme, C.: Nutritional basis of growth failure in children and adolescents with Crohn's disease. Gastroenterology, 76:720–727, 1979.

80. Layden, T., Rosenberg, I., Nemehausky, B., et al.: Reversal of growth arrest in adolescence with Crohn's disease after parenteral alimentation. Gastroenterology, 70:1017–1021, 1976.

81. Kirschner, B.S., Voinchet, O., and Rosenberg, I.H.: Growth retardation in inflammatory bowel disease. Gastroenterology, 75:504–511, 1978.

82. McCaffery, T.D., Nasr, K., Lawrence, A.M., and Kirsner, J.B.: Severe growth retardation in children with inflammatory bowel disease. Pediatrics, 45:386–393, 1970.

83. Tenore, A., Burman, W.F., Parks, J.S., and Bongiovinni, A.M.: Basal and stimulated serum growth hormone concentrations in inflammatory bowel disease. J. Clin. Endocrinol. Metab., 44:622–628, 1977.

84. Gotlin, R.W., and Dubois, R.S.: Nyctohemeral growth hormone levels in children with growth retardation and inflammatory bowel disease. Gut, 14:191–195, 1973.

85. McCaffery, T.D., Nasr, K., Laurence, A.M., and Kirsner, J.B.: Effect of administered human growth hormone on growth retardation in inflammatory bowel disease. Am. J. Dig. Dis., 9:411–416, 1974.

86. Solomons, N.W., Rosenberg, I.H., Sanstead, H.H.,

and Vo-Khactu, K.P.: Zinc deficiency in Crohn's disease. Digestion, *16*:87–95, 1977.

87. Atwell, J.D., and Duthie, H.L.: The absorption of water, sodium and potassium from the ileum of humans showing the effects of regional enteritis. Gastroenterology, *46*:16–22, 1964.

88. Ammon, H.V., and Phillips, S.F.: Inhibition of ileal water absorption by intestinal fatty acids. J. Clin. Invest., *53*:205–210, 1974.

89. Coyne, M.J., Bonorris, G.G., Chung, A., Cowley, D., and Schoenfield, L.J.: Propranolol inhibits bile acid and fatty acid stimulation of cyclic AMP in human colon. Gastroenterology, *73*:971–974, 1977.

90. Gaginella, T.S., Chadwick, V.S., Bebongie, J.C., Lewis, J.C., and Phillips, S.F.: Perfusion of rabbit colon with ricinoleic acid: Dose related mucosal injury, fluid secretion, and increased permeability. Gastroenterology, *73*:95–101, 1977.

91. Snape, W.J., Schiff, S., and Cohen, S.: Effect of deoxycholic acid on colonic motility in the rabbit. Am. J. Physiol., *238*:G321–G325, 1980.

92. Cummings, J.H., James, W.P.T., and Wiggins, H.S.: Role of the colon in ileal resection diarrhea. Lancet, *1*:344–347, 1973.

93. Smidy, F.G., Gregory, S.D., Smith, I.B., and Goligher, J.C.: Fecal loss of fluid, electrolytes and nitrogen in colitis before and after ileostomy. Lancet, *1*:14–19, 1960.

94. Caprilli, R., Vernia, P., Colaneri, O., and Torsoli, A.: Blood pH: A test for assessment of severity in proctocolitis. Gut, *17*:763–769, 1976.

95. Hawker, P.C., McKay, J.S., and Turnberg, L.A.: Electrolyte transport across colonic mucosa from patients with inflammatory bowel disease. Gastroenterology, *79*:508–511, 1980.

96. Rask-Madsen, J., Hammersgaard, E.A., and Knudsen, E.: Rectal electrolyte transport and mucosal permeability in ulcerative colitis and Crohn's disease. J. Lab. Clin. Med., *81*:342–353, 1973.

97. Duthie, H.L., Watts, J.M., deDombal, F.T., and Goligher, J.C.: Serum electrolyte and colonic transfer of water and electrolytes in chronic ulcerative colitis. Gastroenterology, *47*:525–530, 1964.

98. Harris, J., and Shields, R.: Absorption and secretion of water and electrolytes by the intact human colon in diffuse untreated proctocolitis. Gut, *11*:27–33, 1970.

99. Rampton, D.S., Sladen, G.E., Bhakoo, K.K., Heinzelmann, D.I., and Youlten, L.J.F.: Rectal mucosal prostaglandin E release and electrolyte transport in ulcerative colitis. Gut, *21*:591–596, 1979.

100. Milton-Thompson, G.J., Cummings, J.H., Newman, A., Billings, J.A., and Miscewicz, J.J.: Colonic and small intestinal response to intravenous prostaglandin $F_{2\alpha}$ and E_2 in man. Gut, *16*:42–46, 1975.

101. Campieri, M., Lanfranchi, G.A., Bazzocehi, G., Brignola, C., Corazza, G., Cortini, M., Michelini, M., and Labé, G.: Salicylate other than 5-aminosalicylic acid ineffective in ulcerative colitis (letter). Lancet, *2*:993, 1978.

102. Barot, L.R., Rombeau, J.L., Feurer, I.D., and Mullen, J.L.: Caloric requirements in patients with inflammatory bowel disease. Ann. Surg., *195*:214–218, 1982.

103. Barot, L.R., Rombeau, J.L., Steinberg, J.J., Crosby, L.O., Feurer, I.D., and Mullen, J.L.: Energy

expenditure in patients with inflammatory bowel disease. Arch. Surg., *116*:460–462, 1981.

104. Lehr, L., Schober, O., Hundeshagen, H., and Pichlmayr, R.: Total body potassium depletion and the need for pre-operative nutritional support in Crohn's disease. Ann. Surg., *96*:709–714, 1982.

105. Worming, H., Mullertz, S., Thaysen, E.H., and Rang, H.O.: pH concentration of pancreatic enzymes in aspirates from the human duodenum during digestion of a standard meal in patients with intestinal disorders. Scand. J. Gastroenterol., *2*:81–89, 1967.

106. Farivar, S., Fromm, H., Schindler, D., McJunkin, B., and Schmidt, F.: Tests of bile acid and vitamin B_{12} metabolism in ileal Crohn's disease. Am. J. Clin. Pathol. *73*:69–74, 1980.

107. Aarbakke, J., and Schjonsby, H.: Value of urinary simple phenol and indican determinations in the diagnosis of the stagnant loop syndrome. Scand. J. Gastroenterol., *11*:409–414, 1976.

108. Giannella, R.A., Rout, W.R., and Toskes, P.P.: Jejunal brush border injury and impaired sugar and amino acid uptake in the blind loop syndrome. Gastroenterology, *67*:965–974, 1974.

109. Mellors, A.J., Nahrwold, D.L., and Rose, R.C.: Ascorbic acid flux across the mucosal border of guinea pig and human ileum. Am. J. Physiol., *233*:274–279, 1977.

110. Rose, R.C.: Water-soluble vitamin absorption in the intestine. Ann. Rev. Physiol., *233*:274–279, 1977.

111. Wagonfeld, J.B., Gerant, H.K., Hall, J.C., Holt, H., Vander Horst, J., and Rosenberg, I.H.: Quantitative analysis of skeletal growth, demineralization and vitamin D status in patients with inflammatory bowel disease (abstract). Gastroenterology, *68*:1065, 1975.

112. Cox, T.M., and O'Donnell, M.W.: Studies on the binding of iron by rabbit intestinal membranes. Biochem. J., *194*:753–759, 1981.

113. Main, A.N.H., Hall, M.J., Morgan, R.J., MacKenzie, J.F., Shenkin, A., Fell, G.S., and Russell, R.I.: Magnesium status and intravenous requirements in patients with chronic inflammatory bowel disease during intravenous nutrition. Gut, *23*:981–984, 1981.

114. Main, A.N.H., Morgan, R.J., Russell, R.I., Hall, M.J., MacKenzie, J.F., Shenkin, A., and Fell, G.S.: Magnesium deficiency in chronic inflammatory bowel disease and requirements during intravenous nutrition. J.P.E.N., *5*:15–19, 1981.

115. Levine, S.R., Crowley, T.F., and Hai, H.A.: Hypomagnesemia and ventricular tachycardia. A complication of ulcerative colitis and parenteral hyperalimentation in a non-digitalized non-cardiac patient. Chest, *81*:244–246, 1982.

116. Frazier, T.G., Mucha, M.E., Rush, I.M., Trull, E.J., Culson, S.A., and O'Connor, J.A.: Hypomagnesemia: Higher risk using total parenteral nutrition in the treatment of patients with malignancies. J. Surg. Oncol., *13*:35–38, 1980.

117. Sandiford, J.A., and Alexander, R.: Zinc deficiency in Crohn's disease. J. R. Coll. Surg. Edin., *26*:357–359, 1981.

118. Grand, R.J., and Colodny, A.H.: Increased requirement for magnesium during parenteral therapy for granulomatous colitis. J. Pediatr., *81*:788–790, 1972.

119. Tiommy, E., Horwitz, C., Graff, E., Rosen, P., and Gilat, T.: Serum zinc and taste acuity in Tel-Aviv

patients with inflammatory bowel disease. Am. J. Gastroenterol., 77:101–103, 1982.

120. Underwood, E.J.: Trace Elements in Human and Animal Nutrition, 4th ed. New York, Academic Press, 1977, pp. 196–242.

121. McClain, C., Soutor, C., and Zieve, L.: Zinc deficiency: A complication of Crohn's disease. Gastroenterology, 78:272–279, 1980.

122. Main, A.N.H., Hall, M.J., Russell, R.I., Fell, G.S., Mills, P.R., and Shenkin, A.: Clinical experience with zinc supplementation during intravenous nutrition in Crohn's disease: Value of serum and urine measurements. Gut, 23:981–984, 1982.

123. Mills, P.R., and Fell, G.S.: Zinc and inflammatory bowel disease. Am. J. Clin. Nutr., 32:2172–2173, 1979.

124. Solomons, N.W., and Rosenberg, I.H.: Zinc and inflammatory bowel disease. Am. J. Clin. Nutr., 34:1447–1448, 1981.

125. Wohman, S.L., Anderson, G.H., Marliss, E.B., and Jeejeebhoy, K.N.: Zinc in total parenteral nutrition: Requirements and metabolic effects. Gastroenterology, 76:458–467, 1979.

126. Solomons, N.W., Layden, T.J., Rosenberg, I.H., Vo-Khactu, K., and Sandstead, H.H.: Plasma trace metals during parenteral alimentation. Gastroenterology, 70:1022–1025, 1976.

127. Weser, E.: Total parenteral nutrition and bowel rest in inflammatory bowel disease (editorial). Gastroenterology, 79:1337, 1980.

128. Dean, R.E., Campos, M.M., and Barrett, B.: Hyperalimentation in the management of chronic inflammatory intestinal disease. Dis. Colon Rectum, 19:601–604, 1976.

129. Milewski, P.J., and Irving, M.H.: Parenteral nutrition in Crohn's disease. Dis. Colon Rectum, 23:395–400, 1980.

130. Anderson, D.L., and Boyce, H.W.: Use of parenteral nutrition in the treatment of advanced regional enteritis. Am. J. Dig. Dis., 18:633–640, 1973.

131. Fischer, J.E., Foster, G.S., and Abel, R.M.: Hyperalimentation as primary therapy for inflammatory bowel disease. Am. J. Surg., 125:165, 1973.

132. Reilly, J., Ryan, J.A., Strole, W., and Fischer, J.E.: Hyperalimentation in inflammatory bowel disease. Am. J. Surg., 131:192–200, 1976.

133. Vogel, C.M., Corwin, T.R., and Baue, A.E.: Intravenous hyperalimentation in the treatment of inflammatory diseases of the bowel. Arch. Surg., 108:460–467, 1974.

134. Eisenberg, H.W., Turnbull, R.B., and Weakley, F.L.: Hyperalimentation as preparation for surgery in transmural colitis (Crohn's disease). Dis. Colon Rectum, 17:469–475, 1974.

135. Greenberg, G.R., Haber, G.B., and Jeejeebhoy, K.N.: Total parenteral nutrition (TPN) and bowel rest in the management of Crohn's disease. Gut, 12:828, 1976.

136. Fazio, V.W., Kodner, I., Jagelamn, D.G., Turnbull, R.B., and Weakley, F.L.: Parenteral nutrition as primary therapy or adjunctive treatment. Dis. Colon Rectum, 19:574–578, 1976.

137. Harford, F.J., and Fazio, V.W.: Total parenteral nutrition as primary therapy for inflammatory disease of the bowel. Dis. Colon Rectum, 21:555–557, 1978.

138. Mullen, J.L., Hargrove, W.C., Dudrick, S.J., Fitts, W.T., and Rosato, E.F.: Ten years experience with intravenous hyperalimentation and inflammatory bowel disease. Ann. Surg., 187:523–529, 1978.

139. Elson, C.O., Layden, T.J., Nemchausky, B.A., Rosenberg, J.L., and Rosenberg, I.H.: An evaluation of total parenteral nutrition in the management of inflammatory bowel lesion. Dig. Dis. Sci., 25:42–48, 1980.

140. Holm, I.: Benefits of total parenteral nutrition (TPN) in the treatment of Crohn's disease and ulcerative colitis. Acta. Chir. Scand., 147:271–276, 1981.

141. Shiloni, E., and Freund, H.R.: Total parenteral nutrition in Crohn's disease. Is it a primary or supportive mode of therapy? Dis. Colon Rectum, 26:275–278, 1983.

142. Müller, J.M., Keller, H.E., and Pichlmaier, H.: Total parenteral nutrition as the sole therapy in Crohn's disease—a prospective. Br. J. Surg., 70:40–43, 1983.

143. Lochs, H., Marosi, L., Ferenci, P., and Hortnagl, H.: Has total bowel rest a beneficial effect in the treatment of Crohn's disease? Clin. Nutr., 2:61–64, 1983.

144. Truelove, S.C., Lee, E.G., Willoughby, C.P., and Kettlewell, M.G.W.: Further experience in the treatment of severe attacks of ulcerative colitis. Lancet, 2:1086–1088, 1978.

145. Dickinson, R.J., Ashton, M.G., Axon, A.T.R., Smith, R.C., Yeung, C.K., and Hill, G.L.: Controlled trial of intravenous hyperalimentation and total bowel rest as an adjunct to the routine therapy of acute colitis. Gastroenterology, 79:1199–1204, 1980.

146. Rombeau, J.L., Barot, L.R., Williamson, C.E., and Mullen, J.L.: Preoperative total parenteral nutrition and surgical outcome in patients with inflammatory bowel disease. Am. J. Surg., 143:139–143, 1982.

147. Spelgren, K.N., Rombeau, J.L., Casey, J.J., and Treasure, R.L.: A complication of direct right atrial catheterization for total parenteral nutrition. J.P.E.N., 5:164–165, 1981.

148. Fouin-Fortunet, H., Lequernec, L., Erlinger, S., Lerebours, E., and Colin R.: Hepatic alterations during total parenteral nutrition in patients with inflammatory bowel disease: A possible consequence of lithocholate toxicity. Gastroenterology, 82:932–937, 1982.

149. Boss L.P., and Weterman, I.T.: TPN in Crohn's disease. World J. Surg., 4:163–166, 1980.

150. Capron, J.P., Gineston, J.L., Herve, N.A., and Braillon, A.: Metronidazole in prevention of cholestasis associated with total parenteral nutrition. Lancet, 1:446–447, 1983.

CHAPTER 22

Intravenous Nutrition for Acute and Chronic Pancreatitis

BRIAN J. ROWLANDS

The pancreas produces both exocrine and endocrine secretions that are important in the digestion of nutrients from the gastrointestinal tract and in the regulation of carbohydrate homeostasis.[1] In addition, it has a role in the maintenance of homeostasis within the lumen of the bowel—regulation of intestinal growth and immune function—and in calcium absorption and balance.[2] Diseases of the pancreas may interfere with the production of pancreatic exocrine and endocrine secretions, leading to impairment of digestion, absorption, and assimilation of nutrients from the gastrointestinal tract, or may produce symptoms of anorexia, nausea, and vomiting, which further reduce nutrient intake. In these circumstances, parenteral nutrition may be used to replace nutrient deficits and to maintain energy and protein requirements, in order to enable tissue repair and reduce morbidity and mortality. In patients with acute and chronic pancreatitis or pancreatitis complicated by pseudocyst, abscess, or fistula formation, reducing the oral nutrient intake to a minimum and supplying all nutrient requirement via the intravenous route is safe, well tolerated, maintains optimum metabolic and nutritional status,[3] and may be beneficial to pancreatic function and morphology. In this chapter, the etiology of acute and chronic pancreatitis, the common nutritional abnormalities seen in these conditions, the data from animal experiments that form the basis for clinical management with intravenous nutrients, and the results of studies published in the literature are discussed.

ETIOLOGY AND PATHOPHYSIOLOGY OF PANCREATITIS

Social and economic factors are important in the development of pancreatic disease and influence the incidence of acute and chronic pancreatitis and their resultant morbidity and mortality.[4]

Acute Pancreatitis

The most common predisposing factors in the pathogenesis of acute pancreatitis are sustained alcohol abuse and biliary tract disease, the relative frequencies depending on the population studied.[5] Alcohol-associated pancreatitis occurs only after several years of heavy alcohol ingestion, and acute attacks are usually precipitated by heavy drinking "binges." Gallstones are present in 60 per cent of the nonalcoholic patients with acute pancreatitis, and transient obstruction of the pancreatic duct due to passage of a stone through the ampulla of Vater is usually implicated in an attack of acute pancreatitis. Other etiologic factors include trauma; carcinoma of the pancreas or ampulla of Vater; drugs such as corticosteroids, furosemide, thiazides, azathioprine, and estrogens; viral infections; vasculitis and ischemia; pregnancy; type I and type V hyperlipoproteinemia; hereditary factors; and iatrogenic factors such as intra-abdominal surgical procedures, endoscopic retrograde cholangiopancreatography (ERCP) and translumbar aortography.[6] The mechanism by which these factors

401

cause acute inflammation of the pancreas is unclear. Initially there is a release of proteolytic enzymes of the pancreas into the interstitial tissues of the gland and surrounding tissues. These enzymes release other proenzymes—chymotrypsin, the carboxypeptidases, elastase, lysolecithin—which are all vasoactive and highly destructive of tissue. Their release results in edema, hemorrhage, and necrosis of the gland, the movement of large amounts of fluid and plasma into the retroperitoneal tissues, and fat necrosis. The degree of local destruction varies, but extensive necrosis, infection, and abscess formation may ultimately occur. In addition to the local effects, there may be widespread systemic disturbances owing to circulating enzymes and toxins, possibly leading to organ failure in many body systems. These disturbances include hypovolemia, fluid and electrolyte shifts, acid-base inbalance, diffuse intravascular coagulopathy, decreased myocardial contractility, increased peripheral resistance, impaired liver and renal function, hypoxemia, encephalopathy, and disturbance of calcium metabolism. Thus, acute pancreatitis can produce a spectrum of local and systemic effects ranging from a minimally inflamed edematous pancreas to hemorrhagic pancreatitis with extensive local tissue destruction and superadded infection with profound systemic metabolic derangement. The patient with the latter condition represents a considerable clinical challenge, as the acute metabolic illness with its associated increase in metabolic expenditure may occur in the presence of a prior nutritional deficiency due to alcohol consumption, obesity, liver disease, protein malnutrition, or gallstones. Thus, rapid consumption of endogenous protein and fat stores may occur unless vigorous efforts are made as early as possible to provide the daily nutrient requirements for protein and energy substrate via the intravenous route. This is of particular importance in patients who demonstrate, on admission and during their initial 48 hours of hospitalization, several of the signs that have been used as early prognostic indications of the risk of major complications in patients with acute pancreatitis.[7]

Chronic Pancreatitis

The majority of cases of chronic pancreatitis are associated with chronic alcohol consumption or nutritional and metabolic diseases that cause pathologic changes in the gland, consisting of fibrosis, cyst formation, scarring, and calcification, with consequent decrease in enzyme production, impairment of digestion, and malabsorption. The endocrine function of the pancreas is usually disrupted, resulting in glucose intolerance and diabetes mellitus in a large proportion of patients with pancreatic calcification. Large losses of nitrogen and fat in the stool may occur, and vitamin B_{12} malabsorption may develop. Chronic alcohol ingestion may lead to an increase in the protein content of pancreatic juice with precipitation into the ducts of amorphous protein material, which causes ductal obstruction and subsequent inflammation and dilatation.[8] In chronic pancreatitis, as in acute pancreatitis, there is a spectrum of clinicopathologic features, ranging from a condition in which fibrosis predominates, producing a small, firm, usually calcified gland, to a condition in which acinar degeneration and cyst formation are the major features.

Chronic pancreatitis may also occur as a result of hyperlipoproteinemia, inflammatory stricture or neoplasm of the sphincter of Oddi, hyperparathyroidism, and ingestion of a high-fat diet. About 90 per cent of functioning pancreatic exocrine tissue is lost before steatorrhea develops, leading to inadequate absorption of calcium, magnesium, and fat-soluble vitamins. Pain, often severe and associated with ingestion of food, is a common presenting symptom, and together with the anorexia and nausea associated with hyperbilirubinemia, it may lead to a significant voluntary reduction in oral nutrient intake and subsequent malnutrition. Alcoholic consumption has well-known direct effects on the pancreas and liver and may cause hyperlipoproteinemia type IV, which consists of hypertriglyceridemia and elevated plasma high-density and very-low-density lipoproteins associated with obesity, diabetes mellitus, and carbohydrate intolerance as well as effects on the cardiovascular and nervous systems.[9,10] It is against this background that intravenous nutritional support has a role in the management of chronic pancreatitis, because it reduces symptoms due to oral ingestion of nutrients, replenishes existing nutritional deficiencies, and satisfies energy and protein requirements for resolution of the disease process and tissue healing.

GENERAL MANAGEMENT

The most common presenting symptom in both acute and chronic pancreatitis is constant pain in the mid and upper abdomen that radiates into the back and is exacerbated by the ingestion of food and fluids. The pain may be associated with anorexia, nausea, vomiting, and a history of weight loss. Associated presenting symptoms and signs may be jaundice, anemia, gastrointestinal hemorrhage, steatorrhea, diabetes mellitus, and abdominal fullness due to the development of ascites or pancreatic abscess or pseudocyst. The initial management in mild pancreatitis is usually medical, consisting of adequate analgesia, bed rest, antacids, and a fat-free diet, but more aggressive therapy should be instituted if severe pain and vomiting persist or if the patient's general condition begins deteriorating. Surgical intervention may be necessary for complications or failure of response to maximum medical therapy.

Acute Pancreatitis

Initial evaluation should consist of an accurate history (including dietary history), physical examination, and biochemical evaluation, which should include assessment of fluid and electrolyte status and acid-base balance, liver function tests, and measurements of hemoglobin content, hematocrit, and serum calcium and blood glucose levels. If symptoms and signs indicate moderate or severe pancreatitis, the patient should be admitted to a unit where vital signs can be monitored at regular intervals and aggressive support measures such as ventilator support, hemodynamic monitoring via Swan-Ganz catheter, and continuous peritoneal lavage, may be instituted without delay when indicated.

Traditional management for acute pancreatitis includes nasogastric suction and intravenous fluids. There is massive loss of colloid and crystalloid fluid from the inflamed pancreas and retroperitoneum, resulting in the loss of up to 50 per cent of the circulating blood volume in the first 12 hours of illness. These losses should be replaced rapidly with crystalloids, colloid, plasma, and blood transfusion, and the replacement should be monitored by central venous pressure or Swan-Ganz catheter measurements and regular biochemical assessment. Calcium chloride should be given intravenously if the serum calcium level falls. The drop in serum calcium is due to depletions of both ionized calcium and protein-bound calcium, the latter being associated with hypoalbuminemia. The use of nasogastric suction is controversial, although most clinicians use it and its institution often produces prompt symptomatic

improvement through removal of gastric and acid secretions, which otherwise stimulate pancreatic secretion in the fasting patient. For similar reasons, cimetidine has been recommended, but its efficacy is unproven. Other controversial aspects of therapy include the use of systemic antibiotics, anticholinergics, corticosteroids, aprotinin, and glucagon; reports have appeared in the literature both supporting and condemning these therapeutic regimens, but the studies have usually been in patients with mild or moderate acute pancreatitis and there is no consensus on their usefulness in the full spectrum of disease.[6] No controversy exists, however, about the usefulness of adequate and regular analgesia or about an absolute ban on oral ingestion of food and fluids until abdominal pain and tenderness, fever, and leukocytosis have completely subsided. Reinstitution of oral feeding should occur only at this point, beginning with a liquid fat-free diet in small amounts and progressing to a semi-solid diet. If oral feeding is resumed too soon or advanced too quickly, a further exacerbation of acute pancreatitis and complications may result.

In the majority of cases, the preceding measures should produce dramatic clinical improvement and quiescence of the pancreatic inflammation over five to seven days. In severe cases, further therapy may be necessary if the disease fails to respond to massive resuscitation or if clinical and biochemical markers indicate a bad prognosis.[5] Respiratory complications may develop as a result of lung damage, in which there is an increase in pulmonary water content and a decrease in lung compliance. This is probably a direct enzymic effect, but the changes may be due to multiple microemboli or alterations in pulmonary surfactant. Arterial blood gases should be measured at regular intervals and hypoxia treated with oxygen by mask. If hypoxia persists or PaO_2 falls below 60 mm Hg, early endotracheal intubation and positive-pressure ventilation should be considered.[11] Respiratory compromise may persist even after an apparent improvement in pancreatic inflammation. Peritoneal lavage may also be used to remove toxic material in the peritoneal exudate of acute pancreatitis when there is no response to massive resuscitation or clinical and biochemical markers indicate a bad prognosis.[12] This technique is associated with decreased early mortality but may be particularly useful in patients in whom the diagnosis is made at laparotomy, allowing accurate placement of the catheters adjacent to pancreatic tissue.[6,7] If medical management fails, surgical intervention is indicated to confirm the diagnosis and eliminate nonpancreatic causes of deterioration (e.g., ischemic bowel, perforated ulcer), to resect necrotic pancreatic tissue, and to manage complications (e.g., abscess formation, duodenal obstruction, gastrointestinal hemorrhage).[13]

Chronic Pancreatitis

A slow, insidious progression of the disease will occur unless the causative agent is removed. Acute exacerbations of chronic pancreatitis are often precipitated by dietary indiscretion or excessive alcohol intake. An absolute ban on alcoholic consumption is mandatory to allow adequate treatment and nutrition. Diabetes mellitus does not usually require insulin therapy and may be managed with diet or oral hypoglycemic agents. Carbohydrate intake should be restricted in diabetics, and fat intake regulated in the presence of steatorrhea. Protein intolerance is not usually a problem in pancreatitis, although poor protein intake and protein malnutrition may lead to villous atrophy of the small intestine and malabsorption. The optimal maintenance diet is one of high protein and high carbohydrate contents with supplementation of energy and protein intake using oral elemental diets, medium-chain triglycerides, and intravenous nutrition. Pancreatic enzyme replacement, multivitamins, minerals, and trace element replacements are important additions to oral therapy.[14] General measures for the management of acute attacks of pancreatic inflammation are similar to those already discussed.

INTRAVENOUS NUTRITION IN PANCREATITIS

Intravenous nutrition has become an important adjunct to conventional medical and surgical therapy, particularly in patients with acute inflammatory processes of the gastrointestinal tract and previous suboptimal nutritional intake.[15] In acute pancreatitis, its potential benefits are: provision of adequate nutritional intake of protein, energy, vitamins, minerals, and trace elements to satisfy the increased metabolic demands of severe intra-abdominal inflammation; replenishment of previously acquired nutritional deficiencies; and restoration of normal immune function, which is associated with improved morbidity and survival.[15] Optimal supportive management during acute pancreatitis requires elimination of oral nutrient intake and nasogastric aspiration to reduce the stimulatory effect of intraluminal contents on pancreatic secretions. This measure leads to further nutritional compromise, which may be reduced by early nutritional intervention via the intravenous route. There may also be an additional beneficial effect of the nutrient infusion on the pancreatic exocrine secretions, although both animal and clinical studies have failed to clearly distinguish between this direct effect and the role of no oral intake in reducing pancreatic secretions. Maintenance of endogenous body stores of energy and protein are important to sustain the patient throughout the protracted illness that may result from severe acute pancreatitis and to ensure a better candidate for surgical intervention to treat complications such as pancreatic abscess and pseudocyst.

Animal Studies

Clinical observations have shown that intravenous nutrition and bowel rest significantly alter the volume and frequency of bowel movements, reduce the output from enterocutaneous fistulas, and inhibit small bowel peristalsis.[16] These beneficial effects have subsequently been studied in laboratory animals, and several studies have examined the effects of intravenous nutrition on pancreatic function and gastrointestinal secretions.

Johnson and colleagues[17] have shown that parenteral feeding results in significant decreases in the weights of the oxyntic gland area of the stomach, small intestine, and pancreas in association with a reduction in antral gastrin levels. They concluded that an oral intake or the physical presence of food in the gastrointestinal tract was important for maintenance of its structure and of tissue gastrin stores. These effects on the pancreas and small bowel did not occur when pentagastrin was infused simultaneously with intravenous nutrition, suggesting that gastrin may be important in maintaining pancreatic structure.[18] Pavlat and co-workers[19] found rats to show a 50 per cent reduction in the pancreatic acinar nuclear volume together with cell volume and morphologic evidence of lower synthetic activity with intravenous feeding. Dogs maintained on intravenous nutrition for more than 30 days have significant reductions in pancreatic bicarbonate and protein secretions in response to duodenal acidification, secretin, and caerulein.[20] In a study of canine gastric secretion, there was a reduction in basal and stimulated gastrin levels following one month of intravenous feeding.[21] An explanation of the reduction in pancreatic secretions could therefore be depression of the trophic action of gastrin on both the duodenal mucosa and the pancreatic acinar cell.[20, 22] Hamilton and associates[23] showed reduction of gastric, biliary, and pancreatic secretions in response to acute infusions of amino acids and dextrose. They subsequently suggested that both secretin and glucagon may be implicated in the suppression of upper gastrointestinal secretions that occurs with intravenous nutrition and that the dextrose part of the regimen was mainly responsible.[24]

The weight of evidence from animal studies would therefore suggest that the combination of no oral intake and intravenous nutrition reduces pancreatic bicarbonate and enzyme secretions by reducing the functioning pancreatic cell mass and by removing the normal stimuli for secretion. It must be remembered, however, that all these studies were performed in animals with normal pancreatic function and no evidence of pancreatitis. Extrapolation of the results to explain clinical observations of the effect of intravenous nutrition in the management of acute pancreatitis should therefore be made with caution.

Clinical Studies

In 1948, Thomas and Ross[25] were the first clinicians to report the closure of a pancreatic fistula by continuous intravenous support using concentrated dextrose and amino acid solutions. Dudrick and associates[26] subsequently described a patient with a pancreaticoduodenal fistula and autodigestion of the anterior abdominal wall whose fistula ceased draining and closed spontaneously with intravenous hyperalimentation.[26] Further studies have confirmed the efficacy of intravenous nutrition and bowel rest in the management of pancreatic and intestinal fistulas.[27,28] Evidence of its role in the treatment of acute and chronic pancreatitis is sparse, but Feller and co-workers[29] attributed a reduction in overall mortality with acute pancreatitis from 22 to 14 per cent to intra-

venous nutritional therapy. Blackburn and colleagues[30] reviewed the management of several patients who had severe pancreatitis in which a significant acute inflammatory process extended beyond 14 days from admission; they found that aggressive nutritional support was an important adjunct to surgical therapy because it maintained optimal nutritional status throughout the catabolic illness. In a retrospective analysis of 46 patients with acute pancreatitis, Goodgame and Fischer[31] suggested that parenteral nutrition had little effect on the pathophysiology of acute pancreatitis as judged by overall mortality (22 per cent) and the incidence and severity of metabolic and respiratory complications. There was a higher incidence than normal of catheter-associated septicemia in the early phase of acute pancreatitis, but this had no impact on morbidity and survival. Duration of intravenous nutritional support did not influence survival, prompting the researchers to conclude that in acute pancreatitis, nutritional therapy was supportive rather than primary and could be managed with minimal technical problems and metabolic morbidity. More recently, Grant and coworkers[3] have demonstrated the efficacy of total parenteral nutrition in maintaining and improving nutritional status in 121 patients admitted with a variety of pancreatic disorders, including pancreatitis and its complications.

Clinical Management of Intravenous Nutrition

Most patients with acute pancreatitis do not require nutritional support. Symptoms and signs will usually subside over a period of five to seven days, allowing resumption of oral nutrient intake. If they do not, however, intravenous nutrition should be commenced on the fifth post-admission day and should be continued until abdominal pain, nausea, vomiting, and ileus have resolved and biochemical indices have returned toward normal values. When (1) adverse prognostic factors such as age over 55 years, elevated white blood cell count, hypoglycemia, and abnormal liver enzyme readings are present on admission, or (2) clinical deterioration associated with hypoxia, hypocalcemia, elevated blood urea nitrogen, development of base deficit, or excessive fluid sequestration occurs within 48 hours, intravenous nutrition should be started as soon as possible. Patients with such factors (1 or 2 above) usually have a poor prognosis, prolonged hospitalization and rapid nutritional deterioration, making them more susceptible to septic, renal, and pulmonary complications.[5] Aggressive intravenous nutritional support will limit the nutritional deficit but probably does not alter the pathophysiology of the disease.

With information generated from a nutritional assessment profile as a guide to energy and protein needs of the individual patient, an intravenous nutrition regimen for infusion via a central vein is formulated.[15] It is based on the use of hypertonic dextrose as the calorie source and a standard crystalline amino acid solution as the nitrogen source, with the addition of minerals, vitamins, and trace elements to satisfy daily requirements. The regimen is delivered continuously over 24 hours, and adjustments are made to the rate of infusion and nutrient composition on the basis of biochemical monitoring to cope with the problems of renal failure, hepatic impairment, and excessive fluid requirement. Albumin and cimetidine may be added to the infusion, and insulin is used to regulate hyperglycemia. Information from serial nutritional assessments at ten-day intervals may be used to make appropriate adjustments to the regimen as the clinical condition improves or deteriorates.

The nonprotein calorie requirements may be supplied by hypertonic carbohydrate solutions or fat emulsions, but in acute pancreatitis, both should be used with caution and monitored carefully. Dextrose is the carbohydrate calorie source of choice, because it is inexpensive, associated metabolic acidosis is unusual, and hyperglycemia is easily treated with exogenous insulin.[32] In the hypermetabolic patient, nitrogen retention improves as carbohydrate intake increases, provided that total calorie intake matches total metabolic expenditure, and additional nitrogen sparing may be achieved with exogenous insulin.[33,34] The latter can usually be added to the intravenous nutrients, but if diabetic ketoacidosis develops, the regimen should be stopped and the abnormality corrected with peripheral insulin infusion and appropriate isotonic fluid administration. Daily insulin requirements in severe acute pancreatitis may be very high.

The daily dosage of fat emulsion should not exceed 2.5 gm/kg body weight or constitute more than 60 per cent of the total calorie intake. Fat emulsions have limitations as calories sources in hypermetabolic patients, but some fat should always be given to avoid essential fatty acid deficiency when prolonged intravenous nutrition is anticipated. Theoretic objections to the use of fat emulsions in acute pancreatitis have been raised because of the presence of hypertriglyceridemia and hyperlipoproteinemia. However, Silberman and colleagues[35] have shown lipid-based parenteral nutrition to be safe and efficient in 11 patients with acute pancreatitis. The regimen was well tolerated, and nutritional indices improved. There was no significant hyperlipemia before or during lipid infusion, and no exacerbations of pancreatitis were attributable to the intravenous regimen. Grundfest and associates[36] found no increase in volume or enzyme content of pancreatic fistula output during infusion of fat emulsion.

Fat emulsions may also have an advantage as calorie sources when respiratory complications develop secondary to pancreatitis. Askanasi and co-workers[37] have shown that administration of a large glucose load to catabolic and septic patients does not suppress net fat oxidation as it does in the starved, depleted patient and that there is an increase in oxygen consumption, a continuation of fat oxidation, and an increase in the conversion of glucose to glycogen. These processes are associated with increased CO_2 production, however, and the excess CO_2 has to be excreted by the lungs and may precipitate respiratory distress when pulmonary function is already impaired. Glucose may cause an additional physiologic stress that does not occur with fat, but the latter must be used with caution in respiratory distress or "shocked lung," because fat emboli may also compromise gaseous exchange.

Crystalline amino acid solutions should be used to provide the protein requirements of the regimen, and so far there is no information in the literature to suggest that special amino acid formulations, e.g., branched-chain amino acid–enriched solutions, have any advantage over conventional solutions in the management of pancreatitis. Amino acid solutions have not been demonstrated to increase pancreatic enzyme secretions. The development of renal failure should be managed by appropriate adjustments of fluid intake, regular dialysis, and provision of essential and nonessential amino acids and hepatic disorders by appropriate protein, fluid, and sodium adjustments to manage ascites, edema, and encephalopathy. During hypermetabolic illness, the increase in protein requirements exceeds the increase in caloric requirements, and adjustments should be made to the calorie/nitrogen ratio of the regimen to meet these additional demands. Vitamins, trace elements, and minerals are also usually required in greater amounts in these circumstances.[15] In particular, vitamins of the B complex are needed in greater amounts by alcoholics, and magnesium depletion may occur. In the initial phase of the illness, the calcium level may fall dramatically, indicating a bad prognosis. The calcium level should be monitored frequently until the inflammation resolves, and additional calcium should be given by peripheral infusion when indicated.

Intravenous nutrition should be continued until the symptoms abate, ileus resolves, and metabolic derangements return to normal. If exploratory laparotomy is necessary to manage extrahepatic biliary disease, pancreatic abscess or pseudocyst, or gastrointestinal complications, a needle-catheter jejunostomy should be placed at that time. Feeding into the gastrointestinal tract should be introduced either by mouth or by needle-catheter jejunostomy, using fat-free fluid diet initially while intravenous nutrition is maintained. When enteral intake is adequate to maintain nutrition without exacerbating inflammation, the intravenous nutrition may be discontinued.

SUMMARY

Intravenous nutrition is an important adjunct to conventional medical and surgical therapy of acute and chronic pancreatitis, particularly in patients who have evidence of prior malnutrition or in whom a protracted illness and complications are anticipated. Many of these patients can be identified within 48 hours of admission, owing to the demonstration of adverse prognostic criteria or failure of the inflammation to respond to initial supportive therapy. Prolonged ileus that precludes oral nutrition and hypermetabolism that consumes endogenous protein and energy stores may lead to severe nutritional deficit, which may be satisfied by supplying calories, protein, minerals, vitamins, and trace elements via the intravenous route. Clinical and laboratory studies show that a combination of no oral intake and intravenous nutrition reduces pancreatic secretions, although the effect on the pathophysiology of pancreatitis is unknown. The improvements in morbidity and survival rates in pancreatitis have been attributed partially to aggressive intravenous nutritional support started early in the disease process and continued until the inflammation and complications have resolved.

REFERENCES

1. Rowlands, B. J., and Miller, T. A.: The physiology of eating, with particular reference to the role of gastrointestinal hormones in the regulation of digestion. In Rombeau, J. L., and Caldwell, M. D. (eds.): Clinical Nutrition. Vol. I. Enteral and Tube Feeding. Philadelphia, W.B. Saunders Company, 1984, pp. 10–19.
2. Wormsley, K. G.: The secretions of the exocrine pancreas and their control. In Keynes, W. M., and Keith, R. G. (eds.): The Pancreas. London, Heinemann, 1981, pp. 43–67.
3. Grant, J. P., James, S., Grabowski, V., and Trexler, K. M.: Total parenteral nutrition in pancreatic disease. Ann. Surg., 200:627–631, 1984.
4. Sarles, H.: An international survey on nutrition and pancreatitis. Digestion, 9:389–403, 1973.
5. Ranson, J. H. C.: Etiological and prognostic factors in human acute pancreatitis—a review. Am. J. Gastroenterol., 77:633–638, 1982.
6. Trapnell, J. E.: Acute pancreatitis, aetiology and medical management. In Keynes, W. M., and Keith, R. G. (eds.): The Pancreas. London, Heinemann, 1981, pp. 285–303.
7. Ranson, J. H. C.: Acute pancreatitis—Where are we? Surg. Clin. North Am., 61:55–70, 1981.
8. Sarles, H.: Chronic calcifying pancreatitis—chronic alcoholic pancreatitis. Gastroenterology, 66:604–616, 1974.
9. Taylor, K. B., and Anthony, L. E.: Nutritional aspects of alcohol consumption. In Clinical Nutrition. New York, McGraw-Hill, 1983, pp. 489–510.
10. Greenberger, N. J.: Pancreatitis and hyperlipidemia. N. Engl. J. Med., 289:586–587, 1973.
11. Ranson, J. H. C., Turner, J. W., Roses, D. F., Rifkind, K. M., and Spencer, F. C.: Respiratory complications in acute pancreatitis. Ann. Surg., 179:557–566, 1974.
12. Ranson, J. H. C., and Spencer, F. C.: The role of peritoneal lavage in severe acute pancreatitis. Ann. Surg., 187:565–575, 1978.
13. Kune, G. A.: Acute pancreatitis: Surgery and management of complications. In Keynes, W. M., and Keith, R. G. (eds.): The Pancreas. London, Heinemann, 1981, pp. 304–319.
14. Floch, M. H.: Pancreatic diseases. In Nutrition and Diet Therapy in Gastrointestinal Disease. New York, Plenum, 1981, pp. 203–221.
15. Rowlands, B. J., and Dudrick, S. J.: Nutritional support of the infected patient. In Powanda, M. C., and Canonico, P. G. (eds.): Infection: The Physiologic and Metabolic Responses of the Host. Amsterdam, Elsevier/North Holland, 1981, pp. 359–397.
16. Copeland, E. M., and Dudrick, S. J.: Intravenous hyperalimentation in inflammatory bowel disease, pancreatitis and cancer. Surg. Ann. 12:83–101, 1980.

17. Johnson, L. R., Copeland, E. M., Dudrick, S. J., Lichtenberger, L. M., and Castro, G. A.: Structural and hormonal alterations in the gastrointestinal tract of parenterally fed rats. Gastroenterology, 68:1177–1183, 1975.

18. Johnson, L. R., Lichtenberger, L. M., Copeland, E. M., Dudrick, S. J., and Castro, G. A.: Action of gastrin on gastrointestinal structure and function. Gastroenterology, 68:1184–1192, 1975.

19. Pavlat, W. A., Rogers, W., and Cameron, I. L.: Morphometric analysis of pancreatic acinar cells from orally fed and intravenously fed rats. J. Surg. Res., 19:267–276, 1975.

20. Johnson, L. R., Schanbacher, L. M., Dudrick, S. J., and Copeland, E. M.: Effect of long-term parenteral feeding on pancreatic secretion and serum secretin. Am. J. Physiol., 233:E524–E529, 1977.

21. Thor, P. J., Copeland, E. M., Dudrick, S. J., and Johnson, L. R.: Effect of long-term parenteral feeding on gastric secretions in dogs. Am. J. Physiol., 232:E39–E43, 1977.

22. Mayston, P. D., and Barrowman, J. A.: The influence of chronic administration of pentagastrin on the rat pancreas. Q. J. Exp. Physiol., 56:113–122, 1971.

23. Hamilton, R. F., Davis, W. C., Stephenson, D. V., and Magee, D. F.: Effects of parenteral hyperalimentation on upper-gastrointestinal tract secretions. Arch. Surg., 102:348–351, 1971.

24. Towne, J. B., Hamilton, R. F., and Stephenson, D. V.: Mechanism of hyperalimentation in the suppression of upper gastrointestinal secretions. Am. J. Surg., 126:714–716, 1973.

25. Thomas, P. O., and Ross, C. A.: Effect of exclusive parenteral feeding on closure of pancreatic fistula; study made after duodenopancreatic resection for carcinoma of ampulla of Vater. Arch. Surg., 57:104–112, 1948.

26. Dudrick, S. J., Wilmore, D. W., Steiger, E., Mackie, J. A., and Fitts, W. T.: Spontaneous closure of traumatic pancreatoduodenal fistulas with total parenteral nutrition. J. Trauma, 10:542–552, 1970.

27. Weisz, G. M., Moss, G. S., and Folk, F. A.: Parenteral hyperalimentation in management of gastrointestinal fistulas. Can. J. Surg., 15:310–313, 1972.

28. MacFadyen, B. V., Dudrick, S. J., and Ruberg, R. L.: Management of gastrointestinal fistulas with parenteral hyperalimentation. Surgery, 74:100–105, 1973.

29. Feller, J. H., Brown, R. A., Toussant, G. P. M., and Thompson, A. G.: Changing methods in the treatment of severe pancreatitis. Am. J. Surg., 127:196–201, 1974.

30. Blackburn, G. L., Williams, L. F., Bistrian, B. R., Stone, M. S., Phillips, E., Hirsch, E., Clowes, G. H. A., and Gregg, J.: New approaches to the management of severe acute pancreatitis. Am. J. Surg., 131:114–124, 1976.

31. Goodgame, J. T., and Fischer, J. E.: Parenteral nutrition in the treatment of acute pancreatitis: Effect on complications and mortality. Ann. Surg., 186:651–658, 1977.

32. Giddings, A. E. B., Rowlands, B. J., Mangnall, D., and Clark, R. G.: Plasma insulin and surgery. II. Later changes and effect of intravenous carbohydrate. Ann. Surg., 186:687–693, 1977.

33. Long, J. M., Wilmore, D. W., Mason, A. D., and Pruitt, B. A.: Effect of carbohydrate and fat intake on nitrogen excretion during total intravenous feeding. Ann. Surg., 185:417–422, 1977.

34. Woolfson, A. M. J., Heatley, R. V., and Allison, S. P.: Insulin to inhibit protein catabolism after injury. N. Engl. J. Med., 300:14–17, 1979.

35. Silberman, M., Dixon, N. P., and Gisenberg, D.: The safety and efficacy of a lipid-based system of parenteral nutrition in acute pancreatitis. Am. J. Gastroenterol., 77:494–497, 1982.

36. Grundfest, S., Steiger, E., Selinkoff, P., and Fletcher, J.: The effect of intravenous fat emulsions in patients with pancreatic fistula. J.P.E.N., 4:27–31, 1980.

37. Askanasi, J., Weissman, C., Rosenbaum, S. H., Hyman, A. I., Milic-Emili, J., and Kinney, J. M.: Nutrition and the respiratory system. Crit. Care Med., 10:163–172, 1982.

CHAPTER 23

Animal Models in Parenteral Nutrition

KEITH N. APELGREN
PALMER Q. BESSEY
DOUGLAS W. WILMORE

Animal studies have been essential to the development of knowledge in the field of nutrition. Data obtained from these investigations have also aided the understanding of several aspects of human nutrition, such as the definition of the essential amino acids[1, 2] and the toxicity of fat-soluble vitamins.[3] However, most of the information has come from oral feeding experiments. Only recently has information become available from studies utilizing the intravenous route of feeding.

The dictionary definition of *parenteral* includes delivery by any route other than the alimentary tract.[4] Prior to the 20th century, the subcutaneous, intramuscular, intraperitoneal, and even intraosseous (tibia, sternum) routes were occasionally used for nutrient delivery in animal studies as well as in human patients. The current usage of "parenteral" implies intravenous administration—a method of delivery primarily developed in the 20th century. Experimental animal models have played a major role in this development and continue to do so. We will review some of the early studies using animals, describe the major animal models, emphasize pertinent advantages and disadvantages of specific models as they apply to clinical problems, and offer some suggestions for future research.

HISTORY

The earliest reported delivery of intravenous "nutrients" is attributed to Sir Christopher Wren in 1656. Only a few decades after Harvey's demonstration of blood circu-

lation,[5] Wren infused a mixture of wine, ale, and opiates into the vein of a dog by means of a goose quill attached to a pig's bladder.[6] He observed rapid intoxication—the dog survived. During the following two centuries, few studies in parenteral nutrition were performed.[7, 8] By the close of the 19th century and in the early decades of the 20th century, intravenous fluid administration became technically safe. This and other medical advances made it possible to save severely ill patients from early death. Thus emerged a group of patients who were in need of prolonged nutritional support by the parenteral route. The recognition of the importance of nutrition to hospitalized patients evolved simultaneously.

Early Formulations

Animals studies played a key role in solving the problems of delivering intravenous nutrients and in establishing safe techniques for solution formulation and administration. One early problem was the formulation of a safe protein source. Early protein hydrolysates caused severe allergic reactions and even death. The optimal composition of amino acid mixtures was not fully appreciated until the 1930s when all the essential amino acids were defined. It was further realized that various proteins had variable biologic value, depending on each specific composition. During that decade, Elman performed a series of experiments infusing protein hydrolysates first into dogs[9, 10] and then into humans.[11] He was one of the first to demonstrate that positive nitrogen balance could be achieved by the intravenous administration of nutrients. However, 3 to 8 L of fluid were required to provide adequate nutrition to humans. This volume load was often excessive and frequently required the simultaneous administration of diuretics.

Other investigators attempted to develop a calorically dense lipid emulsion that would reduce the high-volume requirement and yet not cause phlebitis when administered by peripheral vein. During the 1920s, Yamakawa and Nomura administered a variety of oils emulsified with various agents and ultimately selected lecithin as the optimal agent.[12] After a safe fat emulsion that could be sterilized had been developed, the only remaining major obstacle was the risk of fat embolism. Infusion of emulsions with particles larger than 2 μ led to trapping in the pulmonary capillaries and respiratory embarrassment. Therefore, this particle size became the limit in the manufacture of lipid emulsions, and it remains so today. Holt and colleagues, working independently during the 1930s, also found that lecithin was the most satisfactory emulsifying agent, and they performed several successful short-term experiments infusing fat emulsions into dogs.[13] Despite these developments, the toxicity of fat emulsions limited their usefulness. Several generations of products were tested before side effects became acceptably low. Wretlind eventually developed a safe product made from soybean oil[14] that could be given by peripheral vein and was metabolized in a manner similar to that of the chylomicrons formed following the ingestion and absorption of orally administered fat.[15]

Fat emulsions were utilized clinically throughout the 1950s. Despite their use, there were increasing numbers of critically ill patients who could not be fed adequately, and the search for a calorically dense, non-phlebitic parenteral nutrient mixture continued. This search was given further impetus when fat emulsions were withdrawn from clinical use in the United States in 1964 because of severe side effects.

Venous Infusion

Dextrose then became the major energy source in intravenous nutrient solutions in the United States. In order to limit the volume of infusion and still supply adequate calories, the dextrose had to be administered as a concentrated solution, which was very hypertonic. This mixture of dextrose and amino acids could not be tolerated when infused by peripheral vein because of severe phlebitis and ultimate thrombosis. Dudrick and coworkers reasoned that delivery into a high-flow central vein could overcome this problem. To test this idea, they placed catheters into the superior vena cavae of beagle puppies and fed them chronically via a swivel infusion apparatus. They showed in dramatic fashion that normal growth and development could be achieved by providing nutrients exclusively by vein.[16, 17] This demonstration, and its successful application in patients, resulted in widespread clinical use of parenteral nutrition. From this experience in patients with various disease processes, questions arose that required further investigation, and animal models played a significant role in providing some important answers.

ADVANTAGES AND LIMITATIONS OF ANIMAL EXPERIMENTATION

Control of Variables, Body Composition Analysis, and Regional Metabolism

One main advantage of using animals for research is the control of variables. In nutritional studies, for example, an animal's metabolism can be perturbed by a variety of controlled experimental conditions, such as injury, tumor growth, or infection. The animal's response to these various situations can be carefully monitored under several conditions of nutrient intake. The effect of nutrients delivered alone and during the perturbed state can be thoroughly studied, and the influences of all factors involved can be determined. These studies, especially the ones utilizing the tumor and injury models, have provided helpful information for the use of parenteral nutrition in patients with similar conditions.

Another advantage of nutritional research using animals is that body composition analyses can be performed at the conclusion of the studies. This is especially important in determining how nutrients are utilized for repletion or maintenance of body tissues. In humans, this can only be studied indirectly by analyzing bodily excretions or by using complex isotopic methods. For example, tumor growth in a depleted individual given parenteral feedings can be studied much more thoroughly in an animal than in a person, because of the ability to perform body composition analysis at various growth stages of the tumor and at various levels of host nutritional status.

One final advantage of animal models is the capability of studying regional metabolism and thus localized substrate effects. In recent years, more complex regional *in vivo* techniques have been developed to answer questions concerning the response of a specific tissue or region, using the analysis of intraregional flux of substrates. For example, the exchange of substrates across the peripheral tissues of the hindquarter has been studied.[18] Similarly, the hepatic veins have been catheterized to study hepatic metabolic processes under altered conditions,[19] and visceral responses to various metabolic perturbations have been studied with an enteric circulation model.[20]

Species Differences and Restraint of Animal Subjects

There are also disadvantages to using animal models for parenteral nutritional research. The first is the relevance of the information gained. There are differences in metabolic pathways between a given animal species and humans. For example, the clearance of intravenously administered fat emulsion is rapid in the dog but is somewhat slower and biphasic in humans.[21] In contrast, primates metabolize lipids similarly to humans when nutrients are administered orally.[22] Essential amino acid requirements are different for different species.

A second major disadvantage of using animals involves the use of restraint. A calm, awake, unrestrained animal is the ideal experimental subject, but most animals need to be restrained in some way during experiments. To restrain an animal without causing stress, a prolonged training period is usually required. If this factor is not considered, an altered hormonal environment may be induced in the newly restrained animal and may alter the metabolic data obtained.[23, 24] One way to solve the restraint problem is to anesthetize the animal. In fact, early studies in parenteral nutrition used anesthetized animals who received infusions over short time periods (up to eight hours). Anesthesia has a variety of effects, depending on the agent used. Regional and total blood flow may be altered, and insulin release may be attenuated.[25] These effects may significantly alter the results of nutritional studies in an unpredictable manner. Thus, the development of techniques for continuous infusion into unanesthetized, minimally restrained animals was a major advance.[16]

Despite these infusion techniques, prolonged, continuous intravenous infusion of nutrients is difficult to accomplish in many animal models. Because of this, the choice of a model for a given experiment may be based more on the animal's docility and good temperament than on its metabolic similarity to humans. Expediency in carrying out an experiment must be balanced against its relevance to human clinical nutrition.

Complications, Nutrient Requirements, and Costs

Catheter sepsis is a potential major complication in the performance of successful chronic animal infusion studies. In short-term animal experiments, considerations for sterility are often not critical, but in chronic studies catheter sepsis may occur and may have significant effects on results and subsequent interpretations.[26] Strict attention to asepsis is mandatory in catheter insertion, in equipment and solution preparation, and in daily fluid administration techniques.

Nutrient requirements vary from species to species and must be considered when designing research projects. Standard texts are available for reference in providing oral nutrients,[22] but extrapolation to parenteral requirements may be difficult. In addition, attention to thermal neutrality and circadian rhythmicity is important in scheduling experiments and in controlling environmental conditions (light, sound, temperature).[27]

The costs of obtaining and maintaining different animal species may be a major limiting factor in choosing a given animal model. Rats are relatively inexpensive and can be housed in a relatively small space. Large numbers can be studied expediently in a short time period. Dogs and primates are more closely related to humans physiologically and phylogenetically, but they are costly to obtain, require more space to house, and take more time to care for and feed.

The study of animals in a perturbed state is often difficult, since sick animals may require intensive care, and the exact quantitation of their clinical course is difficult. These sophisticated experiments require a major commitment of the time and resources of the investigators.

Ethical Concerns

The ethics of animal experimentation have recently been debated. Various individuals and organizations argue that no useful knowledge results from animal experiments and that the animals are treated cruelly, thus harming society because of a collective lowering of sensitivity to all living creatures.[28] Furthermore, animal experimentation is said to usurp the free will of the animal—the researcher, in designing an experimental protocol does not consider the animal's priorities and thus denies the animal a fundamental right.

Conversely, researchers argue that animal experimentation is essential to the advancement of medical knowledge. Although one can use computer simulations as valuable tools in advancing scientific knowledge, objective data must first be collected, and this data has usually come from animal investigations. Furthermore, the theories and techniques developed by computer simulations must then ultimately be confirmed in biologic systems. The Federal Drug Administration (FDA) requires animal studies prior to the use of drugs or parenteral products in humans. Since intravenous nutrient products are regulated by the FDA, parenteral nutrition studies in animals must be performed.

There are safeguards for animals. Standards for their proper care have been established,[29] and they are generally followed. Before accepting papers for publication, major journals require a statement that proper animal care has been provided. Several institutions have established animal experimentation review committees to assure safe and appropriate animal care. In several European countries, detailed legislation has been passed to protect animal rights. Finally, national funding agencies require institutional assurance of proper animal care before a project is funded. Thus, with these safeguards, studies utilizing nutrient infusions in animals can be carried out.

SPECIFIC ANIMAL MODELS

This section describes three major animal models in detail, and serves as a reference for others. The advantages and disadvantages of each will be discussed. More detailed descriptions of the ways in which these models have improved our understanding of specific clinical situations (i.e., cancer, trauma, pregnancy, short-gut syndrome) may be found in other chapters of this book.

The Dog Model

One of the most commonly used models is the dog. From Wren's early studies, through the 19th century, to the landmark chronic infusion studies in the 1960s, the dog has been a preferred model for parenteral nutrition studies. The long-term infusion studies became possible when a chronic infusion apparatus was developed by Vars. He adapted a syringe swivel unit, originally developed by Jacobs,[30] that could tolerate the highly concentrated dextrose solutions at the required infusion rates.[31] In this model, a catheter was placed into the jugular vein of the animal and then advanced into the superior vena cava. The distal end of the catheter was originally brought directly through the neck incision and was protected by a collar. Later, this technique was improved by tunneling the catheter subcutaneously in order for it to exit from the skin of the back in the interscapular area.[17] The dog was fitted with an infusion harness that was placed around the thorax and neck and that absorbed the varying tension of the infusion cable as the animal moved in its cage. This infusion apparatus worked well and was used successfully throughout the 1950s and 1960s. It permitted continuous intravenous infusion and allowed the dog to move around its cage freely (Fig. 23–1). These techniques for chronic infusion were later adapted for use in other animals.

The advantages and disadvantages of using the dog model are listed in Table 23–1. The cost is low in comparison to primates but high in comparison to rats. Dogs are readily available, and their overall temperament usually makes them good animals for study. The dog's size is an important advantage, because it allows frequent blood sampling without volume depletion. In addition, metabolic *in vivo* studies of specific body regions, such as the hindquarter[18] or the splanchnic bed,[20] can be performed. These studies are not possible in smaller animals with currently available techniques. Since dogs are reasonably large at birth, the effects of intravenous feeding on growth can be

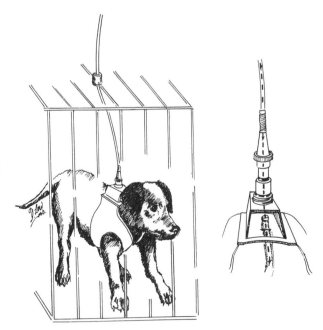

Figure 23–1. Dog model for continuous infusion. *Inset* demonstrates detail of the attachment of the catheter at its exit site.

studied. A germ-free strain of dogs has been developed.[32] The influence of enteric bacteria on metabolic processes can be studied indirectly in these animals. Finally, since the dog has been a popular animal model for many years, there is a large body of metabolic information available, which aids in both the design and interpretation of experiments.

The few disadvantages of using dogs are significant. They are moderately expensive to purchase and feed. They also require considerable space to house. Because dogs are popular pets, there is some objection to their use in experiments. In addition, there is a great hesitancy to use dogs in a perturbed state (such as fasting or injury). Finally, the relevance of data obtained using dogs (as well as other animals) to humans is subject to question. Findings in dogs must ultimately be confirmed in humans.

The Rat Model

A second important animal model is the rat. The technical requirements of chronic infusion are more complicated because of its small size, but most problems have been overcome with well-established techniques. An early approach used the tail vein to gain venous access,[33] but this method was not satisfactory for long-term infusion. Access via the jugular vein in the neck proved more satisfactory. In an early model, the jugular catheter was fixed to the rat's cranium.[34, 35] Although still occasionally used, this technique has largely been abandoned for a system adapted from the dog model in which the central venous catheter is placed via a jugular cut-down and is tunneled to the interscapular area. A harness-cable-swivel system then allows free movement during

Table 23–1. MAJOR ANIMAL MODELS

SPECIES	ADVANTAGES	DISADVANTAGES
Dog	Good temperament; regional studies and multiple blood sampling possible; studies in puppies possible; moderate past information; germ-free model available.	Large space requirements; moderate public resistance; relevance to humans questionable.
Rat	Low cost—little space; large numbers can be studied simultaneously; rapid growth.	Relevance to humans questionable; blood sampling limited; regional studies difficult; duration of infusion limited.
Primate (Monkey)	Simulates humans closely; psychometric studies possible; high intelligence.	High cost; high public resistance; asepsis difficult; bad temperament, large space requirements; restraint usually required; blood sampling limited.

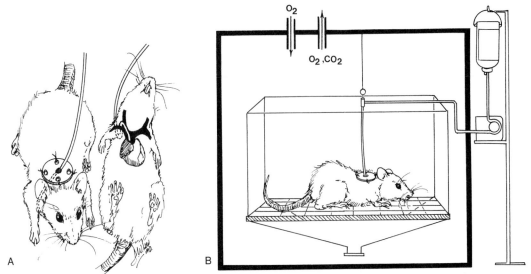

Figure 23–2. Rat model for continuous infusion. A, Dorsal and ventral views. B, Metabolic chamber for measurement of metabolic rate by indirect calorimety and measurement of nitrogen in excreta.

continuous infusion.[36, 37] More recently, the harness has been replaced by a subcutaneously sutured metal button that serves as the stabilizing device for the infusion cable (Fig. 23–2).[38] A further refinement of the model has been the addition of an arterial catheter placed centrally via the carotid artery to allow frequent blood sampling.[39]

The rat model has become the one most frequently used for several reasons. Rats are readily available and cost little to buy and maintain. They can be housed in a small space. There is abundant metabolic data, which aids in designing and interpreting experiments. There is also little public objection to experimentation on rats. A germ-free strain exists.[40] Rats grow rapidly and have a short life cycle. Implanted tumors normally lead to death in six to eight weeks. This is advantageous because short-term experiments (10 to 21 days) represent a significant time period in the animal's life cycle and thus yield significant information. Injury models (burn injury, femoral fracture) have been well described in the rat and are generally acceptable to animal experimentation committees.

The short life cycle and rapid tumor growth may be a disadvantage in that these relatively rapid physiologic and pathologic processes differ significantly from those in humans, so application of results from rat studies to the human condition must be made with caution (see Table 23–1). In vivo regional studies are not currently possible, and frequent blood sampling must be limited in order not to deplete vascular volume. The

recent development of biochemical microanalysis and the technique of reinfusing red cells after removing plasma have partially solved this problem.

The Primate Model

The third major animal model used in parenteral nutrition research is the primate. Chronic chair-restraint models using both the squirrel and Rhesus monkeys have been developed.[41, 42] These models require the animal to sit in a padded chair while being infused (Fig. 23–3). An adaptation period prior to the experimental period is required, and study duration is limited to 14 to 21 days. A freeranging model has recently been achieved by one group of researchers for the Rhesus monkey[42] and by another group for the squirrel monkey.[43] This latter model has been used in the study of circadian rhythms and cyclic enteral feeding.[44] In this model, an intravenous catheter is tunneled to the interscapular area under a nylon mesh jacket. There it is attached to a custom-made cable, which carries the infusion and the monitoring lines to the top of the cage to attach to a swivel (Fig. 23–4). This system has been used continuously for as long as six weeks, but it requires considerable 24-hour maintenance.

The main advantage of the primate model is its phylogenetic similarity to humans. Results of metabolic studies in primates can generally be applied to humans. In addition, the high intelligence of these

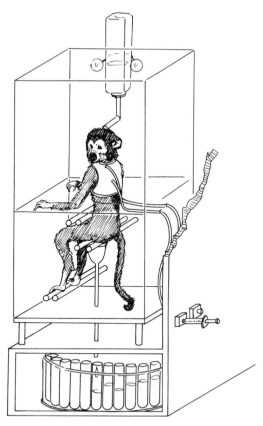

animals theoretically allows the performance of psychometric testing. Thus, the effects of parenteral nutrition regimens on brain development and mental processes could be investigated.

The intelligence and temperament of primates also constitute two of the major disadvantages of their use in intravenous nutritional research. These highly ingenious animals are able to disassemble the most sophisticated devices; the maintenance of a chronic intravenous infusion therefore becomes a formidable task. There are other disadvantages to primate models. The animals are costly, both to purchase and to house. Because they can harbor diseases transmissible to humans, periods of quarantine are necessary to ensure that animals are safe for use. Some species are quite small (the squirrel monkey is 1 kg) and this size precludes regional studies and frequent blood sampling. Maintenance of a long-term sterile system, though difficult in all animal models, is especially difficult in primates. Studies of perturbed states are usually expensive, and public resistance to use of primates is high.

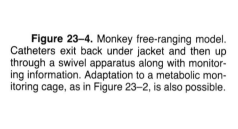

Figure 23–3. Monkey chain model. Catheters exit back under a jacket. No swivel device is used, because the monkey remains sitting. Studies are limited to 14–21 days.

OTHER ANIMAL MODELS

Other animals have been used to study parenteral nutrition. The unique aspects of

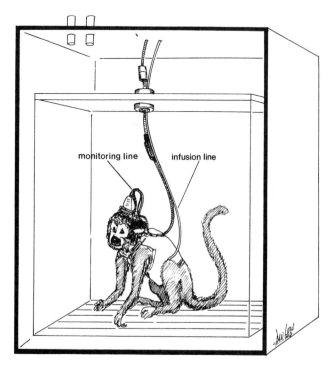

Figure 23–4. Monkey free-ranging model. Catheters exit back under jacket and then up through a swivel apparatus along with monitoring information. Adaptation to a metabolic monitoring cage, as in Figure 23–2, is also possible.

monitoring line   infusion line

several models will be described briefly. Table 23–2 lists appropriate references.

The Rabbit Model

The rabbit has been used both in short-term studies under anesthesia[45] and in a chronic infusion model.[46] Questions of renal and gut function have been addressed; the results obtained are similar to those reported in the dog and the rat.

The Mouse Model

The mouse poses a technical challenge to the ambitious parenteral nutrition investigator. An early technique utilized the inferior vena cava via the tail vein, but this technique was later adapted to the customary chronic infusion model in a minimally restrained animal.[47] This latter model has been published in abstract form only, and it is not yet worked out well. Mice have been used to study the effect of fat infusion on reticuloendothelial cell function following a single intraperitoneal dose of fat emulsion.[48] The very small size of the mouse limits its usefulness in chronic infusion models.

The Sheep Model

Sheep have rarely been used in parenteral nutrition studies. Ruminants have different gut anatomy, physiology, and biochemistry than humans; only specifically designed studies yield results relevant to humans. However, their inability to absorb glucose from the gut makes them unique animals in which to study the effect of intravenous nutrients (especially glucose) on gluconeogenesis. Details of the sheep model can be found in a study defining intravenous

amino acid requirements[49] or in a study examining fetal metabolism.[50]

The Pig Model

A long-term infusion model has also been described in the pig. This animal model has been used to study immune function,[51] general metabolism,[52] and gut irradiation injury.[53]

The Guinea Pig, Cow, and Horse Models

The guinea pig has been used as a source of peritoneal macrophages for *in vitro* studies of the effects of fat emulsion on phagocytic function.[54] The cow has been intravenously fed, both experimentally and therapeutically, for examining gut function and diarrheal illnesses.[55, 56] The infusion system is similar to that used in other animals, but the catheter exits in the posterior neck rather than interscapularly. Finally, horses have been given parenteral nutrition therapeutically in order to treat tetanus[57] or severe diarrhea.[58] However, no experimental studies have been done using the horse as a model.

These models all use central (systemic) veins for infusion. Portal vein infusion models have also been described.[59] Future developments might include the use of an implantable pump so that the animal could be completely free-ranging. Finally, perturbation of the nervous system while studying metabolic processes might provide important information about the fundamental mechanisms of metabolic control.

SUMMARY

Animals have played a major role in the study of parenteral nutrition. Although the first experiment was done in the 17th century, the 20th century has seen the most significant advances. The key development that allowed rapid progress was a technical one, namely, the perfection of a chronic infusion system. More recently, regional flux models have yielded more specific information of metabolic pathways and intraorgan exchange of nutrients, both in simple starvation and in starvation associated with disease states. Further refinements of tech-

Table 23–2. MINOR ANIMAL MODELS

SPECIES	REFERENCE	COMMENTS
Rabbit	45, 56	Renal, gut function
Mouse	47, 48	Technique, immune function
Sheep	49, 50	Pregnancy, metabolism
Pig	51, 52, 53	Irradiation, immunity
Guinea pig	54	Immunity
Cow	55, 56	Gut function
Horse	57, 58	Treatment

niques are likely. Animal models will continue to play an important role in answering major questions relevant to providing safe and effective parenteral nutrition. The dog, rat, and monkey have been the three major animal species used for such studies. Each specific animal model has advantages and disadvantages that must be considered in relation to the goals of the experiment and the available facilities.

The costs of animals and equipment may become a dominant factor in choosing a given animal model as budgetary constraints and expenses play increasingly significant roles in nutritional research. Some experiments may be less expensive and more applicable if performed directly in humans. Thus, a great deal of thought and discussion should precede studies in both humans and animals. However, if important questions cannot be answered by human studies, careful and considerate studies in animals will continue to prove invaluable.

REFERENCES AND SELECTED READINGS

1. Rose, W.C.: Amino acid requirements of man. Fed. Proc., *8*:546, 1949.
2. Rose, W.C.: The nutritive significance of the amino acids. Phys. Rev., *18*:109, 1938.
3. Young, E.A., and Weser, E.: Animal models for enteral feeding of defined formula diets. *In* Rombeau, J.L., and Caldwell, M.D. (eds.): Clinical Nutrition. Vol. 1. Enteral and Tube Feeding. Philadelphia, W. B. Saunders Co., 1983.
4. Dorland's Illustrated Medical Dictionary. Edition 24. Philadelphia, W. B. Saunders Co., page 1102.
5. Annan, G.L.: An exhibition of books on the growth of our knowledge of blood transfusion. Bull. N.Y. Acad. Med., *15*:622, 1939.
6. Macht, S.D.: Three hundred years of parenteral nutrition: the history of intravenous nutritional therapy. Conn. Med., *44*:27, 1980.
7. Foster, M.: Claude Bernard. New York, Longmans Green Co., 1899.
8. Hodder, E.M.: Transfusion of milk in cholera. Practitioner, *10*:14, 1873.
9. Elman, R.: Urinary output of nitrogen as influenced by intravenous injection of a mixture of amino acids. Proc. Soc. Exp. Biol. Med., *37*:610, 1983.
10. Elman, R.: Time factor in retention of nitrogen after intravenous injection of a mixture of amino acids. Proc. Soc. Exp. Biol. Med., *40*:484, 1939.
11. Elman, R., and Weiner, D.O.: Intravenous alimentation with special reference to protein metabolism. J.A.M.A., *112*:796, 1939.
12. Nomura, T.: Experimentelle studien uber intravenuse fettinfusion unter besonder berudesichtigung parenteraler ernahrung. Tohoku J. Exp. Med., *13*:51, 1929.
13. Holt, L.E., Tidwell, H.D., and Scott, T.F.: The intravenous administration of fat. J. Pediatr., *6*:151, 1935.
14. Hallberg, D., Holm, I., Obel, A.L. et al.: Fat emulsion for complete intravenous nutrition. Postgrad. Med. J., *42*:A71, A87, A99, A149, 1967.
15. Hallberg, D.: Elimination of exogenous lipids from the bloodstream. An experimental methodological and clinical study in dog and man. Acta Physiol. Scand. (Suppl.), *65*:254, 1965.
16. Dudrick, S.J., Wilmore, D.W., Vars, H.M. et al.: Long term total parenteral nutrition with growth, development, and positive nitrogen balance. Surgery, *64*:134, 1968.
17. Dudrick, S.J., Steiger, E., Wilmore, D.W., and Vars, H.M.: Continuous long-term intravenous infusion in unrestrained animals. Lab. Anim. Care, *20*:521, 1970.
18. Mitch, W.E.: Amino acid release from the hindquarter and urea appearance in acute uremia. Am. J. Phys., *241*:E415, 1981.
19. Bradley, S.E., Ingelfinger, F.J., Bradley, C.P. et al.: The estimation of hepatic bloodflow in man. J. Clin. Invest., *24*:890, 1945.
20. Katz, M.L., and Bergman, E.N.: Simultaneous measurements of hepatic and portal venous bloodflow in the sheep and dog. Am. J. Phys., *216*:946, 1969.
21. Allen, P.C., and Lee, H.A.: A clinical guide to intravenous nutrition. Blackwell Scientific Publications. London, Spottswoode, Ballantyne & Co., 1969, pages 15 and 16.
22. Mitruken, B.M., Rawnsley, H.M., and Vadehra, D.V. (eds.): Animals for Medical Research. New York, John Wiley & Sons, 1976, pages 552–560.
23. Hume, D.M.: Endocrine and metabolic responses to injury. *In* Schwartz, S.I. (ed.): Principles of Surgery. Chapter 1. New York, McGraw-Hill Book Co., 1960, pages 11–13.
24. Birkhahn, R.H., Bellinger, L.L., Bernardis, L., and Border, J.R.: The stress response in the rat from harnessing for chronic intravenous infusion. J. Surg. Res., *21*:185, 1976.
25. Bessey, P.Q., Black, P.R., Colpoys, M.F. et al.: Barbiturate anesthesia suppresses insulin release. Surg. Forum, *33*:23, 1982.
26. Popp, M.B., and Brennan, M.F.: Long-term vascular access in the rat: importance of sepsis. Am. J. Phys., *241*:H606, 1981.
27. Moore-Ede, M.C., Sulzman, F.M., and Fuller, C.A.: Circadian timing of physiologic systems. *In* The Clocks That Time Us. Cambridge, Massachusetts, Harvard University Press, 1982.
28. Liebert, L.: Animal rights advocates ask ban on use of lost pets for research. The Boston Globe, *224*:5, August 2, 1983.
29. Guide for the Care and Use of Laboratory Animals: DHEW Publication Number (NIH) 80-23, Revised, 1978, Reprinted 1980. Office of Science and Health Reports, DRR/NIH, Bethesda, Maryland, 20205.
30. Jacobs, H.R.D.: An apparatus for constant intravenous injection into unrestrained animals. J. Lab. Clin. Med., *16*:901, 1931.
31. Rhode, C.M., Parkins, W., Tourtellotte, D., and Vars, H.M.: Method for continuous intravenous administration of nutritive solutions suitable for prolonged metabolic studies in dogs. Am. J. Phys., *159*:409, 1949.
32. Levenson, S.M.: The influence of the indigenous microflora on mammalian metabolism and nutrition. J.P.E.N., *2*:78, 1978.
33. Eve, C., and Robinson, S.H.: Apparatus for continuous long-term intravenous infusions in small animals. J. Lab. Clin. Med., *62*:169, 1963.
34. Steffens, A.P.: A method for frequent sampling of

blood and continuous infusion of fluids in the rat without disturbing the animal. Phys. Behav., *4*:833, 1969.

35. Cocchetto, D.M., and Thour, D.B.: Methods for vascular access and collection of body fluids from the laboratory rat. J. Pharm. Sci., *72*:465, 1983.

36. Steiger, E., Vars, H.M., and Dudrick, S.J.: A technique for long-term intravenous feeding in unrestrained rats. Arch. Surg., *104*:330, 1972.

37. Steiger, E., Daly, J.M., Vars, H.M. et al.: Animal research in intravenous hyperalimentation. *In* Cowen, G.S.M., and Sheetz, W.L. (eds.): Intravenous Hyperalimentation. Philadelphia, Lea & Febiger, 1972.

38. Cox, C.E., and Beazley, R.M.: Chronic venous catheterization: a technique for implanting and maintaining venous catheters in rats. J. Surg. Res., *18*:607, 1975.

39. Burt, M.E., Arbeit, J., and Brennan, M.F.: Chronic arterial and venous access in the unrestrained rat. Am. J. Phys., *238*:H599, 1980.

40. Sumi, Y., Hirono, I., Hosaka, S. et al.: Tumor induction in germ-free rats fed bracken. Can. Res., *41*:250, 1981.

41. Hobbs, C.L., Mullen, J.L., Gertner, M.H. et al.: Hyperalimentation in primates. A nutritional model. J.P.E.N., *4*:443, 1980.

42. Wannemacher, R.W., Jr., Kaminski, M.V., Jr., Dinterman, R.E. et al.: Use of lipid calories during pneumococcal sepsis in the Rhesus monkey. J.P.E.N., *6*:100, 1982.

43. Gander, P.H., and Moore-Ede, M.C.: Light-dark masking of circadian temperature and activity rhythms in squirrel monkeys. Am. J. Physiol., *245*:R927–R934, 1983.

44. Apelgren, K.N., Frim, D.M., Gander, P.H. et al.: Effectiveness of cyclic intragastric feeding as a circadian zeitgeber in the squirrel monkey. Physiol. Behav., *34*:335, 1985.

45. Hunt, C.E., Gora, P., and Inwood, R.J.: Pulmonary effects of intralipid: the role of intralipid as a prostaglandin precursor. Prog. Lipid Res., *20*:199, 1981.

46. Eastwood, G.L.: Small bowel morphology and epithelial proliferation in intravenously alimented rabbits. Surgery, *82*:613, 1977.

47. Heller, P.A., Sitren, H.S., Bailey, L.B., and Cerda, J.J.: Total parenteral nutrition in the mouse. Am. J. Clin. Nutr. (Abstract), *35*(6):28, 1982.

48. Fischer, G.W., Hunter, K.W., and Wilson, S.R.: Intralipid and reticuloendothelial clearance. Lancet, *2*:1300, 1980.

49. Asplund, J.M.: A parenteral model to study amino acid requirements of functioning ruminants. Acta Chir. Scand. (Suppl.), *466*:34, 1976.

50. Young, M., Soltesz, G., Noakes, D. et al.: The influence of intrauterine surgery and of fetal intravenous nutritional supplements "in utero" on plasma free amino acid homeostasis in the pregnant ewe. J. Perinatol. Med., *3*:180, 1975.

51. Lindberg, B.W., and Clowes, G.H., Jr.: The effect of hyperalimentation and infused leucine on the amino acid metabolism in sepsis: an experimental study *in vivo*. Surgery, *90*:278, 1981.

52. Hrimmer, W., Pemsel, W., Berg, G. et al.: Methodological and technical problems in long-term infusion therapy using a vena cava catheter. Studies on balanced parenteral nutrition of young miniature pigs. Z. Ernaehrungswiss, *11*:254, 1972.

53. Daburon, F., and Duee, P.H.: Nutritional and clinical aspects of parenteral nutrition in pigs irradiated on the abdomen with supralethal doses. Biomedicine (Express), *25*:385, 1976.

54. Strunk, R.C., Kunke, K., Nagle, R.B. et al.: Inhibition of *in vitro* synthesis of the second (C2) and fourth (C4) components of complement in guinea pig peritoneal macrophages by a soybean oil emulsion. Pediatr. Res., *13*:188, 1979.

55. Sherman, D.M., Hoffsis, G.F., Gingerich, D.A. et al.: A technique for long-term fluid administration in the calf. J. Am. Vet. Med. Assoc., *169*:1310, 1976.

56. Hoffsis, G.F., Gingerich, D.A., Sherman, D.M. et al.: Total intravenous feeding of calves. J. Am. Vet. Med. Assoc., *171*:67, 1977.

57. Greatorex, J.C.: Intravenous nutrition in the treatment of tetanus in horses. Vet. Res., *97*:498, 1975.

58. Gideon, L.: Total nutritional support of the foal. VM-SAC, *72*:1197, 1977.

59. Joyeux, H., Asture, B., Martin, P., and Solassol, C.: Experimental nutrition via the portal vein. Techniques and results. J. Chir. (Paris), *107*:355, 1974.

60. Cuthbertson, D.: Historical background to parenteral nutrition. Acta Chir. Scand. (Suppl.) *498*:1, 1980. A concise review. British viewpoint.

61. Wretlind, A.: Complete intravenous nutrition. Theoretical and experimental background. Nutr. Metab. (Suppl.), *14*:1, 1972. Good extensive review with theoretical explanations.

62. Rhoads, J.E., Vars, H.M., and Dudrick, S.J.: The development of intravenous hyperalimentation. Surg. Clin. North Am., *61*(3):429, 1981. Good clinical review with emphasis on clinical applications.

63. Geyer, R.: Parenteral nutrition. Physiol. Rev., *40*:150, 1960. An excellent review of early work.

64. Kleiber, M.: The Fire of Life. New York, John Wiley & Sons Inc., 1961. A delightful scientific book with sound concepts of interspecies metabolic phenomena.

CHAPTER 24

Enteric Fistulas

JOHN A. RYAN, JR.
BRUCE A. ADYE
ALEX J. WEINSTEIN

The purpose of this chapter is to review the topic of enteric fistulas, with special attention to the role of nutrition in their management. Particular emphasis will be paid to the influence of total parenteral nutrition (TPN) on the treatment and outcome of these conditions.

A fistula is an abnormal communication between two organs. The term derives from the Latin word meaning hollow like a pipe or reed. Enteric fistulas can be categorized in several ways. *External fistulas* are abnormal communications between the gastrointestinal tract and the surface of the body, usually the skin (e.g., colocutaneous or enterocutaneous). *Internal fistulas* are abnormal communications between two internal organs (e.g., colovesical or cholecystoduodenal). Fistulas are also classified as *congenital* or *acquired*, and the latter can be further considered as *spontaneous* (secondary to an inherent disease in the abdomen or gastrointestinal tract) or *traumatic-postoperative-iatrogenic*. This chapter will discuss acquired external gastrointestinal fistulas, with particular emphasis on postoperative fistulas, since they are seen most commonly. Fistulas of the biliary, pancreatic, and urinary systems will not be discussed, but they may occur in conjunction with gastrointestinal fistulas.

Enteric fistulas occur rarely, but they represent major medical and surgical problems that entail high morbidity and mortality, lengthy hospital stays, and high health care costs. They also involve many specialized aspects of modern health care. The patient faces excessive loss of fluids and electrolytes, intra-abdominal sepsis, wound infection, excoriation of the skin, malnutrition, and hemorrhage from the fistula tract—all of which can lead to sequential organ failure and death. As the patient watches the wound disrupt and the enteric contents drain onto the abdominal wall, the full impact of surgical failure may cause psychologic depression and loss of confidence in the surgical team. An organized, rational approach to fistulas is needed in order to understand and overcome the myriad problems. In this chapter, the discussion of fistulas will be divided into five sections: (1) descriptive classification, (2) principles of management, (3) the role of nutritional therapy, (4) the role of operative therapy, and (5) results.

DESCRIPTIVE CLASSIFICATION

An accurate description of a fistula is important in determining the possibility of spontaneous healing and also in making decisions about nutritional management, the timing and need for operation, and the type of operation to be performed. This description is compiled after obtaining a thorough history, physical examination, and laboratory and radiologic examinations, and reviewing previous operations and pathologic data. It may require knowledge gained from invasive radiologic, endoscopic, and surgical procedures. The following is an outline of important factors that should be known in order to adequately describe a fistula:

I. Location
  A. Esophagus
  B. Stomach
  C. Duodenum
  D. Jejunum
  E. Ileum
  F. Colon (specific part)
  G. Involvement of biliary, pancreatic, or urinary systems
  H. Coexisting internal fistulas

II. Diagnosis and Etiology
   A. Spontaneous (perforation of alimentary tract by tumor, inflammation, ischemia, or strangulation that forms an abscess that then penetrates to the body surface)
   B. Traumatic (blunt or penetrating)
   C. Iatrogenic (postoperative)
      1. Unrecognized injury to the enteric wall (enterotomy)
      2. Failure of suture line or anastomosis to heal
         a. Lack of blood supply
         b. Too much tension
         c. Contamination
         d. Foreign body
         e. Lack of hemostasis
         f. Poor technique
         g. Diseased organ
      3. Postoperative abscess that perforates alimentary tract and penetrates to body surface
      4. Erosion of alimentary tract by foreign body, (e.g., drain or stay suture)
      5. Infarction of organ secondary to operative devascularization
      6. Endoscopy—intraluminal injury
III. Local Descriptive Factors of Organ, Tract, and Surface
   A. Organ factors
      1. Condition of organ at site of fistula
         a. Normal
         b. Diseased (cancer, inflammation, radiation, ischemia)
         c. Suture line, anastomosis
      2. Size of hole
      3. Number of holes
      4. Location of hole
         a. Lateral
         b. End
      5. Function of organ in relation to fistula
         a. Distal obstruction
         b. Discontinuity
         c. Reversal of distal organ
      6. Prediction of organ function with spontaneous closure of fistula, (e.g., stenosis with resulting obstruction)
   B. Features of fistula tract
      1. Length
         a. Long
         b. Short—less than 2 cm
         c. Mucosal-cutaneous continuity (epithelialization)
      2. Width
      3. Infection
         a. Abscess (aerobic-anaerobic bacteria)
         b. Unusual pathogens (tuberculosis, actinomycosis, candidiasis)
      4. Number of tracts
      5. Foreign body
         a. Operative (sponge, suture, instrument, device, needle, drains, mesh)
         b. Ingested (e.g., toothpick, pin)
         c. Placed through the fistula (e.g., dressings, facticious manipulation)
      6. Osteomyelitis (bone involvement along the tract)
      7. Neoplasia
   C. Surface factors
      1. Site of exit
         a. Abdominal incision (wound infection, fascial dehiscence, wound hernia)
         b. Drain tract
         c. Peristomal
         d. Virgin skin
      2. Condition of abdominal wall at site of fistula
         a. Normal
         b. Diseased (cancer, infection, radiation)
IV. Miscellaneous Factors
   A. Output
      1. Quantity (high or low output)
      2. Quality
         a. Digestive enzymes (gastric acid, pancreatic juice, bile, succus entericus)
         b. Semisolid, feculent
   B. Chronologic factors
      1. Time from operation
      2. Time from diagnosis of fistula
      3. Time from control of infection
      4. Time from restoration of normal nutrition
   C. Factitious
V. Description of Patient with Enteric Fistula
   A. Age
   B. Sex
   C. Diagnoses detrimental to healing (e.g., obesity, diabetes, collagen vascular disease, or organ failure of heart, lung, liver, or kidney)
   D. Drugs detrimental to healing (e.g., steroids, chemotherapeutic agents, anticoagulants)

E. Nutritional assessment (weight loss, relationship to ideal body weight, serum albumin levels)

F. Previous surgical history

Figures 24–1 to 24–3 depict typical gastroduodenal, small bowel, and colonic fistulas, respectively. Figure 24–2 emphasizes some of the local descriptive factors of the organ, tract, and surface. Complex fistulas require thoughtful description. Figure 24–2*I* shows a small-bowel fistula that followed an emergency resection for severe sigmoid diverticulitis. There is leakage from the drain tract and around the colostomy. A hole in the bladder with urinary leakage complicates the fistula. Figure 24–3*B* demonstrates a complex fistula in a patient with Crohn's disease, which followed removal of an inflamed gallbladder that was adherent to the transverse colon. Note both biliary and feculent drainage, as well as an internal ileocolonic fistula.

PRINCIPLES OF MANAGEMENT

Since most enteric fistulas occur secondary to an operation, the surgeon responsible will be the first to be notified about drainage of feculent contents onto the abdominal wall. Naturally, the surgeon will be discouraged at the failure of the operation and may either ignore the problem or press for immediate surgical repair. Neither of these courses is correct. A fistula demands an urgent but organized approach that takes into account a number of issues. In 1964, Chapman, Foran, and Dunphy outlined definite priorities and a necessary time frame in the treatment of enteric fistulas. Key points included fluid and electrolyte balance, control of fistula drainage, management of infection, attention to nutrition, and decisions about operation.[1] Little has been added in theory to their recommendations, but advances in intensive care, antibiotics, radiology, wound care, intravenous therapy, and nutrition have made

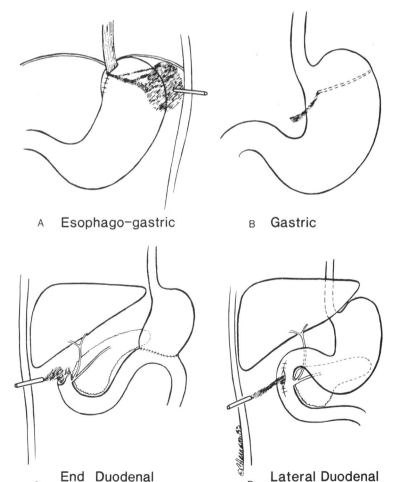

A Esophago–gastric   B Gastric

C End Duodenal   D Lateral Duodenal

Figure 24–1. Gastroduodenal fistulas.

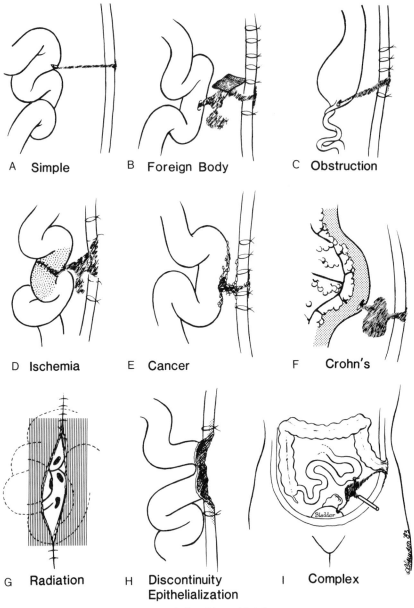

A   Simple   B   Foreign Body   C   Obstruction

D   Ischemia   E   Cancer   F   Crohn's

G   Radiation   H   Discontinuity   I   Complex
                       Epithelialization

Figure 24–2. Small bowel fistulas.

their recommendations easier to accomplish. Our organizational approach to fistula management includes resuscitation, control of drainage and protection of the skin, control of infection, definition of anatomy and descriptive classification, nutritional evaluation and therapy, psychologic support and physical therapy, and operation. Although the areas of importance are listed in the general chronologic order of concern, in practice attention should be given simultaneously to many aspects of fistula care. The health care professionals who may be needed include the surgeon, radiologist, nurse, TPN nurse, enterostomal therapist, housestaff, physical therapist, dietitian, medical consultant, and social worker.

Resuscitation

Intravascular blood volume, fluid and electrolyte requirements, and acid-base balance are of immediate concern, particularly for high-output fistulas (> 500 ml/day). Hematocrit, serum and fistula electrolyte values, arterial blood gases, and total fluid input and output measurements should be obtained immediately and on a periodic basis. Initially most patients should be given nothing by mouth and should be treated with intravenous therapy. Fluid and electrolyte balance will be an ongoing concern over the lengthy period necessary to manage the fistula.

Control of Drainage and Protection of the Skin

The condition of the skin around the surface exit point of the fistula is of emergent concern. Digestive enzymes and bacteria in the effluent may cause maceration, ulceration, and cellulitis of the skin. Before this process starts, the skin can be protected without too much difficulty, but once it is damaged, adequate care becomes increasingly difficult. The most common place for a fistula to exit is through the surgical wound, thus complicating skin protection with the man-

agement of wound infection, fascial dehiscence, and evisceration.

At first recognition of a fistula, we apply Stomahesive to the edges of the skin.[2-4] Stomahesive is a 3-mm-thick wafer of gelatin, pectin, sodium carboxymethylcellulose, and polyisobutylene. It will adhere naturally to dry skin, but it can also be applied to excoriated skin to prevent further damage. It can be cut into any geometric or anatomic pattern necessary to fit the wound and fill crevices and contours in the skin. Karaya paste can also aid in skin protection, but aluminum paste, zinc oxide, karaya powder, and placenta are infrequently used now.

Clear plastic collection bags with adhesive backing that can be cut to match the wound opening are applied to the Stomahesive. The bags collect the fistula drainage, which can then be quantified. Soft sump-suction catheters can be placed into the wound through the bag to help collect volu-

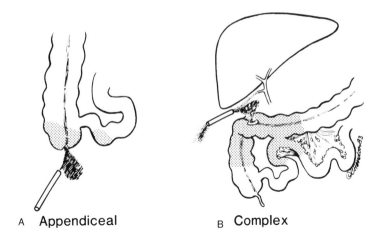

A **Appendiceal**   B **Complex**

Figure 24–3. Colonic fistulas.

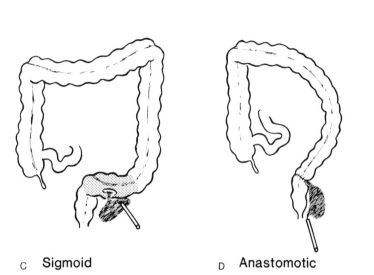

C **Sigmoid**   D **Anastomotic**

minous drainage. The suction catheter should be advanced out of the wound over a period of time. Occasionally, continuous or intermittent drip irrigation of the wound with saline may help clean it and collect the effluent. The ability of trained and experienced enterostomal therapists, whose expertise with colostomy, ileostomy, and urinary diversion procedures can be adapted to uncontrolled enteric fistulas, has proved valuable in wound care. Occasionally, the patient can be positioned using split mattresses or circle beds to elicit gravity as an ally in collecting drainage. The literature is replete with descriptions of suction, irrigation, and collection devices.[5-11] Biologic adhesives and castings of unusual wounds have been reported to help in the management of enteric fistulas, but none of these methods has gained widespread acceptance.[12-15]

Decreasing the volume of fistula drainage may make wound management easier. Initially the patient is given nothing by mouth. Nasogastric drainage is not employed unless gastrointestinal obstruction causes vomiting. Cimetidine will decrease the volume of high-output upper gastrointestinal tract fistulas by decreasing gastric acid production.[16]

Control of Infection

Every external fistula represents some degree of infection as the bacterial contents of the gastrointestinal tract traverse the peritoneal cavity and abdominal wall. The vast majority of fistula deaths occur secondary to sepsis. Therefore, the definition and control of infection becomes a top priority in fistula management.

Physical examination of the wound and abdomen is the first step in the detection of undrained infection. Sometimes the entire subcutaneous wound will need to be opened. At other times, gentle digital examination of the fistula tract will detect abscesses. General abdominal examination, rectal examination, and digital examination of any stoma should be performed to look for intra-abdominal abscesses. Amazingly large collections of pus can be present in the postoperative abdomen without clear-cut physcial signs. Plain films of the chest and abdomen may reveal signs of an elevated diaphragm, pleural effusion, mass effect, abnormal gas bubbles, or bowel obstruction. Computed tomography, ultrasound, and radionuclide scans have vastly improved the detection of the intra-abdominal abscesses.[17] Computed tomographic– or ultrasonic-guided percutaneous drainage of abscesses is to be encouraged whenever appropriate.[18] At other times, formal operative drainage of abscesses will be necessary. Not infrequently the drainage of a postoperative intra-abdominal abscess will lead to the efflux of enteric contents, uncovering the first evidence of a fistula.

Recently, interventional radiologists, using fluoroscopy, have utilized the fistula orifice for fistulography and manipulation of steerable, flexible guide wires and catheters in order to intubate fistulas and to drain intra-abdominal abscesses associated with the fistula tract.[19] With these new imaging methods and drainage techniques, the interventional radiologists have become very important in the control of infection. Often, repeated examinations and manipulations are necessary. No patient should be allowed to succumb when signs of sepsis (such as fever, leukocytosis, mental obtundation, glucose intolerance, or septic shock) are present, without an aggressive search for undrained intra-abdominal infection.

Purulent fistula effluent should be cultured for aerobic and anaerobic bacteria and fungi. Blood cultures should be obtained when signs of sepsis are present. Broad-spectrum antibiotics with anaerobic coverage should be used in conjunction with surgical drainage in the treatment of abscesses, cellulitis, and septicemia. Antibiotics are often used when a fistula first appears, but they should be stopped shortly after control of the fistula is obtained or after the abscess is drained so that resistant organisms are not selected.

Fistula tracts may involve the bony or cartilaginous boundaries of the abdomen, including the xiphoid process, rib cage, iliac crest, pubic bone, and even the spine. The presence of osteomyelitis or bacterial chondritis may affect decisions about surgical debridement and the length of antibiotic therapy.

Fistula patients may be more prone to pneumonia, urinary tract infection, decubitus ulcers, thrombophlebitis, and central venous catheter sepsis.[20,21] These problems, in addition to abdominal sepsis, need to be considered in any evaluation of fever.

Definition of Anatomy and Descriptive Classification

After resuscitation, protection of the skin, and control of infection have been accomplished—hopefully within the first 24 to 48 hours—a more reflective evaluation of the etiology, pathophysiology, and anatomy of the fistula must be documented. The surgeon should attempt to reconstruct the events that led to the fistula so as to have full knowledge of the descriptive classification as suggested in the outline presented previously. Paramount in this endeavor is a review of any previous operative notes and pathology reports. This is particularly necessary when a patient has been transferred to a referral hospital. The accepting physician should not take for granted that a standard operation or disease process has occurred. A review of actual pathologic slides is necessary if confusion about malignancy or inflammatory bowel disease exists.

Occasionally, evaluation of the fistula effluent for amylase, bilirubin, or creatinine, or the oral or rectal administration of charcoal or unabsorbable dyes, such as indigo carmine, can clarify the presence and character of a fistula. Methylene blue dye injected intravenously is excreted in the urine, and if it appears in the wound, it can document urinary tract involvement. Usually, fistulography with water-soluble contrast gives precise information about the location and anatomy of a fistula. Fluoroscopic examinations with barium in the esophagus, stomach, duodenum, small intestine, and colon are often necessary in localizing the fistula, defining anatomy disturbed by prior operation, and documenting coexisting disease. Obviously, the radiologist plays a key role in the definition of the anatomy and the descriptive classification of fistulas, as well as in the detection and drainage of abscesses. The surgeon and the radiologist need to work together, with the surgeon communicating fully to the radiologist about clinical information, suspicions, and what is hoped to be accomplished by each examination. This communication is facilitated if one radiologist who is familiar with gastrointestinal disease and interventional techniques performs all the needed studies and if the surgeon is present for the major examinations. Endoscopy of the gastrointestinal tract for the purpose of biopsy may be important in determining the presence of a disease at a fistula orifice.

Nutritional Evaluation and Therapy

Once a full description of the fistula has been accomplished, decisions about the long-term nutritional management of the patient can be made. The role of nutrition will be considered in detail in the next section of this chapter.

Psychologic Support and Physical Therapy

At this point in the treatment, objective communication with the patient, family, and referring physician can be accomplished. Realistic expectations need to be communicated to the patient and the family about the ultimate prognosis of the fistula, the length of hospitalization, and the possibility of future operations. An overly optimistic or pessimistic view of the patient's condition is unproductive in gaining cooperation or allaying fears. Physical therapy, occupational therapy, and a caring nursing service may be helpful in supporting the patient's morale over the long-term hospitalization.

Rarely, when a fistula with favorable characteristics has not healed despite lengthy hospitalization and multiple operations, factitious manipulation by the patient of the fistula tract must be considered. In these cases, extensive psychologic therapy or preventing the patient from disturbing the fistula by mechanical means may be successful.

Operation

Further on we will discuss the operative therapy of fistulas. Usually definitive operations are postponed for greater than a month to see if the fistula will heal spontaneously under conservative management.

THE ROLE OF NUTRITIONAL THERAPY

This section will examine evidence from the literature to answer the following questions about the nutritional management of patients with fistulas:

1. Does malnutrition contribute to an increased mortality?

2. Does the provision of adequate nutrition improve survival?

3. Does the delivery route of nutrients, either gastrointestinal or intravenous, make a difference in the outcome?

Edmunds and associates reported a 43 per cent mortality rate in 157 patients with enteric fistulas at the Massachusetts General Hospital from 1946 to 1959.[22] Malnourished patients (defined by weight loss greater than 15 lbs and a serum protein level of less than 5.6 gm/dl) had a 61 per cent mortality rate. Patients with colonic fistulas constituted a favorable group, with only a 16 per cent mortality rate; however, when malnutrition was present, 64 per cent of the patients with colonic fistulas died. This paper became a classic in fistula literature because of the correlation of increased mortality with malnutrition. Others have since confirmed this relationship. A report from the same hospital on a total of 119 enteric fistulas in patients from 1960 through 1970 documented 36 patients with severe malnutrition (defined by weight loss greater than 11 kg and a total protein of less than 5 gm/dl with a 28 per cent mortality rate, 68 patients with moderate malnutrition (defined by weight loss of greater than 7 kg or total protein of less than 6 gm/dl, or both) with a 10 per cent mortality rate, and 15 patients without malnutrition with a 7 per cent mortality rate.[23]

Coutsoftides and Fazio reported 174 patients with small-bowel fistulas from the Cleveland Clinic between 1956 and 1976.[24] When weight loss was greater than 15 per cent, mortality was 32 per cent, whereas when weight loss was less than 15 per cent, the mortality rate was 4 per cent. If the serum albumin level was less than 2.5 gm/dl, the mortality rate was 42 per cent, but no patient died if the serum albumin level was greater than 3.5 gm/dl. Patients with high-output fistulas became malnourished because of the loss of nutrients through the fistula, increased metabolic demands associated with sepsis, and poor nutritional intake secondary to decreased appetite and mechanical obstruction. The patient who was least able to obtain nourishment because of the fistula also had the worst prognosis for recovery and healing.

In 1939, Elman and Weiner stimulated interest in intravenous nutrition by reporting the first use of intravenous amino acids (casein hydrolysates) in patients.[25] In 1945, Brunschwig and colleagues described a patient with a high-output postoperative jejunal fistula who was denied oral intake for eight weeks while being treated with intravenous 5 per cent casein hydrolysates and dextrose, which supplied 980 calories intravenously/day.[26] The patient had an average loss of less than 1 gm of nitrogen/day and eventually underwent successful operation. In 1951, Hull and Barnes reported the delivery by peripheral vein of 3 L of 10 per cent dextrose and 1 L of 10 per cent casein hydrolysate, which supplied approximately 1600 calories/day to six patients with small-bowel fistulas.[27] The main benefit was decreased fistula output, and all patients underwent successful operations. Unfortunately, the hypertonicity of these solutions made delivery by peripheral vein difficult, and adequate nutrition could be given for a short time only.

Others were adapting the gastrointestinal tract to help nourish patients with fistulas. In 1956, Smith and Lee reported 11 cases of successful spontaneous closure of duodenal stump fistulas that were treated with continuous nasojejunal feeding of hydrolyzed lactalbumin and dextrose through a small polyethylene catheter.[28]

The papers cited in preceding paragraphs provided anecdotal reports that nourishing patients with enteric fistulas was both possible and beneficial. However, the first real evidence of the benefits of nourishing fistula patients was contained in the report by Chapman, Foran, and Dunphy in 1964.[1] A 45 per cent mortality rate was documented in 56 cases of enteric fistulas that were treated at the University of Oregon. The role of enteric feeding (nasogastric, nasojejunal, transfistula, or jejunal) through small tubes was emphasized. With a combination of enteric tube feedings and intravenous nutrients that included protein hydrolysates, a minimum daily goal of 1600 calories was attempted. Eighteen patients who received optimal nutrition (greater than 1600 calories/day) had a 17 per cent mortality rate, whereas 38 patients who received suboptimal nutrition (less than 1000 calories/day) had a 55 per cent mortality rate. Only 3 of 11 patients (27 per cent) with high-output fistulas who received optimal nutrition died, whereas 13 of 14 patients (93 per cent) with high-output fistulas who received suboptimal nutrition died. Although Edmunds and coworkers had recommended early operation in high-output fistulas to stop the fistula drainage,[22] Chapman, Foran, and Dunphy recommended conservative management emphasizing nutritional maintenance, with operation only in fistulas that did not heal spontaneously.[1]

In 1971, Dunphy's group reported 51 patients from the University of California who were managed with the principles and nutritional goals that had been outlined in the 1964 paper.[29] The overall mortality rate was 12 per cent (gastroduodenal, 23 per cent; small bowel, 14 per cent; colon, 0 per cent). This paper suggested that progress had been made in lowering the mortality rate of fistulas by an organized approach and attention to supplying adequate nutrition.

Roback and Nicoloff confirmed the beneficial effects of supplying nutrients to patients with postoperative small-bowel fistulas irrespective of the need for operation in a review of 55 patients at the University of Minnesota from 1960 through 1970.[30] Patients were separated into good and bad nutritional groups based on whether they had caloric intake of greater than or less than 2500 calories/day. In the good nutritional group, nonoperative cases had a 27 per cent mortality rate (4 of 15), and the operative cases had an 8 per cent mortality (1 of 13). In the bad nutritional group, nonoperative cases had an 81 per cent mortality rate (13 of 16), and the operative cases had a 57 per cent mortality rate (4 of 7). Overall, the good nutritional group had an 18 per cent mortality rate (5 of 28) compared to a 74 per cent mortality rate (17 of 23) in the bad nutritional group.

During these retrospective and uncontrolled studies, the delivery of adequate nutrition was primarily contingent upon the use of the gastrointestinal tract. This often relegated patients with high-output jejunal fistulas, intra-abdominal sepsis, bowel obstruction, inflammatory bowel disease, radiation, and cancer into the groups with inadequate nutrition, and this selection bias in patient grouping, rather than the availability or absence of calories and protein, may have been responsible for the difference in observed mortality rates. Whether the provision of adequate nutrition in fistula patients improved survival could be determined only when it became possible to adequately nourish any patient, regardless of the condition of the gastrointestinal tract.

Dudrick's development of central venous catheterization and solutions of amino acids and hypertonic dextrose for TPN provided the possibility for full nourishment by vein for any patient with an enteric fistula, regardless of other complicating factors.[31] In 1970, Dudrick and colleagues reported three cases of spontaneous closure of traumatic pancreatic and duodenal fistulas with TPN.[32] Dudrick's experience from 1970 through 1972 at the University of Pennsylvania with 78 gastrointestinal fistulas, all of which were treated with TPN, documented a spontaneous closure rate of 70 per cent and a mortality rate of 6 per cent.[33] This was, and remains, the lowest mortality rate in any large series of fistulas, and it stood in stark contrast to the mortality rates of 30 to 45 per cent reported in the era just preceding the development of TPN.[1, 22, 34, 35]

In addition to this dramatic clinical report, experimental evidence in dogs suggested that intravenous hypertonic glucose and amino acids would decrease duodenal secretions by 50 per cent, excretion of bilirubin by 86 per cent, and secretion of amylase by 71 per cent.[36] Hyperosmolality secondary to glucose was responsible for most of the suppression of upper gastrointestinal tract secretions.[37, 38] When dogs with experimental ileal fistulas were treated with TPN instead of regular dog food, there was a reduction in volume and nutrient losses.[39]

Paralleling the development of TPN was the availability of elemental diets composed of amino acids and glucopolysaccharides. Rocchio and associates from Rhode Island reported a four-year experience with 37 enteric fistulas treated primarily with elemental diets by oral or tube feeding, with a 65 per cent spontaneous closure rate and a 16 per cent mortality rate.[40] Voitk and colleagues, from McGill, used elemental diets to nourish 29 patients with enteric fistulas, with a 75 per cent closure rate and a 28 per cent mortality rate.[41] Despite these successful reports and Dunphy's emphasis on enteric feedings in fistula patients, the surgical community had a reluctance to use tube feedings. TPN allowed every fistula patient to receive immediate, full nutrition by vein and gave total rest to the gastrointestinal tract. Tube feedings took longer to arrive at full nutrition and were not practical in all cases. In addition, they stimulated gastrointestinal secretions and required an unpleasant nasal tube. Therefore, in the 1970s most surgeons acquired an automatic reliance on TPN in almost all fistula patients in the belief that it would afford both a high rate of spontaneous closure and a low mortality rate.

Two papers in the late 1970s, however, questioned the contribution of TPN in patients with fistulas. Reber and coworkers analyzed 186 patients with enteric fistulas from the University of California, dividing the experience into two groups.[16] From 1968 through 1971, 82 patients were treated, only 24 per cent of whom received TPN, resulting in a 26 per cent spontaneous closure rate and a 22 per cent mortality rate. In the following period, from 1972 through 1977, 114 patients were treated, with the number of patients receiving TPN increasing to 71 per cent. Despite the increased use of TPN, no statistical difference in the spontaneous closure rate (35 per cent) or mortality rate (22 per cent) existed in this group. This was a further report from the same group led by Dunphy (who had emphasized adequate nutrition as early as 1964), and in those patients not receiving TPN, adequate tube feedings had been delivered. When 41 patients from the first period, who were adequately nourished by tube feeding (greater than 3000 calories/day), were compared to 71 patients from the latter period, who were nourished by TPN, neither mortality (7 per cent versus 14 per cent) nor spontaneous closure rate (22 per cent versus 37 per cent) was significantly different. The authors concluded that TPN *per se* had no impact on fistula mortality and that maintenance of adequate nutrition using enteric feeding was equally effective.[16]

The second paper, by Soeters and associates from the Massachusetts General Hospital, updated the earlier paper of Edmunds and associates. It reviewed 404 patients with enteric fistulas[23] who were grouped into three chronologic eras: 1945 through 1960, 1960 through 1970, and 1970 through 1975. The mortality rates were 43 per cent, 15 per cent, and 21 per cent, respectively. The authors pointed out that the great drop in mortality rate seen in the 1960 to 1970 era came prior to the introduction of TPN and that, in fact,

the addition of TPN did not cause any further improvement in this mortality rate. The authors conceded that the introduction of TPN eased the management of fistula patients and probably increased the rate of spontaneous closure, but it was not responsible for a decrease in the mortality rate.[23]

These two papers are retrospective and uncontrolled reviews comparing arbitrarily grouped patients with many varied types of fistulas over long periods of time. Definitive statements are made about the effect of TPN, but even in the eras when TPN was supposed to have been dominant, only 71 and 57 per cent of the patients received TPN, respectively.[16, 23] However, three well-controlled, albeit retrospective, studies of fistula patients have been published in which patients from the same institution treated in the era just preceding the introduction of TPN were compared to patients who were all treated with TPN in the subsequent era (Table 24–1).[42-44] Similar criteria for patient inclusion in each era were used. In each of these series, a significant increase in the spontaneous closure rate and a significant decrease in the mortality rate were accomplished in patients treated with TPN.

More recently, and because of the availability of intravenous fat emulsions, reports of nutritional management of fistula patients with the use of intravenous amino acids, fat, and glucose—often given by peripheral vein—have recorded excellent results.[45, 46] No clinical comparisons between peripheral and central intravenous nutrition in fistula patients have been published.

The evaluation of the impact of nutritional care on the results of fistula management is limited by the lack of any prospective randomized series comparing types of nutritional treatments. This lack is understandable. The occurrence of fistulas is rare and the presentation is variable so that any prospective trial would take so many years to

Table 24–1. INFLUENCE OF TPN ON OUTCOME OF FISTULAS

UNIVERSITY	TYPE OF FISTULA	CHRONOLOGIC GROUPS	PATIENTS	SPONTANEOUS CLOSURE	MORTALITY
McGill[42]	Small bowel, exclusive of duodenal stump and carcinomatosis	(1960–1973) Pre-TPN With TPN	66 25	27% 56%	33% 8%
Toronto[43]	External alimentary tract including pancreatico-biliary	Pre-TPN (1965–1969) With TPN* (1969–1975)	30 86	34% 81%	40% 9%
Melbourne[44]	High output (> 200 ml/day) gastrointestinal	Pre-TPN (1968–1971) With TPN (1975–1977)	38 35	35% 65%	60% 23%

*In addition to TPN, peripheral hyperalimentation and elemental diets were used.

conduct that the results would become meaningless. Nonetheless, in practical terms, what are the answers to the questions posed at the beginning of this section?

1. Malnutrition is a definite threat to many patients with fistulas unless aggressive measures are instituted to provide adequate nourishment. Parameters of malnutrition (i.e., weight loss and decreased serum albumin levels) have correlated with increased mortality.

2. The ability to provide adequate nourishment to patients with fistulas has almost uniformly been shown to improve the spontaneous closure and mortality rates. This has been demonstrated most clearly when patients treated with TPN are compared with similar patients given no consideration for nutritional replacement (see Table 24–1).

3. The route of administration of nutrients, enteral or parenteral, does not seem to make a difference in the outcome. Excellent results have been reported with either method as long as adequate nutrition has been accomplished. However, not all fistula patients can be successfully managed with enteric feedings. The route of feeding and the choice of nutrients are major decisions that are addressed once a descriptive classification of a fistula has been done.

We prefer, when possible, to use the gastrointestinal tract to nourish fistula patients. The methods are simpler and less expensive, and they lack the serious complications of central venous catheterization.[21] We have had long experience with fine catheters passed into the gastrointestinal tract at various levels in order to deliver elemental diet.[47] No controlled trials have shown elemental diets to be more beneficial than complex liquid diets,[48] but the elemental diets are able to traverse finer catheters, and since these feeding catheters may need to be in position for long periods of time, using the smallest catheter possible leads to the greatest patient comfort and lack of complications. Patients with esophageal and gastric fistulas can be treated by passing a nasal catheter into the stomach or duodenum. Likewise, patients with duodenal fistulas can be nourished through nasojejunal tubes. Occasionally, tubes will need to be positioned over guidewires with the aid of fluoroscopy or they will need to be passed endoscopically.[49] At times, the establishment of a jejunostomy for feeding is indicated.[50] Jejunal fistulas have usually proved to be difficult to manage by the enteral route. Conversely, ileal fistulas that are of low output can be handled either by oral or nasogastric feeding of an elemental or a complete liquid diet. Almost all colonic fistulas can be treated with low-residue oral diets. If a patient with a colonic fistula cannot tolerate an oral diet because of gastrointestinal dysfunction, undrained infection in the abdomen should be suspected.

We reserve TPN for patients with high-output fistulas in the small intestine. TPN is also used in some patients with gastroduodenal fistulas in whom tube placement beyond the fistula cannot be accomplished or in whom tube feeding is not well tolerated. TPN is also preferred in patients in whom aspiration would be a concern if they were tube-fed. We do not view these two feeding methods as competitive and often use them in combination or at different times during the long-term management of fistula patients.

The nutritional needs of a fistula patient should be assessed. Our dietitians use a standard formula to calculate basal energy expenditure (BEE) from the patient's age, sex, height, and weight.[51] We estimate the extra energy requirements necessary for daily activity and the stresses of hypovolemia, fever, infection, or an unhealed wound. In most fistula patients, this rarely is a factor greater than 1.5 times the BEE. Overfeeding the patient with nutrients, particularly those high in glucose, has been shown to lead to abnormal function of the liver, excess carbon dioxide production with pulmonary compromise, and problems of glucose intolerance. By relying on factors of the BEE and by supplying an intravenous diet in which approximately 25 per cent of the calories are in the form of fat emulsions, we have avoided the problems of excess glucose infusion. Our dietitians keep a daily nutritional record in the patient's chart of nutrient intake (total calories, grams of protein, carbohydrate, and fat) and nutrient route (oral, tube, or intravenous) so that we can compare the recommended level with the actual levels taken by the patient.

Two recent reports have documented the role of home TPN in the treatment of complex enteric fistulas.[52, 53] Although this treatment is rarely necessary, an occasional case of fistula associated with multiple operative failures and obliterative peritoneal inflammation complicating short-bowel syndrome, radiation enteritis, Crohn's disease, or proximal small bowel stomas may respond to long-term home TPN with subsequent successful operative repair.

THE ROLE OF OPERATIVE THERAPY

Fistulas that occur spontaneously will likely need an operation to close them because removal of the underlying disease is necessary in curing the fistula. In most of these cases, a lengthy period of conservative management prior to operation is not indicated, but definitive operation should proceed shortly after drainage of any infection. The abdominal cavity will usually prove suitable for operation, with the severe inflammation limited to the area of the fistula alone. Conversely, postoperative fistulas should be given an opportunity to heal spontaneously. Postoperative fistulas occur most often after emergency operations for trauma, hemorrhage, peritonitis, or obstruction. Early major reconstructive operations are usually unwise, since the abdominal cavity will still be recovering from the original operation. Operations for fistulas should be considered in two general categories: (1) resuscitative operations and (2) definitive operations.

1. *Resuscitative operations* have limited goals, namely, to drain infection, to decrease fistula output by establishment of a proximal stoma or, rarely, to establish an avenue for nutrition. They are performed under emergency conditions in patients who may be malnourished and septic. When an intestinal fistula first occurs, its orifice gradually enlarges because of inflammation, edema, and an increase in intraluminal pressure. If no intrinsic or extrinsic factors prevent normal healing, a fistula orifice will first enlarge, then contract, and finally heal. During a resuscitative operation to drain infection, suture repair of the fistula orifice is doomed to failure, since the defect is not a fresh wound, but an infected late manifestation of a previous defect in healing, and it is in the process of enlarging—not contracting. In general, no search for the fistula opening or attempt at resection and reanastomosis should be conducted. Limited dissection or percutaneous radiologic drainage lessens the likelihood of further intestinal damage, which can easily occur when extensive dissection of inflamed, adherent loops of intestine is attempted. If resection of the intestine

and fistula tract is accomplished, proximal diversion as a stoma is safer than anastomosis.[54, 55]

2. *Definitive operations* have the goals of restoring functional continuity of the gastrointestinal tract and eliminating fistula drainage. In the most ideal circumstances, removal of the fistula, restoration of anatomic continuity, and elimination of any underlying disease should be accomplished. Definitive operation should take place electively after complete control of infection is achieved in patients who are well nourished and after an adequate time has been allowed for spontaneous closure. Almost all fistulas that eventually heal spontaneously will do so within one or two months.[16, 56] Further conservative management after this is not warranted except in unusual circumstances. The diagnoses of epithelialization, foreign bodies, radiation enteritis, inflammatory bowel disease, malignancy, distal obstruction, or lack of intestinal continuity make spontaneous closure unlikely. Even in patients with these findings, conservative management without operation for up to a month may be beneficial. Although many papers stress the importance of restoring nutrition prior to operation, in fact many patients with the initial diagnosis of a fistula are well nourished, and rather than restoration, nutritional maintenance is the goal. In contrast, the condition of the peritoneal cavity and control of infection are more cogent reasons for waiting before performing definitive operations so that maturation of the healing process, increased function of the alimentary tract, and total resolution of peritoneal sepsis can occur.

Several types of operations may be used as definitive procedures for fistulas. In Figures 24–4 to 24–6, examples of these operations are illustrated for typical fistulas encountered in the duodenum, small bowel, and colon, respectively.

Types of Operations

1. *Resection* of a segment of the organ and the fistula with anastomosis is the preferred operative treatment for most fistulas of the small bowel and colon (Fig. 24–5A and Fig. 24–6B).[16, 23, 57] In many postoperative abdomens, this may require dissection of the entire intestine in order to identify afferent and efferent loops and eliminate partial ob-

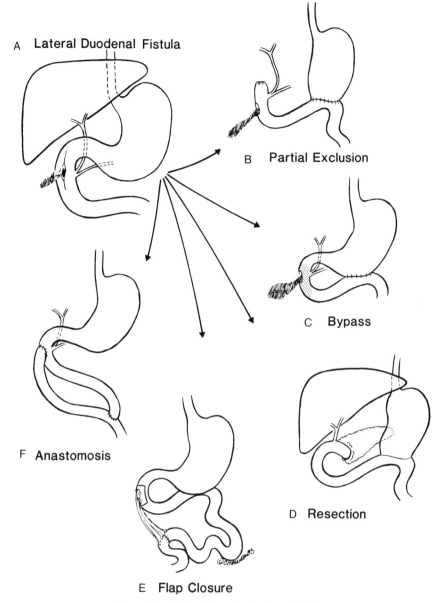

A   Lateral Duodenal Fistula

B   Partial Exclusion

C   Bypass

F   Anastomosis

D   Resection

E   Flap Closure

Figure 24–4. Operations for duodenal fistulas.

structions. In duodenal fistulas, resection would entail pancreaticoduodenectomy and is not indicated unless complex biliary and pancreatic fistulas coexist or an appropriate disease is present in the duodenum (Fig. 24–4D).[58]

2. *Exclusion* of the fistula, total or partial, has historically had particular application for dealing early with spontaneous small bowel fistulas in order to restore nutritive competency and control fistula drainage without contamination of the operative field.[59-61] The abdominal cavity not directly involved with the fistula was usually free for easy identifi-

cation and anastomosis. Currently, since most small bowel fistulas occur postoperatively, the inflamed condition of the peritoneal cavity may make this procedure a difficult one to perform early. Its use as a definitive operation is limited to cases of radiation, Crohn's disease, or malignancy when the surgeon wishes to avoid dissection of the fistula tract (Fig. 24–5B and C).

Exclusion has long been the operation of choice for nonhealing lateral duodenal fistulas (Figure 24–4B).[62] It provides for a decrease in gastric acid production and diversion of the food away from the fistula opening.

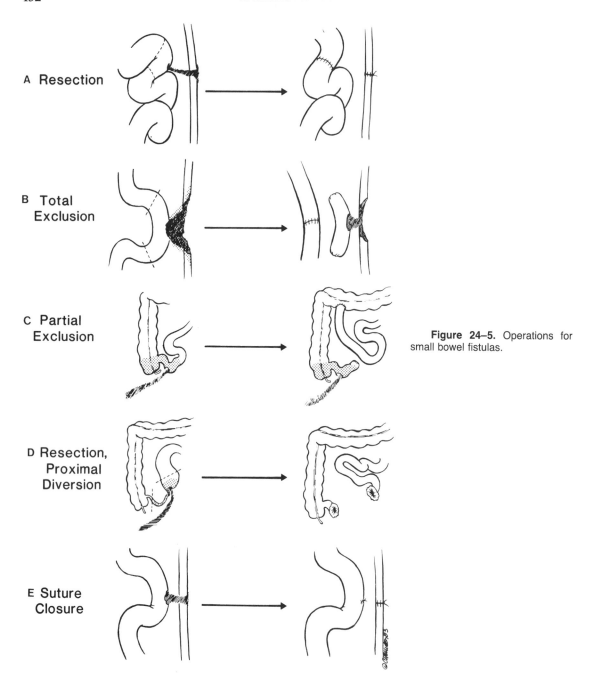

A Resection

B Total Exclusion

C Partial Exclusion

Figure 24–5. Operations for small bowel fistulas.

D Resection, Proximal Diversion

E Suture Closure

Exclusion is also used for fistulas located low in the colon. Figure 24–6D demonstrates a transverse colostomy that effectively excludes a sigmoid fistula. This is usually employed as a staged procedure, with later closure of the colostomy with or without resection of the fistula. It may be a permanent procedure if radiation therapy or metastatic cancer makes dissection in the pelvis unwise. Figure 24–6E demonstrates an end-descending colostomy. It is most often used to per-

manently exclude a fistula associated with metastatic cancer that is not amenable to resection.

3. *Closure* with serosal *patch*,[63, 64] open intestinal *flap* (Fig. 24–4E)[65] or intestinal *anastomosis* to fistula orifice (Fig. 24–4F)[66, 67] have particular application in chronic nonhealing fistulas of the esophagus, stomach, and duodenum.

4. *Proximal diversions with resection* (Fig. 24–5D and 24–6C) are staged operations that

are usually limited to the distal small bowel or colon and involve resection of the organ with the fistula and a proximal stoma. They are indicated mainly when infection or obstruction has not been completely controlled.[54, 55]

5. *Bypass* of the fistula without exclusion has limited use, but excellent results have been reported in lateral duodenal fistulas when partial duodenal obstruction has been present (Fig. 24–4C).[68]

6. *Suture closure* of fistulas (Fig. 24–5E) is condemned by most authorities because they are doomed to failure as emergency procedures and if spontaneous closure has not occurred in chronic situations, there is usually some factor that argues in favor of resection or exclusion. However, certain conditions—such as factitious or short-tract fistulas—may lend themselves to suture closure.

The choice of operation depends on the entire descriptive classification of the fistula. Operative decisions must also be made about the surface exit wound and the location and methods of closure of the laparotomy incision. These decisions require expert surgical experience and judgment. A definitive oper-

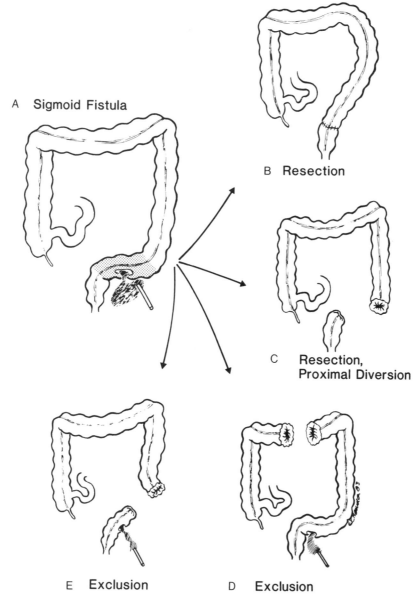

A **Sigmoid Fistula**

B **Resection**

C **Resection, Proximal Diversion**

E **Exclusion**   D **Exclusion**

Figure 24–6. Operations for colonic fistulas.

ation should be planned well in advance and placed on the elective surgical schedule when the surgical team is fresh. The patient should be given a mechanical bowel preparation as well as short-term prophylactic, enteral and systemic antibiotics.

RESULTS

Valid statements about the management and prognosis of fistulas are difficult to make because of the retrospective nature of the literature and the variability in fistula cases. Nonetheless, some generalizations seem true. In the last 25 years, the prognosis of patients with fistulas has improved. In general, the mortality rate from a fistula decreases as its location descends the gastrointestinal tract. Mortality rates for gastroduodenal, small bowel, and colonic fistulas at the Massachusetts General Hospital from 1970 through 1975 were 30 per cent, 25 per cent, and 14 per cent, respectively.[23] These were improvements over the 62 per cent, 54 per cent, and 16 per cent mortality rates seen in the same organs from 1946 through 1959.[22] High-output fistulas have a higher mortality rate than low-output fistulas (30 per cent versus 5 per cent,[24] 40 per cent versus 20 per cent,[56] and 32 per cent versus 6 per cent[69]). Jejunal fistulas have a higher mortality rate than ileal fistulas (38 per cent versus 17 per cent[24]). High mortality rates are seen in patients with cancer (45 per cent,[24] 54 per cent[56]), irradiation (45 per cent,[24] 78 per cent[56]), small bowel obstruction (30 per cent[56]), complicating urinary or biliary fistulas (42 per cent[56]), abdominal wall dehiscence or evisceration (50 per cent,[56] 52 per cent,[24] 60 per cent[69]), and those who are greater than 65 years (65 per cent[56]). Fistula-related deaths are secondary to sepsis or a primary disease (often terminal cancer). Control of sepsis re-

mains the key reversible problem that could lead to further improvement in mortality rates.[16, 23, 70, 71]

Spontaneous closure rates vary considerably, but of fistulas that eventually closed without operation, Reber reported that 91 per cent closed in 30 days after control of infection[16] and Monod-Brocca reported that 80 per cent closed in 40 days from the time of diagnosis.[56] A low spontaneous closure rate occurs in the presence of Crohn's disease (8 per cent), abdominal irradiation (14 per cent), a tract less than 2 cm (17 per cent), and cancer (26 per cent).[16] In the absence of any of these adverse factors, spontaneous closure can be expected in 47 per cent of the patients after infection is controlled.[16] Table 24–2 lists the outcome of small-bowel fistulas reported in the literature.

In summary, external acquired gastrointestinal tract fistulas remain a major problem, with lengthy hospitalization and high morbidity and mortality rates. The current recommended approach is aggressive, organized, and thorough attention to many aspects of patient care, including fluid and electrolyte balance, control of fistula drainage and protection of the skin, early and continued surveillance for intra-abdominal sepsis, nutritional support, allowance of necessary time for resolution of peritoneal inflammation and spontaneous closure, and appropriate operative procedures. An accurate, descriptive classification of each fistula is important in making proper decisions about individual patients and such a classification includes location, etiology, pathology, and anatomic detail. The enterostomal therapist can help greatly in wound management. The radiologist is important both in describing the fistula and controlling infection. Maintaining adequate nutrition either enterally or intravenously has improved outcome and is a major responsibility of those caring for the

Table 24–2. OUTCOME OF EXTERNAL SMALL BOWEL FISTULAS

INSTITUTION	DATES	NO. OF PATIENTS	SPONTANEOUS CLOSURE	MORTALITY RATE
Massachusetts General[22]	1946–1959	46	4%	54%
Oregon[1]	1953–1963	23	NS	65%
California[29]	1964–1971	29	NS	14%
Minnesota[30]	1960–1970	55	40%	31%
Pennsylvania[33]	1970–1972	26	69%	8%
California[16]	1968–1977	120	20%	17%
Leeds[72]	1975–1977	25	60%	20%
Cleveland Clinic[24]	1956–1976	174	NS	22%
Massachusetts General[23]	1970–1975	52	NS	25%

NS = not stated

patient with an enteric fistula. Finally, operation is often necessary, and a variety of procedures are available.

REFERENCES

1. Chapman, R., Foran, R., and Dunphy, J.E.: Management of intestinal fistulas. Am. J. Surg., *108*:157, 1964.
2. Knighton, D.R., Burns, K., and Nyhus, L.M.: The use of stomahesive in the care of the skin of enterocutaneous fistulas. Surg. Gynecol. Obstet., *143*:449, 1976.
3. Gross, E., and Irving, M.: Protection of the skin around intestinal fistulas. Br. J. Surg., *64*:258, 1977.
4. Brubacher, L.L.: To heal a draining wound. R.N., *30*, March, 1982.
5. Firme, C.N., and Paine, J.R.: An improved sump suction drain for the management of gastric and intestinal fistulas. Surgery, *47*:436, 1960.
6. Goldsmith, H.S.: Control of viscerocutaneous fistula by a new suction device. N. Engl. J. Med., *265*:1052, 1961.
7. Gary, E.G., Wolcott, M.W., Meyers, W.H., and Farrell, J.J.: A simplified method of care for gastrointestinal fistulas. Surg. Gynecol. Obstet., *114*:122, 1962.
8. Suriyapa, C., and Anderson, M.C.: A simple device to control drainage from enterocutaneous fistulas. Surgery, *70*:455, 1971.
9. Tribble, D.E.: An improved sump drain-irrigation device of simple construction. Arch. Surg., *105*:511, 1972.
10. MacFarlane, M., and Frawley, J.E.: A technique for drainage of enterocutaneous fistulas. Surg. Gynecol. Obstet., *141*:263, 1975.
11. Westaby, S., McPherson, S., and Everett, W.G.: Treatment of purulent wounds and fistula with an adhesive wound irrigation device. Ann. Roy. Coll. Surg. Engl., *63*:353, 1981.
12. Ota, K.: Closure of viscerocutaneous fistula with adhesives. Arch. Surg., *101*:468, 1970.
13. Sokol, A.B., Michel, S.L., and Morgenstern, L.: Some innovations in the management of enterocutaneous fistulas. Am. Surg., *38*:405, 1972.
14. Streza, G.A., Laing, B.J., and Gilsdorf, R.B.: Management of enterocutaneous fistulas and problem stomas with silicone casting of the abdominal wall defect. Am. J. Surg., *124*:772, 1977.
15. Alm, A., and Elfstrom, J.: Healing of jejunal fistula using a silicone tube and patch. Acta. Chir. Scand., *145*:429, 1979.
16. Reber, H.A., Roberts, C., Way, L.W., and Dunphy, J.E.: Management of external gastrointestinal fistulas. Ann. Surg., *188*:460, 1978.
17. Knochel, J.Q., Koehler, P.R., Lee, T.G. et al.: Diagnosis of abdominal abscess with computed tomography, ultrasound, and ^{111}In leukocyte scans. Radiology, *137*:425, 1980.
18. Gerzof, S.G., Robbins, A.H., Birkett, D.H. et al.: Percutaneous catheter drainage of abdominal abscesses guided by ultrasound and computed tomography. A.J.R., *133*:1, 1979.
19. McLean, G.K., Mackie, J.A., Freiman, D.B. et al.: Enterocutaneous fistula: interventional radiologic management. A.J.R., *138*:615, 1982.

20. Ryan, J.A., Abel, R.M., Abbott, W.M. et al.: Catheter complications in total parenteral nutrition: a prospective study of 200 consecutive patients. N. Engl. J. Med., *290*:757, 1974.
21. Ryan, J.A.: Conditions of total parenteral nutrition. *In* Fischer, J.E. (ed.): Total Parenteral Nutrition. Boston, Little, Brown & Co., 1976, page 55.
22. Edmunds, L.H., Williams, G.M., and Welch, C.E.: External fistulas arising from the gastrointestinal tract. Ann. Surg., *152*:445, 1960.
23. Soeters, P.B., Ebeid, A.M., and Fischer, J.E.: Review of 404 patients with gastrointestinal fistulas. Impact of parenteral nutrition. Ann. Surg., *190*:189, 1979.
24. Coutsoftides, T., and Fazio, V.W.: Small intestine cutaneous fistula. Surg. Gynecol. Obstet., *149*:333, 1979.
25. Elman, R., and Weiner, D.O.: Intravenous alimentation with special reference to protein (amino acid) metabolism. J.A.M.A., *112*:796, 1939.
26. Brunschwig, A., Bigelow, R.R., and Nichols, S.: Intravenous nutrition for eight weeks; partial enterectomy; recovery. J.A.M.A., *129*:441, 1945.
27. Barnes, T.G.: Total intravenous alimentation in the treatment of small bowel fistulas. Ann. Surg., *133*:644, 1951.
28. Smith, D.W., and Lee, R.M.: Nutritional management in duodenal fistula. Surg. Gynecol. Obstet., *103*:666, 1956.
29. Sheldon, G.E., Gardiner, B.N., Way, L.W., and Dunphy, J.E.: Management of gastrointestinal fistulas. Surg. Gynecol. Obstet., *133*:385, 1971.
30. Roback, S.A., and Nicoloff, D.M.: High output enterocutaneous fistulas of the small bowel. Am. J. Surg., *123*:317, 1972.
31. Dudrick, S.J., Wilmore, D.W., Vars, H.M., and Rhoads, J.E.: Can intravenous feeding as the sole means of nutrition support growth in the child and restore weight loss in an adult?—an affirmative answer. Ann. Surg., *169*:974, 1969.
32. Dudrick, S.J., Wilmore, D.W., Steiger, E. et al.: Spontaneous closure of traumatic pancreatoduodenal fistulas with total intravenous nutrition. J. Trauma, *10*:542, 1970.
33. Mac Fadyen, B.V., Dudrick, S.J., and Ruberg, R.L.: Management of gastrointestinal fistulas with parenteral hyperalimentation. Surgery, *74*:100, 1973.
34. Bowlin, J.W., Hardy, J.D., and Conn, J.H.: External alimentary fistulas: analysis of seventy-nine cases, with notes on management. Am. J. Surg., *103*:6, 1962.
35. Lorenzo, G.A., and Beal, J.M.: Management of external small bowel fistula. Arch. Surg., *99*:394, 1969.
36. Hamilton, R.F., Davis, W.C., Stephenson, D.V. et al.: Effects of parenteral hyperalimentation on upper gastrointestinal tract secretions. Arch. Surg., *102*:348, 1971.
37. Towne, J.B., Hamilton, R.F., and Stephenson, D.V.: Mechanisms of hyperalimentation in the suppression of upper gastrointestinal secretions. Am. J. Surg., *126*:714, 1973.
38. Alder, M., Takeshime, T., Dreiling, D.A. et al.: Effects of parenteral hyperalimentation on pancreatic and biliary secretion. Surg. Forum, *26*:445, 1975.
39. Wolfe, B.M., Keltner, R.M., and Willman, V.L.: Intestinal fistula output in regular, elemental and intravenous alimentation. Am. J. Surg., *124*:803, 1972.

40. Rocchio, M.A., Cha, C.M., Haas, K.F. et al.: Use of chemically defined diets in the management of patients with high output gastrointestinal cutaneous fistulas. Am. J. Surg., *127*:148, 1974.

41. Voitk, A.J., Echave, V., Brown, R.A. et al.: Elemental diet in the treatment of fistulas of the alimentary tract. Surg. Gynecol. Obstet., *137*:68, 1973.

42. Himal, H.S., Allard, J.R., Nadea, J.E. et al.: The importance of adequate nutrition in closure of small intestinal fistulas. Br. J. Surg., *61*:724, 1974.

43. Deitel, M.: Nutritional management of external gastrointestinal fistulas. Can. J. Surg., *19*:505, 1976.

44. Thomas, R.J.S., and Rosalion, A.: The use of parenteral nutrition in the management of external gastrointestinal tract fistula. Aust. N.Z. J. Surg., *48*:535, 1978.

45. Kirkpatrick, J.R., and Bouwman, D.L.: Intestinal fistulas: lessons learned from the trauma patient. Compr. Ther., *5*(3):68, 1979.

46. Silberman, H., Granson, M., Fong, G. et al.: Management of external gastrointestinal fistulas with glucose and lipids. Surg. Gynecol. Obstet., *150*:656, 1980.

47. Page, C.P., Ryan, J.A., Huff, R.C. et al.: Continual catheter administration of an elemental diet. Surg. Gynecol. Obstet., *142*:184, 1976.

48. Koretz, R.J., and Meyer, J.H.: Elemental diets—facts and fantasies. Gastroenterology, *78*:393, 1980.

49. Douglas, D.D., and Morrissey, J.F.: New technique for rapid endoscope-assisted intubation of the small intestine. Arch. Surg., *113*:196, 1978.

50. Ryan, J.A.: Jejunal feeding. *In* Fischer, J.E. (ed.): Surgical Nutrition. Boston, Little, Brown & Co., 1983, p. 757–777.

51. Wilmore, D.W.: Energy and energy balance. *In* The Metabolic Management of the Critically Ill. New York, Plenum, 1977, page 1.

52. Byrne, W.J., Burke, M., and Fonkalsrud, E.W.: Home parenteral nutrition: an alternative approach to the management of complicated gastrointestinal fistulas not responding to conventional medical or surgical therapy. J.P.E.N., 3:355, 1979.

53. Oakley, J.R., Steiger, E., Lavery, I.C. et al.: Catastrophic enterocutaneous fistula: the role of home hyperalimentation. Cleve. Clin. Q., *46*:133, 1979.

54. Welch, C.E.: The treatment of combined intestinal obstruction and peritonitis by refunctualization of the intestine. Ann. Surg., *142*:739, 1955.

55. Goligher, J.C.: Resection with exteriorization in the management of faecal fistulas originating in the small intestine. Br. J. Surg., *58*:163, 1971.

56. Monod-Broca, P.: Treatment of intestinal fistulas. Br. J. Surg., *64*:685, 1977.

57. Hill, G.L., and Bambach, C.P.: A technique for the operative closure of persistent external small bowel fistulas. Aust. N.Z. J. Surg., *51*:477, 1981.

58. Musicant, M.E., and Thompson, J.C.: The emergency management of lateral duodenal fistula by pancreaticoduodenectomy. Surg. Gynecol. Obstet., *128*:108, 1969.

59. Keyes, E.L., and Middleman, I.C.: The treatment of fistula and obstruction of the small intestine by complete exclusion. Surg. Gynecol. Obstet., *72*:237, 1941.

60. Harbison, S.P.: The principle of complete exclusion in fistulas of the small intestine. Surgery, *28*:384, 1950.

61. Keyes, E.L.: Hastening operative exclusion for fistula of exteriorized ileum or jejunum. Arch. Surg., *63*:17, 1951.

62. Malangoni, M.A., Madura, J.A., and Jesseph, J.A.: Management of lateral duodenal fistulas: a study of fourteen cases. Surgery, *90*:645, 1981.

63. Wolfman, E.F., Trevino, G., Heaps, D.K. et al.: An operative technic for the management of acute and chronic lateral duodenal fistulas. Ann. Surg., *159*:563, 1964.

64. Camp, T.F., Skinner, D.B., and Connolly, J.M.: Lateral duodenal defects. Am. J. Surg., *115*:291, 1968.

65. Walley, B.D., and Goco, I.: Duodenal patch grafting. Am. J. Surg., *140*:706, 1980.

66. Jones, S.A., and Joergenson, E.J.: Closure of duodenal wall defects. Surgery, *53*:438, 1963.

67. Ujiki, G.T., and Shields, T.W.: Roux-en-Y operation in the management of postoperative fistula. Arch. Surg., *116*:614, 1981.

68. Sandler, J.T., and Deitel, M.: Management of duodenal fistulas. Can. J. Surg., *24*:124, 1981.

69. Sitges-Serra, A., Jaurrieta, E., and Sitges-Creus, A.: Management of postoperative enterocutaneous fistulas: the roles of parenteral nutrition and surgery. Br. J. Surg., *69*:147, 1982.

70. Aquirre, A., Fischer, J.E., and Welch, C.E.: The role of surgery and hyperalimentation in therapy of gastrointestinal-cutaneous fistulae. Ann. Surg., *180*:393, 1974.

71. Fischer, J.E.: The management of high-output intestinal fistulas. Adv. Surg., *9*:139, 1975.

72. Blackett, R.L., and Hill, G.L.: Postoperative external small bowel fistulas: a study of a consecutive series of patients treated with intravenous hyperalimentation. Br. J. Surg., *65*:775, 1978.

CHAPTER 25

Malabsorption and the Short-Gut Syndrome

K. N. JEEJEEBHOY

Resection of the small intestine becomes necessary in a variety of situations, including those resulting from congenital abnormalities, trauma, inflammation, vascular insufficiency, and tumors. In young persons, a frequent cause for bowel resection is Crohn's disease, and in the elderly, a frequent cause is intestinal infarction.

When short lengths of the small bowel are resected, there is little disturbance of bowel function, especially if the ileocecal junction is left intact.

The ability to resect the small intestine without disturbing function is mainly due to the great degree of intestinal reserve in normal humans. In addition, even if intestine is resected in lengths that compromise absorption, adaptation of the remaining bowel to increase function restores the ability to absorb normally. However, when more than 50 per cent of the bowel has been resected, impairment of absorption tends to be prolonged or permanent. The degree of malnutrition that results from bowel resection is thus a function of a number of factors, and simply knowing how much bowel has been resected is not sufficient to predict functional disability.

In any patient with bowel resection, the physician may be called upon to provide a range of nutritional support regimens, depending upon the site and length of resection, the degree of adaptation, and existing disease. Thus, support will change as time allows adaptation of the bowel to proceed.

NORMAL ABSORPTION AND MOTILITY OF THE SMALL INTESTINE

In order to understand the effects of resection it is necessary to review selected aspects of small-bowel function that are relevant to the subsequent clinical effects of resection.

Motility. After eating a meal, transit through the bowel depends upon a complex inter-relationship among the different areas of the gastrointestinal tract that modulate gastric, small-bowel, and colonic motility.

Gastric Emptying. The nature of the chyme entering the small intestine alters gastric emptying. In general, the ingestion of nutrients—especially fat, but also proteins, and to a lesser extent carbohydrates—inhibits gastric emptying. This inhibition depends not only on the stimulation of duodenal receptors but also on receptors that extend down the intestine, so experimental reinfusion of chyme collected from the duodenum into the jejunoileum inhibits gastric motility. Furthermore, it appears that with ingestion of a bigger meal the inhibition is prolonged.[1]

Small Intestine Motility. Small-bowel transit has been studied by the use of non-absorbable isotopes.[2] These studies have shown the striking effect of the ileum in slowing transit. The marker traverses the first 50 per cent of the bowel in a third of the time it takes to pass through the next 30 per cent. Connell[3] has also shown in humans that the passage of chyme through the jejunum is strikingly faster than it is through the distal intestine.

Ileocecal Valve. The nature of the ileocecal valve and its control of intestinal motility is controversial; however, it appears that when the ileum is resected, removal of the valve markedly accelerates small-bowel transit, and reconstruction improves diarrhea and fluid losses under these circumstances.[4, 5]

Colonic Motility. Motility of the gastrointestinal tract is slowest at the level of the colon. The mean transit time through the colon varies widely (between 24 and 150 hours), depending on the fat and fiber content of the diet. Thus, the colon is very important in slowing intestinal transit.

Interdigestive Motility and Secretion. The stomach and small bowel become active periodically when nothing is given by mouth, and they are swept by waves of electrical activity called the interdigestive migratory myoelectrical complexes (MMCs). During these episodes, there is significant secretion of bile and pancreatic juice,[6] which may constitute as much as 30 per cent of the maximal secretion.

Secretion and Absorption of Fluid and Electrolytes. The small bowel receives a total of 5 to 6 L of endogenous secretions/day, about 1 L each of saliva and bile/day, and 1.5 to 3 L of gastric and pancreatic juices/day. Most of this, except for 1 L, is absorbed in the small intestine. The site of absorption depends upon the nature of the meal eaten. With a meat and salad meal, most of it is absorbed high in the jejunum, whereas with a milk and doughnut meal, there is greater water secretion into the bowel, and more is absorbed distally.[7]

The absorption of fluid and electrolytes is significantly different in the three major areas of the intestine—that is, the jejunum, ileum, and colon. These differences depend partly on the nature of the electrolyte transport processes and partly on the permeability of the intercellular spaces. An understanding of these differences is crucial to recognizing the differences in the effect of resecting proximal versus distal bowel and the role of the colon in patients who have undergone intestinal resection.

In general, water absorption is a passive process resulting from the active transport of nutrients and electrolytes. Among the electrolytes, sodium transport is the main process aiding the creation of an electrochemical gradient across the mucosa and also driving the uptake of sugars and amino acids.

There are two main processes that result in the absorption of sodium and chloride. The first is coupled to the absorption of carbohydrates and amino acids, and the second is isotonic sodium chloride absorption. The first process dominates in the jejunum,[8] whereas the second process is of importance in the ileum[9] and the colon.

These mechanisms aid in transporting electrolytes across the intestinal epithelium, and because sodium transport is closely coupled to sugar and amino acid transport, they

also aid in the absorption of nutrients. However, the net effect on the intraluminal contents depends not only on absorption but also on back diffusion through the intercellular junctions. In the jejunum these junctions are "leaky" and thus back diffusion occurs readily, resulting in the maintenance of isotonicity of the jejunal contents. In contrast, the ileal and colonic junctions progressively increase in "tightness" so that back diffusion occurs less readily in these areas, allowing the intraluminal contents to become concentrated with respect to plasma, which conserves fluid from the lumen.

Nutrient Digestion and Absorption. Partially digested gastric contents are mixed with pancreatic secretions and bile in the duodenum. These secretions aid in the digestion of all major nutrients—carbohydrate, protein, and fat. The products of the hydrolysis of triglycerides, beta-monoglycerides and free fatty acids, together with fat-soluble vitamins, are finely dispersed in particles called micelles, which are made up of bile salts. These products of digestion are absorbed by the jejunum, and what remains unabsorbed is taken up by the ileum. Under normal circumstances in humans, absorption of nutrients is completed within the first 150 cm of the bowel.[10] Thus, in the normal individual very little nutrient reaches the ileum.

Unique Functions of the Ileum. The ileum is concerned with the absorption of vitamin B_{12} and bile salts. These functions are unique to this segment of the small intestine and have special implications in patients who have undergone ileal resection. Malabsorption of bile salts in the ileum results in altered digestion and absorption of fat in the jejunum. Normally, the synthesis of bile salts does not equal the demand that fat digestion imposes on them. These needs are met by ileal reabsorption of bile salts, which are then recycled into the jejunum. With ileal resection, bile salts are no longer recycled, and synthesis increases. However, if the loss is total, synthesis never increases sufficiently to meet all the needs throughout the day.

Under these circumstances, bile-salt synthesis adds to the bile-salt pool during the night when the bowel is quiescent, and the first meal of the day results in the bile stored overnight becoming available for the digestion of fat. However, since reabsorption is minimal, the bile-salt pool is depleted, and fat in the subsequent meals is malabsorbed. In addition, the malabsorption of bile acids in patients who have undergone ileal resection results in an increased load of bile salts entering the colon, at which point it reduces the absorption of water and sodium. The deoxybile acids also cause fluid secretion, thus enhancing the fluid and electrolyte losses through the colon.

EFFECTS OF INTESTINAL RESECTION ON MOTILITY

Gastric Motility. It was indicated earlier that the presence of nutrients in the small intestine inhibits gastric motility; thus it is not surprising that small-bowel resection increases the rate of gastric emptying.[11]

Small-Bowel Motility. Since the motility in the jejunum is rapid and in the distal ileum it is slow, proximal bowel resection does not result in an increased rate of intestinal transit.[11] In contrast, after ileal resection the remaining bowel has a very rapid transit rate;[11, 12] thus it is not surprising that when the remaining bowel consists of the jejunum, ^{51}Cr fed as a marker is almost completely excreted within a few hours.[13]

Colonic Motility. The colon is the area of the intestinal tract with the slowest motility. Thus the presence of an intact colon is very important in maintaining a transit rate that is close to normal. Therefore, distal resections that include the colon tend to increase the rate of intestinal transit.

EFFECT OF INTESTINAL RESECTION ON THE ABSORPTION OF FLUID AND ELECTROLYTES

The effect of intestinal resection on fluid and electrolyte absorption will depend upon both the extent of resection and the site. As long as the colon is intact, diarrhea is minimal. Fluid and electrolyte losses will not be excessive unless the fluid load delivered to the colon following small-bowel resection exceeds its reserve capacity or the contents of the small intestine dejecta going into the colon inhibit colonic absorption. Normally the reserve capacity of the colon is about 5 L/day,[14] but both bile salts[15] and free fatty acids[16] alter the ability of the colon to absorb water and sodium. Furthermore, certain forms of vegetable residue and carbohydrate can be degraded by colonic bacteria into titratable acids, which also increase osmotic load and water output.[17, 18]

Thus proximal resection results in little diarrhea, because the ileum can reabsorb the increased fluid and electrolyte load, and any remaining excess is taken up by the colon. The reabsorption of bile salts by intact ileum results in the colon not receiving any substances capable of preventing water and electrolyte absorption. In contrast, when the ileum is resected the colon receives a larger fluid load because the contents are isotonic; furthermore, because bile-salt loss occurs, there are also substances (bile salts, fatty acids, unabsorbed carbohydrate) reaching the colon that reduce the reabsorption of water and electrolytes. These effects result in diarrhea.

If the colon is partially or completely resected, the area of bowel that is capable of taking over the fluid and electrolyte absorption of the resected small bowel is lost. The importance of the colon in modulating the severity of diarrhea following resection has been emphasized in several publications.[19, 20] If both ileum and colon are resected, patients are left with bowel that cannot concentrate luminal contents. In such patients, isotonic water and salt loss is a major problem, resulting in dehydration, hypokalemia, and hypomagnesemia.

EFFECT OF INTESTINAL RESECTION ON NUTRIENT ABSORPTION

The absorption of nutrients occurs throughout the small bowel, so removal of the jejunum alone results in a takeover by the ileum of the absorptive function and little malabsorption.[21] In contrast, resections in excess of only 100 cm of ileum cause steatorrhea.[22] The degree of malabsorption increases with the increasing length of resection,[23] and a variety of nutrients is malabsorbed.[13, 24] The effect of malabsorption on the nutritional status of the patient increases with increased resection. A review of the literature indicates that though there is considerable variability, resections of up to 33 per cent result in no malnutrition, and resections of up to 50 per cent can be tolerated without special aids. However, when resection exceeds 75 per cent of the bowel, nutritional status cannot be maintained without special help.[25-29] When resection results in only a few inches of jejunum remaining, survival is limited and survivors are often nutritionally depleted.[30-35]

Adaptation of the Small Intestine. Following resection, the remaining small intestine hypertrophies and also increases its absorptive function. Flint was the first to demonstrate that following small-bowel resection in humans, a significant increase in villus height occurred, and he computed that the area of the absorptive surface had increased fourfold.[36] Since then, there have been studies in human[37] and animal models[38, 39] demonstrating this phenomenon.

There is an improvement in absorption in animals[40] and humans associated with anatomic changes.[41] The morphologic effects that follow resection seem to be mediated by an increase in cell proliferation[42, 43] and cell migration up the villus. The increased rate of proliferation appears to result from an increase in the size of the crypt zone in which cell replication occurs.[43, 44] Morphologic changes may be responsible for the functional compensation, but in addition, each cell may also show changes in the form of increased sodium-potassium adenosine triphosphatase (ATPase) activity.[45]

There are several possible causes of these functional and morphologic changes. They can be grouped into four major categories: (1) increased workload of the remaining bowel; (2) local nutrition; (3) the effect of endogenous secretion, such as bile and pancreatic juice; and (4) hormonal effects.

When the ileum (which is normally not exposed to a large nutrient load) is transposed to the area of the jejunum, hypertrophy occurs.[46] Such an effect could be due to increased local nutrition or to increased workload. Studies instilling sodium chloride, lactose, and alpha-methylglucoside into intestinal sacs have shown that these non-nutrient agents, which are transported by the mucosa, are very effective in promoting cell proliferation.[47] This supports the concept that increased functional demand, rather than local nutrition, is important for adaptation. Furthermore, since enterally fed amino acids are not taken up by the crypt cell, in which stimulation would be expected to occur,[48] it is unlikely that orally fed amino acids would stimulate mucosal protein synthesis at the site of cell proliferation. In fact, parenterally administered amino acids are taken up by the crypt cells. The role of endogenous secretions in promoting villus hypertrophy has been demonstrated in experiments in which transplantation of the duodenal papilla into the ileum resulted in ileal hyperplasia.[49] Finally, humoral factors have been evoked by observations in parabiotic animals,

in whom intestinal resection in one of the pair resulted in hyperplasia of the intestine in the other.[50] Observations in the human suggest the hormone enteroglucagon as an interesting candidate.[51]

MANAGEMENT OF INTESTINAL RESECTION

Based on the considerations already discussed, the approach to a patient who has undergone intestinal resection depends on the extent of the resection; the presence of continuing intestinal disease, which reduces the functional length of the intestine; the site of resected bowel; and the time for adaptation. The progress of the patient will lead with time to modifications of therapy. However, there is a variety of therapeutic avenues applicable to all patients.

First, these general approaches will be considered, and then the specific applications will be discussed.

General Therapeutic Approaches

Initial Treatment after Resection

Control of Diarrhea. Diarrhea is caused by a combination of increased secretions, increased motility, and osmotic stimulation of water secretion due to malabsorption of luminal contents. Initially diarrhea is controlled by giving the patient nothing by mouth in order to reduce any osmotic component. When there is massive secretion even when the patient is given nothing orally, there may be substantial fluid losses that result from gastric hypersecretion and malabsorbed endogenous secretions stimulated by interdigestive MMCs. Reduction of secretions, especially gastric secretion, can be effected by infusing H_2-blockers. This author prefers to give the H_2-blocker initially as a continuous intravenous (IV) infusion (cimetidine, 300 mg over six hours) rather than as a bolus because of its short half-life. In addition, the use of opiates aids in slowing intestinal propulsion and in increasing ion transport.[52] Loperamide, which acts locally, should be tried in increasing doses. If loperamide is ineffective, codeine or Lomotil (diphenoxylate hydrochloride and atropine) may be tried.

Oral Feeding. The next consideration is to determine the nature and amount of oral feedings. The degree of concern and the rigor of these measures depends upon the extent of bowel resected. In patients who have more than 60 to 80 cm (>15 to 20 per cent of normal length[53, 54]) of their bowel remaining, refeeding should be progressive, with an ultimate view to feeding a normal or modified oral diet. Conversely, in patients who have no small bowel except a duodenum, the initial target should be small liquid feedings. In those patients having intermediate lengths of bowel, progressive feeding should be attempted with the following plan: Initially isotonic, flavored carbohydrate-electrolyte feedings should be given. They contain a mixture of Caloreen, 3.4 per cent; Na^+, 85 mEq/L; K^+, 12 mEq/L; HCO_3^-, 9 mEq/L; and Cl^-, 109 mEq/L. A similar mixture has been shown to be well absorbed by patients with massive resection who were previously dependent on intravenous fluids.[55]

The next stage is to decide whether attempts are to be made to feed a normal diet or to use artificial defined-formula diets. Here again, when resection leaves the patient with more than 60 to 80 cm of small intestine, a normal oral diet should be tried. When attempting such feedings, the patient is given dry solids, with isotonic fluids given one hour after the meal. The separation of solids from liquids is important in view of the marked increase in the speed of gastric emptying noted with resection. Using this approach, we have found that the nature of the diet fed made no difference to the diarrhea or to the total malabsorption in patients with massive resection.[13] In contrast, patients who fail to tolerate a normal diet as indicated and those with a very short bowel should be given a constant infusion of defined-formula diet. The important consideration here is the use of controlled, well-modulated rates of infusion, starting with a diluted diet infused at 25 ml/hour and gradually increasing to full strength at 100 to 125 ml/hour. This procedure ensures that the intestine receives an osmotic load at a constant rate. Furthermore, the rate is modulated depending upon the tolerance of the bowel. Using this approach, we have found that patients who would otherwise need intravenous feeding can be managed entirely by the oral route.

Parenteral Electrolytes and Nutrients. Initially all patients need intravenous fluid and electrolyte replacement, especially sodium chloride, potassium, and magnesium. They are infused to meet needs as judged by a urine flow that would be targeted to exceed 1 L/day and normal serum electrolyte levels, central venous pressure and blood pressure. In particular, there should be no postural drop in blood pressure if hydration is adequate.

The intravenous infusion is gradually decreased as the oral intake is enhanced. The objective is to meet all needs orally, but this may require several weeks of adaptation.

Parenteral Nutrition. In patients in whom the remaining small bowel is less than 60 to 80 cm, parenteral nutrition should be started to avoid the development of malnutrition while oral refeeding is being attempted. Again, parenteral nutrient intake can be gradually reduced as oral intake increases. Often the progress is toward the use of only electrolytes parenterally, whereas other nutrient requirements are met orally. During the administration of parenteral nutrition, an area that is often neglected is the provision of trace elements. We have noted that with small-bowel resection and severe diarrhea, the need for zinc increases to between 12 and 15 mg/day because of endogenous losses.[56] These losses are computed by measuring the volume of intestinal fluid lost/day when nothing is given orally and adding 12 to 13 mg of Zn^{++} for every liter of loss.

Long-term Nutritional Support. This is a dynamic process that should be re-evaluated as the patient adapts. However, there are four possible outcomes:

1. Discharge on normal or modified oral diet, separating solids from liquids.

2. Use of defined formula diets on an ambulatory basis.

3. Oral diet as previously described with parenterally administered electrolytes and fluids.

4. Total, or partial parenteral nutrition with variable oral intake.

The aim should be to progress up the options toward the first in the preceding list. However, it is important to use a system that allows the patient to maintain a normal nutritional status and also be free of serious diarrhea so that he or she is allowed to work and to become socially rehabilitated. For example, it is possible for patients to eat 10 to 12 meals a day, have a similar number of bowel movements—including nocturnal movements, and remain free from parenteral support. However, life for such a person is an oral-anal existence that leaves little time for social or work rehabilitation. The option chosen must avoid such an outcome and permit this rehabilitation. The availability of the options of home enteral[57] and parenteral nutrition[58-60] have revolutionized the outlook for such patients.

Special Considerations Depending on Length and Site of Resection

Jejunal Resection with Intact Ileum and Colon. These patients can be fed immediately and rarely have any problems.

Ileal Resection of Less than 100 cm with Colon Largely Intact. These patients have so-called choleretic diarrhea and are best managed with the use of cholestyramine, 5 gm three times a day. A vitamin B_{12} absorption study should be done, and if abnormal, parenteral vitamin B_{12} should be given, 200 μg/month. Such patients may also have hyperoxaluria[61] because of enhanced colonic absorption of oxalate. They need both a low-oxalate diet and cholestyramine. Since bile salts enhance colonic oxalate absorption, the use of cholestyramine is useful in reducing it.

Ileal Resection of 100 to 200 cm with Colon Largely Intact. These patients have little difficulty in maintaining nutrition with an oral diet, but they have diarrhea because of bile-salt loss into the colon and steatorrhea with fatty acid diarrhea. In such patients, cholestyramine and a fat-restricted diet are useful. In addition, they should receive dietary advice about eating dry meals and separating solids from liquids to reduce diarrhea. Hyperoxaluria and vitamin B_{12} malabsorption should be treated as indicated earlier.

Resection in Excess of 200 cm of Small Bowel and Patients with Lesser Resection Associated with a Colectomy. These patients need the graduated adaptation program indicated under General Considerations earlier, and they will need different regimens, depending on how much bowel is left and on adaptation.

Resection Leaving Less than 60 cm of Small Bowel and Those with only a Duodenum. These patients need parenteral nutrition at home on an indefinite basis. The infusion rate and caloric intake are gradually reduced as normal weight is gained and maintained. The judgment to reduce intravenous feeding is made on the observations that weight gain is occurring beyond desired

limits and that reduced infusion does not result in electrolyte and fluid imbalance.

Remaining Problems. The question of oral micronutrients and vitamin absorption in these patients is an area that needs further study. Although macronutrient requirements can easily be judged by body composition, micronutrient needs and the requirement for oral supplementation have yet to be precisely defined.

REFERENCES

1. Malagelada, J-R.: Gastric, pancreatic and biliary response to a meal. *In* Johnson, L.R. (ed.): Physiology of the Gastrointestinal Tract. New York, Raven Press, 1981, pages 893–924.
2. Summers, R.W., Kent, T.H., and Osborne, J.W.: Effects of drugs, ileal obstruction and irradiation on rat gastrointestinal propulsion. Gastroenterology, *59*:731–739, 1970.
3. Connell, A.M.: Propulsion in the small intestine. Rendic Gastroenterol., 2:38–46, 1970.
4. Singleton, A.O., Redmond, D.C., and McMurray, J.E.: Ileocecal resection and small bowel transit and absorption. Ann. Surg., *159*:690–694, 1964.
5. Ricotta, J., Zuidema, G.D., Gadacz, T.R., and Sadri, D.: Construction of an ileocecal valve and its role in massive resection of the small intestine. Surg. Gynecol. Obstet., *152*:310–314, 1981.
6. Vantrappen, G.R., Peeters, T.L., and Janssens, J.: The secretory component of the interdigestive migrating motor complexes in man. Scand. J. Gastroenterol., *14*:663–667, 1979.
7. Fordtran, J.S., and Locklear, T.W.: Ionic constituents and osmolality of gastric and small-intestinal fluids after eating. Am. J. Dig. Dis., *11*:503–521, 1966.
8. Fordtran, J.S., and Dietschy, J.M.: Water and electrolyte movement in the intestine. Gastroenterology, *50*:263–285, 1966.
9. Turnberg, D.A., Bieberdorf, R.A., Morawski, S.G., and Fordtran, J.S.: Interrelationships of chloride, bicarbonate, sodium and hydrogen transport in human ileum. J. Clin. Invest., *49*:557–567, 1970.
10. Borgstrom, B., Dahlquist, A., Lundh, G., and Sjovall, J.: Studies of intestinal digestion and absorption in the human. J. Clin. Invest., *36*:1521–1536, 1957.
11. Nylander, G.: Gastric evacuation and propulsive intestinal motility following resection of the small intestine in the rat. Acta Chir. Scand., *133*:131–138, 1967.
12. Reynell, P.C., and Spray, G.H.: Small intestinal function in rat after massive resection. Gastroenterology, *31*:361–368, 1956.
13. Woolf, G.M., and Jeejeebhoy, K.N.: Diet for the patient with short bowel syndrome: high fat or high carbohydrate? Gastroenterology. *84*:823–828, 1983.
14. Debongnie, J.C., and Phillips, S.F.: Capacity of the colon to absorb fluid. Gastroenterology, 74:698–703, 1978.
15. Hofmann, A.F., and Poley, J.R.: Cholestyramine treatment of diarrhea associated with ileal resection. N. Engl. J. Med., *281*:397–402, 1969.

16. Binder, H.J.: Fecal fatty acids—mediators of diarrhea? Gastroenterology, 65:847–850, 1973.

17. Williams, R.D., and Olmsted, W.H.: The effect of cellulose, hemicellulose and lignin on the weight of the stool: a contribution to the study of laxation in man. J. Nutr., 11:433–449, 1936.

18. Bond, J.H., and Levitt, M.D.: Fate of soluble carbohydrate in the colon of rats and man. J. Clin. Invest., 57:1158–1164, 1976.

19. Cummings, J.H., James, W.P.T., and Wiggins, H.S.: Role of the colon in ileal-resection diarrhea. Lancet, 1:344–347, 1973.

20. Mitchell, J., Zukerman, L., and Breuer, R.I.: The colon influences ileal resection diarrhea (Abstract). Gastroenterology, 72:1103, 1977.

21. Booth, C.C., Aldis, D., and Read, A.E.: Studies on the site of fat absorption: 2 fat balances after resection of varying amounts of the small intestine in man. Gut, 2:168–174, 1961.

22. Hofmann, A.F., and Poley, J.R.: Role of bile acid malabsorption in the pathogenesis of diarrhea and steatorrhea in patients with ileal resection. I. Response to cholestyramine or replacement of dietary long chain triglyceride by medium chain triglycerides. Gastroenterology, 62:918–934, 1972.

23. Hylander, E., Ladefoged, K., and Jarnum, S.: Nitrogen absorption following small intestinal resection. Scand. J. Gastroenterol., 15:853–858, 1980.

24. Ladefoged, K.: Intestinal and renal loss of infused minerals in patients with severe short bowel syndrome. Am. J. Clin. Nutr., 36:59–67, 1982.

25. Haymond, H.E.: Massive resection of the small intestine: analysis of 257 collected cases. Surg. Gynecol. Obstet., 61:693–705, 1935.

26. McClenahan, J.E., and Fisher, B.: Physiologic effects of massive small intestinal resection and colectomy. Am. J. Surg., 79:684–688, 1950.

27. Trafford, H.S.: Outlook after massive resection of small intestine, with report of 2 cases. Br. J. Surg., 44:10–13, 1956.

28. West, E.S., Montague, J.R., and Judy, F.R.: Digestion and absorption in man with 3 feet of small intestine. Am. J. Dig. Dis., 5:690–692, 1938.

29. Pilling, G.P., and Cresson, S.L.: Massive resection of the small intestine in the neonatal period: report of 2 successful cases and review of the literature. Pediatrics, 19:940–948, 1957.

30. Martin, J.R., Pattee, C.J., Gardner, C., and Marien, B.: Massive resection of small intestine. Can. Med. Assoc. J., 69:429–433, 1953.

31. Kinney, J.M., Goldwyn, R.M., Barr, J.S., Jr., and Moore, F.D.: Loss of the entire jejunum and ileum and the ascending colon. Management of a patient. J.A.M.A., 179:529–532, 1962.

32. Walker-Smith, J.: Total loss of mid-gut. Med. J. Aust., 1:857–860, 1967.

33. Clayton, B.E., and Cotton, D.A.: A study of malabsorption after resection of the entire jejunum and the proximal half of the ileum. Gut, 2:18–22, 1961.

34. Anderson, C.M.: Long-term survival with six inches of small intestine. Br. Med. J., 5432:419–422, 1965.

35. Meyer, H.W.: Sixteen-year survival following extensive resection of small and large intestine for thrombosis of the superior mesenteric artery. Surgery, 51:755–759, 1962.

36. Flint, J.M.: The effect of extensive resection of the small intestine. Johns Hopkins Med. J., 23:127–144, 1912.

37. Porus, R.L.: Epithelial hyperplasia following massive small bowel resection in man. Gastroenterology, 48:753–757, 1965.

38. Booth, C.C., Evans, K.T., Menzies, T., and Street, D.F.: Intestinal hypertrophy following partial resection of the small bowel in the rat. Br. J. Surg., 46:403–410, 1959.

39. Nygaard, K.: Resection of the small intestine in rats III: morphological changes in the intestinal tract. Acta Chir. Scand., 133:233–248, 1967.

40. Stassoff, B.: Experimentelle untersachungen uber die kompensatorischen vorange ker darmresektionen. Beits. Klin. Chir., 89:527–533, 1914.

41. Althausen, T.L., Doig, R.K., Uyeyama, K., and Weiden, S.: Digestion and absorption after massive resection of small intestine; recovery of absorptive function as shown by intestinal absorption tests in 2 patients and consideration of compensatory mechanisms. Gastroenterology, 16:126–139, 1950.

42. Loran, M.R., and Althausen, T.L.: Cellular proliferation of intestinal epithelia in the rat two months after partial resection of the ileum. J. Biophys. Biochem. Cytol., 7:667–672, 1960.

43. Obertop, H., Nundy, S., Malamud, D., and Malt, R.A.: Onset of cell proliferation in the shortened gut. Rapid hyperplasia after jejunal resection. Gastroenterology, 72:267–270, 1977.

44. Cairnie, A.B., Lamerton, L.F., and Steel, G.G.: Cell proliferation studies in the intestinal epithelium of the rat. I. Determination of the kinetic parameters. II. Theoretical aspect. Exp. Cell Res., 39:528–553, 1965.

45. Tilson, M.D., and Wright, H.K.: Augmented ileal sodium and potassium stimulated adenosine triphosphatase after jejunal transposition. Surg. Forum, 21:326–327, 1970.

46. Altmann, G.G., and Leblond, C.P.: Factors influencing villus size in the small intestine of adult rats as revealed by transposition of intestinal segments. Am. J. Anat., 127:15–36, 1970.

47. Clark, R.M.: "Luminal nutrition" versus "functional work-load" as controllers of mucosal morphology and epithelial replacement in the rat small intestine. Digestion, 15:411–424, 1977.

48. Alpess, D.H.: Protein synthesis in intestinal mucosa: the effect of the route of administration of precursor amino acids. J. Clin. Invest., 51:167–173, 1972.

49. Weser, E., Heller, R., and Tawil, T.: Stimulation of mucosal growth in the rat ileum by bile and pancreatic secretions after jejunal resection. Gastroenterology, 73:524–529, 1977.

50. Williamson, R.C.N., Buckholtz, T.W., and Malt, R.A.: Humoral stimulation of cell proliferation in the small bowel after transection and resection in rats. Gastroenterology, 75:249–254, 1978.

51. Gleeson, M.H., Bloom, S.R., Polak, J.M., Henry, K., and Dowling, R.H.: Endocrine tumour in kidney affecting small bowel structure, motility and absorptive function. Gut, 12:773–782, 1971.

52. McKay, J.S., Linaker, B.D., and Turnberg, W.A.: The influence of opiates on ion transport across rabbit ileal mucosa. Gastroenterology, 80:279–284, 1981.

53. Cook, G.C., and Carruthers, R.H.: Reaction of human small intestine to an intraluminal tube and its importance in jejunal perfusion studies. Gut, 15:545–548, 1974.

54. Backman, L., and Hallberg, D.: Small-intestinal length. An intraoperative study in obesity. Acta Chir. Scand., *140*:57–63, 1974.

55. Griffin, G.E., Fagan, E.F., Hodgson, A.J., and Chadwick, V.S.: Enteral therapy in the management of massive gut resection complicated by chronic fluid or electrolyte depletion. Dig. Dis. Sci., *27*:902–908, 1982.

56. Wolman, S.L., Anderson, G.H., Marliss, E.B., and Jeejeebhoy, K.N.: Zinc in total parenteral nutrition: requirements and metabolic effects. Gastroenterology, *76*:458–467, 1979.

57. Main, A.N.H., Morgan, R.J., Hall, M.J., Russell, R.I., Shenkin, A., and Fell, G.S.: Home enteral tube feeding with a liquid diet in the long term management of inflammatory bowel disease

58. Jeejeebhoy, K.N., Zohrab, W.J., Langer, B., Phillips, M. J., Kuksis, A., and Anderson, G. H.: Total parenteral nutrition at home for 23 months, without complication and with good rehabilitation. A study of technical and metabolic features. Gastroenterology, *65*:811–820, 1973.

59. Broviac, J.W., and Scribner, B.H.: Prolonged parenteral nutrition in the home. Surg. Gynecol. Obstet., *139*:24–28, 1974.

60. Shils, M.E.: A program for total parenteral nutrition at home. Am. J. Clin. Nutr., *28*:1429–1435, 1975.

61. Andersson, H., and Jagenburg, R.: Fat-reduced diet in the treatment of hyperoxaluria in patients with ileopathy. Gut, *15*:360–366, 1974.

and intestinal failure. Scott. Med. J., *25*:312–314, 1980.

CHAPTER 26

Intravenous Feeding of the Cancer Patient

STEPHEN F. LOWRY
MURRAY F. BRENNAN

Few applications of intravenous feeding have received more experimental and clinical investigation than that in the tumor-bearing subject. After a decade of extensive clinical experience with parenteral nutrition in the cancer-bearing population, critical questions as to appropriate selection of patients as well as duration of therapy and composition of feeding formulations remain to be answered. The breadth of investigative effort and controversy that surrounds the field of nutritional support in cancer has been summarized in recent national conferences.[1-5]

The earliest justification for intravenous nutritional support in cancer-bearing subjects was extrapolated from observations in cachectic non–tumor-bearing patients in whom positive nitrogen balance, wound closure, and ultimate rehabilitation were effected with intravenous feeding. These observations, coupled with more aggressive multi-modality tumor therapies, appeared to support intravenous feeding (IVF) as a potential therapeutic adjunct in the cancer patient.

This chapter presents an overview of current understanding of the causes and implications of weight loss in cancer patients. Comparisons of the malnutrition in cancer-bearing populations with that observed in other wasting or catabolic states are made. A review of the current applications of complete intravenous feeding, often referred to as total parenteral nutrition (TPN), in the tumor-bearing human is presented. Finally, the metabolic impact of IVF on the nutritional defects of the cancer patient and a summary of prospective clinical trials is discussed.

PROGNOSTIC IMPLICATIONS OF WEIGHT LOSS IN CANCER PATIENTS

It has long been recognized that weight loss, with the associated but variable dissolution of host lean body mass, represents an adverse clinical observation in cancer patients. Among the many presumed systemic effects of malignancy, the anorexia, weight loss, and progressive deterioration of performance status, collectively termed *cancer cachexia*, are perhaps the most frequently observed clinical manifestations. Cancer cachexia often exists without an apparent organic etiology for the failure to ingest or absorb nutrients. Warren[6] observed that 22 per cent of 500 autopsies on cancer-bearing subjects demonstrated no explicable cause of death other than inanition. Recent surveys have documented that weight loss of greater than ten per cent of pre-illness body weight may occur in up to 45 per cent of hospitalized adult cancer patients.[7] Careful nutritional assessment may detect an even greater incidence of subtle malnutrition in such patients.[8-10]

Nutritional surveys of this nature, however, do not clearly distinguish between the propensity of specific tumors to induce cancer cachexia and anorexia-producing effects of antitumor therapy. DeWys and colleagues[11] have addressed this issue in a recent cooperative trial in which 3047 adult patients with 12 types of malignancies were assessed for weight loss prior to the initiation of chemotherapy (Table 26–1). With the ex-

Table 26–1. WEIGHT LOSS IN ADULT CANCER PATIENTS: INCIDENCE AND EFFECT ON SURVIVAL

TUMOR TYPE/LOCATION	TOTAL NO. PATIENTS	PATIENTS WITH WEIGHT LOSS IN PREVIOUS 6 MONTHS (%)			MEDIAN SURVIVAL (WEEKS)		p*
		No Loss	Some Loss	>10% Loss	No Weight Loss	Any Weight Loss	
Pancreas	111	17	83	26	14	12	N.S.
Gastric							
Nonmeasurable	179	17	83	30	41	27	.05
Measurable	138	13	87	38	18	16	N.S.
Colon	307	46	54	14	43	21	.01
Breast	289	64	36	6	70	45	.01
Prostate	78	44	56	10	46	24	.05
Sarcoma	189	60	40	7	46	25	.01
Lung							
Non–small cell	590	39	61	15	20	14	.01
Small cell	436	43	57	14	34	27	.05
Hodgkin's disease							
Favorable	290	69	31	10	—	138	.01
Unfavorable	311	52	48	15	107	55	.01
Acute nonlymphocytic leukemia	129	61	39	4	8	4	N.S.

*N.S. = no significant difference.

(Adapted from DeWys, W. D., Begg, C., Lavin, P. T., et al.: Prognostic effect of weight loss prior to chemotherapy in cancer patients. Am. J. Med., 68:683–690, 1980.)

ception of breast cancer, a significant relationship between weight loss and extent of tumor was not observed. In general, however, weight loss represented a powerful predictor of both performance status and response to therapy. In pediatric tumors, evidence of protein-calorie malnutrition may exist at the time of diagnosis, although efforts to correlate such nutritional factors with survival have not had the success described previously for adult solid tumors.[12, 13]

Another important question is the extent to which nutrition-related decreases in drug or radiation tolerance may cause potential reductions in cure rate. This has been a prominent area of investigation in nutrition repletion studies but has received little documentation in non–nutrition-oriented cancer therapy surveys. Sloan and associates[14] have attempted to define this nutritional component in a series of patients treated with multimodality therapy for soft tissue sarcoma of the head, neck, and trunk.[14] The most significant change in weight (mean ± SD) occurred following surgery (-3.11 ± 1.24 kg) with lesser amounts of weight loss during radiation therapy (-1.58 ± 0.65 kg) or chemotherapy with doxorubicin/cyclophosphamide (-2.8 ± 1.03 kg) or methotrexate ($+1.02 \pm 0.78$ kg). Patients who remained continuously free of disease exhibited stable weight over the entire course of therapy and subsequent adjuvant therapy ($+0.50 \pm 1.70$ kg), whereas patients with resectable, recurrent disease lost weight (-1.20 ± 2.60 kg), and patients who developed disseminated disease exhibited extensive weight loss (-5.80 ± 6.02 kg). These data indicate that a distinct treatment-related effect of anti-tumor therapy does exist, but this effect is usually overcome if treatment is successful.

THE ETIOLOGY OF CANCER CACHEXIA

Cancer cachexia, which encompasses a syndrome of relative hypophagia and progressive deterioration of performance status, implies a systemic effect of malignancy that influences nutrient intake, efficient substrate utilization, and the maintenance of normal host tissue composition. The extent to which weight loss and malnutrition in the cancer subject are a unique form of cachexia or, alternatively, a stress response to the tumor-bearing state that manifests itself in the form of underfeeding or starvation remains controversial. Several areas of investigation are being pursued in an effort to identify the mechanism(s) of cancer cachexia.

Anorexia

Relative hypophagia, evidenced by an inability or voluntary unwillingness to ingest adequate nutrients to sustain integrity of the host carcass mass, eventually represents the dominant element in cancer cachexia. Whether this factor represents a primary response to malignancy or is incited via other anorexia-producing effector mechanisms represents a critical area in both the clinical and research applications of nutritional support in the cancer subject.

Abnormal functioning of the hypothalamic "feeding and satiety" centers has been postulated as a primary cause of cancer cachexia. Experimental destruction of these hypothalamic regions in tumor-bearing rats does not result in alterations of the food intake pattern exhibited by non–tumor-bearing animals with similar lesions, nor do such lesions prevent progressive anorexia in the late stages of tumor growth.[15]

Morrison[16] has experimentally evaluated several interactive feeding control mechanisms that may be mediated, in part, by hypothalamic function. Aside from a persistent hyperphagic response to insulin in the tumor-bearing animal,[16] other hypothalamic responses mediated by catecholaminergic mechanisms appear normal in comparison with the non–tumor-bearing state.[17] A recent report from Krause and associates[18] has postulated a hypothalamic serotonigenic pathway that is mediated by increased blood levels of free tryptophan. Although this hypothesis has not been confirmed by other groups, recent parabiotic experiments would indicate that a peripheral (blood-borne) mechanism is at least partially responsible for the anorexia of cancer cachexia.[19] At this time, however, there is no evidence to support a primary abnormality of hypothalamic function in humans with cancer cachexia.

Several reports have attempted to define the extent of altered gustatory sensation in tumor-bearing subjects. Altered taste perception has been correlated with reduced caloric intake.[20, 21] Further attempts to correlate that taste threshold for specific nutrients with either extent or histologic type of the tumor have not been successful. Many of the subjects evaluated for taste acuity have already exhibited an element of weight loss. As a consequence, micronutrient deficiencies may already exist in such patients. The complex relationship between olfactory sensation and taste has received little serious investigation. At present, altered taste sensation may be considered to exert only a secondary effect in the hypophagia of cancer cachexia.

In addition to changes in taste recognition, visceral receptors sensitive to osmotic, volumetric and chemical effects of nutrients may potentially regulate the amount of food ingested.[22] Failure to correlate the food intake of anorectic patients with upper or lower intestinal malignancy has recently cast doubt on the importance of this mechanism.[23]

Appetite reduction may potentially be regulated by specific central and peripheral recognition systems for glucose,[24, 25] free fatty acids,[26] and amino acids.[27, 28] Abnormalities in the blood level and turnover of these substrates have been identified, but such metabolic perturbations are usually not observed prior to the onset of overt anorexia. Specific tumor types, such as sarcomas, can produce substrate imbalance, as has been demonstrated by increased glucose and amino acid uptake and lactate release across experimental tumors[29] and human tumor-bearing extremities.[30]

Paraneoplastic and Hormonal Causes

It has been postulated that tumors may also produce an anorexigenic peptide. In addition to experimental evidence of a circulating substance that may induce hypophagia,[19] substances have been isolated from the urine of patients with extensive malignant disease[31] that will induce anorexia in non–tumor-bearing animals.

Although it has been well established in the non–tumor-bearing state that appetite may be adversely affected by a variety of hormones, no comprehensive, prospective study of hormone levels or secretion rates in anorexia-prone patients is available. Basal insulin and glucagon levels have been reported from cachectic cancer patients,[32-35] but the interactive effects of hormones, such as catecholamines, insulin, and glucagon, have not been addressed. Such studies would be of great interest to evaluate both the effect of hormones on appetite as well as the alterations of intermediary metabolism outlined later.

Thermogenic Considerations

Negative energy balance resulting from insufficient food consumption is an important manifestation of cancer cachexia. The extent to which this negative energy balance results from potential increases in whole-body energy expenditure of the tumor-bearing subject remains speculative. Some experimental[36, 37] and clinical[38-40] studies have suggested an increased basal energy expenditure in the tumor-bearing host with cachexia. This finding has not been confirmed in animal[41] or human[42, 43] determinations of cancer-bearing subjects prior to the onset of weight loss.

It has been demonstrated that the presence of some tumors may induce an increase in whole-body energy expenditure. Morrison[44] demonstrated a return to normal (non–tumor-bearing) energy expenditure levels in rats within 24 hours of excising Walker 256 carcinomas.[44] In a small group of patients, Arbeit and co-workers[42] have recently demonstrated a linear, tumor volume–related reduction in human energy expenditure following surgical excision of soft part sarcomas (Fig. 26–1). Warnold and associates[39] also suggested that resting (basal) energy expenditure returned toward normal following tumor excision in humans, although energy expenditure was not directly measured in their study.

Studies of absolute energy balance in cancer patients have been limited. These reports have demonstrated a reduction in calorie intake below the predicted levels for energy balance in both diverse[39] and tumor-specific[45] groups.

Animal studies have attempted to define the partition of expended energy between the functional tumor and carcass mass and to determine the energy necessary for the retrieval of food. It has been proposed from these experiments that a progressive decline in eating activity is an important component of experimental cancer cachexia.[46, 47] To what extent a voluntary or asthenia-imposed reduction in eating contributes to early cachexia in cancer patients remains speculative.

Although the assumption that increased whole-body energy expenditure is a contributing factor to cancer-related weight loss appears valid for some tumors, there is no well-documented evidence to suggest that this mechanism is a primary effector of cancer cachexia. Rather, alterations in the basal regulation of energy expenditure appears to correlate best with the extent or stage of tumor burden[42, 48] and reflects an increasing proportion of energy required by the tumor relative to the reduced lean tissue mass of the host.

The mechanism for such alterations in whole-body energy expenditure has not been addressed. Potential mechanisms include a tumor-produced peptide or paraneoplastic hormone[49] and an adrenergic response as observed in other malnourished states,[50, 51] and energy-inefficient substrate cycling (futile cycles) induced by the tumor.[52, 53] Another potential thermogenic phenomenon is an altered core or peripheral temperature response to feeding in the tumor-bearing subject.[54-56] The biochemical regulation of the thermic effect of ingested (or infused) nutrients is a complex phenomenon that will require further elucidation by both calorimetry and hormonal response before a contribution to cancer cachexia can be ascertained.

Psychological Effects

Learned aversion to food may also represent a contributing factor in cachectic patients undergoing radiation treatment[57] or chemotherapy.[58] These alterations may be detected by taste threshold testing and may evolve very early in antitumor therapy. Bernstein and Bernstein[58] have shown that a decreased preference for the diet consumed during active tumor growth may be reversed by the introduction of a novel diet.

IMPACT OF CANCER CACHEXIA ON BODY COMPOSITION AND INTERMEDIARY METABOLISM

Regardless of the mechanism(s) by which relative hypophagia evolves in the

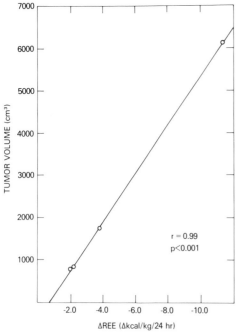

Figure 26–1. Reduction in whole-body resting energy expenditure (REE) in four patients following surgical resection of soft part sarcoma. (*Adapted from* Arbeit, J. M., et al.: unpublished observation.)

tumor-bearing subject, the net result is a dissolution of structural, functional, and energy storage mass in the host. As noted previously, the extent to which such changes are consistent with a malnourished or starvation economy or with a metabolic milieu unique to the cancer-bearing organism remains unsettled. The resolution of this question may have implications for the design of nutritional support regimens specific for the cancer-bearing subject.

Body Composition

The contribution to weight loss in tumor-bearing subjects resulting from the cancer cachexia syndrome or from simple under nutrition and starvation might be revealed by body composition studies of the tumor-bearing host.[59, 60] If for example, a disruptive systemic effect of cancer cachexia is predominant, weight loss should correlate with the extent of tumor and decreased survival, because a disproportionate amount of host tissue loss would derive from the lean tissues of muscle and viscera. Conversely, if simple starvation or undernutrition is the dominant factor in the weight loss, a disproportionate reduction of adipose tissue should be evident.

Recent studies using neutron activation analysis have been undertaken to derive estimates of whole-body composition in both cancer patients and normal volunteers.[61-64] In a series of patients with a variety of hematologic and solid tumors, Cohn and associates[61, 63] observed that body composition in weight-stable patients with hematologic malignancies was no different from that in age-matched controls (Table 26–2). In contrast, however, weight-losing patients with lung, gastrointestinal, and head and neck cancers demonstrated a 13 to 25 per cent reduction in soft tissue mass, primarily from the skeletal muscle compartment. Significant reductions in adipose tissues were not observed until weight loss exceeded ten per cent. Although this study was not controlled for the potential effects of concurrent antitumor therapy, the findings suggest that elements of a delayed or poorly adapted starvation (fat mobilization) body economy may be superimposed upon body composition changes resulting from the presence of cancer.

Intermediary Metabolism

Clarification of the intermediary metabolism of the tumor-bearing subject may provide additional insight into the mechanism of cancer cachexia as well as direct the design of appropriate nutritional support regimens in this population. Extensive animal studies have been performed in an effort to clarify the metabolic interactions between the host and tumor. Such studies have helped to

Table 26–2. BODY COMPOSITION OF NORMAL SUBJECTS AND CANCER PATIENTS AS DETERMINED BY *IN VIVO* NEUTRON ACTIVATION ANALYSIS*

TYPE OF SUBJECTS	TYPE OF MALIGNANCY	NO. OF SUBJECTS	WEIGHT LOSS (%)	LEAN BODY MASS (%)†	MUSCLE LEAN BODY MASS (%)	NON-MUSCLE LEAN BODY MASS (%)	TOTAL BODY FAT (%)
Males							
Normal	—	10	—	75	26	42	24
Cancer-bearing	Hematologic	12	+ 1.6	76	28	38	23
	Lung	6	− 10.7	76	15	54	23
	Gastrointestinal	6	− 19.0	88	14	61	12
	Head and neck	5	− 18.1	84	14	59	17
Females							
Normal	—	10	—	62	11	44	37
Cancer-bearing	Hematologic	8	0	64	13	43	37
	Lung	3	− 24.8	81	0	75	20
	Gastrointestinal	5	− 14.6	74	8	62	26
	Head and neck	6	− 19.5	76	11	57	26

*Compartmental analysis expressed as percentage of current body weight.

†Lean body mass = $\dfrac{\text{total body water}}{0.73}$.

(Adapted from Cohn, S., Gartenhaus, W., Sawitsky, A., et al.: Compartmental body composition of cancer patients by measurement of total body nitrogen, potassium and water. Metabolism, *30*:222–229, 1980.)

Table 26–3. METABOLIC COMPARISON OF STARVED, INJURED, AND TUMOR-BEARING HUMANS*

PARAMETER	STARVED	INJURED	TUMOR-BEARING
Basal metabolic rate	↓ (66)	↓ (67)	↑ (39)
			± (42)
Blood glucose	↓ (65)	↑ (68)	± (32)
Blood lactate	± (69)	↑ (70)	↑ (71)
Serum insulin	↓ (65)	↓ (68)	± (33)
Plasma glucagon	↑ (72)	↑ (68)	± (34)
Total plasma amino acids	↓ (74)	↑ (75)	↓ (76)
Urinary nitrogen excretion	↓ (65)	↑ (77)	± (78)
Glucose tolerance	↓ (65)	↓ (75)	↓ (32)
Whole-body glucose turnover rate	↓ (79)	↑ (80)	↑ (34)
Whole-body glucose recycling			
%	↑ (79)	± (80)	± (34)
Rate	± (79)	↑ (81)	↑ (71)
Whole-body protein turnover	↓ (82)	↑ (83)	± (84,118)
Whole-body protein synthesis	↓ (82)	↑ (83)	± (84,118)
Whole-body protein catabolism	↑ (221)	↑ (83)	± (118)
Gluconeogenesis from alanine	↑ (85)	↑ (86)	↑ (34,87)

* ↑ = a significant increase; ↓ = a significant decrease; ± = either no change or a nonsignificant trend. The numbers in parentheses indicate chapter references.
(Adapted from Brennan, M. F.: Total parenteral nutrition in the cancer patient. N. Engl. J. Med., 30:375–381, 1981.)

elucidate alterations of interorgan substrate flow and the cellular metabolism of both host and tumor tissues. Extrapolation of these data to the human tumor-bearing state, particularly in the presence of weight loss and anti-tumor therapy, must be done with great caution. As a consequence, this discussion focuses upon observations made in the human tumor-bearing state, with an emphasis on those studies that can be contrasted with normal or non–tumor-bearing man.

As noted previously, the contribution of undernutrition or starvation to the weight loss of cancer cachexia is ill-defined. Although metabolic components of starvation are present in the cancer patient, one may also observe similarities to the stress or injured state (Table 26–3).

An intermediary metabolism unique to the cancer-bearing subject has been inferred from an increased competition between the host and tumor tissues for energetic and structural substrate. However, there is *no* evidence to suggest that such a response varies qualitatively from that observed experimentally during rapid growth of nonmalignant tissue[89] or clinically during the early repair of traumatic injury.[90]

Carbohydrate Metabolism

There are numerous reports of carbohydrate intolerance in cancer patients.[32, 33, 35, 91, 92] A variety of clinical and metabolic vectors, including starvation,[93, 94] inactivity,[95, 96] hy-

permetabolic states,[97] and antecedent diet composition,[98] obscure the significance of these observations. In addition to delayed clearance of blood glucose following oral or intravenous challenge, evidence for both a blunted pancreatic insulin secretory response and altered peripheral insulin responsiveness in cancer-bearing host tissue has been obtained.[99] Although the cause of altered insulin responses is unknown, neither tissue insulin receptor function nor insulin-sensitive metabolic pathways other than carbohydrate oxidation or storage is grossly affected.[33, 35] *In vitro* determinations on skeletal muscle from cancer-bearing patients have demonstrated a correlation of reduced glucose carbon incorporation rates into glycogen, lactate, and carbon dioxide to selected enzymes controlling these pathways.[100, 101]

Demonstration of disordered carbohydrate processing may also be observed during whole-body isotope studies of the tumor-bearing human. In the postabsorptive cachectic cancer patient, both glucose turnover (production and utilization)[73, 87, 88, 102] and the rate of glucose carbon recycling are increased[71, 73] (Table 26–4). In addition, both Cori cycle (lactate→glucose) activity[71, 103] and gluconeogenesis from amino acids are increased in cachectic patients.[73, 87] Increased rates of lactate production have also been observed in cancer patients with progressive weight loss.[103, 104] The acceptance of an ongoing, excessive gluconeogenesis from host amino acids to explain the progressive mus-

Table 26–4. POSTABSORPTIVE GLUCOSE AND ALANINE KINETICS IN NORMAL AND
TUMOR-BEARING HUMANS

SUBJECTS	NO. (REFERENCE)	TYPE OF TUMOR	GLUCOSE TURNOVER (mMol/hr)	ALANINE TURNOVER (mMol/hr)	CONVERSION OF ALANINE TO GLUCOSE (%)
Normal	5 (87)	—	31.4	10.9	2.5
(non–tumor-bearing)	6 (88)	—	46.6		
	7 (102)	—	65.4		
Tumor-bearing					
Localized tumors with body weight loss of:	14 (34)	Squamous cell carcinoma of the esophagus			
0–5%			37.3	6.4	4.7
5–10%			42.5	7.3	5.0
10–20%			37.2	6.6	4.8
> 20%			38.8	6.5	3.4
Local/metastatic tumors	12 (88)	Non–oat cell bronchogenic carcinoma	55.7		
	11 (102)	Various solid tumors	77.8		
Metastatic tumors	8 (87)	Various solid tumors	38.6	11.7	5.6

cle wasting of the cachectic patients[34, 87] must be tempered by observations that conversion of alanine to glucose is readily suppressed by small quantities of glucose in normal[86] and cancer-bearing humans[73, 87] but not in sick and septic humans.[86] Certainly, the large quantities of glucose given in IVF central feeding regimens can suppress the conversion of glucose to alanine in cancer-bearing humans.[34]

The increased rates of glucose formation and of inefficient oxidation may be partially ascribed to an obligate glucose consumption by the tumor. Recent *in vivo* studies in sarcoma-bearing patients[30, 42] would support this hypothesis. Whether this glucose substrate inefficiency can be ascribed to other tumor types[103] remains to be elucidated.

The metabolic changes seen in cancer patients do *not* seem to be due to starvation or fasting alone. The increased glucose turnover, gluconeogenesis, and lactate production observed in the cancer cachexia state are the converse of the response seen in a normal starvation-adapted state. However, both whole-body carbohydrate kinetics and peripheral host tissue glucose processing have many elements associated with a stressed adrenergic state. To what extent these mechanisms participate in the glucose metabolism of the cancer patient remains to be answered.

Lipid Metabolism

Terminal oxidation of free fatty acids (FFA) represents the major portion of daily energy expended by the normal human. In addition to existing in the form of triglycerides, which represent the major fuel reserve of the body, free fatty acids are readily taken up from blood for use as fuel by a variety of tissues. The rate of this uptake increases as the plasma FFA/albumin molar ratio increases.[105] An increased FFA/albumin ratio may also increase the rate of gluconeogenesis. That portion of free fatty acids not utilized by peripheral tissues is converted to triglyceride in the liver and secreted as very-low-density lipoproteins (VLDL). The triglycerides in VLDL are processed by the adipose tissue.

Mobilization of adipose fuel from the triglyceride storage as diglyceride and FFA is controlled by a rate-limiting enzyme complex, hormone-sensitive triglyceride lipase. Other lipases complete the conversion to FFA and glycerol. The extent to which intracellular FFA are reesterified or released depends in part on the ability of the adipocytes to fix glycerol (as L-glycerolphosphate) or to generate new glycerol from glucose.[106]

Hormonal factors are important modulators of fat mobilization. Although catecholamines are probably the most important hormone in the lipolytic response, glucagon, growth hormone, and glucocorticoids may also participate. Insulin is the major antilipolytic hormone involved in the regulation of fat mobilization.

During the early transition from the fed to the fasted state, increased lipid mobilization is mediated by increased sympathetic

Table 26–5. RESTING ENERGY EXPENDITURE AND SUBSTRATE OXIDATION RATES IN NON–TUMOR-BEARING AND TUMOR-BEARING HUMANS ($\bar{X} \pm SD$)

SUBJECTS	NO. SUBJECTS	RESTING ENERGY EXPENDITURE (Kcal/kg/day)	OXIDATION RATES (g/kg/day)	
			Carbohydrate	*Fat*
Non–tumor-bearing	10	17.8 ± 2.9	1.66 ± 0.67	1.30 ± 0.29
Tumor-bearing				
Localized tumor	9	21.4 ± 3.7*	1.85 ± 1.03	1.61 ± 0.90
Metastatic tumor	3	24.0 ± 2.6*	1.62 ± 0.35	1.87 ± 0.17*

*p <0.05 versus non–tumor-bearing.
(Adapted from Arbeit, J. M., et al.: Abstract presented at Association for Academic Surgery, 15th Annual Meeting, Chicago, 1981. Localized bony and soft tissue sarcomas and various metastatic solid tumors.)

nerve activity to the adipose tissue and falling levels of insulin. If fasting continues over prolonged periods, obligate glucose-utilizing organs, such as brain, red blood cells, and renal medulla, ultimately decrease their uptake of glucose and begin to utilize lipid energy sources (as ketone bodies).[65, 107, 108] As a consequence of normal starvation adaptation, gluconeogenic precursors such as amino acids are conserved.

Despite the obvious importance of fat mobilization and oxidation to underfed or starved humans, the regulation of this process in the tumor-bearing state is poorly defined. Arbeit and co-workers[222] have determined the fat oxidation rate in selected postabsorptive cancer patients with localized or metastatic disease to equal or exceed that observed in normal controls (Table 26–5). Observations that levels of free fatty acids are similar in normal and tumor-bearing subjects after overnight fast[73, 109] and that suppression of plasma free fatty acid levels by exogenous glucose are qualitatively similar in cancer-bearing and normal humans suggests that the regulation of lipid mobilization is not greatly altered by the tumor-bearing state.[73, 109] Waterhouse and Kemperman[109] observed a slightly higher rate of fatty acid–derived CO_2 production in patients with progressive malignant disease than in weight-stable normals.

As an indirect measure of lipid mobilization, we have used an unlabeled glycerol infusion method to assess glycerol clearance. Despite similar postabsorptive arterial glycerol levels in normal humans and cachectic patients with esophageal or pancreatic cancer, glycerol clearance was significantly lower in the tumor-bearing subjects.[223] These findings suggest that a pattern of fat mobilization similar to that seen in starvation may be important in the later stages of cachectic weight loss. Such observations are consistent

with the timing of adipose tissue dissolution observed in the body composition studies by Cohn and associates[61, 63] (see Table 26–2).

Protein Metabolism

The clinically most evident and functionally most disrupting metabolic abnormality to occur in the tumor-bearing subject is the progressive diminution of host protein stores. Nitrogen balance values in the tumor-bearing subject may be variable even in the presence of overt skeletal muscle wasting.[110-112] As a consequence, study of whole-body or organ-specific nitrogen economy must be controlled for the antecedent nutritional status of the subject and the relationship of protein metabolism to energy expenditure. Many *in vivo* and *in vitro* studies have been performed in cachectic cancer patients after a prolonged period of negative energy balance. As a result, many of these reports are at variance with one another, rendering their interpretation difficult.

It is self-evident that a growing tumor imposes a demand for nitrogen. What is of major importance is the extent to which host nitrogen economy is disrupted in servitude to the tumor "nitrogen trap." *In vitro* isotope studies have demonstrated a greater leucine incorporation into liver protein in tumor-bearing subjects compared with non-tumor bearing patients,[100] whereas the opposite effect has been observed in skeletal muscle.[113] These findings suggest a differential impact upon labile host protein stores. Body composition studies have confirmed the preservation of visceral protein stores even at a point in the cachectic process where skeletal muscle has undergone extensive dissolution[63] (see Table 26–2).

Attempts to define the magnitude of skeletal muscle amino acid release by extremity arterial-venous difference studies have shown variable results when cachectic tumor-bearing subjects are compared with patients with non-malignant malnutrition.[30, 114, 115] A comparison of amino acid flux across a sarcoma-bearing limb has demonstrated greater uptake of some amino acids than in the non–tumor-bearing limb of the same subject.[30] These observations define the potential extent of nitrogen "trapping" by malignant tissue.

In addition to apparent visceral protein conservation, the synthesis of certain secretory proteins may be maintained in cachectic cancer patients. Despite an often lowered serum albumin level, the incorporation of isotope carbon into new albumin is often well-preserved. Fibrinogen and glycoprotein[116] synthesis may also be normal or increased, although the increased turnover of immunoglobulin[117] implies increased synthesis in cancer-bearing humans. To what extent increased synthesis of such acute phase proteins represents merely an appropriate response to increased cannibalism by the tumor or abnormal exogenous losses remains to be elucidated.

The study of whole-body protein kinetics using radioactive and stable isotopes of individual amino acids has achieved increased popularity in the investigation of cancer subjects. Increased rates of protein turnover have been observed after the onset of anorexia in cancer subjects, suggesting that disordered protein metabolism may make a contribution to the abnormal energy expenditure observed in some subjects.[84, 88, 118]

It is the regulation of host protein metabolism that most clearly differentiates cancer cachexia from pure starvation. A growing tumor may obscure the negative nitrogen balance that would result from lean tissue catabolism of starvation or underfeeding in cancer-bearing humans. This would seem to be similar to the nitrogen-conserving starvation state, were it not for the continued high rate of protein turnover and the more linear nature of skeletal muscle dissolution. The observed protein kinetic and compositional changes in cancer cachexia appear more closely aligned to the stressed or post-traumatic state than to starvation (Table 26–6).

Future Considerations

Prospective studies that evaluate both potential anorexia-producing mediators and metabolic abnormalities are necessary to clarify the complex phenomenon of cancer cachexia. Such studies would involve serial evaluation of anorexia-prone populations and would require careful control of both nutritional and therapeutic variables. The weight-losing cancer patient has been likened to a starved individual whose continued abnormal utilization of substrate does not permit effective adaptation to the underfed state. Despite claims to the contrary, there are no data to support a direct cause-and-effect relationship between altered host intermediary metabolism and the relative hypophagia of cancer cachexia. The critical nutritional questions relate to the biologic and clinical efficacy with which these altered metabolic processes can be overcome by intravenous feeding in the cancer patient.

INDICATIONS FOR INTRAVENOUS FEEDING IN CANCER PATIENTS

The adverse effect of weight loss and malnutrition that was observed in many can-

Table 26–6. WHOLE-BODY PROTEIN KINETICS IN NON–TUMOR-BEARING AND TUMOR-BEARING HUMANS ($\bar{X} \pm$ SEM)

SUBJECTS	NO. SUBJECTS	PROTEIN KINETICS (g/kg/day) Turnover	Synthesis	Catabolism	CHAPTER REFERENCE
Non–tumor-bearing					
Normal	3	2.9	2.4		84
Fed	5	3.2 ± 0.1	2.6 ± 0.1	2.0 ± 0.1	221
Fasted for					
12 hours	6	2.1			88
7 days	2	2.5	2.1		84
10 days	5	2.3 ± 0.2	1.7 ± 0.5	2.3 ± 0.2	221
Malnourished	3	3.3 ± 0.6	2.9 ± 0.3		84
Tumor-bearing	7	5.0 ± 0.9	4.3 ± 0.8		84
	18	2.8 ± 0.2	2.2 ± 0.2	2.8 ± 0.2	118
	12	3.2 ± 0.5			88
	11	2.0 – 4.0			224

cer-bearing populations raised considerable hope that aggressive nutritional support of such patients would improve therapeutic outcome. It is now apparent that although intravenous feeding (IVF) may sustain the life of the terminally ill cancer patient for brief periods, the application of IVF must be regarded as a supportive modality. Intravenous nutritional support is indicated in those cancer patients for whom malnutrition represents a distinct adverse predictor for curative or palliative intervention. In cases in which the extent of disease, complications, or responses to therapy preclude successful restoration of functional capacity, the decision to institute IVF must be viewed cautiously. The use of parenteral nutrition with the hope of restoring functional capacity or the "quality of life" is seldom indicated. Prospective follow-up of such patients has demonstrated rapid deterioration in an unsupervised environment.[119-120]

The decision to institute nutritional support must be viewed within the context of the biology of the malignancy. To react to weight loss and malnutrition alone, without considering other available therapeutic options, may lead to prolonged suffering for the patient and increased anguish for the family and physician.

Using the previous considerations, we have become relatively arbitrary in our selection of which patients should receive IVF. Any cancer patient (1) for whom a hospital stay of at least ten days will result in a therapeutic regimen of reasonable expectation for cure or palliation and (2) in whom adequate nutrition cannot or will not be maintained by enteral means should be considered for IVF. Efforts to identify appropriate candidates for IVF should begin at the time of admission and reassessed on a periodic basis. Recent evidence suggests that hospitalization alone will frequently result in progressive undernutrition.[8-10, 121, 122] The failure of many hospitalized patients to maintain a weight-stabilizing diet is multifactorial in origin but probably adds to the weight loss resulting from cancer cachexia.

NUTRITIONAL ASSESSMENT

The current status of nutritional assessment has been well outlined.[123] We have stressed the careful documentation of weight loss in the cancer patient. In the absence of significant edema, serous cavity effusions, or bulky tumor burden, weight loss implies a dissolution of host tissue regardless of the mode by which weight loss occurs. Correlations of antecedent weight loss to mortality following resection of esophageal or colorectal cancer have been made.[124, 125] Some investigators, however, have failed to confirm the usefulness of antecedent weight loss as an independent prognosticator of mortality in the cancer surgery patient.[126]

In addition to losses of structural and energy-storing host tissues, weight loss in the cancer patient may also adversely affect the availability of micronutrients, as has been demonstrated in a large group of hospitalized patients with protein-calorie malnutrition.[10] The quantity and composition of the recently ingested diet should be assessed in an effort both to document the degree of protein-calorie undernutrition and to detect possible taste aversions that may contribute to hypophagia.

By applying anthropometric and biochemical determinants of body composition and protein synthetic capability, several groups have attempted to refine the prognosis of the cancer-bearing subject. Nixon and associates[10] evaluated 54 medical oncology patients with a battery of anthropometric and biochemical studies in order to determine both the extent of malnutrition in this population and the independent prognostic value of each parameter. Only the creatinine/height index accurately predicted early demise ($\leq$70 days) with greater than 90 per cent sensitivity. Preoperative assessment for nutrition-related morbidity and mortality is claimed to be aided by a "prognostic nutritional index" (PNI).[127, 128] An increased PNI was determined to be associated with higher postoperative complication rate and mortality in 100 consecutive cancer patients.[127] Whether such an index will continue to prove useful as a prognosticator of surgical risk remains controversial.

The need for more sophisticated nutritional assessment, such as calorimetric determination of energy expenditure and nitrogen balance, should be dictated by clinical judgement or a failure to achieve the desired results in terms of fluid-free weight gain. Skin test anergy and decreased levels of acute phase proteins and albumin have been correlated with a reduced lean body mass.[129] Reversal of these abnormalities during short-term (less than two weeks) IVF does not document their utility as reliable indicators of *host* lean tissue repletion.[126,130]

THE TECHNIQUE OF INTRAVENOUS FEEDING IN THE CANCER PATIENT

Vascular Access

In cancer patients who are to be fed intravenously, careful attention to the details of catheter insertion and maintenance is required. Patients with advanced cachexia and therapy-related reduction in immune function may be particularly prone to catheter-related septic complications. Certain cancer populations, especially those with lymphoproliferative malignancy, may demonstrate specific cell-mediated immune deficiency in the absence of overt malnutrition.[131] Malnutrition may further aggravate myelotoxicity of some antitumor agents.[132] Risk factors also include a reduction of hemostatic components, and it is our policy to administer fresh platelets immediately prior to percutaneous central venous catheter insertion if the blood platelet count is below 50,000/ml.

The subclavian vein is the most effective site for catheter insertion. The internal and external jugular veins have been utilized for catheter insertion but are suboptimal unless the catheter is tunneled over the clavicle to exit at an infraclavicular site.[133] Because of an increased infectious and thrombotic complication rate, neither the basilic vein nor the saphenofemoral system should be used except to temporize until a more permanent catheter insertion can be effected.

Placement of Silastic catheters of the Hickman or Broviac design are increasingly used for long-term drug therapy and nutritional support in cancer patients. Although the safety of simultaneous or cyclical use of a single catheter for therapy and nutritional support has resulted in a low catheter sepsis rate,[134] such a practice should be done under close supervision. Simultaneous use of two Silastic catheters for purposes of therapy and nutritional support is our preferred alternative.[135] Only limited experience with the percutaneous insertion or permanent Silastic catheters is reported but it may replace more formal surgical procedures in some settings.[136]

Complications related to long-term central venous catheterization may be anticipated in the cancer population.[137] Febrile episodes are very common when the absolute neutrophil count is less than 500/mm[3]. This value is not an indication of catheter sepsis and need not mandate withdrawal of the line.[138,139] A useful technique in IVF cancer patients, in whom the suspicion of catheter sepsis is low, has been the replacement of a new feeding catheter over a commercially available flexible, stainless steel guidewire.[138] Unless another manifestation of sepsis, particularly the onset of glucose intolerance, is observed, our policy has been one of careful observation and frequent culture of all potential sources of fever. In the event of overt evidence of sepsis or a positive blood or catheter tip culture result, removal of the feeding catheter is mandatory. The patient will not be harmed by discontinuation of IVF for 24 to 48 hours, at which point there are sufficient clinical data to initiate treatment of any infectious source and permit confident re-institution of parenteral nutrition.

A four to five per cent incidence of clinically evident subclavian vein thrombosis may be anticipated during parenteral nutrition.[137] The incidence of subclinical thrombosis, detectable by contrast or radionuclide venography, however, approaches an incidence of 25 to 30 per cent.[140-142] The initial observations that Silastic catheters might reduce the incidence of thrombosis seen with the use of polyvinyl chloride catheters[143] has not been substantiated.[142] The implications of subclavian vein thrombosis, particularly in patient populations requiring prolonged or repeated central venous access, have prompted the investigation of the addition of low-dose heparin to the intravenous feeding solution.[141,142]

Nutritional Requirements

Despite the known derangements of intermediary metabolism occurring in the tumor-bearing organism, an intravenous feeding regimen specifically designed for the cancer patient has not been developed. The goal of attaining host protein anabolism must be accomplished with a nonprotein calorie source and an appropriately balanced amino acid source. Documentation that this goal is achieved in tumor-bearing populations is often contradictory.

Calories

Provision of adequate nonprotein calories to induce and sustain protein synthesis

Table 26–7. PATTERN OF MINERAL RETENTION DURING INTRAVENOUS FEEDING OF MALNOURISHED NON–TUMOR-BEARING AND TUMOR-BEARING HUMANS ($\bar{X} \pm SD$)

SUBJECTS	Δ NITROGEN (gm/day)	Δ PHOSPHORUS (gm/day)	Δ POTASSIUM (mEq/day)	Δ SODIUM (mEq/day)	Δ CHLORIDE (mEq/day)	Δ MAGNESIUM (mEq/day)
Non–tumor-bearing* (Ratio per gm N per day)*†	4.6 ± 1.8 (1.0)	0.27 ± 0.13 (0.06)	18.9 ± 6.5 (3.0–4.1)	23.4 ± 5.8 (3.7–5.1)	17.7 ± 4.9 (2.7–3.8)	11.9 ± 4.0 (2.6)
Tumor-bearing* (Ratio per gm N per day)*	5.1 ± 3.8 (1.0)	0.13 ± 0.19 (0.03)	18.7 ± 12.7 (3.7)	19.5 ± 7.4 (3.8)	12.6 ± 6.1 (2.5)	3.2 ± 5.9 (0.6)

*Study of nine cancer patients with various solid tumors and five non-cancer patients during ten to 14 days of IVF. Cancer patients did *not* receive anti-tumor therapy during this period. (Data from Nixon, D. W., Lawson, D. K., Kutner, M., et al.: Hyperalimentation of the cancer patient with protein-calorie malnutrition. Cancer Res., 41:2038–2045, 1981.)

†Study of 11 non–tumor-bearing patients. (Data from Rudman, D., Millikan, W. J., Richardson, T. J., et al.: Elemental balances during intravenous hyperalimentation of underweight adult subjects. J. Clin. Invest., 55:94–104, 1975.)

is of paramount importance. Positive nitrogen balance may be achieved in nutritionally depleted subjects at daily nonprotein calorie infusion rates of 35 to 50 kcal/kg,[144-146] but recent studies have demonstrated the potential risks of excessive carbohydrate infusion in depleted subjects with limited pulmonary reserve.[147] Excessive lactate production may also occur in some tumor-bearing populations.[71,148] Although not directly applicable to the tumor-bearing population, observations that an upper limit of carbohydrate oxidation exists even in hypermetabolic states[149] should be considered. As a consequence of these observations, we have adopted a policy of defining the upper limit of carbohydrate infusion at $\simeq 7$ mg/kg/min. This permits a glucose calorie infusion rate of 33 to 35 kcal/kg/day. Additional nonprotein calorie requirements can be effectively met by the infusion of lipid emulsion.

Concerns that nonprotein calorie supply will partition more favorably to the tumor have not been uniformly substantiated by animal experiments.[150-154] Of recent interest, however, is the experimental observation of an improved host protein metabolism using IVF regimens containing increased amounts of lipid.[155] Such an observation might be anticipated by the increased rates of fat oxidation obtained in cancer patients.[109] At present, these results should not dictate alterations in the IVF formulation most familiar to the clinician.

however, recent prospective studies in cancer patients have documented positive nitrogen balance in cancer patients at an infusion level of 0.2 to 0.3 gm/kg/day of nitrogen during IVF.[34,146,156] As noted previously, however, this apparent accrual of nitrogen does not provide evidence that normal body composition is being restored. Nonspecific whole-body ^{40}K levels have been noted to increase during IVF of cancer patients,[118] but the pattern of minerals retained under such circumstances does not reflect the composition to be expected in normal lean tissue synthesis (Table 26–7).[146] Clarification of the role of IVF in restoring or maintaining host lean tissue stores must await the results of current prospective studies using such techniques as neutron activation analysis and extremity amino acid flux.[115]

In addition to the use of standard balanced amino acid formulations for IVF in cancer-bearing humans, there has been recent interest in the use of branched-chain amino acid–enriched formulas to reduce postoperative lean tissue catabolism. Although such studies have demonstrated an apparent advantage in the stressed patients with[158] and without[159] cancer, their use in the cancer patient undergoing extended therapy has not been evaluated. Until intracellular imbalances or excessive oxidation of such amino acids can be documented, the generalized acceptance of such special formulations cannot be recommended.

Nitrogen

In the non–tumor-bearing, unstressed state, nitrogen retention can be improved by increasing nonprotein calorie supply. Under the constraints of limiting calorie infusion,

Electrolytes

The electrolyte requirements of the intravenously fed cancer patient have previously been reviewed.[160] With the exception of those patients for whom excessive losses (by diarrhea, fistulas, or intestinal drainage), organ failure, or paraneoplastic syndromes result in definable extracellular fluid composition changes, the electrolyte composition of the IVF regimen need not vary from that employed in non-neoplastic disease states. As noted previously (see Table 26–7),[144–146] the restoration of normal host lean tissue will result in the retention of electrolytes in a fixed proportion to nitrogen. For each gram of nitrogen retained, 3.5 to 5.1 mEq of *sodium*, 3.1 to 4.1 mEq of *potassium*, and 2.7 to 3.9 mEq of *chloride* will be retained. Rudman and colleagues[144] have recommended that malnourished subjects receiving IVF should be given 0.74 mEq sodium, 0.65 mEq potassium, and 0.56 mEq chloride per kilogram of ideal body weight per day. For practical purposes, the provision of $\simeq$ 50 mEq sodium, $\simeq$ 40 mEq potassium, and $\simeq$ 40 mEq chloride per liter of parenteral nutrition formula will clearly meet (or exceed) the electrolyte needs of most tumor-bearing patients. Twice-weekly serum electrolyte determinations are indicated to guide electrolyte replacement.

The requirements for *calcium* and *phosphorus* in the IVF cancer patient have recently been clarified. Sloan and associates[161] have observed consistent calcium balance at intakes of more than 15 mEq/day. This balance was achieved, however, in the presence of hypercalciuria (>20 mEq/day) in 34 per cent of the 151 patients studied. Whether such hypercalciuria may ultimately contribute to nephrotoxicity in the patient receiving chemotherapy and/or antibiotic therapy remains unclear, although frank renal stone disease has been seen rarely in patients receiving TPN for one to three months. Phosphorus balance was also achieved at daily intakes of 15 mMol (0.47q) or more.[161] Rudman and colleagues[144] previously recommended a daily infusion of 0.58 mMol per kilogram of *ideal body weight*, but this level now appears excessive on the basis of recent data. In practical terms, the inclusion of 10 to 12 mMol of phosphate per liter of IVF fluid should prevent deficiencies of this critical element.

The intake of *magnesium* necessary for normal protein synthesis is not well defined. Nixon and co-workers[146] recently suggested that depleted, non–tumor-bearing subjects will retain 2.6 mEq of magnesium with each gram of nitrogen accrued. If 5 to 10 grams of nitrogen are retained per day, magnesium infusion should be at least 13 to 26 mEq/day.

The retention of magnesium in cancer-bearing subjects was much lower, however; $\simeq$ 0.6 mEq was retained per gram of nitrogen.[146]

Vitamins and Trace Minerals

Because much of the information about vitamin repletion during IVF has been obtained in the adult cancer patient,[162,163] these requirements do not need further elaboration. Repletion of several vitamins and cofactors, such as vitamin D[162,163] and choline,[164] are undergoing investigation to establish guidelines.

Addition of *iron* to IVF regimens has been safely performed, but the quantities required have not been precisely defined.[165] The restoration of serum iron may be intimately related to the mobilization of iron stores during anabolism.[166]

Trace mineral supplementation has been extensively reviewed. In particular, the requirement for *zinc* in cancer patients has been thoroughly documented.[167,168] Studies of zinc repletion in cancer-bearing humans have not suggested that maintenance requirements differ from those reported in non–tumor-bearing subjects during IVF. Many cancer patients will have undergone numerous periods of therapy-related undernutrition and stress that may predispose to subclinical zinc deficiency. Such patients should receive a higher level of zinc supplementation ($\simeq$ 80 μg/kg/day) to restore and maintain normal blood zinc concentrations.[168] Patients with positive zinc balance may demonstrate an improved glucose tolerance mediated by increased insulin secretion.[169]

Copper supplementation should be routinely given to prevent hematologic manifestations of a copper deficiency syndrome. We have previously documented a positive whole-body copper balance at infusion rates of $\simeq$ 65 μg/kg/day.[168] Such an increased level of copper may be necessary to achieve balance during concurrent zinc supplementation, because the two metals compete for tissue binding sites.

Chromium supplementation, although probably not necessary during abbreviated periods of IVF, should be included in parenteral nutrition formulas for patients receiving long-term (more than six to eight weeks) or home intravenous nutrition. An association of glucose intolerance, peripheral neuropathy, and metabolic encepholopathy with chromium deficiency has been suggested.

Chromium appears to function as a "glucose tolerance factor" that may be critical to effective binding of insulin to receptor sites.

Selenium deficiency, manifested as myalgia, muscle tenderness, and possible cardiac failure, is rare in patients receiving short-term parenteral nutrition. Decreased plasma selenium levels are often observed during prolonged courses of home parenteral nutrition. Prospective studies of selenite repletion are under way to define the requirements for this metal. Supplemental daily doses of 50 μg/day or more can restore low plasma selenium levels to normal within two weeks.[170] Care in the filtering and storage of selenium-supplemented intravenous feeding solutions is necessary to prevent instability of this metal.

Essential Fatty Acids

The provision of 3.2 per cent or more of total caloric intake as intravenous fat emulsion will prevent essential fatty acid deficiency in tumor-bearing humans.[171,172] In practical terms, a twice-weekly infusion of 500 ml of a 10 per cent lipid emulsion will provide a sufficient source of essential fatty acids. There is no evidence to suggest that fatty acid requirements are higher in the presence of active tumor proliferation or during antitumor therapy.

There is increasing interest in the utilization of parenteral lipid emulsions as a non-protein energy source. Numerous reports have attested to the clinical efficacy of increasing the calorie ratio of lipid to dextrose in order to induce and sustain nitrogen balance in depleted[145,173] and hypermetabolic[173] non–tumor-bearing populations. This observation has not been adequately confirmed in tumor-bearing subjects.

METABOLIC INFLUENCE OF INTRAVENOUS FEEDING IN CANCER PATIENTS

Rigorous proof that parenteral nutrition can effectively reverse or ameliorate the catabolic influences of cancer cachexia or antitumor therapy would favor an aggressive posture in the selection of patients for such treatment. Unfortunately, documentation of a favorable biologic impact of IVF on the cancer population is limited. Numerous investigations of host tissue repletion and substrate flux have been reported in the parenterally nourished tumor-bearing animal. Although these studies have often reported restoration of host lean tissue mass[150,153] and improved tolerance to some antitumor therapies,[174] experimental nutritional intervention studies during the terminal stages of tumor growth must be extrapolated cautiously to the host-tumor relationship in human malignancy.

In addition to considerations relative to the host organism, the potential for stimulation of tumor growth by nutritional intervention has been delineated in animal studies.[152,154,175] This caveat may, in theory, represent a deterrent to the use of aggressive nutritional support in the cancer patient, but no clinical case of enhanced tumor growth during IVF has been documented.[4]

This discussion is confined to those controlled, clinical studies that have evaluated the biologic efficacy of intravenous nutrition in tumor-bearing humans. A critical appraisal of IVF technology, when applied to human malignancy, is hampered by the inability of most research methods to distinguish effectively between host and tumor responses to feeding. Despite the increasing application of isotope tracer techniques for the study of substrate turnover and of neutron activation to assess alterations of body composition, the impact of the tumor is not clearly defined.

Body Composition

Although the reversal of weight loss may often be observed during intravenous feeding of cancer patients, the composition of the restored weight may not reflect lean tissue accrual. Traditional methods of defining lean tissue accrual have relied on nitrogen balance studies. Careful balance studies in tumor-bearing patients have documented apparent nitrogen retention in clinically stable subjects receiving IVF during chemotherapy[146] or radiation therapy.[118] The conclusions drawn from these studies, however, are strikingly different with respect to the question of lean tissue restoration. Burt and colleagues[118] observed weight gain (p<0.05) and a statistically insignificant increase in whole body ^{40}K readings after two weeks of IVF in patients receiving radiation therapy for *localized* esophageal carcinoma.[118] The observed positive nitrogen balance and a reduction in urinary 3-methylhistidine excretion suggested a

Table 26–8. IMPACT OF INTRAVENOUS FEEDING ON PROTEIN METABOLISM IN PATIENTS WITH ESOPHAGEAL CANCER*

	WEIGHT (kg)	WHOLE-BODY ^{40}K (gm)	NITROGEN BALANCE (mg/kg/day)	3-METHYLHISTIDINE EXCRETION (μMol/kg/day)
Before IVF	60	100	− 99	2.5
During IVF	63	104	+ 26	1.9
p	<.05	NS	<.05	<.05

*From study of 11 patients who received radiation therapy to the mediastinum during two weeks of IVF. (Data from Burt, M. E., Stein, T. P., and Brennan, M. F.: A controlled randomized trial evaluating the effects of enteral and parenteral nutrition on protein metabolism in cancer-bearing man. J. Surg. Res., 34:303–314, 1983.)

favorable impact on host lean tissue mass (Table 26–8). Nixon and co-workers,[146] on the other hand, have studied patients with metastatic colorectal cancer who were receiving IVF before and during chemotherapy; although they also observed a positive nitrogen balance during these periods, they were unable to document a pattern of mineral and electrolytes retention that might be anticipated from host lean tissue restoration (see Table 26–7). The observed differences in mineral retention may be related to the extent of disease, but failure of such controlled studies to conclusively affirm the benefits of IVF on body composition suggests that more sophisticated techniques, such as neutron activation analysis and nuclear magnetic resonance, may be necessary for resolution of this important question. Such studies are currently under way in several medical centers, and their results may influence current guidelines for both the extent and methods of IVF in the cancer patient.

Intermediary Metabolism

Recent controlled studies have clarified the impact of intravenous nutrition on important pathways for nutrient processing. Isotope tracer studies have suggested that the biologic effects of IVF on intermediary pathways appear to be beneficial in terms of the desired result but have raised questions as to the cost of such benefits in terms of host energy expenditure (Table 26–9).[196]

Carbohydrate Metabolism

During periods of caloric deficiency, the contribution to enhanced gluconeogenesis from products of partial glucose degradation

Table 26–9. METABOLIC RESPONSE TO INTRAVENOUS FEEDING OF STARVED, INJURED, AND TUMOR-BEARING HUMANS*

PARAMETER	STARVED	INJURED	TUMOR-BEARING
Blood glucose	↑ (177)	↑ (86)	↑ (34)
Serum insulin	↑ (177)	↑ (178)	↑ (34)
Insulin/glucose ratio	± (177)	↓ (68)	± (34)
Plasma glucagon	↓ (177)	± (68)	± (179)
Total plasma amino acids	↑ (177)	↑ (178)	↑ (179)
Urinary nitrogen excretion	↑ (177)	↑ (81)	↑ (157)
Nitrogen balance	+ (177)	+ − (81)	+ (157)
Whole-body glucose turnover rate		↑ (81)	↑ (34)
Whole-body glucose recycling %		± (81)	± (34)
Rate		↑ (81)	↑ (34)
Whole-body protein turnover	↓ (180) ↑ (221)	↑ (181)	↑ (118)
Whole-body protein synthesis	↓ (180) ± (221)	↑ (181)	↑ (118)
Whole-body protein catabolism	↓ (180, 221)	↓ (181)	↓ (118)
Gluconeogenesis from amino acids	↓ (86)	↓ (86)	↓ (34)

* ↑ = an increase; ↓ = a decrease, + = positive; − = negative; ± = no change. The numbers in parentheses indicate chapter references.

(Adapted from Brennan, M. F.: Total parenteral nutrition in the cancer patient. N. Engl. J. Med., 305:375–381, 1981.)[196]

Table 26–10. IMPACT OF INTRAVENOUS FEEDING ON CARBOHYDRATE METABOLISM

PARAMETER	BEFORE IVF (μMol/kg/min)	DURING IVF (μMol/kg/min)	CHANGE (%)	REFERENCE
Glucose turnover	15.8	33.5	+ 128	148*
	11.0	45.7	+ 415	34†
Endogenous glucose production	11.0	11.0	0	34†
Glucose oxidation rate	5.5	15.7	+ 202	148*
Cori cycle rate	6.4	3.8	− 41	148*

*Study of eight patients with various metastatic solid tumors.
†Study of 11 patients with localized esophageal cancer.

(i.e., lactate) or from carcass amino acids (i.e., alanine) represents an energy inefficiency and functionally debilitating process. In the post-traumatic setting or during episodes of sepsis, the gluconeogenic process is not readily reversed by small quantities of exogenous glucose.[86] Recent investigations of suppression of gluconeogenesis by infusion of glucose have failed to demonstrate a similarity between cancer cachexia and trauma or sepsis. In contrast to the observation of nonsuppressibility of gluconeogenesis in the trauma or sepsis setting by low-dose glucose infusion,[86] Waterhouse and associates[87] have shown (using ^{14}C alanine as the precursors) that gluconeogenesis is readily suppressed at low and high dextrose infusion rates. This observation was confirmed in esophageal cancer patients during a two-week course of IVF.[34]

The fate of infused glucose during IVF is poorly defined. The glucose turnover rate has been shown to increase during intravenous nutritional support of the cancer patient. Whole-body glucose turnover rate has been reported to increase by between 128 per cent (using ^{14}C glucose tracer)[148] and 415 per cent (using ^{3}H-glucose tracer)[34] (Table 26–10). Whether such discrepancies in turnover rate are a reflection of the tracer isotope, the clinical status of the patients, tumor histology, or composition and rate of IVF remain to be clarified.

To what extent this increased rate of glucose turnover (production and utilization) occurs in the host or the tumor is unknown. Tumor-related anerobic glycolysis may theoretically account for a portion of the increased glucose processing,[103,104] but a 41 per cent decrease in Cori cycle activity (lactate→ glucose) has been observed during IVF of patients with metastatic colorectal carcinoma.[148]

The provision of any nonprotein caloric source is intended to provide oxidative substrate for protein synthesis. Evidence to support appropriate oxidative utilization of glucose during IVF in cancer subjects is limited. During intravenous nutritional support, Holroyde and associates[148] observed a 202 per cent increase in the glucose oxidation rate. This observation suggests that the infused glucose was effectively utilized for energy-yielding metabolism, but complete oxidation could account for only 47 per cent or less of body glucose turnover. The fate of infused glucose not directly oxidized has not been established, but it most likely contributes to futile cycle activity (referred to previously) and is also converted to fat.

Protein Metabolism

Maintenance or restoration of host protein mass represents the fundamental goal in IVF of the cancer patient. Clinical studies relating the efficacy of IVF to favorably impact on the protein economy of the tumor-bearing subject are limited. Such studies have utilized whole-body isotope tracer techniques, which fail to distinguish between the protein kinetic changes occurring in the host and the tumor. Using a constant infusion of ^{15}N-glycine, Norton and co-workers[84] studied seven cachectic cancer patients with a variety of tumor types. They observed a basal (pre-IVF) state of increased protein turnover consistent with observations reported by others (Table 26–11).[88,118] In response to seven to ten day of IVF, no significant change in the rate of whole-body protein synthesis was observed but increased protein turnover was noted. The positive nitrogen balance was attributed to reduced protein catabolism, but this value was not reported. An improvement in protein synthesis, with a concomitant reduction of protein catabolism and urinary 3-methylhistidine excretion, has recently been reported to have occurred during IVF of patients with esophageal carcinoma (see Table 26–8).[118] Mullen and co-workers[176] have reported that there is no apparent stimulation of human gastrointes-

Table 26–11. IMPACT OF INTRAVENOUS FEEDING ON PROTEIN KINETICS IN NON–TUMOR-BEARING AND TUMOR-BEARING HUMANS ($\bar{X} \pm$ SEM)

	WHOLE-BODY PROTEIN KINETICS (gm of protein per kg per day)						
	Flux		Synthesis		Catabolism		
SUBJECTS	BEFORE IVF	DURING IVF	BEFORE IVF	DURING IVF	BEFORE IVF	DURING IVF	REFERENCE
Non–tumor-bearing							
Normal starved patients*	2.3 ± 0.2	2.9 ± 0.1	1.7 ± 0.2	1.7 ± 0.1	2.3 ± 0.2	1.1 ± 0.1	221
Malnourished patients†	3.3 ± 0.6	3.1 ± 0.6	2.9 ± 0.3	2.1 ± 0.4	—	—	84
Tumor-bearing							
Localized tumors‡	2.8 ± 0.4	4.0 ± 0.7	2.2 ± 0.5	2.6 ± 1.0	2.8 ± 0.6	2.4 ± 1.0	118
Localized or metastatic tumors†	5.0 ± 0.9	5.6 ± 0.5	4.3 ± 0.8	4.2 ± 0.5	—	—	84

*Group of five normal volunteers who underwent ten days of starvation followed by ten days of IVF.

†Two groups: three malnourished hospitalized patients with benign disease and seven cancer patients with localized/regional or metastatic solid tumors.

‡Group of 11 patients with esophageal cancer.

tinal malignancies when protein synthesis rates of host and tumor tissues are measured during IVF. Until host organ arteriovenous flux studies and/or *in vivo* tissue protein synthesis can demonstrate that the nontumor protein mass is repleted during IVF, the biological efficacy of IVF to restore lean tissue mass, particularly in the face of toxic antitumor therapies, remains unproven.

Lipid Metabolism

Despite the increased application and theoretic appeal of lipid as a nonprotein calorie source during IVF of cancer patients, this area has received little critical attention. Plasma free fatty acid (FFA) levels appear to decrease appropriately in cancer populations receiving glucose-based intravenous nutrition.[109] Demonstration that the decreased FFA levels are secondary to a decreased turnover rate has not been reported in these patients.

Summary

Whereas the ability of intensive nutritional support to overcome the protein catabolism present in most non–tumor-bearing populations appears certain, documentation that such a favorable response occurs in tumor-bearing patients is generally lacking. A positive nitrogen balance has been observed during IVF, and near total suppression of alanine to glucose conversion has been documented. These beneficial effects, however, do not accrue without an increase in energy

cost, especially in terms of glucose and protein turnover. The questions (1) whether current techniques of IVF in the cancer patient are optimal and (2) to what extent changes in administered substrate composition or adjuvant anabolic procedures can effectively alter the balance in favor of the host remain to be answered.

CLINICAL EFFICACY OF INTRAVENOUS FEEDING IN CANCER PATIENTS

The appropriate utilization of IVF in the cancer patient must ultimately be judged by its impact on clinical management. Early retrospective studies suggested that the weight-losing cancer subject would be more responsive to antitumor therapy if nutritional support was employed.[177-190] Although the concept that maintenance or restoration of host tissue during antitumor therapy appeared intuitively correct, there is a lack of rigorous proof to document either lean tissue restoration or altered clinical response to most antitumor therapies during IVF. There is continuing debate regarding the role of aggressive intravenous nutritional support in tumor-bearing populations.[4,191-194]

Several factors compound the current controversy regarding the appropriate role of IVF in tumor-bearing populations. When *optimal* therapeutic response rate is minimal, the expectation of a prospective clinical study to statistically document improvement in response and clinical outcome by the addition of IVF is inappropriate. The potential impli-

Table 26–12. RESULTS OF RANDOMIZED TRIALS OF INTRAVENOUS FEEDING IN CANCER PATIENTS RECEIVING RADIATION THERAPY*

TUMOR TYPE OR LOCATION†	NO. PATIENTS	LENGTH OF IVF (days)	PERCENTAGE OF PLANNED RADIATION DOSE GIVEN	MORTALITY (%)	MEDIAN SURVIVAL (WEEKS)
Ovarian carcinoma[199, 200]					
IVF	42	NR	NR	NR	39
No IVF	39	—	NR	NR	36
Pelvic carcinoma[201]					
IVF	11	NR	92	45	NR
No IVF	9	—	101	33	NR
Abdominal or pelvic tumor in a child[211]					
IVF	11	42	91	9	>12
No IVF	12	—	82	8	>12
Abdominal or pelvic tumor in a child[202]					
IVF	11‡	44	100	27§	>12
No IVF	14‡	—	100	29§	>12

*NR = not reported.
†Superscript numbers indicate chapter references.
‡14 of these patients also reported in reference 211.
§These patients expired within three to 36 months after completion of therapy; all patients survived therapy period.

cations of previous therapy or acquired malnutrition on response rates and the failure of most nutritional indices to clearly reflect a reversal of malnutrition serve only to complicate the interpretation of clinical results.

Many prospective randomized trials have been undertaken. The results of 21 prospective clinical trials have been reported in sufficient detail to allow analysis.

Radiation Therapy

The utility of adjunctive parenteral nutrition in patients undergoing radiation therapy has not been widely studied (Table 26–12). Body weight has increased during IVF in patients receiving radiation for pelvic carcinomas,[199–203] but neither delivery of the planned radiation dosage[201,203] nor survival was favorably affected by IVF.

Chemotherapy

At least 13 prospective, randomized trials of IVF and chemotherapy in patients with a variety of hematologic and solid tumors have been reported (Table 26–13). Weight was maintained during chemotherapy and IVF in several studies.[139,202–204,207, 209–213] However, no improvement in ability to deliver the planned dosage of chemother-

apy,[206,208-211,213] the infectious morbidity of therapy,[139,207] and a reduction in requirements for transfused blood products[139,206] were also noted. A single study suggested that white blood cell nadir was higher in parenterally nourished patients,[204] but this finding has not been observed by other groups.[139,206] Response to chemotherapy[139,204,205,207-213] and survival have *not* been favorably affected in IVF patients when compared with controls, and in one study, survival was significantly lower in IVF patients than in controls.[208]

Surgery

Early studies of preoperative and/or postoperative IVF in patients undergoing tumor surgery failed to demonstrate an improvement over conventional treatment with respect to postoperative death and major complication rate (Table 26–14).[214-220] These studies did observe a maintenance or increase in body weight[214,215,218] and serum albumin[216,217] and a decreased incidence of wound infection.[214,215]

Müller and associates[126] have recently documented statistically lower rates of major postoperative complications and mortality in patients with resectable gastrointestinal malignancy who received IVF for ten days preoperatively. It is of interest to note that these patients were *not* stratified for antecedent

Table 26–13. RESULTS OF RANDOMIZED TRIALS OF INTRAVENOUS FEEDING IN CANCER PATIENTS RECEIVING CHEMOTHERAPY*

TUMOR LOCATION AND/OR TYPE†	NO. PATIENTS	LENGTH OF IVF (DAYS)	PERCENTAGE OF PLANNED CHEMOTHERAPY DOSE GIVEN	PERCENTAGE OF EVALUABLE RESPONSE		WHITE BLOOD CELL COUNT NADIR ($\times 10^3$)	MORTALITY (%)	MEDIAN SURVIVAL (WEEKS)
				Complete	Partial			
Acute leukemia[203]								
IVF	11	30–70	NR	NR	NR	NR	NR	NR
No IVF	12	—	NR	NR	NR	NR	NR	NR
Diffuse lymphoma[198, 206]								
IVF	17	14–16	88	NR	NR	2.3	NR	ND
No IVF	19	—	85	NR	NR	2.0	NR	
Lung								
Adenocarcinoma[213]								
IVF	19	25	NR	0	15	1.7	11	22
No IVF	24	—	NR	11	28	1.5	4	40
Non–oat cell[205]								
IVF	14	14–19	NR	0	14	NR	NR	11
No IVF	13	—	NR	0	23	NR	NR	12
Small cell[207]								
IVF	21	42	NR	85	15	0	24	ND
No IVF	28	—	NR	59	41	0	32	
Small cell[210]								
IVF	10	NR	NR	83	NR	0.6	NR	NR
No IVF	9	—	NR	80	NR	0.8	NR	NR
Squamous[204]								
IVF	13	31	NR	0	31	2.5	NR	NR
No IVF	13	—	NR	0	8	1.5‡	NR	NR
Testis—Stage III[209]								
IVF	16	18–48	NR	63	25	0.9	NR	60
No IVF	14	—	NR	79	14	0.9	NR	60
Metastatic Bone[212]								
IVF	10	14	80	NR	NR	NR	20	NR
No IVF	10	—	55	NR	NR	NR	20	NR
Colon[208]								
IVF	20	24	NR	NR	NR	NR	NR	11
No IVF	25	—	NR	NR	NR	NR	NR	44
Sarcoma[139, 198]								
IVF	14	NR	NR	NR	NR	ND	0	NR
No IVF	18	—	NR	NR	NR		27	NR

*NR = not reported; ND = no difference between IVF and No IVF groups at time of most recent report.
†Superscript numbers indicate chapter references.
‡p <0.05 versus IVF group.

Table 26–14. RESULTS OF RANDOMIZED TRIALS OF INTRAVENOUS FEEDING IN PATIENTS UNDERGOING MAJOR SURGERY FOR MALIGNANCY*

TUMOR LOCATION†	NO. PATIENTS	DURATION OF IVF (DAYS)			POSTOPERATIVE RESULTS		
		Preoperative	Postoperative	Total	Major Complications (%)	Wound Infections (%)	Mortality (%)
Esophageal[218]							
IVF	10	5–7	None	13–14	NR	0	NR
No IVF	5	—	—	—	NR	20	NR
Esophageal/gastric[214, 218]							
IVF	38	7–10	None	7–10	NR	8	16
No IVF	36	—	—	—	NR	31‡	22
Esophageal/gastric[219]							
IVF	10	7–10	7–10	7–10	NR	NR	0
No IVF	10	—	—	—	NR	NR	10
Gastrointestinal[216, 217]							
IVF	30	2–3	10	12–13	13	NR	7
No IVF	26	—	—	—	19	NR	8
Gastrointestinal[220]							
IVF	12	5–14	Variable	5–14	17	17	0
No IVF	9	—	—	—	11	22	0
Gastrointestinal[126]							
IVF	66	10	Variable	10	17	21	5
No IVF	59	—	—	—	32‡	25	19‡

*NR = not reported.
†Superscript numbers indicate chapter references.
‡p <0.05 versus IVF group.

weight loss or evidence of malnutrition. This fact may suggest that the impact of therapy (surgery), rather than nutritional status, was the major determinant of postoperative outcome in these patients.

Implications of Clinical Trial Results

If confirmed, the observation that *preoperative* IVF is of distinct survival benefit to the patient may have major implications in the management of surgical patients.[126] Until that time, however, the routine use of preoperative IVF should be confined to patients unable to sustain lean body mass by enteral or oral feeding.

Although IVF has not been documented in the preceding studies to affect favorably either responses to therapy or survival in patients receiving radiation therapy or chemotherapy, efforts to define the role of intravenous nutritional support in the individual cancer patient are continuing. The selection for IVF of patients who are undergoing chemotherapy or radiation therapy remains a matter of clinical judgement. When therapy response rates and nutritional morbidity are high, IVF should be instituted until the host can recover from the side effects of antitumor therapy. The corollary to observations in the surgical patient that nutritional "repletion" prior to effective antitumor therapy may improve survival or morbidity represents an attractive, but unproven hypothesis.[210]

Extended Periods of IVF and Home IVF

A single study has documented longer survival in patients with untreated, widespread ovarian or gastrointestinal carcinoma who received IVF than in conventionally treated patients.[200] Whether performance status can be restored or improved in such patients, however, has not been documented. As a consequence, the utilization of prolonged periods of parenteral nutrition, particularly in the outpatient setting, cannot be *routinely* justified in the anticipation of restoring patients to a "treatable" status. The use of prolonged and/or home parenteral nutrition is indicated in those patients for whom enteral nutrition is not feasible *and* in whom antitumor therapy has clearly been successful.

In summary, there is clear evidence that in *individual* patients with cancer, IVF can prevent death from starvation and decrease the morbidity of treatment. In addition, positive effects on the intermediary metabolism of glucose and amino acids have been demonstrated. In selected patients, usually those responding to antineoplastic treatment, lean tissue mass and body strength have been restored. When heterogeneous patient groups receiving varying treatment regimens are studied in rigorous clinical trials, only those patients undergoing surgery for gastrointestinal neoplasia have benefited significantly from the addition of adjuvant IVF.

REFERENCES

1. Milder, J.W. (ed.): Nutrition and Cancer Therapy. Cancer Res., 37:2327–2471, 1977.
2. Nutrition in Cancer. Cancer, 43:1955–2161, 1979.
3. Kisner, D.L., and DeWys, W.D. (eds.): The Nutrition of the Cancer Patient. Cancer Treat. Rep., 65:(Suppl. 5):1–158, 1981.
4. Brennan, M.F., and Copeland, E.M. (eds.): Panel report on nutritional support of patients with cancer. Am. J. Clin. Nutr., 34:1199–1205, 1981.
5. DeWys, W.D. (ed.): Pediatric Cancer and Nutrition Workshop. Cancer Res. (Suppl.), 42:699s–781s, 1982.
6. Warren, S.: The immediate causes of death in cancer. Am. J. Med. Sci., 184:610–615, 1932.
7. Shils, M.E.: Principles of nutritional support. Cancer, 43:2093–2102, 1979.
8. Bistrian, B.R., Blackburn, G.L., Vitale, J., et al.: Prevalence of malnutrition in general medical patients. J.A.M.A., 235:1567–1570, 1976.
9. Bistrian, B.R., Blackburn, G.L., Hallowell, E., et al.: Protein status of general surgical patients. J.A.M.A., 230:858–860, 1974.
10. Nixon, D.W., Heymsfield, S.B., Cohen, A.E., et al.: Protein calorie undernutrition in hospitalized cancer patients. Am. J. Med., 68:683–690, 1980.
11. DeWys, W.D., Begg, C., Lavin, P.T., et al.: Prognostic effect of weight loss prior to chemotherapy in cancer patients. Am. J. Med., 69:491–497, 1980.
12. Rickard, K.A., Grosfield, J.L., Kirksey, A., et al.: Reversal of protein-energy malnutrition in children during treatment of advanced neoplastic disease. Ann. Surg., 190:771–781, 1979.
13. Rickard, K.A., Baehner, R.L., Coates, T.D., et al.: Supportive nutritional intervention in pediatric cancer. Cancer Res. (Suppl.), 42:766s–773s, 1982.
14. Sloan, G.M., Maher, M.M., and Brennan, M.F.: Nutritional effects of surgery, radiation therapy, and adjuvant chemotherapy for soft tissue sarcomas. Am. J. Clin. Nutr., 34:1094–1102, 1981.
15. Baillie, P., Millar, F.K., and Pratt, A.W.: Food and water intakes and Walker tumor growth in rats with hypothalamic lesions. Am. J. Physiol., 209:293–300, 1965.
16. Morrison, S.D.: Feeding response of tumor-bearing rats to insulin and insulin withdrawal and the contribution of autonomous tumor drain to cachectic depletion. Cancer Res., 42:3642–3647, 1982.
17. Leibowitz, S.F.: Catecholaminergic mechanisms for control of hunger. In Novin, D., Wyrwicki, W., and Bray, G. (eds.): Hunger: Basic Mechanisms and Clinical Applications. New York, Raven Press, 1976, pp. 1–18.
18. Krause, R., Humphrey, C., von Meyenfeldt, M., et al.: A central mechanism for anorexia in cancer: A hypothesis. Cancer Treat. Rep. (Suppl.), 65:15–21, 1981.
19. Mordes, J.P., and Rossini, A.A.: Tumor-induced anorexia in the Wistar rat. Science, 213:565–567, 1981.
20. DeWys, W.D.: Abnormalities of taste as a remote effect of a neoplasm. Ann. N.Y. Acad. Sci., 230:427–434, 1974.
21. DeWys, W.D., and Walters, K.: Abnormalities of taste sensation in cancer patients. Cancer, 36:1888–1896, 1975.
22. Novin, D.: Visceral mechanisms in the control of food intake. In Novin, D., Wyrwicki, W., and Bray, G. (eds.): Hunger: Basic Mechanisms and Clinical Implications. New York, Raven Press, 1976, pp. 357–367.
23. Trant, A.S., Serin, J., and Douglas, H.O.: Is taste related to anorexia in cancer patients? Am. J. Clin. Nutr., 36:45–58, 1982.
24. Mayer, J.: Glucostatic mechanism of regulation of food intake. N. Engl. J. Med., 249:13–16, 1953.
25. Mayer, J.: Regulation of energy intake and the body weight: The glucostatic theory and the lipostatic hypothesis. Ann. N.Y. Acad. Sci., 63:15–43, 1955.
26. Oomura, Y.: Significance of glucose, insulin and free fatty acids on the hypothalamic feeding and satiety neurons. In Novin, D., Myrwicki, W., and Bray, G.A. (eds.): Hunger: Basic Mechanisms and Clinical Implications. New York, Raven Press, 1975, pp. 145–157.
27. Mellinkoff, S.M., Franklin, M., Boyle, D., and Griepel, M.: Relationship between serum amino acid concentration and fluctuations in appetite. J. Appl. Physiol., 8:535–538, 1956.
28. Leung, P.M.B., and Rogers, Q.R.: Food intake regulation by plasma amino acid pattern. Life Sci., 8:1–9, 1969.
29. Gullino, P.M., Grantham, F.H., and Courtney, A.H.: Glucose consumption by transplanted tumors in vivo. Cancer Res., 27:1031–1040, 1967.
30. Norton, J.A., Burt, M.E., and Brennan, M.F.: In vivo utilization of substrate by human sarcoma-bearing limbs. Cancer, 45:2934–2939, 1980.
31. Barai, B., and DeWys, W.: Assay for presence of anorexic substance in urine of cancer patients. Proc. Am. Soc. Clin. Oncol., 21:378, 1980.
32. Marks, P.A., and Bishop, J.S.: The glucose metabolism of patients with malignant disease and of normal subjects as studied by means of an intravenous glucose tolerance test. J. Clin. Invest., 36:254–264, 1957.
33. Lundholm, K., Holm, G., and Scherstén, T.: Insulin resistance in patients with cancer. Cancer Res., 38:4665–4670, 1978.
34. Burt, M.E., Gorschboth, C., and Brennan, M.F.: A controlled, prospective randomized trial evaluating the metabolic effects of enteral and parenteral nutrition in the cancer patient. Cancer, 49:1092–1102, 1982.
35. Schein, P.S., Kisner, D., Haller, D., et al.: Cachexia of malignancy. Potential role of insulin in nutritional management. Cancer, 43:2070–2076, 1979.
36. Mider, G.B., Fenninger, L.D., Haven, F.L., et al.: The energy expenditure of rats bearing Walker carcinoma 256. Cancer Res., 11:731–736, 1951.
37. Pratt, A.W., and Putney, F.K.: Observations on the energy metabolism of rats receiving Walker

256 transplants. J. Natl. Cancer Inst., 20:173–187, 1958.

38. Waterhouse, C., Fenninger, L.D., and Keutmann, E.H.: Nitrogen exchange and caloric expenditure in patients with malignant neoplasms. Cancer, 4:500–514, 1951.

39. Warnold, I., Lundholm, K., and Scherstén, T.: Energy balance and body composition in cancer patients. Cancer Res., 38:1801–1807, 1978.

40. Bozzetti, F., Pagnoni, A.M., and DelVecchio, M.: Excessive caloric expenditure as a cause of malnutrition in patients with cancer. Surg. Gynecol. Obstet., 150:229–234, 1980.

41. Popp, M.B., Brennan, M.F., and Morrison, S.D.: Resting and activity energy expenditure during total parenteral nutrition in rats with methylcholanthrene induced sarcoma. Cancer, 49:1212–1220, 1982.

42. Arbeit, J.M., Lees, D.E., Corsey, R., and Brennan, M.F.: Determination of resting energy expenditure in patients with and without extremity sarcomas. Proc. Am. Assoc. Cancer Res. Am. Soc. Clin. Oncol., 22:194-A, 1981.

43. Knox, L.S., Crosby, L.O., Feurer, I.D., et al.: Energy expenditure in malnourished cancer patients. Ann. Surg., 197:152–162, 1983.

44. Morrison, S.D.: Partition of energy expenditure between host and tumor. Cancer Res., 31:98–107, 1971.

45. Costa, G., Bewley, P., Aragon, M., and Siebold, J.: Anorexia and weight loss in cancer patients. Cancer Treat. Rep., 65(Suppl. 5): 3–7, 1981.

46. Morrison, S.D.: Limited capacity for motor activity as a cause for declining food intake in cancer. J. Natl. Cancer. Inst., 51:1535–1539, 1973.

47. Morrison, S.D.: Control of food intake during growth of a Walker 256 carcinosarcoma. Cancer Res., 33:526–528, 1973.

48. Steinberg, J.J., Crosby, L.O., Feurer, I.D., et al.: Indirect calorimetry and cancer patients. Proc. Am. Soc. Clin. Oncol., 21:377, 1980.

49. Theologides, A.: Anorexia producing intermediary metabolites. Am. J. Clin. Nutr., 29:552–558, 1976.

50. Landsberg, L., and Young, J.B.: Fasting, feeding and regulation of the sympathetic nervous system. N. Engl. J. Med., 298:1295–1301, 1978.

51. Ramirez, A., Fletes, L., Mizraki, L., and Parra, A.: Daily urinary catecholamine profile in marasmus and kwashiorkor. Am. J. Clin. Nutr., 31:41–45, 1978.

52. Burt, M.E., Lowry, S.F., Gorschboth, C., and Brennan, M.F.: Metabolic alterations in a non-cachectic animal tumor system. Cancer, 47:2138–2146, 1981.

53. Holroyde, C.P., Gabuzda, T.G., Putnam, R.C., et al.: Altered glucose metabolism in metastatic carcinoma. Cancer Res., 35:3710–3714, 1975.

54. Stevenson, J.A.F., Box, B.M., and Wright, R.B.: The effect of a cold environment on malignant anorexia. Can. J. Biochem. Physiol., 41:531–532, 1963.

55. Strominger, J.L., and Brobeck, J.R.: A mechanism of regulation of food intake. Yale J. Biol. Med., 25:383–390, 1953.

56. Welle, S., Lilavivat, U., and Campbell, R.G.: Thermic effect of feeding in man: Increased plasma norepinephrine levels following glucose but not protein or fat consumption. Metabolism, 30:953–958, 1981.

57. Smith, J.C., and Blumsack, J.T.: Learned taste aversion as a factor in cancer therapy. Cancer Treat. Rep., 65(Suppl. 5): 37–42, 1981.

58. Bernstein, I.L., and Bernstein, I.D.: Learned food aversions and cancer anorexia. Cancer Treat. Rep., 65:(Suppl. 5):43–47, 1981.

59. DeWys, W.D.: Anorexia in cancer patients. Cancer Res., 37:2354–2358, 1977.

60. DeWys, W.D.: Pathophysiology of cancer cachexia: Current understanding and areas for future research. Cancer Res. (Suppl.), 42:721s–726s, 1982.

61. Cohn, S.H., Vartsky, D., Yasumura, S., et al.: Compartmental body composition based on total body nitrogen, potassium and calcium. Am. J. Physiol., 239:E524–530, 1980.

62. Burke, M., Bryson, E.I., Kark, A.E., et al.: Dietary intakes, resting metabolic rate, and body composition in benign and malignant gastrointestinal disease. Br. Med. J., 26:211–215, 1980.

63. Cohn, S.H., Gartenhaus, W., Sawitsky, A., et al.: Compartmental body composition of cancer patients by measurement of total body nitrogen, potassium and water. Metabolism, 30:222–229, 1980.

64. Cohn, S.H., Gartenhaus, W., Vartsky, D., et al.: Body composition and dietary intake in neoplastic disease. Am. J. Clin. Nutr., 34:1997–2004, 1981.

65. Cahill, G.F., Jr., Herrera, M.G., Morgan, A.P., et al.: Hormone-fuel interrelationships during fasting. J. Clin. Invest., 45:1751–1769, 1966.

66. Benedict, F.G.: A study of prolonged fasting. (Carnegie Institute of Washington Publication No. 203). Washington, D.C., Carnegie Institute, 1915.

67. Long, C.L., Schaffel, N., Geiger, J.W., et al.: Metabolic response to injury and illness: Estimation of energy and protein needs from indirect calorimetry and nitrogen balance. J.P.E.N., 3:462–466, 1979.

68. Meguid, M.M., Brennan, M.F., Aoki, T.T., et al.: Hormone-substrate interrelationships following trauma. Arch Surg., 109:776–783, 1974.

69. Owen, O.E., and Reichard, G.A., Jr.: Human forearm metabolism during progressive starvation. J. Clin. Invest., 50:1536–1545, 1971.

70. Harken, A.H.: Lactic acidosis. Surg. Gynecol. Obstet., 142:593–606, 1976.

71. Waterhouse, C.: Lactate metabolism in patients with cancer. Cancer, 33:66–71, 1974.

72. Marliss, E.B., Aoki, T.T., Unger, R.H., et al.: Glucagon levels and metabolic effects in fasting man. J. Clin. Invest., 49:2256–2270, 1970.

73. Brennan, M.F.: Nutritional support of the patient with cancer. In DeVita, V., Hellman, S., and Rosenberg, S.A. (eds.): Principles and Practice of Oncology. Philadelphia, J.B. Lippincott, 1985, pp. 1907–1915.

74. Felig, P., Owen, O.E., Wahren, J., and Cahill, G.F., Jr.: Amino acid metabolism during prolonged starvation. J. Clin. Invest., 48:584–594, 1969.

75. Dahn, M., Kirkpatrick, J.R., and Bouwman, D.: Sepsis, glucose intolerance, and protein malnutrition: A metabolic paradox. Arch. Surg., 115:1415–1418, 1980.

76. Rudman, D., Vogler, W.R., Howard, C.H., et al.: Observations on the plasma amino acids of patients with acute leukemia. Cancer Res., 31:1159–1165, 1971.

77. Moore, F.D.: Metabolic Care of the Surgical Patient. Philadelphia, W.B. Saunders, 1959.

78. Mider, G.B.: Some aspects of nitrogen and energy metabolism in cancerous subjects: A review. Cancer Res., 11:821–829, 1951.

79. Streja, D.A., Steiner, G., Marliss, E.B., and Vranic, M.: Turnover and recycling of glucose in man during prolonged fasting. Metabolism, 26:1089–1098, 1977.

80. Wolfe, R.R., Durkot, M.D., Allsop, J.R., et al.: Glucose metabolism in severely burned patients. Metabolism, 28:1031–1039, 1979.

81. Wilmore, D.W., Aulick, H.L., and Goodwin, C.W.: Glucose metabolism following severe injury. Acta Chir. Scand.(Suppl.), 498:43–47, 1980.

82. Winterer, J., Bistrian, B.R., Bilmazes, C., et al.: Whole body protein turnover, studied with ^{15}N-glycine, and muscle protein breakdown in mildly obese subjects during a protein-sparing diet and a brief total fast. Metabolism, 29:575–581, 1980.

83. Birkhahn, R.H., Long, C.L., Fitkin, D., et al.: Effects of major skeletal trauma on whole body protein turnover in man measured by L-[1,^{14}C]-leucine. Surgery, 88:294–300, 1980.

84. Norton, J.A., Stein, T.P., and Brennan, M.F.: Whole body protein turnover studies in normal humans and malnourished patients with and without cancer. Ann. Surg., 31:94–96, 1980.

85. Felig, P., Pozefsky, T., Maliss, E., and Cahill, G.F., Jr.: Alanine: Key role in gluconeogenesis. Science, 167:1003–1004, 1970.

86. Long, C.L., Kinney, J.M., and Geiger, J.W.: Non-suppressibility of gluconeogenesis by glucose in septic patients. Metabolism, 25:193–201, 1976.

87. Waterhouse, C., Jeanpetre, N., and Keilson, J.: Gluconeogenesis from alanine in patients with progressive malignant disease. Cancer Res., 39:1968–1972, 1979.

88. Heber, D., Chlebowski, R.T., Ishibashi, D.E., et al.: Abnormalities in glucose and protein metabolism in noncachectic lung cancer patients. Cancer Res., 42:4815–4819, 1982.

89. Karlberg, I., Edstrom, S., Ekman, L., et al.: Metabolic host reaction in response to the proliferation of non-malignant cells versus malignant cells in vivo.. Cancer Res., 41:4154–4161, 1981.

90. Clowes, G.H.A., Jr., Randall, H.T., and Cha, C-J.: Amino acid and energy metabolism in septic and traumatized patients. J.P.E.N., 4:195–203, 1980.

91. Jasani, B., Donaldson, L.J., Ratcliff, J.G., et al.: Mechanism of impaired glucose tolerance in patients with neoplasia. Br. J. Cancer, 38:287–292, 1978.

92. Marks, P.A., and Bishop, J.S.: Studies on carbohydrate metabolism in patients with neoplastic disease. II: Response to insulin administration. J. Clin. Invest., 38:668–672, 1959.

93. Genuth, S.M.: Effects of prolonged fasting on insulin secretion. Diabetes, 15:798–806, 1966.

94. Cahill, G.F., Jr., Herrera, M.G., Morgan, A.P., et al.: Hormone fuel interrelationships during fasting. J. Clin. Invest., 45:1751–1769, 1966.

95. Lipman, R.L., Schnure, J.J., Bradley, E.M., et al.: Impairment of peripheral glucose utilization in normal subjects by prolonged bed rest. J. Lab. Clin. Med., 8:221–223, 1970.

96. Lipman, R.L., Raskin, P., Love, T., et al.: Glucose intolerance during decreased physical activity in man. Diabetes, 21:101–107, 1972.

97. Gump, F.E., Long, C.L., Killian, P., et al.: Studies of glucose intolerance in septic injured patients. J. Trauma, 14:378–388, 1974.

98. Smith, S.R., Edgar, P.J., Pozefsky, T., et al.: Insulin secretion and glucose tolerance in adults with protein-calorie malnutrition. Metabolism, 24:1073–1084, 1975.

99. Lundholm, K., Bylund, A-C., and Scherstén, T.: Glucose tolerance in relation to skeletal muscle enzyme activities in cancer patients. Scand. J. Clin. Lab. Invest., 37:267–272, 1977.

100. Lundholm, K., Edstrom, S., Ekman, L., et al.: A comparative study of the influence of malignant tumor on host metabolism in mice and man. Cancer, 42:453–461, 1978.

101. Bylund, A-C., Holm, G., Lundholm, K., et al.: Incorporation rate of glucose carbons, palmitate carbon and leucine carbon into metabolites in relation to enzyme activities and RNA levels in human skeletal muscles. Enzyme, 21:39–52, 1976.

102. Lundholm, K., Edstrom, S., Karlbert, I., et al.: Glucose turnover, gluconeogenesis from glycerol and estimation of net glucose cycling in cancer patients. Cancer 50:1142–1150, 1982.

103. Holroyde, C.P., Axelrod, R.S., Skutches, C.L., et al.: Lactate metabolism in patients with metastatic colorectal cancer. Cancer Res., 39:4900–4904, 1979.

104. Waterhouse, C.: Lactate metabolism in patients with cancer. Cancer, 33:66–71, 1974.

105. Spector, A.A., and Steinberg, D.: The utilization of unesterified palmitate by Ehrlich ascites tumor cells. J. Biol. Chem., 240:3747–3753, 1965.

106. Reshef, L., Hanson, R.W., and Bollard, E.J.: A possible physiological role for glycerol neogenesis in rat adipose tissue. J. Biol. Chem., 245:5979–5984, 1970.

107. Owen, O.E., Morgan, A.P., Kemp, H.G., et al.: Brain metabolism during fasting. J. Clin. Invest., 46:1589–1595, 1967.

108. Cahill, G.F., Jr.: Starvation in man. N. Engl. J. Med., 282:668–675, 1970.

109. Waterhouse, C., and Kemperman, J.H.: Carbohydrate metabolism in subjects with cancer. Cancer Res., 31:1273–1278, 1971.

110. Terepka, A.R., and Waterhouse, C.: Metabolic observations during the forced feeding of patients with cancer. Am. J. Med., 20:225–238, 1956.

111. Pareira, M.D., Conrad, E.J., Hicks, W., and Elman, R.: Clinical response and changes in nitrogen balance, body weight, plasma proteins, and hemoglobin following tube feeding in cancer cachexia. Cancer, 8:803–808, 1955.

112. Peden, J.C., Jr., Bond, L.F., and Maxwell, M.: Comparative protein repletion in cancer and non-cancer cachexia with special reference to changes in blood volume and total circulating plasma protein and hemoglobin. Am. J. Clin. Nutr., 5:305–315, 1957.

113. Lundholm, K., Bylund, A-C., Holm, G., and Scherstén, T.: Skeletal muscle metabolism in patients with malignant tumor. Eur. J. Cancer, 12:465–478, 1976.

114. Clarke, E.F., Lewis, A.M., and Waterhouse, C.: Peripheral amino acid levels in patients with cancer. Cancer, 42:2909–2913, 1978.

115. Bennegård, K., Edén, E., Ekman, L., et al.: Metabolic balance across the leg in weight-losing cancer patients compared to depleted patients without cancer. Cancer Res., 42:4293–4299, 1982.

116. Rudman, D., and Chawla, R.K.: A new system of cancer related antigens: Biochemical properties and clinical applications. Clin. Res., 25:525A, 1977.

117. Waterhouse, C.: Gammaglobulin production and

light-chain metabolism in patients with metastatic cancer. Cancer Res., 35:987–990, 1975.

118. Burt, M.E., Stein, T.P., and Brennan, M.F.: A controlled randomized trial evaluating the effects of enteral and parenteral nutrition on protein metabolism in cancer-bearing man. J. Surg. Res., 34:303–314, 1983.

119. Zaren, H., and Lerner, H.: Review of 100 consecutive total parenteral nutritional support patients on an oncology unit. Proc. Am. Soc. Clin. Oncol., 23:C-228, 1982.

120. Jeffers, S.L., and Mequid, M.M.: Use of total parenteral nutrition in terminally ill oncology patients. Clin. Res., 30:245A, 1982.

121. Hill, G.L., Pickford, I., Young, G.A., et al.: Malnutrition in surgical patients. An unrecognized problem. Lancet, 1:689–691, 1977.

122. Weinsier, R.L., Hunker, E.M., Krundiek, C.L., and Butterworth, C.E., Jr.: Hospital malnutrition: A prospective evaluation of general medical patients during the course of hospitalization. Am. J. Clin. Nutr., 32:418–426, 1979.

123. Grant, J.P., Custer, P.B., and Thurlow, J.: Current techniques of nutritional assessment. Surg. Clin. North Am., 61:437–463, 1981.

124. Conti, S., West, J.P., and Fitzpatrick, H.D.: Mortality and morbidity after esophagogastrectomy for cancer of the esophagus and cardia. Am. J. Surg., 43:92–96, 1977.

125. Hickman, D.M., Miller, R.A., Rombeau, J.L., et al.: Serum albumin and body weight as predictors of post-operative course in colorectal cancer. J.P.E.N., 4:314–316, 1980.

126. Müller, J.M., Dienst, C., Brenner, U., and Pichlmaier, H.: Preoperative parenteral feeding in patients with gastrointestinal carcinoma. Lancet, 1:68–71, 1982.

127. Buzby, G.P., Mullen, J.L., Matthews, D.C., et al.: Prognostic nutritional index in gastrointestinal surgery. Am. J. Surg., 139:160–167, 1980.

128. Mullen, J.L., Buzby, G.P., Matthews, D.C., et al.: Reduction of operative morbidity and mortality by combined pre-operative and post-operative nutritional support. Ann. Surg., 192:604–613, 1980.

129. Shizgal, H.M., and Forse, R.A.: Protein and calorie requirements with total parenteral nutrition. Ann. Surg., 192:132–139, 1980.

130. Dickinson, R.J., Ashton, M.G., Axon, A.T.R., et al.: Controlled trial of intravenous hyperalimentation and total bowel rest as an adjunct to the routine therapy of acute colitis. Gastroenterology, 79:1199–1204, 1980.

131. Lamb, D., Pilney, F., Kelly, W.D., et al.: A comparative study of the incidence of anergy in patients with carcinoma, leukemia, Hodgkin's disease and other lymphomas. J. Immunol., 89:555–558, 1962.

132. Bolducci, L., Little, D.D., Glover, N.S., et al.: Granulocyte reserve in cancer and malnutrition. Clin. Res., 30:243A, 1982.

133. Benotti, P.N., Bothe, A., Jr., Miller, J.D.B., and Blackburn, G.L.: Safe cannulation of the internal jugular vein for long term hyperalimentation. Surg. Gynecol. Obstet., 144:574–576, 1977.

134. Frye, D., Buzdar, A., Hortobagyi, G.N., et al.: Complications of prolonged control venous catheter use in treatment of metastatic breast cancer. Am. Soc. Clin. Oncol., 22:C-223, 1982.

135. Raaf, J.H.: Two Broviac catheters for intensive long-

136. Linos, D.A., and Mucha, P.: A simplified technique for the placement of permanent control venous catheters. Surg. Gynecol. Obstet., 154:248–249, 1982.

137. Mullen, J.L.: Complications of total parenteral nutrition in the cancer patient. Cancer Treat. Rep., 65(Suppl. 5):107–113, 1981.

138. Maher, M.M., Henderson, D.K., and Brennan, M.F.: Central venous catheter exchange in cancer patients during total parenteral nutrition. Nat. Intrav. Ther. Assoc., 5:54–60, 1982.

139. Shamberger, R.C., Pizzo, P.A., Goodgame, J.T., Jr., et al.: The effect of total parenteral nutrition on chemotherapy induced myelosuppression. Am. J. Med., 74:40–48, 1983.

140. Burt, M.E., Dunnick, N.R., Krudy, A.G., et al.: Prospective evaluation of subclavian vein thrombosis during total parenteral nutrition by contrast venography. Clin. Res., 29:264A, 1981.

141. Fabri, P.J., Mirtallo, J.M., Ruberg, R.L., et al.: Incidence and prevention of thrombosis of the subclavian vein during total parenteral nutrition. Surg. Gynecol. Obstet., 155:238–240, 1982.

142. Brismar, B., Hordstedt, C., Jacobson, S., et al.: Reduction of catheter-associated thrombosis in parenteral nutrition by intravenous heparin therapy. Arch. Surg., 117:1196–1199, 1982.

143. Welch, G.W., McKeel, D.W., Silverstein, P., and Walker, H.L.: The role of catheter composition in the development of thrombophlebitis. Surg. Gynecol. Obstet., 138:421–426, 1974.

144. Rudman, D., Millikan, W.J., Richardson, T.J., et al.: Elemental balances during intravenous hyperalimentation of underweight adult subjects. J. Clin. Invest., 55:94–104, 1975.

145. Jeejeebhoy, K.N., Anderson, G.H., Nakhooda, A.F., et al.: Metabolic studies in total parenteral nutrition with lipid in man. Comparison with glucose. J. Clin. Invest., 57:125–136, 1976.

146. Nixon, D.W., Lawson, D.H., Kutner, M., et al.: Hyperalimentation of the cancer patient with protein-calorie undernutrition. Cancer Res., 41:2038–2045, 1981.

147. Askanazi, J., Carpentier, Y.A., Elwyn, D.H., et al.: Influence of total parenteral nutrition on fuel utilization in injury and sepsis. Ann. Surg., 119:40–46, 1980.

148. Holroyde, C.P., Myers, R.N., Smink, R.D., et al.: Metabolic response to total parenteral nutrition in cancer patients. Cancer Res., 37:3109–3114, 1977.

149. Wolfe, R.R., O'Donnell, T.F., Jr., Stone, M.D., et al.: Investigation of factors determining the optimal glucose infusion rate in total parenteral nutrition. Metabolism, 29:892–900, 1980.

150. Popp, M.B., Morrison, S.D., and Brennan, M.F.: Total parenteral nutrition in a methylcholanthrene-induced rat sarcoma model. Cancer Treat. Rep., 65(Suppl. 5):137–143, 1981.

151. Goodgame, J.T., Jr., Lowry, S.F., and Brennan, M.F.: Nutritional manipulations and tumor growth. II: The effects of intravenous feeding. Am. J. Clin. Nutr., 32:2285–2294, 1979.

152. Cameron, I.L., and Pavlat, W.A.: Stimulation of growth of a transplantable hepatoma in rats by parenteral nutrition. J. Natl. Cancer Inst., 56:597–602, 1976.

153. Daly, J.M., Copeland, E.M., and Dudrick, S.J.:

Effects of intravenous nutrition on tumor growth and host immunocompetence in malnourished animals. Surgery, *84*:655–658, 1978.

154. Cameron, I.L.: Effect of total parenteral nutrition responses in rats. Cancer Treat. Rep., *65*(Suppl. 5):93–99, 1981.

155. Buzby, G.P., Mullen, J.L., Stein, T.P., et al.: Host-tumor interaction and nutrient supply. Cancer, *45*:2940–2948, 1980.

156. Lowry, S.F., and Brennan, M.F.: Abnormal liver function during parenteral nutrition: Relation to infusion excess. J. Surg. Res., *26*:300–307, 1979.

157. Brennan, M.F., and Burt, M.E.: Nitrogen metabolism in cancer patients. Cancer Treat. Rep., *65*(Suppl. 5):67–78, 1981.

158. Daly, J.M., Mihranian, M.H., Kehoe, J.E., et al.: Effects of postoperative infusion of branched chain amino acids on nitrogen balance and forearm muscle substrate flux. Surgery, *94*:151–158, 1983.

159. Mazuski, J., Blanc, P., Wolf, W., et al.: Nitrogen retention is proportionate to branched chain load, with no effect on proteolysis. Presented at Assoc. for Academic Surgery, 1983.

160. Blackburn, G.L., Maim, B.S., Bistrain, B.R., et al.: The effect of cancer on nitrogen, electrolyte, and mineral metabolism. Cancer Res., *37*:2348–2353, 1977.

161. Sloan, G.M., White, D.E., and Brennan, M.F.: Calcium and phosphorous metabolism during total parenteral nutrition. Ann. Surg., *197*:1–6, 1983.

162. Lowry, S.F., Goodgame, J.T., Jr., Maher, M.M., and Brennan, M.F.: Parenteral vitamin requirements during intravenous feeding. Am. J. Clin. Nutr., *31*:2149–2158, 1978.

163. Kirkemo, A.K., Burt, M.E., and Brennan, M.F.: Serum vitamin level maintenance in cancer patients on total parenteral nutrition. Am. J. Clin. Nutr., *35*:1003–1009, 1982.

164. Burt, M.E., Hanin, I., and Brennan, M.F.: Choline deficiency associated with total parenteral nutrition. Lancet, *2*:638–639, 1980.

165. Peters, M.L., Maher, M.M., and Brennan, M.F.: Minimal IV iron requirements in TPN. J.P.E.N., *4*:601, 1980.

166. Stead, N.W., Curtas, M.S., and Grant, J.P.: Enhanced mobilization of iron from body stores in malnourished patients during intravenous nutritional support. Surg. Gynecol. Obstet., *154*:321–325, 1982.

167. Lowry, S.F., Goodgame, J.T., Jr., Smith, J.C., et al.: Abnormalities of zinc and copper during total parenteral nutrition. Ann. Surg., *189*:120–128, 1979.

168. Lowry, S.F., Smith, J.C., and Brennan, M.F.: Zinc and copper replacement during total parenteral nutrition. Am. J. Clin. Nutr., *34*:1853–1860, 1981.

169. Wolman, S.L., Anderson, G.H., Marliss, E.B., et al.: Zinc in total parenteral nutrition: Requirements and metabolic effects. Gastroenterology, *76*:458–467, 1979.

170. Batist, G., Katki, A., Norton, J., et al.: Sequential selenium dependent enzyme activity in patients on long term parenteral nutrition. J.P.E.N., *6*:575, 1982.

171. Barr, L.H., Dunn, G.D., and Brennan, M.F.: Essential fatty acid deficiency during total parenteral nutrition. Ann. Surg., *193*:304–311, 1980.

172. Goodgame, J.T., Jr., Lowry, S.F., and Brennan, M.F.: Essential fatty acid deficiency in total par-

enteral nutrition: Time course of development and suggestions for therapy. Surgery, *84*: 271–277, 1978.

173. Nordenstrom, J., Askanazi, J., Elwyn, D.H., et al.: Nitrogen balance during total parenteral nutrition. Glucose vs. fat. Ann. Surg., *197*:27–33, 1983.

174. Steiger, E., Oram-Smith, J.C., Miller, E., et al.: Effects of nutrition on tumor growth and tolerance to chemotherapy. J. Surg. Res., *18*:146–468, 1975.

175. Popp, M.B., Wagner, S.F., and Brito, O.J.: Host and tumor responses to increasing levels of intravenous nutritional support. Surgery, *94*: 300–308, 1983.

176. Mullen, J.L., Buzby, G.P., Gertner, M.H., et al.: Protein synthesis dynamics in human gastrointestinal malignancies. Surgery, *87*:331–338, 1980.

177. Wolfe, B.M., Culebras, J.M., Sim, A.J.W., et al.: Substrate interaction in intravenous feeding: Comparative effects of carbohydrate and fat on amino acid utilization in fasting man. Ann. Surg., *186*:518–540, 1977.

178. Dale, G., Young, G., Latner, A.L., et al.: The effect of surgical operation on venous plasma free amino acids. Surgery, *81*:295–301, 1977.

179. Waterhouse, C., Clarke, E.F., Heinig, R.E., et al.: Free amino acid levels in the blood of patients undergoing parenteral alimentation. Am. J. Clin. Nutr., *32*:2423–2429, 1979.

180. Sim, A.J.W., Wolfe, B.M., Young, V.R., et al.: Glucose promotes whole body protein synthesis from infused amino acids in fasting man: Isotopic demonstration. Lancet, *1*:68–72, 1979.

181. Herrmann, V.W., Clarke, D., Wilmore, D.W., and Moore, F.D.: Protein metabolism: Effect of disease and altered intake on the stable ^{15}N curve. Surg. Forum, *31*:92–94, 1980.

182. Copeland, E.M., III, MacFayden, B.V., Jr., Lanzotti, V.J., et al.: Intravenous hyperalimentation as an adjunct to cancer chemotherapy. Am. J. Surg., *129*:167–173, 1975.

183. Schwartz, G.F., Green, H.L., Bendon, M.L., et al.: Combined parenteral hyperalimentation and chemotherapy in the treatment of disseminated solid tumors. Am. J. Surg., *121*:169–173, 1971.

184. Ford, J.H., Jr., Dudan, R.C., Bennet, J.S., et al.: Parenteral hyperalimentation in gynecologic oncology patients. Gynecol. Oncol., *1*:70–75, 1972.

185. Dematteis, R., and Hermann, R.E.: Supplementary parenteral nutrition in patients with malignant disease. Guidelines to patient selection. Cleve. Clin., *40*:139–145, 1973.

186. Assa, J., Schramek, A., Barzilai, A., et al.: Intravenous hyperalimentation for the onco-surgical patient. J. Surg. Oncol., *1*:239–244, 1974.

187. Copeland, E.M., MacFayden, B.V., Jr., and Dudrick, S.J.: Intravenous hyperalimentation in cancer patients. J. Surg. Res., *16*:241–247, 1974.

188. Copeland, E.M., MacFayden, B.V., Jr., MacComb, W.S., et al.: Intravenous hyperalimentation in patients with head and neck cancer. Cancer, *35*:606–611, 1975.

189. Lanzotti, V.J., Copeland, E.M., III, George, S.L., et al.: Cancer chemotherapeutic response and intravenous hyperalimentation. Cancer Chemother. Rep., *59*:437–439, 1975.

190. Copeland, E.M., MacFayden, B.V., Jr., and Dudrick, S.J.: Effect of intravenous hyperalimentation on established delayed hypersensitivity in the cancer patient. Ann. Surg., *184*:60–64, 1976.

191. Copeland, E.M., Souchon, E.A., MacFayden, B.V.,

Jr., et al.: Intravenous hyperalimentation as an adjunct to radiation therapy. Cancer, *39*:609–616, 1977.

192. Filler, R.M., Jaffe, N., Cassady, J.R., et al.: Parenteral nutritional support in children with cancer. Cancer, *39*:2665–2669, 1977.

193. Frazier, T.G., Copeland, E.M., Khalil, K.G., et al.: Intravenous hyperalimentation as an adjunct to colon interposition for carcinoma of the esophagus. Cancer, *39*:410–412, 1977.

194. Ruberg, R.L.: Intravenous hyperalimentation in head and neck tumour surgery: Indications and precautions. Br. J. Plast. Surg., *30*:151–153, 1977.

195. Deitel, M., Vasic, V., and Alexander, M.A.: Specialized nutritional support in the cancer patient: Is it worthwhile? Cancer, *41*:2359–2363, 1978.

196. Brennan, M.F.: Total parenteral nutrition in the cancer patient. N. Engl. J. Med., *305*:375–382, 1981.

197. Copeland, E.M.: Intravenous hyperalimentation and chemotherapy: An update. J.P.E.N., *6*:236–239, 1982.

198. Levine, A.S., Brennan, M.F., Ramu, A., et al.: Controlled clinical trials of nutritional intervention as an adjunct to chemotherapy, with a comment on nutrition and drug resistance. Cancer Res., *42*:774s–778s, 1982.

199. Solassol, C., and Joyeux, H.: Artificial gut with complete nutritive mixtures as a major adjuvant therapy in cancer patients. Arch Chir. Scand. (Suppl.), *494*:186–187, 1979.

200. Solassol, C., Joyeux, H., and Dubois, J.B.: Total parenteral nutrition (TPN) with complete nutritive mixtures: An artificial gut in cancer patients. Nutr. Cancer, *1*:13–18, 1979.

201. Valerio, D., Overett, L., Malcolm, A., et al.: Nutritive support for cancer patients receiving abdominal and pelvic radiotherapy: A randomized prospective clinical experiment of intravenous versus oral feeding. Surg. Forum, *29*:145–148, 1978.

202. Ghavimi, F., Shils, M.E., Scott, B.F., et al.: Comparison of morbidity in children requiring abdominal radiation and chemotherapy, with and without total parenteral nutrition. J. Pediatr., *101*:530–537, 1982.

203. Coquin, J.Y., Maraninchi, D., Gastaut, J.A., et al.: Parenteral nutrition in chemotherapy of acute leukemias: preliminary results. J.P.E.N., *4*:437, 1980.

204. Issell, B.F., Valdivieso, M., Zaren, H.A., et al.: Protection against chemotherapy toxicity by IV hyperalimentation. Cancer Treat. Rep., *62*: 1139–1143, 1978.

205. Lanzotti, V., Copeland, E.M., Bhuchar, V., et al.: A randomized trial of total parenteral nutrition (TPN) with chemotherapy for non–oat cell lung cancer (NOCLC). Proc. Am. Soc. Clin. Oncol., *21*:377, 1980.

206. Popp, M.B., Fisher, R.I., Simon, R.M., et al.: A prospective randomized study of adjuvant parenteral nutrition in the treatment of diffuse lymphoma. I: Effect on drug tolerance. Cancer Treat. Rep., *65*(Suppl. 5):129–135, 1981.

207. Valdivieso, M., Bodey, G.P., Benjamin, R.S., et al.: Role of intravenous hyperalimentation as an adjunct to intensive chemotherapy for small cell bronchogenic carcinoma: Preliminary observa-

tions. Cancer Treat. Rep., *65*(Suppl. 5):145–150, 1981.

208. Nixon, D.W., Moffitt, S., Lawson, D.H., et al.: Total parenteral nutrition as an adjunct to chemotherapy of metastatic colorectal cancer. Cancer Treat. Rep., *65*(Suppl. 5):121–128, 1981.

209. Samuels, M.L., Selig, D.E., Ogden, S., et al.: IV hyperalimentation and chemotherapy for state III testicular cancer: A randomized study. Cancer Treat. Rep., *65*:615–627, 1981.

210. Serrou, B., Cupissol, D., Plagne, R., et al.: Parenteral intravenous nutrition as an adjunct to chemotherapy in small cell anaplastic lung carcinoma. Cancer Treat. Rep., *65*(Suppl. 5):151–155, 1981.

211. Donaldson, S.S., Wesley, M.N., Ghavimi, F., et al.: A prospective randomized clinical trial of total parenteral nutrition in children with cancer. Med. Pediatr. Oncol., *10*:129–139, 1982.

212. van Eys, J., Copeland, E.M., Cangir, A., et al.: A clinical trial of hyperalimentation in children with metastatic malignancies. Med. Pediatr. Oncol., *8*:63–73, 1980.

213. Jordan, W.M., Valdivieso, M., Frankman, C., et al.: Treatment of advanced adenocarcinoma of the lung with Ftorofur, Doxorubicin, cyclophosphamide, and Cisplatin and intensive IV hyperalimentation. Cancer Treat. Rep., *65*:197–205, 1981.

214. Williams, R.H.P., Heatley, R.V., and Lewis, M.H.: A randomized controlled trial of preoperative intravenous nutrition in patients with stomach cancer. Br. J. Surg., *63*:667, 1976.

215. Heatley, R.V., Williams, R.H.P., and Lewis, M.H.: Preoperative intravenous feeding—a controlled trial. Postgrad. Med. J., *55*:541–545, 1979.

216. Holter, A.R., Rosen, H.M., and Fischer, J.E.: The effects of hyperalimentation on major surgery in patients with malignant disease: A prospective study. Acta Chir. Scand.(Suppl.), *466*:86–87, 1976.

217. Holter, A.R., and Fischer, J.E.: The effects of perioperative hyperalimentation on complications in patients with carcinoma and weight loss. J. Surg. Res., *23*:31–34, 1977.

218. Moghissi, K., Hornshaw, J., Teasdale, P.R., et al.: Parenteral nutrition in carcinoma of the esophagus treated by surgery: Nitrogen balance and clinical studies. Br. J. Surg., *64*:125–128, 1977.

219. Simms, J.M., Oliver, E., and Smith, J.A.R.: A study of total parenteral nutrition (TPN) in major gastric and esophageal resection for neoplasia. J.P.E.N., *4*:422, 1980.

220. Thompson, B.R., Julian, T.B., and Stremple, J.F.: Perioperative total parenteral nutrition in patients with gastrointestinal cancer. J. Surg. Res., *30*:497–500, 1981.

221. Rose, D., Horowitz, G. D., Jeevanandam, M., et al.: Whole-body protein kinetics during acute starvation and intravenous refeeding in normal man. Fed. Proc. *42*:1070, 1983.

222. Arbeit, J.M., et al.: Abstract presented at Association for Academic Surgery, 15th Annual Meeting, Chicago, 1981.

223. Horowitz, G.D., et al.: Unpublished observations.

224. Carmichael, M.J., Clague, M.B., Keir, M.J., et al.: Whole body protein turnover synthesis and breakdown in patients with colorectal carcinoma. Br. J. Surg., *67*:736–739, 1980.

CHAPTER 27

Parenteral Nutrition and Trauma

PALMER Q. BESSEY

Trauma is a major health problem in industrialized society. Some 160,000 individuals die each year in the United States as the result of injuries.[1] Trauma is the leading cause of death for persons from one to 44 years of age and the third leading cause of death for persons of all ages, following cardiovascular diseases and cancer. However, because trauma affects young people disproportionately, it claims as many years of productive life (under age 65) as cardiovascular diseases and cancer combined.[2] Trauma also maims and cripples. For every person who dies following injury, two are permanently disabled. The financial cost to society, including acute and chronic care, lost productivity, and property damage, has been estimated to be some $63 billion annually.

Approximately one-half of the deaths due to trauma occur within one hour of injury.[3, 4] These are usually due to severe lacerations of the brain or great vessels. Occasionally, patients survive these injuries if they receive almost immediate definitive care. However, such occurrences are usually limited to urban settings with well-developed pre-hospital services and designated and dedicated trauma centers. Under those conditions, as many as 20 per cent of patients who arrive in the emergency department with only minimal signs of life may leave the hospital alive and neurologically intact.[5] Another 30 per cent of trauma deaths occur within three or four hours of injury. These are generally due to ongoing hemorrhage and brain injuries. Patients with these injuries also benefit from a well-developed regional trauma care system in which the most severely injured patients are quickly identified and transported to a dedicated trauma center for definitive care. The remaining proportion of deaths occur several days or weeks after injury and early care. The patients often die with multiple organ system failure and sepsis. The mechanisms involved in the development of this syndrome are poorly understood, but they are related at least temporally to the body's responses to injury.

The care of injured patients has improved over the past decade. Those communities that have developed organized, regional trauma care systems have witnessed a marked improvement in early results.[6] Long-term survival of critically ill and injured patients has also improved.[7, 8] Some of the responsible factors may include the proliferation of critical care units and improved techniques of hemodynamic monitoring and ventilatory support. Thus, precise and effective management of shock, fluid and electrolyte balance, and respiratory failure is commonly possible. In addition, techniques of parenteral nutrition have been perfected over the last 15 years, so that aggressive nutritional support also plays a major role in the comprehensive care of the injured or critically ill patient.

The purpose of this chapter is to present a general approach to the nutritional support of injured and critically ill patients and to indicate the important role that parenteral nutrition plays. The approach is based on our current understanding of several characteristic and predictable biochemical and physiologic alterations that occur in patients following injury, and that are known collectively as the metabolic response to injury. Some aspects of this response are discussed in more detail in Chapter 28.

THE METABOLIC RESPONSE TO INJURY

Injury results in profound metabolic alterations, beginning at the time of injury and persisting until wound healing and recovery are complete, some several months or years later.

Time Course—Ebb and Flow

Sir David Cuthbertson,[9] a Scottish biochemist, was one of the first to study the response to injury in a systematic way. In addition to characterizing many of the features of the response, he described its evolution over time. The early phase of the response, characterized by decreased oxygen consumption, lowered body temperature, and vasoconstriction, Cuthbertson called the "ebb" phase.[10] It lasts usually 24 to 36 hours and, after successful resuscitation, gives way to a "flow" phase, characterized by increased metabolic rate and body temperature and accelerated nitrogen loss. Francis Moore[11] further described the temporal characteristics of convalescence. He described an "injury phase," corresponding to both the ebb and the flow phases of Cuthbertson. The injury phase ends rather abruptly, and a "turning point" can be observed clinically. The patient definitely feels and appears improved and begins to take an interest in his or her surroundings. This is an important development following operation or injury, because it generally heralds the end of a period of intense metabolic activity and the beginning of a period of net anabolism during which lean body mass is replenished. Finally, a long period of gradual fat gain completes the period of convalescence.

The major therapeutic concern during the ebb phase of the injury response is the support and stabilization of the patient's pulmonary and cardiovascular function. Metabolic and nutritional supports become important therapeutic considerations during the flow phase, when metabolic activity is most intense. Spontaneous nutritional intake is usually adequate thereafter to meet the patient's nutritional requirements. Understanding of the metabolic response to injury in the flow phase is fundamental to any plan of nutritional support of injured patients. The major characteristics of that response include hypermetabolism, elevated body temperature, accelerated protein breakdown and nitrogen loss, and alterations in amino acid and carbohydrate metabolism.

Hypermetabolism

The metabolic rate is a measure of heat loss from the body. Conversion of potential energy into useful work in biologic systems is an inherently inefficient process associated with a partial loss of energy as heat. Thus, the metabolic rate can be considered to reflect overall physiochemical or metabolic activity. In humans and animals, all energy ultimately comes from the oxidation of organic fuels. Thus, heat loss is related to the consumption of oxygen and the production of carbon dioxide. Metabolic rate can be determined directly by measuring the amount of heat lost from a subject over time (direct calorimetry) or it can be calculated from measurements of oxygen consumption and carbon dioxide production (indirect calorimetry). Metabolic rates determined by both techniques under basal conditions are comparable.[12] Indirect methods require less elaborate equipment than direct methods and have been more widely utilized in the evaluation of critically ill patients. The relationship between metabolic rate (MR), oxygen consumption ($\dot{V}O_2$), and carbon dioxide production ($\dot{V}CO_2$) is given by the equation below.[13]

If the metabolic rate of a normal subject is determined under "basal" conditions—in the early morning after a 10- to 12-hour fast in a semi-darkened, quiet, thermoneutral environment, when the subject is rested, reclining, comfortable, calm, and familiar with the apparatus—the value is known as the basal metabolic rate (BMR). This value is reproducible and also predictable within $\pm$ 12 per cent[14] on the basis of age, sex, and body size. If the metabolic rate of an injured patient is determined under basal conditions, it will generally be greater than the BMR predicted; this increase is known as *hypermetabolism*. The degree of hypermetabolism—the increase in metabolic rate determined under basal conditions—is proportional to the severity of injury.[15] The severity appears to be related to the amount of tissue injured. This phenomenon is seen graphically in burn victims, in whom the amount of tissue injured can be

$$\text{MR (kcal/m}^2\text{/hr)} = \frac{[3.9 \times \dot{V}O_2 \text{ (L/min)} + 1.1 \times \dot{V}CO_2 \text{ (L/min)}] \times 60 \text{ (min/hr)}}{\text{Body Surface Area (m}^2)}$$

quantitated by the extent of body surface area that is burned. Metabolic rate under basal conditions increases with increasing burn size, i.e., with increasing injury severity (see Figure 28–2).

Hypermetabolism is associated with other injuries and critical illness as well (Table 27–1, Fig. 27–1).[16] Although massive burn injuries elicit more intense hypermetabolic responses than most other injuries, there appears to be an upper limit to the response of about twice the basal metabolic rate.[15] In contrast, most elective operations elicit only a small degree of hypermetabolism.[17] Elective surgery does result in a wound and is thus a form of injury. However, the amount of tissue damaged is relatively very small, and excellent perioperative care minimizes pain and prevents hypovolemia, acidosis, and hypoxia. Traumatic injury and elective surgery are metabolically quite different.

Whole-body oxygen consumption is related to cardiac output. Hypermetabolic patients demonstrate clinical signs of increased output, including a widened pulse pressure, mild tachycardia, and hyperdynamic peripheral pulses. In hypermetabolic burn patients, both cardiac index and oxygen consumption are proportional to injury severity,[18] increasing with burn size to a maximum plateau. However, oxygen consumption and blood flow are not closely coupled in certain regional vascular beds. In patients with major burns of one leg, Wilmore and associates[18]

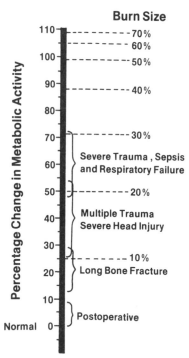

Figure 27–1. The effect of injury on metabolic activity measured under basal conditions. (*Adapted from* Wilmore, D. W.: The Metabolic Management of the Critically Ill. New York, Plenum Medical, 1977, p. 149. *Includes data from* Clifton, G. L., Robertson, C. S., et al.: The metabolic response to severe head injury. J. Neurosurg., 60:687–696, 1984.)

Table 27–1. EFFECTS OF INJURY ON METABOLIC RATE

INJURY	INCREASE IN METABOLIC ACTIVITY (%)	"STRESS FACTOR"
Elective operation	0–5	1.0 –1.05
Peritonitis	5–25	1.05–1.25
Long bone fracture	15–30	1.15–1.30
Multiple trauma	30–55	1.30–1.55
Severe head injury	30–50	1.30–1.50
Multiple trauma and sepsis	50–75	1.50–1.75
Burns		
10%	25	1.25
20%	50	1.50
30%	70	1.70
40%	85	1.85
50%	100	2.0
75%	100–110	2.0–2.1

(Adapted from Wilmore, D. W.: The Metabolic Management of the Critically Ill. New York, Plenum Medical, 1977, pp. 34–36; and Clifton, G. L., Robertson, C. S., Grossman, R. G., et al.: The metabolic response to severe head injury. J. Neurosurg., 60:687–696, 1984.)

found blood flow to the injured limb to be at least two times greater than flow to the uninjured leg. Flow was proportional to the extent of local injury and was directed to the surface wound rather than the underlying muscle.[19] Leg oxygen consumption increased with total body surface injury and represented a fairly constant six per cent of total oxygen consumption. However, despite the difference in flow between the injured and uninjured extremities, oxygen consumption was similar in both, suggesting that blood flow to the wound serves some purpose other than oxygen delivery.

Oxygen consumption by the kidney and splanchnic bed have also been shown to increase in concert with total oxygen consumption.[20] Blood flow to the splanchnic bed increases proportionately to total body flow.[21] The increases in splanchnic and wound blood flows account in large part for the increase in cardiac output in hypermetabolic patients. Renal blood flow correlates best with solute load[21] rather than oxygen consumption. By assuming that myocardial blood flow and

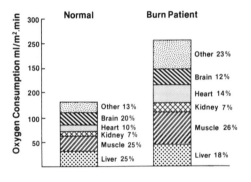

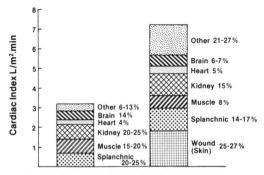

Figure 27–2. Regional distribution of oxygen consumption and cardiac index in normal subject and in hypermetabolic burn patient. (*Adapted from* Wilmore, D. W., and Aulick, L. H.: Metabolic changes in burned patients. Surg. Clin. North Am., *58*:1173–1187, 1978.)

oxygen consumption increase in proportion to the increase in cardiac output, it has been possible to partition both cardiac output and total oxygen consumption among a variety of regional vascular beds (Fig. 27–2).[22]

Alterations in Body Temperature

Body temperature is typically elevated in patients following injuries. Cuthbertson observed "post-traumatic fever" in patients with fractures in the absence of apparent infections.[23] This alteration also appears to be determined by injury severity.[24] Classically, an increase in body temperature has been associated with an increase in metabolic rate—approximately ten per cent per degree above 37°C. (Q_{10} effect).[25] However, this effect could account for only a small portion of the increase in metabolic rates of severely injured patients.[26] One proposed explanation for the increase in metabolic rate seen in patients with burns and other open wounds is that it is a response to an increased rate of heat loss through open wounds. Metabolic studies of burn patients conducted at several

ambient temperatures demonstrated that core and skin temperatures as well as metabolic rate remained elevated in injured patients at all temperatures.[27] The patients were internally warm, not externally cold. Furthermore, when burn patients were allowed to select their own most comfortable environmental temperature, they invariably selected warmer temperatures than controls.[24] Even at thermoneutrality, metabolic rate and core temperatures remained elevated. These observations indicate that there is an upward adjustment in central temperature set point in response to injury.

Accelerated Protein Breakdown and Nitrogen Loss

Perhaps the paramount feature of the injury response is marked protein catabolism with increased urinary nitrogen loss. On the basis of associated urinary losses of phosphorus and sulphur and the marked muscle wasting commonly observed in injured patients, Cuthbertson[28] concluded that the source of the increased nitrogen loss was skeletal muscle. Further studies utilizing a rat fracture model indicated that muscle that was either injured itself or in the vicinity of the fracture could not account for the nitrogen loss observed.[29] It was suggested that the loss of nitrogen resulted from a generalized process. These concepts have been supported by more recent data on the excretion of 3-methylhistidine, a compound formed from histidine after its incorporation into the muscle proteins, actin and myosin.[30] With protein degradation, 3-methylhistidine is released and excreted unchanged by the kidneys. In patients with burns,[31] trauma,[32] and infections,[33] an increased excretion of 3-methylhistidine has also been observed. Thus, a generalized acceleration in the breakdown of muscle protein is a major cause of post-traumatic protein loss. In addition, there may be actual loss of tissue due to injury and autolysis, loss of blood or exudate from the wound, and loss of muscle protein due to disuse atrophy.[34, 35]

Cuthbertson[23] noted that the time course of the increased nitrogen loss was distinctive. Nitrogen excretion peaked several days after injury and gradually returned toward normal over several weeks. Furthermore, he found that the increased nitrogen loss closely followed the increase in metabolic rate—they both reached a peak at about the same time after injury and gradually returned toward normal. Soroff and colleagues[36] and later Wilmore[37] reported the same phenomenon in burn patients—nitrogen excretion peaked several days after injury and gradually returned toward normal as the wounds healed. Kinney[38] observed the same effect in patients following a variety of injuries. In addition, the intensity of the nitrogen loss was proportional to the severity of injury—the more severe the injury, the greater the nitrogen loss (Table 27–2). Thus, accelerated protein breakdown is similar to other responses to injury.

Nitrogen balance is thought to reflect the difference between whole-body protein synthesis and breakdown. Overall protein metabolic activity, protein turnover, has been determined in tracer studies utilizing ^{15}N-labeled amino acids in a variety of conditions. These techniques invoke the concept of a free amino acid pool *to which* nitrogen is added by protein breakdown and by nitrogen intake and *from which* nitrogen is removed both by protein synthesis and by nitrogen excretion.[39] Assuming that the total amino acid nitrogen of the pool is constant, turnover is the total amount of nitrogen that enters or leaves the pool. During the flow phase following injury, protein turnover has been found to be increased.[40] Through combining turnover data with nitrogen intake and excretion values, estimates of total protein synthesis and catabolism may be made. These estimates indicate that both synthesis and catabolism may be increased following injury.[41] Levenson and co-workers[42] performed body composition studies utilizing a burned rat model and found that the incorporation of labeled

Table 27–2. MEAN DAILY NITROGEN LOSS DURING THE FIRST TEN DAYS FOLLOWING INJURY (VARIABLE AMOUNTS OF NUTRIENT INTAKE)

INJURY	CUMULATIVE N LOSS (gm/10 days)
Minor operation	24
Major operation	50
Peritonitis	136
Lone bone fracture	115
Multiple trauma	150
Major burn	170
Severe head injury	200

(Adapted from Wilmore, D. W.: The Metabolic Management of the Critically Ill. New York, Plenum Medical, 1977, p. 149; and Clifton, G. L., Robertson, C. S., Grossman, R. G., et al.: The metabolic response to severe head injury. J. Neurosurg., *60*:687–696, 1984.)

amino acids into various protein tissues after injury was greater than or equal to that in controls. In addition, when the animals were given labeled amino acid prior to injury, the loss of tag from protein tissue after burn was more rapid than in controls. Thus, injury increases whole-body protein activity in part by increasing protein catabolism. Protein synthesis is not suppressed following injury but in fact may be increased.

Post-Traumatic Amino Acid Metabolism

Plasma amino acid concentrations have been determined in a variety of critically ill and injured patients in an effort to identify alterations specific to the postinjury response. The findings have been variable. Although some studies have found a generalized hypoaminoacidemia following injury,[43] others have reported elevations of certain of the amino acids.[44-47] Elevated concentrations of phenylalanine, an essential amino acid that is not metabolized in muscle, have been reported frequently following injury and critical illnesses. The concentration ratio of phenylalanine and tyrosine has been proposed as an indicator of the severity of muscle protein catabolism.[48] The branched-chain amino acids (BCAA), leucine, isoleucine, and valine, are of particular interest because they are oxidized primarily in muscle,[49] unlike other amino acids, which are largely metabolized by liver. Both elevated[44, 50, 51] and decreased[43, 46] plasma concentrations have been reported following injury. The variation in the findings of these several investigations may be due to differences in analytic methodology, patient selection, or intercurrent treatment.[52]

Although amino acid concentrations in plasma are readily determined, they may not reflect quantitative alterations in the total amino acid pool. It has been estimated that as much as 80 per cent of the body's free amino acid pool is found in skeletal muscle.[53] Concentrations of free amino acids in intracellular water may be as much as 30 times greater than in plasma,[54] amounting to some 86.5 gm total for a 70-kg man. On the basis of muscle biopsy data from normal human subjects, the essential amino acids combined constitute only 8.4 per cent of the total intracellular pool, whereas the nonessential amino acid, glutamine, constitutes some 61 per cent.[54] Glutamine, glutamate, and alanine together constitute 79 per cent of the total pool.

Following starvation, inactivity,[51] elective operation,[55] trauma,[51, 56] and sepsis,[52] intracellular glutamine concentration falls. These findings suggest that a decrease in intracellular glutamine concentration may be a typical feature of the response to critical illness.[52] In addition, it would appear that it is a graded response,[57] reflecting the severity of injury. Increases in intracellular and plasma concentrations of phenylalanine, tyrosine, alanine, and the BCAA have also been observed following injury.[52, 55] This pattern of muscle intracellular amino acid concentrations is little affected by intravenous nutrition.[58] During convalescence, the increased essential amino acid concentrations return toward normal, but the decrease in intracellular glutamine persists.[52] Of note is the fact that none of the currently available amino acid mixtures for parenteral nutrition contains glutamine.[59]

The *in vitro* studies of Garber and co-workers[60] demonstrated that glutamine and alanine constitute as much as 70 per cent of the amino acids released from skeletal muscle. This finding indicated intracellular transformation of other amino acids. Furthermore, the relative amounts of alanine and glutamine released depended on amino acid availability.[61] Aulick and Wilmore[62] measured amino acid release from the lower extremities of patients with major burns and compared it to control values. The net total release of amino acid nitrogen, based on the ten amino acids measured, was five times greater in the patients than in controls. Alanine was the only single amino acid whose release was significantly different in the two groups. However, glutamine release was not determined. Alanine release was related to burn size and oxygen consumption, but not to the extent of leg burn, i.e., local injury. Other studies demonstrated that the increased peripheral release was matched by an increased uptake across the splanchnic bed.[20] The splanchnic exchange of alanine in noninfected burn patients was three to four times greater than in postabsorptive, normal controls.

Alterations of Carbohydrate Metabolism

Hyperglycemia and impaired glucose tolerance following injury have long been recognized[63] and gave rise to the term *diabetes of injury*. Although insulin concentrations may be disproportionately low immediately following injury, they are normal or elevated following resuscitation.[64] In addition, the insulin response to a glucose challenge is not impaired.[65] Several studies have documented increased rates of hepatic (endogenous) glucose production following injury.[20, 66, 67] In addition, glucose disappearance has been found to be increased under basal conditions in injured patients.[68] This increased glucose "flow" was proportional to injury severity and decreased toward normal during convalescence.

Both lactate and alanine can serve as precursors for hepatic glucose production.[69] The hepatic uptake of these substances is increased following injury.[20] In the periphery, glucose uptake increases as a function of the extent of local burn injury.[18] It correlates well with blood flow but not with oxygen consumption. Lactate release is also proportional to local injury severity and closely matches glucose uptake. Thus, the wound appears to consume glucose, which is metabolized via glycolysis to lactate, a process that does not require oxygen.

Under fasting conditions, patients recovering from moderate injury have elevations of both plasma glucose and serum insulin concentrations (Table 27–3). However, the elevations are disproportionate, suggesting an alteration in the normal glucose and insulin interactions. Black and associates[70] quantitated these alterations in seriously injured patients utilizing glucose and insulin clamp techniques. A variety of insulin infusions were administered while euglycemia was maintained. At all doses studied and at comparable insulin concentrations, total body glucose disposal was lower in patients than in normal controls (Fig. 27–3). When fixed hyperglycemia was achieved, an exaggerated insulin response was observed in the

Table 27–3. BASAL GLUCOSE AND INSULIN CONCENTRATIONS (MEAN ± SEM)

SUBJECTS	GLUCOSE CONCENTRATION (mg/dl)	INSULIN CONCENTRATION (μU/ml)
Normals (n = 49)	78 ± 1	12 ± 1
Trauma patients (n = 19)	104 ± 2	17 ± 2
p	<0.02	<0.01

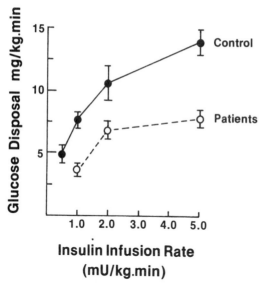

Figure 27-3. Total body glucose disposal under conditions of hyperinsulinemia and euglycemia in normals and in nonseptic trauma patients 5 to 14 days following injury. (*Adapted from* Black, P. R., Brooks, D. C., Bessey, P. Q., et al.: Mechanisms of insulin resistance following injury. Ann. Surg., *196*:420–435, 1982.)

patients, but glucose disposal was significantly depressed. These studies provided quantitative evidence of insulin resistance following injury. Brooks and colleagues[71] determined glucose uptake by uninjured forearm muscle in both patients recovering from injury and normal controls. Despite similar conditions of hyperinsulinemia and euglycemia, uptake was lower in patients than in controls, demonstrating that peripheral tissue, principally skeletal muscle and fat, is a major site of post-traumatic insulin resistance.

Interorgan Substrate Flux

The metabolic processes of the injury response involve principally three tissue beds: liver, skeletal muscle, and the wound. The liver produces glucose in increased amounts. The glucose is transported to the wound, where it is metabolized anaerobically. The lactate produced is transported back to the liver, where it is recycled to glucose, a process requiring energy and producing heat. Skeletal muscle takes up little glucose even though both glucose and insulin concentrations are elevated. Fat oxidation would appear to be the main energy source.[72] Muscle protein breaks down at an accelerated rate. Over 50 per cent of the nitrogen is

released as alanine and glutamine. Alanine is taken up by the liver and converted to new glucose, but the nitrogen is lost as urea. Glutamine may be actively taken up by the gut for conversion to alanine[73] or transported to the kidney, where it serves as a buffer of increased acid excretion associated with protein breakdown.[74] All of these reactions are associated with increased oxygen consumption and heat production and are proportional to the severity of the injury.

The wound appears to have a principal, controlling role in this scheme. The wound robs the host of blood supply and induces profound metabolic alterations. The host breaks down its own lean tissues, releasing amino acids that serve as precursors for acute-phase protein synthesis and wound repair and as substrate for gluconeogenesis to support the wound's energy requirements.[20] As the wound heals, this heightened metabolic activity abates.

Regulation

How the wound controls the host's physiology is not well understood. However, a variety of metabolically active substances have been implicated as mediators of the metabolic response to injury. The concentrations of several hormones are increased following injury, including cortisol,[75] glucagon,[76] and the catecholamines.[77, 78] Hypermetabolism has been shown to be related to urinary catecholamine excretion,[79] and hypercortisolemia and hyperglucagonemia have been shown to be related to injury severity.[75, 76] The response to injury cannot be adequately explained by the actions of any of these hormones alone. However, when cortisol, glucagon, and epinephrine were administered to normal, uninjured subjects in doses that achieved elevations similar to those seen following injury, the principal alterations of the injury response were reproduced.[80] Thus, the altered post-traumatic endocrine environment appears to have a dominant role in the regulation of the response to injury.

Inflammatory cells that participate actively in wound healing can produce one or more substances that exert metabolic effects. Interleukin-1 is one such substance or class of substances. It induces fever and increases acute phase protein synthesis.[82] Recently, Baracos and co-workers[83] reported that interleukin-1 stimulated muscle proteolysis in vitro. Clowes and associates[84] have identified a polypeptide from the serum of septic patients that also induced *in vitro* skeletal muscle proteolysis. The role of such substances *in vivo* has yet to be clarified.

CARING FOR THE INJURED PATIENT

To ensure the best results possible, care of the injured patient follows certain priorities.[85] Immediate recognition and treatment of life-threatening conditions is the first priority. Airway, breathing, and access to the circulation—the "A B Cs" must be assured. Then hemorrhage is controlled and shock is treated; this goal may require an emergency operation if the bleeding is internal. Following these life-saving measures, attention is directed toward identification and definitive treatment of all injuries. Disrupted organs and tissues are repaired, fractures are reduced and fixed either internally or externally, and open wounds are debrided and closed primarily or after a delay to assure wound viability. In many cases, it may be possible to accomplish definitive repair and treatment quickly. Then the metabolic response to injury may be minimal as long as no complications intervene. Many penetrating injuries fall into this category. For example, a stab wound to the heart is certainly a life-threatening injury, but if rapid, definitive repair can be accomplished, the victim will survive and may recover sufficiently to be discharged in a matter of a few days.

However, it may not be possible to complete definitive repair for several days or weeks following some injuries, such as severe blunt trauma, extensive soft tissue injuries, and burns. In these cases the metabolic responses may be particularly intense or prolonged. Attention must be paid not only to management of the wound but also to the physiologic support of the patient. Although comprehensive support of all organ systems is important, our focus here is on metabolic and nutritional support.

Metabolic Support of the Injured Patient

Overall Goals

The goal of all trauma care is to return the injured patient to an active role in society in a safe and timely manner. The clinician intervenes as necessary in order to provide an optimal environment for the processes of healing and recovery. Intervention may involve oxygenation and mechanical ventilation, cardiovascular pharmacologic support, and careful management of fluid, electrolyte, and acid-base balances. Additional stresses that could increase metabolic demands should be avoided. Patients should be kept warm and free of pain and anxiety, and appropriate precautions against septic complications should be taken. Because the wound appears to have a controlling role in the injury response, timely, definitive treatment of all wounds and injuries is strategically important. Finally, exogenous substrate—nutrition—should be provided to reduce the draft on the body's energy and protein stores.

Nutritional Goals

Hypermetabolism and increased protein breakdown result in an accelerated rate of loss of the body cell mass. Unless protein and calories are provided in amounts sufficient to match demands, net loss of lean tissue will ensue. The consequences of weight loss depend on its extent. If loss is limited to less than 10 per cent of preinjury body weight, little disability is observed.[86] However, a severe loss (40 per cent of preinjury body weight) is usually fatal.[8] Weight loss between these limits in a previously healthy individual is associated with increased debility and risk of mortality and morbidity.[88] Thus, a primary goal of nutritional support following injury is to limit net weight loss during convalescence to less than 10 per cent of preinjury body weight.[7]

In the classic study by Benedict,[89] a healthy but starved subject lost 10 per cent of his initial body weight in 11 days. During this time, the subject's metabolic rate *decreased* about 10 per cent also.[90] Injured patients have an *increased* metabolic rate, and if totally starved would lose 10 per cent of their lean weight in less than 11 days. Because of the exigencies of assessment, resuscitation, and early trauma care and because of the potential complicating metabolic effects of aggressive feeding during this unstable period, nutritional support is not begun immediately following injury. Thus, virtually all injured patients sustain a period of posttraumatic starvation. Practically, nutritional support can usually be started two to four days after injury. Although hypocaloric feedings may slow the rate of net catabolism, the operational goal of nutritional support in injured patients is nutritional maintenance or balance.

Estimating Nutritional Requirements

To achieve nutritional maintenance, energy and nitrogen substrate (calories and protein) should be provided in amounts equivalent to the caloric requirements (energy expenditure or heat loss) and to the nitrogen losses of the patients. Post-traumatic hypermetabolism is a graded response; that is, its intensity is a function of injury severity. It is possible to estimate reliably total energy requirements on the basis of age, sex, body size, and injury severity. First, the basal metabolic rate is determined. Several acceptable standards are available to the clinician for this determination. The standards of Fleisch[91] are reproduced in Table 27–4. The standard metabolic rate for age and sex should be multiplied by a "stress factor" to account for the degree of hypermetabolism expected on the basis of injury severity (see Table 27–1). The stress factor is a multiplier for standard basal metabolic rate that reflects the degree of hypermetabolism due to the disease process. After multiplying this value by body surface area (based on preinjury weight and height) and by 24 hours, an additional 25 per cent should be added to

account for minimal activity and the specific dynamic action (SDA) of feeding.[92] The resulting value is the estimated total daily caloric requirement. Duke and coworkers[17] have shown that 15 to 20 per cent of the daily energy expenditure is derived from protein. Thus, 15 to 20 per cent of the estimated total daily caloric requirement should be provided as protein. That value is divided by four to calculate the protein requirement in grams. The result represents a non-protein calorie/nitrogen ratio of 142:1 to 100:1.

Example. A 25-year-old woman has been thrown approximately 10 yards from a car when it went off the road. She has sustained closed head injury with loss of consciousness at the scene; blunt chest trauma with multiple rib fractures on the right side and a severe pulmonary contusion; a severe pelvic fracture with disruption of the pubic symphysis and right sacroiliac joint and fractures of the right superior and inferior pubic rami, a compression fracture of the first lumbar vertebra, and a midshaft fracture of the right tibia. It is now 60 hours following her accident. She wakens and is responsive to verbal commands. Her hemodynamics are satisfactory, and there is no obvious ongoing hemorrhage. Her chest x-ray shows gradual clearing of the right pulmonary contusion, but she still requires mechanical ventilation and positive airway pressures to maintain adequate gas exchange. External pelvic fixation has been applied, and her right leg has been casted. She will probably require open reduction and internal fixation of the spine. It has been elected to defer further evaluation of the vertebral fracture (myelography and computed tomography) and possible operative fixation until her pulmonary status improves. She will require nutritional support. Her nutritional requirements should be estimated using preinjury height of 64 inches and weight of 113 lbs (51.36 kg).

1. From Table 27–4, the standard metabolic rate for a 25-year-old woman is 35.2 kcal/m²/hr.

2. From Figure 27–1 and Table 27–1, the "stress factor" for this woman with multiple injuries would be expected to be 1.4. Multiplying the standard metabolic rate by 1.4 yields 49.3 kcal/m²/hr, which would be her expected metabolic rate determined under basal conditions.

3. On the basis of preinjury height and weight, her body surface area (BSA) can be determined from a standard nomagram (Figure 27–4) or from the formula of DuBois,[93] which is:

$$BSA\ (m^2) = Ht^{0.725}\ (cm) \times Wt^{0.425}\ (kg) \times 0.007184$$

In this example the body surface area is 1.52 m².

4. Her caloric requirement can now be calculated. Basal needs are determined to be:

$$49.3\ kcal/m^2/hr \times 1.52\ m^2 \times 24\ hr/day = 1798\ kcal/day.$$

Table 27–4. STANDARD METABOLIC RATES

AGE (years)	METABOLIC RATE (kcal/m²/hr)	
	Females	*Males*
1	53.0	53.0
5	48.4	49.3
10	42.5	44.0
15	37.9	41.8
20	35.3	38.6
25	35.2	37.5
30	35.1	36.8
35	35.0	36.5
40	34.9	36.3
45	34.5	36.2
50	33.9	35.8
55	33.3	35.4
60	32.7	34.9
65	32.2	34.4
70	31.7	33.8
75	31.3	33.2
80	30.9	33.0

(Adapted from Fleisch, A.: Le métabolisme basal standard et sa détermination au moyen du Metabocalculator. Helv. Med. Acta, *18*:23–44, 1951.)

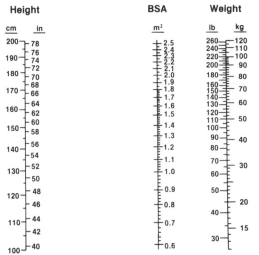

Figure 27–4. Nomogram for determination of body surface area (BSA) based on formula of Dubois.[93] (See text.) With a straight edge, one connects the subject's height on the left scale with his/her weight on the right and reads the body surface area (m²) on the middle scale.

Increasing this value 25 per cent to account for minimal hospital activity and feeding effects (SDA) yields:

$$1798 \text{ kcal/day} \times 1.25 = 2248 \text{ kcal/day}$$

as the estimated total caloric requirement for this injured woman.

5. Of this total, 15 to 20 per cent should be provided as protein. That is,

$$(0.15–0.2) \times 2250 \text{ kcal/day} = 338–450 \text{ kcal/day}.$$

Because 1 gm of protein yields 4 kcal when oxidized, her protein requirement is 85 to 113 gm/day.

Nonprotein Calories

Both carbohydrates and fat may be utilized as nonprotein energy substrate. In simple starvation, glucose is well known to have a pronounced protein-sparing effect.[94] Long and colleagues[95] administered glucose and fat in a variety of combinations to burn patients receiving a fixed amount of protein. Glucose was much more effective than fat in reducing nitrogen excretion when provided in amounts less than the caloric requirement. Reduction of nitrogen excretion was most sensitive to increasing amounts of glucose up to approximately 60 per cent of total caloric requirements. Black and associates[70] found in trauma patients that there was a limit to the amount of glucose that could be removed from the circulation. They provided

a fixed hyperglycemic challenge to both patients and normal controls. Glucose disposal in controls increased steadily throughout the study, but patients demonstrated a fixed level of disposal that was less than that in controls (Fig. 27–5). This value, 6 to 7 mg/kg/min, represented approximately 60 per cent of the patients' estimated caloric requirements. Wolfe and co-workers[96] administered varying amounts of glucose to burn patients and measured glucose oxidation utilizing isotopic techniques. They found that no additional oxidation of glucose occurred when infusion rates were increased above 6 mg/kg/min. Thus, following injury there is a limit to the effective utilization of glucose as an energy source. This limit appears to represent about 50 to 60 per cent of the total caloric requirement. Carbohydrate (glucose) should be a part of a nutritional support regimen because of its beneficial effects on protein economy and should constitute 50 to 60 per cent of total calories.

Example Continued. For the patient described previously, the carbohydrate content of nutritional support can be calculated as:

$$0.6 \times 2250 \text{ kcal/day} = 1350 \text{ kcal/day}$$

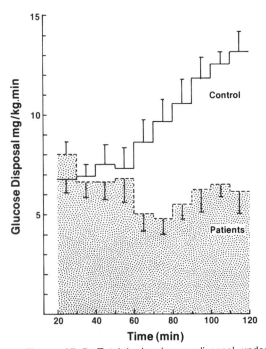

Figure 27–5. Total body glucose disposal under conditions of fixed hyperglycemia (125 mg/dl above basal) in normals and nonseptic trauma patients 5–13 days following injury. (*Adapted from* Black, P. R., Brooks, D. C., Bessey, P. O., et al.: Mechanisms of insulin resistance following injury. Ann. Surg., *196*:420–435, 1982.)

Oral carbohydrate provides 4 kcal/gm. Glucose for intravenous administration is a monhydrate and yields less heat—3.4 kcal/gram. Thus, 338 gm of oral carbohydrate or 397 gm of intravenous glucose would provide the required 1350 kcal.

The remaining 20 to 25 per cent of total caloric requirement may be made up by protein, carbohydrate, or fat. If additional protein is administered, urea production will increase and BUN may rise. In subjects with impaired renal function these increases will contribute to uremia.

If additional carbohydrate is provided, it may give rise to significant hyperglycemia, requiring exogenous insulin for control. Black and associates[70] were able to increase glucose disposal in injured patients to a maximum of 9 to 10 mg/kg/min during euglycemia by infusing large doses of insulin. However, extra quantities of glucose may be associated with respiratory and hepatic dysfunction.

Alternatively, fat may be provided. Fat constitutes 20 to 30 per cent of calories in many of the commonly used enteral nutrition products. Lipid emulsions are available for intravenous administration. Nordenstrom and co-workers[99] supported injured patients with parenteral nutrition in which glucose and intravenous lipid emulsion provided roughly equal amounts of the caloric load. Lipid was indeed utilized as an energy source by the patients, but oxidation did not correlate with plasma clearance. Goodenough and Wolfe[100] provided 30 per cent of calories to burn patients as intravenous lipid and measured free fatty acid and energy metabolism. Fat oxidation accounted for about 25 per cent of the energy expenditure, but most of the fat oxidized appeared to come from endogenous stores. Thus, it was suggested that exogenous intravenous lipid is not directly utilized as an energy source but maintains endogenous fat stores. The administration of both glucose and fat is more physiologic than of glucose alone.[101] The administration of lipid emulsions has been associated with a variety of complications in the past. However, with products currently available, the incidence of these complications should be exceedingly rare,[101] especially if the emulsion is administered over eight to 12 hours. Yet there are recent data from animal and *in vitro* human studies suggesting that lipid emulsion may be associated with abnormalities in neutrophil function and bacterial clearance.[102] The clinical significance of these observations has not been determined.

Feeding the Patient

It is generally accepted that if the gastrointestinal tract is functional, it should be used for nutritional support.[103-105] For many trauma victims, the GI tract is not available because of direct injury, postoperative ileus, ileus due to retroperitoneal hematoma or vertebral fractures, obligatory periods of starvation accompanying multiple diagnostic and operative procedures, or multisystem failure and sepsis. For these patients, nutritional support may be provided utilizing parenteral techniques. Starvation is no longer obligatory following injury. The route of feeding depends on the patient's injuries and the requirements of his or her further care.

Peripheral vein parenteral nutrition may be utilized occasionally in some groups of injured patients to reduce the rate of net catabolism. It may also be useful to supplement oral or enteral feedings. However, the increased calorie and nitrogen requirements of injured patients usually necessitate hypertonic solutions and central vein feedings. Highly concentrated intravenous nutrients are available to the pharmacist, so the clinician has considerable flexibility in designing the parenteral solution. The intravenous regimen should deliver the required amounts of calories and nitrogen in a fluid volume that is appropriate for the patient's cardiopulmonary and renal status. In addition, electrolytes, minerals, and vitamins should be provided. The solutions should be administered via a central vein catheter that is placed, utilizing sterile technique, specifically and exclusively for the administration of TPN. The details of catheter placement, electrolyte and mineral balance, and vitamin therapy are presented elsewhere in this book.

Example Continued. The goal for nutritional support of the young woman presented in this example would be nutritional maintenance. Her pelvic and vertebral fractures most likely will result in ileus for several days. In addition, if she undergoes instrumentation of her spine, the ileus will probably recur. Thus, parenteral nutrition, specifically central vein total parenteral nutrition, is advisable. She requires a total of 2250 kcal/day, of which at least 1350 kcal should be provided as glucose (397 gm) and 338 to 450 kcal as protein (85 to 113 gm). "Standard" TPN solution contains 250 gm glucose and 42.5 gm amino acids in one bottle (usually more than one liter owing to other additives). Two and one-half bottles of this solution would meet the protein requirement (106 gm). This volume would also contain 625 gm of glucose, which would provide 2125 glucose kcal. The total calories delivered would be 2549 kcal. This is an acceptable regimen, provided that the patient could tolerate the high glucose load and that hyperglycemia could be controlled. Intravenous lipid emulsion would be indicated to prevent fatty acid deficiency.[106] One bottle of the 10 per cent emulsion twice a week would be sufficient.

Alternatively, a regimen containing both fat and glucose as energy sources could be utilized. A mixture of 600 ml of an 8.5 per cent amino acid solution and 400 ml of 50 per cent dextrose would provide 51 gm of protein and 680 kcal of glucose per bottle. Two bottles of this solution would deliver 102 gm of protein and 1360 kcal of glucose. One bottle (500 ml) of 10 per cent lipid emulsion daily would provide an additional 550 kcal for a total of 2318 kcal. This regimen would require the same fluid volume administration as the glucose-only regimen. The total glucose load would be less, and hyperglycemia probably would not be a problem.

Special Considerations

Immobilization

Injured patients commonly spend a variable amount of time immobilized. Patients requiring in-line traction or those with spinal cord or peripheral nerve injuries may have a particularly prolonged period of immobilization. Normal subjects at complete bed rest or immobilized demonstrate a net loss of nitrogen, calcium, and sulfur even though they consume a normally adequate diet.[107, 108] Inactivity also alters intracellular amino acid concentrations.[51] The whole-body losses have been reduced, however, by massage and passive exercise[109] or by use of an oscillating bed.[110] Thus, isometric exercises and physical therapy may help maintain muscle tone and mass and are important components of comprehensive trauma care.

Brain Injury

Severe head injury with underlying damage of the brain is a common cause of death and disability from trauma.[4] The influence of an injury to the brain on the metabolic response to injury is complicated in part because the brain may play a central integrating role in the genesis and regulation of the injury response. Accordingly, Wilmore and colleagues[111] found that a patient with a burn injury and electrocerebral silence on electroencephalography was not hypermeta-

bolic. Dempsey and co-workers[112] measured energy expenditures in patients with severe head injuries and found them to be 40 per cent above predicted values. Barbiturate coma eliminated this hypermetabolic response[112] and reduced nitrogen excretion.[113] Clifton and associates[114] found a marked but highly variable hypermetabolic response in patients with severe isolated head injuries and coma. They concluded that head injury was equivalent metabolically to a 20 to 30 per cent burn injury or multiple trauma with sepsis. Incompletely controlled seizure activity or posturing may also affect nutritional requirements. Posturing alone may increase oxygen consumption 40 per cent.

Nutritional Monitoring

The use of changes in body weight, serum albumin, and anthropometric parameters to assess the adequacy of nutritional support is complicated by changes in the fluid compartments of the body.[115] Fluid resuscitation invariably results in an expansion of the extracellular fluid space and a positive sodium balance. Starvation itself may also alter the relative amount of extracellular fluid.[87] In the presence of an expanded extracellular fluid compartment, the serum albumin concentration does not reflect either total body protein content or nitrogen balance.[116] Thus, changes in body weight and serum albumin may be influenced more by sodium and fluid balance than by nitrogen balance. With nutritional support, if the patient's course is relatively uncomplicated, the serum albumin concentration may increase while body weight decreases in association with a negative sodium balance. However, if the course is complicated, for example by sepsis, then sodium balance may be positive, weight will increase, and the serum albumin concentration will remain low or decrease further, despite positive nitrogen balance.

For most patients, nutritional requirements may be estimated reliably. In complicated cases or when convalescence is not satisfactory, further assessment may be helpful. Indirect calorimetry may be performed utilizing a variety of techniques.[117] One of the simplest is the determination of oxygen consumption with a spirometer in a closed circuit.[118] If a thermodilution pulmonary artery catheter is present, oxygen consumption may be calculated as the product of the difference in systemic arterial and pulmonary arterial (mixed venous) oxygen content and cardiac output—although the combined measurement errors make this calculation imprecise. It is usually impossible to achieve completely basal conditions in the modern intensive care unit, but several variables may be controlled. All nutrient intake should be stopped for several hours prior to measurement. The determination should be made in the early morning, and the patient should be kept quiet, comfortable, and warm. To calculate metabolic rate (MR) from oxygen consumption ($\dot{V}O_2$) alone, a conversion factor of 4.86 kcal/L of O_2 (RQ = 0.85)[119] may be used:

$$MR \text{ (kcal/m}^2\text{/hr)} = \frac{4.86 \, \dot{V}O_2 \text{ (L/min)} \times 60 \text{ min/hr}}{BSA \text{ (m}^2)}$$

The resulting rate should be within three per cent of the value that would be obtained if carbon dioxide production were also known. This value (kcal/min) can be multiplied by 24 hr/day and 1.25 to determine total daily caloric requirements.

Nitrogen balance may also be helpful. Determination of total nitrogen excretion is not readily available in most clinical settings, but the determination of urinary urea nitrogen may be readily performed by the clinical laboratory. Although urea nitrogen may compose less than 50 per cent of the total urinary nitrogen in prolonged starvation,[120] under normal conditions it accounts for as much as 90 per cent of the total. In critically ill patients receiving nutritional support, urinary urea nitrogen (UUN) was found to compose 70 to 80 per cent of total urinary nitrogen over a wide range of values.[121] Under normal conditions, GI and skin losses are thought to account for approximately 2 gm of nitrogen per day.[37] GI losses may be increased in the presence of diarrhea, nasogastric suction, or fistula drainage. In the presence of a major burn or large granulating wound, several grams of nitrogen may be lost in the wound exudate.[122] In general, nitrogen loss (N loss) may be estimated as follows:

N loss (gm/day) =
$$\frac{24\text{-hr UUN (gm/day)}}{0.75} + (2\text{--}4 \text{ gm})$$

Nitrogen balance (N bal) may then be calculated:

N bal (gm/day) =
$$\frac{\text{Protein intake (gm/day)}}{6.25} - N \text{ loss}$$

FUTURE DIRECTIONS

The preceding approach to the nutritional support of injured patients can achieve the goal of nutritional maintenance in most cases, and net weight loss may be limited to less than ten per cent of the preinjury weight. Current investigations may modify this approach in the future. Improved understanding of regulatory mechanisms may lead to therapies that could alter the intensity or nature of the response to injury and so modify the consequent metabolic demands and nutritional requirements. Studies of regional metabolism may identify altered requirements for specific nutrients in certain tissues and disease states. In that case, modifications of nutrient supply might have clinical benefit.[123-125] An example of particular current interest is nutritional support with branched-chain amino acid–enriched parenteral and enteral nutritional preparations.

Branched-Chain Amino Acids

The three branched-chain amino acids (BCAA) are metabolized primarily in muscle, unlike other amino acids, which are processed largely by the liver.[49] The deaminated carbon chains may enter the Krebs cycle, providing substrate for oxidative phosphorylation. Odessey and co-workers[126] demonstrated that alanine production by skeletal muscle in vitro was related to oxidation of BCAA. Thus, the BCAA may be utilized by muscle for energy, and the nitrogen released as alanine.

Ryan and associates[127] and O'Donnell and colleagues[128] have presented data suggesting that muscle relies increasingly on BCAA as energy substrate during critical illness. Muscle is thought to break down its own protein to provide BCAA for energy, releasing the other amino acids in increased amounts for processing by the liver and for excretion. The provision of exogenous amino acids containing BCAA in excess of normal proportions has thus been proposed as a strategy to reduce net muscle catabolism.[129] In addition, investigations of muscle protein metabolism in vitro have suggested that the BCAA may have a regulatory function as well, so that exogenous BCAA might exert a modulating effect on post-traumatic metabolic responses.[130] However, Askanazi and co-workers[52] and Vinnars and associates[55] have found increased rather than decreased intracellular concentrations of BCAA following injury, suggesting that endogenous BCAA are readily available for intracellular metabolic processes.

Cerra and colleagues[131] administered isocaloric, isonitrogenous intravenous feedings containing various amounts of BCAA to critically ill patients in a randomized trial. Positive nitrogen balance was observed sooner with the solutions containing the increased BCAA than with those of standard composition. In addition, nitrogen retention appeared to be related to BCAA dose.[132] Urinary 3-methylhistidine excretions did not differ between groups, suggesting that the increase in nitrogen balance observed reflected increased protein synthesis. Bonau and associates[133] showed that the apparent nitrogen-sparing effect of BCAA-enriched solutions depends more on the ratios of the individual BCAA than on the total amount. These studies all utilized whole-body measurements and plasma concentrations of amino acids. The relationship between the positive nitrogen balance observed and the composition of the intracellular amino acid pool was not defined. In addition, these studies did not report any differences in clinical outcome.

Utilizing a standardized catabolic animal model, Johnson and co-workers[134] demonstrated that skeletal muscle uptake of BCAA was related to BCAA dose but that this effect was small and transitory. Additionally, there were no differences in nitrogen balance and skeletal muscle intracellular free amino acid concentrations between animals receiving BCAA-enriched solutions and those receiving standard mixtures. Thus, in these studies the BCAA-enriched solutions had little more anticatabolic effect than standard, balanced solutions. Furthermore, Dudrick and associates[135] observed that BCAA-enriched feedings in an injured rat model resulted in delayed fracture healing, implying a detrimental effect.

In summary, the effects of BCAA-enriched nutritional support of injured and critically ill patients reported to date have been modest and of undetermined clinical benefit. The utility of these and other special nutritional preparations in critical illness will continue to be an area of active investigation.

CONCLUSION

This chapter has presented a general approach to the nutritional support of injured

patients. The objective is to assure that the patient receives sufficient energy and protein substrate to satisfy the increased caloric and nitrogen demands of the injury response. Because of the availability of parenteral nutrition, this objective may be met even in the patient with ineffective gastrointestinal function. In practice, a variety of nutrition support modalities may be used during recovery from injury (Fig. 27–6). After resuscitation and stabilization, parenteral nutrition may be initiated. When GI motility returns, as evidenced by the passage of flatus and stool, oral intake may be resumed. Enteral feedings may replace parenteral nutrition to ensure adequate caloric and nitrogen intake until the patient is able to meet his or her full nutritional requirements by spontaneous oral feeding, including regular meals and nutritional supplements.

The goal of nutritional maintenance may be met in virtually all patients through utilization of standard techniques and readily available nutritional products. Energy and nitrogen balance may be maintained throughout most of the period of convalescence. Maintaining the balance does not reduce the demands of post-traumatic metabolism.[136] Rather, energy and nitrogen substrate are provided to meet heightened demands and so reduce the draft on the patient's lean tissue and energy reserves. ^{15}N-turnover studies indicate that vigorous nutritional support in critically ill patients increases protein synthesis to keep pace with accelerated protein catabolism[137] and so achieves nitrogen balance.

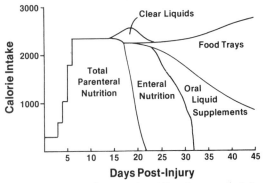

Nutritional Support Following Multiple Trauma in a 25 y.o. Woman

Figure 27–6. Course of nutritional support of the multiple-injured patient used as an example in the text. Total parenteral nutrition is one component of comprehensive nutritional management of critically ill patients.

With current techniques, appropriate nutritional support may be provided with a low incidence of complications.[138] The major determinant of clinical outcome then becomes the patient's primary injury or disease process. Thus, in the care of critically ill and injured patients, nutritional support is not a substitute for early, definitive closure of wounds, repair of injuries, and treatment of infections.

REFERENCES

1. Trunkey, D.D.: On the nature of things that go bang in the night. Surgery, 92:123–132, 1982.
2. Centers for Disease Control: Annual summary 1982: Reported morbidity and mortality in the United States. Morbidity Mortality Wkly. Rep., 31:111, 1983.
3. Trunkey, D.D.: Trauma. Sci. Am., 249:28–35, 1983.
4. Baker, C.C., Openheimer, L., Stephenson, B., et al.: Epidemiology of trauma deaths. Am. J. Surg., 140:144–150, 1980.
5. Baker, C.C., Caronna, J.J., and Trunkey, D.D.: Neurologic outcome after emergency room thoracotomy for trauma. Am. J. Surg., 139:677–681, 1980.
6. West, J.G., Cales, R.H., and Gazziniga, A.B.: Impact of regionalization. Arch. Surg., 118:740–744, 1983.
7. Wilmore, D.W., and Kinney, J.M.: Panel report on nutritional support of patients with trauma or infection. Am. J. Clin. Nutr., 34:1213–1222, 1981.
8. Curreri, P.W., Luterman, A.D., Braun, D.W., Jr., and Shires, G.T.: Burn injury: analysis of survival and hospitalization time for 937 patients. Ann. Surg., 192:472–478, 1980.
9. Cuthbertson, D.P.: The metabolic response to injury and its nutritional implications: Retrospect and prospect. J.P.E.N., 3:108–129, 1979.
10. Cuthbertson, D.P.: Post-shock metabolic response. Lancet, 1:433–437, 1942.
11. Moore, F.D.: Getting well: The biology of surgical convalescence. Ann. N.Y. Acad. Sci., 73:387–400, 1958.
12. Atwater, W.O., and Benedict, F.G.: Experiments on the metabolism of matter and energy in the human body. U.S.D.A. Office of Experimental Stations Bulletin, Publication No. 136, 1903.
13. Ben-Porat, M., Sideman, S., and Burstein, S.: Energy metabolism rate equation for fasting and postabsorptive subjects. Am. J. Physiol., 244:R764–769, 1983.
14. DuBois, E.F.: Basal Metabolism in Health and Disease. Philadelphia, Lea & Febiger, 1936, pp. 163–165.
15. Wilmore, D.W., Long, J.M., Mason, A.D., Jr., et al.: Catecholamines: Mediator of the hypermetabolic response to thermal injury. Ann. Surg., 180:653–669, 1974.
16. Wilmore, D.W.: The Metabolic Management of the Critically Ill. New York, Plenum Medical, 1977, pp. 33–35.
17. Duke, J.H., Jorgensen, S.B., Broell, J.R., et al.: Contribution of protein to caloric expenditure following injury. Surgery, 68:168–174, 1970.
18. Wilmore, D.W., Aulick, L.H., Mason, A.D., and Pruitt, B.A., Jr.: Influence of the burn wound on local and systemic responses to injury. Ann. Surg., 186:444–458, 1977.
19. Aulick, L.H., Wilmore, D.W., Mason, A.D., Jr., and Pruitt, B.A., Jr.: Muscle blood flow following thermal injury. Ann. Surg., 188:778–782, 1978.
20. Wilmore, D.W., Goodwin, C.W., Aulick, L.H., et al.: Effect of injury and infection on visceral metabolism and circulation. Ann. Surg., 192:491–504, 1980.
21. Aulick, L.H., Goodwin, C.W., Becker, R.A., and Wilmore, D.W.: Visceral blood flow following thermal injury. Ann. Surg., 193:112–116, 1981.
22. Wilmore, D.W., and Aulick, L.H.: Metabolic changes in burned patients. Surg. Clin. North Am., 58:1173–1187, 1978.
23. Cuthbertson, D.P.: Observations on disturbance of metabolism produced by injury to the limbs. Q. J. Med., 25:233–246, 1932.
24. Wilmore, D.W., Orcutt, T.W., Mason, A.D., Jr., and Pruitt, B.A., Jr.: Alterations in hypothalamic function following thermal injury. J. Trauma, 15:697–703, 1975.
25. Wilmore, D.W.: The Metabolic Management of the Critically Ill. New York, Plenum Medical, 1977, p. 29.
26. Aulick, L.H., Hander, E.H., Wilmore, D.W., et al.: The relative significance of thermal and metabolic demands on burn hypermetabolism. J. Trauma, 19:559–566, 1979.
27. Wilmore, D.W., Mason, A.D., Jr., Johnson, D.W., and Pruitt, B.A., Jr.: Effect of ambient temperature on heat production and heat loss in burn patients. J. Appl. Physiol., 38:593–597, 1975.
28. Cuthbertson, D.P.: The disturbance of metabolism produced by bony and non-bony injury, with notes on certain abnormal conditions of bone. Biochem. J., 24:1244–1263, 1930.
29. Cuthbertson, D.P., McGirr, J.L., and Robertson, J.S.M.: The effect of fracture of bone on the metabolism of the rat. Q. J. Exp. Physiol., 29:13–25, 1939.
30. Young, V.R., and Munro, H.N.: N$^\tau$-Methylhistidine (3-methylhistidine) and muscle protein turnover: An overview. Fed. Proc., 37:2291–2300, 1978.
31. Bilmazes, C., Kien, C.L., Rohrbaugh, D.K., et al.: Quantitative contributors by skeletal muscle to elevated rates of whole-body protein breakdown in burned children as measured by 3-methylhistidine output. Metabolism, 27:671–676, 1978.
32. Williamson, D.H., Farrell, R., Kerr, A., and Smith, R.: Muscle protein catabolism after injury in man as measured by urinary excretion of 3-methylhistidine. Clin. Sci. Molec. Med., 52:527–533, 1977.
33. Long, C.L., Schiller, W.R., Blakemore, W.S., et al.: Muscle protein catabolism in the septic patient as measured by 3-methylhistidine excretion. Am. J. Clin. Nutr., 30:1349–1352, 1977.
34. Cuthbertson, D.P.: The physiology of convalescence after injury. Br. Med. Bull., 3:96–102, 1945.
35. Threlfall, C.J., Stoner, H.B., and Galasko, C.S.B.: Patterns in the excretion of muscle markers after trauma and orthopedics surgery. J. Trauma, 21:140–147, 1981.
36. Soroff, H.S., Pearson, E., and Artz, C.P.: An estimation of the nitrogen requirements for equilibrium in burned patients. Surg. Gynecol. Obstet., 112:150–172, 1961.

37. Wilmore, D.W.: Nutrition and metabolism following thermal injury. Clin. Plastic Surg., 1:603–619, 1974.

38. Kinney, J.M.: Energy deficits in acute illness and injury. In Morgan, A.P. (ed.): Proceedings of a Conference on Energy Metabolism and Body Fuel Utilization. Cambridge, Harvard University Press, 1966, p. 174.

39. Picou, D., and Taylor-Roberts, T.: The measurement of total protein synthesis and catabolism and nitrogen turnover in infants on different amounts of dietary protein. Clin. Sci., 36:283–296, 1969.

40. Birhahn, R.H., Long, C.L., Fitkin, D., et al.: Effects of major skeletal trauma on whole body protein turnover in man measured by L-[1, ^{14}C]-leucine. Surgery, 88:294–308, 1980.

41. Kien, C.L., Young, V.R., Rohrbaugh, D.K., and Burke, J.F.: Increased rates of whole body protein synthesis and breakdown in children recovering from burns. Ann. Surg., 187:383–391, 1978.

42. Levenson, S.M., Pulaski, E.J., and del Guerico, L.R.M.: Metabolic changes associated with injury. In Zimmerman, L.M., and Levine, R. (eds.): Physiological Principles of Surgery, 2nd ed. Philadelphia, W.B. Saunders, 1964, pp. 5–7.

43. Everson, T.C., and Fritschel, M.J.: The effect of surgery on the plasma levels of the individual essential amino acids. Surgery, 31:226–232, 1952.

44. Levenson, S.M., Howard, J.M., and Rosen, H.: Studies of the plasma amino acids and amino conjugates in patients with severe battle wounds. Surg. Gynecol. Obstet. 101:35–47, 1955.

45. LaBrasse, E.H., Beech, J.A., McLaughlin, J.S., et al.: Plasma amino acids in normal humans and patients with shock. Surg. Gynecol. Obstet., 125:516–520, 1967.

46. Cerra, F.B., Siegel, J.H., Border, J.R., et al.: Correlations between metabolic and cardiopulmonary measurements in patients after trauma, general surgery, and sepsis. J. Trauma, 19:621–629, 1979.

47. McMenam, R.H., Birkhahn, R., Oswald, G., et al.: Multiple systems failure: I. The basal state. J. Trauma, 21:99–114, 1981.

48. Wannemacher, R.W., Jr.: Key role of various individual amino acids in host response to infection. Am. J. Clin. Nutr., 30:1269–1280, 1977.

49. Adibi, S.A.: Metabolism of branched chain amino acids in altered nutrition. Metabolism, 25:1287–1302, 1976.

50. Wedge, J.H., DeCampos, R., Kerr, A., et al.: Branched chain amino acids, nitrogen excretion and injury in man. Clin. Sci. Molec. Med., 50:393–399, 1976.

51. Askanazi, J., Elwyn, D.H., Kinney, J.M., et al.: Muscle and plasma amino acids after injury: The role of inactivity. Ann. Surg., 188:797–803, 1978.

52. Askanazi, J., Carpentier, Y.A., Michelson, C.B., et al.: Muscle and plasma amino acids following injury: Influence of intercurrent infection. Ann. Surg., 792:78–85, 1980.

53. Munro, H.N.: Free amino acid pools and their role in regulation. In Munro, H.N. (ed.): Mammalian Protein Metabolism, Vol. 4, New York, Academic Press, 1970, p. 299.

54. Bergstrom, J., Furst, P., Noree L-O., and Vinnars, E.: Intracellular free amino acid concentration in human muscle tissue. J. Appl. Physiol., 36:693–697, 1974.

55. Vinnars, E., Bergstrom, J., and Fuerst, P.: Influence of the post-operative state on the intracellular free amino acids in human muscle tissue. Ann. Surg., 182:665–671, 1975.

56. Fuerst, P., Bergstrom, J., Chao, L., et al.: Influence of amino acid supply on nitrogen and amino acid metabolism in severe trauma. Acta Chir. Scand. (Suppl.), 494:136–138, 1979.

57. Wilmore, D.W., Black, P.R., and Muhlbacher, F.: Injured man: Trauma and sepsis. In Winters, R.W. (ed.): Nutritional Support of the Seriously Ill Patient. New York, Academic Press, 1983, pp. 33–52.

58. Askanazi, J., Fuerst, P., Micheken, C.B., et al.: Muscle and plasma amino acids after injury: Hypocaloric glucose vs. amino acid infusion. Ann. Surg., 191:465–472, 1980.

59. McEvoy, G.K. (ed.): American Hospital Formulary Service Drug Information '84. Bethesda, American Society of Hospital Pharmacists, Inc., 1984, pp. 972–974.

60. Garber, A.J., Karl, I.E., and Kipnis, D.M.: Alanine and glutamine synthesis and release from skeletal muscle. I: Glycolysis and amino acid release. J. Biol. Chem., 251:826–835, 1976.

61. Garber, A.J., Karl, I.E., and Kipnis, D.M.: Alanine and glutamine synthesis and release from skeletal muscle. II: The precursor role of amino acids in alanine and glutamine synthesis. J. Biol. Chem., 251:836–843, 1976.

62. Aulick, L.H., and Wilmore, D.W.: Increased peripheral amino acid release following burn injury. Surgery, 85:560–565, 1979.

63. Howard, J.M.: Studies of the absorption and metabolism of glucose following injury. Ann. Surg., 141:311–326, 1955.

64. Allison, S.P., Hinton, P., and Chamberlain, M.J.: Intravenous glucose-tolerance, insulin, and free-fatty acid levels in burned patients. Lancet, 2:1113–1116, 1968.

65. Wilmore, D.W., Mason, A.D., Jr., and Pruitt, B.A., Jr.: Insulin response to glucose in hypermetabolic burn patients. Ann. Surg., 183:314–320, 1978.

66. Long, C.L., Spencer, J.L., Kinney, J.M., and Geiger, J.W.: Carbohydrate metabolism in man: Effect of electric operations and major injury. J. Appl. Physiol., 31:110–116, 1971.

67. Wolfe, R.R., Durkot, M.J., Allsop, J.R., and Burke, J.F.: Glucose metabolism in severely burned patients. Metabolism, 28:1031–1039, 1979.

68. Wilmore, D.W., Mason, A.D., and Pruitt, B.A., Jr.: Alterations in glucose kinetics following thermal injury. Surg. Forum, 26:81–83, 1975.

69. Ruderman, M.B.: Muscle amino acid metabolism and gluconeogenesis. Ann. Rev. Med., 26:245–258, 1975.

70. Black, P.R., Brooks, D.C., Bessey, P.Q., Wolfe, R.R., and Wilmore, D.W.: Mechanisms of insulin resistance following injury. Ann. Surg., 196:420–435, 1982.

71. Brooks, D.C., Bessey, P.Q., Black, P.R., Aoki, T.T., and Wilmore, D.W.: Post-traumatic insulin resistance in uninjured skeletal muscle. J. Surg. Res., 37:100–107, 1984.

72. Askanazi, J., Carpentier, Y.A., Elwyn, D.H., et al.: Influence of total parenteral nutrition on fuel utilization in injury and sepsis. Ann. Surg., 191:40–46, 1980.

73. Souba, W.W., and Wilmore, D.W.: Postoperative alteration of arteriovenous exchange of amino acids across the gastrointestinal tract. Surgery, 94:342–350, 1983.

74. Pitts, R.F.: Renal regulation of acid base balance. *In* Physiology of Kidney and Body Fluids, 3rd ed. Chicago, Year Book Medical Publishers, 1974, pp. 217–241.

75. Vaughan, G.M., Becker, R.A., Allen, J.P., Goodwin, C.W., and Mason, A.D., Jr.: Cortisol and corticotrophin in burned patients. J. Trauma, 22:263, 1982.

76. Wilmore, D.W., Lindsey, C.A., Moylan, J.A., Faloona, G.R., Pruitt, B.A., and Unger, R.H.: Hyperglucagonaemia after burns. Lancet, 1:73–75, 1974.

77. Jaattela, A., Alho, A., Avikainen, V., et al.: Plasma catecholamines in severely injured patients: A prospective study of 45 patients with multiple injuries. Br. J. Surg., 62:177–181, 1975.

78. Davies, C.L., Newman, R.J., Molyneux, S.G., and Grahame-Smith, D.G.: The relationship between plasma catecholamines and severity of injury in man. J. Trauma, 24:99–105, 1984.

79. Harrison, T.S., Seaton, J.F., and Feller, I.: Relationship of increased oxygen consumption to catecholamine excretion in thermal burns. Ann. Surg., 165:169–172, 1967.

80. Bessey, P.Q., Watters, J.M., Aoki, T.T., and Wilmore, D.W.: Combined hormonal infusion simulates the metabolic response to injury. Ann. Surg., 200:264–281, 1984.

81. Dinarello, C.A., and Wolff, S.M.: Molecular basis of fever in humans. Am. J. Med., 72:799–819, 1982.

82. Wannemacher, R.W., Pekarek, R.S., Thompson, W.C., et al.: A protein from polymorphonuclear leukocytes (LEM) which affects the rate of hepatic amino acid transport and synthesis of acute phase globulins. Endocrinology, 96:651–659, 1975.

83. Baracos, V., Rodeman, H.P., Dinarello, C.A., and Goldberg, A.L.: Stimulation of muscle protein degradation and prostaglandin E_2 release by leukocytic pyrogen (interleukin-1): A mechanism for the increased degradation of muscle proteins during fever. N. Engl. J. Med., 308:553–558, 1983.

84. Clowes, G.H.A., George, B.C., Villee, C.A., and Saravis, C.A.: Muscle proteolysis induced by a circulating peptide in patients with sepsis or trauma. N. Engl. J. Med., 308:545–552, 1983.

85. Initial assessment and management. *In* Committee on Trauma: Trauma Life Support Course for Physicians—Student Manual. Chicago, American College of Surgeons, 1984, pp. 5–14.

86. Daws, T.A., Consolazio, C.F., Hilty, S.F., et al.: Evaluation of cardiopulmonary function and work performance in man during caloric restriction. J. Appl. Physiol., 33:211–217, 1972.

87. Levenson, S.M., and Seifter, E.: Starvation; metabolic and physiologic responses. *In* Fischer, J.E. (ed.): Surgical Nutrition. Boston, Little, Brown, 1983, pp. 423–478.

88. Studley, H.O.: Percentage of weight loss: A basic indicator of surgical risk in patients with chronic peptic ulcer. J.A.M.A., 106:458–460, 1936.

89. Benedict, F.G.: A Study of Prolonged Fasting. Publication No. 203. Washington, D.C., The Carnegie Institution of Washington, 1915, pp. 69–82.

90. Benedict, F.G.: A Study of Prolonged Fasting. Publication No. 203. Washington, D.C., The Carnegie Institution of Washington, 1915, pp. 384–391.

91. Fleisch, A.: Le métabolisme basal standard et sa détermination au moyen du Metabocalculator. Helv. Med. Acta, 18:23–44, 1951.

92. Wilmore, D.W.: The Metabolic Management of the Critically Ill. New York, Plenum Medical, 1977, p. 37.

93. DuBois, E.F.: Basal Metabolism in Health and Disease. Philadelphia, Lea & Febiger, 1936, pp. 125–144.

94. Gamble, J.L.: Physiological information gained from studies on the life raft ration. Harvey Lect., 1947, pp. 247–273.

95. Long, C.L., Spencer, J.L., Kinney, J.M., and Geiger, J.W.: Carbohydrate metabolism in normal man and effect of glucose infusion. J. Appl. Physiol., 31:102–109, 1971.

96. Wolfe, R.R., O'Donnell, T.F., Jr., Stone, M.D., et al.: Investigation of factors determining optimal glucose infusion rate in total parenteral nutrition. Metabolism, 29:892–900, 1980.

97. Askanazi, J., Elwyn, D.H., Silverberg, P.A., et al.: Respiratory distress secondary to a high carbohydrate load: A case report. Surgery, 87:596–598, 1980.

98. Sheldon, G.F., Peterson, S.R., and Sanders, R.: Hepatic dysfunction during hyperalimentation. Arch. Surg., 113:504–508, 1978.

99. Nordenstrom, J., Carpentier, Y.A., Askanazi, J., et al.: Metabolic utilization of intravenous fat emulsion during total parenteral nutrition. Ann. Surg., 196:221–231, 1982.

100. Goodenough, R.D., and Wolfe, R.R.: Effect of total parenteral nutrition on free fatty acid metabolism in burned patients. J.P.E.N., 8:357–366, 1984.

101. JeeJeebhoy, K.N., and Marliss, E.B.: Energy supply in total parenteral nutrition. *In* Fischer, J.E. (ed.): Surgical Nutrition. Boston, Little, Brown, 1983, pp. 645–662.

102. Fischer, G.W., Wilson, S.R., Hunter, K.W., and Mease, A.D.: Diminished bacterial defenses with Intralipid. Lancet, 2:819–820, 1980.

103. Matarese, L.E.: Enteral alimentation. *In* Fischer, J.E. (ed.): Surgical Nutrition. Boston, Little, Brown, 1983, pp. 719–755.

104. MacBurrey, M.M., and Wilmore, D.W.: Rational decision-making in nutritional care. Surg. Clin. North Am., 31:571–582, 1981.

105. Mochizuki, H., Trocki, O., and Dominioni, L.: Mechanism of prevention of post-burn hypermetabolism and catabolism by early enteral feeding. Ann. Surg., 200:297–310, 1984.

106. Wilmore, D.W.: The Metabolic Management of the Critically Ill. New York, Plenum Medical, 1977, pp. 188–190.

107. Howard, J.E., Parson, W., Eisenberg, K., et al.: Studies on fracture convalescence. I.: Nitrogen metabolism after fracture and skeletal operation in healthy males. Bull. Johns Hopkins Hosp., 75:151–168, 1944.

108. Deitrick, J.E., Wheldon, G.D., and Shorr, E.: The effects of immobilization upon various metabolic and physiologic functions of normal men. Am. J. Med., 4:3–36, 1948.

109. Cuthbertson, D.P.: Certain effects of massage on the metabolism of convalescing fracture cases. Q. J. Med., 25:401–408, 1932.

110. Wheldon, G.D., Deitrick, J.E., and Shorr, E.: Modifications of the effects of immobilization upon metabolic and physiologic functions of normal men by the use of an oscillating bed. Am. J. Med., 6:684–711, 1949.

111. Wilmore, D.W., Taylor, J.W., Handler, E.W., et al.: Central nervous system function following thermal injury. *In* Wilkinson, A.W., and Cuth-

bertson, D.P. (eds.): Metabolism and the Response to Injury. Chicago, Year Book Medical Publishers, 1976, pp. 274–286.

112. Dempsey, D.T., Guenter, P., Crosby, L.O., et al.: Barbiturate therapy and energy expenditure in head trauma. Presented at 42nd annual meeting of the American Association for the Surgery of Trauma, Colorado Springs, 1982.

113. Fried, R., Dempsey, D., and Guenter, P.: Barbiturates improve nitrogen balance in patients with severe head trauma (abstract). J.P.E.N., 8:86, 1984.

114. Clifton, G.L., Robertson, C.S., Grossman, R.G., et al.: The metabolic response to severe head injury. J. Neurosurg., 60:687–696, 1984.

115. Elwyn, D.H., Bryan-Brown, C.W., and Shoemaker, W.C.: Nutritional aspects of body water dislocations in postoperative and depleted patients. Ann. Surg., 182:76–85, 1975.

116. Starker, P.M., Gump, F.K., Askanazi, J., et al.: Serum albumin levels as an index of nutritional support. Surgery, 91:194–199, 1982.

117. Johnson, R.E., Norton, A.C., Kinney, J.M., et al.: Indirect calorimetry—methods and applications in man. In Kinney, J.M. (ed.): Assessment of Energy Metabolism in Health and Disease—Report of the First Ross Conference on Medical Research. Columbus, Ross Laboratories, 1980, pp. 32–62.

118. Wilmore, D.W.: The Metabolic Management of the Critically Ill. New York, Plenum Medical, 1977, pp. 11–14.

119. Peters, J.P., and Van Slyke, D.D.: Quantitative Clinical Chemistry: Interpretations, 2nd ed. Baltimore, The Williams & Wilkins Company, 1946, p. 9.

120. Cahill, G.F., Jr.: Starvation in man. N. Engl. J. Med., 282:668–675, 1970.

121. Naftel, B., Hill, O.R., and Bessey, P.Q.: Monitoring nitrogen balance in hypermetabolic patients. In preparation.

122. Moore, F.D., Langohr, J.L., Ingerbretsen, M., and Cope, O.: The role of exudate losses in the protein and electrolyte imbalance of burned patients. Ann. Surg., 132:1–19, 1950.

123. Border, J.R., Chenier, R., McMenamy, R.H., et al.: Multiple systems organ failure: Muscle fuel deficit with visceral protein malnutrition. Surg. Clin. North Am., 56:1147–1167, 1976.

124. Sapir, D.G., Walser, M., Moyer, E.D., et al.: Effects of α-ketoisocaproate and of leucine on nitrogen metabolism in postoperative patients. Lancet, 1:1010–1014, 1983.

125. Deneke, S.M., Gershoff, S.N., and Fanburg, B.L.: Potentiation of oxygen toxicity in rats by dietary protein or amino acid deficiency. J. Appl. Physiol., 54:147–151, 1983.

126. Odessey, R., Khairallah, E.A., and Goldberg, A.L.: Origin and possible significance of alanine production by skeletal muscle. J. Biol. Chem., 249:7623–7629, 1974.

127. Ryan, N.T., Blackburn, G.L., and Clowes, G.H.A., Jr.: Differential tissue sensitivity to elevated endogenous insulin levels during experimental peritonitis in rats. Metabolism, 23:1081–1089, 1974.

128. O'Donnell, T.F., Jr., Clowes, G.H.A., Jr., Blackburn, G.L., et al.: Proteolysis associated with a deficit of peripheral energy fuel substrates in septic man. Surgery, 80:192–200, 1976.

129. Blackburn, G.L., Moldawer, L.L., Usui, S., et al.: Branched chain amino acid administration and metabolism during starvation, injury, and infection. Surgery, 86:307–315, 1979.

130. Buse, M.G., and Reid, S.S.: Leucine: A possible regulator of protein turnover in muscle. J. Clin. Invest., 56:1250–1261, 1975.

131. Cerra, F.B., Upson, D., Angelico, R., et al.: Branched chains support postoperative protein synthesis. Surgery, 92:192–199, 1982.

132. Cerra, F.B., Mazuski, J., Teasley, K., et al.: Nitrogen retention in critically ill patients is proportional to branched chain amino acid load. Crit. Care Med., 11:775–778, 1983.

133. Bonau, R., Ang, S., Jeevanandam, M., and Daly, J.M.: High branched chain amino acid solutions: Relationship of composition to efficacy (abstract). J.P.E.N., 8:91, 1984.

134. Johnson, D.J., Kapadia, C.R., Jiang, Z-M., et al.: Branched chain amino acid supplementation fails to reduce post-traumatic protein catabolism. Surg. Forum, 35:102–105, 1984.

135. Dudrick, S.J., Matheny, R.G., and O'Donnell, J.J.: Effect of enriched branched chain amino acid solutions in traumatized rats (abstract). J.P.E.N., 8:86, 1984.

136. Wilmore, D.W., Curreri, P.W., Spitzer, K.W., et al.: Supranormal dietary intake in thermally injured hypermetabolic patients. Surg. Gynecol. Obstet., 132:881–886, 1971.

137. Hermann, V.M., Clarke, D., Wilmore, D.W., and Moore, F.D.: Protein metabolism: Effect of disease and altered intake on the stable ^{15}N curve. Surg. Forum, 31:92–96, 1980.

138. Apelgren, K.N., Malloy, D.F., See-Young, L., et al.: Safe maintenance parenteral nutrition in critically ill surgical patients. Presented at the 68th Annual Clinical Congress, American College of Surgeons, Chicago, 1982.

CHAPTER 28

Parenteral Nutrition in Thermal Injuries

CLEON W. GOODWIN

The metabolic response to severe injury characteristically manifests as a biphasic reaction.[1] The *ebb phase* immediately follows injury and is characterized by circulatory instability and poor tissue perfusion. It gives way to the *flow phase*, which is characterized by heightened total body blood flow and metabolic activity. Although elective surgical procedures elicit a minimal increase, major trauma and infection cause substantial elevation of metabolic expenditure (Fig. 28–1).[2, 3] However, large thermal injuries cause the greatest degree of hypermetabolism, which may exceed twice resting levels and may approach the limits of the injured patient's physiologic reserve.[4] The clinical manifestations of marked hypermetabolism are increased energy expenditure and erosion of body mass and must be counterbalanced by intensive nutritional support. Provision of nutrients by enteral techniques is safest and practical in most burned patients, but complications associated with burn injury may preclude use of the gut and dictate reliance on parenteral techniques. Postburn alterations in water and electrolyte requirements must be integrated into planning of parenteral nutrition formulations; the increase in water requirements actually may facilitate the administration of the increased nutrients required by burned patients. The use of parenteral nutrition is associated with a number of complications, most of which can be avoided by use of rigorous implementation protocols and experienced personnel.

METABOLIC RESPONSE TO THERMAL INJURY

Following adequate resuscitation of the severely burned patient, metabolic rate rises and is accompanied by an increase in total body oxygen consumption that is proportional to the extent of injury (Fig. 28–2).[4, 5] Total-body blood flow increases in concert with the rise in oxygen consumption, reaching a plateau level that may exceed two to three times that in uninjured subjects.[6, 7] Regional blood flow to the visceral organs increases following the onset of postburn hypermetabolism, but its fraction of total flow

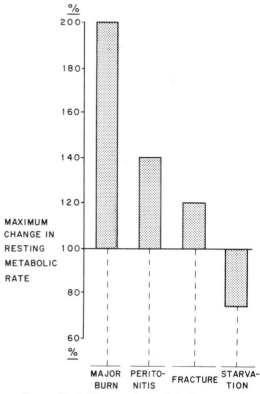

Figure 28–1. The magnitude of the hypermetabolic response to severe burns exceeds that associated with other injuries and infection. Hypometabolism is characteristic of starvation.

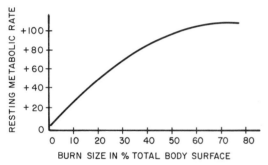

Figure 28–2. Relationship between metabolic rate and burn size. The metabolic response in burned patients is related to the extent of injury and reaches its maximum during the second week after injury. (*From* Wilmore, D. W., Long, J. C., Mason, A. D., Skreen, R. W., and Pruitt, B. A.: Catecholamines: Mediator of the hypermetabolic response to thermal injury. Ann. Surg., *180*:653, 1974, with permission.)

remains unchanged or is only slightly increased.[8] Concomitant visceral oxygen utilization, although increased, maintains an unchanged or slightly elevated proportion of total-body oxygen consumption. Although skeletal muscle appears to be an important source of carbon chains following injury, this role following thermal injury is performed without altering blood flow from preinjury levels.[9] By contrast, blood flow to the burn wound is markedly exaggerated in relation to total-body blood flow, but oxygen consumption is insignificantly elevated.[10] The burn wound appears to utilize primarily anaerobic intermediary mechanisms to effect wound repair.

With the onset of postburn hypermetabolism, heat production is elevated, and burned patients commonly exhibit elevated core and skin temperatures and higher core-to-skin heat transfer coefficients.[4] Central thermoregulation appears to be altered in burned patients, with an upward shift of the temperature of maximal comfort and least metabolic expenditure. The patients seem to be internally warm and not externally cold.[11] Attempts to modulate the hypermetabolic response by externally heating thermally injured patients above temperatures of thermoneutrality do not decrease the metabolic rate. Evaporation of one milliliter of water requires approximately 0.58 kcal of heat. Because thermal injury abolishes the water vapor barrier function of skin, evaporative water loss through the burn wound has been suggested as the etiology of the hypermetabolic response.[12–17] However, coverage of the burn wound with water-impermeable dressing under environmentally controlled conditions reduced evaporative water loss but produced only a modest reduction in metabolic rate.[18] Although animal studies indicate that caloric intake increases metabolic response over that expected from the specific dynamic action of the nutrients, such findings have not been demonstrated in burned patients.[19, 20] Only a small fraction of the hypermetabolic response can be ascribed to the endogenous specific dynamic action of accelerated protein breakdown.[21] The Q_{10} effect of hyperpyrexia accounts for only a modest fraction of postburn hypermetabolism, and the augmented heat production following injury is a consequence of an elevated metabolic state, not of increased thermoregulatory drives.[22]

Catecholamines appear to be the major mediators of the hypermetabolic response to thermal injury.[4] Adrenergic activity is related to the extent of burn injury and to total-body blood flow and oxygen consumption. In burned patients, adrenergic blockade of beta, but not alpha, receptors blunts many of the manifestations of hypermetabolism, including the rises in metabolic rate, ventilation, pulse rate, and free fatty acids. Conversely, many of the metabolic changes in burned patients can be reproduced by administering beta-adrenergic agonists to normal subjects.[24] Increased thyroid hormone activity does not appear to explain the higher metabolic response in patients with large burns.[25] Although levels of total T_3 and T_4 may be depressed and of reverse T_3 elevated following injury, the unbound metabolically active forms ("free" T_3 and T_4) are normal in stable, hypermetabolic burned patients.[26] These free fractions fall only when the patient becomes septic and clinically deteriorates. That adequate thyroid function may be necessary to facilitate physiologic adaptation by the severely burned patient to postinjury metabolic demands is demonstrated by the apparent relationships among plasma levels of T_3, T_4, and catecholamines.[27, 28] Burn injury alters adrenal activity by abolishing the normal diurnal variations in glucocorticord concentrations, but these hormones do not appear to influence metabolic activity directly and play only a permissive role in relation to the catecholamines.[29]

Nitrogen loss increases following thermal injury, and 80 to 90 per cent of the nitrogen appears in the urine as urea, which may exceed 40 gm/day in fed patients with severe burns.[30] Skin losses of nitrogen through the burn wound may account for 20 to 25 per cent of total daily nitrogen loss.[31] Over a wide range of metabolic responses, varying from those of normal, uninjured subjects to those of severely burned patients, body protein contributes a constant 15 to 20 per cent of the energy required to meet metabolic needs.[32] Measurement of whole-body protein turnover in burned patients indicates that although protein breakdown proceeds at accelerated rates, protein synthesis also continues, albeit at slower rates.[33] Alterations in nitrogen economy in regional organ beds are reflected by changes in nitrogen transfer as amino acids. Following severe burns, peripheral amino acids, principally alanine and glutamine, are released in increased quantities into the circulation.[34] Alanine appears to act as a carrier of nitrogen from muscle to liver and is derived from the transamination of pyruvate from branched-chain amino acids.[35] Skeletal muscle is the primary source of nitrogen lost in the urine, and muscle proteolysis is reflected by the increased excretion of creatinine and 3-methylhistidine.[36]

The major sources of three-carbon precursors for new glucose production by the liver are the wound and skeletal muscle. The wound utilizes glucose by anaerobic glycolytic pathways, producing large amounts of lactate as end-product. The wound meets its high glucose requirements through high glucose delivery rates, which arise from the enhanced circulation to the wound. In the liver, lactate is extracted and is utilized for new glucose production by the Cori cycle.[37] Concomitantly, alanine and other glucogenic amino acids also contribute to increased gluconeogenesis.[8, 38] Increased ureagenesis parallels the rise in hepatic glucose output. Peripheral amino acids and wound lactate account for approximately one-half to two-thirds of new glucose produced by the liver.[39] The mild hyperglycemia characteristically observed in the hypermetabolic burned patient is a consequence of accelerated glucose flow arising from increased hepatic glucose production, not from decreased peripheral utilization.[40–42]

Because glucose obtained by gluconeogenic pathways is ultimately derived from protein stores, depletion of body protein during periods of starvation leads to energy deficits and malfunctioning of glucose-dependent energetic processes at the cellular level. Active transport mechanisms responsible for maintaining transmembrane ionic gradients in erythrocytes are deranged in catabolic, thermally injured patients.[43] The abnormal sodium and potassium gradients in red blood cells can be reversed by providing high-caloric levels of carbohydrate (glucose). Hepatic clearance of indocyanine green, an energy-dependent active transport process, is decreased in severely injured patients when energy normally supplied as glucose is replaced by an isocaloric glucose-free source.[44] Glucose-insulin solutions correct the "sick cell syndrome" in burned patients, who exhibit a prompt natriuresis and nonosmotic diuresis when metabolic requirements for energy are met by glucose.[45]

NUTRITIONAL IMPLICATIONS OF THE POSTBURN METABOLIC RESPONSE

Energy requirements and nitrogen loss parallel energy expenditure and are determined by the severity of injury. To preserve body integrity following large burns, greater quantities of calories and nitrogen are necessary. The intake of nitrogen alone spares protein and improves nitrogen balance following injury. The addition of nonprotein calories to the source of nitrogen further improves nitrogen balance and allows more calories to be utilized for restoration of nitrogen balance. Energy and protein thus cooperatively contribute to this improvement in protein economy. Following parenteral administration, nitrogen balance on a fixed amino acid formulation is determined by energy content; conversely, nitrogen content determines nitrogen balance on a fixed energy formulation.[46] The addition of glucose to a carbohydrate-free diet enhances amino acid incorporation into protein with no change in the rate of protein catabolism.[47] Following injury, the individual effects of glucose and amino acids on nitrogen equilibrium appear to operate by at least two different mechanisms.[48] Amino acid administration accelerates synthesis of visceral and muscle protein without affecting the rate of protein breakdown. Glucose depresses whole-body protein breakdown and decreases the total amino acid pool, exerting little effect on protein synthesis. Both mechanisms improve nitrogen balance, and both glucose and nitrogen should be components of the nutritional regimen for severely injured, catabolic patients. Initial studies in animal models suggest that the utilization of branched-chain amino acid solutions following major surgery and trauma leads to improved nitrogen conservation and decreased muscle catabolism, but the efficacy of these formulations in burned patients remains to be demonstrated.[49]

The role of fat as a source of nonprotein calories depends on the extent of injury and associated metabolic response. When hypercaloric diets not containing nitrogen are administered, carbohydrate is more effective than fat in sparing body protein when each calorie source is used alone. The reduction in nitrogen excretion by parenteral fat emulsions is accounted for by the glycerol content of the fat emulsions.[50, 51] In patients with small burns, chronic illness, or recent elective surgery, fat and carbohydrate, when combined with protein, produce equal improvements in nitrogen balance.[52-55] In a study of severely hypermetabolic burned patients receiving constant doses of amino acid (11.7 gm/m^2/day), carbohydrate decreased nitrogen excretion, but equicaloric doses of fat (as lipid emulsions) failed to exert a similar effect.[56] The small improvement in nitrogen balance was due to the free glycerol present in the emulsion. The administration of insulin to this group of patients further decreased nitrogen loss. In contrast to the response of starved-adapted patients, the signals that increase skeletal muscle proteolysis and gluconeogenesis in hypermetabolic patients override the ability to adapt to starvation by developing ketosis, decreasing nitrogen excretion, reducing energy expenditure, and utilizing lipid substrates.[57]

NON-NUTRITIONAL METABOLIC SUPPORT MEASURES

Metabolic expenditure can be minimized by blunting a variety of stressful stimuli, as follows:

Warm Environment. Thermally injured patients, particularly children, have difficulty maintaining body temperature in cold environments; because of an apparent change in hypothalamic set point, burned patients require higher ambient temperatures for comfort.[58] The temperature of thermal neutrality in severely burned patients is 30 to 31°C, approximately four degrees higher than that in normal subjects.[59] Warming burned patients to this level decreases metabolic rate and corresponding energy requirements (Fig. 28–3).[60, 61] Thermal blankets, radiation reflectors, and heat lamps may be required to maintain the patient's temperature above 37°C.

Analgesics. Pain accompanies wound manipulation and other care procedures. Such pain accentuates metabolic expenditure, and controlled administration of narcotics will reduce metabolic rate in such patients.[24] Adequate analgesia and sedation should be provided so that patients will have periods of uninterrupted rest.

Treatment of Hypovolemia, Dehydration, and Sepsis. Because hypovolemia, dehydration, and sepsis are potent stimuli of catecholamine secretion, appropriate volume replacement and antibiotic administration should be utilized as indicated. Systemic infection accentuates erosion of body mass, and additional calories must be supplied to maintain nitrogen balance at the same level obtained on lower caloric intake before infection.[46]

Anabolic Hormones. Human growth hormone increases nitrogen retention when administered with adequate calories and nitrogen.[62] Improved nitrogen balance is reflected by increased retention of potassium, phosphorus, and amino acids. The actions of exogenous growth hormone appear to be mediated by the effects of increased insulin secretion on carbohydrate metabolism.

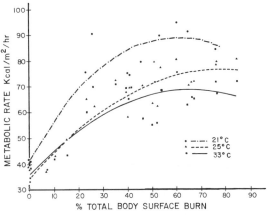

Figure 28–3. Relationship between metabolic rate and burn size at three ambient temperatures. Resting metabolic rate is minimized in a thermal neutral environment. Cooling accelerates metabolic rate and increases energy requirements.

Physical Activity. Lack of activity promotes muscle wasting and atrophy. Vigorous physical therapy promotes preservation of muscle bulk, and supervised activity must be provided continuously on a daily basis to all patients requiring prolonged hospitalization. Skeletal traction and air-fluidized beds encourage immobility and loss of lean body mass. These patients are usually capable of simple isometric exercises.

Wound Closure. Meticulous wound care and expeditious wound closure are the most effective measures of limiting the injury and its associated metabolic sequelae.

EFFECT OF BURN INJURY ON NUTRITIONAL SUPPORT

Patients with burns larger than 30 per cent of the body surface (BSA) have increased nutritional requirements that are proportioned to the size of injury. Associated injuries, such as fractures, accentuate these requirements. Such patients require long-term hospitalization, and a complete feeding program should be integrated into their total care plans from the outset. Operative procedures interrupt feeding schedules and should be organized so that maximal benefit is obtained from each procedure; each excision of the burn wound generally is limited to 20 per cent of the body surface because of the associated massive blood loss and length of anesthesia. Local debridement of the burn can be carried out with narcotic analgesia without interrupting feeding schedules. Intercurrent sepsis alters hepatic gluconeogenesis and impairs glucose tolerance, increasing the difficulty of administering the high-calorie solutions required by these patients.

Nutrient Requirements

Calories

A number of methods are available for estimating calorie requirements. On the basis of a comparison of percentage weight changes with daily calorie consumption for adult patients with a wide range of burn sizes, ideal daily calorie intake can be estimated by the following formula:[63]

kcal/day = 25 kcal/kg + 40 kcal/% BSA burned

More frequently used is the Harris-Benedict equation, which predicts basal energy expenditure on the basis of body size and age; a multiple of this equation is used to predict energy requirements in burned patients.[30] Daily calorie needs for patients with extensive burns may be estimated quite conveniently as 2000 to 2200 kcal per square meter of body surface area.[30] Since the proportional increase in metabolic rate plateaus in patients with burns exceeding 60 to 70 per cent of body surface, this last formula closely predicts requirements for a wide range of burn sizes. For difficult-to-assess patients, indirect calorimetry is helpful. The goal of nutritional support is to provide sufficient calories to meet energy expenditure and maintain lean body mass. Supranormal caloric support, although achievable in burned patients, may initiate lipogenesis and is potentially hazardous.

Nitrogen

Nitrogen requirements of burned patients exceed those of uninjured subjects, but specific guidelines are less precise for nitrogen than for calorie support. The ratio of nitrogen to energy intake (nitrogen/calorie ratio, gm/kcal) needed to achieve nitrogen equilibrium is lower in critically ill patients.[64] Injured hypermetabolic patients demonstrate inefficient utilization of administered protein and have an effective nitrogen/calorie ratio between 1:100 and 1:200, with an optimal around 1:150. Higher proportions of nitrogen intake, in animal studies, improve nitrogen balance but have no effect on body weight.[65] Higher nitrogen intake does not improve survival and may cause fatty infiltration of the liver following thermal injury.[65, 66] Thus, a nitrogen/calorie ratio of 1:150 appears to be a satisfactory guideline for determining nitrogen requirements in hypermetabolic patients and can be conveniently estimated as 15 grams per square meter of body surface area in patients with large burns.[30]

Vitamins

Vitamin requirements in critically ill hypermetabolic patients remain poorly defined. The fat-soluble vitamins (A, D, E, and K) are stored in fat depots and are slowly depleted with prolonged parenteral feeding. The water-soluble vitamins (B complex and C) are not stored in appreciable amounts and are depleted rapidly. Care must be taken to ensure that all vitamins are supplemented. The dosage guidelines recommended by the Nutritional Advisory Group of the American Medical Association (NAG/AMA) are reasonable for burned patients unless symptoms of deficiency occur.[67] Ascorbic acid plays an essential role in wound repair, and plasma levels are frequently depressed in burned patients.[68] Therefore, it seems prudent to supplement the NAG/AMA formulation with 250 to 500 mg of vitamin C daily. Larger doses may cause diarrhea and renal stone formation and will interfere with laboratory results.[69] Excessive doses of vitamins A and D produce toxic symptoms, and monitoring of serum levels is misleading if the concentrations of the vitamin carrier proteins are decreased, as commonly occurs in critically ill patients.

Trace Minerals

Even less is known about trace mineral requirements following thermal injury. Zinc is an important cofactor in wound repair, and zinc deficiency has been documented in burned patients.[70, 71] Following injury in an animal model, zinc and other trace minerals seem necessary for nitrogen retention, but these elements may only reflect nitrogen balance and have little direct influence.[72, 73] Periodic measurements of zinc, copper, manganese, and chromium levels provide the best guidelines for replacement dosages. Trace elements are present in varying concentrations as contaminants in parenteral amino acid solutions.

Fats. As discussed previously, fat appears to be an ineffective calorie source for the maintenance of nitrogen equilibrium and lean body mass in hypermetabolic patients with large burns. Patients with only moderate elevations of metabolic rate can utilize lipid calories efficiently; however, such individuals rarely require parenteral nutrition, and table food or defined formula diets contain all necessary fat nutrients. When fat is omitted from nutritional solutions of patients receiving total parenteral nutrition for prolonged periods, essential fatty acid deficiency may develop.[74-76] This deficiency manifests as dermatitis, hemolytic anemia, thrombocytopenia, impaired wound healing, loss of hair, and early death. Although no exact requirement is known, two to four per cent of daily energy requirement should consist

of linoleic acid. A triene/tetraene ratio in tissue fats greater than 0.4 indicates essential fatty acid deficiency, but such determinations are not practical clinically.[77]

Water and Electrolyte Requirements

Thermal injury destroys the water vapor barrier of skin, and the wound becomes a free water surface with unimpeded evaporative loss. Evaporative water loss can be estimated by the following formula:[78, 79]

$$\text{Water loss (ml/hr)} = (25 + \% \text{ BSA burned}) \times \text{BSA (m}^2)$$

However, environmental conditions in burn centers vary considerably, and evaporative water loss measured at 2.0 to 3.1 ml/kg body weight/% burn more accurately reflects the magnitude of daily fluid losses in burned patients.[17] Deficits of 6 to 10 L/day are not uncommon, and relatively dilute carbohydrate–amino acid solutions may satisfy daily nutritional and water requirements. Fluid replacement is best guided by daily determinations of body weight and serum sodium and osmolal concentrations. Through calculation of evaporative loss and desired urinary output, hourly infusion rates can be predicted; most adults with large burns require 200 to 250 ml/hr of fluid.

Once the huge sodium load received during resuscitation has been excreted (usually by seven to ten days after burn), adult sodium requirements are 1 to 2 mEq/kg daily. This figure may be altered drastically by certain aspects of burn care, such as use of silver nitrate dressings, which cause severe loss of not only sodium but also chloride, calcium, and potassium.[80] Hypokalemia is common after resuscitation and is associated with large losses in the urine. Such losses are accentuated by the use of mafenide acetate, a carbonic anhydrase inhibitor, as a topical antimicrobial wound agent.[81] Losses of 300 to 600 mEq/day may occur and must be replaced. Potassium moves intracellularly with glucose and amino acids and is retained in a ratio of 3 mEq of potassium for each gram of nitrogen synthesized as protein. Higher quantities of phosphorus are required when glucose intake is increased; approximately 20 to 25 mEq of phosphorus are needed for each 1000 kcal of energy administered.[82] Frequent determinations of serum sodium, potassium, chloride, calcium, magnesium, and phosphorus levels are the best clinical guides to electrolyte replacement.

Initiating Nutritional Support

No attempt is made to meet predicted nutritional requirements of acutely burned patients during the period of resuscitation and hemodynamic instability. Resuscitation is carried out by giving glucose-free balanced electrolyte solutions.[77] The infusion of glucose at this time results in marked hyperglycemia.[41] Most of the infused fluid is lost into injured tissues, and the resulting edema is reflected by weight gains of 10 to 20 per cent of preinjury weight by the end of the first postburn day. Ileus develops soon after injury and precludes use of the gastrointestinal tract for either resuscitation or feeding. After 48 to 72 hours, tissue fluid begins to be reabsorbed and excreted, and the patient returns to preinjury weight by the seventh to tenth postburn day. After fluid mobilization has returned weight to near preinjury levels and electrolyte requirements have stabilized, nutritional support can be instituted; these conditions usually are met between the fifth and tenth postburn days. Institution of full nutritional support at an earlier time, when massive fluid shifts and electrolyte fluctuations are occurring, complicates fluid management, is unnecessarily dangerous, and produces no demonstrable improvement in nutritional status.

Conditions Requiring Parenteral Nutrition

Most patients with even large thermal injuries can be successfully fed enterally.[83] However, certain aspects of burn injury render the gastrointestinal tract unsuitable for nutritional repletion, and affected patients require parenteral nutrition.

Immediately following injury, patients with burns covering more than 30 per cent of body surface commonly develop *ileus*. With successful resuscitation and subsequent resolution of edema, gastrointestinal function recovers, usually between the third and fifth postburn days.[84] Return of colon motility is much slower than of small bowel activity following trauma.[85–88] The early return of small bowel function often allows early feed-

ing of burned patients following surgery.[89] However, certain thermally injured patients, particularly the elderly and those with massive burns or inhalation injury, experience a prolonged period of paralytic ileus following thermal injury, and bowel activity may not return until after the second postburn week. When such patients are identified, parenteral nutrition should be instituted until intestinal function returns.

Sepsis, which may occur at any time during hospitalization, is associated with ileus and severe glucose intolerance, and such symptoms initially may be the only clinical evidence of this complication.[8, 41, 90] Previously tolerated feedings often must be discontinued while hyperglycemia is being controlled and the patient resuscitated. Ileus commonly persists, and nutrition is reinstituted by the parenteral route, often requiring large doses of insulin.

The gastrointestinal tract is a major target organ of the altered pathophysiologic response following burn injury. Complications uniquely associated with large burn injury include stress ulceration of the stomach and duodenum (Curling's ulcer), pancreatitis, acalculous cholecystitis, non-occlusive ischemic enterocolitis, superior mesenteric artery syndrome, and pseudo-obstruction of the colon. Any of these complications may preclude use of the gastrointestinal tract for dietary support and require parenteral alimentation to meet nutritional goals.

Curling's ulcer manifests as a spectrum of lesions in the stomach and duodenum. As verified by serial endoscopic examinations, punctate hemorrhages and shallow mucosal erosions occur soon after injury in up to 90 per cent of patients with burns of more than 35 per cent of body surface. With current prophylactic measures, these lesions do not progress unless sepsis or respiratory failure intervenes.[91, 92] Gastric acid secretion plays a primary role in this disease, but its participation is quite complex.[93–95] The results of a controlled randomized trial of antacids and placebo have demonstrated definitively the beneficial effects of continuous gastric acid neutralization: the major complications of Curling's ulcer, perforation and hemorrhage have virtually disappeared.[96] Cimetidine is equally effective in preventing Curling's ulcer.[97]

Acute *pancreatitis* may occur in patients with extensive burns, with an incidence as high as 35 per cent in patients requiring treatment in an intensive care unit.[98] Measurement of amylase excretion rate appears to be the most sensitive laboratory diagnostic study. Treatment is directed toward general supportive measures, nasogastric drainage, and parenteral alimentation.

Acute *acalculous cholecystitis* in burned patients occurs as two distinct clinical syndromes. In one form, the gallbladder is infected by hematogenous seeding from a primary source in the septic patient (usually from the invaded burn wound).[99] The other form occurs in critically ill burned patients who have developed marked dehydration, ileus, or pancreatitis. Almost all of these patients are hyperosmolar, and sepsis usually is not the inciting event. The gallbladder and its fluid in this latter presentation are often sterile. Physical examination is difficult in these patients, who may be obtunded and have painful abdominal burn wounds. Jaundice and complaints of abdominal pain in conscious patients suggest acalculous cholecystitis, and such patients should be evaluated by ultrasonography and computerized axial tomography. Once the diagnosis is made, cholecystectomy is indicated to avoid rupture of the gallbladder.

Nonocclusive ischemic enterocolitis is being increasingly recognized in severely burned patients with multisystem organ failure.[94] The lesions in the distal small bowel and colon clinically and histologically resemble those of Curling's ulcer in the upper gastrointestinal tract. These lesions bleed and perforate less often, but if the patient recovers, healing of the bowel occurs with stricture formation. Patients who develop these lesions should be put at bowel rest and fed by parenteral techniques.

Burned patients who experience marked weight loss may develop *superior mesenteric artery syndrome*. The superior mesenteric artery obstructs the transverse portion of the duodenum, and enteral alimentation becomes impossible. Gastric decompression and vigorous parenteral nutrition have reduced the need for operative intervention from 42 to 11 per cent.[100]

Pseudo-obstruction of the colon occurs in approximately one per cent of thermally injured patients.[101] All affected patients have nonpainful abdominal distension. After barium enema proves the absence of mechanical obstruction, the patient should be treated initially with tube decompression and par-enteral fluids and calories. Laparotomy and cecostomy may be necessary in cases that do not respond to conservative therapy.

PARENTERAL NUTRITION IN BURNED PATIENTS

The unique features of parenteral nutrition in burned patients relate to the large quantity of calories that must be administered, the constant risk of infection from the continued presence of necrotic burn wound, and the associated need for frequent changes of venous access. The goal of nutritional support in the critically ill burned patient is to achieve energy and nitrogen balance. As these patients stabilize, gain wound coverage, and return to normal activities, metabolic needs decrease, and diets that previously met only maintenance requirements now provide positive balances of nitrogen and energy. At this time, such supranormal diets may be tolerated safely and allow the patient to restore lost fat and lean body mass. It cannot be stressed too forcefully that every patient should receive nutritional support according to the classic hierarchy of alimentation. Oral and nonoral enteral techniques should be utilized if possible before one resorts to parenteral nutrition. Enteral alimentation is safer and, as indicated previously, is successful in the majority of hospitalized burned patients.

Components of Parenteral Solutions

Carbohydrates

Glucose is the carbohydrate most commonly used as a calorie source. It is readily available, inexpensive, and well tolerated in high concentrations after a period of adaptation. Complete oxidation of glucose yields 4.1 kcal/gm. Because fructose may precipitate lactic acidosis, hypophosphatemia, hyperuricemia, and liver dysfunction, it is rarely used.

Lipids

Parenteral emulsions are available in 10 and 20 per cent concentrations (Table 28–1). Because triglycerides exert little osmotic activity, glycerol is added in a 2.5 per cent concentration to provide sufficient osmolarity to the solutions. The two concentrations pro-

Table 28–1. COMPOSITION OF COMMERCIAL 10 PER CENT FAT EMULSIONS

COMPOSITION	INTRALIPID	LIPOSYN
Lipid (%)		
Triglycerides	10 (soybean oil)	10 (safflower oil)
Phospholipids	1.2 (egg)	1.2 (egg)
Glycerol	2.5	2.5
Fatty acids (%)		
Linoleic acid (C 18:2)	55	77
Oleic acid (C 18:1)	26	13
Palmitic acid (C 16:0)	9	7
Others	10	3
Osmolarity (mOsm/L)	280	300
Calories (kcal/ml)		
	1.1	1.1

vide 1.1 kcal/ml and 2 kcal/ml, respectively. Although the recommended dosage for adults is 2.5 gm/kg/day, up to 4 gm/kg/day is well tolerated for prolonged periods by younger patients receiving over 50 per cent of calorie requirements as fat.[102] In patients requiring prolonged parenteral nutrition, lipid emulsions effectively prevent essential fatty acid deficiencies.[74] The major essential fatty acid in both commercial preparations is linoleic acid, and 500 ml of 10 per cent lipid emulsion infused two to three times weekly meets most patients' requirements.

A number of adverse reactions may accompany the use of fat emulsions. All are rare and abate with reduction or cessation of the infusate. Pyrogenic reactions, thrombocytopenia, and hyperlipidemia occur in less than one per cent of patients. Pulmonary diffusing capacity may fall with rapid administration of an emulsion to a patient with pre-existing pulmonary insufficiency.[103] Fat deposition and microgranuloma formation in the liver may occur but are not predictably associated with liver dysfunction.[104] The available emulsions contain high concentrations of phosphate and must be used with caution in patients with renal failure.

Nitrogen

Nitrogen currently is administered by a wide variety of crystalline amino acid solutions. New solutions directed toward specific disease states appear almost daily, and practically every amino acid combination is available. Despite claims to the contrary, no specific formulation has been proved to be superior for nitrogen repletion in hypermetabolic burned patients. Albumin provides a usable but prohibitively expensive source of nitrogen. It is rapidly degraded, and its amino acid constituents are added to the body nitrogen pool. If given in sufficient quantities, exogenous albumin can achieve nitrogen balance.[105]

Vitamins

Parenteral vitamins are supplied by a variety of commercial preparations whose composition is based on empiric standards. Most do not contain a full spectrum of vitamins, and familiarity with the concentrations in each formulation is essential. One preparation (MVI-12) contains all the vitamins except K in doses meeting the guidelines of the Nutrition Advisory Group of the American Medical Association for maintenance requirements (Table 28–2).[67]

Routes of Administration

Peripheral vein infusion in the severely burned patient is never successful as the sole mode of nutritional support.[46] Peripheral administration of hypertonic solutions is associated with the rapid onset of thrombophlebitis. The so-called peripheral protein-sparing regimens supply only a small fraction of calories needed by badly burned patients.[106, 107] Protein sparing is not a unique

Table 28–2. VITAMIN REQUIREMENTS FOR DAILY MAINTENANCE

VITAMIN (units)	INFANTS AND CHILDREN <11 YEARS	OLDER CHILDREN AND ADULTS
A (IU)	2300	3300
D (IU)	400	200
E (IU)	7.0	10
K (mg)	0.2	—
Ascorbic acid (mg)	80	100
Thiamine (mg)	1.2	3
Riboflavin (mg)	1.4	3.6
Niacin (mg)	17	40
Pyridoxine (mg)	1	4
Pantothenic acid (mg)	5	15
Folic acid (μg)	140	400
B_{12} (μg)	1	60
Biotin (μg)	20	60

(From Shils, M. E.: Parenteral multivitamins: Time for changes. Bull. Parenter. Drug Assoc., *30*:226, 1976, with permission.)

feature of amino acids alone, and the effect of amino acids is not related to endogenous fat mobilization.[108, 109] In general, this technique does not totally reverse negative nitrogen balance, and most of the administered amino acid is catabolized and excreted as urea.[110] Parenteral infusion either by peripheral vein or by central vein can be used to supplement the enteral intake of burned patients with inadequate gastrointestinal function. Combined enteral and parenteral feeding is the most common use of the intravenous alimentation in the burned patient. In many patients, only a limited volume can be enterally infused before large residuals begin to accumulate. Because of the large evaporative losses and associated fluid requirements, nutritional goals can be met by concomitant administration of isosmotic parenteral solutions.[46] Total parenteral nutrition (TPN) by continuous central vein infusion is the only means of meeting complete nutritional requirements when enteral feeding is not feasible.

Formulations of TPN Solutions

The daily diet utilizing TPN can be constructed easily by following a logical sequence of calculations.

1. Determine the patient's daily fluid requirements.

2. Determine the patient's energy requirements (by direct measurements or by nomograms that reflect the effect of burn injury severity).[111]

3. Decide on optimal nitrogen/calorie ratio. This ratio is 1:150 for critically ill, hypermetabolic burned patients. Nitrogen is administered as crystalline amino acids.

4. Distribute glucose and amino acids evenly in the fluid to be administered.

5. Add vitamins, electrolytes, and essential fatty acids as indicated by known daily requirements and timely laboratory determinations.

The fluid volume and energy requirements of most severely burned patients result in nutrition solutions containing approximately 1 kcal/ml. Solutions should be prepared in a special section of the hospital pharmacy department by a pharmacist who is a member of a multidisciplinary team with primary responsibility for advanced hospital nutrition support techniques. The glucose and amino acid portions should not be combined until shortly before use. If the two ingredients are allowed to remain mixed for prolonged periods, they combine to form glucosamines (Maillard reaction), which discolor the solutions and bind zinc and copper following infusion.[112]

Administration of Parenteral Fluids

The introduction of central venous cannulation techniques provided the technical means to administer hypertonic parenteral solution for complete nutrition.[113, 114] Although the catheter can be introduced safely through the internal jugular and external jugular veins, the infraclavicular subclavian vein is the most popular approach for long-term parenteral nutrition.[115–117] Central venous cannulation is not a technique that should be carried out by occasional users, especially in critically burned patients who lack the additional physiologic reserve to respond to associated complications of the insertion.[118] Rather, vascular access is the responsibility of the experienced burn center surgeon (more than 1000 insertions) who uses these techniques daily.

Catheter insertion is a sterile procedure, and the operator should wear a gown, gloves, and a mask.[117, 119, 120] Adequate preparation of the skin before insertion is the most effective means of limiting catheter-related infection.[121] Insertion sites closer to the midline than described in the original literature ensure a higher success rate and lower incidence of complications of subclavian vein catheterization.[122] Following insertion, the catheter is advanced into the vena cava. Intrusion of the catheter into the cardiac chambers is associated with a high incidence of endocarditis in burned patients, and roentgenograms must verify that this break in technique has not occurred.[123, 124]

Because the risk of catheter-related infection in burned patients rises markedly with time, central venous catheters should be replaced every 48 to 72 hours.[125, 126] Catheter tips should be cultured in conjunction with simultaneously drawn blood cultures.[127] Application of antibiotic ointments to the insertion site and intravenous line filters do not affect the incidence of infection.[121, 128, 129] In addition to the approaches to the superior vena cava, the requirement for frequent cannula changes in the burned patients mandates use of the inferior vena cava via the femoral vein. This route is associated with a higher incidence of infection and thrombosis and should be used only as a temporary expedient when tributaries of the superior cava are difficult to cannulate.[130]

Hypertonic solutions are administered by infusion pumps beginning at relatively slow infusion rates (1 L/24 hr.). Gradually, the infusion rate is increased to the maximal levels of fluid and energy requirements. The speed with which the infusion rate can be increased is determined by the patient's glucose tolerance. With each increment, small doses of insulin may be administered subcutaneously or may be added to the infusion to facilitate normoglycemia. Later, as the patient's endogenous insulin production increases, exogenous insulin may be decreased or eliminated.

Monitoring Patient Response to Nutritional Regimens

The high incidence of associated dangerous complications necessitates frequent monitoring of the hypermetabolic burned patient receiving a high-calorie diet. In addition, a systematic monitoring protocol facilitates assessment of nutritional status. The patient's nutrient and fluid needs must be reviewed daily and correlated with laboratory data (Table 28–3).

Tests of immunocompetence and carrier protein, although useful in chronically ill patients, have not yet been demonstrated to predict nutritional status in burned patients.[132, 133] The best measures for assessing the adequacy of nutritional support in burned patients are body weight, nitrogen balance, and calorie counts. Standard anthropometric measurements, such as triceps skinfold thickness, arm-muscle circumference, and creatinine/height index, are valuable for patients with chronic diseases but often are unusable in burned patients who have extensive skin wounds and, frequently, amputations. Change in body weight is the most easily quantified index of metabolic balance. The magnitude and duration of weight loss are related directly to the extent of burn injury.[134] Weight loss is not obligatory and can be reversed with vigorous nutritional support. Rapid changes in weight almost always arise from alterations in body water balance. An increase in weight exceeding 0.4 kg/day in an adult indicates water accumulation. Comparison of intake and output rec-

Table 28–3. MONITORING SEVERELY BURNED PATIENTS RECEIVING PARENTERAL NUTRITION

VARIABLE	FREQUENCY OF MONITORING IN THE FIRST WEEK
Energy balance	
Weight	Daily
Indirect calorimetry	As needed
Fluid balance	
Volume of infusate	Daily
Oral intake (if any)	Daily
Urinary output	Daily
Other losses	Daily
Metabolic variables	
Blood measurements:	
Plasma electrolytes (Na^+, K^+, Cl^-)	Daily
Blood urea nitrogen	Daily
Creatinine	Daily
Osmolarity	Daily
Total calcium and inorganic phosphate	3× weekly
Glucose	Daily
Liver profile	3× weekly
Total protein and fractions	2× weekly
Acid-base status	As indicated
Hemoglobin	Daily
Prothrombin time	Weekly
Magnesium	2× weekly
Triglyceride	Weekly
Urine measurements	
Glucose	4–6× daily
Specific gravity or osmolarity	2–4× daily
Urea (for balance studies)	As indicated
Creatinine	Daily
Sodium	Daily
Potassium	Daily
Prevention and detection of infection	
Clinical observations (activity, temperature, symptoms)	Daily
WBC and differential counts	As indicated
Cultures	As indicated

ords with weight changes allows accurate estimates of lean body mass alteration in most situations. Long-term trends are most useful.

Nitrogen balance studies reflect alterations in body protein stores. Nitrogen balance is the algebraic sum of daily intake and loss of nitrogen. Intake is easily quantified, but nitrogen loss is difficult to determine in burned patients because of the difficulty of measuring losses through the burn wound.[31] Calorie counts are carried by the dietician and dietary technicians working with the nutrition support team. When they are combined with daily weight determinations and nitrogen balance studies, the overall effectiveness of nutritional support in preserving or restoring body mass can be assessed on a

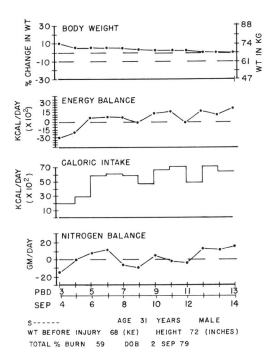

Figure 28–4. Computerized monitoring chart of nutritional status of the burned patient. Such charts posted by bedside provide constant reminder to the patient and nursing staff of the importance of adequate nutrition.

continuous basis (Fig. 28–4). Computer monitoring of nutritional support provides a means for accurate record-keeping and for quality control and evaluation of techniques and diets.[135] The data files store information about each nutrient, laboratory data, patient condition, and associated complications.

Complications of Parenteral Nutrition
(Table 28–4)

Mechanical Complications

Mechanical complications related to catheter malposition usually are not hazardous to the patient initially. Instead of turning down into the superior vena cava, the cannula inserted through the subclavian vein may pass into the internal jugular vein or, rarely, into the opposite subclavian vein. Before infusion of hypertonic fluids, the misplaced catheter should be repositioned into the superior vena cava, where maximal flow and dilution of infusate occur.

Pneumothorax is the most common and potentially most dangerous mechanical complication. As with most of the mechanical complications, the incidence of pneumothorax is related to physician experience with

catheter placement. The incidence of pneumothorax following subclavian catheterization by members of an experienced nutrition support team is commonly less than one or two per cent. Excessive bleeding can occur in patients with severe thrombocytopenia (platelet count less than 25,000/ml), and if central venous catheterization is imperative, platelet transfusions should be administered.

Transient phrenic nerve paralysis, air embolism, and hydromediastinum may occur less frequently following superior vena cava cannulation.[136–138] Most potential complications can be prevented or detected early by adhering to strict insertion protocols and by obtaining a postinsertion roentgenogram.

Infectious Complications

The most serious late complication of TPN is catheter sepsis, which is defined as a febrile episode that is unexplained by another identifiable septic focus and that is relieved by removal of the catheter. Although patients receiving TPN often have diseases and are receiving medications that predispose them to infection, the adherence to a strict protocol of catheter care can reduce the incidence of catheter sepsis to under five per cent. With rare exception, the central venous cannula should not be used for hemodynamic moni-

Table 28–4. MECHANICAL AND INFECTIOUS COMPLICATIONS OF CENTRAL VEIN CATHETERIZATION

Mechanical	Pneumothorax
	Hemothorax
	Arterial or venous laceration
	Air embolism
	Cardiac perforation and tamponade
	Hydromediastinum
	Subclavian vein or superior vena cava thrombosis
	Catheter embolism
	Pulmonary embolism
	Thoracic duct laceration
	Cardiac arrhythmias
	Subcutaneous emphysema
	Nerve injury (brachial plexus, phrenic, vagus)
	Improper catheter location
Infectious	Endocarditis
	Septic thrombophlebitis
	Septic embolism
	Septicemia arising from contaminated catheter or contaminated parenteral solution

toring, the infusion of blood products, blood sampling, or the administration of medications or other parenteral agents. Parenteral solutions are excellent culture media and should be freshly prepared or refrigerated until used. Members of the *Klebsiella*, *Enterobacter*, and *Serratia* genera have a unique ability to grow in hypertonic nutrition fluids, and episodes of septicemia produced by contaminated solutions have been reported.[139, 140] Although *Candida* species are the most common agents causing septicemia in the general patient population, staphylococci and gram-negative organisms more frequently do so in burned patients.[125, 141]

The most dangerous catheter-related infectious complication is suppurative thrombophlebitis.[125, 142, 143] Local signs of infection are present in only 35 per cent of affected patients. Mortality is high, and treatment requires removal of the cannula, appropriate antibiotics, and excision of the involved peripheral vein. In recent years, central venous cannulation has been used with increasing frequency for fluid administration; this trend seems to have reduced the incidence of suppurative thrombophlebitis (Fig. 28–5).[125] Obviously, an infected central vein is not amenable to surgical excision; antibiotics and systemic anticoagulation are required for prolonged periods.

Metabolic Complications

A large number of metabolic complications have been associated with the admin-

istration of specific nutrients; the major complications are listed in Table 28–5.

Hyperglycemia, the most common complication, is accentuated by sepsis, hypovolemia, hypokalemia, and certain drugs. Pronounced hyperglycemia leads to glycosuria and an osmotic diuresis, resulting in dehydration and hyperosmolarity. Hyperglycemia following the institution of TPN is treated with exogenous insulin and/or a reduction in the rate of glucose administration. Often, hyperglycemia can be avoided by slowly increasing the daily glucose dose to the desired caloric levels, allowing the pancreas to adapt gradually to new endogenous insulin requirements. If this regimen is unsuccessful, insulin is administered in dosages usually determined by the degree of glycosuria. If the patient has a high renal threshold for glucose, which can be determined by simultaneously obtained blood glucose concentrations, or if the patient has diabetes mellitus with a known insulin requirement, proportionately higher doses of insulin will be needed. Except in patients with diabetes mellitus, ketonemia and ketonuria do not often accompany, and are largely prevented by, the use of hypertonic glucose and rarely occasion the need for additional insulin. If the severely stressed patient receiving TPN becomes hyperglycemic with glycosuria and dehydration, it is virtually impossible to treat the hyperglycemia without first correcting the deficit of free water and intravascular volume. Correction requires using five per cent dextrose solutions and restoring electro-

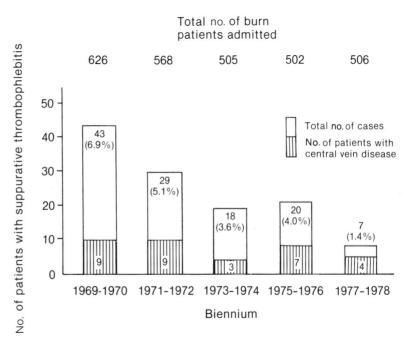

Figure 28–5. Incidence of suppurative thrombophlebitis. Note the declining incidence of this complication with increasing utilization of central venous cannulation for vascular access.

Table 28–5. METABOLIC COMPLICATIONS OF TOTAL PARENTERAL NUTRITION

COMPLICATION(s)	POSSIBLE CAUSE(s)	SOLUTION(s)
Glucose-related		
Hyperglycemia, glycosuria, hyperosmolar dehydration	Excessive rate of infusion of glucose; inadequate endogenous insulin; sepsis; glucocorticoids; hypokalemia	Reduce glucose infusion rate; administer insulin; utilize fat emulsion as portion of calories; replace potassium; correct fluid deficit
Ketoacidosis (rare)	Inadequate endogenous insulin response; insufficient exogenous insulin therapy	Give insulin; reduce glucose administration
Postinfusion (rebound) hypoglycemia	Persistence of increased insulin secretion rates by islet cells following abrupt cessation of hypertonic glucose infusions	Administer 5 to 10% glucose before discontinuing infusions
Respiratory failure	Increased triglyceride synthesis following calorie excess	Reduce glucose infusion rate; utilize fat emulsion as portion of calories
Fat-related		
Pyrogenic reaction	Fat emulsion	Exclude other causes of fever
Altered coagulation	Hyperlipemia	Remeasure coagulation after fat has cleared from bloodstream
Hyperlipemia	Rapid infusion; decreased clearance	Decrease of rate of infusion; reassess after lipid has cleared from bloodstream
Impairment of liver function	Possibly fat emulsion, but more likely underlying disease process	Exclude other causes of hepatic dysfunction
Essential fatty acid deficiency	Absence or inadequate administration of essential fatty acid, especially of linoleic acid; vitamin E deficiency	Give parenteral lipid emulsions
Amino acid-related		
Hyperchloremic acidosis	Excessive chloride content of some crystalline amino acid solutions	Administer Na^+ and K^+ as acetate or lactate salts
Hyperammonemia	Deficiencies of specific amino acids in TPN solutions, especially arginine; primary liver disease	Reduce total amino acid intake; administer specific amino acid (arginine)
Prerenal azotemia	Excessive amino acid infusion with inadequate nonprotein calories	Reduce amino acid intake; increase glucose calories
Amino acid imbalance	Optimal amino acid mixtures not yet determined for specific disease processes	Utilize low concentrations (2 to 3%) of amino acids; experimental amino acid solutions

lyte balance. The azotemia often associated with hyperglycemic, hyperosmolar dehydration readily responds to fluid replacement. Glucose-free solutions containing insulin should not be used in most cases, because sudden and unexpected hypoglycemia may occur. When the patient's fluid and electrolyte abnormalities have returned to normal levels and body weight is restored, TPN can be resumed slowly, with additional insulin, if necessary.

The consequences of carbohydrate overload have not been defined specifically in burned patients. Carbohydrate loads in excess of estimated energy requirements have been implicated as a cause of liver function impairment in burned patients.[56, 143] Hepatic dysfunction may occur during TPN administration.[144] Affected patients develop jaundice without pruritus or prominent hepatomegaly. Although the serum bilirubin may be substantially elevated (exceeding 10 mg/dl), alkaline phosphatase usually exhibits a mild and transient rise. Liver histology reflects fatty infiltration and intrahepatic cholestasis. The hepatic steatosis secondary to TPN may be treated by lowering the glucose concentration of the infusate or by administering glucose-free amino acid solutions. Even less well defined in hypermetabolic patients is the adverse effect of excess carbohydrate on pulmonary function. When carbohydrate is administered in quantities that exceed metabolic expenditure, fat is synthesized and respiratory quotient exceeds unity. Carbon dioxide production at this point greatly accelerates, requiring increasing respiratory exchange to eliminate this gas. In critically ill patients, this series of events may precipitate respiratory failure and necessitate ventilatory assistance.[145-147] However, attempts to raise the respiratory quotient above unity in severely burned patients by administering greatly excessive calories have been unsuccessful.[20]

When lipids are omitted from the diet for more than one to two weeks, unsaturated fatty acid deficits occur and cause a characteristic deficiency syndrome.

The hyperammonemia associated with protein hydrolysates and the metabolic acidosis associated with the hydrochloride salts of amino acids are now rarely encountered. Occasionally, these complications, as well as azotemia, occur in infants and small children receiving large volumes of amino acid solutions deficient in histidine and arginine.[148] These disorders can be treated by ensuring that adequate nonprotein calories are administered with amino acids (which should include histidine and arginine) or by decreasing the rate of administration of the amino acid solutions.

Vitamin overdoses (especially of A and D) and deficiencies are avoided by the daily administration of recommended allowances and by clinical laboratory assessment. Daily calcium requirements vary, but the amount given must prevent bone demineralization while avoiding soft tissue calcification. Increased protein intake and immobilization accentuate calcium loss in the urine. Hypercalcemia may be caused by excessive vitamin D, phosphate deficiency, inactivity, and overzealous calcium administration. Phosphate deficiency usually arises from inadequate administration. Sudden infusion of a large glucose load (as with the inappropriate institution of TPN) may elicit a profound drop in serum phosphate; conversely, hyperphosphatemia may occur when glucose administration is reduced.[149] Adequate phosphate intake is essential for nitrogen retention, with approximately 85 mg of phosphate required for each gram of nitrogen incorporated.[150] Severe hypophosphatemia (less than 1.0 mg/kl) causes reduced erythrocyte concentrations of 2,3-diphosphoglycerate, increased oxygen affinity for hemoglobin, hemolytic anemia, altered phagocytosis, hyperventilation, seizures, and coma.[151]

Magnesium, for which there is a well-established requirement, is frequently overlooked in planning of TPN. The administration of amphotericin, carbenicillin, and other drugs accentuate urinary magnesium losses, which must be replaced. Because magnesium is an intracellular cation, serum magnesium determinations may not reflect acute losses. Balance studies calculated from urine and drainage collections will provide a more accurate quantification of daily magnesium requirements.

REFERENCES

1. Cuthbertson, D.P., and Tilstone, W.J.: Metabolism during the postinjury period. Adv. Clin. Chem., 12:1, 1969.
2. Gump, F.E., Partin, P., and Kinney, J.M.: Oxygen consumption and caloric expenditure in surgical patients. Surg. Gynecol. Obstet., 137:499, 1973.
3. Long, C.L.: Energy balance and carbohydrate metabolism in infection and sepsis. Am. J. Clin. Nutr., 30:1301, 1977.
4. Wilmore, D.W., Long, J.C., Mason, A.D., Skreen, R.W., and Pruitt, B.A., Jr.: Catecholamines: Mediator of the hypermetabolic response to thermal injury. Ann. Surg., 180:653, 1974.
5. Gump, F.E., and Kinney, J.M.: Energy balance and weight loss in burned patients. Arch. Surg., 103:442, 1971.
6. Gump, F.E., Price, J.B., Jr., and Kinney, J.M.: Blood flow and oxygen consumption in patients with severe burns. Surg. Gynecol. Obstet., 130:23, 1970.
7. Wilmore, D.W., Aulick, L.H., Mason, A.D., Jr., and Pruitt, B.A., Jr.: Influence of the burn wound on local and systemic responses to injury. Ann. Surg., 186:444, 1977.
8. Wilmore, D.W., Goodwin, C.W., Aulick, L.H., Powanda, M.C., Mason, A.D., Jr., and Pruitt, B.A., Jr.: Effect of injury and infection on visceral metabolism and circulation. Ann. Surg., 192:491, 1980.
9. Aulick, L.H., Wilmore, D.W., Mason, A.D., Jr., and Pruitt, B.A., Jr.: Muscle blood flow following thermal injury. Ann. Surg., 188:778, 1978.
10. Aulick, L.H., Wilmore, D.W., Mason, A.D., Jr., and Pruitt, B.A., Jr.: Influence of the burn wound on peripheral circulation in thermally injured patients. Am. J. Physiol., 233:H520, 1977.
11. Wilmore, D.W., Orcutt, T.W., Mason, A.D., Jr., and Pruitt, B.A., Jr.: Alterations in hypothalamic function following thermal injury. J. Trauma, 15:697, 1975.
12. Roe, F.C., Kinney, J.M., and Blair, C. Water and heat exchange in third degree burns. Surgery, 56:212, 1964.
13. Gump, F.E., and Kinney, J.M.: Caloric and fluid losses through the burn wound. Surg. Clin. North Am., 50:1235, 1970.
14. Birke, G., Carlson, L.A., von Euler, V.S., Lilledahl, S.O., and Plantin, L.O.: Lipid metabolism, catecholamine excretion, basal metabolic rate, and water loss during treatment of burns with warm dry air. Acta Chir. Scand., 138:321, 1972.
15. Neely, W.A., Petro, A.B., Holloman, G.H., Rushton, F.W., Turner, D.M., and Hardy, J.D.: Researches on the cause of burn hypermetabolism. Ann. Surg., 179:291, 1974.

16. Caldwell, F.T.: Energy metabolism following thermal burns. Arch. Surg., *111*:181, 1976.

17. Harrison, H.N., Moncrief, J.A., Duckett, J.W., and Mason, A.D.: The relationship between energy metabolism and water loss from vaporization in severely burned patients. Surgery, *56*:203, 1964.

18. Zawacki, B.F., Spitzer, K.W., Mason, A.D., and Johns, L.A.: Does increased evaporative water loss cause hypermetabolism in burned patients? Ann. Surg., *171*:236, 1970.

19. Wolfe, R.R., Durkot, M.J., Clarke, C.C., Bode, H.H., and Burke, J.F.: Effect of food intake on hypermetabolic response to burn injury in guinea pigs. J. Nutr., *110*:1310, 1980.

20. Wilmore, D.W., Curreri, P.W., Spitzer, K.W., Mason, A.D., Jr., and Pruitt, B.A., Jr.: Supranormal dietary intake in thermally injured hypermetabolic patients. Surg. Gynecol. Obstet., *132*:881, 1971.

21. Gusberg, R.J., Scholz, P.M., Gump, F.E., and Kinney, J.M.: Can protein breakdown explain the increased calorie expenditure in injury and sepsis? Surg. Forum, *24*:79, 1973.

22. Aulick, L.H., Hander, E.H., Wilmore, D.W., Mason, A.D., Jr., and Pruitt, B.A., Jr.: The relative significance of thermal and metabolic demands on burn hypermetabolism. J. Trauma, *19*:559, 1979.

23. Harrison, T.S., Seaton, J.F., and Feller, I.: Relationship of increased oxygen consumption to catecholamine excretion in thermal burns. Ann. Surg., *165*:169, 1967.

24. Taylor, J.W., Hander, E.W., Skreen, R., and Wilmore, D.W.: The effect of central nervous system narcosis on the sympathetic response to stress. J. Surg. Res., *20*:313, 1976.

25. Cope, O., Nardi, G.L., Quijano, M., Rovit, R.L., Stanbury, J.B., and Wight, A.: Metabolic rate and thyroid function following acute thermal trauma in man. Ann. Surg., *137*:165, 1953.

26. Becker, R.A., Wilmore, D.W., Goodwin, C.W., Jr., Zitzka, C.A., Wartofsky, L., Burman, K.D., Mason, A.D., and Pruitt, B.A., Jr.: Free T_4, free T_3, and reverse T_3 in critically ill, thermally injured patients. J. Trauma, *20*:713, 1980.

27. Becker, R.A., Vaughan, G.M., Goodwin, C.W., Jr., Ziegler, M.G., Harrison, T.S., Mason, A.D., Jr., and Pruitt, B.A., Jr.: Plasma norepinephrine, epinephrine, and thyroid hormone interactions in severely burned patients. Arch. Surg., *115*:439, 1980.

28. Becker, R.A., Vaughan, G.M., and Goodwin, C.W., Jr., Ziegler, M.G., Zitzka, C.A., Mason, A.D., Jr., and Pruitt, B.A., Jr.: Interactions of thyroid hormones and catecholamines in severely burned patients. Rev. Infect. Dis., *5*:908, 1983.

29. Vaughan, G.M., Becker, R.A., Allen, J.P., Goodwin, C.W., and Mason, A.D., Jr.: Cortisol and corticotrophin in burned patients. J. Trauma, *22*:263, 1982.

30. Wilmore, D.W.: Nutrition and metabolism following thermal injury. Clin. Plast. Surg., *1*:603, 1979.

31. Soroff, H.S., Pearson, E., and Artz, C.P.: An estimation of the nitrogen requirements for equilibrium in burned patients. Surg. Gynecol. Obstet., *112*:159, 1961.

32. Duke, J.H., Jorgensen, S.B., Broell, J.R., Long, C.L., and Kinney, J.M.: Contribution of protein to caloric expenditure following injury. Surgery, *68*:168, 1970.

33. Kien, C.L., Young, V.R., Rohrbaugh, D.K., and Burke, J.F.: Increased rates of whole body protein synthesis and breakdown in children recovering from burns. Ann. Surg., *187*:383, 1978.

34. Aulick, L.H., and Wilmore, D.W.: Increased peripheral amino acid release following burn injury. Surgery, *85*:560, 1979.

35. Odessey, R., Khairallah, E.A., and Goldberg, A.L.: Origin and possible significance of alanine production by skeletal muscle. J. Biol. Chem., *23*:7623, 1974.

36. Bilmazes, C., Kien, C.L., Rohrbaugh, D.K., Vady, R., Burke, J.F., Munro, H.N., and Young, V.R.: Quantitative contribution by skeletal muscle to elevated rates of whole-body protein breakdown in burned children as measured by N^+-methyl-histidine output. Metabolism, *27*:671, 1978.

37. Felig, P.: The glucose-alanine cycle. Metabolism, *22*:179, 1973.

38. Gump, F.E., Long, C.L., Geiger, J.W., and Kinney, J.M.: The significance of altered gluconeogenesis in surgical catabolism. J. Trauma, *15*:704, 1975.

39. Goodwin, C.W., Jr., Aulick, L.H., Powanda, M.C., Wilmore, D.W., and Pruitt, B.A., Jr.: Glucose dynamics following severe injury. Eur. Surg. Res. 12(Suppl. 1):126, 1980.

40. Long, C.L., Spencer, J.L., Kinney, J.M., and Geiger, J.W.: Carbohydrate metabolism in man: Effect of elective operations and major injury. J. Appl. Physiol., *31*:110, 1971.

41. Wilmore, D.W., Mason, A.D., Jr., and Pruitt, B.A., Jr.: Impaired glucose flow in burned patients with gram-negative sepsis. Surg. Gynecol. Obstet., *143*:720, 1976.

42. Wilmore, D.W., Mason, A.D., Jr., and Pruitt, B.A., Jr.: Insulin response to glucose in hypermetabolic burn patients. Ann. Surg., *183*:314, 1976.

43. Curreri, P.W., Wilmore, D.W., Mason, A.D., Jr., Newsome, T.W., Asch, M.J., and Pruitt, B.A., Jr.: Intracellular cation alterations following major trauma: Effect of supranormal caloric intake. J. Trauma, *11*:390, 1971.

44. McDougal, W.S., Wilmore, D.W., and Pruitt, B.A., Jr.: Glucose-dependent hepatic membrane transport in nonbacteremic and bacteremic thermally injured patients. J. Surg. Res., *22*:697, 1977.

45. Allison, S.P., Hinton, P., and Chamberlain, M.J.: Intravenous glucose-tolerance, insulin, and free-fatty acid levels in burned patients. Lancet, *2*:1113, 1968.

46. McDougal, W.S., Wilmore, D.W., and Pruitt, B.A., Jr.: Effect of intravenous near isosmotic nutrient infusions on nitrogen balance in critically injured patients. Surg. Gynecol. Obstet., *145*:408, 1977.

47. Sim, A.J.W., Young, V.R., Wolfe, B.M., Clarke, D., and Moore, F.D.: Glucose promotes whole-body protein synthesis from infused amino acids in fasting man. Lancet, *1*:68, 1979.

48. Moldawer, L.L., O'Keefe, S.J.D., Bothe, A., Bistrian, B.R., and Blackburn, G.L.: In vivo demonstration of nitrogen-sparing mechanisms for glucose and amino acids in the injured rat. Metabolism, *29*:173, 1980.

49. Freund, H., Yoshimura, N., Lunetta, L., and Fischer, J.E.: The role of the branched-chain amino acids in decreasing muscle catabolism in vivo. Surgery, *83*:611, 1978.

50. Brennan, M.F., Fitzpatrick, G.F., Cohen, K.H., and Moore, F.D.: Glycerol: Major contributor to the short term protein sparing effect of fat emulsions in normal man. Ann. Surg., *182*:386, 1975.

51. Brennan, M.F., and Moore, F.D.: An intravenous fat emulsion as a nitrogen sparer: Comparison with glucose. J. Surg. Res., 14:501, 1973.

52. Silberman, H., Freehauf, M., Fong, G., and Rosenblatt, N.: Parenteral nutrition with lipids. J.A.M.A., 238:1380, 1977.

53. Jeejeebhoy, K.N., Anderson, G.H., Nakhooda, A.F., Greenberg, G.R., Sanderson, I., and Marliss, E.B.: Metabolic studies in total parenteral nutrition with lipid in man. J. Clin. Invest., 57:125, 1976.

54. Gassaniga, A.B., Bartlett, R.H., and Shobe, J.B.: Nitrogen balance in patients receiving either fat or carbohydrate for total intravenous nutrition. Ann. Surg., 182:163, 1975.

55. Elwyn, D.H., Kinney, J.M., Gump, F.E., Askanazi, J., Rosenbaum, S.H., and Carpenter, Y.A.: Some metabolic effects of fat infusions in depleted patients. Metabolism, 29:125, 1980.

56. Long, J.M., Wilmore, D.W., Mason, A.D., Jr., and Pruitt, B.A., Jr.: Effect of carbohydrate and fat intake on nitrogen excretion during total intravenous feeding. Ann. Surg., 185:417, 1977.

57. Birkhahn, R.H., Long, C.L., Fitkin, D.L., Busnardo, A.C., Geiger, J.W., and Blakemore, W.S.: A comparison of the effects of skeletal trauma and surgery on the ketosis of starvation in man. J. Trauma, 21:513, 1981.

58. Wilmore, D.W., Long, J.M., Mason, A.D., Jr., and Pruitt, B.A., Jr.: Stress in surgical patients as a neurophysiologic reflex response. Surg. Gynecol. Obstet., 142:257, 1976.

59. Wilmore, D.W., Mason, A.D., Jr., Johnson, D.W., and Pruitt, B.A., Jr.: Effect of ambient temperature on heat production and heat loss in burn patients. J. Appl. Physiol., 38:593, 1975.

60. Crowley, L.V., Seifter, E., Kriss, P., Rettura, G., Nakao, K., and Levenson, S.M.: Effects of environmental temperature and femoral fracture on wound healing in rats. J. Trauma, 17:436, 1977.

61. Cuthbertson, D.P., Dell, G.S., Smith, C.M., and Tilstone, W.J.: Metabolism after injury. I: Effects of severity, nutrition, and environmental temperature on protein, potassium, zinc and creatinine. Br. J. Surg., 59:68, 1972.

62. Wilmore, D.W., Moylan, J.A., Jr., Bristow, B.F., Mason, A.D., Jr., and Pruitt, B.A., Jr.: Anabolic effects of human growth hormone and high caloric feedings following thermal injury. Surg. Gynecol. Obstet., 138:875, 1974.

63. Curreri, P.W., Richmond, D., Marvin, J., and Baxter, C.R.: Dietary requirements of patients with major burns. J. Am. Diet. Assoc., 65:415, 1974.

64. Long, C.L., Crosby, F., Geiger, J.W., and Kinney, J.M.: Parenteral nutrition in the septic patient: Nitrogen balance, limiting plasma amino acids, and calorie to nitrogen ratios. Am. J. Clin. Nutr., 29:380, 1976.

65. Dominioni, L., Trocki, O., Fang, C.H., and Alexander, J.W.: Nitrogen balance and liver changes in burned guinea pigs undergoing prolonged high-protein enteral feeding. Surg. Forum, 34:99, 1983.

66. Markley, K., Smallman, E., and Thornton, S.W.: The effect of diet protein on late mortality. Proc. Soc. Exp. Biol. Med., 135:94, 1970.

67. Shils, M.E.: Parenteral multivitamins: Time for changes. Bull. Parenter. Drug Assoc., 30:226, 1976.

68. Lund, C.C., Levenson, S.M., and Green, R.W.: Ascorbic acid, thiamine, riboflavin and nicotinic acid in relation to acute burns in man. Arch. Surg., 55:557, 1946.

69. Smith, H.L., and Posner, E.: Large ascorbic acid intake. N. Engl. J. Med., 287:412, 1972.

70. Pories, W.J., Henzel, J.H., Rob, C.G., and Strain, W.H.: Acceleration of wound healing in man with zinc sulfate given by mouth. Lancet, 1:7482, 1967.

71. Larson, D.L., Maxwell, R., Abston, S., and Dobrkovsky, M.: Zinc deficiency in burned children. Plast. Reconstr. Surg., 46:13, 1970.

72. Thompson, H.J., Griminger, P., and Evans, J.L.: Effect of dietary copper, manganese, and zinc on nitrogen equilibrium and mineral distribution subsequent to trauma in mature rats. J. Nutr., 106:1421, 1976.

73. Cuthbertson, D.P. Morrison, C., Fleck, A., Queen, K., Bissent, R.S., Husain, S.L., and Fell, G.S.: Urinary zinc levels as an indication of muscle catabolism. Lancet, 1:280, 1973.

74. Caldwell, M.D., Jonsson, H.T., and Othersen, H.B., Jr.: Essential fatty acid deficiency in an infant receiving prolonged parenteral alimentation. J. Pediatr., 81:894, 1972.

75. Helmkamp, G.M., Wilmore, D.W., Johnson, A.A., and Pruitt, B.A., Jr.: Essential fatty acid deficiency in red cells after thermal injury: Correction with intravenous fat therapy. Am. J. Clin. Nutr., 26:1331, 1973.

76. McCarthy, M.C., Cottam, G.L., and Turner, W.W.: Essential fatty acid deficiency in critically ill surgical patients. Am. J. Surg., 142:747, 1981.

77. Rivers, J.P.W., and Frankel, T.L.: Essential fatty acid deficiency. Br. Med. Bull., 37:59, 1981.

78. Pruitt, B.A., Jr.: Advances in fluid therapy and the early care of the burned patient. World J. Surg., 2:139, 1978.

79. Warden, G.D., Wilmore, D.W., Rogers, P.W., Mason, A.D., Jr., and Pruitt, B.A., Jr.: Hypernatremic state in hypermetabolic burn patients. Arch. Surg., 106:420, 1973.

80. Moyer, C.A., Brentano, L., Gravens, D.L., Margraf, H.W., and Monafo, W.W.: Treatment of large human burns with 0.5% silver nitrate solution. Arch. Surg., 90:812, 1965.

81. White, M.G., and Asch, M.J.: Acid-base effects of topical mafenide acetate in the burned patient. N. Engl. J. Med., 284:1281, 1971.

82. Sheldon, G.F., and Grzyb, S.: Phosphate depletion and repletion: Relation to parenteral nutrition and oxygen transport. Ann. Surg., 182:683, 1975.

83. Larkin, J.M., and Moylan, J.A.: Complete enteral support of thermally injured patients. Am. J. Surg., 131:722, 1976.

84. Kirksey, T.D., Moncrief, J.A., Pruitt, B.A., Jr., and O'Neill, J.A.: Gastrointestinal complications in burns. Am. J. Surg., 116:627, 1968.

85. Woods, J.H., Erickson, L.W., Condon, R.E., Schulte, W.J., and Sillin, L.F.: Postoperative ileus: A colonic problem. Surgery, 84:527, 1978.

86. Wilson, J.P.: Postoperative motility of large intestines in man. Gut, 16:689, 1975.

87. Glucksman, D.L., Kalser, M.H., and Warren, W.D.: Small intestinal absorption in the immediate postoperative period. Surgery, 60:1020, 1966.

88. Postoperative ileus (editorial). Lancet, 2:1186, 1978.

89. Page, C.P., Ryan, J.A., Jr., and Haff, R.C.: Continual catheter administration of an elemental diet. Surg. Gynecol. Obstet., 142:184, 1976.

90. Pruitt, B.A., Jr., and Goodwin, C.W.: Burns: In-

cluding cold, chemical and electrical injuries. *In* Sabiston, D.C., Jr.: Davis-Christopher Textbook of Surgery, 12th ed. Philadelphia, W.B. Saunders, 1981, pp. 287–316.

91. Czaja, A.J., McAlhany, J.C., and Pruitt, B.A., Jr.: Acute gastroduodenal disease after thermal injury. An endoscopic evaluation of incidence and natural history. N. Engl. J. Med., *291*:925, 1974.

92. Czaja, A.J., McAlhany, J.C., and Pruitt, B.A., Jr.: Gastric acid secretion and acute gastroduodenal disease after burns. Arch. Surg., *111*:243, 1976.

93. Rosenthal, A., Czaja, A.J., and Pruitt, B.A., Jr.: Gastrin levels and gastric acidity in the pathogenesis of acute gastroduodenal disease after burns. Surg. Gynecol. Obstet., *144*:232, 1977.

94. Goodwin, C.W., and Pruitt, B.A., Jr.: The massive burn with sepsis and Curling's ulcer. *In* Hardy, J.D. (ed.): Critical Surgical Illness, 2nd ed. Philadelphia, W.B. Saunders, 1980, pp. 211–233.

95. Pruitt, B.A., Jr., and Goodwin, C.W.: Stress ulcer disease in the burned patient. World J. Surg., *5*:209, 1981.

96. McAlhany, J.C., Czaja, A.J., and Pruitt, B.A., Jr.: Antacid control of complications from acute gastroduodenal disease after burns. J. Trauma, *16*:645, 1976.

97. McElwee, H.P., Sirinek, K.R., and Levine, B.A.: Cimetidine affords protection equal to antacids in prevention of stress ulceration following thermal injury. Surgery, *84*:113, 1978.

98. Goodwin, C.W., and Pruitt, B.A., Jr.: Increased incidence of pancreatitis in thermally injured patients: A prospective study. Proc. Am. Assoc. Surg. Trauma, 1981, vol. 13, p. 106.

99. Munster, A.M., Goodwin, M.N., and Pruitt, B.A., Jr.: Acalculous cholecystitis in burned patients. Am. J. Surg., *172*:965, 1970.

100. Lescher, T.J., Sirinek, K.R., and Pruitt, B.A., Jr.: Superior mesenteric artery syndrome in thermally injured patients. J. Trauma, *9*:567, 1979.

101. Lescher, T.J., Teejarden, D.K., and Pruitt, B.A., Jr.: Acute pseudo-obstruction of the colon in thermally injured patients. Dis. Colon Rectum, *21*:618, 1978.

102. Hansen, L.M., Hardie, W.R., and Hidalgo, J.: Fat emulsion for intravenous administration: Clinical experience with Intralipid 10%. Ann. Surg., *184*:80, 1976.

103. Wilmore, D.W., Moylan, J.A., Helmkamp, G.N., and Pruitt, B.A., Jr.: Clinical evaluation of 10% intravenous fat emulsion for parenteral nutrition in thermally injured patients. Ann. Surg., *178*:503, 1973.

104. Thompson, S.W.: Hepatic toxicity of intravenous fat emulsion. *In* Meng, H.C., and Wilmore, D.W., (eds.): Fat Emulsions in Parenteral Nutrition. Chicago, American Medical Association, 1976, pp. 90–95.

105. Allen, J.G., Stemmer, E., and Head, L.R.: Similar growth rates of litter mate puppies maintained on oral protein with those on the same quantity of protein as daily intravenous plasma for 99 days as only protein source. Ann. Surg., *144*:349, 1958.

106. Blackburn, G.L., Flatt, J.P., Clowes, G.H., Jr., O'Donnell, T.F., and Hensle, T.E.: Protein sparing therapy during periods of starvation with sepsis or trauma. Ann. Surg., *177*:588, 1973.

107. Blackburn, G.L., Flatt, J.P., Clowes, G.H., and O'Donnell, T.E.: Peripheral intravenous feeding with isotonic amino acid solutions. Am. J. Surg., *125*:447, 1973.

108. Greenberg, G.R., Marliss, E.B., Anderson, G.H., Langer, B., Spence, W., Tovee, E.B., and Jeejeebhoy, K.N.: Protein-sparing therapy in postoperative patients. N. Engl. J. Med., *294*:1411, 1976.

109. Felig, P.: Intravenous nutrition: Fact and fancy. N. Engl. J. Med., *294*:1455, 1976.

110. Wolfe, B.M., Culebras, J.M., Sim, A.J., Ball, M.R., and Moore, F.D.: Substrate interaction in intravenous feeding. Ann. Surg., *186*:518, 1977.

111. Wilmore, D.W.: The Metabolic Management of the Critically Ill. New York, Plenum Medicals, 1977, pp. 21–36.

112. Dudrick, S.J., and Wilmore, D.W.: Long-term parenteral feeding. Hosp. Practice, *3*:65, 1968.

113. Aubaniac, R.: Une nouvelle voie d'injection ou du poncture vieneuse: La voie sous-claviculare. Sem. Hop. Paris, *28*:3445, 1952.

114. Wilson, J.N., Grow, J.B., DeMay, C.V., Prevedel, A., and Owens, J.: Central venous pressure in optimal blood volume maintenance. Arch. Surg., *85*:563, 1952.

115. Mogil, R., DeLaurentis, D., and Rosemund, G.: The infraclavicular vein puncture. Arch. Surg., *95*:320, 1967.

116. Dudrick, S.J., Wilmore, D.W., Vars, H.N., and Rhoads, J.E.: Can intravenous feeding as the sole means of nutrition support growth in the child and restore weight loss in the adult? An affirmative answer. Ann. Surg., *169*:974, 1969.

117. Wilmore, D.W., and Dudrick, S.J.: Safe long-term venous catheterization. Arch. Surg., *98*:256, 1969.

118. Bernard, R.W., and Stahl, W.M.: Subclavian vein catheterizations: A prospective study. I. Noninfectious complications. Ann. Surg., *173*:184, 1971.

119. Maki, D.G.: Preventing infection in intravenous therapy. Hosp. Pract., *11*:95, 1976.

120. Herbst, C.A.: Indications, management, and complications of percutaneous subclavian catheters: An audit. Arch. Surg., *113*:1421, 1978.

121. Jarrad, M.M., and Freeman, J.B.: The effect of antibiotic ointments and antiseptics on the skin flora beneath subclavian catheter dressings during intravenous hyperalimentation. J. Surg. Res., *22*:521, 1977.

122. Borja, A.R., and Hinshaw, J.R.: A safe way to perform infraclavicular subclavian vein catheterization. Surg. Gynecol. Obstet., *130*:673, 1970.

123. Sasaki, T.M., Panke, T.W., Dorethy, J.F., Lindberg, R.B., and Pruitt, B.A., Jr.: The relationship of central venous and pulmonary artery catheter position to acute right-sided endocarditis in severe thermal injury. J. Trauma, *19*:740, 1979.

124. Baskin, T.W., Rosenthal, A., and Pruitt, B.A., Jr.: Acute bacterial endocarditis: A silent source of sepsis in the burned patient. Ann. Surg., *184*:618, 1976.

125. Pruitt, B.A., Jr., McManus, W.F., Kim, S.H., and Treat, R.C.: Diagnosis and treatment of cannula-related intravenous sepsis in burn patients. Ann. Surg., *191*:546, 1980.

126. Goldman, D.A., Maki, D.G., and Rhame, F.S.: Guidelines for infection control in intravenous therapy. Ann. Intern. Med., *79*:848, 1973.

127. Maki, D.G., Weise, C.E., and Sarafin, H.W.: A semiquantitative culture method for identifying intravenous catheter-related infection. N. Engl. J. Med., *296*:1306, 1977.

128. Zinner, S.H., Denny-Brown, B.C., and Braun, P.: Risk of infection with intravenous indwelling catheters. Effect of antibiotic ointment. J. Infect. Dis., *120*:616, 1969.

129. Collin, J., Tweedle, D.E.F., and Venables, F.L.: Effect of millipore filters on complications of intravenous infusions: Prospective clinical trial. Br. Med. J., *4*:456, 1973.

130. Warden, G.D., Wilmore, D.W., and Pruitt, B.A., Jr.: Central venous thrombosis: A hazard of medical progress. J. Trauma, *13*:620, 1973.

131. Bistrian, B.R., Blackburn, G.L., Sherman, M., and Scrimshaw, N.S.: Therapeutic index of nutritional depletion in hospitalized patients. Surg. Gynecol. Obstet., *141*:512, 1975.

132. Beisel, W.R., Edelman, R., Nauss, K., and Suskind, R.M.: Single-nutrient effects on immunologic function. J.A.M.A., *245*:53, 1981.

133. Mullen, J.L., Buzby, G.P., Waldman, M.T., Gertner, M.H., Hobbs, C.L., and Rosato, E.F.: Prediction of operative morbidity and mortality by preoperative nutritional assessment. Surg. Forum, *30*:81, 1979.

134. Newsome, T.W., Mason, A.D., Jr., and Pruitt, B.A., Jr.: Weight loss following thermal injury. Ann. Surg., *178*:215, 1973.

135. McLaurin, N.K., Goodwin, C.W., Zitzka, C.A., and Hander, E.W.: Computer generated graphic evaluation of nutritional status in critically injured patients. J. Am. Diet. Assoc., *82*:49, 1983.

136. Obel, I.W.P.: Transient phrenic nerve paralysis following subclavian venipuncture. Anesthesiology, *33*:369, 1970.

137. Flanagan, J.P., Gradisar, I.V., and Gross, R.J.: Air embolus: A lethal complication of subclavian venipuncture. N. Engl. J. Med., *281*:488, 1969.

138. Adar, R., and Aozes, M.: Hydromediastinum. J.A.M.A., *214*:372, 1970.

139. Maki, D.G., and Martin, W.T.: Nationwide epidemic of septicemia caused by contaminated infusion products. J. Infect. Dis., *131*:267, 1975.

140. Maki, D.G., Anderson, R.L., and Shulman, J.A.: In-use contamination of intravenous infusion fluid. Appl. Environ. Microbiol., *28*:778, 1974.

141. Goldman, D.A., and Maki, D.G.: Infection control in total parenteral nutrition. J.A.M.A., *233*:1360, 1973.

142. Stein, J.M., and Pruitt, B.A., Jr.: Suppurative thrombophlebitis—a lethal iatrogenic disease. N. Engl. J. Med., *282*:1452, 1970.

143. Burke, J.F., Wolfe, R.R., Mullany, C.J., Matthews, D.W., and Bier, D.M.: Glucose requirements following burn injury. Ann. Surg., *190*:274, 1979.

144. Sheldon, G.F., Petersen, S.R., and Saunders, R.: Hepatic dysfunction during hyperalimentation. Arch. Surg., *113*:504, 1978.

145. Askanazi, J., Rosenbaum, S.H., Hyman, A.I., Foster, R.J., Milic-Emili, J., and Kinney, J.M.: Effects of total parenteral nutrition on gas exchange and breathing patterns. Crit. Care Med., *7*:125, 1979.

146. Askanazi, J., Rosenbaum, S.H., Hyman, A.I., Silverbery, P.A., Milic-Emili, J., and Kinney, J.M.: Respiratory changes induced by the large glucose loads of total parenteral nutrition. J.A.M.A., *243*:1444, 1980.

147. Askanazi, J., Elwyn, D.H., Silverberg, P.A., Rosenbaum, S.H., and Kinney, J.M.: Respiratory distress secondary to a high carbohydrate load: A case report. Surgery, *87*:596, 1980.

148. Heird, W.C., Bell, D.B., Driscoll, J.M., Jr., Grebin, B., and Winters, R.W.: Metabolic acidosis resulting from intravenous alimentation mixtures containing synthetic amino acids. N. Engl. J. Med., *287*:943, 1972.

149. Sheldon, G.F., and Grzyb, S.: Phosphate depletion and repletion: Relation to parenteral nutrition and oxygen transport. Ann. Surg., *182*:683, 1975.

150. Rudman, D., Millikan, W.J., Richardson, T.J., Boxler, T.J., Stackhouse, W.J., and McGarrity, W.C.: Elemental balances during intravenous hyperalimentation of underweight adult subjects. J. Clin. Invest., *55*:94, 1975.

151. Knochel, J.P.: The pathophysiology and clinical characteristics of severe hypophosphatemia. Arch. Intern. Med., *137*:203, 1977.

CHAPTER 29

The Neurologic or Neurosurgical Patient

MARTIN H. SAVITZ
BYRON YOUNG

The indications for parenteral therapy in the neurologic or neurosurgical patient who has become acutely obtunded are not well recognized. As long as the gastrointestinal tract is normal, external feedings via nasogastric tube or gastrostomy should provide adequate nutrition in patients who are chronically comatose because of craniocerebral trauma, cerebrovascular accident, intracranial mass lesion, or neuromuscular disease.[45] Ileus in an unresponsive patient is far more likely to be caused by direct abdominal trauma or spinal cord injury than by intrinsic autonomic dysfunction. Vagal nerve deficits resulting from progressive bulbar palsy, amyotrophic lateral sclerosis, multiple sclerosis, lateral medullary syndrome, pseudobulbar palsy, vertebrobasilar aneurysm, infiltrating brainstem tumor, or basilar skull fracture may produce dysphagia, but interruption of gut function is rare.

CHRONIC CEREBRAL EDEMA

Nutritional disturbances are not usually considered very important in the postoperative care of the neurosurgical patient. Because most significant changes occur within the first week following craniotomy, it has even been suggested that no concerted effort is needed to correct the imbalances of fluid, electrolytes, and nitrogen metabolism.[50, 51] However, on admission many patients with intracranial lesions are in a state of poor nutrition because of an inadequate dietary intake prior to hospitalization.[15] The catabolic status generally presents as a simple weight loss rather than clinically evident cachexia, and initial routine laboratory tests may reveal only mild hyponatremia and hypoalbuminemia. The institution of fluid restriction, osmotic diuretics, and steroid therapy further alters the water, mineral, and protein balance. Mechanical decompression provides favorable circumstances for the resolution of cerebral edema subsequent to excision of a tumor from the intracranial cavity. Some patients do not make the desired progress until long after the expected period of brain swelling from operative trauma has elapsed.

Mount Sinai Hospital Study
Unsuspected Nutritional Failure

Shoemaker and coworkers[39] reported the rapid onset of postoperative dishydration or water maldistribution in 17 of the 602 cases admitted in 1971 to the Mount Sinai Hospital surgical intensive care unit. Two neurosurgical patients in this study and eight more patients over the next two years went into a neurasthenic decline during a prolonged recovery period following craniotomy. Consistent with the accepted therapy for cerebral edema, they were treated primarily with steroids, osmotic diuretics, and fluid restriction. Body compartment measurements demonstrated a depletional state with an expanded extracellular space and an intracellular deficit that was proportionally greater than the weight loss. Hyponatremia, hypoalbuminemia, low blood volume, and intestinal malabsorption were also observed. Six of these ten patients died; treatment in the remaining four patients was then entirely directed toward reversal of the previously unsuspected nutritional failure.[9, 37]

The patients who were studied entered

508

the hospital with symptoms and signs of an intracranial mass; the diagnosis was confirmed by cerebral angiography. Preoperatively they were all in fair condition; postoperatively they recovered more slowly than expected, becoming weak and unable to eat and responding only to painful stimuli. There was considerable weight loss, but they did not look wasted. In each case, funduscopic examination was negative, lumbar puncture revealed normal cerebrospinal fluid pressure, and no clinical signs of increased intracranial pressure (ICP) were observed. None of the patients was suffering from an airway problem, and blood gases were persistently within normal limits. Repeat angiography showed the cerebral vasculature to be intact, excluded hematoma formation, and demonstrated mild hemispheric swelling.

Each of the four patients was at first unable to take more than an 800-calorie tube feeding without developing diarrhea and a negative water balance. It was elected to feed the patients intravenously with a standard hyperalimentation regimen; protein hydrolysate and dextrose solutions with conventional additives were administered through centrally placed silicone catheters. Blood volume deficits and hypoalbuminemia were initially treated with blood transfusions and 5 per cent albumin. Throughout this period of intravenous alimentation, tube feedings, and later oral feedings, were continued and increased as gastrointestinal function improved. Intravenous feeding was employed until the patient could manage an oral diet of more than 2000 calories; tube feeding was also discontinued within the same interval.

Data Collection

Daily intake and output of water, sodium, and potassium were measured until the patient's diet was too varied to make an accurate determination possible. Weights were taken every day before breakfast. Full routine biochemical and hematologic testing was performed twice a day.

Plasma volume was measured by the indicator dilution technique with ^{125}I-labeled human serum albumin. Blood volume was calculated as the plasma volume divided by one minus the corrected hematocrit expressed as a per cent. The volume of dilution of ^{82}Br was used as an estimate of the extracellular fluid, and dilution of heavy water was used as a measure of total body water.

The intracellular fluid was computed as the difference between total body and extracellular water.

Case Histories

Case One. A 59-year-old man (Fig. 29–1) underwent occipital craniectomy for removal of a recurrent hemangioblastoma of the cerebellum. For the first three postoperative days, a ventilator was required because of central apnea. When tube feedings were instituted, diarrhea ensued. Five weeks later, his weight had dropped from 85 to 65 kg, and since he was in true coma and appeared to be dying, discharge from the intensive care unit was contemplated. Although he lost less than one quarter of his normal body weight, his intracellular space had halved. His extracellular space had expanded to give him a normal amount of body water for his current weight. The serum albumin level was 2.5 gm/dl, the serum sodium level was 129

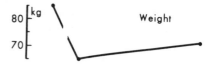

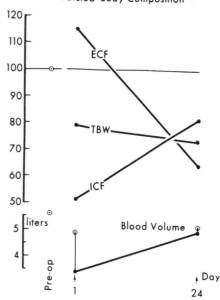

Figure 29–1. Case 1. Note progressive increase in intracellular fluid (ICF) and decrease in extracellular fluid (ECF) in relation to total body water (TBW). Predicated norms for blood volume are represented by small circles, and deficits, by vertical lines.

mEq/L, the hematocrit was 27 per cent, and the blood volume was 72 per cent of that expected. The response to a 4000-calorie intravenous hyperalimentation diet was dramatic. Over five days, he absorbed 700 mEq of potassium. By the 16th day, he could drink from a cup and took cognizance of his surroundings by demonstrating open hostility toward his mother. By the 24th day, he could make pleasant conversation, even telling humorous anecdotes. There was an acceptable increase in intracellular fluid, and he was able to ambulate with only mild ataxia.

Case Two. A 39-year-old woman (Fig. 29–2) underwent frontal craniotomy for clipping of a left anterior communicating aneurysm. Over the first three postoperative days, she developed drowsiness, right hemiplegia, and aphasia. Angiography documented left-middle cerebral artery spasm. Three weeks later, she was unarousable and had lost 11 kg. Repeat angiography revealed only hemispheric swelling. Her serum albumin level was 2.8 gm/dl, and the serum sodium level was 128 mEq/L. She was placed on a 3000-

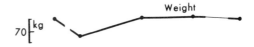
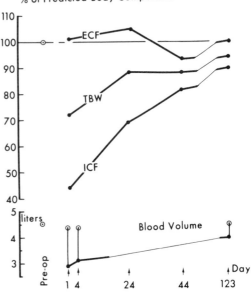

Figure 29–3. Case 3. Note the two-fold increase in intracellular fluid (ICF) without remarkable weight change. ECF, extracellular fluid; TBW, total body water.

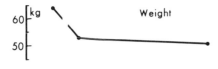
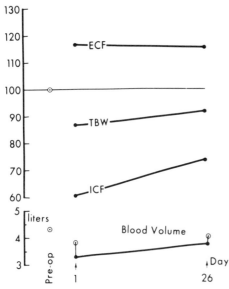

Figure 29–2. Case 2. Note 2.2-L increase in intracellular fluid (ICF) despite 3-kg weight loss. ECF, extracellular fluid; TBW, total body water.

calorie parenteral diet, and for five days she had a positive potassium balance of 550 mEq. She then awoke suddenly, kissed her husband, and cried when shown photographs of her children. She continued to take considerable nutrition by mouth, regained use of her right side, and was discharged from the hospital.

Case Three. A 60-year-old woman (Fig. 29–3) underwent left craniotomy for removal of a tentorial meningioma. Her wound failed to heal, and she was treated with antibiotics for two episodes of meningitis. During the first two postoperative weeks, mechanical support of her respiration was necessary. After a full month of standard intravenous fluid replacement, there was a 70 per cent deficit in expected intracellular space. Her serum albumin level had risen from 1.3 to 1.6 gm per dl. A 4000-calorie parenteral diet was begun and continued until an oral intake of 2000 calories was possible without diarrhea. She had an intermittently positive potassium balance averaging 20 mEq/day. After two weeks of hyperalimentation, her incision could be reclosed surgically. By the third week, she was sitting out of bed, became very talkative, and fed herself. At the end of

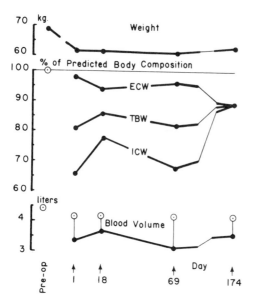

Figure 29–4. Case 4. Note the one-third increase in intracellular fluid (ICF) without remarkable weight change. ECF, extracellular fluid; TBW, total body water.

10 weeks of nutritional therapy, her space measurements were in the normal range, and she could walk with minimal assistance. Her memory improved, and she regained her sense of humor.

Case Four. A 56-year-old woman (Fig. 29–4) underwent left frontotemporal craniotomy for excision of a convexity meningioma with hyperostosis, followed two weeks later by a right frontal craniotomy for removal of a parasellar meningioma. She had a residual left hemiplegia and remained febrile and somnolent for five weeks. Her weight had fallen from 70 to 60 kg, and her intracellular space was 66 per cent of that expected. Her serum sodium level was 128 mEq/L. A 3000-calorie parenteral diet was instituted. During the first 10 days, she had a positive potassium balance of 300 mEq/L. She was then able to sit up in a chair and absorb tube feedings. Two weeks of antibiotic therapy were required for an infected subclavian catheter site. After one month of hyperalimentation, her intercellular fluid returned to 88 per cent of that expected. She was alert and able to eat by herself. At 10 weeks, active physical therapy was begun. Her left hemiplegia resolved over a three-month period, and a left cranioplasty was performed. She was discharged from the hospital and resumed her preoperative plans of separating from her husband.

Pathology of Cerebral Edema

Electron microscopy has shown that edema in gray matter is characterized by swelling of the cellular elements.[27] The hydrops is more evident in the perivascular feet of astrocytes and dendrites than in the oligodendroglia. Alterations of virtually all cytoplasmic organelles occur, but the mitochondria are the earliest to be affected. In marked contradistinction, the edematous fluid in white matter is extracellular, with evolving expansion of the Virchow-Robin spaces. Separation and vacuolization of the myelin sheath, as well as formation of lacunae in the cytoplasm of oligodendrocytes, are regularly observed. The regions of the brain that normally have a high water content—arcuate zone, corpus callosum, and internal capsule—exhibit minimal disruption.[18]

Biochemical analysis of edematous tissue adjacent to human brain tumors has contributed further to an understanding of the basic pathology of cerebral edema.[35] Determinations of water content confirm that the increase in volume of the white matter (25 per cent) is about three times that of the cortex (8.6 per cent). The edematous fluid accumulated within the cerebral cortex has an amazingly high sodium concentration of 280 mEq/L, whereas the concentration in swollen white matter is about 125 mEq/L. The loss of potassium from the affected gray matter is about one third of the sodium increase. Studies of the energy stores in human edematous cortex reveal that the concentrations of creatine phosphate and adenosine triphosphate are low, whereas adenosine diphosphate and monophosphate and inorganic phosphate are greater than normal. The lowered level of glucose and the corresponding rise of lactate are additional evidence of anaerobic glycolysis and tissue hypoxia consistent with mitochondrial dysfunction. The buildup of free fatty acids from the breakdown of lipids further impairs oxidative phosphorylation and neuronal function.[36]

Followup Application

Soon after completion of the study of neurosurgical patients with unsuspected nutritional failure,[9, 37] the radioactive tracer [82]Br became unavailable for clinical use. Space compartment volumes could not be accurately computed. Nevertheless, the syndrome of chronic cerebral edema following craniotomy has virtually been eliminated at Mount Sinai Hospital by early postoperative therapy with a full high-calorie diet.

HEAD TRAUMA

Severe head injury is associated with a massive systemic metabolic insult. Calculations of the caloric requirements of head-injured patients show a significant correlation between the severity of brain damage and energy requirements.[28] Profound catabolism in the head-injured patient has been confirmed by several studies.[5, 10, 20, 29-31, 41, 48] Decerebrate patients may require 4500 kcal/24 hours, an amount similar to the metabolic demands of patients with major burn injuries.[8, 11] Schiller and colleagues[38] have attributed at least part of the catabolism associated with head injuries to the widespread use of steroids; head-injured patients receiving steroids excreted an average of 25.5 gm/day of nitrogen.

Nutritional support for acutely head-injured patients has conventionally been provided via the enteral route and has been delayed until good gastrointestinal function returned in the postinjury period.[15] Many patients receive no nutritional support for 6 to 10 days after injury. Despite the widespread recognition of the potential for nutritional deficiency, few attempts at providing early parenteral nutritional support in head-injured patients have been reported.[1, 42] Blackhorn and Cunitz[5] found a favorable energy balance when parenteral nutrition was used in patients who had suffered head trauma.

University of Kentucky Medical Center Study

Total Parenteral Versus Standard Enteral Nutrition

Thirty-eight head-injured patients admitted to the neurosurgical service of the University of Kentucky Medical Center were randomly assigned to receive total parenteral nutrition (TPN) or standard enteral nutrition (SEN).[34] Assignment was made within 48 hours of admission. Eligibility for entry into the study was restricted to patients who had penetrating missile wounds or blunt head trauma causing intracranial hematomas, a major focal neurologic deficit, unconscious-

ness, or a combination of these conditions. Cases with severe extracranial injuries that were expected to alter metabolic demands or to delay use of SEN, such as abdominal organ injury, were excluded.

Twenty patients assigned to the TPN group were started on the parenteral nutrition regimen within 48 hours after admission. Synthetic amino acids and hypertonic dextrose solutions were administered by electronic infusion control through a percutaneous infraclavicular subclavian vein catheter. The TPN solution contained 42.5 gm/L synthetic amino acids and 25 per cent dextrose, electrolytes, and vitamins. Trace elements were also added to the solution. To supply essential fatty acids and additional calories, 250 to 500 ml/day of 10 per cent soybean oil emulsion were given. In addition to the laboratory tests done on all study patients for comparative data collection, TPN patients were closely monitored to prevent the metabolic or septic complications that are common with this form of therapy. When required, insulin was used to control hyperglycemia.

Eighteen SEN patients were given feedings via nasogastric tube as soon as such feedings could be tolerated. The tube-feeding preparation used for all SEN patients was a high-nitrogen product consisting of 42 gm of protein/L, 10.8 gm of fat/L, and 185 gm of carbohydrates/L. More than 100 per cent of the United States Department of Agriculture's recommended daily dose of vitamins and minerals was supplied in each 1500 calories. Digestive capability was assessed by determining the presence or absence of bowel sounds and the amount of gastric residual every two hours.[4] Tube feeding was begun when bowel sounds were present, and the gastric residual volume was less than 100 ml/hour. The patient's head was kept at a 30-degree angle, and feeding was given through a No. 9 French polyurethane feeding tube to decrease the possibility of gastric reflux and aspiration.

Collection of Data

Calorie and nitrogen requirements were calculated with the goal of achieving a positive or zero nitrogen balance. Calculations were based on the patient's body surface area (derived from weight and height), age, sex, and severity of injury.[19, 49] Both groups were given maintenance intravenous fluids over and above nutritional solutions as required. Assessment of nutritional status included measurements of triceps skinfold and midarm muscle circumference, serum albumin levels, total iron-binding capacity and transferrin, total lymphocyte count, delayed hypersensitivity skin testing (*Trichophyton*, streptokinase-streptodornase, mumps, and *Candida* test antigens), nitrogen excretion, and daily calorie and nitrogen intake. Other factors that were monitored included fluid intake and output, the use of a respirator, the frequency of nosocomial infection, the use of antibiotics, serum glucose levels, the daily temperature peak, the use of dexamethasone, patient mortality, the length of stay in the intensive care unit, and the number of days hospitalized.

Nutritional data were collected on all cases until death or for 18 days of hospitalization. Survival and functional recovery were monitored for up to one year following admission to the study. Patients were managed with intraventricular pressure monitoring, dexamethasone, surgery, and barbiturates, as indicated, to control intracranial hypertension. The Glasgow Coma Scale (GCS)[44] was used daily to grade the level of consciousness for all patients. The highest GCS score in the first 24 hours and the daily GCS score thereafter were used for grading the level of consciousness. Functional recovery was evaluated by an attending neurosurgeon who was not aware of the nutritional support regimen: grading was good (resumed normal activities), moderately disabled (disabled but independent), or vegetative (unresponsive and speechless).[25]

Categoric data were analyzed using chi-square tests or Fisher's exact test if expected cell frequencies were low. Continuous data were analyzed using an independent samples t-test. Data that were collected sequentially over time were analyzed using a repeated-measure analysis of variance. The data derived by treatment-group interaction were used to test whether the change over time was the same for the two treatment groups.

Baseline admission data were similar for both the TPN and the SEN groups (Table 29–1). The only statistically significant difference noted was the mean peak temperature during the first 24 hours of hospitalization, 38.6° C in the TPN group compared with 38°C in the SEN group (p = 0.02). There was no significant difference in the mean GCS score for the two groups as determined by the highest GCS score in the first 24 hours (p = 0.52, Table 29–2).

Eight (44 per cent) of the 18 SEN patients died during the 18 days of data collection, whereas no patient on TPN therapy died during this period (Table 29–2). This difference between groups was highly significant (p < 0.0001). During the inhospital followup period of up to 83 days, one additional patient from the SEN group died and three TPN patients died. However, there was still a highly significant difference in the inhospital deaths, with the TPN patients faring better (p = 0.002, Table 29–2). Of the 18 SEN patients, death occurred in one patient with a low GCS score, in four patients with intermediate GCS scores, and in three patients with high GCS scores. The patient with the low GCS score died four days after admission

Table 29–1. CLINICAL DATA AND NUTRITIONAL PARAMETERS*

CLINICAL DATA	SEN PATIENTS (MEAN ± SD)	TPN PATIENTS (MEAN ± SD)	p VALUE
No. of cases	18	20	
Age (yr)	34.9 ± 3.76	29.2 ± 4.12	0.32
Height (cm)	177.8 ± 2.39	174.2 ± 3.67	0.42
Weight (kg)	59.3 ± 6.99	58.5 ± 6.69	0.94
Urine urea nitrogen (initial 24 hr)	15.9 ± 1.08	18.0 ± 1.24	0.24
Serum albumin (gm/dl)	3.82 ± 1.88	3.72 ± 1.58	0.67
Transferrin (mg/dl)	258.1 ± 15.31	276.8 ± 23.35	0.50
Total lymphocyte count (cells/mm³)	1350 ± 199	1427 ± 211	0.79
Triceps skin-fold (cm)	16.0 ± 1.17	13.3 ± 1.04	0.10
Midarm muscle circumference	25.1 ± 0.73	26.4 ± 0.79	0.24
Peak temperature during first 24 hrs.	38.0 ± 0.2	38.6 ± 0.2	0.02

*Admission data for patients receiving standard enteral nutrition (SEN) and total parenteral nutrition (TPN).

Table 29–2. ANALYSIS OF DEATHS BY HIGHEST GCS SCORE WITHIN 24 HOURS AFTER ADMISSION*

| PATIENT GROUP | GCS SCORE | | | TOTAL CASES | ADMISSION GCS SCORE (MEAN ± SD) |
	3 to 4	5 to 7	≥8		
SEN patients					7.2 ± 0.60
No. of patients	2	8	8	18	
Deaths by 18 days	1	4	3	8†	
Deaths 18 to 83 days	1	0	0	1	
Total deaths	2	4	3	9‡	
TPN patients					
No. of patients	1	10	9	20	7.7 ± 0.56
Deaths by 18 days	0	0	0	0†	
Deaths 18 to 83 days	1	1	1	3	
Total deaths	1	1	1	3‡	

*GCS = Glasgow Coma Scale; SEN = standard enteral nutrition; TPN = total parenteral nutrition.
Significance: † = p<0.0001; ‡ = p<0.02.

secondary to elevated ICP. Three of the four patients with intermediate GCS scores who died developed sepsis, but brain injury was considered the primary cause of death for all four patients. Of the three patients with high GCS scores, two died primarily of sepsis; the third was also septic, but died from the effects of elevated ICP.

To avoid bias, mean GCS scores for 18 days were evaluated separately for survivors and nonsurvivors. The peak GCS score in the first 24 hours was not statistically different for the 18-day survivors and all the study patients (7.2 and 7.7 for SEN and TPN patients, respectively) (Table 29–2). The improvement in the GCS score over time was the same for both groups of 18-day survivors (an increase of 4.9 and 4.6 for the SEN and TPN groups, respectively). Patients receiving TPN had high mean GCS scores on all but three of the study days (Fig. 29–5). Mean GCS scores of the patients surviving 102 days

were not substantially different from those of 18-day survivors in both groups. There was no significant difference between groups in patients receiving barbiturates or dexamethasone.

At discharge, one of nine SEN patients and three of 17 TPN patients were in a vegetative state. Four of nine SEN patients and 12 of 17 TPN patients were severely disabled. There were two SEN patients and one TPN patient in each of the moderately disabled and good condition categories. A year after injury, one additional death had occurred in the SEN group, but there were no additional deaths in the TPN group. At that time, no SEN patients and two TPN patients were in a vegetative state. One SEN patient and two TPN patients remained severely disabled, and four SEN patients and seven TPN patients were moderately disabled. Good recovery resulted in five TPN patients and three SEN patients. One TPN

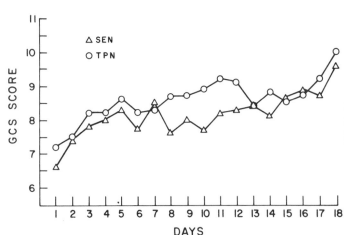

Figure 29–5. Change in Glasgow Coma Scale (GCS) score over the 18-day study period for head-injured patients receiving total parenteral nutrition (TPN) and standard enteral nutrition (SEN).

Table 29–3. CONDITION OF 20 TPN AND 18 SEN PATIENTS AT DISCHARGE AND AT ONE YEAR POSTINJURY*

CLINICAL CONDITION	TPN PATIENTS		SEN PATIENTS	
	At Discharge	At One Year†	At Discharge	At One Year
Good recovery	1	5	2	3
Moderate disability	1	7	2	4
Severe disability	12	2	4	1
Vegetative state	3	2	1	0
Dead	3	3	9	10

*TPN = total parenteral nutrition; SEN = standard enteral nutrition.
†One patient was lost to followup review.

patient was lost to followup review (Table 29–3). There was no significant difference in days spent in the hospital between groups of 18-day survivors (49.4 and 52.6 days for SEN and TPN patients, respectively), and there was also no significant difference in the number of days spent on a respirator between groups of 18-day survivors (10.3 and 10.4 days for SEN and TPN patients, respectively).

A highly significant difference in nitrogen intake was recorded for the SEN and TPN groups (p = 0.002, Fig. 29–6A). The changeover time of calorie intake between the two groups was also different (p = 0.001, Fig. 29–6B). The mean intake/day for the TPN group was 1750 calories and 10.2 gm of nitrogen for the 18-day study period. The mean intake for the SEN group was 685 calories and 4 gm of nitrogen/day, not including calories obtained from isotonic intravenous fluids (5 per cent dextrose). The calculated average minimum requirement for both groups, to assure weight maintenance and a zero to positive nitrogen balance, was 2600 calories and 6.7 gm of nitrogen. Because of the greater intake of nitrogen in the TPN group, the overall nitrogen balance was significantly different for the groups (−17.6 and −10.9 gm/24 hours for the SEN and TPN groups, respectively) (p = 0.002, Fig. 29–6A). A mean of 0.35 gm/kg/day of nitrogen was excreted by both groups. A peak nitrogen excretion of 0.41 gm/kg on day 10 in the SEN group was recorded. Both groups remained in negative nitrogen balance through day 16 of the study period (Fig. 29–6A).

A greater overall average decrease in serum transferrin values over time was seen in the SEN group when compared with the TPN group (−26.6 and −6.9 per cent, respectively) (p = 0.6, Table 29–4). The greater decrease of serum albumin over time for the SEN group did not vary significantly from the TPN patients (p = 0.75, Table 29–4). There was also no substantial difference over

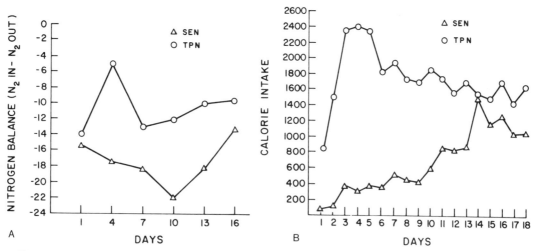

Figure 29–6. Nitrogen balance data *(A)* and mean caloric intake *(B)* for patients receiving total parenteral nutrition (TPN) and standard enteral nutrition (SEN) over the study period.

Table 29–4. CHANGES IN SERUM TRANSFERRIN AND SERUM ALBUMIN IN SEN AND TPN PATIENTS DURING THE STUDY PERIOD*

FACTORS	DAYS AFTER INJURY						p VALUE
	1	4	7	10	13	16	
Mean transferrin (mg/dl)							
SEN	258	231	195	203	190	208	NS
TPN	277	236	229	260	249	229	NS
% Change transferrin (mg/dl)							
SEN		−16.8	−24.7	−32.0	−33.3	−33.8	p=0.06
TPN		−4.3	−5.4	+2.9	−9.6	−17.9	
Mean albumin (gm/dl)							
SEN	3.8	3.1	2.5	2.4	2.3	2.3	NS
TPN	3.7	3.1	2.8	2.7	2.8	2.7	
% Change albumin (gm/dl)							
SEN		−17.0	−32.6	−33.2	−35.4	−41.2	NS
TPN		−16.3	−25.0	−24.2	−23.4	−25.5	

*SEN = standard enteral nutrition; TPN = total parenteral nutrition. NS = not significant.

time in the total lymphocyte counts between groups, even though TPN patients had higher mean values on most days. There was an overall mean total lymphocyte value of 1582 cells/mm³ for TPN patients and 1410 cells/mm³ for SEN patients.

Reactions to skin-test antigens for energy screening were measured weekly. There was a greater percentage of positive reactions to antigens among TPN patients than among SEN patients, despite similar dexamethasone therapy for both groups. This difference was significant on day 7, with 14.3 per cent positive reactions for the SEN group and 41.2 per cent positive reactions for the TPN group (p < 0.04, Fig. 29–7A). The percentage of positive reactions was highest for both groups on day 14 when the percentage of patients on steroids was lowest (Fig. 29–7 B).

Mean serum glucose levels were compared between groups. These levels were highest for TPN patients through day 10 (p = 0.01). After day 11, glucose levels were higher in the SEN group. The change of glucose levels over time was different between the two groups (p = 0.008). The difference in daily levels between groups is not clinically significant, since the actual difference in glucose concentrations between TPN and SEN patients ranged from 11.5 to 44 mg/dl (midrange 27.75 mg/dl). The osmolar contributions of these differences are minimal (range 0.63 to 2.4 mOsm).

For most days, the mean body temperature was higher in the SEN group; however, TPN patients had higher temperatures on enough days to show up as a significant day-by-group interaction (p = 0.01). The decrease over time of the triceps skinfold measurement was significantly less dramatic for TPN patients (p = 0.005). Midarm muscle circumference decreases were the same over time for the two groups.

Conclusions

The prospective randomized study of head-injured patients found a highly significant difference in survival at 18 days (p < 0.001) between patients begun on TPN ad-

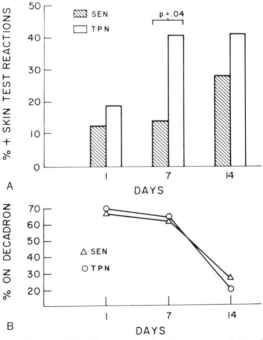

Figure 29–7. Bar graph of skin test reactivity of patients receiving standard enteral nutrition (SEN) and total parenteral nutrition (TPN) calculated with steroid usage.

ministered by a central vein within 48 hours of injury and those begun on SEN when the gastrointestinal tract recovered function. Age, height, weight, mean GCS scores, and nutritional status at the time of entry into the study were not significantly different for the SEN and TPN groups. On this basis, the improved survival rate seen in the TPN patients may be attributable to the early parenteral feedings.

The GCS is an objective and reproducible means of quantifying neurologic impairment and of predicting likely outcome of head-injured patients. Previous studies reported that more than 95 per cent of head-injured patients with an initial GCS score of 8 or higher survive, which contrasts with a 67 per cent survival rate when GCS scores are 5 to 7, and only a 10 per cent survival rate when scores are 3 or 4.[52] All categories closely approximated these predictions, except for the patients receiving TPN who had GCS scores of 5 to 7 and a mortality rate of 10 per cent. Although the incidence is not significantly different (p < 0.10) from predicted outcome, a trend toward improved survival was demonstrated. Furthermore, 90 per cent of the TPN group with GCS scores of 5 to 7 had a good outcome compared to only 50 per cent of cases with GCS scores of 5 to 7 in previous studies.[52] The predominant beneficial effect of early parenteral nutrition seems to be in patients classified as having intermediate GCS scores (5, 6, or 7).

The goal of nutritional support is to provide nutrients to sustain visceral protein levels and immunologic competence and to provide material for healing or replacement of injured tissue. The serum transferrin and serum albumin levels and the total lymphocyte count declined in both the SEN and TPN groups over the study period, but the percentage of decrease was greater in the SEN group, reaching statistical significance with the serum transferrin level (p < 0.006). Likewise, the triceps skinfold decrease was significantly less in the TPN group (p = 0.01). The data suggest that the TPN patients should have better immunologic competence on a nutritional basis than the SEN patients. A significantly greater percentage of positive responses to skin-test antigen was observed on day 7 in the TPN patients when compared with the SEN patients (p < 0.004). The difference may have clinical importance in that five of the eight deaths that occurred within 18 days in the SEN group were either attributed to or associated with sepsis.

The catabolic effect of head injury and its treatment is apparent in the nitrogen balance data. A mean value of 0.35 gm/kg/day of nitrogen was excreted by both groups, which is equivalent to 24.5 gm/day for a 70-kg man; the figure closely matches the nitrogen excretion previously reported by Schiller and coworkers.[38] This nitrogen wastage was partially offset during the first 14 days by the significantly higher calorie and nitrogen intake of the TPN group when compared with the SEN group (p < 0.0001). Both groups remained in negative nitrogen balance through day 16, though the TPN group maintained a significantly smaller negative nitrogen balance than did the SEN group (p = 0.002, Fig. 29–6A). The differences may have been critical, since seven of the eight deaths in the SEN group occurred in the first 14 days.

Although eight patients in the SEN group died during the 18-day study period, whereas no deaths occurred in the TPN group during that period, there was no significant difference at 13 days following injury in the number of patients with a favorable outcome (death, vegetative state, or severely disabled). Thirteen patients had unfavorable outcomes in the SEN group versus 15 in the TPN group. One year after injury, however, only 7 of the 15 TPN patients having an unfavorable outcome at 18 days remained in this category. The administration of TPN prevented early death, thereby seeming to provide the opportunity for eventual neurologic recovery in a high proportion of cases. The basis for the favorable outcome may be the enhanced immunologic response to infection by the nutritionally supported patient. The overall results justify the routine provision of TPN to the head-injured patient.

COMPLICATIONS OF PARENTERAL ALIMENTATION

Hyperosmolar, hyperglycemic, nonketotic coma is a potentially fatal complication of intravenous hyperalimentation.[14] Since clinical recognition may be difficult, especially postoperatively, emphasis must be placed on prevention. Careful monitoring of glucose levels in both blood and urine should provide an early indication for the institution of insulin therapy.

Hypophosphatemia following parenteral alimentation may also be progressively associated with paresthesias, lethargy, dysarthria, muscle flaccidity, dyspnea, seizures, and coma, even though serum electrolyte and glucose levels and acid-base balance are within normal limits; the pathophysiology of this syndrome is only poorly understood.[13, 33, 40] The administration of sodium phosphate restores the serum levels to the normal range, but it does not improve the clinical condition of the patient. Reducing the supply of calories leads to a disappearance of symptoms and a rise in the serum phosphate level.

In addition to metabolic sequelae, complications involving the central nervous system may be caused by the catheters that are inserted for intravenous hyperalimentation. Thrombophlebitis of the right external jugular vein that was cannulated for TPN resulted in thrombosis of dural sinuses in one adult patient.[46] Attempted use of a scalp vein in one infant allowed the accidental infusion of protein hydrolysate and lipid emulsion into the subarachnoid space; arachnoiditis, venous sinus occlusion, and cortical atrophy were found at autopsy.[2] During a 12-month period, 3 of 12 infants treated at one medical center developed signs of increased ICP following the institution of intravenous hyperalimentation via catheters inserted into the internal jugular vein; the pathogenesis was not clearly defined, but chronic decrease in the venous drainage of cerebral blood was a suggested mechanism.[32]

SPECIAL CONSIDERATIONS

The benefits of tracheostomy in comatose patients requiring respiratory assistance are well established.[16, 17, 43] Since the surgical neck wound tends to become infected, placement of central venous lines and even shunt tubing may be more difficult. Insertion of long intravenous catheters via cubital or brachial puncture avoids the potentially contaminated cervical region. In cases of posttraumatic hydrocephalus requiring ventriculoperitoneal shunting, subcutaneous tunneling through the right side of the neck is the preferred route; prophylactic antibiotics are particularly indicated in the presence of tracheostomy.

Systemic effects of even remote infections may worsen post-traumatic encephalopathy.[21] Careful observations of the tracheal flora, bacteruria induced by indwelling Foley catheters, and the inflammation around insertion sites of central venous lines should be standard procedures in all patients receiving TPN.[12] Early treatment of cultured pathogens can avert the additional metabolic stress of sepsis in the neurologically compromised patient.

SUMMARY

The pathophysiology of unremitting cerebral edema involves a generalized metabolic derangement. Debilitating disease, trauma, or surgery can result in a rapid deterioration of the nutritional status of patients.[3, 6, 22, 23, 26, 39, 47] The resulting malnutrition can be a factor in suboptimal responses to therapy and ultimately to the patient's chances for survival.[7, 9, 21, 24, 37] Conventional therapy is not directed toward the continuous supply of metabolically produced energy required for the support of normal glial and neuronal structure and activity. Early treatment of protein, water, and mineral imbalances provides optimal circumstances for return of neural function in the severely edematous brain.

REFERENCES

1. Allison, S.P.: Metabolic aspects of intensive care. Br. J. Anaesth., 49:689–696, 1977.
2. Beaumont, E., Malin, S., and Meng, R.: Accidental intracranial hyperalimentation infusion. J.P.E.N., 6:532–533, 1982.
3. Bistrian, B.R., Blackburn, G.L., Hallowell, E. et al.: Protein status of general surgical patients. J.A.M.A., 230:858–860, 1974.
4. Bistrian, B.R., Blackburn, G.L., Vitale, J. et al.: Prevalence of malnutrition in general medical patients. J.A.M.A., 235:1567–1570, 1976.
5. Blackhorn, J., and Cunitz, G.: Parenteral nutrition in patients with head injuries. Unfallheilkd., 81:673–680, 1980.
6. Bollet, A.J., and Owens, S.: Evaluation of nutritional status of selected hospitalized patients. Am. J. Clin. Nutr., 26:931–938, 1973.
7. Bozzetti, F., Terno, G., and Longoni, C.: Parenteral hyperalimentation and wound healing. Surg. Gynecol. Obstet., 141:712–714, 1975.
8. Bryan-Brown, C.W., and Kaufman, H.H.: Personal communication, March 1, 1984.
9. Bryan-Brown, C.W., Savitz, M.H., Elwyn, D.N. et al.: Cerebral edema unresponsive to conventional therapy in neurosurgical patients with unsuspected nutritional failure. Crit. Care Med., 1:125–129, 1973.
10. Cambria, S., and Gambardella, G.: Significance of parenteral hyperalimentation in patients with severe brain stem lesions. Acta Anaesthesiol. Ital., 27:913–920, 1976.
11. Clifton, G.L., Robertson, C.S., Grossman, R., et al.: The metabolic response to severe head injury. J. Neurosurg., 60:687–696, 1984.
12. Copeland, E.M., III, MacFadyen, B.V., Jr., McGown, C. et al.: The use of hyperalimentation in patients with potential sepsis. Surg. Gynecol. Obstet., 138:377–380, 1974.

13. Derr, R.F., and Zieve, L.: Etiology of hyperalimentation coma. N. Engl. J. Med., *288*:1080–1081, 1973.
14. Doromal, N.M., and Canter, J.W.: Hyperosmolar hyperglycemia nonketotic coma complicating intravenous hyperalimentation. Surg. Gynecol. Obstet., *136*:729–732, 1973.
15. Drew, J.H., Koop, C.E., and Grigger, R.P.: A nutritional study of neurosurgical patients. With special reference to nitrogen balance and convalescence in the postoperative period. J. Neurosurg., *4*:7–15, 1947.
16. Dunsmore, R.H., Scoville, W.B., Reilly, F. et al.: Tracheotomy in neurosurgery. J. Neurosurg., *10*:228–232, 1953.
17. Echols, D.H., Llewellyn, R., Kirgis, H.D. et al.: Tracheotomy in the management of severe head injuries. Surgery, *28*:801–811, 1950.
18. Feigin, I.: Sequences of pathological changes in brain edema. *In* Klatzo, I., and Seitelberger, F. (eds.): Brain Edema. New York, Springer-Verlag, 1967.
19. Fleisch, A.: Le metabolisme basal standard et sa determination au moyen du "metabocalculator." Helv. Med. Acta, *18*:23–44, 1951.
20. Gadisseux, P., Ward, J.D., Young, H.F. et al.: Nutrition and the neurosurgical patient. J. Neurosurg., *60*:219–232, 1984.
21. Gordon, J.E., and Scrimshaw, N.S.: Infectious disease in the malnourished. Med. Clin. North Am., *54*:1495–1508, 1970.
22. Hill, G.L., Blackett, R.L., Rickford, I. et al.: Malnutrition in surgical patients. An unrecognized problem. Lancet, *1*:689–692, 1977.
23. Holter, A.R., and Fischer, J.E.: The effects of perioperative hyperalimentation on complications in patients with carcinoma and weight loss. J. Surg. Res., *23*:31–34, 1977.
24. Irvin, T.T., and Hunt, T.K.: Effect of malnutrition on colonic healing. Ann. Surg., *180*:765–772, 1974.
25. Jennett, B., and Bond, M.: Assessment of outcome after severe brain damage. A practical scale. Lancet, *1*:480–484, 1975.
26. Leevy, C.M., Cardi, L., Frank, O. et al.: Incidence and significance of hypovitaminemia in a randomly selected municipal hospital population. Am. J. Clin. Nutr., *17*:259–271, 1965.
27. Long, D.M., and Hartmann, J.F.: The ultrastructure of human cerebral edema. J. Neuropath. Exper. Neurol., *24*:150–151, 1965.
28. Lutz, H., Peter, K., and VanAckern, K.: Total parental alimentation in neurosurgical and neurological patients. *In* Manni, C., Magalini, S.I., and Serascio, E. (eds.): Total Parenteral Alimentation. Amsterdam, Excerpta Medica, 1976.
29. Manelli, J.C., Francois, G., Bimar, J. et al.: EEG changes in certain types of coma with prolonged parenteral feeding. Rev. EEG Neurophysiol. Clin., *5*:283–288, 1975.
30. Mazzarella, B., DeMari, M.B., Cafaggi, G. et al.: Parenteral feeding in prolonged cerebral-vascular coma. Rass. Int. Clin. Terap., *54*:831–840, 1971.
31. McLaurin, R.L., King, L., Tutor, F.T. et al.: Metabolic response to intracranial surgery. Surg. Forum, *10*:770–773, 1959.
32. O'Tuama, L.A., Kirkman, H.N., and James, P.M.: Raised intracranial pressure after hyperalimentation. Lancet, *2*:2101, 1973.
33. Prins, J.G., Schrijver, H., and Staghouwer, J.H.: Hyperalimentation, hypophosphataemia, and coma. Lancet, *1*:1253–1254, 1973.

34. Rapp, R.P., Young, B., Twyman, D. et al.: The favorable effect of early parenteral feeding on survival in head-injured patients. J. Neurosurg., *58*:906–912, 1983.
35. Reulen, H.J., Medzihradsky, F., Enzenback, R. et al.: Electrolytes, fluids and energy metabolism in human cerebral edema. Arch. Neurol., *21*:517–525, 1969.
36. Sato, K., Yamaguchi, M., Mullan, S. et al.: Brain edema, a study of biochemical and structural alterations. Arch. Neurol., *21*:413–424, 1969.
37. Savitz, M.H., Bryan-Brown, C.W., Elwyn, D.H., et al.: Postoperative nutritional failure and chronic cerebral edema in neurosurgical patients. Mt. Sinai J. Med., *45*:394–401, 1978.
38. Schiller, W.R., Long, C.L., and Blakemore, W.S.: Creatinine and nitrogen excretion in seriously ill and injured patients. Surg. Gynecol. Obstet., *149*:561–566, 1979.
39. Shoemaker, W.C., Bryan-Brown, C.W., Quigley, L. et al.: Body fluid shifts in depletion and poststress states and their correction with adequate nutrition. Surg. Gynecol. Obstet., *136*:371–374, 1973.
40. Silvis, S.E., and Paragas, P.D.: Paresthesias, weakness, seizures, and hypophosphatemia in patients receiving hyperalimentation. Gastroenterology, *62*:513–520, 1973.
41. Simon, J.: Parenteral feeding in cerebrocranial injuries. Prakt. Anaesth., *12*:1–9, 1977.
42. Stern, W.E.: Preoperative evaluation: complications, their prevention and treatment. *In* Youmans, J.P. (ed.): Neurological Surgery. Philadelphia, W.B. Saunders Co.,1982.
43. Taylor, G.W., and Austin, G.M.: Treatment of pulmonary complications in neurosurgical patients by tracheostomy. Arch. Otolaryngol., *53*:386–392, 1951.
44. Teasdale, G., and Jennett, B.: Assessment of coma and impaired consciousness. A practical scale. Lancet, *2*:81–84, 1974.
45. Twomey, P.L., and St. John, J.M.: The neurologic patient. Rombeau, J. (ed.): Clinical Nutrition. Vol. 1. Enteral and Tube Feeding. Philadelphia, W.B. Saunders Co., 1980.
46. Van DeMortel, I., Degauque, C., and Thibaut, A.: Thrombosis of cerebral venous sinuses due to a catheter for parenteral nutrition. J. Neurol. Neurosurg. Psychiat., *66*:458–459, 1983.
47. Weinsier, R.L., Hunker, E.M., Krumdieck, C.L., et al.: Hospital malnutrition. A prospective evaluation of general medical patients during the course of hospitalization. Am. J. Clin. Nutr., *32*:418–426, 1979.
48. White, R.K.: Aspects and problems of total parenteral alimentation in the neurosurgery patient. *In* Manni, C., Magalini, S.I., and Serascio, E. (eds.): Total Parenteral Alimentation. Amsterdam, Excerpta Medica, 1976.
49. Wilmore, D.W.: The Metabolic Management of the Critically Ill. New York, Plenum Medical Books, 1977.
50. Wise, B.L.: Preoperative and Postoperative Care in Neurological Surgery. Springfield, Illinois, Charles C Thomas, 1972.
51. Wise, B.L.: Fluid and Electrolytes in Neurological Surgery. Springfield, Illinois, Charles C Thomas, 1965.
52. Young, B., Rapp, R.P., Norton, J.A. et al.: Early prediction of outcome in head injured patients. J. Neurosurg., *54*:300–303, 1981.

CHAPTER 30

The Use of Total Parenteral Nutrition in the Treatment of Anorexia Nervosa*

JAMESON FORSTER

Total parenteral nutrition (TPN) has become part of the armamentarium of today's practicing physician, whatever his or her specialty. Recently, a new specialty has been included, that of psychiatry, with the realization that patients with anorexia nervosa can be effectively and safely fed on intravenous nutrition.[1, 2] In this chapter, the role of TPN in the treatment of anorexia nervosa will be discussed by first describing the disease itself, then by reviewing the available data concerning the effects of TPN on these patients, and ending by exploration of the future of this treatment modality. For the sake of brevity, the terms *anorexia* and *anorectic* will be used throughout this chapter to refer to that particular form of anorexia seen in the disease anorexia nervosa.

HISTORY

The disease anorexia nervosa has afflicted women for several centuries. In 1554, chlorosis or "the disease of virgins" was first described.[3] Afflicted women suffered from amenorrhea and anemia in addition to severe malnutrition. This illness shares many of the features of anorexia nervosa, including age and sex incidence, amenorrhea, anorexia, and alterations in mental state.[3] If not actually the same disorder, anorexia nervosa may at least be the modern version of chlorosis.

Throughout the last several centuries, fasting women have been objects of medical and societal curiosity. The first reported case was in 1613.[4] Although some of these women were apparently impostors who used their "fasting" as attention-getting devices, most had an element of psychologic disease and would be classified today as anorectics.[4]

In 1689, Richard Morton described what is now considered the classic case of anorexia nervosa when he wrote of a 16-year-old woman who "fell into a total suppression of the monthly courses for a multitude of cares and passions of her mind."[2] In this description, the features of anorexia nervosa were identified as psychologic unrest, amenorrhea, and malnutrition.

It was not, however, until late in the 19th century that the term *anorexia nervosa* was used by Sir William Gull. He and Charles Lasegue in France provided precise clinical descriptions of the disease and emphasized a psychologic explanation for the altered eating behavior.[5] Treatment at that time included separation from family, rest, nourishment, and supportive therapy.

Early in the 20th century, Simmonds reported a case of pituitary cachexia in an emaciated woman.[6] This association led many to incorrectly label patients with extreme weight loss, such as anorectics, as suffering from Simmonds' disease or hypopituitarism. The psychic component of anorexia nervosa was neglected while patients were treated with pituitary gland extract.

---

*I want to thank Dr. Barry Fogel for his critical comments regarding this chapter.

In 1930, Berkman reported on a large series of patients treated at the Mayo Clinic who had a diagnosis of anorexia nervosa and concluded that the disease was secondary to a psychic disturbance producing a physiologic disorder and not *vice versa.*[7] In 1939, Richardson expressed doubt about the association between hypopituitarism and anorexia in reviewing his treatment of six cases of malnourished women.[8] He had prescribed pituitary hormones in treating the first three patients and found dubious improvement. In fact, autopsy of one patient failed to reveal any abnormalities in either the adrenal or pituitary gland. He concluded that the diagnosis of Simmonds' disease should be made by exclusion of other causes of inanition, especially anorexia nervosa. He admonished others to treat anorectic patients for their neuroses and inanition before resorting to hormonal therapy.

In 1949, Sheehan and Summers sought to clarify the cause of weight loss occurring during the syndrome of hypopituitarism.[9] They correlated the pathologic changes seen in the pituitary gland and the general pathologic changes of the body and discovered that hypopituitarism was infrequently associated with malnutrition. In fact, the nutritional status of patients with severe hypopituitarism was no different from that of healthy individuals. These authors concluded that there was no justification to suppose that anorexia nervosa was due to functional hypopituitarism.

Despite agreement that the underlying problem in anorexia nervosa was psychologic and not hormonal, investigators in the 1950s and early 1960s disagreed on the type of psychologic conflict. Each author emphasized his or her own area of expertise. For the last 30 years, the disease has been viewed as a compulsive neurosis, an organic neurosis, hysteria, psychosis, and, psychoanalytically, as an expression of aversion to sexuality.[5]

Hilda Bruch began the modern era of treatment of anorexia nervosa when she identified three pathognomonic psychologic traits of anorectics that distinguished them from other patients with psychologic disease and weight loss: (1) distortion of body image, (2) disturbance in the accuracy of perception or cognitive interpretation of stimuli arising within the body, and (3) a paralyzing sense of ineffectiveness.[10] She labeled patients with these problems as true anorectics; all others were labeled atypical anorectics. Additionally, she noted little psychoanalytic therapeutic success in this disease and found improvement only when she was able to arouse awareness in the patients about their disease. With these two insights—that anorexia nervosa is a disease separable from other psychologic disturbances and that its treatment involves methodologies other than psychoanalysis—the modern era of the understanding and treatment of anorexia began.

PATIENT CHARACTERISTICS

The following research criteria proposed by Feighner[11] are commonly accepted guidelines for the diagnosis of anorexia nervosa (the first five criteria are required):

1. Age of onset prior to 25 years.
2. Anorexia with accompanying weight loss of at least 25 per cent of original body weight.
3. A distorted, implacable attitude toward eating, food, or weight that overrides hunger, admonitions, reassurance, and threats, for example, denial of illness with failure to recognize nutritional needs; apparent enjoyment in losing weight with an overt manifestation that food refusal is a pleasurable indulgence; a desired body image of extreme thinness, with overt evidence that it is rewarding to the patient to achieve and maintain this state; and unusual hoarding or handling of food.
4. No known medical illness that could account for the anorexia and weight loss.
5. No other known psychiatric disorder, with particular reference to primary affective disorders, schizophrenia, and obsessive-compulsive and phobic neuroses.
6. At least two of the following manifestations: amenorrhea, lanugo, bradycardia (persistent resting pulse of 60 or less), periods of overactivity, episodes of bulimia, or vomiting (may be self-induced).

However, some authors still include patients older than 25 years[12] and patients with a degree of weight loss less than 25 per cent of ideal body weight when writing about anorexia nervosa.[13, 14] All would agree that the third, fourth, and fifth criteria are the most important.

The incidence of anorexia nervosa worldwide is about 1/100,000 and is increasing.[15, 16] In subgroups, the incidence is higher. One in 200 pubertal white females may be affected.[14] In fact, one severe case/100 cases was found in affluent white English girls 16 to 18 years of age.[17] Women outnumber men by 10 to 20:1.[14, 18, 19]

The disease most commonly affects individuals from the upper socioeconomic class (professional and managerial)[20] and patients with average to above-average intelligence.[14] Premorbidly, they were "good" and compliant children with no discipline problems. In fact, most patients were very conscientious and were interested in sports and games.[20]

The relationship of the child to the family is often pathologic, being enmeshed or overinvolved in more than one third of cases.[20, 21] This state is often coupled with poor parental relationships.[20] Additionally, the parents frequently have or had psychiatric problems. Thus, the family environment of the typical anorectic is far from normal.

Anorexia nervosa appears most frequently following a self-imposed diet, which is often instigated after being teased about obesity.[14] Most patients are slightly overweight at the start of the diet. Once started, however, the diet becomes severe and takes on a value all its own, irrespective of the amount of weight loss. Onset occurs most frequently within seven years of menarche;[20] some patients never experience menarche.

On presentation for medical treatment, most anorectics have been symptomatic for several years[20, 22] and are severely malnourished, with weights approximately 70 per cent of their ideal body weight (range 56 to 100 per cent).[20, 23] Invariably, the women are amenorrheic.[14, 18, 20, 24] All demonstrate some physical sign of severe starvation, including low blood pressure,[8] decrease in body fat,[14] decrease in breast tissue mass,[14] decrease in metabolic rate,[7] lanugo,[19] and hypothermia.[19]

Despite their starved appearance, anorectics maintain a normal to above-normal level of activity; 40 per cent are frankly hyperactive.[14, 20] They continue in their studies, often being overachievers. Many are straight-A students. Jogging, long working hours, and behaving in a ritualistic fashion toward food or cleaning are frequent patterns. The eating of food, if tolerated, is often followed by vomiting and may be bulimic in nature (i.e., gorging followed by vomiting).

LABORATORY EVALUATIONS

Metabolic and endocrine evaluations of anorectics reveal a diverse pattern of abnor-

malities that appear related to the degree of starvation and that respond to refeeding by normalizing. The most well-known hormonal abnormality in anorexia nervosa is amenorrhea, which affects almost all patients. Evaluation of the pituitary-ovarian axis has brought to light many alterations in both hormonal levels and the hormonal response to releasing factors. Yet the precise cause of the amenorrhea remains elusive.[25]

Patients with anorexia nervosa have a low serum concentration of luteinizing hormone (LH), but they usually have a normal serum concentration of follicle-stimulating hormone (FSH).[26, 27] In addition, the sleep-wake pattern of LH is frequently infantile (has no episodic variation) or pubertal (shows marked episodic secretion only at night).[28, 29] The secretion of both LH and FSH in response to luteinizing hormone–follicle-stimulating hormone releasing hormone (LH–FSH-RH) is impaired;[27] the LH response shows a greater reduction than the FSH response.[30–32] Serum and urinary estrogen concentrations are below normal;[23, 26] moreover, the pattern of metabolites is changed. The serum concentration of estriol is increased, whereas estrone and estradiol concentrations are decreased.[27, 31, 33]

Improvement in the malnutrition of the anorectic is associated with the correction of both serum hormonal concentration and the hormonal response. Menstrual cycles resume in more than half of patients who improve with therapy and gain weight.[31, 34] In a group of anorectics studied before and after weight gain, the serum concentrations of both LH and FSH increased with weight gain and were linearly related to the per cent of standard weight.[31] With improved nutrition, the sleep-wake pattern of LH secretion shifts toward the adult pattern (episodic secretion throughout the day).[28, 29] The response of LH and FSH to LH–FSH-RH became more exaggerated than in controls (mature women), and is similar to the pattern seen in prepubertal women.[31] Finally, mean basal estradiol concentrations rose to within normal range in patients who gained up to 80 per cent or more of standard weight.[31]

The mean LH and FSH concentrations have been measured in a male anorectic and were found to be below the lower limits of normal. With weight gain, the hormonal concentrations increased to within normal limits. The testosterone serum concentration remained in the low-normal range regardless of weight gain.[35] In women anorectics, testosterone concentrations are increased and fall with weight gain.[24]

The pituitary-thyroid axis is also altered in patients with anorexia nervosa. Afflicted individuals appear clinically hypothyroid, with bradycardia, constipation, and hypothermia, yet they rarely have delayed relaxation of deep tendon reflexes and never have been found to have myxedema or resistant anemia.[14, 36] Investigation of serum hormonal concentrations has revealed decreased triiodothyronine (T_3) but normal concentrations of thyroid-stimulating hormone (TSH) and thyroxine (T_4).[14, 26, 37] In addition, concentrations of reverse triiodothyronine (rT_3), a peripherally formed inactive isomer of T_3, are increased in patients suffering from anorexia nervosa.[37] TSH release responds less than normally to stimulation by thyrotrophin-releasing hormone (TRH).[37] With refeeding, both the concentration of T_3 and the magnitude of the response of TSH to TRH promptly increase to normal ranges.[37] The observed changes in thyroid metabolism in patients with anorexia nervosa are thought to be adaptive to malnutrition and a "homeostatic protective adjustment at the cellular level."[35]

Adrenocortical function has been considered to be normal in anorexia nervosa.[23] The concentration of adrenocorticotropic hormone (ACTH) is within normal limits.[23] However, recent precise determination of serum cortisol concentrations has shown them to be high and without diurnal variation.[25, 26] In addition to high serum concentrations of cortisol, urinary free cortisol secretion was found to be increased, and cortisol production rates were in the high-normal range.[25, 38] Recovery from anorexia nervosa was found to be associated with a marked decrease in cortisol production and a return to normal of serum cortisol concentrations.[25, 38] These findings are consistent with the hypothesis that in anorexia nervosa the activity of the hypothalamic-pituitary-adrenal axis is increased and the adrenal glands are unusually responsive to ACTH stimulation.[25]

Other pituitary hormones are variably affected in anorexia nervosa. The basal prolactin secretion rate, the prolactin response to stimulus, and the prolactin sleep-wake rhythm are normal.[32, 39] The basal plasma growth hormone concentration may be higher in anorectics than in controls.[18, 26] The ability to secrete free water is impaired in anorectics.[40] Recently, arginine vasopressin has been found to be in low concentration in the cerebrospinal fluid and plasma of anorec-

tics and to respond erratically to a saline challenge.[41] With normalization of weight, normal responsiveness of vasopressin to a saline challenge is regained.[41]

Further abnormalities are found in pancreatic function. In particular, glucose tolerance is impaired and is associated with higher than normal concentrations of insulin. With weight gain, the glucose tolerance test shows improvement, and the serum insulin concentrations decrease.[23]

In summary, anorectics have many hormonal abnormalities. None of these changes appears specific to anorexia nervosa itself.[42, 43] In fact, weight loss alone has been shown to produce the same hormonal changes as those seen in patients with anorexia nervosa.[44] Also, it is well known that body composition (fat stores in particular) is a determinant of reproductive ability.[45] Therefore, correction of the malnutrition may return both hormonal concentrations and response to within reference ranges. However, in long-term followup of greater than five years, only about 50 per cent of anorectics who do well by any criteria regain their menstrual cycles.[34] Indeed, LH concentrations may not necessarily return to normal ranges even if ideal weight is achieved.[25] This fact and the observation that anorectics frequently lose their menstrual cycles before they become malnourished have influenced one author to conclude that there may be a primary disturbance in the hypothalamus.[46]

NUTRITIONAL ASSESSMENT

Nutritional assessment of patients with anorexia nervosa reveals a marked degree of weight loss, down to 50 per cent of their ideal body weight. The patients appear uniformly cachectic. They have depressed anthropometric indices with marked muscle and fat wasting. A recent study of a group of 22 anorectics (21 female, 1 male) found the average triceps skinfold thickness to be 27 per cent of normal and the midarm muscle circumference to be 69 per cent of standard.[47]

On hospital admission, anorectics have a normal hemoglobin concentration and hematocrit;[47, 48] however, with hospital treatment, the hemotocrit falls, suggesting a relative initial hemoconcentration.[48]

Although the average white blood cell count was normal in 22 anorectics, 8 of the individuals, or 40 per cent, had values less than the lower limit of normal.[47] This finding has been confirmed.[48] Skin-test reactivity has been found to be depressed in anorectic patients and appears to be dependent on the degree of malnutrition as determined by anthropometric measurements.[47] Yet anorectics have a normal to above normal *in vitro* response to mitogen stimulation and a normal per cent of T lymphocytes[49] as well as a normal hemagglutinin-titer response following vaccination to influenza.[50] Additionally, bone marrow neutrophil reserves are normal in anorexia nervosa.[47] Overall, anorectics appear to have a normal incidence of infections. A population of 68 hospitalized anorectics had the same number of infectious events as an age- and sex-matched group of patients with other psychiatric diseases.[47]

Vitamin deficiencies have been rarely reported in anorexia nervosa despite the accompanying marked malnutrition. Possibly the patients protect themselves by their consumption of fruit and green vegetables. Plasma folic acid concentrations were measured and found normal in 30 women with the disease, though the range was very large.[51] The variability probably resulted from widely differing diets and degrees of weight loss. Plasma cholesterol levels were elevated and returned to normal values with weight gain.[51] Hypercarotenemia is a frequent finding and is thought to be diet-related.[14] In a recent study of 30 patients with anorexia nervosa, which was designed to test the hypothesis that zinc deficiency is related to hypercarotenemia through a defect in vitamin A metabolism, carotene concentrations were confirmed to be significantly higher in the anorectics than in a control group of 32 laboratory employees.[51] However, these patients were also found to have normal concentrations of both vitamin A and retinol-binding protein (RBP). Thus, a defect in vitamin A metabolism was unlikely to be the cause of the increased concentrations of carotene. Although the authors did report one patient whose increased intake of apricot juice was clearly the cause of her hypercarotenemia, they concluded that in general the etiology of this abnormality remains undetermined.[51]

In patients with anorexia nervosa, both plasma concentrations of zinc and urinary zinc excretion were found to be depressed.[51] Again, individual values varied greatly, depending on the intake of vitamin and mineral supplements. Plasma copper concentrations were also statistically lower than in the control group of laboratory employees.[51] Serum iron concentrations were within normal limits.[51]

Despite the cachexia, patients with anorexia nervosa on the average have normal visceral protein status (i.e., normal concentrations of serum proteins, including total protein, albumin, and transferrin).[23, 40, 47, 49] Albumin and total protein serum levels were normal in two studies,[47, 51] yet individuals may have markedly low levels on presentation. Average calculated transferrin concentrations were within normal limits,[47, 51] but were statistically lower than in a control group of laboratory employees.[51] RBP plasma concentrations were measured and found to be no different from those in a control group, as were ceruloplasmin concentrations.[51]

The average patient with anorexia nervosa presents a classic undernutritional form of malnutrition, similar to marasmus, characterized by depressed anthropometric indices, normal visceral protein status, and anergy.[52, 53] Despite long-term decreased food intake, anorectics are able to survive because on the average they consume a diet that gives them 1000 kcal/day and a relatively normal amount of protein, approximately 41 gm in 24 hours.[23, 40] This diet maintains an anorectic patient in a quasi-steady state. Because the body's fat stores are required to provide only a small portion of the total energy expenditure, the patient's body can tolerate this semi-starvation for a long period. However, the patient continues to lose body cell mass and becomes more at risk each day from starvation-induced morbidity and mortality.

PSYCHOLOGIC THERAPY

Many different modalities have been used in the treatment of anorexia nervosa, depending on what is considered the dominant pathologic process.[13] At the beginning of this century, hormonal manipulation with pituitary extracts was the treatment of choice, since the underlying pathology was thought to be hypopituitarism. The therapy changed radically with the realization that all cachexia is not hypopituitarism and that the disease was partly psychologic in origin. Using classic psychoanalysis, the psychiatrist sought to give the patient insight into the disease. Classic psychoanalysis was uniformly met with defeat, since the patients appeared to have difficulty knowing what they felt themselves.[10, 15]

For the last 20 years, therapy for anorexia nervosa has included the combined approach of nutritional and psychiatric modalities. According to most therapists, refeeding is the first step to recovery, since starvation has a major effect on psychic function and may interfere with the ability to integrate new understanding.[54-56] The methods employed vary from dietary counseling to TPN, with some form of behavior modification being the most prevalent.[12, 55, 57-59] Along with receiving nutritional therapy, the patients are treated for their psychologic difficulties. Specific regimens vary, but usually the patient receives individual psychotherapy, group therapy, and family therapy. Each case is individualized. Patients with severe anorexia are often hospitalized to remove them from the enmeshment found at home; some psychiatrists, however, try to keep their anorectic patients out of the hospital as long as possible.[21, 60] Although electroconvulsive therapy and leukotomy have been used for severe cases, they are rarely part of current therapy.[13]

Psychotropic drugs have been used as primary therapy in the treatment of anorexia nervosa.[61, 62] In a review of the literature, lithium, cyproheptadine (a serotonin antagonist), and tricyclic antidepressants were found to be the most useful of all drugs studied in promoting weight gain and improving patients' moods.[61] However, the effects of these agents are not always consistent from one report to another, and the improvement noted is often minimal and of short duration. Psychotropic drugs have also been employed during psychotherapy when a patient's severe anxiety or depression interferes with full participation.[12]

OUTCOME

The initial outcome of treatment is generally favorable and may be independent of the initial therapeutic modality used.[39, 63] Despite the specter of starvation, death occurs in only about six per cent of cases (an average of many followup studies).[34, 63] The causes of death include suicide, electrolyte imbalances, gastric dilatation, and, terminally, overwhelming infection.[64-67] In long-term followup of up to 50 years, anorectics continue to succumb to their disease and appear not to have a normal life expectancy.[63] The majority of anorectics had gained weight at followup (average of five years), though only about 50 per cent had experienced return of menstrual function.[34] Despite weight gain, patients continue to be concerned about their body weight, and their eating patterns rarely return to normal. Overall, 49 per cent of those admitted were completely recovered at followup, 31 per cent experienced some improvement in weight, and 18 per cent were unchanged.[63] Psychiatrically, however, anorectics continue to have marked problems. They deal poorly in both the psychosexual and psychosocial spheres,[34, 63] yet they are extremely good workers.[34]

Prognostic factors have been identified that relate patient characteristics to poor outcome in anorexia nervosa.[68, 69] They include prior hospitalizations, prior hospitalization treatment failures, denial of illness, inactivity, loss of appetite, and psychosexual immaturity.[68, 69] Other negative prognostic factors include long duration of illness, older age of onset, lower weight, and lower social class.[68] At four to eight years after initial presentation, psychosocial development has been found to be prognostically important. Impaired social adjustment (lack of friends) and a poor or disturbed relationship with the parents (extensive dependence) were associated with poor outcome at followup.[68] Thus, an anorectic with a favorable outcome would be expected to have had no previous hospitalizations for the illness, be overactive, have less denial of illness, have less psychosexual immaturity, and readily admit to having an appetite.[69]

NUTRITIONAL THERAPY

The nutritional therapy of anorexia has encompassed all avenues of alimentation. By far, the majority of patients are able to take food by mouth once their psychologic therapy has started.[14] In fact, some researchers concentrate their attention on psychotherapy and do not even show concern about the patient's eating, assuming that once the patient is better good nutritional intake will follow.[70] In hospitalized patients, weight gain is enforced in a variety of ways. Behavior modification by contingency management has consistently been very successful. In this therapy, the patients enter a contract in which they are required to gain a set amount of weight daily in order to have access to the social activities of the ward.[12] Another approach has patients take extra liquid food supplements if weight gain is not sufficient.[58] In most reported programs, the weight gain sought is approximately one-half lb. daily. The diet usually consists of regular hospital fare, though formulas are currently playing a larger role.[57] Because of complications associated with refeeding such starved individuals, one group has limited the total calories consumed to 125 per cent of basal requirements for the first week, 150 per cent for the second week, 200 per cent for the third week, and unlimited calories for the fourth week.[57] Approximately 5000 to 7000 extra calories are needed for each kilogram of weight gained.[71]

In the past, tube feeding was used for severely malnourished or recalcitrant individuals.[14, 18] In 1968, however, a report of a death following aspiration while the patient was receiving nutritional support with tube feeding led to the reluctance of investigators to use this modality.[64] Additionally, anorectics were thought to have adverse psychologic reactions to nasogastric tubes. A recent report from France documented very favorable results in treating 14 anorectics (average per cent of ideal body weight was 65 per cent) with tube feedings.[72] They noted excellent weight gain, improvement in nutritional assessment parameters, and resumption of adequate oral intake with no complications.

THE HISTORY OF TPN USE

Until recently, few reports have discussed the treatment of anorectics with TPN, despite the theoretic and practical advantages of this modality.[73] A literature search has revealed five papers documenting 19 cases (Table 30–1).[1, 2, 74–76] One additional case is included of a patient who was treated with peripheral intravenous nutrition.[77]

The first reported use of TPN in the treatment of anorexia nervosa was in 1972. Finkelstein, in a letter to the *Journal of the American Medical Association*, reported two patients who had psychologic disturbances and cachexia and required parenteral nutrition for treatment.[74] Whether these patients actually had anorexia nervosa is unknown, since they were both older, 44 and 50 years, and since the brief descriptions paint a picture of psychosis. However, neither patient responded to the treatment regimens of psychotherapy, electroconvulsive therapy, anabolic steroids, phenothiazines, and narcostimulation treatments. Behavior modification apparently was not used. Both patients refused to eat and both had starved themselves to marked cachexia. One had developed starvation edema and hypokalemia. No mention was made of the degree of weight loss. Parenteral nutrition was successful in achieving weight gain. One patient regained her normal weight and returned to work. The other patient had marked improvement of her "bodily functions," and the "features of anorexia nervosa disappeared completely."[74] However, she had not returned to her premorbid life at the time of the report.

In the Japanese literature, mention is made of feeding an anorectic patient with an intravenous fat emulsion via peripheral vein combined with tube feeding.[77] The patient was a 32-year-old woman. The diagnosis of anorexia nervosa was made according to three criteria: (1) the weight loss resulted from refusal to eat normally, (2) no organic reason was identified for the weight loss, and (3) cachexia was of long duration. The patient's weight on hospital admission was 26 kg (normal weight was 40 kg). Nutritional treatment included intravenous administration of a 10 per cent fat emulsion, 500 ml daily, plus intravenous administration of 400 ml of Proteamin XT and 100 ml of 40 per cent glucose. In addition to her intravenous feed-

Table 30–1. TPN USE IN ANOREXIA NERVOSA

DATE	NO.	SEX	TYPE	COMPLICATIONS	WEIGHT GAIN	PSYCHIATRIC IMPROVEMENT	REF. NO.
1972	2	F	Atypical	NS	Yes	Yes	64
1974	1	F	Atypical	NS	Yes	NS	66
1977	1	F	Typical	NS	Yes	Yes	67
1980	4	F	Typical	NS	Yes	Yes	1
1981	11	F, 10 M, 1	Typical	Liver function test elevations, hypophosphatemia, death, pneumothorax	Yes	NS	2

NS = not stated.

ings, she also ate. However, when she developed nausea and vomiting, tube feedings were begun. Total intake increased from 1000 kcal to 2300 kcal/day with institution of tube feedings. During her treatment, her liver function values increased, and for reasons that are unclear, they later reverted to normal. No mention was made of other complications that were possibly due to the intravenous alimentation. The patient gained weight, was weaned to total oral intake, and left the hospital improved. Nine months after her treatment, she had further increased her weight, and her anorexia nervosa was reported "cured."

In 1974, an eight-year-old anorectic was given TPN for four weeks to evaluate the rate of fat clearance.[75] She was given Intralipid 20 per cent, Vamin, and glucose at a rate of 120 kcal/kg/day. The patient tolerated the regimen well and did not suffer from acetonuria, acidosis, coagulopathy, or liver function test abnormalities. Her weight increased at a rate of about 1 kg/week. No mention was made of the effect TPN had on her disease.

The third reported case of anorexia nervosa treated with TPN was published in 1977 and described a typical anorectic who developed acute tubular necrosis following two episodes of hypotension secondary to severe malnutrition.[76] She was given D50 and 2.13 per cent Fre-Amine for 15 days. On the fourth day of that regimen, she began to eat once again. She improved clinically. Her creatinine and blood urea nitrogen (BUN) levels decreased, and her ankle edema disappeared. At one-and-a-half years after hospitalization, she was "a well adjusted, well fed, and attractive adolescent."[76]

In 1980, a study of the use of TPN in treating severe anorectics was published.[1] All subjects were typical anorectics who were unresponsive to behavior modification, family therapy, and psychotherapy, and all were severely malnourished, weighing, on the average, 59 per cent of their ideal body weight. They were treated with TPN for 12 to 44 days and gained an average of 2.5 kg/week. No complications were reported. In addition to the benefits of weight gain, all the patients showed marked mood improvements, allowing psychotherapy. The patients continued to gain weight. Followup at 5 to 16 months revealed that the patients weighed 88 to 106 per cent of their ideal body weight.

A retrospective review of 11 typical an-orectics treated with TPN focused on the problems encountered in this therapy as experienced over 11 years.[2] The patients treated were unresponsive to standard treatment or had extreme weight loss. All patients on TPN for longer than one week gained weight during TPN at a rate of 2.5 kg/week. Their hospital stay was longer than that of the majority of anorectics but was no different from a control group of anorectics matched for age, sex, and per cent of ideal body weight. Although no long-term followup data are available, the patients continued to gain weight in the hospital after the TPN was terminated, and when compared with non–TPN-treated anorectics, they did not have increased hospital readmissions (unpublished observations). Complications did occur. Almost all patients showed some elevation of liver enzymes, one had a pneumothorax, and one had arthritis. Two patients developed severe hypophosphatemia, and one of them died. These two patients were given TPN when the technique was new and the complication of hypophosphatemia was unknown. Recent practice has all but eliminated this problem. No information was given concerning the effect TPN had on the psychologic disease in these patients.

SUMMARY OF TPN USE

In summary, TPN has been used infrequently but effectively in the treatment of the severely anorectic patient. In one university teaching hospital, about one anorectic a year has been so treated since the technique of TPN first became available.[2] Most patients experienced weight gain, psychologic improvement, and minimal complications (Table 30–1).

The criteria for the use of TPN have included intractability to other therapy, worsening psychologic state, and extreme weight loss.[1, 2] If the experience at one university teaching hospital can be generalized, about 10 per cent of anorectics admitted would fulfill one or more of these criteria and would benefit from TPN.[2]

TPN improves the nutritional status of anorectics. Weight is gained at a rate of 2.5 kg/week.[1, 2] Other anthropometric indices—the triceps skinfold thickness and the midarm muscle circumference—increase under TPN therapy.[78] Visceral protein status improves as evidenced by increases in the serum concentrations of albumin[2, 78] and transferrin.[78] Additionally, certain complement components (C_{3b} amplification loop proteins, C_3, factor B, β-1H, and C_{3b}INA) showed significant increases with 22 days of TPN.[78]

The most exciting feature in the use of TPN has been the observed improvement in the patient's mental status.[1] It is well known that starvation has profound psychologic effects. Participants in a study of experimental starvation became increasingly concerned about food, lost interest in social and sexual matters, and grew moody and depressed.[79] Thus, some of the psychologic turmoil of patients with anorexia nervosa may result from starvation alone. Weight gain or even a change in the nutrient concentration of plasma appears to diminish the obstructing psychologic effects of starvation and facilitates psychotherapy.[1]

There have been severe complications associated with the use of TPN in anorectics. However, these problems, both metabolic and catheter-related, are well recognized and, under the auspices of a nutritional support service, would be reduced. As would be expected with depletion of intracellular ions (potassium, phosphorus, magnesium, zinc) secondary to starvation, marked alterations in serum concentrations of these ions can occur during refeeding. In particular, hypophosphatemia has been reported and eliminated with the routine addition of phosphate to TPN solutions and with careful monitoring of serum phosphate levels. Pneumothorax occurs infrequently with insertion of the catheter; its incidence is related to the experience of the operator and the degree of emaciation of the patient. Thus, only the experienced members of a nutritional support service team should insert the subclavian lines in these patients. Liver function abnormalities relate to fatty infiltration of the liver, which is a complication of high-carbohydrate loads. This implies that, despite their severe cachexia, anorectics should be refed slowly at first, working up to high-energy loads after a few weeks.

DISCUSSION

The use of TPN, an invasive nutritional technique, in the treatment of anorexia nervosa disagrees with current therapeutic prejudices.[14, 18] First, there is concern that TPN, being a form of forced feeding, may interfere with the psychologic state of the patient and worsen the disease.[14, 18] The patient may consider TPN an intrusion into her space and further proof that she has no control over her environment. The use of TPN may thus be associated with longer hospital admissions, increased anxiety or depression during administration, or recurrence of the disease after TPN use. As previously stated, in a retrospective study of a group of 11 patients with anorexia nervosa, patients continued to gain weight after TPN was stopped, they had the same length of hospital admission as comparably sick orally fed anorectics, and they did not have an increased rate of readmission.[2] In fact, patients on TPN had improved moods and improved receptivity to psychotherapy, not the reverse.[1]

Second, TPN may be considered a dangerous form of nutritional therapy fraught with complications.[18] A recent review did emphasize the complications associated with the administration of TPN, including death, electrolyte abnormalities, pneumothorax, and liver function abnormalities.[2] However, this study examined 11 years of use during which time the technique of TPN was perfected. Current practice has all but eliminated the electrolyte and liver function abnormalities in the practice of intravenous nutrition therapy (see Chapter 17).

Third, TPN has been said to be expensive.[80] Although no study has specifically looked at the relative expense of oral refeeding versus TPN, recent studies seem to indicate that patients fed with TPN can be treated with psychotherapy earlier than would have been the case had they been fed orally. This observation suggests that in the future, the hospital stays of patients treated with TPN might be reduced. A shortened hospital stay would help defray the cost of TPN. Also, if TPN could prevent an occasional oral refeeding death, the cost differential would be lessened even more.

Fourth, since most patients with anorexia nervosa can be refed orally, TPN may be superfluous in a modern treatment facility.[58] This contention is correct for approximately 90 per cent of patients with anorexia nervosa admitted to the hospital. However, 10 per cent are severe anorectics who steadfastly refuse to eat adequately, are severely malnourished, or show worsening of their psychologic disease despite intense therapy.[1, 2, 80] These individuals require immedi-

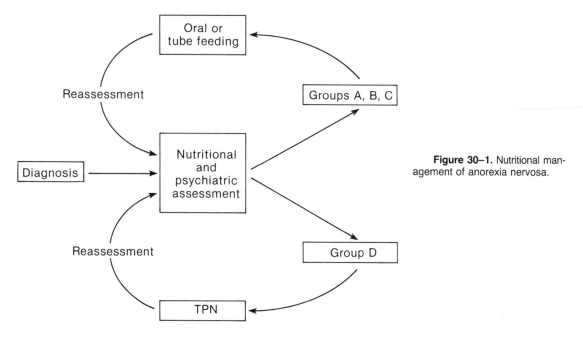

Figure 30–1. Nutritional management of anorexia nervosa.

ate nutritional therapy. Although tube feeding has been used in the past and continues to have popularity in some people's hands,[71] refeeding by means of the gastrointestinal tract may in itself be dangerous. Many of the deaths that occur in anorectics are secondary to complications involved in oral refeeding. Such complications include acute gastric dilatation[65–67] and aspiration.[64] The patient who died following aspiration was fed by tube; acute gastric dilatation followed refeeding by mouth.

The benefits of TPN are several—the nutritional status of the patient is improved reliably and rapidly, the technique avoids the complications associated with refeeding by mouth, and the psychologic outlook of the patient is improved.

Including TPN in the armamentarium for treating the patient with anorexia nervosa allows the health provider to remain confident that the patient is being nourished while being treated psychiatrically. Despite its proven ability to improve their mental status, TPN should not as yet be offered to all anorectics. In the mildly starved individual, behavior modification works well.

Thus, it would seem reasonable that TPN may be integrated into the treatment of anorexia nervosa in the manner shown in Figure 30–1. After the diagnosis of anorexia nervosa is made, the patient should be assessed nutritionally (i.e., by dietary history, body composition, and serum concentrations of albumin and transferrin)[52] and psychiatrically (i.e., by the number of previous admis-

sions, family history, intractability, and so on).[68, 69] Following initial nutritional and psychiatric assessment, the patient would fall into one of the four groups shown in Table 30–2: normal or favorable assessment in both areas (Group A), depressed or unfavorable assessment in both areas (Group D), or a combination of the two conditions (Group B or C). If the patient is severely malnourished and has an unfavorable psychiatric future (a severe anorectic; i.e., in Group D), the patient should be considered for TPN. For patients who fall into Groups A, B, or C, oral or tube feedings should be tried. Once the initial therapy has been chosen, routine reassessment (e.g., weekly) is required to identify crossovers. For instance, patients in Group D who are responding to therapy may be able to be switched to oral feedings, or some patients in one of the other three groups may regress and refuse to eat and could thereby benefit from TPN. Under this schema, the nutritional well-being of the anorectic is assured by initial assessment and careful followup.

The methodology of TPN administration is outlined in this volume and includes a nutritional support service and the frequent

Table 30–2. ASSESSMENT GROUPINGS

GROUP	A	B	C	D
Nutritional assessment	Normal	Depressed	Normal	Depressed
Psychiatric assessment	Favorable	Favorable	Unfavorable	Unfavorable

monitoring of laboratory parameters. In particular, the patient should be followed carefully for electrolyte abnormalities (especially potassium and phosphate levels), congestive heart failure,[81, 82] and vitamin deficiencies. Because of their severe muscle wasting, these patients may be more susceptible than normal patients to complications associated with catheter insertion. Infectious complications are particularly severe in individuals who have little or no reserve. Additionally, TPN should be started with low glucose and amino acid concentrations and advanced slowly to protect the patient from massive electrolyte shifts and liver damage.

Under the careful eyes of a nutritional support team, TPN has a useful role in the treatment of severe anorectics, from both a nutritional and a psychologic viewpoint. Knowing the benefits of TPN on the psychologic status of anorectics, less severely ill patients may be helped by TPN if its administration produces a faster acceptance of psychotherapy than does behavior modification, thus reducing the length of hospitalization. This issue would be addressed by a study comparing the hospital course of two groups of anorectics randomly assigned to TPN or oral diet, and by following both their psychologic status and nutritional parameters. Long-term followup of these groups would help define the potential benefits accrued by more rapid return to normal weight.

REFERENCES

1. Maloney, M.J., and Farrell, M.K.: Treatment of severe weight loss in anorexia nervosa with hyperalimentation and psychotherapy. Am. J. Psych., *137*:310–314, 1980.
2. Pertschuk, M.J., Forster, J., Buzby, G., and Mullen, J.L.: The treatment of anorexia nervosa with total parenteral nutrition. Biol. Psychol., *16*:539–550, 1981.
3. Loudon, I.S.L.: Chlorosis, anaemia, and anorexia nervosa. Br. Med. J., *281*:1669–1675, 1980.
4. Morgan, H.G.: Fasting girls and our attitudes to them. Br. Med. J., 2:1652–1655, 1977.
5. Lucas, A.R.: Toward the understanding of anorexia nervosa as a disease entity. Mayo Clin. Proc., *56*:254–264, 1981.
6. Simmonds, M.: Ueber Hypophysisschwund mit todlichem Ausgang. Deutsch. Med. Wochenschr., *40*:322–323, 1914.
7. Berkman, J.M.: Anorexia nervosa, anorexia, inanition, and low basal metabolic rate. Am. J. Med. Sci., *180*:411–424, 1930.
8. Richardson, H.B.: Simmonds' disease and anorexia nervosa. Arch. Intern. Med., *63*:1–28, 1939.
9. Sheehan, H.L., and Summers, V.K.: The syndrome of hypopituitarism. Q. J. Med., *18*:319–378, 1949.
10. Bruch, H.: Perceptual and conceptual disturbances in anorexia nervosa. Psychosom. Med., *24*:187–194, 1962.
11. Feighner, J.P., Robins, E., Guze, S.B., Woodruff, R.A., Winokur, G., and Munoz, R.: Diagnostic criteria for use in psychiatric research. Arch. Gen. Psychiatry, *26*:57–63, 1972.
12. Pertschuk, M.J.: Behavior therapy: Extended followup. *In* Vigersky, R.A. (ed.): Anorexia Nervosa. New York, Raven Press, 1977.
13. Piazza, E., Piazza, N., and Rollins, N.: Anorexia nervosa: Controversial aspects of therapy. Compr. Psychiatr., *21*:177–189, 1980.
14. Schwabe, A.D., Lippe, B.M., Chang, R.J., Pops, M.A., and Yager, J.: Anorexia nervosa. Ann. Intern. Med., *94*:371–381, 1981.
15. Bruch, H.: Anorexia nervosa: Therapy and theory. Am. J. Psychiatr., *139*:1531–1538, 1982.
16. Jones, D.J., Fox, M.M., Babigian, H.M., and Hutton, H.E.: Epidemiology of anorexia nervosa in Monroe County, New York: 1960–1976. Psychol. Med., *42*:551–558, 1980.
17. Crisp, A.H., Palmer, R.L., and Kakocy, R.S.: How common is anorexia nervosa? A prevalence study. Br. J. Psychiatry, *128*:549–554, 1976.
18. Drossman, D.A., Ontjes, D.A., and Heizer, W.D.: Anorexia nervosa. Gastroenterology, *77*:1115–1131, 1979.
19. Warren, M.P., and VandeWiele, R.L.: Clinical and metabolic features of anorexia nervosa. Am. J. Obstet. Gynecol., *117*:435–449, 1973.
20. Crisp, A.H., Hsu, L.K.G., Harding, B., and Hartshorn, J.: Clinical features of anorexia nervosa. J. Psychosom. Res., *24*:179–191, 1980.
21. Minuchin, S., Rosman, B.L., and Baker, L.: Psychosomatic Families: Anorexia Nervosa in Context. Cambridge, Harvard University Press, 1978.
22. Bruch, H.: Eating Disorders: Obesity, Anorexia Nervosa, and the Person Within. New York, Basic Books, 1973.
23. Kanis, J.A., Brown, P., Fitzpatrick, K., Hibbert, D.J., Horn, D.B., Nairn, I.M., Shirling, D., Strong, J.A., and Walton, H.J.: Anorexia nervosa: A clinical, psychiatric, and laboratory study. Q. J. Med., *43*:321–338, 1974.
24. Halmi, K.A.: Anorexia nervosa: Recent investigations. Ann. Rev. Med., *29*:137–148, 1978.
25. Weiner, H.: Abiding problems in the psychoendocrinology of anorexia nervosa. Report of the 4th Ross Conference on Medical Research: Understanding Anorexia Neurosis and Bulimia. Columbus, Ohio, Ross Laboratories, 1983.
26. Hurd, H.P., Palumbo, P.J., and Gharib, H.: Hypothalamic-endocrine dysfunction in anorexia nervosa. Mayo Clin. Proc., *52*:711–716, 1977.
27. Halmi, K.A., and Sherman, B.M.: Gonadotropin response to LH-RH in anorexia nervosa. Arch. Gen. Psychiatry, *32*:875–878, 1975.
28. Pirke, K.M., Fichter, M.M., Lund, R., and Doerr, P.: Twenty-four hour sleep-wake pattern of plasma LH in patients with anorexia nervosa. Acta Endocrinol., *92*:193–204, 1979.
29. Boyar, R.M., Katz, J., Finkelstein, J.W., Kapen, S., Weiner, H., Weitzman, E.D., and Hellman, L.: Anorexia nervosa: Immaturity of the 24-hour luteinizing hormone secretory pattern. N. Engl. J. Med., *291*:861–865, 1974.

30. Sherman, B.M., Halmi, K.A., and Zamudio, R.: LH and FSH response to gonadotropin-releasing hormone in anorexia nervosa: Effect of nutritional rehabilitation. J. Clin. Endocrinol. Metab., *41*:135–142, 1975.

31. Beaumont, P.J.V., George, G.C.W., Pimstone, B.L., and Vinik, A.I.: Body weight and the pituitary response to hypothalamic releasing hormones in patients with anorexia nervosa. J. Clin. Endocrinol. Metab., *43*:487–496, 1976.

32. Isaacs, A.J., Leslie, R.D.G., Gomez, J., and Bayliss, R.: The effect of weight gain on gonadotrophins and prolactin in anorexia nervosa. Acta Endocrinol., *94*:145–150, 1980.

33. Baranowska, B., and Zgliczynski, S.: Enhanced testosterone in female patients with anorexia nervosa: Its normalization after weight gain. Acta Endocrinol., *90*:328–335, 1979.

34. Hsu, L.K.G.: Outcome of anorexia nervosa. Arch. Gen. Psychiatry, *37*:1041–1046, 1980.

35. McNab, D., and Hawton, K.: Disturbances of sex hormones in anorexia nervosa in the male. Postgrad. Med. J., *57*:254–256, 1981.

36. Moshang, T., and Utiger, R.D.: Low triiodothyronine euthyroidism in anorexia nervosa. *In* Vigersky, R.A. (ed.): Anorexia Nervosa. New York, Raven Press, 1977.

37. Leslie, R.D.G., Isaacs, A.J., Gomez, J., Raggatt, P.R., and Bayliss, R.: Hypothalamo-pituitary-thyroid function in anorexia nervosa: Influence of weight gain. Br. Med. J., *2*:526–528, 1978.

38. Walsh, B.T., Katz, J.L., Levin, J., Kream, J., Fukushima, D.K., Weiner, H., and Zumoff, B.: The production rate of cortisol declines during recovery from anorexia nervosa. J. Clin. Endocrinol. Metab., *53*:203–205, 1981.

39. Giusti, M., Mazzocchi, G., Mortara, R., Mignone, D., and Giordano, G.: Prolactin secretion in anorexia nervosa. Horm. Metab. Res., *13*:585–586, 1981.

40. Russell, G.F.M.: Metabolic, endocrine, and psychiatric aspects of anorexia nervosa: Sci. Basis Med. Ann. Rev., :236–255, 1969.

41. Gold, P.W., Kaye, W., Robertson, G.L., and Ebert, M.: Abnormalities in plasma and cerebrospinal-fluid arginine vasopressin in patients with anorexia nervosa. N. Engl. J. Med., *308*:1117–1123, 1983.

42. Fichter, M.M., Doerr, P., Pirke, K.M., and Lund, R.: Behavior, attitude, nutrition, and endocrinology in anorexia nervosa. Acta Psychiatr. Scand., *66*:429–444, 1982.

43. Vigersky, R.A., and Loriaux, D.L.: Anorexia nervosa as a model of hypothalamic dysfunction. *In* Vigersky, R.A. (ed.): Anorexia Nervosa. New York, Raven Press, 1977.

44. Vigersky, R.A., Andersen, A.E., Thompson, R.H., and Loriaux, D.L.: Hypothalamic dysfunction in secondary amenorrhea associated with simple weight loss. N. Engl. J. Med., *297*:1141–1145, 1977.

45. Frisch, R.: Food intake, fatness, and reproductive ability. *In* Vigersky, R.A. (ed.): Anorexia Nervosa. New York, Raven Press, 1977.

46. Russell, G.F.M.: Anorexia nervosa. Proc. R. Soc. Med., *58*:811–814, 1965.

47. Pertschuk, M.J., Crosby, L.O., Barot, L., and Mullen, J.L.: Immunocompetency in anorexia nervosa. Am. J. Clin. Nutr., *35*:968–972, 1982.

48. Bowers, T.K.: Leukopenia in anorexia nervosa. Arch. Intern. Med., *138*:1520–1523, 1978.

49. Golla, J.A., Larson, L.A., Anderson, C.F., Lucas, A.R., Wilson, W.R., and Tomasi, T.B.: An immunological assessment of patients with anorexia nervosa. Am. J. Clin. Nutr., *34*:2756–2762, 1981.

50. Armstrong-Esther, C.A., Crisp, A.H., Lacey, J.H., and Bryant, T.N.: An investigation of the immune response of patients suffering from anorexia nervosa. Postgrad. Med. J., *54*:395–399, 1978.

51. Casper, R.C., Kirschner, B., Sandstead, H.H., Jacob, R.A., and Davis, J.M.: An evaluation of trace metals, vitamins, and taste function in anorexia nervosa. Am. J. Clin. Nutr., *33*:1801–1808, 1980.

52. Blackburn, G.L., Bistrian, B.R., Maini, B.S., Schlamm, H.T., and Smith, M.F.: Nutritional and metabolic assessment of the hospitalized patient. J.P.E.N., *1*:11–22, 1977.

53. Jellife, D.B.: The assessment of the nutritional status of the community. Geneva, WHO Monograph Series No. 53, 1966.

54. Bruch, H.: Treatment in anorexia nervosa. Int. J. Psychoanal. Psychother., *9*:303–312, 1982–1983.

55. Nillius, S.J.: Weight and the menstrual cycle. Report of the 4th Ross Conference on Medical Research: Understanding Anorexia Nervosa and Bulimia. Columbus, Ohio, Ross Laboratories, 1983.

56. Russell, G. F. M.: The current treatment of anorexia nervosa. Br. J. Psychiatry, *138*:164–166, 1981.

57. Halmi, K.A., Powers, P., and Cunningham, S.: Treatment of anorexia nervosa with behavior modification. Arch. Gen. Psychiatry, *32*:93–96, 1975.

58. Maxmen, J.S., Siberfarb, P.M., and Ferrell, R.B.: Anorexia nervosa: Practical initial management in a general hospital. J.A.M.A., *229*:801–803, 1974.

59. Wulliemier, F., Rossell, F., and Sinclair, K.: La therapie comportementale de l'anorexie nervose. J. Psychosom. Res., *19*:267–272, 1975.

60. Reinhart, J.B., Kenna, M.D., and Succop, R.A.: Anorexia nervosa in children: Outpatient management. Am. Acad. Child Psychiatr., *11*:114–131, 1972.

61. Johnson, C., Stuckey, M., and Mitchell, J.: Psychopharmacological treatment of anorexia and bulimia, review and synthesis. J. Nerv. Mental Dis., *171*:524–534, 1983.

62. Rockwell, J.K., Ellinwood, E.H., Dougherty, G.G., and Brodie, H.K.H.: Anorexia nervosa: Review of current treatment practices. South. Med. J., *75*:1101–1107, 1982.

63. Schwartz, D.M., and Thompson, M.G.: Do anorectics get well? Current research and future needs. Am. J. Psychiatry, *138*:319–323, 1981.

64. Browning, C.H., and Miller, S.I.: Anorexia nervosa: A study in prognosis and management. Am. J. Psychiatry, *124*:1128–1132, 1968.

65. Bruch, H.: Death in anorexia nervosa. Psychosom. Med., *33*:135–144, 1971.

66. Saul, S.H., Dekker, A., and Watson, C.G.: Acute gastric dilatation with infarction and perforation: Report of fatal outcome in patient with anorexia nervosa. Gut, *22*:978–983, 1981.

67. Browning, C.H.: Anorexia nervosa: Complications of somatic therapy. Compr. Psychiatry, *18*:399–403, 1977.

68. Hsu, L.K.G., Crisp, A.H., Harding, B.: Outcome of anorexia nervosa. Lancet, *1*:61–65, 1979.

69. Halmi, K.A., Goldberg, S.C., Casper, R.C., Eckert, E.D., and Davis, J.M.: Pretreatment mediators of outcome in anorexia nervosa. Br. J. Psychiatry, *134*:71–78, 1979.

70. Goetz, P.L., Succop, R.A., Reinhart, J.B., and Miller, A.: Anorexia nervosa in children: A follow-up study. Am. J. Orthopsychiatry, 47:597–603, 1977.
71. Walker, J., Roberts, S.L., Halmi, K.A., and Goldberg, S.C.: Caloric requirements for weight gain in anorexia nervosa. Am. J. Clin. Nutr., 32:1396–1400, 1979.
72. Richard, J.L., Bringer, J., Mirouze, J., Monnier, L., and Bellet, M.H.: Intérêt de l'alimentation entérale à faible débit continu dans le traitement de l'anorexie mentale. Ann. Nutr. Metab., 27:19–25, 1983.
73. Fischer, J.E.: Hyperalimentation. Adv. Surg., 11:1–69, 1977.
74. Finkelstein, B.A.: Parenteral hyperalimentation in anorexia nervosa. J.A.M.A., 219:217, 1972.
75. Forget, P.P.F.X., Fernandes, J., and Begemann, P.H.: Enhancement of fat elimination during intravenous feeding. Acta Paediatr. Scand., 63:750–752, 1974.
76. Hirschmann, G.H., Rao, D.D., and Chan, J.C.M.: Anorexia nervosa with acute tubular necrosis treated with parenteral nutrition. Nutr. Metab., 21:341–348, 1977.

77. Akamatsu, K., Nishizaki, T., Endo, H., and Taketa, K.: A case of anorexia nervosa improvement following intravenous administration of fat emulsion (Intralipid) combined with tube feeding. J. Jap. Soc. Intern. Med., 61:274–281, 1972.
78. Wyatt, R.J., Farrell, M., Berry, P.L., Forristal, J., Maloney, M.J., and West, C.D.: Reduced alternative complement pathway control protein levels in anorexia nervosa: Response to parenteral alimentation. Am. J. Clin. Nutr., 35:973–980, 1982.
79. Keys, A., Brozek, J., Henschel, A., Mickelsen, O., and Taylor, H.L.: The Biology of Human Starvation. Minneapolis, University of Minnesota Press, 1950.
80. Drossman, D.A.: Anorexia nervosa: A comprehensive approach. Adv. Int. Med., 28:339–361, 1979.
81. Gottdiener, J.S., Gross, H.A., Henry, W.L., Borer, J.S., and Ebert, M.E.: Effects of self-induced starvation on cardiac size and function in anorexia nervosa. Circulation, 58:425–433, 1978.
82. Powers, P.S.: Heart failure during treatment of anorexia nervosa. Am. J. Psychiatry, 139:1167–1170, 1982.

CHAPTER 31

Parenteral Nutrition in the Septic Patient*

HERBERT R. FREUND

THE METABOLIC RESPONSE TO INJURY AND SEPSIS

The metabolic response to injury is a characteristic and apparently purposeful set of events that accommodate the need of the injured organism. This response is followed by healing and a return to bodily and social integrity. The essentials of this unique neuroendocrine metabolic activation are characterized by the stimulation of catecholamine secretion, which, in turn, stimulates glucagon secretion and inhibits pancreatic secretion and peripheral activity of insulin. Increased adrenocorticotropic hormone (ACTH) production stimulates the adrenocortical production and release of glucocorticoids. Increases in renin, angiotensin, aldosterone, and antidiuretic hormone (ADH) result in sodium and water retention. The catecholamines synergize with the corticosteroids and glucagon to cause a rapid breakdown of muscle protein, an increased urinary nitrogen loss (accompanied by an increased excretion of sulfur, phosphorus, potassium, and magnesium), gluconeogenesis from protein, and an acceleration of fat oxidation, but to a limited degree only. The overall negative nitrogen balance is the result of mildly increased whole-body protein synthesis and even further increased protein breakdown rates.

Sepsis, the systemic response to an infecting agent, is basically a metabolic process that ranges from changes of little clinical significance to severe metabolic derangements culminating in multiorgan failure and

death, which is apparently the result of the inhibition of adenosine triphosphate (ATP) production.

Sepsis is a major catabolic insult, leading to increased muscle breakdown and nitrogen loss. This progressive proteolysis is accompanied by modified carbohydrate and fat metabolism, limiting the availability of energy at a time when the body is in desperate need of easily accessible energy. The result is proteolysis and amino acid oxidation to supply energy needs. The source of most of the mobilized protein is muscle tissue, whereas visceral protein is apparently spared.

Glucose Metabolism

The alterations in glucose metabolism include hyperglycemia that increases with increasing glucose loads and is resistant to insulin administration,[1, 2] an increased rate of gluconeogenesis that is nonsuppressable by exogenous glucose,[3, 4] and a progressive rise in lactate and pyruvate levels while the lactate/pyruvate ratio remains constant.

This apparent "stress diabetes" or "diabetes of injury" has been long recognized[1] and is characterized by appropriate or even higher than expected plasma insulin concentrations in response to the hyperglycemia.[2] It appears that insulin resistance exists in peripheral tissues and is primarily limited to the muscle. According to Black and associates.[5] it is probably a postreceptor defect. Recently, Wichterman and colleagues suggested that insulin resistance occurs in the liver rather than in skeletal muscle.[6] Clowes and coworkers suspected a circulating substance of moderate molecular size to be the cause of insulin resistance.[1] Keenan and

*Supported in part by grants from the Chief Scientist of the Israel Ministry of Health, Ministry of Defense, and the Joint Research Fund of the Hebrew University and Hadassah.

associates[7] were able to initiate insulin and energy substrate responses similar to those observed during infection by injecting rats with rabbit leukocyte endogenous mediator. Long, studying patients with major injury or sepsis, found a threefold increase in glucose pool size, turnover, and oxidation rates.[3] Major injury and sepsis caused a greater increase in glucose synthesis relative to its rate of removal by oxidation and conversion to fat.[3] The substrates for this increased glucose turnover are presumably amino acids, glycerol, lactate, and pyruvate. Gump and coworkers found that among 20 amino acids studied, alanine uptake predominated and was associated with increased hepatic production of glucose and urea.[8] Using ^{14}C-alanine, a twofold increase in the conversion of alanine to glucose was found in septic patients. Furthermore, this increased gluconeogenesis was observed while patients received a constant glucose infusion at normal hepatic glucose production rates, indicating that the controlling mechanism for glucose synthesis is modified.[4]

Infected rats and monkeys showed an accelerated turnover, utilization, and production rate of glucose. Rates of gluconeogenesis were also significantly elevated, with the gluconeogenic capacity decreasing only during agonal stages of sepsis.[9] Recently, Black and associates, looking into the mechanisms of insulin resistance following injury, found the maximal rate of glucose disposal reduced in trauma patients and the clearance rate of insulin almost twice normal in injury.[5]

Glucose intolerance was found to be associated with a high mortality rate, whereas glucose tolerance in sepsis was associated with improved survival.[10, 11] These are all facts to be considered when providing hyperalimentation for the septic patient and will be discussed in more detail later in this chapter.

Fat Metabolism

There is some confusion as to the effect of infection on fat metabolism. This confusion is the result of using different animal species and a variety of infecting organisms. The deranged fat metabolism includes inappropriately high[12, 13] or low[14, 15] levels of free fatty acids relative to existing glucose levels or normal fasting and increased fat turnover. Triglyceride levels are high and rise progressively, whereas triglyceride clearance decreases.[12, 16] High glucose levels, which would normally suppress fatty acid oxidation in liver and muscle, do not do so in injury.[17] In the face of a very high glucose intake, net fat oxidation persists in the hypermetabolic septic patient.[17] Initially, ketone-body production is maintained. However, abnormalities soon appear, with an increase in the β-hydroxy-butyrate/acetoacetate ratio caused by a fall in acetoacetate. In animal studies, different trends in ketone-body levels were noted. In the infected rat, Wannemacher found a reduced ketogenic capacity of the liver, with fatty acids shuttling away from β-oxidation and ketogenesis toward triglyceride production.[18] As death approaches, ketone bodies fall to a nondetectable range. Some studies indicate there is a decreased utilization of fat.[1, 13] Kinney's group, studying the effect of nutritional therapy on the utilization of fat emulsion in injured, infected, or depleted patients, found that triglyceride utilization is stimulated in the septic state, causing plasma free fatty acids to increase with 419 kcal/day of fat oxidized, even though carbohydrate intake was in excess of energy needs.[19] Similarly, intravenous fat emulsions are readily utilized and will be discussed later on in this chapter.

Protein Breakdown

The origin of the fuel deficit is still uncertain. Clowes and coworkers,[1] and many others, claim the deficit occurs as a result of insulin resistance, preferentially in the muscle. Border and colleagues implicated a deficiency of carnitine.[3] Another possibility is the presence of intracellular metabolic blocks that lead to decreased substrate utilization and low oxygen consumption from nonutilization.[20] Muscle biopsies in septic patients[21] and kidney and liver specimens from septic rats[22] documented decreased levels of ATP, with increased levels of adenosine diphosphate (ADP) and adenosine monophosphate (AMP) consistent with a progressive inhibition of substrate entry into the Krebs' cycle at multiple points. The decreased oxygen consumption from nonutilization of substrate results in the hemodynamic and physiologic abnormalities and derangements of sepsis. Processes that require oxidized nicotinamide-adenine dinucleotide (NAD+) at the mitochondrial level are suspected to cause these metabolic blocks.[20]

To meet the energy fuel deficit that occurs in sepsis, protein is oxidized. Duke and colleagues calculated that an increased proportion of needed calories are derived from protein sources.[23] This is also supported by the increased urinary nitrogen loss and the mean respiratory quotient in the range of 0.83 to 0.85. A considerable number of data are now available that point toward skeletal muscle as the source of most of the mobilized protein. In patients with skeletal trauma, Long and associates found that whole-body protein breakdown was increased by 73 per cent, whereas the muscle contribution to this whole-body breakdown rate ranged from 60 to 65 per cent.[24] Simultaneous with the increased protein degradation, there is also increased protein synthesis, but not to the same degree as degradation.[25] The excessive use of muscle protein for energy and the synthesis of vital proteins results clinically in a decreasing muscle mass, weight loss, increased urinary nitrogen loss and negative nitrogen balance, anergy and predisposition to infection and sepsis, impaired wound healing, and, finally, multiple-system organ failure and death. Depending on the severity of injury or sepsis, body protein is catabolized at a rate of 75 to 150 gm/day, resulting in a loss of up to 300 to 600 gm of lean body mass/day. In addition to being economically wasteful, muscle protein breakdown also leads to a relative deficiency of essential amino acids, in particular the branched-chain amino acids (BCAAs), which are selectively, preferentially, and extensively utilized by muscle as an energy source and substrate for gluconeogenesis.

BCAA Formulations

The BCAAs valine, leucine, and isoleucine are the only amino acids that have a branch in their skeleton, which makes their structure unique. Furthermore, they are the only amino acids that are oxidized principally by skeletal muscle.[26–31] The rate of oxidation of BCAAs in muscle is stimulated by fasting, hormonal influences, stress, diabetes, and other conditions associated with muscle protein wasting and negative nitrogen balance. Oxidation of the BCAAs supplies energy to the muscle and nitrogen (and possibly also the carbon skeleton) for the glucose-alanine cycle and muscle glutamine synthesis.[31–38] Recent in vitro experiments have also ascribed regulatory functions to the BCAAs in the muscle. Fulks and colleagues suggested that the BCAAs promote protein synthesis and reduce protein degradation in a dose-dependent fashion.[39] Odessey and associates showed that the BCAAs inhibit net protein breakdown in muscle and stimulate *de novo* synthesis of alanine and glutamine, thus offering energy substrate for the liver, kidney, and gut.[31] Buse and Reid suggested that leucine might act as a regulator of protein turnover in skeletal muscle by inhibiting protein degradation and promoting protein synthesis.[27] Walser's group achieved prolonged and improved nitrogen conservation during fasting, injury, and hepatic encephalopathy by the administration of alpha-keto analogues of the BCAAs.[39–41, 56] Sherwin infused leucine in fasting obese subjects, with improvement in nitrogen balance but unchanged 3-methyl-histidine excretion, suggesting stimulation of muscle protein synthesis.[42]

As a result of our ongoing research interest in the etiology and therapy of hepatic encephalopathy, we investigated the use of a special amino acid formulation that was relatively rich in BCAAs. Primarily, our intention was to take advantage of the BCAAs' ability to compete at the blood-brain barrier. However, it became evident that both animals and patients achieve nitrogen equilibrium when infused with this special amino acid formulation[43, 43a, 43b] and that the nitrogen balance and amount of solution infused are negatively correlated to plasma, brain, and cerebrospinal fluid (CSF) levels of aromatic amino acids,[44] suggesting a reduced muscle protein breakdown. Keeping in mind the in vitro studies of Goldberg and his group[30, 35] and Buse and her group,[27] we assumed that if the BCAAs are also functioning as regulators of muscle protein synthesis and degradation (in addition to being primarily oxidized by skeletal muscle and being used for gluconeogenesis), they might be useful in the postinjury and septic state, in which protein catabolism is one of the major sources of the body's energy.

We used a standard rat-injury model in which we performed laparotomy and jugular vein cannulation that resulted in a mean negative nitrogen balance of 250 mg/day. By infusing a solution containing 35 per cent BCAAs in five per cent dextrose or the three BCAAs alone in five per cent dextrose, we achieved nitrogen equilibrium.[45] The addition of 25 per cent dextrose did not result in significantly greater protein-sparing,[46] suggesting that in the presence of large doses of BCAAs little additional protein-sparing may be achieved by carbohydrate. Infusion of the three BCAAs alone promoted not only nitrogen equilibrium but also normalization of plasma and muscle amino acid patterns, suggesting an inhibition of amino acid flux from the muscle, which was observed when using other less-BCAA-enriched amino acid formulations. By comparing the infusion of alanine to the infusion of BCAAs in the postinjury state, we were able to conclude that the production of alanine in and of itself cannot completely explain the nitrogen-conserving effect of the BCAAs.[47]

Following the preceding experiment, we infused each of the BCAAs and alanine separately, and using ^{14}C-tyrosine we were able to demonstrate that all three BCAAs improve the fractional synthesis rate (FSR) in the liver, that only valine improves the FSR in the muscle, and that all three BCAAs and alanine decrease the total body protein breakdown rate.[48] Similar results were also reported by Blackburn's group in sepsis and pancreatitis rat models receiving BCAAs alone or BCAA-enriched amino acid formulations.[49-51] These results suggested that the nitrogen-conserving quality of amino acid formulations in the postinjury rat might be improved by increasing the amount of BCAAs. We therefore set out to determine the minimum amount of BCAAs needed to exert their beneficial effect so that we could create a balanced amino acid formulation containing enough BCAAs combined with adequate amounts of all other essential and nonessential amino acids.

The results of nitrogen balances, plasma amino acid patterns, and plasma albumin levels finally pointed toward a 45 per cent BCAA-containing balanced amino acid formulation as the most favorable one for the postinjury state.[51a]

Clinical studies with BCAA-enriched amino acid formulations were started in the early 1970s by Fischer's group in Boston, who were studying patients with chronic cirrhosis and hepatic encephalopathy. Our experience with 63 such patients who were treated with a BCAA-enriched formulation demonstrated nitrogen equilibrium during the infusion of 80 to 100 gm of amino acids/day, with a significant correlation among the amount of nitrogen infused, nitrogen balance, and the ratio of BCAAs/aromatic amino acids. Furthermore, discriminant analysis revealed that the improvement in encephalopathy grade

correlated well with the amount of calories and nitrogen infused.[43] These clinical findings have now been repeatedly confirmed in an increasing number of patients in Europe, Japan, and the United States.[43a-c]

We initiated clinical studies with BCAAs in injury by examining 35 adult patients undergoing moderate operative injury.[52] Infusion of the three BCAAs alone in glucose resulted in nitrogen equilibrium for the first five postoperative days, similar to two other more balanced amino acid formulations tested (Fig. 31–1). Similar results were seen in seven patients receiving 16 per cent, 50 per cent, or 100 per cent BCAAs.[53] Patients receiving a complete amino acid formulation containing 50 per cent BCAAs developed the least-negative nitrogen balance. With the increase in BCAA contribution to total amino acid intake, there was an increase in total protein flux and efficiency of amino acid utilization. In prospective randomized trials of postoperative and septic patients, Cerra and colleagues found that patients receiving a balanced amino acid mixture containing 50 per cent BCAAs retained more nitrogen, faster and at a lower nitrogen input, suggesting stimulation of protein synthesis.[54, 82a]

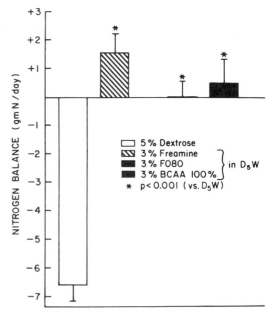

Figure 31–1. Nitrogen balance in four groups of postoperative patients given infusions of 5 per cent dextrose only or 5 per cent dextrose and a formulation containing 22, 35, or 100 per cent branched-chain amino acids. (*From* Freund, H. R., Hoover, H. C., Atamian, S., and Fischer, J. E.: Infusion of the branched chain amino acids in post-operative patients: anticatabolic properties. Ann. Surg., *190*:18–23, 1979, with permission.)

Furthermore, improvement in nitrogen balance was directly correlated to BCAA load. Since this improvement was not accompanied by a reduction in 3-methyl-histidine excretion, the mechanism does not appear to be the result of an effect on proteolysis. Moreover, the administration of a branched-chain–enriched formula effectively supported visceral protein synthesis, particularly transferrin, and improved immune competence and absolute lymphocyte count.[81, 82] Initial clinical studies in patients undergoing elective moderate to severe surgical procedures proved the new branched-chain–enriched amino acid solution containing 45 per cent BCAAs to be safe and nitrogen-sparing.[55, 55a] Walser, studying keto analogues in patients undergoing abdominal surgery, found the infusion of keto-leucine reduces muscle protein breakdown and urea nitrogen excretion and attenuates the fall in liver-synthesized proteins.[56]

Recently, in a prospective randomized study, Muggia-Sullam and colleagues demonstrated that severely stressed or septic patients who were infused with branched-chain–enriched amino acid formulations exhibited an improved nitrogen balance, a normalized plasma amino acid pattern, and an increase in serum transferrin, retinol binding protein, prealbumin, and albumin levels.[56a]

Plasma Amino Acid Patterns

Looking at sepsis as the most extreme form of injury, we studied the plasma amino acid pattern of 40 patients suffering overwhelming (mainly abdominal) sepsis. Sepsis was characterized by an increase in aromatic amino acids (phenylalanine and tyrosine) and the sulfur-containing amino acids (taurine, methionine, and cystine). Alanine, aspartic acid, glutamic acid, and proline were also elevated but to a lesser degree. The BCAAs were within normal limits, as were glycine, serine, threonine, lysine, histidine, and tryptophan. Patients who did not survive sepsis had higher levels of aromatic and sulfur-containing amino acids when compared with those patients who survived. Furthermore, patients surviving sepsis had higher levels of alanine and BCAAs (Fig. 31–2).[57]

This apparent close relationship between the basic deranged energy metabolism in sepsis and a deranged plasma amino acid pattern received further confirmation by using the plasma amino acid changes as predictors of the severity of sepsis and the patient's final outcome. Using stepwise discriminant analysis,[58] the combination of cystine, methionine, phenylalanine, isoleucine, leucine, and valine correctly predicted the severity of sepsis, as determined by the presence and grade of septic encephalopathy, in 82 per cent of patients without encephalopathy and in 86 per cent of patients with encephalopathy (average of 84 per cent). Similarly, the combination of arginine, cystine, methionine, isoleucine, tyrosine, phenylalanine, and alanine determined correctly the patient's final outcome in 79 per cent of the

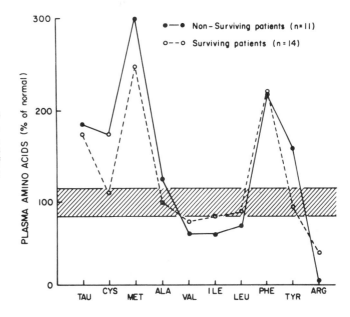

Figure 31–2. Plasma amino acid patterns in surviving and non-surviving septic patients. (*From* Freund, H. R., Atamian, S., Holroyde, J., and Fischer, J. E.: Plasma amino acids as predictors of the severity and outcome of sepsis. Ann. Surg., *190*:571–576, 1979, with permission.)

survivors and in 91 per cent of the nonsurvivors for an average of 84 per cent. Following these results, we infused 25 severely septic patients with an amino acid formulation that was poor in aromatic amino acids and enriched in BCAAs (35 or 42 per cent). During infusion of BCAA-enriched amino acid formulations in septic patients, encephalopathy disappeared concomitantly with a significant drop in plasma levels of methionine, phenylalanine, cystine, and tyrosine, whereas the BCAAs and alanine remained normal or a bit above normal. Similar results were presented by Lohlein and associates using a 45 per cent BCAA-enriched amino acid formulation.[59] Cerra and colleagues found clearly elevated serum proline levels in septic patients. These increased proline levels correlated well with lactate levels and total peripheral resistance.[20] In septic patients who were closer to death, there were increasingly higher plasma levels of glutamate ammonia, ornithine, and proline, substances involved in the hepatic pathway of proline metabolism. Furthermore, plasma concentrations of lactate, pyruvate, and proline had a significantly inverse correlation with total peripheral resistance and oxygen consumption. Proline levels were a good indicator of mortality in sepsis.[20]

Muscle protein breakdown to satisfy energy requirements in a state of inadequate fuel supply results in the release into the circulation of large amounts of various amino acids, with the exception of the BCAAs, which the muscle itself is able to oxidize and use for gluconeogenesis. Since muscle contains only 20 per cent of its amino acid composition as BCAAs, a substantial release of amino acids occurs during periods in which oxidation of BCAAs is accelerated. The oxidation of BCAAs serves to supply the muscles' own energy requirements, as well as the nitrogen and perhaps even the carbon skeleton for alanine synthesis and gluconeogenesis, since the alanine so produced in the muscle is transferred to the liver and used for glucose production.[33] The increased production of alanine not only serves as a source for hepatic gluconeogenesis but also as a mechanism to shuttle nitrogen back to the liver for deamination through the urea cycle, and it explains in part the increased nitrogen excretion. Furthermore, production of alanine permits the complete oxidation of leucine, isoleucine, and valine, yielding 42, 43, and 32 ATP/mole, respectively, so that the

BCAA cycle may provide up to 25 times more ATP than the Cori cycle and fill the energy deficit in muscle.[31]

The utilization of BCAAs for muscle energy and the utilization of alaline for gluconeogenesis explain the normal plasma BCAA levels and the only mildly elevated levels of alanine in our patients. Of the remaining amino acids released into the circulation as a result of muscle proteolysis, the aromatic and sulfur-containing amino acids, as well as proline, cannot be utilized by the muscle but have to be metabolized by the liver. McMenamy and coworkers, studying the splanchnic substrate balances in a severely septic patient, found rising plasma proline levels that were associated with increasing splanchnic clearance of proline, pointing toward a release of proline from the periphery, most likely from muscle.[60]

During infection, protein synthesis in the liver is reduced because of the early hepatic dysfunction that occurs in sepsis[12, 20, 57, 61] and because of the low pool of essential amino acids like the BCAAs that are utilized to satisfy muscle energy requirements. The net end result of muscle protein breakdown and the efflux of amino acids, coupled with relative hepatic incompetence, is an excessive accumulation of all the unused amino acids in plasma, as evidenced by the "catabolic" pattern of amino acids in our patients' plasma.[57, 58] The only exceptional values were the BCAAs and alanine, utilized by muscle for energy and gluconeogenesis, which were present at normal or near-normal levels. The differences in plasma amino acid patterns in surviving and nonsurviving septic patients might indicate a better-preserved hepatic reserve and function (lower aromatic and sulfur-containing amino acid levels) and better maintenance of overall energy metabolism (normal BCAA levels). The clinical implications and practicalities of managing injured and septic patients, in view of this deranged metabolism, will be discussed later in this chapter.

METABOLIC REQUIREMENTS DURING SEPSIS

With the advent of parenteral nutrition, it became possible in recent years to supply energy and nitrogen to the injured or septic patient. However, it soon became apparent that in sepsis it is not only a matter of quantity—namely, an excessive need for energy and nitrogen—but also of quality. The septic patient in whom the metabolic response to injury is a very special and distinct neuroendocrine set of events needs specialized nutritional support. There is glucose intolerance, difficulty in utilizing fat tissue, protein breakdown for energy, essential amino acid wasting, and loss of important ingredients for protein synthesis. All this happens at a time when the septic patient is in desperate need of nitrogen and calories. The present discussion follows the first part of this chapter and is based on the present-day knowledge and data of what should and could be offered as nutrition to the septic patient. It is important to remember that this is a new and dynamic field of interest and research in which progress is made continuously.

Calories

The increase in resting energy expenditure in sepsis may reach up to 60 per cent above normal. The normal response to a carbohydrate load in excess of energy expenditure is a rise in the nonprotein respiratory quotient (RQ) to 1 or above. This indicates that the main substrate being oxidized for energy is glucose. A nonprotein RQ above 1 indicates conversion of glucose to fat. In the infected hypermetabolic patient, the administration of twice the resting energy expenditure as carbohydrate will result in an RQ lower than 1, indicating the continued utilization of endogenous fat for energy. High glucose levels, which would normally suppress fatty acid oxidation in liver and muscle, do not do so in trauma. Studies in Kinney's laboratory indicate that net fat oxidation persists in the hypermetabolic patient in the face of very high glucose intake.[17, 62–64] Glucose cannot be converted to fat and there is excessive glycogen deposition, increased sympathetic drive, increased glucose oxidation, and increased resting expenditure.[17] Elwyn and coworkers, studying the effect of increased glucose load in injury, found that (1) plasma glucose concentrations are maintained at the already high level associated with trauma but are not significantly increased, (2) rates of glucose oxidation and nonoxidative metabolism increase proportionately with intake, (3) there is an abnormally high rate of glycogen deposition that is proportional to glucose intake, (4) gluconeogenesis from protein is abnormally high but can be completely suppressed with an intake of approximately 600 gm glucose/day, (5) glucose recycling with glycogen or glycerol, or both, is increased with increasing intake. Carpentier and coworkers, studying the effect of hypercaloric glucose infusions on lipid metabolism of injured and septic patients, found that glycerol turnover (unidirectional triglyceride breakdown) during the infusion of both D5W or hypercaloric TPN exceeding energy requirements was similarly elevated. This is in contrast to a 62 per cent decrease in glycerol turnover observed in depleted patients during a similar carbohydrate load.[62] This means that despite high glucose and insulin levels during TPN, triglyceride breakdown continued, probably the result of high catecholamine release. In the septic state, 419 kcal/day of fat was oxidized even though carbohydrate intake was in excess of energy needs.[64] Patients who are hypermetabolic with high urinary norepinephrine excretion seem to respond to a glucose load by a further increase in norepinephrine, which apparently offsets the rise in insulin that is expected to occur in response to the glucose load of TPN. This results in a high resting value of lipolysis, which is minimally suppressed by the administration of TPN. The rise in free fatty acid levels and oxidation inhibits muscle glucose utilization and oxidation while it enhances the conversion of glucose to glycogen. It seems as if endogenous fat may serve as a preferential substrate in injury and sepsis.[64] Nordenstrom and associates, studying patients with major injury, infection, or nutritional depletion, found that fat emulsions were readily utilized (similar to endogenous lipids) as an energy substrate, suggesting that fat is a useful caloric source in TPN.[65]

Considerable controversy exists as to the fate of parenterally administered fat and its effect on protein-sparing and lean body mass catabolism in injury and sepsis. Jeejeebhoy and associates compared amino acids and glucose with amino acids and a combination of glucose and fat.[66] They found no difference in nitrogen balance between the two groups of stable patients. Elwyn and colleagues found that in depleted adult patients receiving TPN based on glucose and amino acids, the substitution of fat emulsion for one third of the glucose calories proved as effective as glucose in maintaining positive nitrogen balance.[67] Long and coworkers detected no nitrogen-sparing effect of Intralipid in five injured patients.[68] Data of Woolfson and associates[69] indicate that fat emulsions have nitrogen-sparing effects in patients who have undergone operation, but not in severely hypercatabolic patients. Using body composition determinations, carbohydrate proved more efficient than lipid calories.[70] In injured rats, Intralipid and glucose that was infused without any added protein exhibited an identical nitrogen-conserving quality. However, when amino acids were added, glucose exhibited a decisively better nitrogen-conserving quality than isocaloric amounts of Intralipid (Fig. 31–3).[71] Similarly, in severely stressed rats, Souba and associates found that fat was unable to spare nitrogen.[34] Nordenstrom and colleagues, studying traumatized and septic patients, found a similar nitrogen-sparing effect for the glucose group and for the mixed glucose-fat group.[73] To further confuse the fat-glucose controversy, recent reports from Kinney's group indicate that in certain trauma or sepsis patients, administering large amounts of glucose may be undesirable in many ways. TPN with glucose significantly increases norepinephrine excretion and modestly increases resting energy expenditure, both of which do not occur when using the lipid system (50 per cent glucose and 50 per cent lipids).[74] Cate-

cholamines stimulate glucagon secretion and inhibit insulin production, causing a further deterioration in the metabolic state of the septic patient.[64] Furthermore, acutely ill patients receiving glucose as the only caloric source in TPN exhibited an up to 75 per cent increase in CO_2 production.[75] This increase in CO_2 production is secondary to both an increased O_2 consumption and an increase in RQ.[64] In a patient with compromised pulmonary function and respiratory distress, difficulty in weaning from mechanical ventilation and cardiovascular stress may be precipitated by the increase in CO_2 production and O_2 consumption.[76] In these patients, the use of the lipid system was associated with less CO_2 production and no increase in catecholamine secretion or basic metabolic expenditure.

Thus, the controversy over the efficacy of fat as a caloric source seems to continue, and it can best be summarized by stating that "depending on the patient's pathophysiologic state and the proportion of lipid in the diet, this substance may have a nitrogen-conserving effect that ranges from nothing to one equal that of glucose."[67] Therefore, it seems logical to limit glucose intake in the septic patient to 50 per cent or a maximum of 75 per cent of the total caloric intake and to provide the remainder of the diet in the form of fat emulsions.

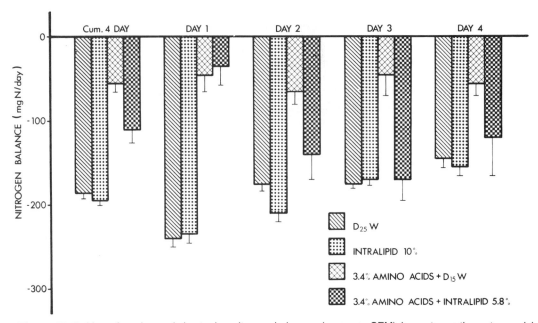

Figure 31–3. Mean four-day and day-to-day nitrogen balances (mean ± SEM) in postoperative rats receiving parenteral nutrition for 96 hours with 25 per cent glucose or 10 per cent Intralipid without amino acids, or 3.4 per cent amino acids with either 15 per cent glucose or 5.8 per cent Intralipid.

Insulin

Studies on insulin secretion after injury have shown that catecholamine-mediated suppression of insulin secretion in the acute phase of injury is followed by a period of insulin resistance. Black and associates,[5] using the hyperglycemic glucose clamp in injured patients, found a maximal rate of glucose uptake of 6 mg/kg/minute. In a 70-kg patient, this would provide about 2400 glucose kcal/day. Using the euglycemic insulin clamp, insulin stimulation increased the maximal rate of glucose disposal to 9 mg/kg/minute or 3600 kcal of carbohydrate/day in a 70-kg patient. When infusing very high concentrations of insulin, the rate of glucose disposal ranged maximally at 8 to 9 mg/kg/minute,[5] or the direct oxidation of glucose reached a plateau as the infusion rate in human patients exceeded 5 mg/kg/minute,[77] confirming the limit in glucose metabolism following injury, even at supraphysiologic insulin concentrations.[5, 77] Independent of its effect on carbohydrate metabolism, there are reports claiming that insulin favorably affects protein metabolism, resulting in improved nitrogen balance.[68] This nitrogen-sparing effect of insulin may be due to its stimulatory effect on protein synthesis[77, 78] or to its inhibition of muscle protein breakdown.[69] Others showed that insulin promotes muscle protein anabolism and storage through improvement in amino acid uptake and transport, protein synthetic activity, peptide chain formation, and ribosomal protein aggregation. We use insulin routinely in our TPN solutions. In septic patients, we combine a lower glucose concentration with increased amounts of insulin in an attempt to overcome glucose intolerance.

Amino Acids

Sepsis is a metabolic disorder that is characterized by the abnormal processing of substrate and an abnormal demand of substrate for energy and protein metabolism. The metabolic problem in sepsis appears to be mitochondrial in origin and one of progressive energy deficit for cellular processes caused by a progressive inability to use glucose, fat, and, ultimately, amino acids. The energy production economy appears to become progressively protein-based, with an increasing reliance on BCAAs. Since BCAAs are preferentially catabolized in the muscle, they are used primarily and extensively during sepsis. The amino acids that the periphery cannot catabolize are released to be returned to the liver. Eventually, however, the liver is also affected, which is manifested, among other things, by progressively rising levels of aromatic and sulfur-containing amino acids, proline, and a few other amino acids.[20, 57] Since the body relies primarily on protein breakdown, specifically on BCAA utilization, it is reasonable to offer both quantitatively and qualitatively specialized amino acid formulations as nutritional support. It seems necessary to administer a BCAA-enriched balanced amino acid formulation at up to 2.5 to 3.5 gm/kg/day. Recently, Clowes and associates[79] demonstrated that despite giving septic patients what was considered adequate TPN—2.1 gm protein/kg/day and 45 kcal/kg/day—there was a continuous peripheral release of amino acids, suggesting that requirements for certain amino acids were not satisfied.

Following extensive previous animal studies concerning the use and effectiveness of BCAAs in injury,[45–48, 52] experimental work by Gimmon and associates[51a, 80] determined that the appropriate amino acid formulation in injury is a solution containing adequate amounts of essential and nonessential amino acids and 45 per cent BCAAs. In moderately injured patients, nitrogen equilibrium was maintained by the infusion of 1.7 gm/kg of protein equivalent containing 45 per cent BCAAs mixed with 5 or 25 per cent glucose.[55, 55a] By infusing a 35 per cent BCAA-enriched amino acid formulation, we were able to normalize the deranged plasma amino acid pattern of sepsis.[57] Recently, Cerra and coworkers, in a series of clinical trials, found that BCAAs support protein synthesis without affecting proteolysis in injury.[54, 81, 82] Furthermore, nitrogen retention was proportional to the BCAA load, with maximal effect around 50 per cent.[82a] Applying this modified metabolic support to patients with sepsis, administering BCAAs at 1 to 1.5 gm/kg/day as part of a 45 to 50 per cent BCAA-enriched amino acid formulation resulted in an improved nitrogen balance, increased total lymphocyte count, reversal of anergy, stimulation of chemotaxis, increased transferrin levels, and decreased 3-methyl-histidine excretion. Furthermore, the oxygen consumption index and lactate levels decreased, whereas total peripheral resistance increased.[81, 82a, 92]

Similar beneficial effects are reported by Muggia-Sullam and associates[56a] in a prospective randomized study of intensive care and septic patients. Recently, interest has been generated in the effect of malnutrition, injury, and sepsis on anergy, immunologic parameters, predisposition to infection, and cancer and on the effect of nutritional support and repletion. Alexander and co-workers[83] found that in severely burned children, supplementation of a normal dietary regime with excess protein of high biologic value resulted in improved immunologic parameters, a decrease in the number of bacteremic days, and a significantly improved survival. The high-protein group received 4.9 gm protein/kg/day with a calorie/nitrogen ratio of 110:1, compared to the control group receiving 3.8 gm protein/kg/day at a calorie/nitrogen ratio of 151:1. In addition, many positive correlations of immunologic parameters and individual amino acids were found to exist and await further investigation.[83] In a number of excellent papers published over recent years, Barbul and colleagues called attention to and proved the special role and beneficial effect of arginine on wound healing and thymus and immunostimulation. In studies on animals injured by bilateral femoral fractures, thymic function—as assessed by thymic size, the number of thymic lymphocytes, and the ability of thymic lymphocytes to respond to mitogenic stimulation—was impaired. Dietary supplementation with one per cent arginine largely prevented or minimized these post-trauma dysfunctions.[84] In addition, dietary arginine supplementation significantly increased thymic weight, cellularity, and T-cell blastogenic responsiveness in uninjured rats. Supplemental dietary arginine in healthy humans stimulated in vitro lymphocyte reactivity.[85]

Thus it seems that in the injured septic patient the amount of protein supplied should be increased to about 3 gm/kg/day, and the standard amino acid formulations should be modified so as to include about 45 per cent BCAAs and arginine, and perhaps a few other as yet unknown amino acids that might prove important for the survival of the septic patient.

Calorie/Nitrogen Ratio

Considering the glucose intolerance, the insulin resistance, and the increasing dependence on protein of the septic hypermetabolic patient, the calorie/nitrogen ratio of intravenous nutrition solutions should be modified. The glucose load should be reduced by using a 10 to 15 per cent glucose solution and by increasing the exogenous insulin intake. When liver and kidney function allow, protein intake should be increased to 2.5 to 3.5 gm/kg/day. This combination will result in a calorie/nitrogen ratio of 80 to 100:1 instead of the 150 to 200:1 routinely used for TPN in stable patients.

Electrolytes, Minerals, Vitamins, and Trace Elements

The neuroendocrine activation that results from injury is reflected also in the metabolism of water and electrolytes. Injury reduces urinary sodium and the excretion of water as a result of increased secretion of ACTH, renin, angiotensin, aldosterone, and ADH. Appropriate amounts of electrolytes and minerals are added to the TPN solutions as needed by each patient. By doing so, we are able to offer the patient every milliliter of fluid needed and tolerated as TPN while supplying protein, calories, and all electrolyte and mineral needs. Most recommended dietary allowances for vitamins are based on the needs of normal, healthy humans. However, there are very few data available on the special needs arising from injury or infection. Because vitamin deficiencies and imbalances—particularly of water-soluble vitamins—can occur early in injured or septic patients, vitamin supplementation should begin as soon as TPN is started, and it is an integral part of almost all TPN formulas. There seems to be no additional need for fat-soluble vitamins in injury.[86] However, the water-soluble vitamins are needed in 5 to 20 times the amounts recommended in normal persons.[86] Currently, we are using a commercial multivitamin preparation that contains both water- and fat-soluble vitamins, which is based on the AMA's nutrition advisory group statement. The only additional vitamin that is needed is vitamin K, 10 mg intramuscularly once a week. At the present time, trace elements that are recognized as essential for humans include iron, iodine, cobalt, zinc, copper, chromium, manganese, selenium, and molybdenum. Other trace elements, such as vanadium, tin, silicon, and arsenic, are believed to be essential for humans; however, at present there are insufficient data to recommend their use in TPN. There is very little information regarding trace element requirements during or as a result of injury and sepsis. The only information available concerns zinc, which is lost in considerable quantities whenever muscle protein breakdown occurs. Currently, we are routinely adding zinc (5 to 10 mg), copper (1 to 2 mg), and chromium (10 to 20 μg) to TPN solutions.

Essential Fatty Acids

Despite our difficulties in defining the absolute role of fat as a caloric source in injury and sepsis, there is no doubt that fat should be administered early in the course of TPN to prevent essential fatty acid deficiency. Essential fatty acid deficiency and the resultant prostaglandin deficiency[87] can occur early, particularly in depleted or injured patients.[88] To satisfy the need for essential fatty acids, 4 to 10 per cent of the total caloric intake should be supplied as fat.

Summary

To summarize the metabolic requirements in sepsis and how to satisfy them, a general guideline is offered:

1. Avoid excess energy and large amounts of glucose.
2. To meet energy expenditure, provide energy as a mixture of glucose and fat.
3. Keep the calorie/nitrogen ratio at about 100:1.
4. Use large amounts of protein. Whenever possible infuse 2.5 to 3.5 gm amino acids/kg/day.
5. Use a balanced amino acid formulation modified to contain 45 per cent BCAAs.
6. Nutritional manipulation and support is an integral part of the treatment of sepsis. However, remember it is only an adjunct to cardiovascular and respiratory support, intensive care and monitoring, antibiotics, and surgical drainage.

SPECIFIC ORGAN AND SYSTEM DERANGEMENTS DURING SEPSIS

The metabolic derangements of sepsis discussed in the previous part of this chapter describe a general phenomenon. However, certain organs and systems are either more sensitive or their failure is more crucial for the survival of the septic patient. These metabolic derangements of vital organs sometimes culminate in what has been termed in recent years *multiple-system organ failure*. In this unique and very often lethal syndrome, essential organ systems—such as lungs, kidneys, liver, heart, brain, gastrointestinal tract, as well as others—are compromised or damaged and finally fail. It is assumed that the target organelles are the mitochondria that fail in ATP production, thus leading to nonoxidative catabolic pathways and the failure of substrate utilization for ATP production.[89] A brief discussion of metabolic derangements and their treatment in some of the more commonly affected systems follows.

Liver Failure

Alterations in hepatic function are central to the metabolic derangements and adjustments occurring in sepsis. Infection and sepsis impair the liver's ability to respond to the increased metabolic demands by altering hepatocyte function. This is evident by increased mitochondrial membrane permeability, diminished active transport of indocyanine green, and decreased liver ATP levels. Experimental endotoxemia results in mitochondrial structural damage. The functional correlates of endotoxin mitochondrial injury are diminished respiratory control, indicating uncoupling of oxidation from phosphorylation, and a fall in state III respiration, indicating inefficient ATP production.[90] In an abdominal sepsis rat model[89] and in endotoxin-treated dogs,[93] decreased levels of ADP and ATP in liver and kidney were found in addition to progressive depression of reticuloendothelial function, elevation of serum enzyme levels, and hepatocellular dysfunction manifested by a progressive depression in the hepatocyte membrane transport of indocyanine green.[92, 93]

Eventually, the process will affect hepatic metabolism, manifesting itself by the nonsuppressibility of hepatic gluconeogenesis by exogenous glucose and hyperinsulinemia,[4] hepatic insulin resistance,[6] and deranged hepatic uptake of amino acids, with progressively rising levels of proline and aromatic and sulfur-containing amino acids.[20, 57, 58] This hepatic failure is poorly reflected in the standard tests of liver function: bilirubin, serum glutamic oxaloacetic transaminase

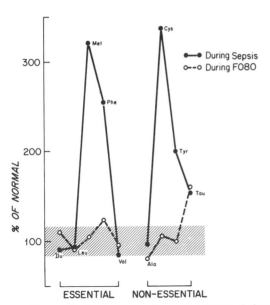

Figure 31–4. Plasma amino acid patterns during sepsis and during the infusion of septic patients with a formulation enriched with branched-chain amino acids (F080). (*From* Freund, H. R., Ryan, J. A., and Fischer, J. E.: Amino acid derangements in patients with sepsis: Treatment with branched-chain amino acid enriched infusions. Ann. Surg., *188*:423–430, 1978, with permission.)

(SGOT), LDH, or alkaline phosphatase levels.[61] The plasma amino acid profile appears to provide a much earlier and more sensitive index of hepatic insufficiency in sepsis.[20, 57, 58] This relative hepatic insufficiency requires a specific and rational metabolic support, consisting of a decreased carbohydrate load and a specialized amino acid formulation enriched with BCAAs. The use of such formulations in injured and septic patients results in improved nitrogen balance, normalization of the plasma amino acid pattern (Fig. 31–4), and reversal of hepatic or septic encephalopathy.[43, 52–55, 57, 81, 82] In animal studies, the infusion of BCAAs even resulted in the improvement of the fractional synthesis rate of mixed liver protein.[48, 49] A more extensive and detailed review of nutritional support in liver failure can be found in another chapter of this volume.

Renal Failure

The kidneys are usually the first organ or system to be affected and eventually fail in sepsis. The mortality rate in patients with sepsis and acute renal failure is extremely high and may reach 50 to 70 per cent. Acute renal failure, independent of the septic process, rapidly causes severe metabolic derangements and adds to the severe catabolism and hypermetabolism that are already present. In recent years it has been repeatedly shown that the combination of hemo- or peritoneal dialysis and aggressive and specific nutritional support will reduce mortality and morbidity in this group of patients, provided that the septic focus causing acute renal failure is eliminated.

The metabolic derangements and nutritional requirements in renal failure are the subjects of another presentation in this volume. We would like to provide a brief overview of the use of TPN in septic patients suffering from acute renal failure. There are currently two main approaches to the administration of TPN in acute renal failure. One approach uses hypertonic glucose and preparations of low quantities of nitrogen in the form of essential amino acids alone. This approach is based on the assumption that urea can be reutilized for the synthesis of nonessential amino acids. With this approach, serum urea and potassium decreased, survival improved, the duration of renal failure decreased, and recovery of renal function was promoted.[94] However, recent evidence has suggested that the capacity to reutilize urea for the synthesis of nonessential amino acids is limited, indicating that the quantity of amino acids necessary to promote a neutral or positive nitrogen balance may be greater than previously suspected. Furthermore, the marked catabolism and mortality of patients with acute renal failure who are in need of TPN suggests the need for infusing larger amounts of both essential and nonessential amino acids. Here, too, large amounts of hypertonic glucose (45 per cent) are used to increase energy intake in the face of hypermetabolism and fluid restriction. The optimal energy intake, caloric source, and calorie/nitrogen ratio for patients with renal failure are as yet undetermined. In this form of therapy, frequent treatment with dialysis is required because of the greater nitrogen and fluid load. The optimal composition of the amino acid solution for acute renal failure is still a matter of debate. Studies of plasma and muscle amino acid patterns indicate that the minimum requirements for essential amino acids, as suggested by Rose for healthy subjects, cannot be directly applied in uremia. The BCAAs, particularly valine, are often reduced in plasma and muscle, indicating increased requirements. There is also evidence that histidine and perhaps also tyrosine should be included.

At present, TPN for the injured septic patient with renal failure should consist of maintenance levels (55 to 60 gm/day) of a mixture of a balanced amino acid formulation (essential and nonessential) with one of the commercially available essential amino acid formulations in 45 per cent glucose and insulin. This way we take into consideration the special requirements of both sepsis and renal failure. We administer all the protein and calories required and dialyze accordingly. Only when dialysis is not required or is hazardous do we use essential amino acids alone in 45 per cent glucose to try to postpone the need for dialysis as much as possible.[94]

Septic Encephalopathy

Patients with sepsis often manifest symptoms of encephalopathy, including irritability, disorientation, confusion, somnolence, obtundation, stupor, and even frank coma. These symptoms are similar to those seen in hepatic encephalopathy, in which a causal relationship has been demonstrated between the degree of encephalopathy and

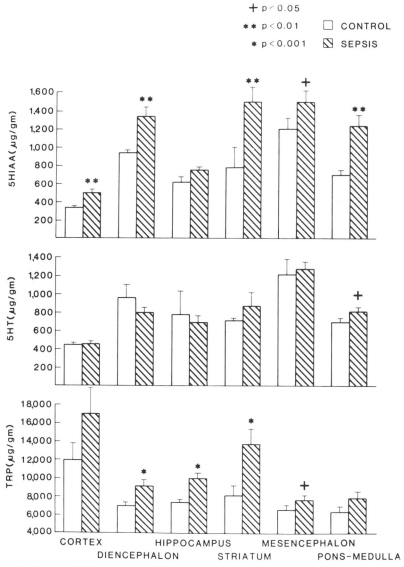

Figure 31–5. Tryptophan (TRP), serotonin (5HT), and 5-hydroxyindoleacetic acid (5HIAA) levels in different brain regions in control and septic rats with septic encephalopathy infused with 5 per cent dextrose.

plasma, CSF, or brain levels of aromatic amino acids, and a disturbed profile of neurotransmitters.[95] Furthermore, in both hepatic and septic encephalopathy, a deranged function of the blood-brain barrier neutral amino acid transport system occurs,[95, 96] with increased uptake of neutral amino acids, mainly the aromatic amino acids. Discriminant analysis of the presence or absence of encephalopathy in septic patients and of some of their plasma amino acid levels revealed an 84 per cent correct classification by using plasma levels of cystine, methionine, phenylalanine, isoleucine, leucine, and valine,[58] pointing to the close and significant relationship of the aromatic amino acids and BCAAs to septic encephalopathy. Studying brain neurotransmitters in septic rats undergoing cecal ligation and puncture, we found the most consistent change to be the accumulation of indoleamines with increased brain tryptophan levels, resulting in enhanced metabolism of serotonin (5HT), increased production of 5-hydroxyindoleacetic acid (5HIAA), and a high 5HT/5HIAA ratio in all brain regions studied (Fig. 31–5). These changes in the serotonergic line of neurotransmitters can affect behavior both directly, as inhibitory neurotransmitters, and via their anatomic and neurophysiologic effects in other brain areas and other lines of neurotransmitters—such as dopamine, particularly in the striatum and hippocampus.[96a] Infusion of branched-chain–enriched amino acid formulations had a beneficial effect on the brain amino acid and neurotransmitter profile.[96a] Our somewhat limited experience with the infusion of a BCAA-enriched amino acid formulation to septic patients resulted in normalization of the plasma amino acid pattern and reversal of encephalopathy.[57, 58] In our experience, reversal of encephalopathy is usually indicative of a better prognosis.

Heart Failure

It is generally accepted that the heart will ultimately fail in sepsis. However, its possible contributory role is still in debate. Some claim heart failure is observed only late during sepsis, as a result of deranged hemodynamics leading to inadequate coronary perfusion. Others assume the heart is primarily affected in sepsis and fails relatively early as a general metabolic-toxic phenomenon, exerting a negative inotropic effect. We

investigated the effect of abdominal sepsis and of different amino acid formulations on the systolic properties and coronary flow of normal and septic rat hearts.[97, 97a] In our experiments, septic hearts demonstrated a decrease in developed force and force velocity when compared to normal hearts.

These systolic properties improved during perfusion with all solutions tested, pointing toward a mechanical washout effect of a "toxic" substance. On top of this mechanical washout effect of all amino acid formulations tested, there was a distinct, greater improvement in systolic properties when an amino acid formulation was used that contained 42 per cent BCAAs (compared to 15 and 100 per cent BCAA formulations) (Fig. 31–6). These results correspond with in vitro and in vivo studies that claim that protein turnover in heart muscle is positively affected by the provision of amino acids,[98] particularly BCAAs[99] or even metabolites of BCAAs.[100] Thus, it seems that the failing heart in sepsis will benefit from nutritional support, particularly by amino acid formulations that are rich in BCAAs.

Respiratory Failure

Severe respiratory failure resulting from injury or sepsis is a well-known cause of mortality and morbidity in the surgical patient. Respiratory failure is brought about by acute alterations in the integrity of the pulmonary microvascular and alveolar membranes. The usual sequence of events is a high pressure or permeability injury to the microvascular membrane that results in interstitial edema with an eventual disruption of the alveolar membrane and alveolar flooding. Because the direct causes for the syndrome are as yet unknown, no specific therapy exists, and treatment is symptomatic. In addition, very little is known about the role of nutrition in respiratory failure. We owe to Starling the dictum that the heart and respiratory muscles are spared during starvation and malnutrition. However, over the years a number of experiments and studies have demonstrated a reduction in heart size, lung weight, and diaphragm mass in proportion to the reduction in body weight during malnutrition.[101] Furthermore, starvation progressively diminished vital capacity, decreased lung protein synthesis, and caused a marked increase in respiratory infection rate.[102] Cur-

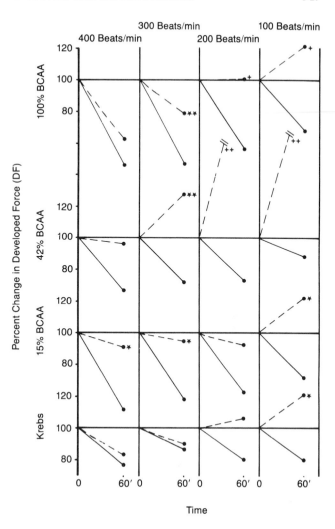

Figure 31–6. Percentage of change in force velocity (df/dt) during 60 minutes of Langendorff perfusion of normal and septic rat hearts paced at 100, 200, 300, and 400 beats/minute and perfused with Krebs + Glucose or Krebs + Glucose + amino acid formulations containing 15, 42, or 100 per cent branched-chain amino acids (BCAA). (*From* Freund, H. R., Dann, E. J., Burns, F., and Hassin, Y.: The effect of branched-chain amino acids on systolic properties of the normal and septic isolated rat heart. Arch. Surg., *120*:483–488, 1985, with permission.)

rently, there are insufficient data on the optimum form and amount of nutritional intake for patients with pulmonary insufficiency. Furthermore, the nutritional requirements of the lung, particularly the injured lung, are also unknown as yet. However, we do know that malnutrition is deleterious to the lungs and should be avoided by early and aggressive nutritional support. The limiting factor is fluid restriction. In order to make the fluid intake limitation compatible with adequate caloric and protein intake, a more concentrated solution containing 4.25 to 5 per cent amino acids in 35 per cent dextrose is used. This enables the administration of almost 3000 calories in a total volume of 2000 ml/day. As already mentioned, there is increased CO_2 production and O_2 consumption in patients receiving glucose as the primary source of nonprotein calories, resulting in cardiovascular and respiratory stresses.[76] In addition,

there is a failure in septic patients for glucose to completely suppress lipolysis or fat oxidation, with a marked increase in urinary norepinephrine excretion.[19] These facts necessitate modifications in nutritional support. Some centers prefer to cut down on the amount of glucose infused, increase the amount of amino acids, and utilize a 50:50 mixture of fat and carbohydrate. The result might be, for example, a solution containing 5 to 7 per cent amino acids, 10 to 15 per cent glucose, and about 5 per cent fat (wt/vol).

Host Defense Derangements

Injury and sepsis are followed by decreased host resistance as evidenced by a decreased number of T-lymphocytes, an impaired ability of peripheral blood lymphocytes to undergo blastogenic transformation in response to mitogens, impaired lymphocyte chemotaxis, impaired neutrophil chemotaxis, impaired monocyte function, and many other immunologic derangements. This in vitro immunologic depression correlated with a clinical state of anergy, which, in turn, is associated with significantly increased rates of sepsis and mortality, particularly in surgical patients.[103] Among the few therapeutic modalities available to boost immune function, nutritional support is the main one. Animal and clinical data have shown that nutritional repletion can reverse cellular and humoral function, reverse anergy, and decrease morbidity and mortality.[103, 104]

PRACTICAL CONSIDERATIONS OF TPN IN THE SEPTIC PATIENT

The prime therapy for sepsis is early and prompt eradication of the septic focus. Support therapy includes specific bactericidal antibiotics; cardiovascular, respiratory, and renal support therapy; and nutritional support therapy specific for the nutritional requirements and derangements of the septic patient.

Nutritional support is aimed at the replenishment of body cell mass, minimizing future catabolism and losses, and maintaining or improving deranged functions such as host resistance, wound healing, respiratory failure, and many other functions that have already been discussed earlier in this chapter.

Indication

It is important to stress that sepsis, being a strong catabolic and hypermetabolic stimulus, is an absolute indication for TPN. Unfortunately, there are still many clinicians who suspend initiation of TPN in the septic patient, claiming the risk of TPN catheter infection to be greater in septic patients. This claim, to the best of our knowledge, has never been actually proved, and patients suffering ongoing sepsis do not have a higher incidence of TPN catheter sepsis. Furthermore, cancer patients on TPN with diminished host resistance[105] or patients receiving TPN as an adjunct to bone marrow transplantation or aggressive chemotherapy do not have an increased rate of catheter-related sepsis,[106] nor is there an increased colonization of their catheters from septic focuses somewhere else in the body.

Recently, Bjornson and associates[107] demonstrated that colonization of TPN catheters by organisms present on the skin at the catheter insertion site occurred twice as frequently as colonization by the hematogenous route and that colonization by organisms present at the insertion site occurred only after a threshold number of organisms was reached. This threshold number can probably be held under control and sepsis avoided by proper management of the insertion site, which will be discussed later.

Solution

The optimal composition of a nutritional support solution for sepsis remains unclear. From what is known so far, the appropriate substrate support of the septic patient requires (1) increased intake of amino acids to approximately 2.5 to 3.5 gm/kg/day; (2) a balanced amino acid formulation enriched to 45 to 50 per cent with BCAAs; (3) a decreased glucose load (a 15 per cent glucose solution at a total carbohydrate intake of 15 to 25 kcal/kg/day is well tolerated); (4) utilization of mixed fuel (fat and carbohydrate).

Technical Considerations

Complications related to the act of placing the TPN catheter or to the mere presence of a foreign body in a large vein are not more common in septic patients than in the general TPN population. Although complications are more common in the subclavian approach, we prefer it because management and long-term safe maintenance are easier for both patient and team.

Metabolic Considerations

The management of the septic patient is certainly different from the management of the general TPN population. Disorders of glucose metabolism, in particular hyperglycemia, are much more common and can become life-threatening if untreated, leading to hyperglycemic hyperosmolar, nonketotic coma. As stated before, lower concentrations of glucose, in the range of 15 per cent, should not be exceeded. The rest of the needed caloric intake should be administered as fat (currently there are at least three commercially available fat emulsions on the market). The use of insulin in high concentrations is advocated, though many believe it is futile because of the insulin resistance that characterizes sepsis. In the general TPN population, it is our practice to start infusing at the rate of 60 ml/hour and increase the infusion rate by 20 ml/hour every 24 to 48 hours. In sepsis we sometimes start with only 40 ml/hour and increase the infusion rate even more slowly, depending on glucose tolerance, which is checked by blood and urine glucose levels.

Deficiency states during TPN are becoming quite uncommon with accumulated knowledge and experience. This statement is correct for electrolytes, vitamins, and most trace elements. However, it must be remembered that for certain vitamins, mainly vitamins B and C, there are increased requirements during sepsis. Further exceptions are zinc and copper. Zinc is lost in excess amounts during muscle breakdown, and the suggested daily recommended amount should therefore be increased by 50 to 100

per cent during sepsis. Zinc requirements must be considered together with copper requirements. The role of chromium in the glucose tolerance riddle of sepsis is as yet unsettled. Essential fatty acid deficiency and the resultant prostaglandin deficiency occur early during TPN,[87] particularly in depleted or injured patients.[88] To prevent essential fatty acid deficiency, we usually offer 4 to 10 per cent of the total caloric intake as fat. In sepsis, in which we make greater use of fat as a caloric source, essential fatty acid deficiency should be very rare.

Liver Function

Derangements of liver function are common in both TPN and sepsis. A broad spectrum of liver function derangements has been reported to occur during TPN in 26 to 90 per cent of adult patients and in as many as 84 per cent of pediatric patients with all types and amounts of protein sources, caloric sources, caloric/nitrogen ratios, and carbohydrate/fat ratios. The causes for these biochemical and morphologic lesions are as yet

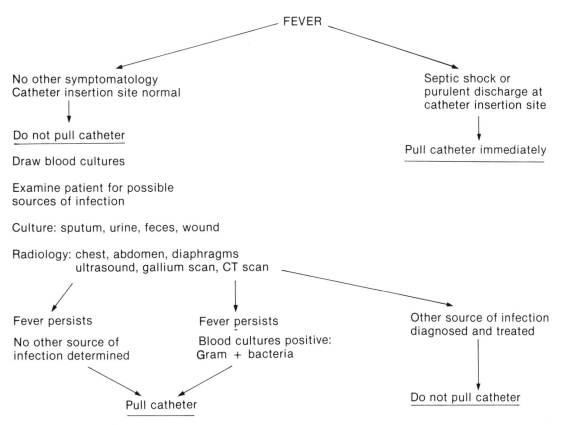

Figure 31–7. Guidelines for management of the central venous catheter in a patient with spiking fever during TPN.

poorly understood, and many as yet un-proven etiologies have been proposed. The liver function failure of sepsis has been treated earlier in this chapter in the discussion on multiple organ failure. It is sometimes evident only on more sophisticated and sensitive tests, such as plasma amino acid patterns, and is not evident on routine liver function tests. To the best of our current knowledge, there is not a greater risk of liver function derangement or failure in septic patients on TPN. Also, based on our current knowledge of the different beneficial effects and mechanisms of action of the BCAAs in liver failure, injury, and sepsis,[43, 44, 48, 49, 52–55, 57, 80–82, 95] we would like to advocate once more the use of balanced amino acid formulations containing 45 to 50 per cent BCAAs combined with a balanced mixture of glucose and fat as caloric sources. Recently, experimental work suggested a beneficial effect of metronidazole in reducing TPN-associated fatty infiltration of the liver.[90a]

Infection Control

The infection rate during TPN ranges from 1.8 to 7 per cent, a surprisingly low rate considering the many predisposing factors for infection these patients have. Among the factors predisposing to catheter sepsis, we find primarily improper attention to protocol of catheter insertion, intravenous tubing, bottle and filter changes, and routine insertion site dressing changes. In our own experience[91] and in that of others,[107] it has been found that it is generally skin microorganisms, mainly gram-positive staphylococci, originating at the catheter's site of entry and advancing along the catheter into the bloodstream, that are responsible for TPN catheter sepsis. Furthermore, a recent study proved that colonization of catheters by organisms present at the insertion site occurs only after a threshold number of more than 10^3 of a bacterial- or fungal-colony-forming unit was reached.[107] This is the rationale for the strict adherence to catheter insertion site care and dressing change, which we strongly advocate in all patients. If strict protocols for TPN are followed, there seems to be no increased tendency for line sepsis in patients who are already septic for some other reason. The only problem for the clinician is to recognize and distinguish TPN catheter sepsis, which necessitates removal of the TPN line, from other common causes of sepsis. Until recently, we used to remove every TPN catheter promptly upon the appearance of fever of unexplained origin during TPN. This way, three to four "innocent" catheters used to be pulled for every catheter responsible for infection.[91] At present, when a patient on TPN develops a fever, the hyperalimentation bottle, tubing, and filter are changed, blood cultures are drawn, and a thorough search is made for obvious sources of fever, such as pulmonary infection, urinary tract infection, wound infection, or intra-abdominal abscess (Fig. 31–7). Only if no other source of sepsis is found and fever persists, or blood cultures show gram-positive bacteria, is the line pulled and the tip cultured (Fig. 31–7). The catheter should be removed immediately if the patient goes into septic shock, if candidemia is suspected, or if a purulent discharge at the catheter insertion site is obvious. In most instances, the infection will clear once the infected catheter has been removed. It is our practice to wait approximately 24 hours for the infection to clear before replacing the TPN line.

REFERENCES

1. Clowes, G. H. A., O'Donnel, T. F., Blackburn, G. L., and Maki, T. N.: Energy metabolism and proteolysis in traumatized and septic man. *In* Clowes, G. H. A. (ed.): Response to Infection and Injury. Surg. Clin. North Am., 56:1169, 1976.
2. Wilmore, D. W.: Carbohydrate metabolism in trauma. Clin. Endocrinol. Metab., 5:731, 1977.
3. Long, C. L.: Energy balance and carbohydrate metabolism in infection and sepsis. Am. J. Clin. Nutr., 30:1301, 1977.
4. Long, C. L., Kinney, J. L., and Geiger, J. W.: Nonsuppressibility of gluconeogenesis by glucose in septic patients. Metabolism, 25:193, 1976.
5. Black, P. R., Brooks, D. C., Bessey, P. Q., Wolfe, R. R., and Wilmore, D. W.: Mechanisms of insulin resistance following injury. Ann. Surg., 196:420, 1982.
6. Wichterman, K. A., Chaudry, I. H., and Baue, A. E.: Studies of peripheral glucose uptake during sepsis. Arch. Surg., 114:740, 1979.
7. Keenan, R. A., Moldawer, L. L., Sakamoto, A., Blackburn, G. L., and Bistrian, G. L.: Effect of leukocyte endogenous mediator(s) on insulin and substrate profiles in the fasted rat. J. Surg. Res., 33:151, 1982.
8. Gump, F. E., Long, C. L., Geiger, J. W., and Kinney, J. M.: The significance of altered gluconeogenesis in surgical catabolism. J. Trauma, 15:704, 1975.
9. Wannemacher, R. W., Beall, F. A., Canonico, P. G., Dinterman, R. E., Hadick, C. L., and Neufeld, H. A.: Glucose and alanine metabolism during bacterial infections in rats and Rhesus monkeys. Metabolism, 39:201, 1980.

10. Dahn, M., Bouwman, D., and Kirkpatrick, J.: The sepsis-glucose tolerance riddle: a hormonal explanation. Surgery, 86:423, 1979.

11. Hinshaw, L. B., Peyton, M. D., Archer, L. T., Black, M. R., Coalson, J. J., and Greenfield, L. J.: Prevention of death in endotoxin shock by glucose administration. Surgery, 139:851, 1974.

12. Yaidyamath, N., Oswald, G., Trietley, G., Weissenhoffer, W., Moritz, E., McMenamy, R. H., Birkhahn, R., Yuan, T. F., and Border J. R.: Turnover of amino acids in sepsis and starvation. Effect of glucose infusion. J. Trauma, 16:125, 1976.

13. Neufeld, H. A., Kaminski, M. V., and Wannemacher, R. W.: Effect of inflammatory and non-inflammatory stress on ketone bodies and free fatty acids in rats. Am. J. Clin. Nutr., 30:1357, 1977.

14. Clowes, G. H. A., O'Donnell, T. F., Ryan, N. T., and Blackburn, G. L.: Energy metabolism in sepsis: treatment based on different patterns in shock and high output stage. Ann. Surg., 179:684, 1974.

15. Ryan, N. T., Blackburn, G. L., and Clowes, G. H. A.: Differential tissue sensitivity to elevated endogenous insulin levels during experimental peritonitis in rats. Metabolism, 23:1081, 1974.

16. Cerra, F. B., Siegel, J. H., McMenamy, R. H., and Border, J. R.: Hormonometabolic profiles in trauma, general surgery and sepsis. J. Trauma. In press.

17. Elwyn, D. H.: Nutritional requirements of adult surgical patients. Crit. Care Med., 8:9, 1980.

18. Wannemacher, R. W., Pace, J. G., Beall, F. A., Dinterman, R. E., Petrella, V. J., and Neufeld, H. A.: Role of the liver in regulation of ketone body production during sepsis. J. Clin. Invest., 64:1565, 1979.

19. Askanazi, J., Carpentier, Y. A., Elwyn, D. H., Nordenstrom, J., Jeevanandam, M., Rosenbaum, S. H., Bump, F. E., and Kinney, J. M.: Influence of total parenteral nutrition on fuel utilization in injury and sepsis. Ann. Surg., 191:40, 1980.

20. Cerra, F. B., Caprioli, J., Siegel, J. H., McMenamy, R. P., and Border, J. R.: Proline metabolism in sepsis, cirrhosis and general surgery. Ann. Surg., 190:577, 1979.

21. Bergstrom, J., Bostrous, H., Furst, P., et al.: Preliminary studies of energy rich phosphagens in critically ill patients. Crit. Care Med., 4:197, 1976.

22. Chaudry, I. H., Wichterman, K. A., and Baue, A. E.: Effect of sepsis on tissue adenine nucleotide levels. Surgery, 85:205, 1979.

23. Duke, J. H., Jorgensen, S. B., Long, C. L., and Kinney, J. M.: Contribution of protein to caloric expenditure following injury. Surgery, 68:168, 1970.

24. Long, C. L., Birkhan, R. H., Geiger, J. W., and Blakemore, W. S.: Contribution of skeletal muscle protein in elevated rates of whole body protein catabolism in trauma patients. Am. J. Clin. Nutr., 34:1087, 1981.

25. Long, C. L., Jeevanandam, M., Kim, B. M., and Kinney, J. M.: Whole body protein synthesis and catabolism in septic man. Am. J. Clin. Nutr., 30:1340, 1977.

26. Buse, M. G., and Buse, J.: Effect of free fatty acids and insulin on protein synthesis and amino acid metabolism of isolated rat diaphragms. Diabetes, 16:753, 1967.

27. Buse, M. G., and Reid, M.: Leucine, a possible regulator of protein turnover in muscle. J. Clin. Invest., 58:1251, 1975.

28. Manchester, K. L.: Oxidation of amino acid by isolated rat diaphragm and the influence of insulin. Biochem. Biophys. Acta, 100:295, 1965.

29. Miller, L. L.: The role of the liver and non-hepatic tissues in the regulation of free amino acid levels in blood. In Holden, J. J. (ed.): Amino Acid Pools. Amsterdam, Elsevier Publishing Co., 1962, page 708.

30. Odessey, R., and Goldberg, A. L.: Oxidation of leucine by rat skeletal muscle. Am. J. Physiol., 223:1376, 1972.

31. Odessey, R., Khairallah, E. A., and Goldberg, A. L.: Origin and possible significance of alanine production by skeletal muscle. J. Biol. Chem., 249:7623, 1974.

32. Felig, P., Pozefsky, T., Marliss, E., and Cahill, G. F.: Alanine: Key role in gluconeogenesis. Science, 167:1003, 1970.

33. Felig, P. L.: The glucose alanine cycle. Metabolism, 22:179, 1973.

34. Garber, A. J., Karl, I. E., and Kipnis, D. M.: Metabolic interrelationship and factors controlling skeletal muscle protein degradation and the selective synthesis and release of alanine and glutamine. In Clinical Nutrition Update—Amino Acids. American Medical Association, 1977, page 10.

35. Goldberg, A. L., and Odessey, R.: Oxidation of amino acids by diaphragms from fed and fasted rats. Am. J. Physiol., 223:1384, 1972.

36. Marliss, E. B., Aoki, T. T., Pozefsky, T., et al.: Muscle and splanchnic glutamine and glutamate metabolism in postabsorptive and starved man. J. Clin. Invest., 50:814, 1971.

37. Ruderman, N. B., and Berger, M.: The formation of glutamine and alanine in skeletal muscle. J. Biol. Chem., 249:5500, 1974.

38. Wahren, J., Felig, P., and Hagenfeldt, L.: Effect of protein ingestion on splanchnic and leg metabolism in normal men and in patients with diabetes mellitus. J. Clin. Invest., 57:987, 1976.

39. Fulks, R. M., Li, J. B., and Goldberg, A. L.: Effects of insulin glucose and amino acids on protein turnover in rat diaphragm. J. Biol. Chem., 250:280, 1975.

40. Sapir, D. G., and Walser, M.: Nitrogen sparing induced early in starvation by infusion of branched chain keto-acids. Metabolism, 26:301, 1977.

41. Herlong, H. E., Maddrey, W. C., and Walser, M.: Treatment of portal-systemic encephalopathy with ornithine salts of branched-chain ketoacids. In Holm, E. (ed.): Amino Acid and Ammonia Metabolism in Hepatic Failure. Germany, Verlag Gerhard Witzstrock, 1982, pages 114–148.

42. Sherwin, R. W.: Effect of starvation on the turnover and metabolic response to leucine. J. Clin. Invest., 61:1471, 1978.

43. Freund, H., Dienstag, J., Lehrich, J., Yoshimura, N., Bradford, R. R., Rosen, H., Atamian, S., Slemmer, E., Holroyde, J., and Fischer, J. E.: Infusion of branched-chain enriched amino acid solution in patients with hepatic encephalopathy. Ann. Surg., 196:209, 1982.

43a. Cerra, F. B., Cheung, N. K., Fischer, J. E., Kaplowitz, N., Schiff, E. R., Dienstag, J. L., Mabry, C. D., Leevy, C. M., and Kiernan, T.: A multicenter trial of branched chain enriched amino acid infusion in hepatic encephalopathy (Abstract). Hepatology, 2:699, 1982.

43b. Cerra, F. B., McMillen, M., Angelico, R., Cline, B., Lyons, J., Faulkenbach, L. A., and Paysinger, J.: Cirrhosis, encephalopathy, and improved results with metabolic support. Surgery, 94:612, 1983.

43c. Rossi Fanelli, F., Riggio, O., Cangianco, C., Cascino, A., Concilis, De D., Stortoni, M., and Giunchi, G.: Branched chain amino acids vs. lactulose in the treatment of hepatic coma. Dig. Dis. Sci., 27:929, 1982.

44. Rosen, H. M., Soeters, P. B., James, J. H., and Fischer, J. E.: Influences of exogenous intake and nitrogen balance on plasma and brain aromatic amino acid concentration. Metabolism, 27:393, 1978.

45. Freund, H., Yoshimura, N., Lunetta, L., and Fischer, J.E.: The role of the branched chain amino acids in decreasing muscle catabolism in vivo. Surgery, 83:611, 1978.

46. Freund, H. R., Yoshimura, N., and Fischer, J. E.: The effect of branched chain amino acids and hypertonic glucose infusion on post-injury catabolism in the rat. Surgery, 87:401, 1980.

47. Freund, H.R., Yoshimura, N., and Fischer, J.E.: The role of alanine in the nitrogen conserving quality of the branched chain amino acids in the post-injury state. J. Surg. Res., 29:23, 1980.

48. Freund, H.R., James, J.H., and Fischer, J.E.: Nitrogen sparing mechanisms of singly administered branched-chain amino acids in the injured rat. Surgery, 90:237, 1981.

49. Blackburn, G.L., Moldawer, L.L., Usui, S., Bothe, A., O'Keefe, S.J.D., and Bistrian, B.R.: Branched chain amino acid administration and metabolism during starvation, injury and infection. Surgery, 86:307, 1979.

50. Sakamoto, A., Moldawer, L.L., Usui, S., Bothe, A., O'Keefe, S.J.D., and Blackburn, G.L.: In vivo evidence for the unique nitrogen sparing mechanisms of branched chain amino acid administration. Surg. Forum, 30:67, 1979.

51. Sakamoto, A., Moldawer, L.L., Bothe, A., Bistrian, B.R., and Blackburn, G.L.: Are the nitrogen sparing mechanisms of branched chain amino acid administration really unique? Surg. Forum, 31:99, 1980.

51a. Gimmon, Z., Freund, H.R., and Fischer, J.E.: The optimal branched chain to total amino acid ratio in the injury-adapted amino acid formulation. J.P.E.N., 9:133, 1985.

52. Freund, H.R., Hoover, H.C., Atamian, S., and Fischer, J.E.: Infusion of the branched chain amino acids in post-operative patients: anticatabolic properties. Ann. Surg., 190:18, 1979.

53. Blackburn, G.L., Desai, S.P., Keenan, R.A., Bentley, B.T., Moldawer, L.L., and Bistrian, B.R.: Clinical use of branched chain amino acid enriched solutions in the stressed and injured patient. In Walser, M., and Williamson, J.R. (eds.): Metabolism and Clinical Implications of Branched-Chain Amino and Keotacids. New York, Elsevier-North Holland, 1981, pages 521–526.

54. Cerra, F. B., Upson, D., Angelico, R., Wiles, C., Lyons, J., Faulkenbach, L., and Paysinger, J.: Branched chain support post-operative protein synthesis. Surgery, 92:192, 1982.

55. Kern, K.A., Bower, R.H., Atamian, S., Matarese, L.E., Ghory, M.J., and Fischer, J.E.: The effect of a new branched chain enriched amino acid solution on post-operative catabolism. Surgery, 92:780, 1982.

55a. Bower, R.H., Kern, K.A., and Fischer, J.E.: Use of branched chain amino acid-enriched solutions in patients under metabolic stress. (In press.)

56. Walser, M.: Nitrogen sparing effects of branched chain keto acids. In Kleinberger, G., and Deutsch, E. (eds.). New Aspects of Clinical Nutrition. Basel, S. Karger Verlag, 1983, pages 319–324.

56a. Muggia-Sullam, M., Bower, R.H., Hurst, J.M., La France, R., and Fischer, J.E.: Infusion of branched chain amino acid enriched solutions in severely traumatized and septic patients: A prospective randomized study. Submitted for publication.

57. Freund, H.R., Ryan, J.A., and Fischer, J.E.: Amino acid derangements in patients with sepsis: treatment with branched chain amino acid rich infusions. Ann. Surg., 188:423, 1978.

58. Freund, H.R., Atamian, S., Holroyde, J., and Fischer, J.E.: Plasma amino acids as predictors of the severity and outcome of sepsis. Ann. Surg., 190:571, 1979.

59. Lohlein, D., Donay, F., Lehr, L., Pahlow, J., and Pichlmayer, R.: Correction of amino acid imbalances in patients with septic peritonitis by treatment with branched chain amino acid enriched solutions (Abstract). J.P.E.N., 4:433, 1980.

60. McMenamy, R.H., Border, J.R., Cerra, F.B.,et al.: Splanchnic substrate balances and biochemical changes during sepsis. In press.

61. Cerra, F.B., Siegel, J.H., Border, T.R., Wiles, J., and McMenamy, R.R.: The hepatic failure of sepsis: Cellular versus substrate. Surgery, 86:409, 1979.

62. Carpentier, Y.A., Askanazi, J., Elwyn, D.H., Jeevanandam, M., Gump, F.E., Hyman, A.I., Burr, R., and Kinney, J.M.: Effects of hypercaloric glucose infusion on lipid metabolism in injury and sepsis. J. Trauma, 19:649, 1979.

63. Elwyn, D.H., Kinney, J.M., Jeevanandam, M., Gump, F.E., and Braell, J.R.: Influence of increasing carbohydrate intake on glucose kinetics in injured patients. Ann. Surg., 190:117, 1979.

64. Askanazi, J., Carpentier, Y.A., Elwyn, D.H., Nordenstrom, J., Jeevanandam, M., Rosenbaum, S.H., Gump, F.E., and Kinney, J.M.: Influence of total parenteral nutrition on fuel utilization in injury and sepsis. Ann. Surg., 191:40, 1980.

65. Nordenstrom, J., Carpentier, Y., Askanazi, J., Robin, A.P., Elwyn, D.H., Hensel, T.W., and Kinney, J.M.: Metabolic utilization of intravenous fat emulsion during total parenteral nutrition. In press.

66. Jeejeebhoy, K.N., Anderson, G.H., Nakhooda, A.F., Greenberg, G.R., Sanderson, I., and Marliss, E.B.: Metabolic studies in TPN with lipid in man. J. Clin. Invest., 57:125, 1976.

67. Elwyn, D.H., Kinney, J.M., Gump, E.E., Askanazi, J., Rosenbaum, S.H., and Carpentier, Y.A.: Some metabolic effects of fat infusions in depleted patients. Metabolism, 29:125, 1980.

68. Long, J.M., Wilmore, D.W., Mason, A.D., and Pruitt, B.A.: Effect of carbohydrate and fat intake on nitrogen excretion during total intravenous feeding. Ann. Surg., 185:417, 1977.

69. Woolfson, A.M.J., Heatley, R.V., and Allison, S.P.: Insulin to inhibit protein catabolism after injury. N. Engl. J. Med., 300:14, 1979.

70. Shizgal, H.M., and Forse, R.A.: Protein and calorie requirements with TPN. Ann. Surg., 192:562, 1980.

71. Freund, H.R., Yoshimura, N., and Fischer, J.E.: Does intravenous fat spare nitrogen in the injured rat? Am. J. Surg., 140:377, 1980.

72. Souba, W.W., Long, J.M., and Dudrick, S.J.: Energy intake and stress as determinants of nitrogen excretion in rats. Surg. Forum, 29:76, 1978.

73. Nordenstrom, J., Askanazi, J., Elwyn, D.H., Martin, P., Carpentier, Y.A., Robin, A.P., and Kinney, J.M.: Nitrogen balance during TPN: Glucose versus fat. Acta Chir. Scand. (Suppl.), 510:159, 1982.

74. Nordenstrom, J., Jeevanandam, M., Elwyn, D.H., Carpentier, Y.A., Askanazi, J., Robin, A., and Kinney, J.M.: Increasing glucose intake during TPN increases norepinephrine excretion in trauma and sepsis. Clin. Physiol., 1:525, 1981.

75. Askanazi, J., Nordenstrom, J., Rosenbaum, S.H., Elwyn, D.H., Hyman, A.I., Carpentier, Y.A., and Kinney, J.M.: Nutrition for the patient with respiratory failure. Anesthesiology, 54:373, 1981.

76. Askanazi, J., Elwyn, D.H., and Silverberg, P.A.: Respiratory distress secondary to the high carbohydrate load of TPN. Surgery, 87:596, 1980.

77. Burke, J.F., Wolfe, R.R., Mullany, L.J., Mathews, D.E., and Bier, D.M.: Glucose requirements following burn injury. Ann. Surg., 190:274, 1979.

78. Manchester, R.L.: Sites of hormonal regulation of protein metabolism. In Munro, H.N. (ed.): Mammalian Protein Metabolism. Vol. 4, New York, Academic Press, 1970, pages 229–238.

79. Clowes, G.H., Heideman, M., Lindberg, B., Randall, H.T., Hirsch, E.F., Cha, C.J., and Martin, H.: Effects of parenteral alimentation on amino acid metabolism in septic patients. Surgery, 88:531, 1980.

80. Freund, H.R., Gimmon, Z., and Fischer, J.E.: Nitrogen sparing effects and mechanisms of branch-chain amino acids in the injured rat. Clin. Nutr., 1:137, 1982.

81. Cerra, F.B., Mazuski, J.E., Chute, E., et al.: Branched chain metabolic support: A prospective randomized, double blind trial in surgical stress. Ann. Surg., 199:286, 1984.

82. Cerra, F.B.: Influence of nutrition on the outcome of septic patients. In Kleinberger, G., and Deutsch, E. (eds.): New Aspects of Clinical Nutrition. Basel, Switzerland, S. Karger, 1983, pages 136–145.

82a. Cerra, F.B., Mazuski, J.E., Teasley, K., Nuwer, N., et al.: Nitrogen retention in critically ill patients is proportional to the branched chain amino acid load. Crit. Care Med., 11:775, 1983.

83. Alexander, J.W., MacMillan, B.G., Stinnett, J.D., Ogle, C.K., Bozian, R.C., Fischer, J.E., Oakes, J.B., Morris, M.J., and Krummel, R.: Beneficial effects of aggressive protein feeding in severely burned children. Ann. Surg., 192:505, 1980.

84. Barbul, A., Wasserkrug, H.L., Seifter, E., Rettura, G., Levenson, S.M., and Efron, G.: Immunostimulatory effects of arginine in normal and injured rats. J. Surg. Res., 29:228, 1980.

85. Barbul, A., Sisto, D.A., Wasserkrug, H.L., and Efron, G.: Arginine stimulates lymphocyte immune response in healthy human beings. Surgery, 90:244, 1981.

86. Gann, D.S., and Robinson, H.B.: Salt, water and vitamins. In Ballinger, W.F., et al. (eds.): Manual of Surgical Nutrition. Philadelphia, W.B. Saunders Co., 1975, pages 79–90.

87. Freund, H.R., Floman, N., Schwartz, B., and Fischer, J.E.: Essential fatty acid deficiency in total parenteral nutrition: Detection by changes in intraocular pressure. Ann. Surg., 190:139, 1979.

88. McCarthy, M.C., Cottam, G.L., and Turner, W.W.: Essential fatty acid deficiency in critically ill surgical patients. Am. J. Surg., 142:747, 1981.

89. Chaudry, I.H., Wichterman, K.A., and Baue, A.E.: Effect of sepsis on tissue adenine nucleotide levels. Surgery, 85:205, 1979.

90. DePalma, R.G., Glickman, M.H., Hartman, P., and Robinson, A.V.: Prevention of endotoxin-induced changes in oxidative phosphorylation in hepatic mitochondria. Surgery, 82:68, 1977.

90a. Freund, H.R., Muggia-Sullam, M., LaFrance, R., Enrione, E.B., Popp, M.B., Bjornson, S.H., and Fischer, J.E.: A possible beneficial effect of metronidazole in reducing TPN-associated liver function derangements. J. Surg. Res., in press.

91. Colley, R., Wilson, J., Kapusta, E., Atamian, S., Freund, H., Hopkins, C., and Fischer, J.E.: Does fever mean infection in central TPN? (Abstract)J.P.E.N., 3:32, 1979.

92. Chaudry, I.H., Schleck, S., Clemens, M.G., Kupper, T.E., and Baue, A.E.: Altered hepatocellular active transport: an early change in peritonitis. Arch. Surg., 117:151, 1982.

93. McDougal, W.S., Heimburger, S., Wilmore, D.W., and Pruitt, B.A.: The effect of exogenous substrate on hepatic metabolism and membrane transport during endotoxemia. Surgery, 84:55, 1978.

94. Abel, R.M., Beck, C.H., Abbott, W.M., Ryan, J.A., Barnett, G.O., and Fischer, J.E.: Improved survival from acute renal failure following treatment with intravenous essential 1-amino acids and glucose. New Engl. J. Med., 228:265, 1973.

95. Freund, H.R., and Fischer, J.E.: Hepatic failure. In Hill, G.L. (ed.): Nutrition and the Surgical Patient. London, Churchill Livingstone, 1981, pages 201–218.

96. Jeppsson, B., Freund, H.R., Gimmon, Z., James, T.H., Von Meyenfeldt, M.F., and Fischer, J.E.: Blood-brain barrier derangement in sepsis: cause of septic encephalopathy. Am. J. Surg., 141:136, 1981.

96a. Freund, H.R., Muggia-Sullam, M., LaFrance, R., and Fischer, J.E.: Brain neurotransmitter derangements during abdominal sepsis and septic encephalopathy in the rat. J. Surg. Res., 38:267, 1985.

97. Freund, H.R., Dann, E.J., Burns, F., and Hassin, Y.: The effect of branch-chain amino acids on systolic properties of the normal and septic isolated rat heart. Arch. Surg., 120:483, 1985.

97a. Markovitz, L.J., Dann, E.J., Hasin, Y., and Freund, H.R.: The different effects of branched chain amino acids on systolic properties of the normal and septic isolated rat heart. Surg. Forum, 34:361, 1983.

98. Morgan, H.E., Earl, D.C.N., Broadus, A., Wolpert, E.B., Geiger, K.E., and Jefferson, L.S.: Regulation of protein synthesis in heart muscle: effect of amino acid levels on protein synthesis. J. Biol. Chem., 246:2152, 1971.

99. Morgan, H.E., Chua, B.H.L., Boyd, T.A., and Jefferson, L.S.: Branched chain amino acids and the regulation of protein turnover in heart and skeletal muscle. *In* Walser, M., and Williamson, J.R. (eds.): Metabolism and Clinical Implications of Branched Chain Amino and Keto Acids. New York, Elsevier-North Holland, 1981, pages 217–226.

100. Tischler, M.E., Desautels, M., and Goldberg, A.L.: Does leucine, leucyl-tRNA, or some metabolite of leucine regulate protein synthesis and degradation in skeletal and cardiac muscle? J. Biol. Chem., *257*:1613, 1982.

101. Arora, N.S., and Rochester, D.F.: Effect of general nutritional and muscular state on the human diaphragm. Am. Rev. Resp. Dis., *115*:84, 1977.

102. Askanazi, J., Wissman, C., Rosenbaum, S.H., Hyman, A.I., Milic-Emili, J., and Kinney, J.M.: Nutrition and the respiratory system. Crit. Care Med., *10*:163, 1982.

103. Meakins, J.L., Pietsch, P., Bubenick, O., Kelly, R., Rode, H., Gordon, J., and MacLean, L.D.: Delayed hypersensitivity: indicator of acquired failure of host defenses in sepsis and trauma. Ann. Surg., *186*:241, 1974.

104. Dionigi, R., Zonta, A., Dominioni, L., Gnes, F., and Ballabio, A.: The effect of TPN on immunodepression due to malnutrition. Ann. Surg., *185*:467, 1977.

105. Copeland, E.M., MacFadyen, B.V., McGown, C., and Dudrick, S.J.: The use of hyperalimentation in patients with potential sepsis. Surg. Gynecol. Obstet., *138*:377, 1974.

106. Larson, E.B., Wooding, M., and Hickman, R.O.: Infectious complications of right atrial catheters used for venous access in patients receiving intensive chemotherapy. Surg. Gynecol. Obstet., *153*:369, 1981.

107. Bjornson, H.S., Colley, R., Bower, R.H., Duty, V.P., and Fischer, J.E.: Association between the number of microorganisms present at the catheter insertion site and colonization of the central venous catheter in patients receiving total parenteral nutrition. Surgery, *92*:720, 1982.

CHAPTER 32

Physiologic and Nutritional Implications of Abnormal Hormone-Substrate Relations and Altered Protein Metabolism in Human Sepsis

JOHN H. SIEGEL

CARDIOVASCULAR ASPECTS OF SEPSIS

The septic process induces an abnormal pattern of cardiovascular dynamics that appears to originate in the specific disorder of intermediary metabolism occurring in sepsis. Hemodynamic manifestations of severe human sepsis can be characterized as demonstrating a rise in cardiac output associated with a disproportionate fall in peripheral vascular resistance, so that a net decrease in vascular tone (the pressure/flow relationship of the body) occurs (Fig. 32–1).[1, 6–8] The central manifestations of this hyperdynamic septic response are evidenced by an increase in cardiac ejection fraction (which is enhanced by the disproportionate fall in peripheral resistance) and by a shift in the Starling relationship to a higher output per unit of left ventricular end-diastolic volume (Fig. 32–2). There is also a decrease in the ventilation/perfusion ratio ($\dot{V}_A/\dot{Q}/_T$) and an increase in respiratory dead space (V_D/V_T).[9] In association with this evidence of a ventilation/perfusion maldistribution, there is an increase in pulmonary shunt ($\dot{Q}_S/\dot{Q}_T$).[4, 9]

These cardiovascular and respiratory abnormalities have also been shown to closely relate to evidence of peripheral metabolic dysfunction.[1, 7]

Previous studies using multivariable analytic techniques have demonstrated that with the development of a hyperdynamic cardiovascular state, the severely ill septic patient can be seen to pass through two different phases, metabolic adequacy and insufficiency.[1, 4, 7] The first of these phases (Fig. 32–3A), which has been characterized as the septic A state, shows an increased oxygen consumption in association with a rise in flow and a decrease in peripheral vascular resistance. In this phase, myocardial contractile function is quite good, and there is no evidence of significant metabolic acidosis, as reflected in the arterial or mixed venous blood pH. As the septic process proceeds, a pathologic hyperdynamic state evolves. This septic B state (Fig. 32–3B) is characterized by a narrowing of the arteriovenous oxygen difference that is disproportionate to the rise in flow, and an absolute decrease in oxygen consumption. During this phase, the peripheral pressure/flow dynamics are seen to be-

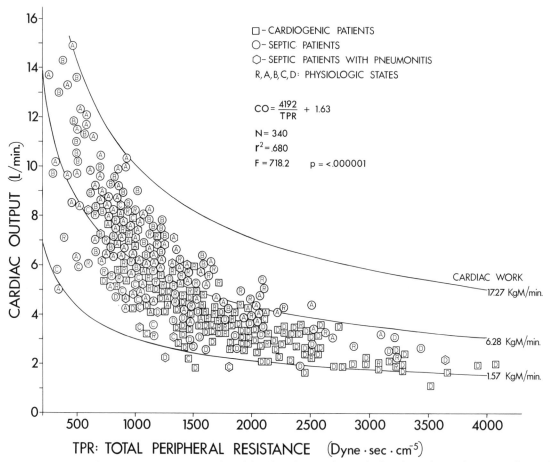

Figure 32–1. Cardiac output *versus* total peripheral resistance in surgical patients in septic, nonseptic, and cardiogenic shock. Lines of constant cardiac work are shown. Individual patient points are labelled by physiologic state (R, A, B, C and D) as described in text. Septic patients in physiologic states A and B are seen to have increased cardiac output at reduced total peripheral resistance and are shown to do increased quantities of flow-related cardiac work (normal 6 kg/min). (*From* Siegel, J. H., Cerra, F. B., Coleman, B., Giovannini, I., Shetye, M., Border, J. R., and McMenamy, R. H.: Physiological and metabolic correlations in human sepsis. Surgery, *86*:164, 1978, with permission.)

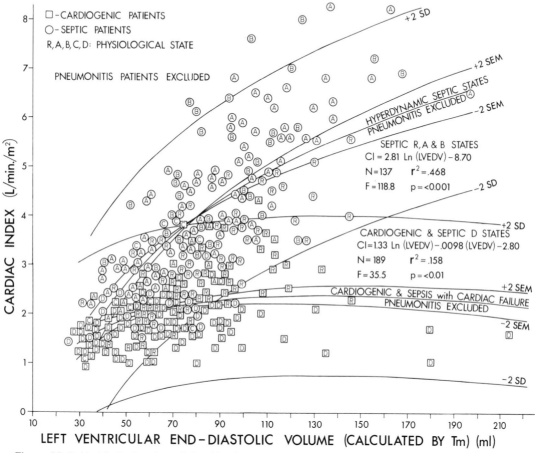

Figure 32–2. Ventricular function relationships in septic and nonseptic surgical patients. This figure demonstrates the relationship between cardiac index and left ventricular end-diastolic volume in hyperdynamic septic A and B patients compared with nonseptic cardiogenic patients and patients with septic cardiogenic decompensation. In the hyperdynamic septic states, patients with A and B sepsis are seen to have left-shifted ventricular function relationships; patients in an R state are normodynamic. These R state patients fall between the cardiogenic D state patients and the hyperdynamic septic A and B state patients. In general, patients with B state sepsis appear to have the highest cardiac output for a given left ventricular end-diastolic value, because of the lower TPR and reduced afterload to cardiac ejection. (*From* Siegel, J. H., Cerra, F. B., Coleman, B., Giovannini, I., Shetye, M., Border, J. R., and McMenamy, R. H.: Physiological and metabolic correlations in human sepsis. Surgery, *86*:164, 1979, with permission.)

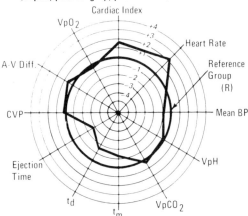

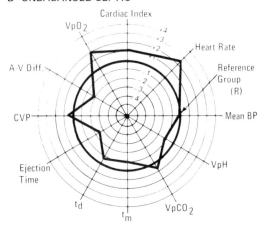

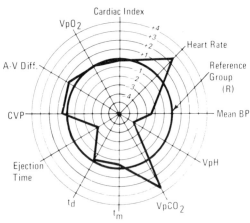

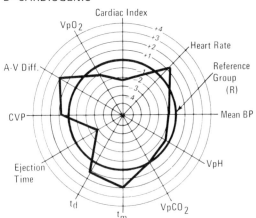

Figure 32–3. Physiologic state classifications in compensated stress (A state), metabolically decompensated sepsis (B state), decompensated sepsis with septic ARDS (C state), and nonseptic cardiogenic decompensation (D state). In each figure, the individual variables—cardiac index (CI), heart rate, mean blood pressure (BP), mixed venous pH (VpH), mixed venous pCO$_2$ (VpCO$_2$), cardiac mixing time from which the ejection fraction is calculated (t$_m$), cardiac pulmonary blood flow mean transit time (t$_d$), systolic ejection time, right atrial pressure (CVP), arteriovenous oxygen content difference (A-V Diff.), and mixed venous oxygen tension (VpO$_2$)—have been normalized by the mean and standard deviations in a control group (R state) of patients who had neither sepsis, stress, trauma, cardiogenic decompensation, nor cirrhotic liver disease. The mean values are shown by the dark perfect circle; each standard deviation of the indicated variable is shown by a light circle increasing or decreasing from the mean of the control R state. (*From* Siegel, J. H., Cerra, F. B., Peters, D., Moody, E., Brown, D., McMenamy, R. H., and Border, J. R.: The physiologic recovery trajectory as the organizing principle for the quantification of hormonometabolic adaptation to surgical stress and severe sepsis. *In* Schumer, W., Spritzer, J. J., and Marshall, B. E. (eds.): Advances in Shock Research. New York, Alan R. Liss, 1979, pp. 177–203, with permission.)

come strikingly abnormal, and the greatest degree of reduction in vascular tone occurs (see Fig. 32–1). There is also evidence of the development of a metabolic acidosis, which may be partly compensated for by respiratory alkalosis. When this peripheral metabolic failure is associated with an extreme degree of abnormality in pulmonary $\dot{V}_A/\dot{Q}_T$ and $\dot{Q}_S/\dot{Q}_T$ (C state), combined respiratory and metabolic acidosis occurs, with rapid decompensation and death. In addition, the patient with B

state sepsis appears to be more vulnerable to the development of high-output myocardial failure with deterioration of myocardial function, reduction in ejection fraction, and development of a secondary state of septic myocardial depression, producing a low flow decompensation (D state) superimposed on the metabolic insufficiency B state (Fig. 32–4).[1, 9] At any moment in the clinical time course, the similarity of a given patient's condition to each of these prototype mean states can be established as a "state distance" in a multidimensional physiologic space.[1–5] This allows a precise quantification of the nature and severity of the pathophysiologic process.

PHYSIOLOGIC AND METABOLIC CORRELATIONS

Evidence that the physiologic state is a manifestation of fundamental metabolic abnormalities has been presented by Siegel[6] and associates[1] and others.[10–12] In particular, physiologic patterns reflect a more fundamental set of abnormalities in glucose, amino acid, and fat metabolism.[1, 4, 6, 9, 13] Figure 32–5 shows the patterns of abnormalities in the circulating blood of glucose metabolites, branched-chain amino acids (BCAA), aromatic amino acids (AAA), amino acids involved in urea synthesis, fat metabolites and ketone bodies, and glucose-regulating hormones, as they relate to the abnormalities of cardiovascular function and the state distance ratios (D/A and C/B). The means of sets of observations on three groups of patients

(traumatic nonseptic, septic A state, and septic B state) are compared with regard to the magnitude of their standard deviational differences (SD) from the means of a group of control elective general surgical patients in the R state of accommodation (the perfect circle at zero standard deviations). A physiologically important alteration seems likely for a mean change of ±1 SD from control. The nonseptic traumatized patients show increased cardiac index (CI) and oxygen consumption per m² (O_2CI) associated with reduced circulating levels of BCAA, AAA, and the precursors of urea, with normal or slightly elevated levels of urea and glucose. There are also normal levels of triglycerides, free fatty acids (FFA), ketones and the glucose-regulating hormones glucagon and insulin.

In contrast, as sepsis progresses from compensated A state to the unbalanced B state, which appears clinically to be associated with evidence of hepatic decompensation as part of the septic multiple organ failure (MOF) syndrome, progressively more abnormal pressure/flow relations are associated with a fall in oxygen consumption and

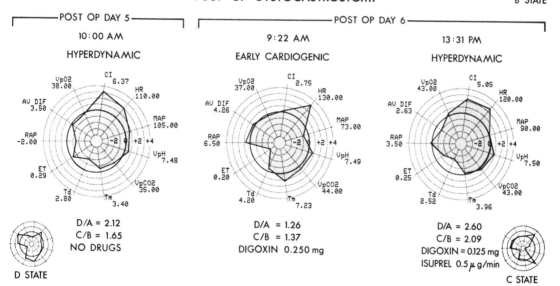

Figure 32–4. Development of myocardial depression in conjunction with the sepsis transition from a hyperdynamic septic A state with increased oxygen consumption (postoperative day 5) to transient myocardial depression in early D state (postoperative day 6, 9:22 A.M.). This development results from the development of septic metabolic insufficiency (postoperative day 6, 13:31 P.M.), which was revealed when the myocardial depression was treated by inotropic agents. Figures in corners represent prototypic A, B, C, and D states, as shown in Figure 32–3. (From Siegel, J. H., Giovannini, I., and Coleman, B.: Ventilation:perfusion maldistribution secondary to the hyperdynamic cardiovascular state as the major cause of increased pulmonary shunting in human sepsis. J. Trauma, 19:432, 1979, with permission.)

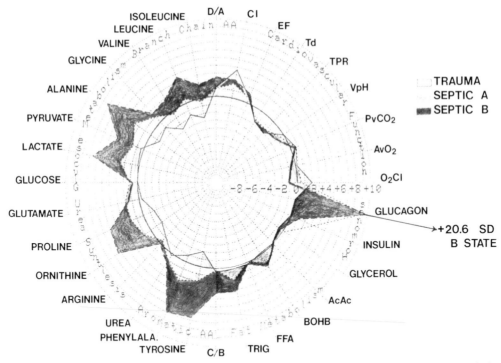

Figure 32–5. Pattern of abnormalities in amino acids, glucose precursors, fat metabolites, insulin and glucagon, cardiovascular parameters, and oxygen consumption as a function of classification into nonseptic trauma, septic A state, and septic B state. Perfect circle represents the R state control means, with scale of standard deviations from control in each variable. The pattern shows increasing levels of branched-chain amino acids, glucose metabolites, urea precursors, aromatic amino acids, and fat metabolites associated with rise in glucagon as oxygen consumption (O₂CI) falls in transition from septic A to septic B state. (*From* Siegel, J. H., Cerra, F. B., Coleman, B., Giovannini, I., Shetye, M., Border, J. R., and McMenamy, R. H.: Physiological and metabolic correlations in human sepsis. Surgery, *86*:164, 1979, with permission.)

a metabolic acidosis. In this B state, one sees a progressive rise in BCAA with a marked increase in the levels of the NH₃⁺ carrier amino acids alanine and glycine.[1, 10] Pyruvate and lactate rise proportionately,[1] as does the level of circulating glucose as O₂CI decreases (Fig. 32–6). Urea and all the amino acids and intermediates of urea synthesis (proline, ornithine, arginine, etc.) rise, even without any evidence of renal failure.[1, 12] However, the most marked abnormalities in amino acid metabolism are seen in the increases in aromatic amino acids (AAA) phenylalanine and tyrosine.[1, 7, 10] Under these circumstances, Siegel and colleagues[7] have observed an increase in octopamine that appears directly correlated with the fall in vascular tone and represents specific biochemical evidence of hepatocyte dysfunction. The levels of the sulfur-containing amino acid methionine and its metabolic catabolic product α-aminobutyric acid also rise in B state sepsis, further evidence of abnormal hepatic catabolism of amino acids.[11] Triglycerides rise to extremely high levels even though FFA levels remain

similar to those seen in trauma; there is a progressive elevation in the ratio between reduced and oxidized ketone bodies, owing to a rise in β-hydroxybutyric acid (BOHB) with normal or low levels of acetoacetate (AcAc), but absolute ketone levels tend not to rise. The most striking differences from the nonseptic traumatic injured state lie in the distorted pattern of insulin and glucagon. Glucagon levels rise to more than 20 SD above normal in B state septics with lesser rises in insulin, (see Fig. 32–5), so that the glucagon/insulin ratio progressively increases.[1, 11] The mean values for the circulating levels of these hormones and substrates also are shown in Figure 32–6, which displays the metabolic pathways for oxidative catabolism in an idealized hepatocyte as well.

SEPTIC AUTOCANNIBALISM

As B state progression occurs, so does the phenomenon of *septic autocannibalism*,[10] which is highly correlated with a fatal out-

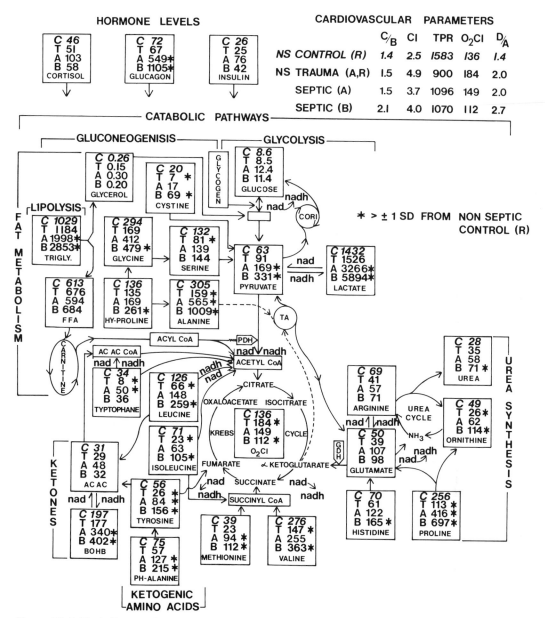

Figure 32–6. Block diagram of plasma levels of stress hormones, glucose precursors, gluconeogenic and ketogenic amino acids as well as urea synthesis precursors from nonseptic trauma patients and septic A and B state patients. These levels are related to cardiovascular values and oxygen consumption levels. (*From* Siegel, J. H., Cerra, F. B., Coleman, B., Giovannini, I., Shetye, M., Border, J. R., and McMenamy, R. H.: Physiological and metabolic correlations in human sepsis. Surgery, 86:164, 1979, with permission.)

come. In septic autocannibalism, the normal dependence of the circulating levels of many amino acids, and especially the BCAA and the NH_3^+ carrier amino acids alanine and glycine, on the quantity of exogenously administered amino acids is lost. In these mostly B state patients (or A state patients close to a B state transformation by state distance ratios), more valine and isoleucine appear than can be accounted for by the administered nutrition (Fig. 32–7).[10] These high "endogenous" BCAA levels ocur simultaneously with increased levels of AAA, proline, and methionine, and are correlated with increases in alanine and glycine.[1, 10, 12] This finding suggests enchanced muscle catabolic release of protein-derived amino acids at a time of increased utilization of BCAA. Such high "endogenous" BCAA levels are not prevented by very large quantities of adminis-

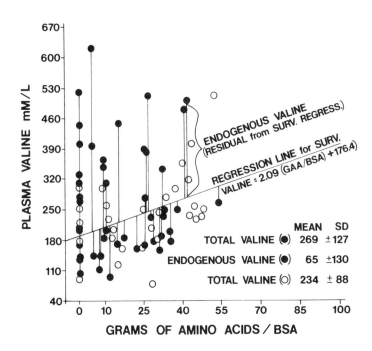

Figure 32–7. Estimation of increased endogenous plasma valine values in septic deaths (●) computed as residuals from the regression for grams of amino acid per day per square meter body surface area in septic survivors (○). Increase in the net plasma value levels in nonsurvivors suggests increased muscle catabolism. (*From* Cerra, F. B., Siegel, J. H., Border, J. R., and McMenamy, R. H.: The hepatic failure of sepsis: Cellular vs. substrate. Surgery, *86*:409, 1979, with permission.)

tered CHO calories and amino acids as TPN. Moreover, there appears to be differential utilization of BCAA under these conditions, with impaired valine and isoleucine utilization but increased utilization of leucine.[10] This clinical observation is compatible with the leucine utilization studies reported by Clowes and associates[14] in isolated skeletal muscle from septic animals and humans. Differential utilization of BCAA under conditions of B state deterioration, in which metabolic acidosis occurs, may reflect preference for one pathway of BCAA access into the Krebs cycle over another, perhaps because of limited availability of cofactors such as oxidized NAD^+, which plays a critical role in the BCAA ketoacid oxidation pathways.[15, 16]

SEPTIC MULTIPLE-ORGAN FAILURE

The patterns of nonutilization seen in the B state septic process suggest a major pathologic alteration in the normal interorgan regulation of substrate and fuel-energy metabolism. Figure 32–8 illustrates a suggested hypothesis for the failure mechanisms altering the normal muscle-liver–adipose tissue cycle of organ metabolism. In this conceptual model,[6] the septic insult initiates an as yet unknown factor that may be related to some aspect of the process of complement activation–complement cascade or subsequent

kinin formation[17, 18] and that causes proteolysis and BCAA catabolism in skeletal muscle.[1, 10, 20] It has been suggested recently that this proteolysis inducing factor (PIF) may be an active fragment of interleukin I.[14] The neuroendocrine response to injury is apparently enhanced, with increased release of glucagon, corticosteroids, and catecholamines.[1, 21–24] The muscle catabolism releases muscle amino acids in quantities proportionate to their concentrations in actin and myosin.[25–27] However, the muscle itself uses mainly BCAA effectively as metabolic substrates.[26] Also, as sepsis progresses into B state, only leucine may be fully utilized.[10] These BCAA are converted to their respective ketoacids, which then enter the Krebs tricarboxylic acid (TCA) cycle for oxidation[15] (see Fig. 32–8). The NH_3^+ liberated by ketoacid formation in muscle is detoxified by transamination with pyruvate derived from muscle glucose-6-PO_4, or glycogen, to form the carrier amino acids alanine and glycine.[15, 16] These carrier amino acids, which are significantly increased in sepsis,[1] are transported via the blood to liver and kidney, where the transamination is reversed and alanine plus α-ketogluterate yields pyruvate and glutamate.[15, 16] Glutamine, which is also formed in muscle, is transported to kidney and gut and transaminated to alanine, some of which also returns to liver.

In the nonseptic patient, the major part of the pyruvate produced by this transport mechanism appears to be oxidized via acetyl-CoA to the TCA cycle, and oxygen consumption rises. However, in the septic patient, especially as B state sepsis progresses (see Figs. 32–5 and 32–8), there is evidence of a diversion of pyruvate into gluconeogenic pathways, with a higher level of equilibration with lactate (see Fig. 32–6).[1] In the septic liver, a significant fraction of the glucose-6-PO$_4$ produced by gluconeogenesis is apparently hydrolized, producing glucose,[28-30] which is then transported via the circulating blood to the visceral organs and skeletal muscle. This increased gluconeogenesis may account for the hyperglycemia seen in sepsis (see Fig. 32–8).

The nongluconeogenic amino acids liberated by muscle catabolism are also transported to the liver and the kidney for oxidative catabolism and urea synthesis.[28] However, as B state sepsis develops, there appears to be impairment of the complete oxidation of the group of amino acids entering into the TCA cycle via glutamate to α-ketoglutarate, perhaps because of inhibition of glutamate dehydrogenase (GDH). Consequently, proline and the related ureagenic precursor amino acids increase,[12]

even though urea synthesis is also increased—accounting for the uremia of sepsis. In the specific case of the AAA, tyrosine and phenylalanine, the impairment of oxidative catabolism is very great. Not only do the circulating levels of these substances rise, but there is evidence that false neurotransmitter by-products, such as octopamine,[7] also rise perhaps accounting for the close relationship of the abnormal vascular tone and $\dot{V}_A/\dot{Q}_T$ abnormalities to the rise in AAA.[7]

The abnormalities of function in the third major organ of substrate fuel production, adipose tissue (see Fig. 32–8), appear to be correlated with the pathophysiologically increased levels of glucagon and may also be modulated by the rise in corticosteroids and catecholamines. The net result is increased peripheral lipolysis and the hypertriglyceridemia of sepsis. Because FFA and glycerol levels are not increased above those seen in nonseptic trauma, increased triglyceride breakdown into these two by-products is likely occurring, with enhanced utilization but incomplete oxidation, since O$_2$ and CO$_2$ fall. Glycerol seems to be a significant gluconeogenic precursor in the septic patient,[29] and FFA, especially the carnitine-dependent

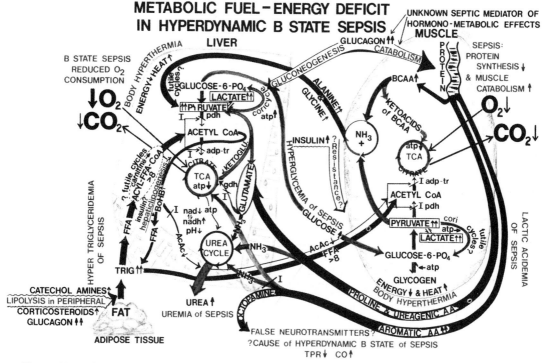

Figure 32–8. Hypothesis for abnormal interorgan regulation of substrate-energy metabolism in hyperdynamic B state sepsis. (*From* Siegel, J. H.: Relations between circulatory and metabolic changes in sepsis. Ann. Rev. Med., *32*:175, 1981, with permission.)

long-chain components, may be converted to the acyl-FFA-CoA form. A distortion of the normal mechanisms may explain the peculiar manifestations of the B state septic process, in which oxidative metabolism decreases as various catabolic breakdown products and energetic fuel substrates increase in the plasma. The hepatic aspect could occur by virtue of the known inhibitory and stimulatory actions of long-chain FFA acting through the medium of acyl-FFA-CoA esters[31] in the presence of the increased gluconeogenic precursors alanine, pyruvate, lactate, and glycerol. These may be modulated by the peripheral protein catabolic, gluconeogenic, and lipolytic actions of the elevated glucagon levels.[31–37] The possible inhibitory action of these acyl-FFA-CoA esters and of increased acetyl CoA and NADH on hepatic pyruvate dehydrogenase (PDH)[6] might be expected to reduce pyruvate entry into the TCA cycle, and the concomitant stimulation of pyruvate carboxylase activity,[35] which initiates gluconeogenesis, would make glucose synthesis dependent on the concentration of pyruvate, which is increased as B state sepsis develops[1] (see Figs. 32–6 and 32–8). The increased glucagon levels may also cause enhancement of gluconeogenesis, by stimulating the second key gluconeogenesis step, the conversion of pyruvate and oxaloacetate to phosphoenolpyruvate.[34] The combination of altered activity of these glucose oxidizing and gluconeogenic regulating enzymes, plus the increased peripheral BCAA conversion to alanine by skeletal muscle in sepsis, enhances the net gluconeogenesis from alanine.[33] In addition, it has been speculated that these acyl-FFA-CoA esters inhibit adenine nucleotide translocase (ADP-tr) in mitochondria and act as regulators for conversion of acetyl CoA into aceto-acetate (AcAc), which is then reduced to β-hydroxybutyrate (BOHB), rather than into citrate formation and oxidation via the TCA cycle.[31, 38]

Other possibly important effects of long-chain acyl-FFA-CoA esters are the inhibition of the malate-aspartate shuttle and the related transport of H^+ ions across the mitochondrial membrane, resulting in a decreased mitochondrial redox potential.[31] Also, the increased level of lactate in the presence of lactate dehydrogenase may influence H^+ availability in the cytoplasmic portion of the cell.[39] This would produce intracellular and intramitochondrial acidosis and a tendency to saturate the nicotinamide ad-

enine dinucleotide hydrogen acceptor, so that NADH rather than NAD^+ would occur in preponderance.[39] The lack of a hydrogen acceptor in the presence of a reduced redox potential may be responsible for the lack of oxidation of BOHB to acetoacetate seen in the septic process and may account for the rising BOHB/AcAc ratio.[1] In addition, many of the critical enzymes in amino acid catabolism depend on NAD ⇆ NADH or NADP ⇆ NADPH,[15] especially glutamate dehydrogenase (GDH) as well as key enzyme systems for the oxidation of leucine, isoleucine, valine, and tryptophan. This dependence on an available free hydrogen acceptor co-enzyme may well account for the generalized impairment of amino acid metabolism that occurs late in the B state, in which all amino acid levels, including BCAA, rise as a preterminal event.[1] All of these factors would tend to reduce the amount of substrate entering the TCA cycle. The expected fall in oxygen consumption and CO_2 production appears to occur as the transition from A to B septic state develops.[1]

An additional critical consideration in the septic process is this: When oxidative metabolism and therefore ATP synthesis are declining, two processes that are extremely competitive for hepatic ATP, namely, urea synthesis and gluconeogenesis,[40] are increasing. At the reduced level of oxygen-consumption in the septic B state patient, it is possible that a major fraction of the already diminished ATP produced is being diverted into these two synthetic cycles rather than supporting other catabolic metabolic pathways and protein synthesis, which are also energy dependent. Indeed, preliminary observations suggest that the synthesis of acute-phase proteins and immunologic proteins decreases and that skin test hypersensitivity is reduced even to the point of complete anergy in B state sepsis. Also, gluconeogenesis is extremely wasteful of ATP, produces more heat and a net reduction in energy, and may be related to the body hyperthermia characteristic of sepsis.

Another possible futile cycle is the diversion of acetyl-CoA away from oxidation and/or ketone synthesis[22, 38] into hepatic lipogenesis. The cycle also involves a diversion of citrate into the cytosol for condensation with cytosolic acetyl-CoA to form malonyl CoA. As a result, there may be resynthesis of FFA and triglycerides rather than fat oxidation from glucose-derived carbons.[38] This

**INFLUENCE OF NUTRITIONAL FUEL ON RQ
IN SEPSIS**

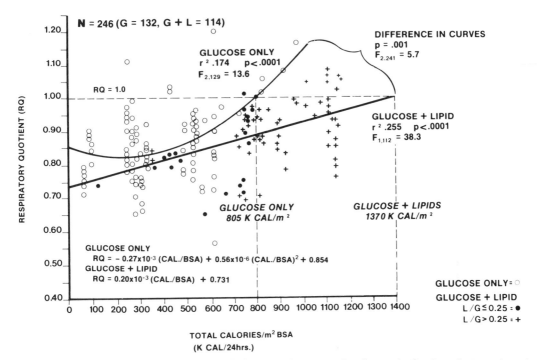

Figure 32–9. Influence of different nutritional fuels on respiratory quotient in sepsis. Septic patients evaluated on glucose only TPN versus glucose plus lipid TPN. The individual regressions and differences between the regressions for glucose only and glucose plus lipid curves are highly significant by Scheffe's method. These data suggest greater oxidative benefit from lipid-containing nutritional support in sepsis. (*From* Nanni, G., Siegel, J. H., Coleman, B., Fader, P., and Castiglione, R.: Increased lipid fuel dependence in the critically ill septic patient. J. Trauma, 24:14–30, 1984, with permission.)

change may account for the histologic fatty degeneration seen in the livers of patients dying with severe sepsis. This concept is also supported by clinical observations that when the B state septic patient dies, there is evidence of marked muscle catabolism with wasting of all skeletal muscle, at a time when peripheral adipose tissue fat deposits remain prominent, and there is marked hepatic fat deposition.

In spite of evidence of enhanced lipogenesis, the septic patient shows evidence of a preferential oxidation of administered lipids over glucose.[13] As shown in Figure 32–9, septic patients receiving glucose plus lipids (at a mean lipid/glucose calorie ratio > .47) maintain a respiratory quotient (RQ) of less than 1.0 at higher total caloric inputs (< 1370 kcal/m²BSA/24 hrs vs < 805 kcal/m²BSA/24 hrs) than septic patients receiving only glucose as a fuel source.[13] In septic patients receiving only glucose fuel, at a lower caloric

load than when lipid is added to the glucose fuel, the RQ increase to more than 1.0 suggests that some oxidatively engendered energy must be diverted into net lipogenesis rather than into other energy-dependent functions (e.g., hepatic protein synthesis or xenobiotic detoxification reactions). Because (1) lipid oxidation, which is a mitochondrial process liberating energy (ATP), and (2) lipid synthesis, which is a cytosolic process consuming energy, have different enzyme systems, cofactors, and hormonal regulators, it may be possible to influence the net balance between them so as to maximize energy synthesis available for more critical processes, if the pattern of hormonal influence in sepsis is known and understood. For example, the high levels of glucagon, catecholamine, and cortisol may stimulate peripheral lipolysis, but hepatic lipogenesis is stimulated by insulin,[41] which may also stimulate some forms of hepatic protein synthesis. This makes it important to consider the biochemical mechanisms of lipid synthesis and oxidation and their hormonal control.[42]

BIOCHEMICAL MECHANISMS AND A HYPOTHESIS FOR OXIDATIVE PRIORITY OF LIPIDS IN SEPSIS

On the basis of known biochemical pathways and their mechanisms for control,[13, 42] it seems reasonable to assume that in nonseptic individuals, administered glucose, facilitated by but not dependent on insulin, enters the hepatocyte by phosphorylation to glucose-6-phosphate (glucose-6-P) and then is converted to pyruvate through the glycolytic enzyme sequence.[30, 42–45] The pyruvate formed may be oxidized or recycled back around the irreversible energetic steps of glycolysis by entering the gluconeogenic pathway for resynthesis of glucose-6-P. This latter compound can re-enter the glycolytic mechanism, can be converted to glycogen, or can be hydrolyzed to yield plasma glucose. The critical step in this process is the initial carboxylation of pyruvate, an ATP-using reaction catalyzed by *pyruvate carboxylase*, a glucagon-regulated enzyme.

In the main, however, pyruvate is acted on by the complex enzyme system known as *pyruvate dehydrogenase* to produce an oxidative decarboxylation to acetyl-CoA with liberation of a CO_2 molecule.[42] Acetyl-CoA is the key compound from which the critical oxidative or synthetic pathways emanate. Conversion of acetyl-CoA to citrate provides entry into the mitochondrial Krebs or tricarboxcylic acid (TCA) cycle for oxidation. The TCA cycle is the source of the major ATP generation through electron transport as O_2 is bound to the substrate carbons and CO_2 is formed. This process regulates cellular oxygen consumption ($\dot{V}O_2$) and CO_2 production ($\dot{V}CO_2$) and is a major determinate of the RQ.

As the synthetic focal point, acetyl-CoA carbons can be used to form ketones for peripheral tissue oxidation, or they can be diverted into fatty acid (FFA) synthesis (lipogenesis). The process of FFA synthesis involves the diversion of intramitochondrial citrate into the cytosol for formation of extramitochondrial acetyl-CoA and conversion by *acetyl-CoA carboxylase* into malonyl-CoA, which serves to add 2-carbon units to the elongating FFA chain via microsomal *FFA synthetase*.[38, 42] This process is controlled by the availability of citrate and ATP and appears to be regulated inversely by the level of cyclic AMP.[42] Because insulin lowers cyclic AMP, it stimulates lipogenesis.

Under nonseptic conditions, administered or endogenous lipids, which are transported in plasma as chylomicrons, are broken down into glycerol and FFA. The former can be oxidized glycolytically to pyruvate, and the FFA enters the cell and the mitochondria via a carnitine carrier mechanism.[38, 42, 46] These FFA are activated to acyl-FFA-CoA derivatives, which are substrates for catabolism by the beta-oxidation enzymes to acetyl-CoA. Whereas the enzymes for FFA synthesis are located in the cytosol, those for FFA oxidation are present only in the mitochondria.[42] This structural separation, as well as the need for different co-factors, allows for different mechanisms of control. The acyl-FFA-CoA derivatives have been shown to inhibit nucleotide translocation from mitochondria[32] and thus possibly to regulate the activity of pyruvate dehydrogenase. More important PDH regulators are ATP and the levels of the products of pyruvate oxidation, acetyl-CoA and NADH.[42] Whereas glucagon stimulates both glycogenolysis and gluconeogenesis,[32, 33] insulin facilitates the entry of glucose through the cell membrane into the glycolytic process so that more acetyl-CoA and citrate are formed.[42] It also stimulates the key carboxylase enzyme system that controls lipogenesis.[38]

The activation, enhancement, or inhibition of these naturally occurring metabolic pathways to different degrees, by alteration of the levels of substrate flux and hormonal regulators, may account for the differential response to administered lipids in septic and nonseptic critically ill patients. Tulikoura and colleagues[47] studied the effect of parenteral nutrition on the levels of circulating insulin and glucagon. They found that in nonseptic malnourished surgical patients, the administration of glucose-only TPN solution produced a significant increase in plasma insulin (IRI) and in plasma glucagon (IRG), but the increase in insulin was more prominent so that the IRI/IRG ratio rose to more than twice the control level. In contrast, a glucose-plus-lipid TPN solution produced a much smaller rise in insulin, with no significant change in glucagon levels, so that the IRI/IRG ratio rose to a much smaller extent; also, growth hormone levels actually declined. Furthermore, nonseptic injury has been shown to result in a more easily controlled peripheral muscle catabolic process that often can be suppressed by glucose-only TPN.[48–51] In nonseptic injury, the substrate flow of gluconeogenic amino acids to the liver, although above normal, may not be excessive, and rising insulin levels would be expected to inhibit lipoprotein lipase and reduce endogenous FFA mobilization from adipose tissue.[52–56] In addition, this pattern of hormone and substrate interaction in nonseptic patients receiving glucose-only TPN would be expected both to increase glucose utilization and to enhance gluconeogenesis moderately and thus to raise plasma glucose levels. However, the substantial rise in insulin at a higher-than-normal IRI/IRG ratio would also favor lipogenesis, and thus one might expect a higher RQ at any calorie level than in septic patients, as has been found in several studies.[13, 56, 57]

Severe sepsis activates a very complex set of hormone-substrate effects. Siegel and colleagues[1] have shown that septic patients have an excessive rise in plasma glucagon (up to 20 SD above the level in nonseptic surgical patients), so that although plasma insulin also rises (three to four SD), the IRI/IGI ratio is reversed, with a dominant glucagon effect. At these plasma glucagon levels, the pharmacologic rather than physiologic actions of glucagon may become dominant, and there does appear to be excessive gluconeogenesis as well as possibly enhanced lipoprotein lipase activity, so that fat mobilization occurs. These effects may also be enhanced by increases in catecholamines[58] and glucocorticoids,[1] which are also elevated. In addition, there appears to be a markedly increased muscle proteolysis.[1, 10, 28, 49] This septic autocannibalism[10] appears to release large quantities of gluconeogenic amino acids, especially alanine, from the transamination of the ammonia moiety from muscle branched-chain amino acids to muscle pyruvate. These gluconeogenic amino acids are transported to the liver, where they may overload the glycolytic mechanism and increase hepatocellular pyruvate[1] and possibly the products of pyruvate oxidation; acetyl-CoA increases, and NAD is converted to NADH[38] as lactate also rises.[1] These regulators of pyruvate dehydrogenase (PDH) rise, and there may be increases in the acyl-FFA-CoA regulators derived from increased lipolysis as well. The increased substrate flux combined with inhibition of PDH would be

expected to enhance the glucagon-stimulated gluconeogenic activity by diverting a larger fraction of the increased pyruvate production to glucose synthesis; indeed, plasma glucose rises to very high levels in the septic patient.

Sepsis has also been shown to alter FFA and ketone synthesis.[21, 22] Pace[38] has demonstrated in an experimental study that ketone body formation is reduced and hepatic lipogenesis is increased by bacterial peritonitis. These data are in agreement with the septic changes in ketone and FFA levels noted by Siegel and colleagues,[1] in humans. Neufeld and associates[21] have suggested that the high insulin levels may be responsible for preferential lipogenesis rather than ketogenesis in sepsis. Because fat oxidation and fat synthesis are separately controlled, it is of interest to see that data from Nanni and co-workers[13] suggest that fat oxidation may be enhanced in sepsis. Also, other carnitine-transported substrates such as acetyl-carnitine appear to be utilized to a greater degree in septic patients than in nonseptic surgical patients.[46]

The mechanisms just described may account for the poorer oxidative response to a glucose-only caloric load than to glucose-plus-lipid TPN. When glucose alone is infused in sepsis, it simply adds another source of pyruvate to an already increased hepatic pyruvate pool, thus increasing the substrate input to an already glucagon-stimulated gluconeogenic process, with resultant hyperglycemia. Insulin levels are also high, however, and may be further increased by glucose; therefore, although the pyruvate oxidation products may also increase somewhat, they most probably partially inhibit pyruvate dehydrogenase. This would reduce pyruvate-derived mitochondrial acetyl-CoA and ultimately diminish complete glucose oxidation. Nevertheless, there is evidence that cytosolic acetyl-CoA levels may still be high and that therefore the insulin-stimulated lipogenesis can still proceed at a high rate with citrate derived from other acetyl-CoA sources and from the quantity of pyruvate that can undergo oxidative decarboxylation by PDH. As a result, the net glucose oxidation versus net lipogenesis falls, and the RQ rises to more than 1.0.

When infused lipids are added to a glucose-only TPN, however, there is no evidence that FFA transport or beta oxidation is impaired, as long as carnitine levels are adequate.[38, 46] Also, the insulin rise seen with glucose-only fuels may be damped by

FFA.[47, 59] As a result of these factors, FFA-derived mitochondrial acetyl-CoA would be expected to increase, thus promoting oxidation of TCA intermediates and consequent ATP generation. Also, as ATP and cyclic AMP (cAMP) increase, the rise in cAMP will tend to reduce the lipogenic stimulus induced by insulin. This would have the effect of decreasing citrate diversion to FFA synthesis, thereby enhancing mitochondrial acetyl-CoA and citrate oxidation. Since the oxidative pathways for FFA are independent of the rate of gluconeogenic activity,[38, 42] they would be expected to increase as a function of the magnitude of the lipid load. Furthermore, because the major inhibitors of pyruvate dehydrogenase are the levels of acetyl-CoA, NADH, and possibly the acyl-FFA-CoA derivatives,[42] the better these substrate inhibitors are oxidized (especially if NAD^+ regeneration occurs), the more glucose-derived pyruvate can be converted to mitochondrial acetyl-CoA and thus oxidized. These interactions at the control sites for substrate oxidation may account for the apparently greater utilization rate of glucose when glucose-plus-lipid rather than glucose-only TPN is used in septic patients.

All of these speculations as to the mechanism of lipid enhancement of oxidative metabolism in sepsis need testing by specific tracer methods. Regardless of mechanism, however, the advantage of glucose-plus-lipid TPN over glucose-only TPN in sepsis seems clear and should motivate further clinical studies in this area.

SEPSIS-INDUCED ALTERATIONS IN HEPATIC PROTEIN SYNTHESIS AND THE MULTIPLE-ORGAN FAILURE SYNDROME

The progressive failure of oxidative utilization of catabolically increased levels of carbohydrate and amino acid substrates that occurs in the septic B state is paralleled by clinical and biochemical evidence of hepatic involvement in the septic process.[7] These processes are in turn associated with protein synthetic and immunologic abnormalities as characteristic features of the so-called multiple-organ failure (MOF) syndrome.

Clinical and experimental investigations of a variety of body proteins lead to the inescapable conclusion that a resetting of the body priorities in protein synthesis occurs

after trauma, inflammation, or sepsis.[61–64] In particular, there is a major alteration in the rate of synthesis and the equilibration levels of a number of acute phase hepatic secretory proteins,[61] which may be of great importance with regard to how successfully the injured or septic host can achieve compensation to pathophysiologic stress. Indeed, the clinical study of Nazari and colleagues[65] using cluster analysis techniques developed from previous classification studies of sepsis by Friedman and associates,[2] strongly suggests that the pattern of acute-phase plasma protein abnormalities has a high discriminant value for ascertaining the risk of development of postoperative sepsis and may also be a significant predictor of death from sepsis in the malnourished host who requires surgical intervention. In particular, low serum transferrin has been correlated with increased risk of sepsis.[66]

The hepatic response to systemic injury in producing a rapid increase in synthesis of acute phase (AP) proteins at the expense of nutritional carrier proteins such as albumin and transferrin has been well described in both experimental and clinical settings.[61–66] In brief, trauma or nonseptic inflammation produces a 50- to 100-fold increase in serum levels of C-reactive protein (CRP) in humans, the calculated mean initial rates of increase being 0.270 mg/ml/hr.[68] Other acute-phase hepatic secretory plasma proteins have also been noted to rise after acute myocardial infarction (sterile inflammation)—haptoglobin (>250 per cent), fibrinogen (>225 per cent), orosomucoid ($\cong$200 per cent), alpha$_1$ antitrypsin (>150 per cent), ceruloplasmin (>150 per cent), and complement C_3 (>125 per cent)—whereas albumin (<75 per cent), transferrin (<75 per cent), and prealbumin (<50 per cent) have been shown to fall from control levels.[62, 63]

Although little has been done in sepsis, experimental studies of turpentine inflammation by Schreiber and associates[64] in a rat model using ^{14}C-leucine incorporation as a means of estimating the synthesis rates of some of these AP proteins have shown maximum ^{14}C-leucine incorporation rates to albumin to decrease to 40 per cent of control in 24 hours, and the AP proteins all to rise—transferrin (>30 per cent), fibrinogen (>200 per cent), alpha$_1$-acid glycoprotein (>900 per cent) and acute-phase alpha$_1$-protein (>3000 per cent)—although the initial levels of the alpha$_1$-proteins were very low.

These differential rates suggest a marked alteration in the prioritization of synthesis of these hepatic proteins, because the same hepatic intracellular pool of ^{14}C-leucine has been shown to be used for the biosynthesis of all hepatic plasma proteins.[64] The half-life ($T_{1/2}$ of each of these proteins is different and varies as a function of the differences in total pool size and utilization rate for each, but the distribution space is similar, implying that the fall in total body albumin as the acute-phase proteins increase represents a true diversion of amino acids to different synthetic priorities. Similar changes have been noted in humans[62, 63] in whom albumin synthesis appears to be compromised in favor of production of acute-phase proteins that may be critical for survival.

The clinical importance of the acute-phase proteins is somewhat controversial, but CRP has been implicated as an activator of complement and as a stimulator of leukocyte phagocytosis.[69–70] Fibrinogen has a wide range of functions essential to an adequate response to injury and infection.[61] It plays a major role in coagulation and the control of hemorrhage. Fibrin deposition in extravascular locations supplies a matrix for fibroblasts in wound healing, promotes leukocyte and macrophage migration, and forms a substrate for proteolytic enzymes needed for wound clean-up and bacterial destruction. However, excess fibrinogen may predispose to intravascular coagulation, thrombophlebitis, and pulmonary embolization; and fibrin degradation by-products have anticoagulant properties that may be important in disseminated intravascular coagulation (DIC), which can be a feature of the MOF syndrome. Haptoglobin (Hp) binds free hemoglobin (Hg), preventing renal toxicity and facilitating catabolism, and the HpHg complex has peroxidase activity.[61] Ceruloplasmin has ascorbate oxidase activity and may help to maintain the circulatory levels of serotonin, epinephrine, and ascorbic acid. It also may be a free radical scavenger, and it plays an important role in permitting proper function of the respiratory chain electron transport by acting as the copper carrier to cytochrome oxidase.[61] Ceruloplasmin also oxidizes ferrous ion to the ferric form for binding with apotransferrin.[61] The function of the alpha$_1$-acid glycoprotein (orosomucoid) is more obscure, but evidence has been presented that suggests it may inhibit transformation of prothrombin into thrombin and thus may help

to prevent increased coagulation in inflammation or sepsis.[61]

Alpha$_1$-antitrypsin (α_1-AT) may be an especially important AP protein because (1) it inhibits leukocyte proteases and (2) by inhibiting lysosomal enzymes liberated during the inflammatory response, it may help limit the vascular and tissue injury incurred during the septic process. Evidence that α_1-AT may be important in limiting the auto-injury potential of the inflammatory response is derived from studies of patients with genetic α_1-AT deficiency states who develop chronic obstructive pulmonary disease of an inflammatory nature.[61]

Other acute-phase proteins, whose site of origin is in some cases less clear but that also rise in inflammatory processes, are complements C_3 and C_4, IGM, and the opsonic fibronectins; also, split products of C_3 (C_3a) have been implicated (as has C_5a) as interfering with complement dependent neutrophil opsonophagocytosis.[71] IGM, which may be hepatic in origin, and opsonic fibronectin (OF), which may be derived from endothelium or RE cells, are also important for successful control of bacterial sepsis, and OF deficiencies after injury or infection have been shown to be associated with an increased incidence of mortality from sepsis.[72]

This list is far from complete, yet in conjunction with another important set of observations about AP proteins, it serves to develop a hypothesis that severe sepsis alters the normal inflammatory acute-phase protein defense response. The related observations are that hormone deficiency states and severe malnutrition states have been noted to alter the levels and synthesis rates of albumin and some of the other acute-phase proteins. Several studies have shown that hepatic C_3 is particularly sensitive to nutritional depletion.[73] Diabetes (insulin deficiency) lowers synthesis of hepatic secretory proteins, which can be restored by insulin.[74] Abnormal patterns of human AP proteins are seen in malnutrition and sepsis,[65] and amino acid deficiencies have been noted to result in decreased or abnormal AP protein synthesis.[75] Recently, a set of very elegant experiments on embryonic chick hepatocytes grown in a hormone-free medium[60] have shown a hepatocyte biphasic protein synthetic response to insulin. The early AP protein responders in terms of increased synthesis were albumin, alpha$_1$-globulin M, prealbumin C, alpha$_1$-antitrypsin, and alpha$_2$-

macroglobulin. The later synthesis responders to insulin administration were fibrinogen, plasminogen, and the lipoproteins. No response was seen for transferrin or alpha$_2$-acid glycoprotein. These data suggest that hormone-substrate interactions (especially insulin and glucagon ratios), which are known to be modified by progressive sepsis,[1] may play an important role in modifying the rate or priority of hepatic acute-phase protein synthesis. They also suggest the possibility that the progressive energy defect of late sepsis may be the cause of the AP and other protein synthesis defects (via pathophysiologic feed back from the abnormal byproducts or effectors), and these in turn may lead to the host defense failures that further reduce the substrate-energy balance, thus leading to an uncontrolled MOF state of septic deterioration.

The energy defect of sepsis, due to the competition for cellular high-energy sources by a variety of processes that are or may be accelerated in sepsis (increased cellular and mitochondrial transport of Ca^{++}, proteolysis, gluconeogenesis, ureagenesis, and lipogenesis), is likely to be a major factor.[76, 77] Also, an unbalanced amino acid pattern is produced by the enhanced septic muscle proteolysis and increased muscle oxidation of BCAA to support muscle TCA energetics;[78] the possibility that this pattern may alter the requirement priorities for hepatic AP protein synthesis from the normal post-trauma or inflammatory response pattern to an abnormal septic one[79] needs to be quantitatively explored. Such AP protein reprioritization in turn may have several important consequences:

1. If critical hepatic AP protein synthesis related to leukocyte bacterial opsonization or killing is impaired, host control of infection may also be impaired.

2. Increases in fibrinogen or decreases in AP protein coagulation inhibitors may promote DIC.

3. Reduction in alpha$_1$-antitrypsin and other hepatic AP protein lysozyme inhibitors may potentiate tissue damage and abscess formation from infectious organisms of otherwise low toxicity.

4. Reduction in hepatic AP proteins with free radical scavenger or reducing capability may potentiate host cell injury from leukocyte superoxides.

5. Reduction in hepatic lipoprotein synthesis may prevent lipids produced by the increased insulin-induced hepatic lipogenesis from being extruded from the cell and thus may reduce the amount of plasma FFA that is in a protein-bound form suitable for peripheral oxidation. Because ketogenesis is reduced and peripheral glucose oxidation is impaired at a post-insulin receptor level, failure to introduce a suitable alternative fuel into the circulation could result in a vicious circle of an uncontrolled oxidation of muscle-derived BCAA and increased muscle proteolysis. Also, if hepatic lipids are not extruded from the cell, they would tend to increase in concentration in the hepatocytes with fatty degeneration, and toxic lipid binding to cell and mitochondrial membranes could occur, because these types of membrane deformations appear to be ultrastructural features of excessive lipid deposition in the absence of lipid oxidation.[80]

6. Increased complement activation and cascade without normal control responses may produce more toxic by-products, which further alter leukocyte or hepatocyte functions, thereby enhancing the vicious circle of hepatic and host failure.

IMPLICATIONS FOR NUTRITIONAL SUPPORT

The implications for parenteral nutritional support in severe sepsis are that the composition of energetic fuels for energy utilization must be tailored to the pattern of biochemical utilization.

Early in the process—or in the recovery state from a serious septic insult, when the patient's adaptive state of metabolic compensation demonstrates a hyperdynamic A or R state response with increased oxygen consumption—a balanced amino acid mixture is not only well tolerated but may be necessary for the full range of protein synthesis needs. Glucose oxidation is generally increased,[30] but because gluconeogenesis is enhanced and the balance between glucose oxidation and lipogenesis favors the latter,[38] glucose calories should be limited to about 800 to 1000 kcal/m^2 BSA/24 hr.[13, 44, 47, 51] Lipid oxidation appears favored under most conditions in severe sepsis; therefore, lipid calories should represent between 30 and 50 per cent of the total nonprotein caloric mixture.[13] However, there is no evidence that hypercaloric mixtures of lipid and glucose together need to be greater in amount than that required to increase the RQ to 1.0. Indeed, total daily caloric inputs that increase RQ to more than 1.0 may be wasteful of energy, and they certainly increase CO_2 production disproportionately, an effect that will be deleterious in the septic patient with an ARDS syndrome.[56] A total calorie input of 1400 to 1500 kcal/m² BSA/24 hr would appear adequate for most needs in the septic patient[13] (possibly excluding those with severe body burns, in whom the excessive evaporative heat loss may require higher caloric expenditure than sepsis alone).

In the B state septic patient, or in the patient in whom transition from A to B state is occurring, oxygen consumption falls below cellular energetic needs,[1, 8] and gluconeogenesis, which is already stimulated by glucagon and catecholamines,[33, 58] appears to be enhanced owing to the excessive muscle proteolysis and its resultant alanine and glycine precursor load.[1, 10, 20, 25, 27] Consequently, glucose calories should be restricted to 500 to 800 kcal/m² BSA/24 hr and lipid calories increased to 50 to 60 per cent of the estimated total-body calorie requirement, because the RQ in these patients is quite low,[13, 57] indicating a greater relative dependence on lipid oxidation for energy generation. Unfortunately, these types of septic patients also show evidence of a markedly increased hepatic lipogenesis with a resultant hypertriglyceridemia.[1] Serum triglycerides must be carefully monitored six to eight hours after lipid administration, and if serum triglycerides reach very high levels, lipid administration may have to be reduced even though total caloric input may also fall. Administered glucose is also very poorly tolerated by these patients, and hyperosmolar nonketotic hyperglycemia is common.

In these B state patients, the possibility of using simple ketogenic fuels with a carnitine carrier may be useful.[46] Acetyl carnitine has been explored by Castegneto and associates (personal communication), but this work is still in too preliminary a stage for any definitive recommendation to be made.

The B state patient also appears to be unable to utilize most of the proteolytically released muscle amino acids, especially the aromatic amino acids, proline, and the sulfur-containing amino acids.[1, 10–12, 20, 26, 78] False neurotransmitter by-products of tyrosine metabolism (octopamine) have been shown to increase to pathophysiologic levels and may be responsible for the reduction in vascular tone and the lethargy or coma seen in B state patients.[7] Conversely, the oxidation of branched-chain amino acids appears to be relatively well preserved until very late in the septic process.[26, 78] Skeletal muscle, heart, and liver can use branched-chain amino acids, especially leucine, for energy generation, and the modicum of ATP that results from their oxidation may be the critical factor in keeping other essential transport, detoxification, and protein-synthetic processes going. The implications of this hypothesis are that a TPN mixture rich in branched-chain amino acids (up to 50 per cent of total amino acids) and poor in aromatic amino acids, with a low glucose content and a relatively high lipid content, appears to be the best approach, justified by our present state of ignorance. It is hoped that the future holds a more sophisticated view of substrate utilization and that newer types of energetic fuel mixtures that can be more favorably oxidized by the metabolically impaired septic host will be developed.

REFERENCES

1. Siegel, J. H., Cerra, F. B., Coleman, B., Giovannini, I., Shetye, M., Border, J. R., and McMenamy, R. H.: Physiological and metabolic correlations in human sepsis. Surgery, 86:164, 1979.
2. Friedman, H. P., Goldwyn, R. M., and Siegel, J. H.: The use and interpretation of multivariable methods in the classification of stages of serious infectious disease processes in the critically ill. In Elashoff, R. (ed.): Perspectives in Biometrics. New York, Academic Press, 1975, pp. 81–122.
3. Siegel, J. H., Goldwyn, R. M., and Friedman, H. P.: Pattern and process in the evolution of human septic shock. Surgery, 70:232, 1971.
4. Siegel, J. H., Cerra, F. B., Peters, D., Moody, E., Brown, D., McMenamy, R. H., and Border, J. R.: The physiologic recovery trajectory as the organizing principle for the quantification of hormonometabolic adaptation to surgical stress and severe sepsis. In Adv. Shock Res., 2:177, 1979.
5. Siegel, J. H., Cerra, F. B., Moody, E. A., Shetye, M., Garr, L., Shubert, M., Browne, D., and Keane, J. S.: The effect on survival of critically ill and injured patients of an ICU teaching service organized about a computer-based physiologic CARE system. J. Trauma, 20:558, 1980.
6. Siegel, J. H.: Relations between circulatory and metabolic changes in sepsis. Ann. Rev. Med., 32:175, 1981.
7. Siegel, J. H., Giovannini, I., Coleman, B., Cerra, F. B., and Nespoli, A.: Pathologic synergy in cardiovascular and respiratory compensation with cirrhosis and sepsis: A manifestation of a common metabolic defect. Arch. Surg., 117:225, 1982.
8. Siegel, J. H., Greenspan, M., and DelGuercio, L. R. M.: Abnormal vascular tone, defective oxygen

transport and myocardial failure in human septic shock. Ann. Surg., 165:504, 1967.

9. Siegel, J. H., Giovannini, I., and Coleman, B.: Ventilation:perfusion maldistribution secondary to the hyperdynamic cardiovascular state as the major cause of increased pulmonary shunting in human sepsis. J. Trauma, 19:431, 1979.

10. Cerra, F. B., Siegel, J. H., Coleman, B., Border, J. R., and McMenamy, R. H.: Septic autocannibalism: A failure of exogenous nutritional support. Ann. Surg., 192:570, 1980.

11. Cerra, F. B., Siegel, J. H., Border, J. R., and McMenamy, R. H.: The hepatic failure of sepsis: Cellular vs. substrate. Surgery, 86:409, 1979.

12. Cerra, F. B., Caprioli, J., Siegel, J. H., Border, J. R., and McMenamy, R. H.: Abnormal proline metabolism in human sepsis: Evidence of specific metabolic blocks. Ann. Surg., 190:577, 1979.

13. Nanni, G., Siegel, J. H., Coleman, B., Fader, P., and Castiglione, R.: Increased lipid fuel dependence in the critically ill septic patient. J. Trauma, 24:14, 1984.

14. Clowes, G. H. A., Jr., George, B. C., Villee, C. A., and Sarovis, C. A.: Muscle proteolysis induced by a circulating peptide in patients with sepsis or trauma. N. Engl. J. Med., 308:545, 1983.

15. Rosenberg, L. E., and Scriver, C. R.: Disorders of amino acid metabolism. In Bondy, P. K., and Rosenberg, L. E. (eds.): Duncan's Diseases of Metabolism. Philadelphia, W. B. Saunders, 1974, pp. 465–653.

16. Felig, P.: Amino acid metabolism in man. Ann. Rev. Biochem., 44:933, 1975.

17. Schumer, W., Erve, P. E., and Miller, B.: Immune response in septic shock. Therapeutic implications. In Nyhus, L., and Schumer, W. (eds.): Treatment of Shock: Principles and Practice. Philadelphia, Lea & Febiger, 1974, pp. 141–153.

18. Beisel, W. R., and Sobocinski, P. Z.: Endogenous mediators of fever-related metabolic and hormonal responses. In Lipton, J. M. (ed.): Fever. New York, Raven Press, 1980, pp. 39–48.

19. O'Donnell, T. F., Clowes, G. H. A., Jr., Blackburn, G. L., Ryan, N. T., Benotti, P. N., and Miller, J. D.: Proteolysis associated with deficit of peripheral energy fuel substrates in septic man. Surgery, 80:192, 1976.

20. Clowes, G. H. A., Jr., Randall, H. T., Cha, C. J. M., Tyan, B. A., and Hirsch, E.: Amino acid and energy metabolism in septic and traumatized patients. J.P.E.N., 4:195, 1980.

21. Neufeld, H. A., Pace, J. G., Kaminski, M. W., George, D. T., Jahrling, P. B., Wannemacher, R. W., and Beisel, W. R.: A probable endocrine basis for the depression of ketone bodies during infections or inflammatory state in rats. Endocrinology, 107:596, 1980.

22. Neufeld, H. S., Pace, J. G., Kaminski, M. W., Sobocinski, P., and Crawford, D. J.: Unique effects of infectious or inflammatory stress on fat metabolism in rats. J.P.E.N., 6:511, 1982.

23. Liddell, M. J., Daniel, A. M., MacLean, L. D., and Shisgal, H. M.; The role of stress hormones in the catabolic metabolism of shock. Surg. Gynecol. Obstet., 149:822, 1979.

24. Wilmore, D. W., Moyland, J. A., Jr., Lundsey, C. A., Falonna, G. R., Unger, R., and Pruitt, B. A., Jr.: Hyperglucagonemia following thermal injury: Insulin and glucagon in the post traumatic catabolic state. Surg. Forum, 24:99, 1973.

25. George, B. C., Clowes, G. H. A., Jr., Heidman, M., Saravis, C., and Ryan, M. T.: Muscle glucose and amino acid metabolism in fasting normal and septic states. Fed. Proc., 39:818, 1980.

26. Freund, H. R., Ryan, J. A., Jr., and Fischer, J. E.: Amino acid derangements in patients with sepsis: Treatment with branched chain amino acid rich infusions. Ann. Surg., 188:423, 1978.

27. Askanazi, J., Carpenter, Y. A., Michelsen, C. B., Elwyn, D. H., Furst, P., Gump, F., and Kinney, J. M.; Muscle and plasma amino acids following injury: Influence of intercurrent infection. Ann. Surg., 192:78, 1980.

28. Beisel, W. R., and Wannemacher, R. W.: Gluconeogenesis, ureagenesis and ketogenesis during sepsis. J.P.E.N., 4:277, 1980.

29. Long, C. L., Spencer, J. L., Kinney, J. M., and Geiger, J. W.: Carbohydrate metabolism in man: Effect of elective operations and major injury. J. Appl. Physiol., 31:110, 1971.

30. Long, C. L.: Energy balance and carbohydrate metabolism in infection and sepsis. Am. J. Clin. Nutr., 30:1301, 1977.

31. Shrago, E., Shug, A., and Elson, C.: Regulations of cell metabolism by mitochondrial transport systems. In Hanson, R. W., and Mehlman, M. A. (eds.): Gluconeogenesis: Its Regulation in Mammalian Species. New York, John Wiley & Sons, 1976, pp. 221–238.

32. Lefebvre, P.: Glucagon and lipid metabolism. In Lefebvre, P., and Unger, R. H. (eds.): Glucagon: Molecular Physiology, Clinical and Therapeutic Implications. New York, Pergamon, 1972, pp. 109–119.

33. Chiasson, J. L., Cook, J., Liljenquist, J. E., and Lacy, W. W.: Glucagon stimulation of gluconeogenesis from alanine in the intact dog. Am. J. Physiol., 227:19, 1974.

34. Tilgham, S. M., Hanson, R. W., and Ballard, F. S.: Hormonal regulation of phosphoenopyruvate carboxykinase (GTP) in mammalian tissues. In Hanson, R. W., and Mehlman, M. A. (eds.): Gluconeogenesis: Its Regulation in Mammalian Species. New York, John Wiley & Sons, 1976, pp. 47–91.

35. Barritt, J. G., Zander, G. L., and Utter, M. F.: The regulation of pyruvate carboxylase activity in gluconeogenic tissues. In Hanson, R. W., and Mehlman, M. A. (eds.): Gluconeogenesis: Its Regulation in Mammalian Species. New York, John Wiley & Sons, 1976, pp. 3–46.

36. Unger, R. H.: Glucagon and the insulin:glucagon ratio in diabetes and other catabolic illnesses. Diabetes, 20:834, 1971.

37. Unger, R. H.: Pancreatic glucagon in health and disease. Adv. Intern. Med., 17:265, 1971.

38. Pace, J. G.: Fatty acid metabolism and ketogenesis during a streptococcus pneumonal infection in the rat. Dissertation, George Washington Universtiy, 1980.

39. Williamson, J. R.: Role of anion transport in the regulation of metabolism. In Hanson, R. W., and Mehlman, M. A., (eds.): Gluconeogenesis: Its Regulation in Mammalian Species. New York, John Wiley & Sons, 1976, pp. 165–220.

40. Krebs, H. A., Lund, P., and Stubbs, M.: Interrelations between gluconeogenesis and urea synthesis. In Hanson, R. W., and Mehlman, M. A. (eds.): Gluconeogenesis: Its Regulation in Mammalian Species. New York, John Wiley & Sons, 1976, p. 269–291.

41. Shreeve, W. W.: Effect of insulin on the turnover of plasma carbohydrates and lipids. Am. J. Med., *40*:724, 1966.

42. Coleman, J. E.: Metabolic interrelationships between carbohydrates, lipids and proteins. *In* Bondy, P. K., and Rosenberg, L. E. (eds.): Metabolic Control and Disease. Philadelphia, W. B. Saunders, 1980, pp. 161–274.

43. Long, C., Kinney, J. M., and Geiger, J. W.: Non-suppressibility of gluconeogenesis by glucose in septic patients. Metabolism, *25*:193, 1976.

44. Wolfe, R. R., O'Donnell, T. F., Jr., Stone, M. D., et al.: Investigation of factors determining the optimal glucose infusion rate of total parenteral nutrition. Metabolism, *29*:89, 1980.

45. Wolfe, R. R., Allsop, J. R., and Burke, J. F.: Glucose metabolism in man: Responses to intravenous glucose infusion. Metabolism, *28*:210, 1979.

46. Nanni, G., Castagneto, M., Pittiruti, M., et al.: Influence of carnitine on the metabolic response to injury and sepsis. *In* Progressive Care of Acutely Ill and Injured. Chichester, John Wiley & Sons, 1982.

47. Tulikoura, I., Liewendahl, K., Taskinen, M. R., et al.: Effect of parenteral nutrition on the blood levels of insulin, glucagon, growth hormone, thyroid hormones and cortisol in catabolic patients. Acta Chir. Scand., *148*:315, 1982.

48. Blackburn, G. L., and Wolfe, R. R.: Clinical biochemistry and intravenous hyperalimentation. *In* Alberti, K. G. M. M., and Price, C. P. (eds.). Recent Advances in Clinical Biochemistry. Edinburgh, Chuchill-Livingstone, 1981, pp. 197–228.

49. Dudrick, S. J., and Rhoads, J. E.: Metabolism in surgical patients: Protein, carbohydrate and fat utilization by oral and parenteral routes. *In* Sabiston, D. C., Jr. (ed.): Davis-Christopher Textbook of Surgery, 12th ed. Philadelphia, W. B. Saunders, 1981, pp. 144–171.

50. Long, J. M., III, Wilmore, D. W., Mason, A. D., Jr., et al.: Effect of carbohydrate and fat intake on nitrogen excretion during total intravenous feeding. Ann. Surg., *185*:417, 1977.

51. Rutten, P., Blackburn, G. L., Flatt, J. P., et al.: Determination of optimal hyperalimentation infusion rate. J. Surg. Res., *18*:477, 1975.

52. Carpenter, Y. A., Askanazi, J., Elwyn, D. A., et al.: Effects of hypercaloric glucose infusion on lipid metabolism in injury and sepsis. J. Trauma, *19*:649, 1979.

53. Elwyn, D. H., Kinney, J. M., Gump, F. E., et al.: Metabolic and endocrine effects of fasting followed by infusion of five-percent glucose. Surgery, *90*:810, 1981.

54. Jeejeebhoy, K. N., Anderson, G. H., Nakhooda, A. F., et al.: Metabolic studies in total parenteral nutrition with lipid in man. Comparison with glucose. J. Clin. Invest., *57*:125, 1976.

55. Long, C. L., Spencer, J. L., Kinney, J. M., et al.: Carbohydrate metabolism in man: Effect of elective operations and major injury. J. Appl. Physiol., *31*:110, 1971.

56. Robin, A. P., Askanazi, J., Cooperman, A., et al.: Influence of hypercaloric glucose infusions on fuel economy in surgical patients; a review. Crit. Care Med., *9*:680, 1981.

57. Nanni, G., Pittiruti, M., Giovannini, I., et al.: Prognostic value of exchange ratio in critically ill patients. Urg. Chir. Comm., *4*:101, 1981.

58. Wilmore, D. W., Long, J. M., Mason, A. D., Jr., et al.: Catecholamines: Mediators of the hypermetabolic response to thermal injury. Ann. Surg., *180*:653, 1974.

59. Coran, A. G., Cryer, P. E., and Horwitz, D. L.: Effect of intravenously administered fat on serum insulin levels. Am. J. Clin. Nutr., *25*:131, 1972.

60. Liang, T. J., and Grieninger, G.: Direct effect of insulin on the synthesis of specific plasma proteins; Biphasic response of hepatocytes cultured in serum and hormone-free medium. Cell Biol., *78*:6972, 1981.

61. Koj, A.: Acute-phase reactants. *In* Allison, A. C. (ed.): Structure and Function of Plasma Proteins, Vol. 1. London, Plenum Press, 1974, pp. 73–125.

62. Turner, M. W., and Hulme, B.: The plasma proteins: An introduction. London, Pitman Medical and Scientific Pub., 1975, p. 129.

63. Blomback, B., and Hanson, L. A.: Plasma Proteins. New York, John Wiley & Sons, 1979, pp. 351–354.

64. Schreiber, G., Howlett, G., Nagashima, M., Millership, A., Martin, H., Urban, J., and Kotler, L.: The acute phase response of plasma protein synthesis during experimental inflammation. J. Biol. Chem., *257*:10271, 1982.

65. Nazari, S., Dionigi, R., Comodi, I., Dionigi, P., and Campani, M.: Pre-operative prediction and quantification of septic risk caused by malnutrition. Arch. Surg., *117*:266, 1982.

66. Smale, B. F., Busby, G. P., Mullen, J. L., and Rosato, E. F.: Prognostic value of serum transferrin in the surgical patient. Surg. Forum, *32*:112, 1981.

67. Aulick, L. H., and Wilmore, D. W.: Increased peripheral amino acid release following burn injury. Surgery, *85*:560, 1979.

68. Kushner, I., Broder, M. L., and Karp, D.: Control of the acute phase response. J. Clin. Invest., *61*:235, 1978.

69. Kaplan, M. H., and Volanakis, J. E.: Interactions of C-reactive protein complex is with the complement system I: Consumption of human complement associated with the reaction of C-reactive protein with pneumococcal C-polysaccharide and with the choline phosphatides, lecithin and sphingomyelin. J. Immunol., *112*:2135, 1974.

70. Siegel, J., Osmond, A. P., Wilson, M. F., and Gewurz, H.: Interactions of C-reactive protein with the complement system. II: C-reactive protein–mediated consumption of complement by poly-L-lysine polymers and other polycations. J. Exp. Med., *142*:709, 1975.

71. Ogle, J. D., Ogle, C. K., and Alexander, J. W.: Inhibition of neutrophil function by a degradation product of C₃. Surg. Forum, *32*:37, 1981.

72. Lanser, M. E., and Saba, T. M.: Decreased resistance to *Staphylococcus aureus* by opsonic fibronectin depletion. Surg. Forum, *32*:54, 1981.

73. Alexander, J. W., Stinnett, J. D., and Ogle, C. K.: Nonspecific immunologic defense mechanisms in nutritional assessment. *In* Levinson, S. M. (ed.): Nutritional Assessment—Present Status, Future Directions and Prospects. Columbus, Ohio, Ross Laboratories, 1981, pp. 116–117.

74. Peavy, D. E., Taylor, J. M., and Jefferson, L. S.: Correlation of albumin production rates and albumin mRNA levels in livers of normal, diabetic, and insulin-treated diabetic rats. Proc. Natl. Acad. Sci. U.S.A., *75*:5879, 1978.

75. Flaim, K. E., Peavy, D. E., Everson, W. V., and Jefferson, L. S.: The role of amino acids in the regulation of protein synthesis in perfused rat

liver. I. Reduction in rates of synthesis resulting from amino acid deprivation and recovery during flow-through perfusion. J. Biol. Chem., *257*:2932, 1982.

76. Villalobo, A., and Lehninger, A. L.: Inhibition of oxidative phosphorylation in ascites tumor mitochondria and cells by intramitochondrial Ca^{2+}. J. Biol. Chem., *255*:2457, 1980.

77. Rossi, C. S., and Lehninger, A. L.: Stoichiometry of respiratory stimulation, accumulation of Ca^{++} and phosphate, and oxidative phosphorylation in rat liver mitochondria. J. Biol. Chem., *239*:3971, 1964.

78. Blackburn, G. L., Moldawer, L. L., Usui, S., Bothe, A. Jr., O'Keefe, S. J. D., and Bistrian, B. R.: Branched chain amino acid administration and metabolism during starvation, injury and infection. Surgery, *60*:307, 1979.

79. Sganga, G., Siegel, J. H., Brown, G., Coleman, B., Wiles, C. E., Belzberg, H., Wedel, S., and Placko, R.: Reprioritization of hepatic plasma protein release in trauma and sepsis. Arch. Surg., *120*:187, 1985.

80. Liedthe, J. A., Nellis, S., and Neely, J. R.: Effect of excess free fatty acids on mechanical and metabolic function in normal and ischemic myocardium in swine. Circ. Res., *43*:652, 1978.

CHAPTER 33

Nutritional Support and the Cardiac Patient

RONALD M. ABEL

Although the presence of severe cardiac disease should not preempt nutritional support when indicated, priorities of care based on *immediate* threat to life have generally placed nutritional considerations near the bottom of the list of clinical problems. There may be indirect impediments to aggressive treatment of nutritional disorders in severely ill patients with heart disease. For example, "nutritional assessment" *per se* is nearly never part of the routine admission and management policies in most coronary care units throughout the country. Nutritional aspects of most practices of cardiology consist of understanding the need for sodium restriction in patients with hypertension or congestive heart failure and an occasional warning about the dietary content of saturated fats and cholesterol for patients with arteriosclerotic heart disease. The vast majority of patients with heart disease in this country suffer from arteriosclerosis, a disease usually not associated with identifiable undernutrition. The rare patient with long-standing congestive heart failure and cardiac cachexia is seen less and less commonly in the United States. Surgeons and gastroenterologists who provide specialized techniques of nutritional support for most patients may compromise the goal of providing adequate nutrients because of a fear of complications resulting from parenteral nutritional support in patients with advanced heart disease.

As the patient population with concomitant heart disease and nutritional inadequacies enlarges, nutritional support in such patients emerges as a more prevalent problem. With an increase in life expectancy in North America, the average age of the hospitalized patient and hence of the potential candidate for parenteral nutritional support in cardiac disease has also increased. For example, at the Newark Beth Israel Medical Center, an average-sized urban institution, a 19.2 per cent increase in hospital admissions over age 65 was noted during the years 1974 to 1981 (Table 33–1).

Because cardiovascular disease occurs with greater prevalence with age, one might anticipate that in an older population of hospitalized patients with a variety of medical and surgical diseases, the incidence of concomitant heart disease would also rise. Clinical and technical advances in cardiovascular surgery particularly have exposed a population of older patients with severe heart disease to conditions requiring aggressive nutritional support in order to achieve clinical success. Successful surgical management of ruptured abdominal aortic aneurysms, urgent open heart surgery for consequences of acute myocardial infarction, successful procedures for dissections of the aorta, and the inevitable postoperative complications of cerebral and other organ system impairment have created a large population of critically ill patients in need of continued metabolic

Table 33–1. ADMISSIONS OF PATIENTS OVER 65 YEARS TO THE NEWARK BETH ISRAEL MEDICAL CENTER, 1974–1981*

YEAR	ADMISSIONS
1974	2,629
1975	2,623
1976	2,818
1977	2,766
1978	2,829
1979	2,934
1980	2,965
1981	3,133

*Total bed capacity of 540 remained unchanged during this period.

575

and nutritional support. The major clinical experience in management of patients with severe heart disease comes from cardiac surgical centers. When subjected to the catabolic stress of surgery, cardiac surgical patients frequently demonstrate difficulty in weaning from respiratory support, presumably because of continued musculoskeletal weakness and chronic illness. Poor wound healing following cardiac surgery is common in older patients, undoubtedly owing to the insidious development of protein-calorie malnutrition, which so frequently occurs in the elderly. Because the alternative to nutritional support is starvation, a state that precludes recovery from major catabolic illnesses, the goal of the nutritionist, cardiologist, and cardiac surgeon is to provide efficacious and safe nutritional support to patients with severely diseased hearts.

Congestive heart failure is characterized by a decrease in cardiac output and increases in ventricular filling pressures. Each of these hemodynamic mechanisms results in metabolic and endocrine changes that cause the fluid and electrolyte alterations associated with congestive heart failure. For example, decreased cardiac output depresses renal perfusion, with a resultant release of renin from the juxtaglomerular apparatus. The increase in angiotensin I and its conversion to angiotensin II are associated with greater aldosterone secretion. The resultant retention of sodium and water by the kidney, combined with a stronger tendency toward kaliuresis, is characteristic of the renal changes associated with untreated congestive heart failure. Renal excretion of sodium is minimal unless treated with diuretics.

The larger blood volume that results produces passive congestive changes in other organs, more notably the liver, the kidneys themselves, and the splanchnic bed. The effects of passive congestion on the gastrointestinal tract have been thought to explain, in part, the development of cardiac cachexia (see later discussion).

The water retention, which is almost always in excess of sodium, usually results in dilutional hyponatremia. With the extremely rare exception of the truly sodium-depleted patient, such as an individual on chronic diuretic therapy for prolonged periods or the patient with excessive sodium losses through a surgical wound or gastrointestinal tract drainage, it can generally be predicted that patients with both heart failure and signs of peripheral edema with hypo-

natremia are *both* sodium- and water-overloaded. The general approach to this type of patient, as outlined later, should enable even the most congested patient to be fed *regardless* of the degree of fluid and electrolyte abnormality.

CARDIAC CACHEXIA

Nutritional considerations in patients with severe cardiac illness differ, depending upon the baseline nutritional status of each patient. At one end of the spectrum are patients with normal nutritional status but severe cardiac illness who are then subjected to an acute catabolic stress in association with interference with normal nutritional intake. These patients, by and large, constitute the surgical population of patients undergoing cardiac or noncardiac operative procedures, in whom an indication for parenteral nutritional support arises in the postoperative period. Another large group of patients are those with so-called cardiac cachexia, a specific form of protein-calorie malnutrition that results in a baseline pre-stress state of nutritional inadequacy. When these patients are further subjected to a major catabolic stress such as an operative procedure or a serious illness, adverse clinical consequences can occur.

Cardiac cachexia has been described classically as a wasting disease associated with chronic congestive heart failure, most commonly exemplified in this country by chronic rheumatic valvular heart disease. The mechanism of this specific form of protein-calorie malnutrition is multifactorial in etiology and may vary from patient to patient. The pathogenesis of cardiac cachexia, as outlined by the classic work of Pittman and Cohen,[1] includes at least four mechanisms that may account for the undernourished state: anorexia, malabsorption due to increased nutrient losses, a relatively hypermetabolic state, and impaired delivery of nutrients and oxygen at the cellular level. Heymsfield and co-workers[2] presented an elegant explanation of these pathogenetic mechanisms, suggesting that cellular hypoxia due to a decrease in cardiac output deprives cellular tissue of nutrient blood flow and hence causes cellular atrophy (Fig. 33–1). Other mechanisms of cardiac cachexia relate to the chronic passive congestion, in which an increase in venous pressure leads to hepatic engorgement and transmission of elevated hepatic venous pres-

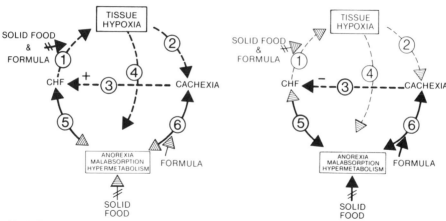

Figure 33–1. Proposed mechanisms and nutritional sensitivity of cardiac cachexia are shown. The panel on the left espouses the view that tissue hypoxia is central to the pathogenesis of cardiac cachexia. Tissue "stagnant anoxia" not only reduces cellular nutrient blood flow and waste removal but also purportedly causes anorexia and malabsorption. These abnormalities are considered adaptive, in that the demand for ventricular output is minimized by (1) decreasing food intake and (2) reducing the total mass of oxygen-consuming lean tissues. According to this model, hyperalimentation would be blocked or inefficient owing to hypoxia and might adversely affect cardiac performance. The panel on the right presents an alternative view, in which tissue hypoxia is considered relatively unimportant, and the cachexia-producing mechanisms anorexia, malabsorption, and hypermetabolism are now the focus. These are considered CHF epiphenomena, which hypothetically further impair cardiac function by limiting the myocardial nutrient supply required for optimum performance. Hyperalimentation using specially prepared solutions should correct lean tissue deficits in cardiac cachexia and improve CHF if this model is correct. (*From* Heymsfield, S. B., Smith, J., Redd, S., and Whitworth, H. B., Jr.: Nutritional support in cardiac failure. Surg. Clin. North Am., *61:*635–652, 1981, with permission.)

sure to the portal system. This elevation can cause congestion of gastric and small intestine mucosa, which may develop into frank postprandial distress and early feelings of satiety.[3] Furthermore, Heymsfield and co-workers[2] suggest that tissue hypoxia associated with the effects of low cardiac output (forward flow) further compounds the problem of anorexia as a result of inadequate increases in splanchnic blood flow resulting from ingestion of a large meal (see Fig. 33–1). Fat malabsorption secondary to congestive gastroenteropathy has also been suggested as a cause by many investigators.[4]

The hypermetabolism suggested by Pittman and Cohen[1] to result, in part, in cardiac cachexia has never been clearly defined. Indeed, the short-term effects of protein-calorie malnutrition on patients with normal hearts appears to be the production of a hypometabolic state. The findings of the tragic "human experimentations" of World War II revealed that cardiac output, blood pressure, venous pressure, and heart rate decrease in response to chronic starvation.[5, 6, 7]

Another important factor in the pathogenesis of cardiac cachexia is the psychologic response to chronic illness, which frequently results in reactive depression. Patients with deteriorating chronic diseases such as rheumatic valvular heart disease frequently become despondent, and with constant breath-

lessness and poor exercise tolerance, they become withdrawn and emotionally depressed. In addition to the progressive rise in symptom level is the inevitable increase in the amount and frequency of medications that must be ingested. Adverse side effects of digitalis, for example, include anorexia and sometimes frank nausea. The side effects of many of the antihypertensives and diuretics merely compound the problem of assuring an adequate nutritional state in these patients.

THERAPEUTIC CONSIDERATIONS

It has been our experience that unless significant reversal in the degree of cardiac impairment occurs, substantial improvement in the nutritional status in patients with cardiac cachexia is not possible. The problems of reactive depression and anorexia can be ameliorated somewhat by judicious and attentive dietary counseling and antidepressant pharmacologic agents. Altering drug mechanisms and patterns of eating frequently will enable the consumption of higher quantities of nutrient substrates.

Cardiac cachexia has the potential to reverse the cause-and-effect relationship and make the "tail wag the dog," as suggested by Keys and co-workers[8] and by Hottinger and associates.[9] In one series of patients with severe rheumatic heart diseases commonly associated with ventricular hypertrophy, such as aortic stenosis or regurgitation and mitral regurgitation, several individuals with profound cachexia were observed to have unexpected myocardial atrophy.[9] This finding was suggested to result from chronic protein undernutrition. With inhibition of left ventricular hypertrophy, which is the ordinary hemodynamic response to increased ventricular volume or pressure load, significant depression of left ventricular function was observed to occur in the experimental animal[10] and has been suggested by further experimental observations.[11, 12]

My colleagues and I examined the morphologic, biochemical, and hemodynamic effects of acute protein-calorie malnutrition in a canine model in which average cardiac performance in normal dogs was compared with that in matched dogs subjected to short-term semistarvation diets.[11, 12] Following a weight loss of approximately 40 per cent, animals were placed on cardiopulmonary bypass in a preparation yielding isovolumetric left ventricular contractions. From this model the force-velocity, length-tension, and diastolic compliance relationships of the left ventricle were evaluated. Animals subjected to subacute semistarvation were observed to have decreases in the peak developed velocity of contractile element compared with controls at each increment of preload. A decrease in left ventricular compliance was observed in the malnourished animals. We concluded that not only did myofibrillar atrophy occur in the animals subjected to protein-calorie malnutrition (and hence fewer contractile elements were available), but the interstitial edema associated with hypoproteinemia caused an increase in left ventricular wall stiffness. The possibility that a vicious circle occurs in patients with cardiac cachexia, whereby the malnutrition begins to adversely effect cardiac function, was proposed as a possible mechanism for poor results in cachectic patients who underwent cardiac surgery.

In a randomized evaluation of 44 malnourished patients undergoing cardiac surgery, my associates and I[13] observed higher morbidity and mortality than in normally nourished controls. Malnourished patients developed more sepsis and respiratory failure, spent more days in the intensive care unit, and incurred greater hospital costs than nonmalnourished patients. The purpose of the study was to determine whether or not parenteral nutrition administered in the immediate postoperative period would be effective in decreasing the higher morbidity and mortality. Although the treated patients received twice the calories and nitrogen than controls, the overall incidence of complications and the mortality were not improved statistically by early postoperative nutritional support. We concluded that in order to effect improvement in outcome, nutritional repletion must be given preoperatively.

Blackburn and associates[14, 15] suggested that a three-week plan of preoperative nutritional repletion was efficacious in "decreasing" morbidity and mortality in three patients requiring multiple valve replacement. They also suggested that a vicious circle involving cellular hypoxia could result from severe cardiac cachexia in patients with advanced cardiac disability (Fig. 33–2). Sheldon and Peterson[16] noted that marked alterations in oxygen transport occur during periods of protein-calorie malnutrition; these alterations are related not only to primary starvation effects on the heart and lungs but also to a decrease in 2,3-diphosphoglycerate concentrations and a decrease in erythropoiesis.

Although Blackburn and associates[14, 15] suggested that preoperative reversal of cardiac cachexia with aggressive nutritional support was advantageous, it is rarely feasible in actual practice. It is our clinical observation that although a short-term course of seven to ten days of dietary counseling and orally ingested dietary supplements can result in a brief reversal of caloric balance, patients appear to improve only when cardiac function is on the road to recovery. For example, patients with cardiomyopathies or other surgically incorrectable cardiac lesions are generally in a preterminal state once cardiac cachexia ensues. Aggressive parenteral nutrition in such patients has not yielded satisfactory long-term results. Our current recommendation for patients with cardiac cachexia in need of corrective cardiac surgery is to admit them from one to two weeks preoperatively, because aggressive oral dietary intake can generally be improved over the short term. Postoperatively patients are begun on oral feedings as soon as feasible. If patients remain on mechanical ventilators for more than 24 hours or develop an early complication generally associated with poor nutritional intake, total parenteral nutrition is initiated on the second or third postoperative day. Other management considerations

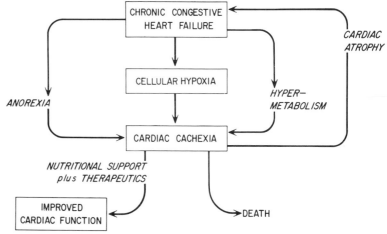

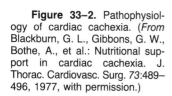

Figure 33–2. Pathophysiology of cardiac cachexia. (*From* Blackburn, G. L., Gibbons, G. W., Bothe, A., et al.: Nutritional support in cardiac cachexia. J. Thorac. Cardiovasc. Surg. 73:489–496, 1977, with permission.)

in the cachectic patients are similar to the following general guidelines.

INDICATIONS FOR NUTRITIONAL SUPPORT IN PATIENTS WITH HEART DISEASE

Nutritional assessment has been extensively outlined in Volume I. The difficulties with nutritional assessment of patients with heart disease are various and interfere with usual concepts of changes in weight for height and anthropometric or even biochemical descriptors ordinarily used to determine adequacy of nutritional status. In the evaluation of patients for a prospective, randomized study on the effects of early postoperative parenteral nutrition,[13] triceps skinfold thickness was not a statistically reliable indicator of nutritional status in clinically malnourished patients. Indeed, a history of a ten-kilogram weight loss in the recent preoperative period was the only valid clinical descriptor. Walesby and co-workers,[17] using as their "gold standard" of nutritional status total body potassium as measured with a whole-body counter, looked critically at 47 randomly selected patients undergoing cardiac surgery. Utilizing body cell mass estimates, they observed a highly significant correlation between body cell mass and fat-free mass as determined by measuring total body fat. Total body fat was measured by the use of skinfold calipers according to the method of Durnin and Womersley.[18] The fat-free mass was then calculated by subtraction of total body fat from body weight. Walesby and co-workers[17] suggested that in patients with a normal packed cell volume who are clinically free of edema, measurements of fat-

free mass could be useful as a bedside indicator of nutritional status.

In a prospectively analyzed group of 100 consecutive adult patients undergoing open heart surgery, however, my associates and I[19] were unable to confirm the usefulness of total body fat measurements as a form of nutritional assessment. We examined anthropometric measurements, including height, weight, percentage of ideal body weight, triceps skinfold thickness, arm muscle circumference, and estimates of total body fat utilizing the techniques just described. Serum albumin and transferrin levels and total lymphocyte count were also evaluated, as was skin cell–mediated immunity as determined by delayed hypersensitivity testing. Right atrial samples were assayed for myocardial glycogen content at the time of surgery. A literal interpretation of our results suggested that heavier, fatter, and larger-muscled patients developed fewer complications than thinner, less fat, and lower-weight counterparts. Although our series was heavily weighted with patients in whom left ventricular function was normal and arteriosclerosis was the underlying disease, there appeared to be no predictive value of nutritional assessment indices in determining postoperative morbidity and mortality in an individual patient. We were able to confirm *retrospectively* that one could identify patient *groups* at greater risk to develop complications on the basis of preoperative group differences in some of these indices. We could not confirm the results of Lolley and co-workers[20] that right atrial glycogen concentrations correlated with postoperative morbidity and mortality; they examined myocardial glycogen levels as a function of myocardial preservation and correlated right atrial glycogen concentrations with postoperative morbidity and mortality. We concluded that nutritional assessment tests performed prior to routine heart surgery were of no value in predicting outcome or guiding nutritional therapy in an individual patient. We did confirm, however, that as a research tool, nutritional assessment provides interesting statistical information for population studies.

In clinical practice, patients evaluated for cardiac surgery should undergo little more than a routine history, physical examination, and serum albumin determination. If the patient gives a history of recent weight loss, and such a loss is confirmed by physical findings (inadequate subcutaneous fat stores, atrophy of the interosseous and thenar muscles), significant clinical evidence for undernutrition probably exists, and when feasible, preoperative nutritional repletion should be undertaken. Hypoalbuminemia is difficult to correct preoperatively because of the danger that rapid volume expansion will result in congestive heart failure.

INDICATIONS FOR PARENTERAL NUTRITION IN PATIENTS WITH CARDIAC ILLNESS

The reasons for instituting total parenteral nutrition in patients with serious heart disease do not differ from those in patients without heart disease. Because many patients with congestive heart failure initially become nutritional problems during an acute phase of cardiac or related illnesses, the setting in which parenteral nutrition is frequently begun is the intensive or coronary care unit. As discussed in detail in Chapters 20, 24, and 34, these indications generally include the following.

Nonfunctioning Gastrointestinal Tract

This category includes bowel fistulas and the prolonged adynamic ileus that can on occasion accompany major surgery or complicated myocardial infarction (primarily diaphragmatic).

Cardiac Cachexia

As in all patients with profound protein-calorie malnutrition, patients with cardiac cachexia who are about to be subjected to a major catabolic stress such as a surgical procedure become candidates for total parenteral nutrition under circumstances that preclude adequate intake by the gastrointestinal tract.

Acute and Chronic Renal Failure

This category includes prerenal azotemia resulting from overzealous diuretic therapy in the management of severe congestive heart failure. Under these circumstances, the use of the essential amino acids and hypertonic dextrose solution would be helpful.[21-24] Acute hepatic insufficiency can be treated with an amino acid solution containing a higher percentage of branched-chain amino acids and a lower percentage of the aromatic amino acids (see Chapter 35).

Indications for Short-Term TPN

This category consists of central nervous system dysfunctions precluding adequate or safe oral intake. They constitute the major indications for total parenteral nutrition in patients recovering from recent open heart or other major cardiovascular surgery. Perioperative stroke due to air emboli or decreased cerebral perfusion frequently results in a stuporous and poorly responsive patient whose central nervous system may remain depressed for several days to weeks. During this period of depressed state of consciousness, patients frequently remain on ventilators because of concomitant respiratory insufficiency. Nasal placement of small feeding tubes to provide defined formula diets in the form of "enteral hyperalimentation" are frequently associated with "blind" endotracheal aspiration of gastric contents. In our hands, total parenteral nutrition has, therefore, been safer for short-term use in such patients. If such a patient requires prolonged endotracheal intubation necessitating tracheostomy, a further hazard exists in the greater possibility of bacterial contamination at the catheter entry site owing to the proximity of tracheal secretions. If the total duration of nutritional support is anticipated to be greater than two weeks, therefore, we would recommend operative placement of a jejunostomy tube to provide long-term nutritional support, minimizing the risk of aspiration pneumonia and catheter-related sepsis.

Indications for TPN in "Medical" Heart Disease

The indications for TPN patients with severe "medical" cardiac disease do not differ substantially from those for patients recently recovered from major cardiovascular surgery.[25] The major difficulties in instituting total parenteral nutrition are physician awareness and identification of nutrition as a problem in the patient with complicated cardiac illness. The octogenarian admitted with acute myocardial infarction, transient heart block, and moderate congestive heart failure further complicated by low-grade pneumonitis ordinarily represents a complex enough constellation of diseases for the physicians to treat. Throughout the period of active diagnosis and therapy, the awareness of inadequate nutritional intake will on occasion come to attention only because of an alert coronary care unit nurse or concerned family members. The inability to eat adequate nutrients or the lack of desire to eat owing to reactive depression following prolonged illness frequently constitutes an indication for total parenteral nutrition, particularly in the elderly.

TECHNICAL CONSIDERATIONS

Percutaneous placement of a subclavian or internal jugular venous cannula is the preferred route of administration for total parenteral nutrition in the adult. In patients with marked congestive heart failure and elevated right cardiac chamber pressures, the usual precautions against introduction of air into the venous circulation should be modified. Specifically, the placement of catheters (see Chapter 15) is usually facilitated by having the patient placed in steep Trendelenburg position in order to distend the great veins of the thoracic outlet, not only to make the structures an easier target but also to prevent introduction of air. In patients with congestive heart failure, not only will a Trendelenburg position not be tolerated because of severe dyspnea, but the procedure is unnecessary. A brief examination of the jugular venous pressure would serve well to guide the operator as to the need for the head-down position. Certainly, a Valsalva maneuver during catheter insertion or tubing change is hazardous for patients with congestive heart failure, and indeed many of them cannot perform the maneuver.

Many patients with severe cardiac disease are anticoagulated either with heparin on a short-term basis or with warfarin. In addition, many patients with arteriosclerotic coronary artery disease are given platelet-inhibiting drugs such as dipyridamole and acetylsalicylic acid. Under these circumstances, hemorrhagic complications of percutaneous catheter placement are more likely. For patients receiving intravenous heparin, it is suggested that the heparin be discontinued for two to three hours immediately prior to catheter placement. For patients receiving warfarin or dicumarol, in whom it is not appropriate to discontinue the anticoagulant to allow the prothrombin time to return toward normal, it is frequently safer to employ the internal jugular venous access route as the first choice, because hemorrhage can be controlled with manual pressure at this site whereas it cannot be for subclavian venipuncture.

In patients with cardiac cachexia who are to undergo open heart procedures and in whom a prolonged period of postoperative nutritional support is anticipated, the intravenous catheter may be inserted at the time of thoracic incision (usually median sternotomy), allowing easier placement of a Silastic tube.

NUTRIENT REQUIREMENTS

The nutritional requirements of patients with heart disease do not differ from those of other patients. Heymsfield and co-workers[2] presented several arithmetic calculations that can be utilized to estimate nutrient requirements.

For the past decade at Newark Beth Israel Medical Center, the concept of standardized formulations for patients receiving total parenteral nutrition has been used. A family of standardized formulations has evolved, including mixtures for "ordinary" patients, patients with severe cardiac disease, those with renal insufficiency, and those with hepatic insufficiency. Daily physician ordering of "tailor-made" intravenous diets lessens the possibility of physician error, improves pharmacy efficiency in compounding the solutions, increases cost efficiency of a total parenteral nutrition program, and facilitates nursing care. The solution currently used as a "cardiac hyperalimentation solution" at the Newark Beth Israel Medical Center is presented in Table 33–2. Because the

Table 33–2. STANDARD ADULT CARDIAC TPN FORMULATION*

FORMULA	
FreAmine III 8.5%	500 ml
Dextrose 70%	500 ml
Magnesium sulfate 4 mEq/ml	2 ml
Potassium acetate 2 mEq/ml	20 ml
Potassium chloride 2 mEq/ml	25 ml
MVI-12 Concentrate	10 ml†
Vitamin C 1000 mg	4 ml†
CONTENT	
Protein equivalent	39 gm
Dextrose	350 gm
Magnesium	8 mEq
Potassium	50 mEq
Acetate	20 mEq
Chloride	30 mEq
Phosphate	10 mM
Sodium	5 mEq
MVI-12 Concentrate	10 ml†
Vitamin C 1000 mg	4 ml†
Insulin	Added as indicated

*This solution provides approximately 1.370 Kcal and 6.5 Gm nitrogen.
†Vitamins are added only to the first bottle of the day.

net glucose concentration of this solution is approximately 35 per cent, exogenous insulin therapy is frequently required, and as with ordinary patients, insulin is to be added directly to the intravenous nutrient solutions.

MANAGEMENT CONSIDERATIONS FOR TPN IN PATIENTS WITH SEVERE CARDIAC ILLNESS

The major deviation from standard total parenteral nutrition therapy in these patients is the need to restrict total sodium and water administration. Because the absolute osmolarity of intravenous nutrient solutions is not an issue when the central venous route is used, the general rule has been to provide nutrients in as high a concentration as practically and economically feasible so as to minimize the possibility of fluid overload. In our experience, total parenteral nutritional support in adult patients with heart disease is not possible to achieve through peripheral veins. In subsequent discussion, therefore, all forms of total parenteral nutrition consist of infusion of highly concentrated nutrient solutions via a central catheter with the tip lying in the superior vena cava.

In patients with normal renal and hepatic function, it is rarely necessary to restrict total water intake to less than 1500 ml/day. The usual patient with left ventricular dysfunction requiring digitalis and diuretic therapy can generally be allowed to ingest between 1500 and 2500 ml/day. In patients unable to eat who require total parenteral nutrition, judicious increments in diuretics can enable higher volumes of calorie-rich nutrient solutions to be administered, provided that no significant decrement in renal function occurs. Loss of non–calorie-containing endogenous fluids such as those through nasogastric drainage can be replaced on a milliliter-for-milliliter basis with intravenous nutritional fluids. Furthermore, cardioactive drugs such as positive inotropic agents, peripheral vasodilating agents, and antibiotics should be infused intravenously in concentrated form so as to allow greater "space" for nutrient solutions.

The potent diuretics most commonly used in patients with acute or chronic congestive heart failure act on the renal tubule and loop of Henle, e.g., furosemide. These agents produce a marked water diuresis associated with natriuresis, and kaliuresis and loss of magnesium. Because the ionic effects on cardiac automaticity of hypomagnesemia act synergistically with those of hypokalemia, additional consideration must be given to magnesium salt replacement. Replacement can be achieved by increasing the magnesium sulfate ordinarily present in the cardiac hyperalimentation solution, although this has rarely been necessary. Because many patients in congestive heart failure are also receiving digitalis glycosides for the management of supraventricular arrhythmias or congestive heart failure, the potential added hazards of potassium and magnesium losses in such patients can lead to the development of life-threatening arrhythmias. Potassium salts in dosages up to 200 mEq/day have occasionally been necessary to prevent serious ventricular arrhythmias.

Glucose intolerance occurs more frequently in patients with severe cardiac illness receiving total parenteral nutrition. These patients are more likely to have diabetes mellitus, and the presence of low cardiac output with poor peripheral muscle perfusion results in a further decrease in glucose uptake. The glucose concentration of the suggested cardiac hyperalimentation solution is 35 per cent, so extreme caution must be taken to avoid "runaway" hyperglycemia. The infusion is generally initiated at low infusion rates—between 30 and 50 ml/hr depending on body surface area. If an acceptable range of blood glucose concentration (i.e., below 250 mg/dl) is exceeded even at low rates of infusion, regular (crystalline zinc) insulin in an initial dose of 10 U/bottle should be added. Progressive increases in intravenous insulin additions to the nutrient mixture should occur until an adequate infusion of total non-nitrogen calories (45 kcal/kg/day) is achieved and is maintaining reasonable blood glucose concentration. It has, on occasion, been necessary to add as much as 100 units of regular insulin in each hyperalimentation bottle. During the period that the exogenous insulin requirements are being established, intravenous boluses of regular insulin every four to six hours may become necessary. If the absolute blood glucose concentration exceeds 500 mg/dl during this adjustment period, however, it is generally safest to discontinue total parenteral nutrition temporarily, substituting five per cent dextrose in water for the nutrient mixture until exogenously administered regular insulin can once again bring the blood glucose concentration under control. If these rather simple guidelines are followed, hyperosmolar nonketotic dehydration with coma should not occur.

In patients in whom one can anticipate a relative insulin resistance, such as the insulin-dependent patient with diabetes mellitus, the patient who has acute pancreatitis, hepatic insufficiency, or generalized sepsis, is receiving glucocorticoids, or is in the immediate postoperative hypermetabolic period, total parenteral nutrition therapy should be *initiated* with exogenous insulin in an initial dose of between 15 and 25 U/L.

INTRAVENOUS FAT EMULSIONS

The usual circumstances under which patients with severe heart disease receive total parenteral nutrition consist of nutritional maintenance for a brief time, usually less than three weeks. Because of this time frame, in a personal series of more than 500 patients recently recovering from open heart surgery, my colleagues and I have not encountered a single episode of clinically apparent essential fatty acid deficiency. The use of intravenous fat emulsions to *prevent* this syndrome from occurring in such patients is, therefore, analogous to sending the emperor's new clothes out to the laundry!

The potential usefulness of fat calories as a fuel source is extremely attractive in patients with severe cardiac illness, however.

At a caloric density of 9 kcal/gm, the nutrient density is appealing to patients in whom total fluid volume must be limited. Although controversy exists concerning the optimum percentage of calories derived from fat versus from carbohydrate,[26, 27] intravenous fat emulsions can be used as accessory calorie sources in patients with severe heart disease, provided that the total non-nitrogen caloric contribution does not exceed 30 or 40 per cent.

Although ten per cent soy oil and safflower oil emulsions have been available in the United States and are safe and efficacious, the recent introduction of 20 per cent soy oil emulsion to the American market has led to the availability of even greater caloric density for patients with serious cardiac disease.

Because intravenous fat emulsions are associated with increased free fatty acid concentrations in the plasma, there has been some concern regarding potential adverse cardiac effects.[28-30] Earlier studies by Grimes and Abel[31] indicated that in the anesthetized dog on cardiopulmonary bypass, significant decreases in the force-velocity and length-tension relationships of the left ventricle during isovolumetric beats occurred during infusions of 10 per cent oil emulsions given at rapid rates. Opie[32] and others confirmed that free fatty acids are detrimental during periods of acute myocardial ischemia, because they have negative inotropic effects and increase heart size. It became important to examine the hemodynamic effects of intravenous fat emulsions, therefore, in patients with severe heart disease, primarily myocardial ischemia. Fisch and Abel[33] administered 10 per cent soy and safflower oil emulsions to patients recently recovering from coronary bypass operations at rates between 1.1 and 1.7 mg/kg/min. There were no significant adverse hemodynamic changes in either left ventricular stroke work, cardiac output, or systemic vascular resistance.

In a second study, my colleagues and I[34] found that administration of 20 per cent soy oil emulsion at 2 ml/min (5.25 mg/kg/min) resulted in significant depression of myocardial contractility and in one patient was associated with what appeared to be an episode of myocardial ischemia. We established a dose-response relationship with safe limits for infusion of intravenous fat emulsion that appear to be less than 2.67 mg/kg/min of intravenous fat emulsion. We currently employ intravenous fat emulsions *cautiously* in patients with severe heart disease. Furthermore, because of the more complicated methods of administration and the greater concern about catheter-related sepsis in patients with cardiovascular prosthetic materials, it is our present recommendation to withhold intravenous fat emulsions for the first several weeks following institution of total parenteral nutrition. When such emulsions are to be used, an efficient method appears to be to administer 500 ml of 20 per cent intravenous fat emulsion daily over ten to twelve hours.

SPECIAL SITUATIONS AND COMPLICATIONS

Infective endocarditis poses additional complications when the gastrointestinal tract cannot be utilized to provide an adequate nutritional state. Because starvation, which might occur under these circumstances, is unacceptable and would prevent survival, we have advocated active total parenteral nutritional support. If ongoing bacteremias cannot be controlled by intravenous antibiotics, we recommend change of the intravenous catheter every 72 to 96 hours to avoid secondary contamination of the hyperalimentation catheter. In general, however, institution of specific antimicrobial therapy is associated with the prompt elimination of bacteremia; otherwise, immediate cardiac surgical intervention directed toward the endocarditis itself would be indicated.

The complications that occur in association with total parenteral nutrition in patients with severe cardiac illness do not differ qualitatively from those that occur in ordinary patients. Additional hazards associated with concomitant glucose intolerance, anticoagulation, and bacteremias have been discussed.

In order to ensure adequate nutrient intake to even the most critically ill patient, the physician's confidence becomes a most critical factor. By applying common sense and the guidelines for safe and efficacious care presented here, a situation should never occur in which nutritional support is "contraindicated."

REFERENCES

1. Pittman, J.G., and Cohen, P.: The pathogenesis of cardiac cachexia. N. Engl. J. Med., 271:403–409, 1964.
2. Heymsfield, S.B., Smith, J., Redd, S., and Whitworth, H.B., Jr.: Nutritional support in cardiac failure. Surg. Clin. North Am., 61:635–652, 1981.
3. Jones, R.V.: Fat malabsorption in congestive cardiac failure. Br. J. Med., 1:1276, 1961.
4. Jones, R.V., Heymsfield, S.B., Dawson, A.M., and Isselbacher, K.J.: Fat absorption. Arch. Intern. Med., 107:305–308, 1961.
5. Follis, R.H.: Deficiency Disease. Springfield, Charles C Thomas, 1958, p. 577.
6. Dmochowski, J.R., and Moore, F.D.: Chloroba, Glodowa. N. Engl. J. Med., 293:356–357, 1975.
7. Winick, M.: Hunger Disease. New York, John Wiley & Sons, 1979, p. 125.
8. Keys, A., Brosek, J., Henschel, A., and Mickelson, O.: Laboratory of physiological hygiene. In The Biology of Human Starvation. Minneapolis, University of Minnesota Press, 1950, p. 494.
9. Hottinger, V.A., Esell, O., and Uehlinger, E.: Hungerkronkeit, Hunderodem, Hungertuberkulose. Basel, Benno, Schwabe & Co., 1948, p. 181.
10. Yokota, Y., Ota, K., Ageta, M., Ishida, S., Toshima, H., and Kimura, N.: Effects of low protein diet on cardiac function and ultrastructure of spontaneously hypertensive rats loaded with sodium chloride. Rec. Adv. Stud. Cardiac Struct. Metab., 12:157–162, 1978.
11. Abel, R.M., Alonso, D.R., Grimes, J., Gay, W.A., Jr.: Biochemical, ultrastructural and hemodynamic changes in protein-calorie malnutrition in dogs. Circulation, 56(Suppl. 3):551, 1977.
12. Abel, R.M., Grimes, J.B., Alonso, D., Alonso, M., and Gray, W.A., Jr.: Adverse hemodynamic and ultrastructural changes in dogs' hearts subjected to protein-calorie malnutrition. Am. Heart J., 97:733–744, 1979.
13. Abel, R.M., Fischer, J.E., Buckley, M.J., Barnett, G.O., and Austen, W.G.: Malnutrition in cardiac surgical patients: Results of a prospective randomized evaluation of early postoperative parenteral nutrition. Arch. Surg., 111:45–50, 1976.
14. Blackburn, G.L., Gibbons, G.W., Bothe, A., Benotti, P.N., Harken, D.E., and McEnany, T.M.: Nutritional support in cardiac cachexia. J. Thorac. Cardiovasc. Surg., 73:489–496, 1977.
15. Gibbons, G.W., Blackburn, G.L., Harken, D.E., Valdes, P.J., Morehead, D., and Bistrian, B.R.: Pre- and postoperative hyperalimentation in the treatment of cardiac cachexia. J. Surg. Res., 20:439–444, 1976.
16. Sheldon, G.F., and Peterson, S.R.: Malnutrition and cardiopulmonary functions: Relation of oxygen transport. J.P.E.N., 4:376–383, 1980.
17. Walesby, R.K., Goode, A.W., Spinks, T.J., Herring, A., Ranicar, A.S.O., and Bentall, H.H.: Nutritional status of patients requiring cardiac surgery. J. Thorac. Cardiovasc. Surg., 77:570–576, 1979.
18. Durnin, J.V.G.A., and Womersley, J.: Body fat assessed from total body density and its estimation from skinfold thickness measurement on 481 men and women ages 16–72 years. Br. J. Nutr., 32:77–97, 1974.
19. Abel, R.M., Fisch, D., van Gelder, H.M., and Grossman, M.L.: Should nutritional assessment be performed routinely prior to open heart surgery? J. Thorac. Cardiovasc. Surg., 85:752–757, 1983.
20. Lolley, D.M., Ray, J.F., III, Meyers, W.O., Sautter, R., and Tewsbury, D.A.: Importance of preoperative myocardial glycogen levels in human cardiac preservation. J. Thorac. Cardiovasc. Surg., 78:678–687, 1979.
21. Abel, R.M., Abbott, W.M., and Fischer, J.E.: Intravenous essential L-amino acids and hypertonic dextrose in patients with acute renal failure: Ef-

fects on serum potassium, phosphate and magnesium. Am. J. Surg., *123*:632–638, 1972.

22. Abel, R.M., Beck, C.H., Jr., Abbott, W.M., Ryan, J.A., Jr., Barnett, G.O., and Fischer, J.E.: Treatment of acute renal failure with intravenous administration of essential amino acids and glucose: Results of a prospective double-blind study. Surg. Forum, *23*:77–84, 1972.

23. Abel, R.M., Beck, C.H., Jr., Abbott, W.M., Ryan, J.A., Jr., Barnett, G.O., and Fischer, J.E.: Improved survival from acute renal failure after treatment with intravenous essential L-amino acids and glucose: Results of a double-blind study. N. Engl. J. Med., *288*:695–699, 1973.

24. Abel, R.M., Abbott, W.M., Beck, C.H., Jr., Ryan, J.A., Jr., and Fischer, J.E.: Essential L-amino acids for hyperalimentation patients with disordered nitrogen metabolism. Am. J. Surg., *128*:317–323, 1974.

25. Abel, R.M., Fischer, J.E., Buckley, M.J., and Austen, W.G.: Hyperalimentation in cardiac surgery: A review of sixty-four patients. J. Thorac. Cardiovasc. Surg., *67*:294–300, 1974.

26. Long, J.M., III, Wilmore, D.W., Mason, A.D., Jr., and Pruitt, B.A.: Effect of carbohydrate and fat intake on nitrogen excretion during total intravenous feeding. Ann. Surg., *185*:417–422, 1977.

27. Freund, H., Yoshimura, N., and Fischer, J.E.: Does intravenous fat spare nitrogen in the injured rat? Am. J. Surg., *140*:377–383, 1980.

28. Kjekshus, J.K., and Mjos, O.D.: Effect of inhibition of lipolysis on infarct size after experimental coronary artery occlusion. J. Clin. Invest., *52*:1770–1778, 1973.

29. Opie, L.H., Tansey, M., and Kennelly, B.M.: Proposed metabolic vicious circle in patients with large myocardial infarcts and high plasma-free-fatty-acid concentrations. Lancet, *2*:890–892, 1977.

30. Vik-Mo, H., and Mjos, O.D.: Influence of free fatty acids on myocardial oxygen consumption and ischemic injury. Am. J. Cardiol., *48*:361–365, 1981.

31. Grimes, J.B., and Abel, R.M.: Hemodynamic effects of fat emulsion in dogs. J.P.E.N., *3*:40–44, 1979.

32. Opie, L.H.: Metabolism of free fatty acids, glucose and catecholamines in acute myocardial infarctions. Relation to myocardial ischemia and infarct size. Am. J. Cardiol., *36*:938–953, 1975.

33. Fisch, D., and Abel, R.M.: Hemodynamic effects of intravenous fat emulsions in patients with heart disease. J.P.E.N., *5*:402–405, 1981.

34. Abel, R.M., Fisch, D., and Grossman, M.L.: Hemodynamic effects of intravenous 20% soy oil emulsion following coronary bypass surgery. J.P.E.N., *7*:534–540, 1983.

CHAPTER 34

Nutrition in Acute Renal Failure

EBEN I. FEINSTEIN

Acute renal failure presents a difficult challenge in nutritional therapy. It may occur in many clinical settings and is of concern to the internist, surgeon, obstetrician, and pediatrician. In the patient who was in previous good health without other serious complicating illnesses, acute renal failure is a serious but potentially reversible disorder. In the setting of multiple organ system failure, such as in patients with extensive trauma, acute renal failure aggravates the many other metabolic and circulatory disturbances that are present.

Dialysis therapy, either hemodialysis or peritoneal dialysis, is frequently required and has greatly improved the management of acute renal failure. It is clear, however, that despite the use of dialysis, the overall mortality rate from acute renal failure has not been affected to any degree when compared with the improved mortality rate in chronic renal failure.[1, 2] Since dialysis therapy has reduced or eliminated the mortality from electrolyte disturbances and fluid overload, it is safe to say that most patients with acute renal failure do not die of uremia but rather from associated complications such as infection and poor wound healing. Nutritional therapy has an important role to play in improving the ability of the body to repair cellular damage and in maintaining the body's defense mechanisms.[3, 4]

The nutritional support of patients with acute renal failure requires an understanding of basic nutritional concepts that apply to many hospitalized patients and of the specific problems that are peculiar to acute uremia. In this chapter, the latter subject will receive the most attention.

ETIOLOGY

The perturbations in electrolyte balance and other metabolic homeostatic mechanisms that occur in renal disease have been reviewed in Chapter 21. To begin this discussion it is necessary to define the patient groups in question. Acute renal failure is a syndrome of diverse etiology. It occurs in association with or following infectious diseases—for example, poststreptococcal glomerulonephritis. Many inflammatory glomerular diseases may cause acute renal failure. Vascular diseases and conditions of the lower urinary tract that obstruct the flow of urine are also important causes of acute renal failure. The main concern in this chapter, however, is with the diseases that cause acute tubular necrosis. Strictly speaking, this entity is a pathologic diagnosis that has come to be used clinically to represent the acute renal failure caused by nephrotoxins or impaired renal perfusion. It is this form of acute renal failure that is frequently seen in postoperative and septic patients.

The severity of the renal dysfunction that is seen with acute tubular necrosis varies widely. Commonly, patients who have aminoglycoside-induced acute renal failure do not have oliguria. They are seen by medical or surgical services, and their degree of catabolism may be mild. At the other extreme, the trauma patient is usually a surgical patient who is oliguric and has a marked degree of catabolism. The first type of patient is likely to be able to eat, whereas the trauma patient will almost certainly require parenteral nutrition. Clearly, a different management approach should be expected in these different types of patients.

CATABOLISM IN ACUTE RENAL FAILURE

The catabolic state of acute renal failure may vary from mild to marked. The significance of the degree of catabolism lies in its prognostic implications and its effect on the deranged nitrogen metabolism of uremia. Hypercatabolic patients are likely to have delayed wound healing, impaired immune responsiveness, and in general a prolonged and difficult clinical course. Their chances for recovery and survival may also be reduced. The increased rate of protein breakdown will also produce an accelerated rate in the rise of blood urea nitrogen and may necessitate more frequent dialysis treatments.

The evidence for catabolism in acute renal failure is clear, yet the reasons for it remain the subject of ongoing investigations. The obvious clinical manifestations of protein breakdown are seen in the weight loss and clinical wasting that occur. In extreme cases, body weight has fallen 20 kg in three weeks. Estimated protein degradation rates between 100 and 300 gm/day were observed despite parenteral hyperalimentation.[5, 6] Serum total protein and albumin levels were usually low. The fall in serum albumin levels during the period of hyperalimentation was significantly greater in the group of patients exhibiting a high degree of catabolism.[6] In general, plasma amino acid levels are low in patients who are not receiving amino acids, and they tend to remain low or normal despite the infusion of amino acids.[6, 7]

It is clear that acute renal failure *per se* produces accelerated proteolysis, but the mediators of this response are not clearly defined. Factors that are implicated in the catabolic response in acute renal failure include an insufficient intake of calories and amino acids, coexistent catabolic conditions, circulating proteolytic enzymes, increased circulating levels of catabolic hormones (parathyroid hormone, adrenal corticosteroids), insulin resistance, and loss of nutrients during dialysis therapy. Owing to the frequent inability to provide adequate enteral nutrition because of ileus or gastrointestinal injury or surgery, as well as the reluctance to administer large intravenous fluid volumes in oliguria, many patients in the past have not received adequate nutrition. In addition, loss of protein from wounds and fistulae will aggravate nutritional deficits, as may losses of nutrients during dialysis procedures.

Acute renal failure is frequently seen in patients with trauma and sepsis, so it is not surprising that catabolism may be marked. These are conditions in which protein degradation (e.g., as measured by negative nitrogen balance) has been well established.[8] Another disease associated with muscle catabolism is nontraumatic rhabdomyolysis with myoglobinuric acute renal failure. In this case, dramatic rises in serum creatinine, urea nitrogen, potassium, phosphorus, and uric acid levels occur often, reflecting the release of protein, electrolytes, and purines from skeletal muscle.[9]

The mediators of protein breakdown in nonuremic patients with sepsis and trauma are the subject of considerable research efforts. Recently, the existence of a circulating peptide with proteolytic activity has been demonstrated in patients with sepsis and trauma.[10] Clowes and associates were able to correlate levels of this peptide with the release of amino acids from the lower extremities, which is an indication of protein breakdown.[10] With a postulated molecular weight of 4270, this substance would not be small enough to pass across standard hemodialysis membranes and might therefore accumulate in the blood of patients with acute renal failure. A role for increased prostaglandin synthesis in the stimulation of proteolysis has been expounded by Baracos and coworkers.[11] They have shown that interleukin produced by human leukocytes will effect an increase in protein breakdown in isolated muscle preparations. Although it is likely that these mediators of proteolysis found in nonuremic individuals are also active in uremic patients, this remains to be demonstrated.

Of interest in this regard are the studies of Hörl and Heidland. They have described a serum factor, derived from patients with hypercatabolic acute renal failure, that acts as a protease and digests albumin and phosphorylase kinase.[12] Subsequently, they showed that α-2-macroglobulin, an inhibitor of proteases, could reduce the proteolytic activity in the serum of a patient with acute renal failure.[13]

Perturbations in the metabolism of the liver and skeletal tissue contribute greatly to the catabolic state of acute renal failure. The production of urea increases in the isolated livers of uremic animals.[14] Concomitantly, gluconeogenesis is also stimulated. The substrates for ureagenesis are amino acids that are released in increased amounts from skeletal muscle[15, 16] and are taken up at an increased rate by the liver.[17] Among the amino acids showing accelerated release from muscle are alanine, glutamine,[15] phenylalanine, and tyrosine.[16]

The increase in proteolysis does not appear to be accompanied by a rise in the protein synthesis rate.[14, 18] The uptake of certain amino acids by muscle is reduced, and the response to insulin stimulation is lower than in nonuremic animals.[19] This decrease in amino acid transport probably limits substrate availability and may explain, in part, the observation that muscle protein synthesis is reduced. Synthesis of other proteins, such as albumin, is also reduced in uremia.[20]

These observations suggest that some of the amino acids administered to patients in their nutritional regimen are probably taken up by the liver, which is predisposed to a higher rate of ureagenesis. The diminished uptake of amino acids by muscle supports the argument that giving small amounts of amino acids to patients may not provide adequate quantities needed for cell protein synthesis.

There is evidence that hormonal derangements in uremia may contribute to catabolism. Parathyroid hormone is elevated in acute renal failure[21] and is recognized as a catabolic hormone. Recent studies by Garber using rat muscle have shown clearly that proteolysis was increased after two weeks of uremia in animals that received the 1-34 fragment of parathyroid hormone.[22] A role for insulin resistance has been established by the work of Mitch and Clark, in which tyrosine release from the rat hindquarter in uremic rats was increased when compared with controls.[18] Although insulin reduced this release in the control animals, it had little effect in the uremic group. Adrenal corticosteroids may also contribute to protein breakdown in acute uremia, as illustrated in the experiments of Bondy, in which adrenalectomy led to reduced amino acid release.[23]

CLINICAL EXPERIENCE WITH PARENTERAL NUTRITION IN ACUTE RENAL FAILURE

The current nutritional management of acute renal failure is based on clinical studies conducted over the past 20 years. To understand the approach outlined in this chapter, some familiarity with the results of these investigations is necessary. Several general observations are pertinent. The heterogenous nature of acute renal failure makes it difficult to compare the results of one study with another, unless it is clear that similar patients were used by the various investigators. Unfortunately, the data needed to compare groups of patients are infrequently reported. For example, the underlying causes of renal failure, the nature of associated illnesses, and the use of concurrent enteral nutrition is not evident in some reports. The degree of catabolism is also important, but information concerning nitrogen balance or urea nitrogen generation is not consistently reported. Some studies were carried out on groups of patients that were not large enough to allow the demonstration of statistically significant changes in the recovery of renal function or survival. It would also have been helpful if the same nutritional regimens had been used by different investigators. Finally, there are only a few prospective trials in the literature.

Supplying Protein in Acute Renal Failure

In the predialysis era, patients with acute renal failure were prescribed diets in which protein was severely restricted. Calories were provided in the form of candies, butterballs, and syrup.[24] The aim of this regimen was to reduce protein breakdown, as had been suggested by Gamble's work with normal subjects in a "life-raft" situation.[25]

The question of how to provide protein in acute renal failure was addressed by a number of investigators. The works of Giordano[26] and Giovanetti[27] are the most prominent and influential. They advocated a diet in which the protein source consisted of small amounts of high-biologic-value protein. Such protein contains a high proportion of the essential amino acids. It was argued that these amino acids would allow utilization of urea nitrogen in the synthesis of nonessential amino acids. Thus, nitrogen balance would be less negative and net urea generation would decrease. These effects were demonstrated in studies conducted in patients with chronic renal failure.

A similar approach was applied in the treatment of acute renal failure. Berlyne and coworkers reported that clinical improvement and reduced urea production ensued when patients were fed protein of dairy and egg origin in contrast to feeding a protein-free diet.[28] Wilmore and associates applied the idea of using protein of high biologic value to surgical patients who could not eat. They reported that parenteral nutrition with hypertonic glucose and small amounts of essential amino acids produced a positive nitrogen balance and reduced serum levels of urea nitrogen, potassium, and phosphorus. Other clinical effects of the diet included more rapid wound healing and less need for dialysis.[29, 30]

Lee and colleagues were early advocates of the use of soya emulsions as caloric sources.[31, 32] These preparations were available in the United Kingdom several years before they were marketed in the United States. Initial concern over the possibility that the emulsion would interfere with the function of the dialysis membrane was dispelled. Lipemic serum did result: triglyceride elimination from the serum was slowed in acute and chronic renal failure but returned toward normal after dialysis.[32]

Effects of Amino Acid Infusions

The beneficial effects of amino acid infusions have been reported by several groups since the initial work of Wilmore and associates. Baek and coworkers treated patients having postoperative acute uremia with glucose and a protein hydrolysate and compared this group to patients receiving glucose alone. The survival rates were 70 and 40 per cent, respectively.[33] Interpretation of these results is limited because of the lack of information about the patients and the way the treatments were selected. In a retrospective study of prognostic factors in acute renal failure, McMurray and colleagues pointed out that the outcome of patients with severe complications, such as sepsis, was improved when large amounts of a general amino acid solution (essential and nonessential) were given.[34] Another retrospective report attributes a dramatic improvement in survival from acute renal failure to the introduction of total parenteral nutrition (TPN) including essential and nonessential amino acids.[35]

Several prospective studies of parenteral nutrition with amino acids and glucose have been reported. The work of Abel and coworkers has been very influential. In a series of reports,[36–38] including a prospective randomized trial, this group investigated the use

of an essential amino acid formulation in acute renal failure. The rationale for using such a formula was the experience with the protein diet of high biologic value in chronic renal failure. In the prospective trial, 28 patients were treated with 13 gm/day of essential amino acids and hypertonic glucose and were compared to a group of 23 patients who received an isocaloric infusion of hypertonic glucose alone. Patients in whom shock or sepsis was present were not entered in the study. Other diagnoses excluded were congestive heart failure, renal embolic disease, and urinary tract obstruction. The group receiving the essential amino acids experienced a significantly improved recovery rate from the acute renal failure. Although hospital survival was higher in the amino acid group, it was not significantly different from the glucose group. However, a significant improvement in survival was found when the most severely ill patients were assessed separately (Fig. 34–1).[38] The authors also found that the daily rise in serum creatinine concentration was less rapid in the amino acid group and implied that the treatment might have modified the degree of renal function impairment.

Abel and coworkers also showed that infusions of essential amino acids and glucose resulted in a fall in serum potassium, phosphorus, and magnesium levels.[37] These changes occurred without dialysis. Regarding the effects on plasma amino acid concentrations, there was no increase in any of the essential amino acids to levels above the normal range. There were significant increases in the levels of phenylalanine and methionine. These data support the idea that the infused amino acids were rapidly cleared from the circulation to be utilized for protein synthesis or metabolized.[7]

The improved rates of recovery of renal function and survival reported by Abel and colleagues[38] are in contrast to the results of the study by Leonard and associates.[39] In their randomized prospective trial, essential amino acids and hypertonic glucose were again compared with hypertonic glucose alone. The rate of recovery of renal function and the survival rate did not differ in the two treatment groups. The rate of the rise in blood urea nitrogen was decreased in the patients receiving amino acids, but the mean nitrogen balance was negative at 10 gm/day in both groups. Also, in a retrospective analysis of patients treated with a solution similar to that used in the two studies just described,

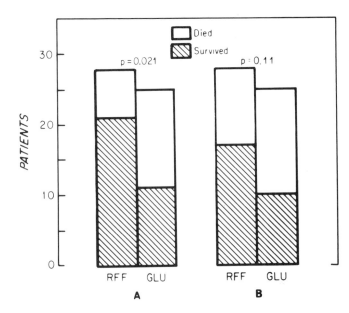

Figure 34–1. Survival rates from acute renal failure *(A)* and overall hospital mortality rates *(B)* in 53 patients treated with either essential L-amino acids and hypertonic glucose (RFF) or hypertonic glucose alone (GLU). *(From Abel, R. M., Beck, C. H., Jr., Abott, W. M., Ryan, J. A., Jr., Barnett, G. O., and Fischer, J. E.: Improved survival from acute renal failure after treatment with intravenous essential L-amino acids and glucose. Results of a prospective double-blind study. N. Engl. J. Med. 288:695–699, 1973, by permission of the New England Journal of Medicine.)*

Sofio and Nicora[40] could not confirm the findings of improved patient survival.

The observation that nitrogen balance remained negative when small amounts of essential amino acids were infused suggests that larger quantities of amino acids might be beneficial in acute renal failure. A prospective controlled trial to investigate this idea was conducted by Feinstein and colleagues.[6] In this protocol, three treatment regimens were compared: (1) hypertonic glucose alone, (2) hypertonic glucose in combination with 21 gm/day of essential amino acids, or (3) hypertonic glucose in combination with 42 gm/day of essential and nonessential amino acids. The mean caloric intake did not differ and ranged from about 2200 to 2700 kcal/day. More patients survived in the essential amino acid group than did in the other two groups, but the groups contained too few patients to make the differences statistically significant. A poor prognosis was seen in patients in whom acute renal failure was due to hypotension or sepsis. Their survival rate was 17 per cent in comparison to the groups whose renal failure was due to other causes (antibiotics, radiocontrast agents, rhabdomyolysis), in which the survival rate was 67 per cent.

Many patients in all three groups were very catabolic. The mean urea nitrogen levels were greater in the essential and nonessential amino acid group when compared with the essential amino acid group (14 gm/day and 6.7 gm/day, respectively). In the majority of patients, the daily nitrogen balance was neg-

ative, often markedly so. Other indications of severe catabolism were the subnormal concentrations of serum total protein, albumin, and transferrin levels. The plasma amino acid concentrations in general were reduced at the end of the study in all three treatment groups.

The results of this therapeutic trial suggested that a higher intake of essential and nonessential amino acids might help to decrease the negative nitrogen balance. In a prospective study of 11 patients (the majority of whom were postoperative or trauma patients), 5 patients were treated with 21 gm of essential amino acids and glucose and 6 patients received essential and nonessential amino acids in variable quantities (to a maximum of 15 gm of nitrogen/day) depending upon their urea nitrogen appearance. The aim was to attempt to match the urea nitrogen appearance and the nitrogen intake. The results of administering a higher amino acid intake included an increase in the mean urea nitrogen appearance for the group and the achievement of nitrogen balance in some patients. However, no patient who received a higher nitrogen intake survived.[41] Once again, this preliminary report has the shortcoming of a very small sample size. As discussed earlier, the need for large groups of well-matched patients is a major obstacle to the search for an optimum nutritional regimen in this disease.

Other reports have failed to show a beneficial effect of essential and nonessential amino acids on recovery and survival. Blackburn and associates investigated the effects of three amino acid regimens. Their uncontrolled study did not show an improvement in the survival rate for patients treated with essential and nonessential amino acids when compared with glucose treatment alone.[42] Freund and coworkers reported a mortality rate of 91 per cent in surgical patients treated with a mean of 3.7 gm of nitrogen/day as essential and nonessential amino acids.[43] The recent report of Mirtallo and coworkers[44] compared the effects of small amounts of essential amino acids versus small amounts of essential and nonessential amino acids in patients with mild acute renal failure. The mean creatinine clearance was high, and no patient received dialysis in their study. There were no differences in mortality, recovery of renal function, or urea nitrogen appearance. These data suggest that there is no advantage to either regimen and could also be used to justify either approach. One must bear in mind that these conclusions do not apply to the patient with more severe renal failure and marked catabolism.

EXPERIMENTAL STUDIES

The contribution of the laboratory to understanding the catabolism of acute renal failure has been reviewed (see earlier). Experimental evidence of catabolism in acute renal failure includes increased hepatic production of glucose and urea; increased urea nitrogen appearance; release of alanine, glutamine, and other amino acids from muscle; resistance to insulin, causing decreased muscle uptake of amino acids, decreased muscle protein synthesis, and an increased ratio of lactate release to glucose uptake. The treatment of animals with experimental acute renal failure has been valuable in furthering our knowledge of the effects of nutrition in this disorder. In rats with bilateral nephrectomy, Sellers and colleagues demonstrated that the addition of glucose to the diet resulted in decreased urea production.[45] Van Buren and coworkers treated nephrectomized dogs with essential amino acids and hypertonic glucose and reported a lower serum urea nitrogen concentration when compared to treatment with glucose alone.[46]

The work of Toback and coworkers has advanced our understanding of the effects of amino acid therapy on the renal response to mercuric chloride injury. The mean serum creatinine concentration in rats with mercuric chloride–induced acute renal failure was significantly lower if the animals were given infusions of glucose and a general formula of amino acids (i.e., essential and nonessential) than if glucose alone was infused.[47] Other experiments support the notion that amino acid therapy results in improved cellular regeneration. The incorporation of ^{14}C-leucine into renal protein was increased. This indicates that the rate of protein synthesis was increased.[48] Treatment with amino acids and glucose also accelerated the rate of ^{14}C-choline incorporation into renal phospholipid (Fig. 34–2).[47] Further studies of phospholipid metabolism, using kidney slices in vitro, showed that synthesis of phosphatidylcholine was enhanced.[49] This observation points to the role of amino acids in increasing the amount of substrate available for phospholipid synthesis.

Some of the results obtained by Toback's group have not been reproduced by other

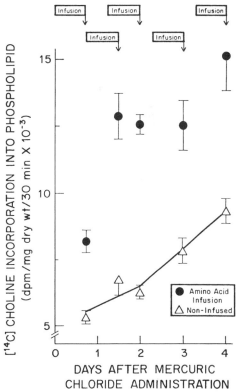

Figure 34–2. Rate of (^{14}C)-choline incorporation into phospholipid in the kidney of rats made uremic with mercuric chloride. The values are expressed as mean ± SEM and are greater in the amino acid–infused animals than in non–amino acid–infused animals at each time. (*From* Toback, F. G.: Amino acid enhancement of renal regeneration after acute tubular necrosis. Kidney Internat. *12*:193–198, 1977, with permission.)

investigators. Oken and coworkers[50] did not demonstrate an improvement in the course of acute renal failure in rats with either the mercuric chloride– or glycerol-induced model. On the contrary, there was increased mortality in the amino acid–treated rats when compared with control rats treated with glucose alone. These different results may be explained in part by differences in experimental design.

NUTRITIONAL REQUIREMENTS IN ACUTE RENAL FAILURE

The goals of nutritional therapy in the patient with acute renal failure are to promote maximum nutritional status and hasten the recovery of renal function without aggravating the metabolic disturbances of the uremic state. The first goal is central to nutritional therapy in general, and to accomplish it a knowledge of the nutritional requirements of the patient is necessary.

Calorie Requirements

The calories required will usually depend upon the underlying cause of acute renal failure and other associated illnesses. The provision of adequate calories is important to meet the energy requirements of the patient and to reduce the amount of protein degraded. In nonuremic patients, the nitrogen released by protein breakdown is excreted in the urine; with renal failure, the nitrogen is retained and leads to an accelerated rise in blood urea nitrogen levels. In a recent study of energy balance, Mault and coworkers[51] found that the resting energy expenditure in patients with acute renal failure in an intensive care unit was 37 per cent above normal. Twenty of the 29 patients studied were in negative cumulative nitrogen balance.

The protein-sparing effect of glucose has been recognized since the studies by Gamble of normal volunteers in a "life raft" situation.[25] Gamble showed that net protein breakdown was diminished by feeding 100 gm of glucose daily. This amount of glucose would, of course, be grossly inadequate for the catabolic stress of acute renal failure. Several groups of investigators have pointed to the improved nitrogen balance that results in acute renal failure when amino acids are administered with increasing amounts of calories.

Abitbol and Holliday treated anuric children with calorie intakes that ranged from 20 to 70 kcal/kg/day, with improvement in the negative nitrogen balance at the higher calorie intake.[52] Blackburn and colleagues studied adults using three treatment regimens consisting of essential amino acids or essential and nonessential amino acids and either 37.5 or 52.2 per cent glucose solutions. The urea nitrogen appearance decreased with each type of treatment in association with higher calorie intake.[42] A direct correlation of calorie intake and estimated nitrogen balance in adults with acute renal failure was reported by Spreiter and colleagues.[53] An increase in amino acid intake to 1 gm/kg/day and calorie intake to 50 kcal/kg/day produced a positive nitrogen balance in these hypercatabolic patients. However, in this study, as in the other reports in which the effect of calorie intake on protein breakdown was assessed, the amounts of amino acids and calories administered were both changed during treatment. Thus, it is not possible to separate the effects of calorie intake alone on catabolism. These reports, together with those in nonuremic patients, would strongly suggest that the provision of adequate calories to catabolic patients is useful in controlling the degradation of protein.

Two major sources of calories are available—hypertonic dextrose solutions and lipid emulsions. The relative merits of these two sources will not be extensively reviewed here. In nonuremic patients undergoing catabolic stress, carbohydrate and lipids are both adequately utilized.[54] Studies of their comparative effects on protein breakdown seem to indicate an advantage for carbohydrate in the most catabolic patients. For example, Long and associates,[55] in studies of severely burned patients, found that lipid was adequately utilized but that its ability to reduce nitrogen output was significantly less than that of glucose. This greater nitrogen-sparing action was also shown by Woolfson and coworkers.[56] There are no studies comparing the effects of fat and carbohydrate in patients with acute renal failure.

Hypertonic glucose solutions and lipid infusions have been successfully used and advocated in acute renal failure. The most commonly used energy source in the literature is hypertonic glucose. A 70 per cent dextrose solution supplies about 2.4 kcal/ml in comparison to 2 kcal/ml for the 20 per cent lipid solutions. When limitations on fluid administration are important, there is an advantage to using a more concentrated calorie source. However, the frequent occurrence of insulin resistance and hyperglycemia when hypertonic glucose is used in acute uremia, and the need for fats as an essential nutrient, make it desirable to use both lipid and glucose in the patient with large caloric requirements. When using lipid emulsions in acute renal failure, one should avoid giving an excessive phosphate load in view of the phosphate content of the solutions. Since triglyceride removal from serum is impaired in chronic renal failure, monitoring the serum triglyceride levels is prudent in the patient with acute renal failure.

Finally, excess production of carbon dioxide occurs when the calories derived from carbohydrate exceed metabolic requirements.[57] Providing part of the energy requirement with lipids will reduce the occurrence of this complication.

The importance of meeting the caloric requirements for the clinical course of the patient is suggested by the fact that patients with renal failure who recovered renal function or survived received more calories than those who did not.[6] In the study of Mault and coworkers, the resting energy expenditure of patients who "survived" long enough to leave the intensive care unit was lower than in the nonsurvivors. Furthermore, "survival" was higher in those patients whose cumulative calorie balance was positive when compared with those patients in whom it was negative. There was no difference between the resting energy expenditure in patients who were in negative as compared with positive calorie balance. Although it is usually easier to administer large volumes of fluid to nonoliguric patients than to oliguric patients, there was no difference in calorie balance between these groups.[51] In summary, it is imperative to meet the caloric requirements of the patient with acute renal failure. Although fluid restrictions have been a limiting factor in the past, newer techniques of dialysis may reduce this concern (see further on).

AMINO ACID REQUIREMENTS IN ACUTE RENAL FAILURE

Essential and Nonessential Amino Acids

The most frequently asked question about nutrition in acute renal failure concerns the choice of amino acid solution: essential amino acids alone or a general solution containing both essential and nonessential amino acids. The answer may be given simply as: both have their indications. Although it is true that evidence can be cited in support of or against the efficacy of either solution, it is a reasonable clinical approach today to prescribe amino acids based upon the clinical condition of the patient.

The original impetus to the use of essential amino acids alone in the treatment of acute renal failure was the observation that small amounts of protein fed to chronic uremia patients reduced the rate of rise of blood urea nitrogen levels. This effect was attributed to the reutilization of urea nitrogen for the synthesis of nonessential amino acids.[58] It now appears that the extent of such reutilization is very limited. Only 3.2 per cent of ^{15}N-labeled urea nitrogen was incorporated into albumin in a study of chronic uremia patients.[59] It is unlikely that the degree of incorporation into protein is significantly greater in acute renal failure.

The work of Kopple and Coburn provided further support for the inadequacy of the low-protein diet in chronic renal failure.[60] Patients who ingested a diet of 20 gm of protein/day had a negative nitrogen balance, which improved to a neutral or positive balance when the diet was changed to 40 gm/day of protein. Similar observations of negative nitrogen balance have been made in patients with acute renal failure who received small amounts of essential amino acids.[6, 39] This might suggest that larger amounts of essential amino acids would be beneficial. Such an approach has resulted in hyperammonemia and marked abnormalities in plasma amino acid concentrations in children.[61] Thus, if large quantities of amino acids (0.5 gm/kg body weight or more) are prescribed, they should be given in a general formula.

Some of the evidence supporting the use of essential and nonessential amino acids has already been considered. The increased rate of renal cellular repair described by Toback and associates[46] was a result of treatment with a general amino acid formula. In chronically uremic rats, nonessential amino acids added to the essential amino acids produced improved growth.[62] Nitrogen balance in normal human subjects ingesting a low-protein diet was improved when nonessential amino acids were included.[63]

One may conclude that the use of essential amino acids in small quantities along with hypertonic glucose results in a reduced rate in the rise of blood urea nitrogen levels, but probably not as a result of nitrogen reutilization. Although this can be an adequate diet for some patients with renal failure, it may not be more beneficial than small amounts of a general formula of amino acids.[44] For the patient with moderate to marked protein catabolism, a general formula should be used.

Another argument for the inclusion of nonessential amino acids relates to the body's ability to synthesize and utilize nonessential amino acids from exogenous essential amino acids. It is likely that individual variations exist in the ability to synthesize certain nonessential amino acids.[64] During stressful situations it would be unwise to rely on these synthetic pathways to provide needed nutrients. Lastly, the movement of amino acids into cells depends upon the mass action effect at the cell membrane surface. Provision of adequate amounts of the necessary amino acids is needed to maintain and augment synthetic processes.[65]

Branched-Chain Amino Acids

Another question to consider, and one that is receiving considerable attention currently, is the role of solutions containing an increased proportion of branched-chain amino acids—leucine, isoleucine, and valine. Leucine, in particular, has a stimulatory effect on protein synthesis and an inhibitory effect on protein degradation. These effects are seen in isolated normal muscle preparations[66, 67] and in rats with sepsis and trauma.[68] Toback found a cellular deficit of leucine in his experimental model of acute renal failure.[48] This was corrected by the infusion of a general amino acid formula. The stimulatory effect of leucine in the uremic rat may depend upon the muscle tested. In one report, leucine stabilized protein synthesis and protein degradation in atrial muscle but not in the diaphragm or soleus muscles.[69] In humans, leucine infusion reduces urinary nitrogen loss during starvation.[70] There is increasing evidence as to the value of infusing amino acid formulations of increased branched-chain composition to postoperative patients.[71, 72] Further studies on the use of these newer formulations in acute renal failure are necessary.

VITAMIN AND MINERAL REQUIREMENTS

Water-soluble vitamins may be lost during dialysis, and it is common practice to administer vitamin B complex and folic acid to patients with chronic renal failure who require dialysis. The daily requirement for pyridoxine is 10 mg/day.[73] It is likely that the requirements in patients with acute renal failure are similar. The use of vitamin C in large amounts has resulted in widespread oxalate deposition in acute renal failure.[74] This side effect is apparently of importance when the vitamin is administered over a prolonged period.

The requirements for fat-soluble vitamins vary. Vitamin A is usually not required and, in fact, elevated levels of the vitamin have been reported in chronically uremic patients.[75] The vitamin D metabolite 25-hydroxycholecalciferol is not usually given, though its level in blood is reduced.[76]

Administration of minerals and electrolytes in acute renal failure requires daily or twice daily monitoring of the serum electrolyte concentrations. It is preferable to adjust the individual amounts of electrolytes infused and not to rely solely on fixed formulations. In the initial period of treatment, serum potassium, phosphorus, and magnesium levels are usually elevated. As treatment with dialysis and TPN proceeds, infusion of potassium and particularly phosphorus becomes necessary to prevent serious depletion.[77]

DIALYSIS

Dialysis therapy is the key element in the modern management of renal failure. Without dialysis, the subject of nutritional support of acute renal failure would not need to be discussed at any great length. As already noted, before dialysis was available many patients were treated with severe protein and fluid restriction. Indeed, one therapeutic goal that was advised was that the patient should lose weight daily, an indication that volume overload was being avoided. At present, with dialysis easily provided at most hospitals, it is practical to give large amounts of fluid to many patients in order to ensure adequate nutrition.

There are two components to dialysis therapy: removal of fluid and diffusion of solute down a concentration gradient. Modern nephrologic practice is to maintain the blood urea nitrogen level at 80 to 100 mg/dl and to control hyperkalemia and hyperphosphatemia by frequent dialysis. Early or prophylactic dialysis is now the rule. The aim is to avoid uremic complications such as bleeding and neurologic disturbances. In patients who require large volumes of nutritional solutions in addition to antibiotics, blood, and other fluid intake, daily dialysis therapy (usually hemodialysis) is mandatory.

Fluid Balance in Dialysis

Although maintenance of fluid balance by dialysis is usually feasible, there are frequently substantial fluctuations in the extracellular fluid volume and osmolality because dialysis is performed for 4 to 5 hours in order to remove the fluid accumulated in the previous 24 hours. Despite intensive dialysis, many patients remain in a positive fluid balance. There are some patients who have hemodynamic instability during hemodialysis, which results in hypotension and limits the ability to remove fluid. A number of techniques are available to facilitate ultrafiltration in such cases. Perhaps the simplest method is sequential ultrafiltration-dialysis. In this technique, the ultrafiltration is performed first by simply applying a high transmembrane pressure across the dialyzer membrane without the presence of dialysis fluid. The rise in plasma oncotic pressure and the higher plasma refilling rate alleviate the hypotensive effect of volume removal. Dialysis is then begun by circulating dialysis fluid and reducing the transmembrane pressure.

The daily fluctuations in fluid volume can be eliminated with the technique of continuous arteriovenous hemofiltration (CAVH). This procedure requires the use of a membrane that is more permeable to water than are conventional hemodialysis membranes. Such a membrane, made of polysulfone, is so permeable that large flux rates are obtained using the hydrostatic pressure generated by the heart without the need for a blood pump as in hemodialysis.[78] As much as 20 L of fluid/day can be removed. By performing continuous ultrafiltration, the removal of urea, creatinine, and other solutes is obtained, and their serum concentrations are controlled.[79] The obvious drawback to this technique is the need for careful monitoring and continuous replacement of fluid volume deficits to prevent hypotension. Also, patients need to receive prolonged heparin infusions, which are dangerous in patients with a bleeding tendency. CAVH, then, is a promising new modality of therapy. However, no significant improvement in survival in critically ill patients has yet been reported.[79, 80]

Nutrient Supplementation in Dialysis

In recent work at our hospital, we have been able to administer glucose and amino acids to patients by adding these nutrients to the hemodialysis fluid.[81] In order to allow for sufficient nutrient uptake, the blood and dialysate flow rates were reduced. At lower flow rates, of course, the clearances during dialysis are lower, and a longer duration of therapy is needed. An advantage of this technique is the ability to provide nutrients without worrying about fluid intake because fluid can be removed during the dialysis.

Losses of nutrients during both hemodialysis and peritoneal dialysis may affect the nutritional state of the patient (Table 34–1).

Table 34–1. NUTRITIONAL EFFECTS OF DIALYSIS THERAPY

LOSSES OF NUTRIENTS
Amino Acids
   Hemodialysis—6 to 9 gm/treatment
   Peritoneal dialysis—0.5 to 0.3 gm/exchange[83]
Protein
   Hemodialysis—none
   Peritoneal dialysis—0.6 ± 0.5 gm/hr of treatment,[85] protein losses increase during episodes of peritonitis
Glucose
   Hemodialysis—28 gm lost during 6 hr dialysis with a glucose-free dialysate[86]
Vitamins
   Hemodialysis and peritoneal dialysis resulting losses of water-soluble vitamins
ABSORPTION OF NUTRIENTS
Glucose
   Peritoneal dialysis—varies with dialysate volume and glucose concentration. 182 ± 61 gm/day of glucose is absorbed daily during continuous ambulatory peritoneal dialysis[87]

Losses of amino acids occur in both forms of treatment.[82, 83] In patients with chronic renal failure, the infusion of 40 gm of amino acids during hemodialysis was accompanied by removal of 12 gm of amino acids in the hemodialysis fluid.[84] Of course, not all of these amino acids were derived from the infusion. The administration of amino acids during hemodialysis to patients with acute renal failure has been reported,[6] but there is no data concerning its specific benefit. It seems reasonable to increase the rate of infusion of amino acids during periods of dialysis therapy, especially in the very catabolic patient.

Protein molecules are too large to cross the hemodialysis membrane but can cross the peritoneal membrane.[85] The amounts of protein removed by peritoneal dialysis require the administration of additional quantities of amino acids or plasma protein. This supplementation is especially critical when peritonitis is present.

Glucose is removed by hemodialysis when glucose-free hemodialysis fluid is used. This has been shown to stimulate gluconeogenesis in the patient with chronic renal failure.[86] The use of a glucose-containing hemodialysis bath will eliminate this problem. Glucose absorption by the patient undergoing peritoneal dialysis is very important. The amount absorbed is a function of the glucose concentration of the dialysis fluid and the volume of fluid infused. In patients with chronic renal failure who are treated with continuous ambulatory peritoneal dialysis, about 180 gm/day of glucose are absorbed.[87]

Finally, water-soluble vitamins are lost during dialysis and a deficiency of some vitamins may result. Vitamin supplementation has already been discussed.

MANAGEMENT OF THE PATIENT

The approach to the nutritional support of the patient with renal failure entails an initial assessment of and subsequent monitoring of the course of therapy (Table 34–1). The most important factors to consider in patient assessment are the degree of catabolism, the nature of any associated diseases, the daily urine volume, the route of nutrient administration, and the type and frequency of any dialysis therapy.

Degree of Catabolism

Among the clues to the presence of a very catabolic state are the nature of the renal insult, the rate of rise of serum urea nitrogen levels, and the urea nitrogen appearance rate. Patients with rhabdomyolysis, extensive abdominal trauma, and septicemia are likely to be more catabolic than patients with antibiotic or other nephrotoxin-related renal failure. However, if nephrotoxic renal failure should occur in an already catabolic situation, the catabolic stress will be aggravated. Daily increments of blood urea nitrogen of 30 to 50 mg/dl are strong evidence of increased protein breakdown if the patient is not receiving large amounts of protein or amino acids. When rhabdomyolysis is present, the rapid rise in serum creatinine, potassium, and phosphorus levels points to extensive muscle cell disruption with release of intracellular contents into the circulation. Other indicators of protein breakdown and inadequate nutrition are similar to those found in nonuremic patients, for example, depressed lymphocyte count and rapid declines in serum albumin and serum transferrin concentrations. Anthropometry is not usually of great help in the initial assessment, but it may substantiate the loss of lean body mass that can occur after one to two weeks of catabolism.

The estimation of urea nitrogen appearance can be done with easily measured clinical data, and it provides the best clinical indication of protein breakdown. The urea nitrogen appearance does not measure the exact amount of urea produced daily because some urea enters an enterohepatic circuit. The urea nitrogen appearance reflects the amount of nitrogen intake, the renal excretion of urea, and the amount of protein degradation. The bulk of urea excretion occurs normally via the urine. When urinary excretion is minimal, as in acute renal failure, urea accumulates and is distributed in the total body water. Since the total body water fluctuates in renal failure because of the decrease in urine formation, the urea nitrogen appearance must take this change in the urea space into account.

The urea nitrogen appearance can be easily calculated during a 24-hour time interval using the equations on the following page. (It is necessary to avoid a time period during which dialysis is performed because urea losses into dialysate are not easily measured.)

(1) Urea nitrogen appearance (gm/day) = change in body urea nitrogen content + urinary urea nitrogen
+ dialysate urea nitrogen

(2) Change in body urea nitrogen (gm/day) = (change in blood urea nitrogen [gm/L] × initial body
weight (kg) × 0.6 L/kg) + (change in body weight [kg] × final blood urea nitrogen (gm/L) × 1 L/kg)

The urea nitrogen appearance is not equal to the total nitrogen output because it does not include nitrogen losses from the integument and the gastrointestinal tract. Nitrogen losses from these routes do not usually vary markedly. This may not be the case, however, when there are increased losses from postoperative drains and fistulae. For clinical purposes, rigorous measurement of nitrogen output is not needed. It can be estimated from the urea nitrogen appearance using the following equation, which is derived from observations in chronic uremia patients.

(3) Nitrogen output = (0.97) (urea nitrogen
appearance) + 1.93 [88]

The urea nitrogen appearance can also be used to estimate nitrogen balance. Since the bulk of nitrogen released by protein degradation is reflected in the urea nitrogen appearance, the difference between it and the nitrogen intake has been used to indicate the nitrogen balance.[6]

Associated Illnesses

There are a number of conditions that are likely to aggravate the catabolic state of the patient and make nutritional therapy more difficult. The use of corticosteroids will increase the rate of rise of blood urea nitrogen levels. For the same reason, tetracyclines should be avoided in acute renal failure. Recurrent infection and septicemia, such as may occur after abdominal trauma, will prolong the duration of marked protein breakdown. The feasibility of infusing large volumes of fluid will be reduced when circulatory overload or congestive heart failure is present. Diabetes mellitus will require extra caution in the use of hypertonic glucose. For these patients, it is advisable to infuse insulin and nutrients via separate pumps.

Urine Volume

The amount of urine produced will affect the amount of nutrient solutions that can be given without the patient developing volume overload or hyponatremia, and it will thus affect the amount of ultrafiltration that is required. In addition to having a higher urine volume, patients with the nonoliguric form of acute renal failure tend to have a higher glomerular filtration rate than do those with oliguric renal failure. As a result, the rate of rise in serum urea nitrogen and creatinine levels will be slower and the need for dialysis will be accordingly decreased. Nonoliguric renal failure may occur with any precipitating factor, but it is more commonly seen in nephrotoxin-related disease.[89] In general, the nonoliguric patient is less catabolic and less difficult to manage.

Route of Nutrient Administration

It is a safe assumption that the sickest patients will not be able to receive adequate enteral nutrition. Even patients who can be fed orally may not receive the amount of nutrition required because of anorexia and nausea. When neither oral nor gastrointestinal tube feedings are adequate or feasible, a parenteral route is necessary. Peripheral infusion of lipid may be used as an adjunct to oral feedings in the patient who cannot ingest enough calories. For most of the very catabolic patients, a central infusion catheter will be required.

Type of Dialysis Therapy

The nutrition requirements will influence the type and amount of dialysis prescribed. Certainly, oliguric patients receiving 2 L or more of fluid daily will require daily ultrafiltration. Peritoneal dialysis can be done continuously, but it is more common to use daily hemodialysis to maintain fluid balance. In addition, in the very catabolic patient, hemodialysis is more effective than peritoneal dialysis in reducing the serum urea nitrogen and potassium levels.

Enteral Nutrition versus TPN
(Table 34–2)

Once the initial assessment of the patient has been made, the nutritional regimen can

HISTORY
  Age
  Complicating chronic illnesses
    Chronic liver disease—may limit amino acid intake
    Chronic obstructive pulmonary disease
    Congestive heart failure—may limit amount of
      fluid administered
  Specific causes of acute renal failure
    Aminoglycoside administration—a frequent cause
      of nonoliguric acute renal failure
    Skeletal muscle trauma—patients may be expected
      to be hypercatabolic
    Radiographic contrast study—a cause of acute
      renal failure, particularly in patients with
      longstanding diabetes mellitus
    Recent abdominal surgery—usually precludes
      enteral nutrition
PHYSICAL EXAMINATION
  Muscle tenderness and swelling
  Abdominal wounds
  Fistulae and abdominal drains
LABORATORY VALUES
  Urinalysis
    Myoglobinuria
    Bacteriuria
  Serum electrolytes
    Sodium
    Phosphorus
    Uric acid
    Calcium
  Serum enzymes
    Creatinine phosphokinase
  Complete blood count
    Lymphocyte count
  Protein
    Total protein
    Albumin
    Transferrin
  Urea nitrogen appearance

be ordered. It is generally agreed that whenever possible nutrition should be provided via the gastrointestinal tract. It is an unusual patient who can be adequately nourished from a hospital diet alone, because of the anorexia that is common in acute renal failure. Supplementation of the diet with specific formulations for these patients is very helpful. Two preparations to consider are Amin-Aid (McGaw Laboratories) or Travasorb Renal (Travenol Laboratories). Amin-Aid provides concentrated dextrose solutions and essential amino acids alone, and Travasorb Renal provides a mixed amino acid formula. Other products that contain a mixed amino acid formula and have high caloric density are Isocal-HCN (Mead-Johnson) and Magnacal (Organon). They are more useful in patients who are undergoing frequent dialysis. All of the formulations mentioned

contain no electrolytes or, at most, small amounts of sodium. Dilution is required initially because of the high osmolality of the solutions.

When the gastrointestinal tract is not a feasible route for the administration of nutrients, it is usually necessary to use a central venous catheter. The technical details of the insertion and care of the catheter system will not be discussed here. The major consideration for TPN in renal failure is to provide the maximal amount of nutrition in the smallest quantity of fluid volume. When a mixed formula of amino acids is called for, we prefer to use a 10 per cent solution, such as Aminosyn 10 per cent (Abbott Laboratories). If this concentration is not available, an 8.5 per cent solution can be used (FreAmine, McGaw Laboratories, or Travasol, Travenol Laboratories). At least 60 per cent of the required calories should be administered in the form of hypertonic dextrose, either a 50 or 70 per cent concentration. A 20 per cent lipid emulsion (Intralipid, Cutter, or Lyposyn, Abbott Laboratories) will provide the remainder of calories and also the needed essential fatty acids.

In patients who are not very catabolic, that is, the urea nitrogen appearance is less than 5 g/day, between 2000 and 2500 kcal/day can be administered in about 1500 ml. A solution of 70 per cent dextrose provides about 2.4 kcal/ml. Thus, 600 ml of 70 per cent dextrose and 400 ml of 5.2 per cent essential amino acid solution will contain about 1500 kcal. The 20 per cent lipid emulsions yield 2 kcal/ml; 250 to 500 ml daily can deliver the remainder of needed calories. This regimen provides 21 gm of amino acids. If the patient is not oliguric and is not receiving large amounts of other intravenous fluids, daily dialysis may not be required to maintain fluid balance.

The patient who has a urea nitrogen appearance in excess of 5 gm/day is likely to be oliguric and to require frequent or daily hemodialysis. In this case, we currently advocate the use of essential and nonessential amino acids in quantities up to 80 gm/day. The calorie intake should be about 40 to 45 kcal/kg body weight. These requirements can be met with 1 L of 70 per cent dextrose solution, 800 ml of 10 per cent amino acids, and 500 ml of lipid emulsion.

Close monitoring of the patient is mandatory with any nutritional regimen (Table 34–3). When large amounts of glucose are being used, a twice-daily or even more fre-

Table 34–3. DAILY MONITORING OF PATIENTS WITH ACUTE RENAL FAILURE

Body Weight
Urine Output
Central Venous Catheter Site
Daily Laboratory Values
  Serum sodium
  Serum potassium
  Serum urea nitrogen
  Serum creatinine
  Serum glucose
  Serum phosphorous
Other Monitoring—Every 2 or 3 days
  Urea nitrogen appearance—every 2 to 3 days
  Nitrogen balance—the difference between
    nitrogen intake and urea nitrogen appearance
Laboratory values
  Serum magnesium
  Prothrombin time
  Serum calcium

quent measurement of blood glucose levels should be ordered. Insulin administration needs to be adjusted accordingly. When good control of blood glucose levels is obtained, daily blood glucose measurements are still needed. If further catabolic stresses supervene, such as septicemia or reoperations to drain an abscess, the previously well-controlled blood glucose level may rise, and increased insulin administration will be needed.

As already noted, potassium, phosphorus, and magnesium are usually not required early in TPN, but after several days the addition of these electrolytes to the infusion are frequently necessary.

When large amounts of a mixed amino acid solution are prescribed, the blood urea nitrogen levels and the urea nitrogen appearance may rise, in part because of the increased nitrogen load. This development may be acceptable in order to provide amino acids to replace those lost in dialysis and replace some of the nitrogen lost as a consequence of the catabolic state.

FUTURE PROSPECTS

The current state of the art in nutrition for patients with acute renal failure is unsatisfactory. A variety of nutrient regimens are in use, and dialysis support is widely available. Yet, as noted at the beginning of this chapter, the mortality rate in acute renal failure remains particularly high in surgical patients and in patients with sepsis and hypotension underlying the renal disease. Future research efforts in this area will need to

address the metabolic perturbations that produce the profound degree of protein breakdown so commonly observed. The use of amino acid solutions with increased proportions of branched-chain amino acids may prove valuable in this regard. The identification of humoral factors that mediate the catabolic response may lead to the development of means of tempering their activity. Finally, when trials of any new mode of therapy are conducted, their design should be such to ensure that the patients treated are well matched in terms of their clinical condition and level of catabolism.

REFERENCES

1. Stott, R.B., Cameron, J.S., Ogg, C.S. et al.: Why the persistently high mortality in acute renal failure? Lancet, 2:75, 1972.
2. Kjellstrand, C.M., Ebben, J., and Davin, T.: Time of death, recovery of renal failure and need for chronic hemodialysis in patients with acute tubular necrosis. Trans. Am. Soc. Artif. Intern. Organs, 27:45, 1981.
3. Bozzetti, F., Terno, G., and Longoni, C.: Parenteral hyperalimentation and wound healing. Surg. Gynecol. Obstet., 141:712, 1975.
4. Bistrian, B.R., Blackburn, G.L., Scrimshaw, M.S. et al.: Cellular immunity in semi-starved states in hospitalized adults. Am. J. Clin. Nutr., 28:1148, 1975.
5. Giordano, C., De Santo, N.G., and Senatore, R.: Effects of catabolic stress in acute and chronic renal failure. Am. J. Clin. Nutr., 31:1561, 1978.
6. Feinstein, E.I., Blumenkrantz, M.J., Healy, M. et al.: Clinical and metabolic responses to parenteral nutrition in acute renal failure—a controlled double-blind study. Medicine, 60:124, 1981.
7. Abel, R.M., Shih, V.E., Abbott, W.M. et al.: Amino acid metabolism in acute renal failure: Influence of intravenous essential L-amino acid hyperalimentation therapy. Am. J. Surg., 180:350, 1974.
8. Herrmann, V.M., Clark, D., Wilmore, D.W. et al.: Protein metabolism: effect of disease and altered intake on the stable 15N curve. Surg. Forum, 31:92, 1980.
9. Koffler, A., Friedler, R.M., and Massry, S.G.: Acute renal failure due to nontraumatic rhabdomyolysis. Ann. Intern. Med., 85:23, 1976.
10. Clowes, G.H.A., Jr., George, B.C., Villee, C.A., Jr. et al.: Muscle proteolysis induced by a circulating peptide in patients with sepsis or trauma. N. Engl. J. Med., 308:545, 1983.
11. Baracos, V., Rodermann, H.P., Dinarello, C.A. et al.: Stimulation of muscle protein degradation and prostaglandin E2 release by leukocyte pyrogen: a mechanism for the increased degradation of the muscle proteins during fever. N. Engl. J. Med., 308:553, 1983.
12. Hörl, W.H., and Heidland, A.: Enhanced proteolytic activity—cause of protein catabolism in acute renal failure. Am. J. Clin. Nutr., 33:1423, 1980.
13. Hörl, W.H., Gantert, C., Auer, I.O. et al.: In vitro inhibition of protein catabolism by alpha-2-mac-

roglobulin in plasma from a patient with post-traumatic acute renal failure. Am. J. Nephrol., 2:32, 1982.

14. Fröhlich, J., Hoppe-Seyler, G., Schollmeyer, P. et al.: Possible sites of interaction of acute renal failure with amino acid utilization for gluconeogenesis in isolated perfused rat liver. Eur. J. Clin. Invest., 7:261, 1977.

15. Mitch, W.E.: Amino acid release from the hindquarter and urea appearance in acute uremia. Am. J. Physiol., 241(6):E415, 1981.

16. Flugel-Link, R.M., Salusky, I., Jones, M. et al.: Protein and amino acid metabolism in the posterior hemicorpus of acutely uremic rats. Am. J. Physiol., 244:E615, 1983.

17. Lacy, W.E.: Effect of acute uremia on amino acid uptake and urea production by perfused rat liver. Am. J. Physiol., 216:1300, 1969.

18. Clark, A.S., and Mitch, W.E.: Muscle protein turnover and glucose uptake in rats with acute uremia. J. Clin. Invest., 72:836, 1983.

19. Arnold, W.E., and Holliday, M.A.: Tissue resistance to insulin stimulation of amino acid uptake in acutely uremic rats. Kidney Int., 16:124, 1979.

20. Grossman, S.B., Yap, S.H., and Shafritz, D.A.: Influence of chronic renal failure on protein synthesis and albumin metabolism in rat liver. J. Clin. Invest., 59:869, 1977.

21. Massry, S.G., Arieff, A.I., and Coburn, J.W.: Divalent ion metabolism in patients with acute renal failure: studies on the mechanism of hypocalcemia. Kidney Int., 5:437, 1974.

22. Garber, A.J.: Effects of parathyroid hormone on skeletal muscle protein and amino acid metabolism in the rat. J. Clin. Invest., 71:1806, 1983.

23. Bondy, P.K., Engel, F.L., and Farrar, B.: The metabolism of amino acids and protein in the adrenalectomized-nephrectomized rat. Endocrinology, 44:476, 1949.

24. Borst, J.G.: Protein catabolism in uremia. Effects of protein-free diet, infection and blood transfusions. Lancet, 1:824, 1948.

25. Gamble, J.L.: Physiological information from studies on the life-raft ration. Harvey Lect., 42:247, 1946–1947.

26. Giordano, C.: Use of exogenous and endogenous urea for protein synthesis in normal and uremic subjects. J. Lab. Clin. Med., 62:231, 1963.

27. Giovanetti, S., and Maggiore, Q.: A low-nitrogen diet with proteins of high biological value for severe chronic uremia. Lancet, 1:1000, 1964.

28. Berlyne, G.M., Bazzard, F.J., Booth, E.M. et al.: The dietary treatment of acute renal failure. Q. J. Med., 36:59, 1967.

29. Wilmore, D.W., and Dudrick, S.J.: Treatment of acute renal failure with intravenous essential L-amino acids: Arch. Surg., 99:669, 1969.

30. Dudrick, S.J., Steiger, E., and Long, J.M.: Renal failure in surgical patients. Treatment with intravenous essential amino acids and hypertonic glucose. Surgery, 68:180, 1970.

31. Lee, H.A., Sharpstone, P., and Ames, A.C.: Parenteral nutrition in renal failure. Postgrad. Med. J., 43:81, 1967.

32. Lee, H.A., Hill, L.F., Ginks, W.R. et al.: Some aspects of parenteral nutrition in the treatment of renal failure. In Berlyne, G.M. (ed.): Nutrition in Renal Disease. Baltimore, The Williams & Wilkins Co., 1968, page 216.

33. Baek, S.M., Makabali, G.G., Bryan-Brown, C.W. et al.: The influence of parenteral nutrition on the course of acute renal failure. Surg. Gynecol. Obstet., 141:405, 1975.

34. McMurray, S.D., Luft, F.C., Maxwell, D.R. et al.: Prevailing patterns and predictor variables in patients with acute tubular necrosis. Arch. Intern. Med., 139:950, 1978.

35. Rainford, D.J.: Nutritional management of acute renal failure. Acta Chir. Scand. (Suppl.) 507:327, 1980.

36. Abel, R.M., Abbott, W.M., and Fischer, J.E.: Intravenous essential L-amino acids and hypertonic dextrose in patients with acute renal failure. Am. J. Surg., 12:631, 1972.

37. Abel, R.M., Abbott, W.M., and Fischer, J.E.: Intravenous essential L-amino acids and hypertonic dextrose in patients with acute renal failure. Effects on serum potassium, phosphate, and magnesium. Am. J. Surg., 123:632, 1972.

38. Abel, R.M., Beck, C.H., Jr., Abbott, W.M. et al.: Improved renal failure after treatment with intravenous essential L-amino acids and glucose. Results of a prospective double-blind study. N. Engl. J. Med., 288:695, 1973.

39. Leonard, C.D., Luke, R.G., and Siegel, R.R.: Parenteral essential amino acids in acute renal failure. Urology, 6:154, 1975.

40. Sofio, C., and Nicora, R.: High calorie essential amino acid parenteral therapy in acute renal failure. Acta Chir. Scand. (Suppl.) 466:98, 1976.

41. Feinstein, E.I., Kopple, J.D., Silberman, H. et al.: Total parenteral nutrition with high or low nitrogen intake in patients with acute renal failure. Kidney Int., 26:S-319, 1983.

42. Blackburn, G.L., Etter, G., and Mackenzie, T.: Criteria for choosing amino acid therapy in acute renal failure. Am. J. Clin. Nutr., 31:1841, 1978.

43. Freund, H., Atamian, S., and Fischer, J.E.: Comparative study of parenteral nutrition in renal failure using essential and non-essential amino acid–containing solutions. Surg. Gynecol. Obstet., 151:652, 1980.

44. Mirtallo, J.M., Schneider, P.J., Mavko, K. et al.: A comparison of essential and general amino acid infusions in the nutritional support of patients with compromised renal function. J.P.E.N., 6:109, 1982.

45. Sellers, A.L., Katz, J., and Marmorstein, J.: Effect of bilateral nephrectomy on urea formation in rat liver slices. Am. J. Physiol., 191:345, 1957.

46. Van Buren, C.T., Dudrick, S.J., Dworkin, L. et al.: Effects of intravenous essential L-amino acids and hypertonic dextrose on anephric beagles. Surg. Forum, 23:83, 1972.

47. Toback, F.G.: Amino acid enhancement of renal regeneration after acute tubular necrosis. Kidney Int., 12:193, 1977.

48. Toback, F.G., Dodd, R.C., Maier, E.R. et al.: Amino acid enhancement of renal protein synthesis during regeneration after acute tubular necrosis. Clin. Res., 27:432a, 1979.

49. Toback, F.G., Teegarden, D.E., and Havener, L.J.: Amino acid–mediated stimulations of renal phospholipid biosynthesis after acute tubular necrosis. 15:542, 1979.

50. Oken, D.E., Sprinkel, F.M., Kirshbaum, B.B. et al.: Amino acid therapy in the treatment of experimental renal failure in the rat. Kidney Int., 17:14, 1980.

51. Mault, J.R., Bartlett, R.H., Dechert, R.E. et al.:

Starvation: a major contribution to mortality in acute renal failure? Trans. Am. Soc. Artif. Intern. Organs, 29:390, 1983.

52. Abitbol, C.L., and Holliday, M.A.: Total parenteral nutrition in anuric children. Clin. Nephrol., 5:153, 1976.

53. Spreiter, S.C., Myers, B.D., and Swenson, R.S.: Protein-energy requirements in subjects with acute renal failure receiving intermittent hemodialysis. Am. J. Clin. Nutr., 33:1433, 1980.

54. Jeejeebhoy, K.N., Anderson, G.H., Nakhooda, A.F. et al.: Metabolic studies in total parenteral nutrition with lipid in man: comparison with glucose. J. Clin. Invest., 57:125, 1976.

55. Long, J.M., Wilmore, D.W., Mason, A.D., Jr. et al.: Fat-carbohydrate interaction: effects on nitrogen-sparing in total intravenous feeding. Surg. Forum, 25:52, 1974.

56. Woolfson, A.M.J., Heatley, R.V., and Allison, S.P.: Insulin to inhibit protein catabolism after injury. N. Engl. J. Med., 300:14, 1979.

57. Ashkanazi, J., Rosenbaum, S.H., Hyman, A.L. et al.: Respiratory changes induced by the large glucose loads of total parenteral nutrition. J.A.M.A., 243:1444, 1980.

58. Giordano, C., De Pascal, C., Balestrieri, C. et al.: Incorporation of urea 15N in amino acids of patients with chronic renal failure on a low nitrogen diet. Am. J. Clin. Nutr., 21:394, 1968.

59. Varcoe, R., Halliday, D., Carson, E.R. et al.: Efficiency of utilization of urea nitrogen for albumin synthesis by chronically uremic and normal man. Clin. Sci. Mol. Med., 48:379, 1975.

60. Kopple, J.D., and Coburn, J.: Metabolic studies of low protein diets in uremia, I: Nitrogen and Potassium. Medicine, 52:583, 1973.

61. Motil, K.J., Harmon, W.E., and Grupe, W.E.: Complications of essential amino acid hyperalimentation in children with acute renal failure. J.P.E.N., 4:32, 1980.

62. Pennisi, A.J., Wang, M., and Kopple, J.D.: Effects of protein and amino acid diets in chronically uremic and control rats. Kidney Int., 13:472, 1978.

63. Swendseid, M.E., Harris, C.L., and Tuttle, S.G.: The effects of sources of nonessential nitrogen on nitrogen balance in young adults. J. Nutr., 71:105, 1960.

64. Bessman, S.P.: The justification theory: the essential nature of the non-essential amino acids. Nutr. Rev., 37:209, 1979.

65. Christensen, H.N.: Mass action effects are indispensable for all amino acids. Nutr. Rev., 34:30, 1976.

66. Fulks, R.M., Li, J.B., and Goldberg, A.L.: Effects of insulin, glucose and amino acids on protein turnover in rat diaphragm. J. Biol. Chem., 250:290, 1975.

67. Buse, M.G., and Reid, S.S.: Leucine—a possible regulator of protein turnover in muscle. J. Clin. Invest., 56:1250, 1975.

68. Blackburn, G.L., Maldawer, L.L., Usui, S. et al.: Branched-chain amino acid administration and metabolism during starvation, injury and infection. Surgery, 86:307, 1979.

69. Kunin, A.S.: Effect of acute renal failure on muscle protein turnover. Clin. Res., 30:245A, 1982.

70. Sherwin, R.S.: Effect of starvation on the turnover and metabolic response to leucine. J. Clin. Invest., 61:1471, 1978.

71. Desai, S.P., Bistrian, B.R., Moldawer, L.L. et al.: Plasma amino acid concentrations during branched-chain amino acid infusions in stressed patients. J. Trauma, 22:747, 1982.

72. Cerra, F.B., Upson, D., Angelico, R. et al.: Branched chains support postoperative protein synthesis. Surgery, 92:192, 1982.

73. Kopple, J.D., Mercurio, K., Blumenkrantz, M.J. et al.: Daily requirements of pyridoxine supplements in chronic renal failure. Kidney Int., 19:694, 1981.

74. Friedman, A.L., Chesney, R.W., Gilbert, E.F. et al.: Secondary oxalosis as a complication of parenteral alimentation in acute renal failure. Am. J. Nephrol., 3:248, 1983.

75. Smith, F.R., and Goodman, D.S.: The effects of diseases of the liver, thyroid, and kidneys on transport of vitamin A in human plasma. J. Clin. Invest., 50:2426, 1971.

76. Pietrek, J., Kokot, F., and Kuska, J.: Serum 25-hydroxyvitamin D and parathyroid hormone in patients with acute renal failure. Kidney Int., 13:178, 1978.

77. Knochel, J.P.: The pathophysiology and clinical characteristics of severe hypophosphatemia. Arch. Intern. Med., 137:203, 1977.

78. Kramer, P., Wiggin, W., Rieger, J. et al.: Arteriovenous hemofiltration: a new simple method for treatment of overhydrated patients resistant to diuretics. Klin. Wochenschr., 55:121, 1977.

79. Kramer, P., Böhler, J., Kehr, A. et al.: Intensive care potential of continuous arteriovenous hemofiltration. Trans. Am. Soc. Artif. Intern. Organs, 28:28, 1982.

80. Olbricht, C., Mueller, C., Schwek, H.J. et al.: Treatment of acute renal failure in patients with multiple organ failure by continuous spontaneous hemofiltration. Trans. Am. Soc. Artif. Intern. Organs, 28:33, 1982.

81. Feinstein, E., Collins, J., Blumenkrantz, M. et al.: Nutritional hemodialysis. In Atsumi, K., Maekawa, M., and Ota, K. (eds.): Progress in Artificial Organs—1983. Cleveland, 1984, p. 421.

82. Kopple, J.D., Swendseid, M.E., Shinaberger, J.H. et al.: The free and bound amino acids removed by hemodialysis. Trans. Am. Soc. Artif. Organs, 14:309, 1973.

83. Berlyne, G.M., Lee, H.A., Giordano, C. et al.: Amino acid loss in peritoneal dialysis. Lancet, 1:1399, 1967.

84. Wolfson, M., Jones, M.R., and Kopple, J.D.: Amino acid losses during hemodialysis with infusion of amino acids and glucose. Kidney Int., 21:500, 1982.

85. Blumenkrantz, M.J., Gahl, G.M., Kopple, J.D. et al.: Protein losses during peritoneal dialysis. Kidney Int., 19:593, 1981.

86. Wathen, R., Keshaviah, P., Hommeyer, P. et al.: The metabolic effects of hemodialysis with and without glucose in the dialysate. Am. J. Clin. Nutr., 31:1870, 1978.

87. Grodstein, G.P., Blumenkrantz, M.J., Kopple, J.D. et al.: Glucose absorption during continuous ambulatory peritoneal dialysis. Kidney Int., 19:564, 1981.

88. Kopple, J.D.: Nutritional therapy in kidney failure. Nutr. Rev., 39:193, 1981.

89. Anderson, R.J., Linas, S.L., Berns, A.S. et al.: Non-oliguric acute renal failure. N. Engl. J. Med. 296:1134, 1977.

CHAPTER 35

Hepatic Indications for Parenteral Nutrition

ROBERT H. BOWER
JOSEF E. FISCHER

The liver is the biochemical center of the body. As the recipient of the portal blood flow, it processes and prepares nutrients for use by the periphery through its complex system of enzymes and metabolic processes. Unfortunately, hepatic insufficiency is a common consequence of critical illness. When the liver fails, multiple metabolic processes become deranged, affecting all phases of body economy.

The liver's capacity for regeneration is well known. Thus, therapy in hepatic failure is supportive to allow time for regeneration to occur. Numerous factors that promote hepatic regeneration have been described, including triiodothyronine, adrenocortical steroids, growth hormone, insulin, glucagon, "ileal factor," and nutrition (Fig. 35–1). Of these, nutrition is most easily manipulated by the physician.[1] The provision of adequate nutrients is important to help sustain hepatic function and promote repair and regeneration.

In hepatic insufficiency, the metabolism of all nutrients is altered. However, it is intolerance to protein, manifested as hepatic encephalopathy, that most severely limits attempts to nourish the patient with a failing liver. Adequate protein synthesis is critical to maintaining all the vital functions during critical illness, including muscular, respiratory, metabolic, immunologic, and host-defense functions. Without adequate protein, the patient has little chance for recovery, yet administration of protein in the conventional fashion may result in encephalopathy and eventually coma.

Hepatic encephalopathy becomes the central problem in the nutritional management of the patient with hepatic insuffi-

ciency. Therapy should be aimed at supplying adequate nutrients and protein to the patient without precipitating encephalopathy. To do so requires an understanding of hepatic encephalopathy and the nature of its cause.

PATHOGENESIS OF HEPATIC ENCEPHALOPATHY

The presentations of hepatic encephalopathy may be subtle and varied, especially in the patient with chronic liver disease upon which is superimposed an acute exacerbation. Clinically, patients may present with mania or psychosis. Other early signs that may be less readily apparent are subtle changes in mood, errors in judgment, reversal of the normal day-night rhythm, and postural disorders such as the flapping tremor known as asterixis.

Prevention and treatment of hepatic encephalopathy require an understanding of its cause. Hypotheses concerning the cause of hepatic encephalopathy generally fall into two categories. The first suggests that the signs and symptoms of hepatic encephalopathy are the result of substances that act either singly or in combination with other substances as central nervous system "toxins." The second category of hypotheses concentrates on derangements of the neurotransmitters in the central nervous system and the amino acids that are their precursors.

The Ammonia Hypothesis

The most prominent of the toxic hypotheses involves ammonia. According to

602

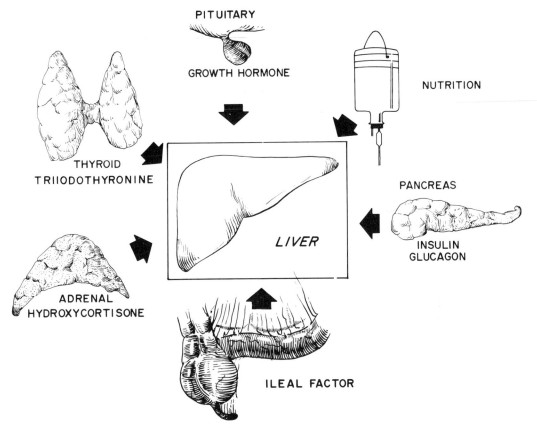

Figure 35–1. Proposed hepatotrophic factors. Of these, nutrition is the most easily manipulated by the clinician.

this hypothesis, ammonia, liberated by gut bacteria, exerts a toxic effect on the central nervous system because of the diseased liver's inability to inactivate it. The mechanism by which ammonia produces encephalopathy, however, remains unclear. The varied manifestations and subtle changes in behavior of patients with encephalopathy make it unlikely that it is the result of a single toxin. Neither is it likely that a deranged energy metabolism would be responsible for such a variety of presentations.

The grade of encephalopathy does not correlate well with venous ammonia concentration. Arterial ammonia levels are only slightly better. Moreover, ammonia concentrations do not correlate with toxicity. Methionine sulfoximine, an inhibitor of glutamine synthesis, increases the level of ammonia in the central nervous system but decreases its toxicity.[2] Conversely, the administration of monoamine oxidase inhibitors decreases blood ammonia levels but increases the grade of encephalopathy.[3] In addition, this hypothesis fails to recognize that as a nitrogen radical, ammonia may be increased because of increased protein catabolism, deamination of amino acids, and generally deranged nitrogen metabolism in the patient with liver failure.[4]

The Synergistic Hypothesis

A synergistic hypothesis involving toxins and metabolic abnormalities has been proposed by Zieve.[5] According to this theory, ammonia, mercaptans, fatty acids, and methanethiols may act synergistically to produce encephalopathy in the presence of the metabolic abnormalities of liver disease. Although experiments have implicated certain of these substances individually, direct evidence that these abnormalities result in encephalopathy is lacking.[6]

The Amino Acid Neurotransmitter Hypothesis

As originally proposed by Fischer and Baldessarini,[7] the amino acid neurotransmitter hypothesis states that in the presence of decreased hepatic function and shunting of blood around the liver, amines or their amino acid precursors escape inactivation by the liver. Their accumulation in the peripheral aminergic nervous system produces the high output–low peripheral resistance syndrome, as well as the hepatorenal syndrome associated with redistribution of blood secondary to loss of peripheral catecholaminergic tone. Their accumulation in the central aminergic system results in symptoms of encephalopathy, coma, and postural disorders of the basal ganglia, such as asterixis.[8] Animal experiments showed decreases in norepinephrine and striatal dopamine in the face of increased levels of the β-hydroxyphenylethylamine neuromodulators or neuroregulators octopamine and phenylethanolamine, and increased levels of indoleamines, including serotonin.[9, 10]

The imbalance of amines in the aminergic nervous system assumes greater importance because of the unique arrangement of the central, primitive, and generally midline aminergic nervous system. Its axons and dendrites end free in the matrix rather than ending in classic synaptic relationships. This system has extensive ramifications and feedback circuits, which suggest a neuromodulatory or neuroregulatory role.[11]

The abnormal concentrations of amines observed in the central nervous system were not simply the result of the amines crossing the blood-brain barrier, but rather were a reflection of a complex series of metabolic derangements in the periphery. In hepatic failure, there is an imbalance of insulin and glucagon, resulting in hyperglucagonemia.[12, 13] Epinephrine and adrenocortical steroids are increased, presumably resulting from a lack of hepatic inactivation.[14] The resulting hormonal milieu of increased glucagon, epinephrine, and adrenocortical steroids favors sustained gluconeogenesis. Catabolism is further increased, since the failing liver is unable to produce glucose or ketone bodies in sufficient quantities to meet the organism's energy needs. In the face of increased energy demands, the branched-chain amino acids (BCAAs) are consumed locally by fat and muscle. The net effect is to decrease the plasma concentration of the BCAAs. The aromatic amino acids are dependent upon the liver for their catabolism. Consequently, in liver failure the concentration of aromatic amino acids rises. Thus, the typical plasma amino acid pattern in liver disease shows increases in those amino acids that are dependent upon the liver for degradation, including phenylalanine, methionine, tyrosine, free (not total) tryptophan, and glutamate. At the same time, there are decreases in the BCAAs that are consumed locally. The altered ratio of aromatic amino acids/BCAAs leads to an excess of aromatic amino acids in the brain. The aromatic amino acids phenylalanine and tyrosine are the metabolic precursors of the β-phenylethylamines, whereas tryptophan is a precursor of the indoleamine serotonin.[13, 15]

The aromatic amino acids, the BCAAs, and methionine and histidine form the large neutral amino acid group. Members of this group compete for a single transport system (System L), which mediates their entry into the brain at the blood-brain barrier.[16] The concentration of amino acids in the brain can be predicted from their plasma competitor ratios using the equation developed by Fernstrom and Faller.[17] In animal experiments, the equation accurately predicted the brain concentration of neutral amino acids in the control animals, but it underestimated the concentrations of neutral amino acids in animals with portacaval anastomosis. The latter group of animals had brain aromatic amino acid concentrations that exceeded the predicted values in a linear fashion (Fig. 35–2).[18]

More recent evidence suggests that there is an alteration in the blood-brain barrier that results in an increased uptake of the neutral amino acids.[19] The differences between the observed and predicted concentrations of aromatic amino acids within the brain of rats with portacaval anastomosis had an excellent correlation with brain glutamine, the metabolite of ammonia.[20] Experiments with isolated brain capillaries from control animals and from animals that had undergone portacaval anastomosis have lent support to the hypothesis that glutamine is exchanged for the neutral amino acids at the blood-brain barrier. Increased levels of glutamine increase the velocity of transport of the neutral amino acids into the brain.[21] It appears, therefore, that ammonia does not have a direct toxic effect on the central nervous system. Instead, its effect is to alter amino acid transport via its metabolite glutamine and thereby alter neurotransmitter metabolism.[20]

The chronic amino acid imbalance in the patient with liver disease leads to threshold disturbances in neurotransmission, which render the brain sensitized to any accentuation of the imbalance. In the pre-encephalo-

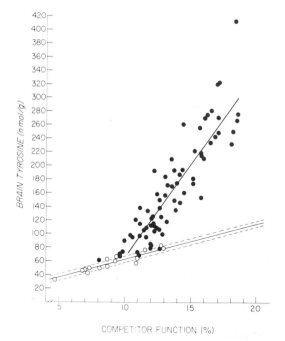

Figure 35–2. The observed brain concentrations of tyrosine compared with the predicted brain concentrations of tyrosine as calculated from the equation of Fernstrom and Faller.[17] The open circles represent sham-operated animals. Their brain concentrations of tyrosine fall within one standard deviation of those predicted. The closed circles represent animals that underwent portacaval anastomosis. Their brain concentrations of tyrosine exceed those predicted in a linear fashion.

an increase in free tryptophan levels secondary to a decrease in serum albumin levels. Aromatic amino acids increase in brain because of decreased plasma competition and increased neutral amino acid uptake (Fig. 35–3).

If any additional stress occurs in the patient with liver disease, the chronic amino acid imbalance may be aggravated and may result in increased neurotransmitter disturbances (Fig. 35–4). Clinical events such as starvation, increased catabolism, sepsis, gastrointestinal bleeding, or overdiuresis increase aromatic amino acid levels or decrease BCAA levels, or both, and may ultimately result in encephalopathy (Fig. 35–5).

Since a central feature of the unified amino acid neurotransmitter hypothesis is that the altered amino acid pattern in plasma is causally related to encephalopathy, nutritional therapy should attempt to decrease plasma levels of aromatic amino acids and increase plasma levels of BCAAs. If this were the case, tolerance to protein administration might increase.

Experiments to test this hypothesis were carried out in animals that had undergone portacaval anastomosis. Hepatic encephalopathy occurred when concentrations of phenylalanine, tyrosine, tryptophan, phenylethamine, octopamine, and 5-hydroxyindoleacetic acid in the cerebrospinal fluid were highest. Infusion of BCAAs and hypertonic dextrose resulted in a return of these substances to normal concentrations, with simultaneous awakening from encephalopathy.[22]

pathic state, plasma BCAAs are decreased, though brain levels remain normal as a result of increased neutral amino acid uptake. Brain tryptophan levels are increased secondary to decreased plasma competition, and there is

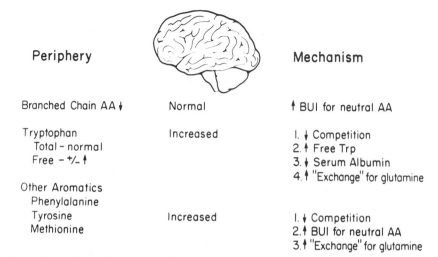

Periphery		Mechanism
Branched Chain AA ↓	Normal	↑ BUI for neutral AA
Tryptophan Total – normal Free – +/– ↑	Increased	1. ↓ Competition 2. ↑ Free Trp 3. ↓ Serum Albumin 4. ↑ "Exchange" for glutamine
Other Aromatics Phenylalanine Tyrosine Methionine	Increased	1. ↓ Competition 2. ↑ BUI for neutral AA 3. ↑ "Exchange" for glutamine

Figure 35–3. Comparison of plasma and brain amino acid levels in the pre-encephalopathic state. Although decreased in the plasma, the branched-chain amino acid levels remain normal in the brain owing to the increased activity of the blood-brain barrier. The brain tryptophan level increases because of the increased free tryptophan in the plasma secondary to decreased albumin binding sites.

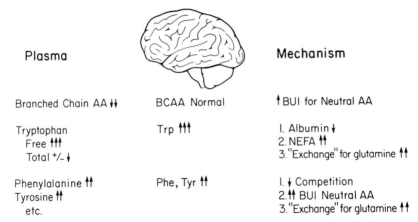

Figure 35–4. Comparison of plasma and brain amino acids in encephalopathy. Branched-chain amino acid levels remain at or near normal in the brain. The brain tryptophan level rises further as a result of decreased serum albumin level and increased serum non-esterified fatty acid levels, probably a glucagon effect, both of which tend to increase the plasma free tryptophan level. Brain aromatic amino acid levels increase owing to decreased competition from the branched-chain amino acids at the blood-brain barrier, increased activity of the blood-brain barrier, and increased exchange for glutamine.

Subsequent experiments performed on dogs with carotid loops demonstrated that infusion of both tryptophan and phenylalanine are required for the production of hepatic coma. When the experiment was repeated with BCAAs added to the infusion, coma did not occur.[23] These findings lend further support to the hypothesis that aromatic amino acids are involved in the production of hepatic encephalopathy and suggest that both deficiency of catecholamines and increased indoleamines are also involved in encephalopathy.

In addition, these findings help to explain the seemingly contradictory finding that intraventricular infusion of octopamine fails to produce coma.[24] Infusion of octopamine alone should result in release of indoleamines as well as catecholamines. Since increased indoleamines appear to be required for encephalopathy, no coma occurs.

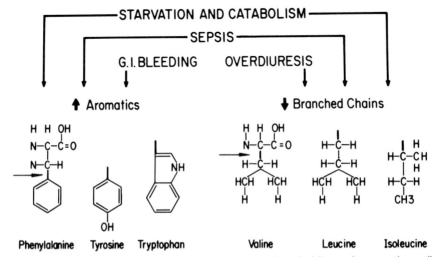

Figure 35–5. The effects of starvation, catabolism, sepsis, gastrointestinal hemorrhage, and overdiuresis on the plasma amino acids. These clinical events accentuate the plasma amino acid imbalance by increasing the aromatic amino acid levels, as occurs in starvation, catabolism, and gastrointestinal hemorrhage, or by decreasing the branched-chain amino acid levels, as occurs in catabolism, sepsis, and overdiuresis.

NUTRITIONAL SUPPORT OF PATIENTS WITH HEPATIC INSUFFICIENCY

Protein Needs

Protein is a critical component of nutrition in patients with hepatic insufficiency, not only for regeneration of the failing liver but also for maintaining other vital functions such as nonspecific host resistance.[25] However, administration of adequate protein frequently results in encephalopathy. Therefore, despite the deranged metabolism of all nutrients, it is hepatic encephalopathy that severely limits the nutritional support of patients with hepatic insufficiency.

Catabolism and increased gluconeogenesis are important contributors to the abnormal amino acid pattern of hepatic insufficiency. The breakdown of skeletal muscle results in increased plasma concentrations of the aromatic acids that are not catabolized by the failing liver. The provision of even modest amounts of protein and adequate calories would not only result in decreased gluconeogenesis, with a consequent decrease in plasma aromatic amino acids, but would also serve to promote protein synthesis, causing intracellular transfer of all amino acids, including the aromatic amino acids.

Despite the need for protein restriction in some patients, a protein-free diet may mimic the amino acid pattern that is seen with a high-protein diet, since gluconeogenesis increases the plasma levels of aromatic amino acids. In rats that had undergone portacaval anastomosis, there was an inverse relationship between the amount of protein infused and the plasma and brain concentrations of aromatic amino acids. Plasma phenylalanine and tyrosine, as well as the false neurotransmitter octopamine, fell as the nitrogen balance became positive.[26]

From these observations, it is apparent that some protein is preferable to no protein at all. Generally, patients with encephalopathy of Grades 0 and 1 who have impaired but stable hepatic function can tolerate moderate amounts of protein if it is given with adequate calories to promote protein synthesis. Approximately 50 per cent of such patients will tolerate 50 to 60 gm of orally administered protein or the intravenous equivalent using a standard, commercially available solution. Thus, rather than starting special hepatic formulations in all patients

with hepatic insufficiency, the first step in a patient with moderate hepatic impairment is to try cautious administration of standard formulas without exceeding 50 to 60 gm of protein equivalent. For those patients who do not tolerate such an approach or who become encephalopathic, a special solution with a modified amino acid pattern has been used.

Types of Nutritional Formulations

In order to normalize the deranged plasma amino acid pattern in hepatic insufficiency, the nutritional solution should theoretically have increased levels of BCAAs and should minimize the administration of aromatic amino acids. In addition to its effect on plasma amino acids, such a BCAA-enriched solution should have additional theoretic advantages:

1. BCAAs promote muscle protein synthesis which favors intracellular transfer of amino acids. However, adequate calories must also be administered.

2. BCAAs generally provide five to seven per cent of the peripheral energy requirements. In the presence of decreased hepatic glucose export and decreased ketone body production, BCAAs may provide a greater percentage of peripheral energy.

3. BCAAs appear to be regulators of amino acid efflux from muscle cells.[27, 28] Increased BCAA concentrations should reduce the efflux of all amino acids from muscle, including the aromatic amino acids.

4. BCAAs form the major competition with aromatic amino acids at the blood-brain barrier. Increasing the concentration of BCAAs at the blood-brain barrier should decrease intracerebral concentrations of aromatic monoamine precursors.

5. Providing exogenous BCAAs should decrease gluconeogenesis and endogenous ammonia production, thereby decreasing brain glutamine levels. Decreased glutamine levels should result in lowering the velocity of neutral amino acid transport.

6. Experiments have suggested that BCAAs act by an as-yet-unknown mechanism to increase hepatic protein synthesis.[29] If this proves to be the case, exogenous administration of BCAAs may accelerate hepatic repair and regeneration.

Experience in treating patients in the United States has largely been limited to a single solution recently made available commercially as HepatAmine (American McGaw Laboratories). It is a BCAA-enriched formula containing 35 per cent BCAAs rather than the 14 to 22 per cent BCAAs found in most standard amino acid solutions. The aromatic amino acids phenylalanine and methionine are reduced, and arginine and alanine are present in increased amounts. The solution is administered with 24 per cent dextrose by the technique of central amino acid hypertonic dextrose parenteral nutrition.

Approximately 80 patients have been treated anecdotally using this solution. Patients could be divided into two groups based upon clinical presentation and amino acid pattern. Most of the patients had chronic liver disease and cirrhosis with acute decompensation caused by gastrointestinal bleeding, overdiuresis, or sepsis that resulted in encephalopathy. These "acute-on-chronic" patients exhibited the classic amino acid pattern with decreased levels of the BCAAs and increased levels of methionine, phenylalanine, tyrosine, aspartate, and glutamate (Fig. 35–6). Approximately 20 of the patients had either viral or drug-induced fulminant hepatitis. This latter group of patients was acutely ill and required other means of supportive care in addition to nutritional support. The amino acid pattern of patients with hepatitis

differs from that of the "acute-on-chronic" patient. A diffuse hyperaminoacidemia was seen in the hepatitis group, with marked increase in the levels of methionine, phenylalanine, tyrosine, and glutamate, with lysine, glycine, and ornithine levels increased as well. The BCAAs in this group were not elevated but were present at normal levels or were slightly reduced (Fig. 35–6). The hyperaminoacidemia of the hepatitis group may be due to the release of amino acids into the circulation from dying hepatocytes.[15]

Coma was present in both groups of patients for a mean of five days before treatment with BCAAs. Both groups were hyperbilirubinemic, with a mean of 13 mg/100 ml for the "acute-on-chronic" patients and 25 mg/100 ml for the patients with hepatitis. Most patients had deranged coagulation patterns.

Criteria for treatment with HepatAmine included hepatic encephalopathy of Grade II or greater, gastrointestinal dysfunction necessitating parenteral nutritional support, and intolerance to commercially available amino acid formulations. The amino acid solution was administered as a 4 per cent solution with 23 per cent dextrose and was begun at a rate of 40 to 60 ml/hour. The infusion rate was increased by 10 to 20 ml/hour daily, according to tolerance, up to

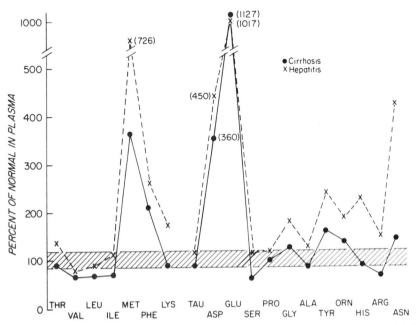

Figure 35–6. Amino acid patterns of patients with acute-on-chronic liver failure and patients with fulminant hepatitis. In the acute-on-chronic group, methionine, phenylalanine, tyrosine, glutamate, and aspartate levels are elevated, but the branched-chain amino acid levels are decreased. The patients with hepatitis show a diffuse hyperaminoacidemia with the exception of the branched-chain amino acid levels, which are normal or slightly decreased.

120 gm of amino acids and 3000 calories daily. These doses of amino acids appeared to be tolerated well.[30]

Results differed between the two patient groups, but were encouraging for both. More than half of the patients improved by at least one grade of encephalopathy (as determined by three independent observers) within 24 to 48 hours. A linear correlation between nitrogen balance and daily intake of HepatAmine was apparent, with nitrogen equilibrium occurring when 75 to 80 gm of amino acids were infused (Fig. 35–7).[30] These results are in agreement with previous studies.[31] There was no correlation between blood ammonia levels and improvement of encephalopathy.

Survival was 45 per cent in the "acute-on-chronic" group and 47 per cent for those with hepatitis. Since patients with fulminant hepatitis have a predicted mortality rate of 80 to 90 per cent from clinical events such as cerebral edema and coagulopathies, this group's survival of 47 per cent may lend support to the theory that increased protein administration improves not only hepatic function but also survival.[30]

Several anecdotal reports from other centers also show improvement in the grade of hepatic encephalopathy with administration of BCAAs.[32–35] Despite anecdotal evidence supporting the benefits of BCAA-enriched solutions, the subtlety and variability of hepatic encephalopathy make randomized prospective studies mandatory in order to prove efficacy.

Prospective Trials

A number of such trials have been reported and appear to show efficacy of BCAA-enriched solutions as compared to standard solutions.[36–39] However, the numbers of patients in various groups suggests that some patient selection was used in assigning patients to treatment groups. Therefore, the randomization is suspect.

At the time of this writing, several properly randomized prospective trials have been reported comparing BCAA therapy to standard forms of therapy. Results have been positive in those trials that have used the BCAA solutions with hypertonic dextrose as the calorie source. The results have been quite different in the two studies that have used intravenous fat emulsions to provide 50 to 70 per cent of the total calories. The stud-

ies, their results, and the possible causes for the differences will now be considered in more detail.

An Italian multicenter randomized prospective trial was completed by Rossi-Fanelli and coworkers.[40] Forty patients with "acute-on-chronic" hepatic encephalopathy or chronic recurrence of hepatic encephalopathy were randomized, with three patients in each group failing to complete the trial. Patients were entered within six hours of the onset of hepatic encephalopathy and were randomized to receive either 60 gm of BCAAs in hypertonic dextrose or isocaloric dextrose and lactulose. Coma reversed itself in 70 per cent of patients in the BCAA group but in only 49 per cent of the lactulose group. Although this represented no statistically significant difference between the groups in the number of patients studied, the trend is in favor of the BCAA group, whose pre-entry parameters suggest they were somewhat sicker than the lactulose group. There was no difference in survival.

Three other randomized prospective trials used an amino acid mixture generally based on F080, which is now HepatAmine. Another Italian trial reported by Fiaccadori randomized patients into three groups of 16 patients each.[41] The first group received conventional therapy with lactulose alone, the second group received a BCAA-enriched complete nutritional solution with hypertonic dextrose, and the third group received both lactulose and the nutritional solution. Coma reversal appeared better in both of the groups that received the BCAA-enriched solution than in the group that received lactulose alone. Five deaths occurred in the group that received lactulose as compared with one death in the BCAA group and no deaths in the group that received both the BCAA-enriched solution and lactulose. This report provides evidence that BCAA therapy may favorably influence survival in patients with acute hepatic encephalopathy.

The randomized prospective trial performed in the United States involved eight centers that contributed 80 patients, by far the largest group entered in a randomized prospective trial.[42, 43] Patients were entered into the trial if they were perceived as requiring nutritional support and if they did not respond to conventional therapy of hepatic encephalopathy within 48 hours. In this double-blind study, patients were randomized to receive either HepatAmine with hy-

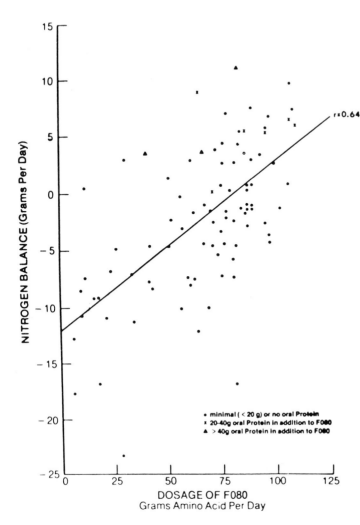

NITROGEN BALANCE VS. DOSE F080
NON-RENAL PATIENTS

r≈0.64

• minimal (< 20 g) or no oral Protein
× 20-40g oral Protein in addition to F080
▲ > 40g oral Protein in addition to F080

NITROGEN BALANCE (Grams Per Day)

DOSAGE OF F080
Grams Amino Acid Per Day

Figure 35–7. Nitrogen balance as a function of dosage of F080 (Hepat-Amine). Nitrogen equilibrium was achieved at approximately 75 gm of administered amino acids per day.

pertonic dextrose or neomycin and isocaloric hypertonic dextrose. The trial had a crossover provision for these seriously ill patients, and patients needed to complete at least 72 hours of therapy to be considered as entering the trial. Global assessment of clinical improvement was significantly better in the HepatAmine group when compared to the neomycin and isocaloric dextrose group. Coma reversal was significantly better in those who received HepatAmine, as measured clinically and electroencephalographically by several neurologists who did not know the type of treatment administered. Of note was the increased survival in the group that received nutritional support (85 per cent) as compared to the group that received neomycin (55 per cent). Deaths resulted, for the most part, from liver failure rather than from gastrointestinal bleeding or other causes.

The Brazilian randomized prospective trial, as reported by Strauss and associates, also compared HepatAmine to neomycin and isocaloric hypertonic dextrose.[44] Only 16 episodes of hepatic encephalopathy were included in each of the two groups, and it is unclear at present how patients were selected and whether they had failed to respond to conventional therapy for hepatic encephalopathy. Coma reversal was faster in the group that received HepatAmine than in the neomycin and isocaloric dextrose group. Two patients died in each group, resulting in no difference in survival.

As previously mentioned, the two trials that have failed to demonstrate the efficacy of BCAA both utilized intravenous fat as the major source of calories. In the study from Montpelier, France, reported by Michel, patients were randomized to receive a conventional amino acid solution containing 20 per cent BCAAs and a high concentration of arginine or a 35 per cent BCAA-enriched solution that contained less arginine.[45] Sixty-seven per cent of the calories were given as intravenous lipid emulsion. The duration of symptoms or time of entrance into the study remain unclear. However, the patients received little or no treatment other than amino acid solutions. No difference in the rate of awakening between the two groups was demonstrated.

A multicenter Swedish and French trial reported by Wahren and coworkers compared a treatment group that received a BCAA solution of 70 per cent leucine with smaller amounts of isoleucine and valine to a control group that received no amino acid supplementation.[46] Fifty per cent of the calories were provided as intravenous lipid emulsion. The results failed to show the efficacy of BCAAs, but the study is marred by high mortality in both treatment and control groups.

Several explanations are possible to explain the differing results obtained with the differing calorie sources. As previously mentioned, experimental evidence suggests that both phenylalanine and tryptophan are required for the production of hepatic coma.[23] Capocaccia and coworkers have demonstrated that free tryptophan levels fall when BCAAs are administered with glucose. However, when the BCAAs are administered with glucose and fat, there is no decrease, and free tryptophan levels may even increase slightly.[47] Another possible explanation involves improved BCAA utilization with glucose as compared with lipid.

In summary, the use of BCAA-enriched solutions administered with hypertonic dextrose in the treatment of hepatic encephalopathy is associated with improvement that is at least as good as conventional therapy utilizing neomycin or lactulose. When BCAA solutions are administered with fat as the major calorie source, efficacy has not been demonstrated. The cause of this discrepancy remains unclear at present.

CHRONIC ENCEPHALOPATHY

Of interest is the small but important group of patients who have chronic encephalopathy as a result of either posthepatitic changes or the presence of an end-to-side portacaval shunt. Such patients may tolerate only 20 gm of protein or less, despite conventional forms of therapy including neomycin and lactulose. Protein tolerance may be increased by the oral administration of BCAAs alone or a BCAA-enriched amino acid mixture with glucose supplied as an elemental diet (Hepatic-Aid, American McGaw Laboratories).

Prospective Trials

A randomized comparison of an elemental supplement, A662, the precursor of HepatAmine, to mixed dietary protein in protein-intolerant patients was reported by Horst and coworkers.[48] Nitrogen balance and encephalopathy were monitored carefully. The BCAA-supplemented patients achieved a positive nitrogen balance equal to that achieved from dietary mixed protein, but they had significantly less hepatic encephalopathy.

Egberts and coworkers showed similar superiority for BCAA supplementation in 22 patients with latent hepatic encephalopathy who were studied in crossover fashion.[49] The BCAAs demonstrated nutritional efficacy as well as improvement of performance in psychometric tests during BCAA administration.

Eriksson and coworkers have interpreted their data on a very small number of patients as demonstrating a negative result with BCAA administration.[50] Interpretation of the psychometric data suggests a trend toward improvement in the BCAA treatment group, which could be significant if continued in a larger group of patients.

The ketoanalogues of the BCAAs also have been found to be useful in patients with protein intolerance.[51] Recent evidence suggests that the ornithine salts of the BCAA ketoanalogues are superior to both the calcium salts of the BCAA ketoanalogues and an equivalent dose of the BCAAs.[45] However, improvement occurred following administration of either BCAA ketoanalogues or BCAA alone. The decrease in ammonia following treatment with the ornithine salts may help to explain the greater efficacy of the ornithine ketoanalogue group, since reduction of ammonia and glutamine, as well as changing the plasma concentration of the BCAAs, will have a greater effect on brain amino acids than changing plasma ratios alone. (See also Chapter 22 of Volume 1.)

SUMMARY

According to the amino acid neurotransmitter hypothesis, the patient with hepatic insufficiency initially suffers from deficient hepatic energy production and a hormonal background that favors catabolism. In the face of sustained gluconeogenesis, aromatic amino acids are released from the breakdown of skeletal muscle. In hepatic insufficiency, phenylalanine, tyrosine, tryptophan, and methionine accumulate, since their primary site of degradation is the liver. The BCAAs are consumed locally in the absence of adequate energy supplied to the periphery. The resultant amino acid pattern has increased levels of aromatic amino acid monoamine precursors and decreased levels of BCAAs. In addition, free tryptophan accumulates secondary to increased nonesterified fatty acids and decreased serum albumin.

The altered amino acid pattern results in an altered competitor ratio between aromatic amino acids and the BCAAs at the blood-brain barrier. The velocity of the transport system for these neutral amino acids appears accelerated, possibly caused by exchange for glutamine, the central nervous system metabolite of ammonia.

The result is a derangement of the neurotransmitters in the aminergic nervous system with decreased norepinephrine and striatal dopamine, and increased β-hydroxyphenylethylamines and serotonin. The imbalance in neurotransmitters leads to hepatic encephalopathy.

Therapy is aimed at returning the plasma amino acid pattern to normal. This is accomplished through the administration of BCAA-enriched solutions plus adequate calories in an attempt to promote protein synthesis, decrease catabolism, and provide competition for the aromatic amino acids at the blood-brain barrier.

The treatment of hepatic encephalopathy and the nutritional support of the patient with hepatic insufficiency remain controversial. As more randomized trials are performed, there appears to be an increasing body of evidence that shows efficacy for the use of BCAAs in the treatment of hepatic encephalopathy. The ability to modify the plasma amino acid pattern, and thereby increase the ability to administer protein to patients with hepatic insufficiency, should become an important therapeutic modality in the future.

REFERENCES

1. Bucher, N.L.R., and McGowan, J.A.: Regeneration: regulatory mechanisms. In Wright, R., Alberti, K.G.M.M., Karran, S., and Millward-Sadler, G.N. (eds.): Liver and Biliary Disease. Philadelphia: W.B. Saunders Co., 1979, pages 210–221.
2. Warren, K.S., and Schenker, S.: Effect of an inhibitor of glutamine synthesis (methionine sulfoximine) on ammonia toxicity and metabolism. J. Lab. Clin. Med., 64:442–449, 1964.
3. Dawson, A.M., and Sherlock, S.: Effect of an amine oxidase inhibitor on arterial ammonium levels of liver disease. Lancet, 1:1332–1333, 1957.
4. Hoyumpa, A.M., Desmond, P.V., Avant, G.R., Roberts, R.K., and Schenker, S.: Hepatic encephalopathy. Gastroenterology, 76:184–195, 1979.
5. Zieve, F.J., Zieve, L., Doizani, W.M., and Gilsdorf, R.B.: Synergism between ammonia and fatty acids in the production of coma. Implications for hepatic coma. J. Pharm. Exp. Ther., 191:10–16, 1974.
6. Zieve, L.: The mechanism of hepatic coma. Hepatology, 1:360–365, 1981.
7. Fischer, J.E., and Baldessarini, R.: False neurotransmitters and hepatic failure. Lancet, 2:75–80, 1971.
8. Fischer, J.E., and James, J.H.: Treatment of hepatic coma and hepatorenal syndrome: Mechanism of action of L-dopa and aramine. Am. J. Surg., 123:222–230, 1972.
9. Baldessarini, R.J., and Fischer, J.E.: Serotonin metabolism in rat brain after surgical diversion of the portal venous circulation. Nature, 245:25–27, 1973.
10. Dodsworth, J.M., James, J.H., Cummings, M.C., and Fischer, J.E.: Depletion of brain norepinephrine in acute hepatic coma. Surgery, 75:811–820, 1974.
11. Dismukes, K.: New look at the aminergic nervous system. Nature, 269:557–558, 1977.
12. Sherwin, R., Joshi, P., Hendler, R., Felig, P., and Conn, H.O.: Hyperglucagonemia in Laennec's cirrhosis: The role of portal systemic shunting. N. Engl. J. Med. 290:239–248, 1974.
13. Soeters, P.B., and Fischer, J.E.: Insulin, glucagon, amino acid imbalance and hepatic encephalopathy. Lancet, 2:880–882, 1976.
14. Eigler, N., Sacca, L., and Sherwin, R.S.: Synergistic interactions of physiologic investment of glucagon, epinephrine and cortisol in the dog. A model for stress induced hyperglycemia. J. Clin. Invest., 631:114–123, 1979.
15. Rosen, H.M., Yoshimura, N., Hodgman, J.M., and Fischer, J.E.: Plasma amino acid patterns in hepatic encephalopathy of differing etiology. Gastroenterology, 72:483–487, 1977.
16. Wade, L.A., and Katzman, R.: Synthetic amino acids and the nature of L-dopa transport at the blood-brain barrier. J. Neurochem., 25:837–842, 1975.
17. Fernstrom, J.D., and Faller, D.V.: Neutral amino acids in brain: changes in response to food ingestion. J. Neurochem., 30:1531–1538, 1978.
18. James, J.H., Escourrou, J., and Fischer, J.E.: Blood-brain neutral amino acid transport activity is increased after portacaval anastomosis. Science, 200:1395–1397, 1978.
19. Cremer, J.E., Lal, J.C., and Sarna, G.S.: Rapid blood-brain transport and metabolism of butyrate and pyruvate after portacaval anastomosis. J. Physiol. (London), 266:70P–71P, 1977.
20. James, J.H., Jeppsson, B., Ziparo, V., and Fischer,

J.E.: Hyperammonaemia, plasma amino acid imbalance, and blood-brain amino acid transport: A unified theory of portal-systemic encephalopathy. Lancet, 2:772–775, 1979.

21. Cardelli-Cangiano, P., Cangiano, C., James, J.H., Jeppsson, G., Brenner, W., and Fischer, J.E.: Uptake of amino acids by brain microvessels isolated from rats after portacaval anastomosis. J. Neurochem., 36(2):627–632, 1981.

22. Smith, A.R., Rossi-Fanelli, F., Ziparo, V., James, J.H., Perelle, B.A., and Fischer, J.E. Alterations in plasma and CSF amino acids, amines and metabolites in hepatic coma. Ann. Surg., 187:343–350, 1978.

23. Rossi-Fanelli, F., Freund, H., Krause, R., Smith, A.R., James, J.H., Castorina-Ziparo, S., and Fischer, J.E.: Induction of coma in normal dogs by the infusion of aromatic amino acids and its prevention by the addition of branched-chain amino acids. Gastroenterology, 83:664–671, 1982.

24. Zieve, L., and Olsen, R.L. Can hepatic coma be caused by a reduction of brain noradrenaline or dopamine? Gut, 18:688–691, 1977.

25. Alexander, J.W., Macmillan, B.G., Stinnett, J.D., Ogle, C.K., Bozian, R.C., Fischer, J.E., Oakes, J.B., Morris, M.J., and Krummel, R.: Beneficial effects of aggressive protein feeding in severely burned children. Ann. Surg., 192:505–517, 1980.

26. Rosen, H.M., Soeters, P.B., James, J.H., Hodgman, J., and Fischer, J.E.: Influences of exogenous intake and nitrogen balance on plasma and brain aromatic amino acid concentrations. Metabolism, 27:393–404, 1978.

27. Buse, M.G., and Reid, J.: Leucine, a possible regulator of protein turnover in muscle. J. Clin. Invest., 56:1250–1261, 1975.

28. Oddessey, R., and Goldberg, A.L.: Oxidation of leucine by rat skeletal muscle. Am. J. Physiol., 223:1376–1383, 1971.

29. Freund, H.R., James, J.H., and Fischer, J.E.: Nitrogen sparing mechanisms of singly administered branched chain amino acids in the injured rat. Surgery, 90:237–243, 1981.

30. Freund, H., Dienstag, J., Lehrick, J., Yoshimura, N., Bradford, R.R., Rosen, H., Atamian, S., Slemmer, E., Holroyde, J., and Fischer, J.E.: Infusion of branched-chain enriched amino acid solution in patients with hepatic encephalopathy. Ann. Surg., 196:209–220, 1982.

31. Fischer, J.E., Rosen, H.M., Ebeid, A.M., James, J.H., Keane, J.M., and Soeters, P.B. The effect of normalization of plasma amino acids on hepatic encephalopathy in man. Surgery, 80:77–91, 1976.

32. Bouletreau, P., Delafosse, B., Auboyer, C., Motin, J., Crotte, J., and Creyssel, R.: Role of branched-chain amino acids in the encephalopathy of patients with cirrhosis of the liver. In LeFole en Anesthesie et en Reanimation. Journées, d'enseignement post-universitaire d'anesthesie et de reanimation, Paris, 1980.

33. Streibel, J.P., Holm, E., Lutz, H., and Storz, W.: Parenteral nutrition and coma therapy with amino acids in hepatic failure. J.P.E.N., 3:240–246, 1979.

34. Okada, A., Ikeda, Y., Itakura, T., Kim, C.W., Kamata, S., and Kawashima, Y.: Treatment of hepatic encephalopathy with a new parenteral amino acid mixture (Abstract). J.P.E.N., 2:218, 1978.

35. Capocaccia, L, Calcaterra, V., Cangiano, C., Cassano, A., Fiaccadore, F., Gentile, F., Gisinelli, G.,

Pelosu, G., Riggio, O., Rossi-Fanelli, F., Sacchime, D., and Ginchi, G. Therapeutic effects of branched-chain amino acids in encephalopathy: A preliminary study. In Orloff, M.N., Stepa, S., and Ziparo, V. (eds.): Medical and Surgical Problems in Portal Hypertension. London, Academic Press, 1980, pages 239–250.

36. Rakette S, Fischer, M., Reimann, H.J., and Sommoggy, S.V.: Effects of special amino acid solutions in patients with liver cirrhosis and hepatic encephalopathy. In Walser, M., and Williamson, J.R. (eds.): Metabolism and Clinical Implications of Branched-Chain Amino and Ketoacids. New York, Elsevier-North Holland, 1981, pages 419–427.

37. Okada, A., Kamata, S., Kim, C.W., and Kawashima, Y.: Treatment of hepatic encephalopathy with BCAA-rich amino acid mixture. In Walser, M., and Williamson, J.R., (eds.): Clinical Implications of Branched-Chain Amino and Ketoacids. New York, Elsevier-North Holland, 1981, pages 447–452.

38. Egberts, E.H., Hamster, W., Jurgens, P., Schumacher, H., Fondalinski, G., Reinhard, U., and Schomerus, H. Effects of branched-chain amino acids on latent portal systemic encephalopathy. In Walser, M., and Williamson, J.R. (eds.): Metabolism and Clinical Implications of Branched-Chain Amino and Ketoacids. New York, Elsevier-North Holland, 1981, pages 453–464.

39. Holm, E., Streibel, J.P., Moller, P., and Hartmen, M.: Amino acid solutions for parenteral nutrition and for adjuvant treatment of encephalopathy in liver cirrhosis: Studies concerning 120 patients. In Walser, M., and Williamson, J.R. (eds.): Metabolism and Clinical Implications of Branched-Chain Amino and Ketoacids. New York, Elsevier-North Holland, 1981, pages 513–520.

40. Rossi-Fanelli, F., Riggio, O., Cangiano, C., Cascino, A., DeConciliis, D., Merli, M., Stortoni, M., Giunchi, G., and Capocaccia, L.: Branched-chain amino acids vs lactulose in the treatment of hepatic coma: A controlled study. Dig. Dis. Sci., 27:929–935, 1982.

41. Fiaccadori, F., Ghinelli, F., Pedretti, G., Pelosi, G., Sacchini, D., Zeneroli, M.L., Rocchi, E., Gibertini, P., and Ventura, E.: Branched-chain amino acid–enriched solutions in hepatic encephalopathy. A controlled trial. In Capocaccia, L., Fischer, J. E., and Rossi-Fanelli, F. (eds.): Hepatic Encephalopathy in Chronic Liver Failure. New York, Plenum Press, 1984, pp. 311–321.

42. Cerra, F.B., Cheung, N.K., Fischer, J.E., Kaplowitz, N., Schiff, E.R., Dienstag, J.L., Mabry, C.D., Leevy, C.M., and Kiernan, T.: A multicenter trial of branched-chain enriched amino acid infusion (F080) in hepatic encephalopathy (Abstract). Hepatology, 2:699, 1982.

43. Cerra, F.B., Cheung, N.K., Fischer, J.E., Kaplowitz, N., Schiff, E.R., Dienstag, J.L., Bower, R.H., Mabry, C.D., Leevy, C.M., and Kiernan, T.: Disease-specific amino acid infusion (F080) in hepatic encephalopathy: A prospective, randomized, double-blind controlled trial. J.P.E.N., 9:288–295, 1985.

44. Strauss, E., Santos, W.R., DaSilva, C., Lacet, C.M., Capacci, M.L.L., and Bernardini, A.P.: A randomized controlled clinical trial for the evaluation of the efficacy of a [sic] enriched branched chain

amino acid solution compared to neomycin in hepatic encephalopathy. (Abstract) Hepatology, 3:862, 1983.

45. Michel, H., Pomier-Layrargues, G., Duhamel, O., Lacombe, B., Cuilleret, G., and Bellet, H.: Intravenous infusion of ordinary and modified amino-acid solutions in the management of hepatic encephalopathy (Abstract). Gastroenterology, *79*: 1038, 1980.

46. Wahren, J.J., Denis, J., Desurmont, P. et al.: Is I.V. administration of branched-chain amino acids effective in the treatment of hepatic encephalopathy? A multicenter study. Eur. Soc. Paren. Ent. Nutr., *FC47*: 61, 1981.

47. Cangiano, C., Rossi-Fanelli, F., and Capocaccia, L.: Personal communication.

48. Horst, D., Grace, N., Conn, H.O., Schiff, E., Schenker, S., Viteri, A., Law, D., and Atterbury, C.E.: Comparison of dietary protein with an oral, branched chain-enriched amino acid supplement in chronic portal-systemic encephalopathy: a ran-domized controlled trial. Hepatology, 4:279–287, 1984.

49. Egberts, E.H., Schomerus, H., Hamster, W., and Jurgens, P.: Effective treatment of latent portosystemic encephalopathy with oral branched chain amino acids. *In* Capocaccia, L., Fischer, J.E., and Rossi-Fanelli, F. (eds.): Hepatic Encephalopathy in Chronic Liver Failure. New York, Plenum Press, 1984, pp. 351–357.

50. Eriksson, L.S., Persson, A., and Wahren, J.: Branched chain amino acids in the treatment of chronic hepatic encephalopathy. Gut, *23*:801–806, 1982.

51. Maddrey, W.C., Weber, F.L., Coulter, A.W., and Walser, M.: Effects of ketoanalogues of the essential amino acids in portal systemic encephalopathy. Gastroenterology, *71*:190–195, 1976.

52. Herlong, H.F., Maddrey, W.C., and Walser, M.: The use of ornithine salts of branched-chain ketoacids in portal-systemic encephalopathy. Ann. Intern. Med., *93*:545–550, 1980.

CHAPTER 36

Parenteral Nutrition in Pregnancy

MAUREEN MacBURNEY
DOUGLAS W. WILMORE

Since the introduction of parenteral nutrition by central vein infusion 18 years ago, application of this technique has expanded to patients with a wide variety of diseases. Pregnant women are uncommon candidates for intravenous feedings, but, when indicated, parenteral nutrition may be life-saving for both mother and child. The solution should be specifically formulated to satisfy the nutrient requirements of the pregnant woman in order to optimize normal growth and development of the fetus and to minimize potential complications. Because limited knowledge is available in this area, only general guidelines and recommendations can be made at this time. These guidelines are based on information on normal maternal nutrition reported in the literature and our personal experiences in caring for pregnant women. Safe parenteral nutrition can be provided to the pregnant woman so that nutritional deficits will not compromise the outcome for the mother and child.

NUTRITION AND NORMAL PREGNANCY

Nutrition may have a major impact on fetal outcome. Factors such as pre-pregnancy weight, weight gain during pregnancy, pre-pregnancy nutritional status, multiparity, and birth spacing are all known to influence maternal weight gain and fetal survival.[1] In general, a successful outcome can be predicted if the woman weighs at least 45 kg (100 lbs.), is within 10 per cent of her ideal body weight,[2] and is normally nourished at the time of conception. Moreover, the woman should gain approximately 12.5 kg (25 lbs.) throughout the 40 weeks of gestation.[3] The spacing of births in a multiparous woman should be at least one year apart for optimal growth of the infant and adequate repletion of maternal stores.[4]

Weight gain throughout pregnancy is the most important indicator of the adequacy of nutritional state of mother and child. During the first trimester, a weight gain of one to two kilograms (two to five pounds) is generally expected. In the second and third trimesters, a gain of 0.34 to 0.5 kg (0.5 to 1.0 lb) per week has been associated with a normal fetal outcome. The calories required to achieve such weight gain throughout the entire pregnancy have been estimated at approximately 84,000 kcal, which represent the Recommended Dietary Allowances (RDA) for normal women, plus an additional 300 calories per day for each day of pregnancy.[5] Weight gain by the mother is not entirely new tissue, but also represents increases in extracellular fluid, a rise in blood volume, and accumulation of amniotic fluid. The total increase in maternal weight during pregnancy has been partitioned by Pitkin, who has detailed the pattern and components of gestational weight gain.[6] If total weight gain at term is assumed to be 12.5 kg, the maternal components represent approximately 7 kg (15 lb), and the fetal compartment represents about 5.5 kg (12 lb). Although the rate of weight gain of the woman is similar in the last two trimesters, accumulations in the maternal and fetal compartments vary with the duration of pregnancy. During the second trimester, weight gain reflects increases in maternal components, represented by blood volume expansion, growth of the uterus and breasts, and fat storage. By contrast, the third-trimester gain mostly involves growth of the fetus and placenta and an increase in amniotic fluid; maternal tissues and fluids increase to a much smaller degree. Maternal fat stores increase during pregnancy; the average gain is approximately three kilograms (7 lb), but this quantity is highly variable. The amount of protein gained during pregnancy, calculated from nitrogen measurements of the fetus, placenta, and expanded maternal components, amounts to slightly less than one kilogram (2 lb), and whether protein is also stored in maternal liver and skeletal muscle remains controversial.[7, 8] Protein needs can be satisfied by consuming a normal, balanced diet for women plus 30 grams more of protein per day, or approximately 1.3 to 1.7 gm of protein per kg of body weight per day. Additional requirements for vitamins, folic acid, calcium, phosphate, zinc, iron, and magnesium occur during pregnancy, as outlined in the RDA.[5]

MALNUTRITION AND INFANT OUTCOME

Frisch[9] has correlated the relationship between body fat and fecundity and has emphasized that women with minimal body fat stores (or undernourished women) have reduced menstrual periods, ovulate less, and often are unable to conceive. When conception does occur and maternal malnutrition is present, there is a high incidence of fetal demise. If the infant survives, there is an increased probability that the baby will be below normal birth weight.[10] Decreased numbers of brain cells[11] and other congenital anomalies have been associated with poor nutritional status in the first trimester. The relationship to specific nutrient deficits in maternal nutrition has not been clearly established in humans. However, neural tube defects may be associated with subclinical deficiencies of various vitamins and minerals.[12] Maternal iron deficiency has been linked to the development of iron deficiency anemia in the first year of life.[13] Low concentrations of folic acid in the maternal blood have been correlated with reduced birth weight and congenital malformations.[14, 15] Zinc deficiency may cause fetal growth retardation and multiple congenital anomalies.[16–18] Calcium and vitamin D deficiencies may be related in part to neonatal hypocalcemia and rickets.[19] Asymptomatic maternal thiamine deficiency

may cause fatal heart failure in the newborn, i.e., congenital beri beri.[20] All of these examples emphasize that the parasitic capacity of the fetus is limited; maintenance of normal nutrition by the mother is extremely important for the fetus.

During the latter half of pregnancy, the fetus grows rapidly. Malnutrition late in pregnancy may result in increased incidences of prematurity, low birth weight (LBW; less than 2500 gm), and small-for-gestational-age (SGA) infants, and an underdeveloped fetal central nervous system characterized by a decreased brain cell size.[11, 21–23] It is generally believed that nutritional repletion of pregnant women during the second trimester will increase birth weight. However, nutritional intervention studies in large populations have not always improved fetal outcome.[24] The etiology of these discrepancies is not entirely clear. A variety of factors, including patient compliance, affect the results of nutritional intervention trials. Such discrepancies in intervention studies should not lessen the importance of providing adequate nutrition to an individual pregnant woman.

NUTRITIONAL ASSESSMENT IN PREGNANCY

The best assessment of nutritional adequacy during an otherwise normal pregnancy is the health and birth weight of an infant. However, there are few direct measurements available during the pregnancy to assess fetal health. Standards of assessing nutritional status in a nonpregnant woman cannot be used for interpreting data during pregnancy. The normal physiologic changes associated with pregnancy must be considered when nutritional assessments are performed.

Maternal Weight and Weight Gain

Next to a history of LBW infants, low pre-pregnant weight and weight gain during pregnancy are the most significant factors contributing to the development of growth-retarded infants and are the most direct measurements available to predict fetal growth. Birth weight is positively associated with total weight gain in pregnancy, and as birth weight increases to an optimum of 3,400 gm, neonatal morbidity and mortality decrease. Total maternal weight gain below 6.5

kg (14 lbs) should be regarded as weight loss, because the products of conception—the fetus and placenta, amniotic fluid, increased blood volume, and increased weight of the uterus—represent this amount of weight. Thus, with weight gain below this amount, the mother is losing weight from her body tissues and drawing on her own stores of nutrients to nourish the fetus.[25, 26] In marginally nutritionally deficient women, such as growing teenagers, and the chronically or acutely ill, such as women with diabetes, inflammatory bowel disease, or hyperemesis gravidarum, the continuous drain on nutrient stores may seriously compromise both mother and fetus.

Except in the very obese, a total weight gain of less than five kilograms (11 lbs) or gains of less than 0.5 lb per week during the second half of pregnancy, may be detrimental to fetal outcome.[1, 25, 27] In this group of gravidas, the overall incidence of LBW infants is doubled. This finding is significant, since two-thirds of all neonatal deaths occur among LBW infants.[1] The frequency of perinatal deaths and prematurity diminishes as maternal weight gain increases, up to approximately 15 kg (30 lbs). Weight gain beyond this point does not exert any further beneficial effect.[3, 25, 27]

In addition to weight gain during pregnancy, pre-pregnant weight influences infant outcome. Both factors emphasize the importance of maternal body mass on fetal growth. Gravidas with a low pre-pregnancy weight, that is, less than 54.5 kilograms (120 lbs), are at greatest risk for producing a LBW infant. The incidence of LBW infants in this setting continues to increase as pre-pregnancy weight drops below 45.4 kg (100 lbs). Alternately, the impact of inadequate weight gain on fetal outcome may be tempered if maternal pre-pregnancy weight is greater than 54.5

kilograms (120 lbs).[1, 25, 27] It may be that maternal body mass *per se* is more important than absolute weight gain. For example, Eastman and Jackson[25] found that minimal weight gain (less than 4 kg or 8.8 lb) in women who weighed more than 73 kg (160 lbs), resulted in an incidence of LBW babies of only 2.3 per cent. In contrast, women who weighed less than 54.5 kilograms (120 lbs) and gained less than four kilograms had 2.5 times this incidence of LBW infants. However, the overall importance of weight gain during pregnancy should not be underemphasized; in the same study, women who gained less than four kilograms had the highest incidence of LBW infants regardless of their initial body weight. These results have recently been supported by the data of van den Berg (Table 36–1).[1]

In summary, then, short-term total starvation or semi-starvation in a normally nourished pregnant woman provides minimal nutritional stress on the fetus in the first trimester, whereas more extensive deficits, particularly in the latter half of pregnancy, limit infant growth and the development of full genetic potential.

Total maternal body mass, not weight gain alone, may influence fetal growth. Therefore, the fetus of a "lightweight" mother is at greater risk than the fetus of a heavier woman if a feeding problem arises.

Laboratory Assessment

Standard biochemical indices for non-pregnant women are frequently not applicable in pregnancy. Accurate interpretation of laboratory data depends upon a thorough knowledge of the normal physiologic changes associated with pregnancy as well as variations due to laboratory methodology,

Table 36–1. INFLUENCE OF MATERNAL PRE-PREGNANCY WEIGHT AND WEIGHT GAIN ON BIRTH WEIGHT

PRE-PREGNANCY WEIGHT (LBS)	INFANTS <2500 gm (%)		
	Weekly Gain* <0.5 lb	*Weekly Gain* 0.5 to <1.0 lb*	*Weekly Gain* 1.0 lb or more*
<110	14.1	7.8	5.8
110 to <125	8.9	4.2	3.7
125 to <140	5.8	3.6	3.0
140 to <155	4.9	1.8	2.4
155 or more	5.8	1.4	1.6

*After 20 weeks gestation.
(Adapted from van den Berg, B. J.: Maternal variables affecting fetal growth. Am. J. Clin. Nutr., 34:722–726, 1981.)

measurement techniques, and institutional norms. Misinterpretations of these changes may result in misdiagnosis of malnutrition or inappropriate nutritional intervention. Specific criteria for deficiency states in pregnancy are scanty. However, estimates can be made from some selected population studies (Table 36–2).

Two laboratory values frequently used in nutritional assessment are albumin and total iron-binding capacity (TIBC), which reflects serum transferrin levels. In normal pregnancy, serum albumin concentrations fall abruptly in the first trimester, then decline more gradually until weeks 24 to 28, after which there is little change. The total decline in albumin concentration is approximately 1 gm/100 ml.[3, 7, 30]

Serum TIBC levels gradually increase throughout gestation, peaking during the last trimester. This phenomenon occurs regardless of concomitant iron therapy, although the increase is less pronounced in women receiving iron supplements. Normal TIBC in the nonpregnant woman ranges between 250 and 400 μg/100 ml; by the third trimester it may be increased to 500 to 800 μg/100 ml. TIBC levels in iron-supplemented women may increase to 300 to 600 μg/100 ml.[7, 31, 32] An elevated TIBC should not be mistaken for iron deficiency. Women not receiving an iron supplement generally demonstrate a gradual decrease in serum iron during the course of pregnancy, with a concurrent rise in TIBC. The combined effect of decreasing serum iron and the normal rise in transferrin in pregnancy must be evaluated carefully for an accurate diagnosis of iron deficiency. In pregnancy, the most sensitive indicator of iron deficiency is bone marrow iron stores. However, transferrin saturation of 16 per cent or a serum iron level below 60 or 70 μg/100 ml is considered indicative of iron deficiency in pregnancy.[3, 7, 32] Carr[33] demonstrated increases in hemoglobin and transferrin saturation after iron therapy was given to women with less than 20 per cent transferrin saturation. The National Research Council (NRC)[7] therefore recommends maintaining transferrin saturation at greater than 20 per cent.

A depressed TIBC may be due to disease states, such as inflammatory bowel disease and chronic infection. It has been suggested that patients with TIBC of less than 350 μg/100 ml and transferrin saturation of less than 20 per cent be evaluated carefully for other causes of anemia and low transferrin levels.[33]

Other biochemical alterations that commonly occur in pregnancy are fasting hypoglycemia and postprandial hyperglycemia. Fasting blood glucose begins to decrease in

Table 36–2. LABORATORY ASSESSMENT OF NUTRITIONAL STATUS

LABORATORY TEST	NORMAL VALUES*		FINDINGS IN DEFICIENCY STATUS (Pregnant)
	Nonpregnant	*Pregnant*	
Urinary acetone	Negative	Faint positive in A.M.	Positive
Serum total protein (gm/100 ml)	6.5–8.5	6.8	<6[28]
Serum albumin (gm/100 ml)	3.5–5	2.5–4.5[30, 7]	<3.5[28]
Blood urea nitrogen (mg/100 ml)	10–25	5–15	<5
Fasting blood sugar (mg/100 ml)	70–110	65–100[7]	<65[7]
Two-hour postprandial blood sugar (mg/100 ml)	<110	≤120 (plasma)[7]	>120[7]
Serum calcium (mEq/L)	4.6–5.5	4.2–5.2	<4.2 or normal
Serum phosphate (mg/100 ml)	2.5–4.8	2.3–4.6	No change
Alkaline phosphatase (IU/L)	35–48	35–150	No change
Cholesterol (mg/100 ml)	120–290	177–345[7, 37]	—
Triglycerides (mg/100 ml)	33–166	130–400[7, 37]	—
Folic acid (serum) (ng/ml)	5–21	4–14	<4
Vitamin B_{12} (pg/ml)	430–1025	Decreased	Decreased
Hgb	12	>11	<11[28]
Hct	36	33	33
Serum Fe (μg/100 ml)	>50	>60	<60
TIBC (μg/100 ml)	250–400	300–600	<450
% TIBC saturation	30	≥20[7, 32]	<16[7, 32]
Serum zinc (μg/100 ml)	65–115	55–80	±50[29]
Urinary zinc (μg/day)	200–450	200–450	±150[29]

*Superscript numbers indicate chapter references.

(Adapted from Aubrey, R. H., Roberts, A., and Cuenca, V. G.: The assessment of maternal nutrition. Clin. Perinatol., 2:207–219, 1975.)

the first trimester and progresses with advancing gestation. Alternatively, pregnant women demonstrate impaired glucose tolerance on oral glucose tolerance tests, which becomes more pronounced as term approaches.[34–36] Although these changes may be quantified, they frequently fall within the normal range for glucose tolerance.

Hyperlipidemia is also characteristic of pregnancy. The most marked increase observed is the serum triglyceride level, which may be 250 to 400 per cent above normal. Cholesterol and phospholipids each increase an average of 25 per cent but may increase as much as 140 to 180 per cent. These increases in lipids begin at the end of the first trimester and rise progressively until they peak at or just prior to labor. Increases in free fatty acids begin late in the second trimester, reaching maximum levels (up to 200 per cent) at term. Complications associated with hyperlipidemia in pregnancy are rare and appear to have no long-term effects on maternal health.[7, 37]

Biochemical Assessment of Vitamins

Generally, plasma levels of fat-soluble vitamins tend to increase during pregnancy in association with the elevated lipid components. Many water-soluble vitamins demonstrate a decrease in blood levels. The data on normal vitamin metabolism in pregnancy are scarce, and most are subject to the influences of recent dietary intake, vitamin intake, age, parity, season of the year, smoking, sociologic status, and drug-nutrient interactions.

Ascorbic Acid. Plasma levels of vitamin C decline ten to 15 per cent during pregnancy, even in conjunction with vitamin C supplementation.[3, 7] Concentrations at term may be one-half those measured at midpregnancy. There are no generally recognized effects of vitamin C deficiency in pregnancy. However, isolated reports have raised questions regarding low plasma levels of vitamin C and premature rupture of membranes and pre-eclampsia.[38, 39]

Thiamine (B_1). Urinary thiamine excretion decreases during the second and third trimesters. The most pronounced effect occurs during the third trimester, which may reflect an increase in metabolic requirements. Erythrocyte transketolase assay is a more sensitive indicator of thiamine status. An erythrocyte transketolase stimulation of less than 15 per cent is considered to reflect adequate thiamine stores.[7] In a study by Heller and associates,[40] there was no correlation between thiamine status and pregnancy outcome despite a 25 to 30 per cent incidence of thiamine deficiency when judged by nonpregnant standards.

Riboflavin. Urinary excretion of riboflavin increases during the second trimester and decreases in the third trimester. Erythrocyte glutathione reductase activity, a functional parameter of riboflavin status, is comparable in normal pregnant and nonpregnant women.[7]

Niacin. Niacin status is assessed by measurement of the metabolites of nicotinic acid. Urinary excretion of one of these metabolites, N-methyl-nicotinamide, has been observed to increase gradually in the second trimester and to reach a plateau during the third trimester.[7]

Vitamin B_6. Pregnant women often demonstrate biochemical evidence of B_6 deficiency when judged by normal standards for nonpregnant females. During pregnancy, urinary xanthurenic acid excretion following a test dose of tryptophan increases steadily during gestation and by term may be several times higher than that observed in nonpregnant women. A decline in plasma levels of pyridoxal phosphate in serum and blood has also been observed during pregnancy. These changes are generally regarded as a physiologic adjustment to pregnancy; however, a true maternal deficiency state, due to fetal vitamin consumption, may be superimposed upon these "physiologic" alterations; these changes usually occur in late pregnancy.[7, 41]

Vitamin B_{12}. Vitamin B_{12} levels decrease during pregnancy, independent of B_{12} supplementation. Decreases in concentration of approximately 100 pg/ml have been observed. Some of the decrease may be accounted for by depletion of maternal stores; however, it is believed that a large part of the decline is due to changes in B_{12} metabolism.[7, 3] B_{12} levels are also lower in cigarette smokers at all stages of pregnancy.[42]

Folate. Serum folate levels typically fall during pregnancy, especially during the third trimester, and plasma levels at term may be one-half pre-pregnant values. The decrease is most likely due to increased demand for the nutrient.[3, 7] Megaloblastic anemia secondary to folate deficiency occurs most frequently in pregnant women. Those at highest risk for developing folate-induced megaloblastic anemia (1) have low serum or red blood folate levels at the start of pregnancy, (2) have chronic hemolytic states, (3) have tropical sprue or other malabsorption states, (4) are multigravidas, or (5) are receiving anticonvulsant drugs.[43] Folate status should always be assessed in conjunction with vitamin B_{12} measurements.

Vitamin E. Serum tocopherol levels may rise 40 to 60 per cent, starting in the second trimester. This increase is probably related to the elevation in lipid fractions observed in pregnancy.[3, 7]

Vitamin K. Normalization of prothrombin time following vitamin K administration is the best assessment of vitamin K deficiency. Deficiency is rare but may occur in fat malabsorption states, with prolonged antibiotic therapy, or during parenteral nutrition without vitamin K supplementation.[7]

Vitamin A. Serum vitamin A levels tend to decrease early in the first trimester, then gradually increase through later pregnancy.[7] However, reports regarding the specific changes in vitamin A are conflicting. In a recent study by Wallingford and colleagues,[44] no significant differences were found in serum retinol from the tenth to the 33rd week of pregnancy; however, there was a significant increase in amniotic fluid retinol concentration after the 20th week of gestation over that in weeks 16 to 18. Vitamin A toxicity is probably a greater concern in pregnancy; megadoses (greater than 6,000 IU daily) should be avoided.[45]

Vitamin D. Serum levels of 25-hydroxycholecalciferol are basically unchanged in pregnancy, although other factors, such as ethnic and racial background, dietary practices, and season of the year, may cause variations in concentration. Serum alkaline phosphatase levels typically increase with vitamin D deficiency, but these changes should be interpreted with caution in the pregnant woman. Late in pregnancy, serum alkaline phosphatase may rise because of the increased production of placental alkaline phosphatase.[7]

Mineral Assessment

Serum calcium, magnesium, and phosphate all decline during gestation. Serum calcium declines two to ten per cent below pre-pregnant values. This decline occurs in conjunction with a decline in serum proteins and therefore is believed to reflect a decline in bound calcium due to hemodilution. Serum magnesium levels decline seven to 12 per cent below pre-pregnant values. Serum phosphate declines during gestation, although increases may be noted near term.[3, 7]

Trace Element Assessment

Zinc. Several studies indicate that the quantity of zinc consumed by many healthy pregnant women is well below the RDA of 20 mg/day.[29, 46] In one study by Hambridge and coworkers,[18] the dietary zinc intake in the supplemented and unsupplemented groups averaged 11.3 and 10.6 mg/day, respectively, or about 56 per cent of the RDA.[18]

Plasma zinc begins to decline as early as the middle of the first trimester and continues to do so throughout gestation.[7, 18, 46, 47] Even with adequate supplementation, zinc levels drop 20 to 25 per cent below pre-pregnant levels.[7, 18, 29, 47, 48] It has been proposed that this drop is due to increases in blood volume, endogenous estrogens, or fetal needs or the decrease in albumin. However, the decline observed in early pregnancy cannot be attributed to these events, which are more apparent later in pregnancy.[7, 18, 47]

Hambridge and coworkers[18] suggest that standards for plasma zinc levels be established for each month of gestation. Current recommendations are to maintain plasma zinc at 50 μg/100 ml or higher.[7, 29]

Other disease states that are associated with low serum zinc levels but often include no symptoms of zinc deficiency are acute and chronic infections, hypoalbuminemia, endocrine disorders, Crohn's disease, fibrocystic disease with proteinuria, and short bowel syndrome.[7, 49]

Copper. Serum copper level increases progressively during pregnancy, and the rise parallels increasing concentrations of ceruloplasmin, the copper-binding protein. Increases of 1.5 to four times pre-pregnancy levels have been observed.[7, 47] It is speculated that the rise is due to the effects of increased estrogen and progesterone.[41, 47]

Low serum copper levels have been associated with placental insufficiency and intrauterine death.[50] In this setting, however, serum levels do not fall below normal pre-pregnancy levels. The NRC[7] therefore suggests that in the absence of hypoproteinemia, serum levels below the normal range for nonpregnant women are indicative of copper deficiency or abnormal copper metabolism.

Hambridge and Droegemueller[47] studied serum copper levels in 20 well-nourished pregnant women at 16 and 38 weeks' gestation (average). Serum copper levels were above the normal controls (107.4 μg/100 ml) at 16 weeks and increased significantly from 162.4 μg/100 ml at 16 weeks to 192.1 μg/100 ml at 38 weeks, an increase of one to five times normal levels.[47]

Chromium. The importance of chromium in fetal development is not known, although it is present in the human fetus.[49] Hair chromium levels appear to be dependent upon chromium intake, and it is suggested that an acceptable level for hair chromium content in pregnancy is the same as for the nonpregnant woman.[7]

Hambridge and Rodgerson[51] found significantly lower hair chromium levels in parous women than in nulliparous women.[51] In another study, hair chromium levels were decreased but not to significant levels; in the same study, fasting plasma chromium concentrations were the same for nonpregnant women and at 16 and 38 weeks' gestation.[47] Decreases in plasma chromium probably reflect inadequate chromium intake; however, criteria for the biochemical measurement of chromium stores have not been established for routine application.[7]

Manganese. Plasma and hair manganese levels showed minimal variation during pregnancy; however, it is not known whether either of these measurements is a valid index of manganese status.[7, 47]

Iodine. Iodine metabolism is altered as a result of the pregnancy state. Plasma inorganic iodide (PII) and thyroid clearance rates normally diagnostic of iodine deficiency are considered normal in pregnancy. This alteration is due to the increased renal clearance of iodine, which results in a decrease in PII level and an increase in the thyroid clearance of iodine to two to three times above normal in order to achieve a normal uptake of iodine by the thyroid. However, radioiodine studies should not be performed in the pregnant woman owing to the risk of radiation to the fetal thyroid.[7]

Both T_3 and T_4 levels are elevated in pregnancy. Low levels of T_3 and free T_4 may be applicable in the diagnosis of iodine deficiency in pregnancy.[7]

NUTRITIONAL GOALS IN PREGNANCY

Satisfying Nutritional Requirements by Central Venous Feedings

After a careful evaluation of a patient, every attempt should be made to provide nutrient intake by enteral feedings, whether this be through dietary counseling and the provision of food supplements or via the insertion of a nasogastric tube and the initiation of tube feedings. Most often, the patient is referred to a nutrition support service because of failure of standard nutritional intervention. The patient usually presents with failure of weight gain or with weight loss associated with the pregnancy. After initial nutritional assessment, a decision is made by the patient, family, and obstetrician in conjunction with the nutrition support service as to the institution of parenteral feedings. This decision is based on the assessment of the risk of undernutrition to infant and mother, maternal health, and maternal disease state. Once the decision has been made to initiate parenteral feedings, the nutritional goals should be:

1. To achieve a normal rate of weight gain. This goal can be modified according to the overall body size of the mother and is not necessarily directed toward achieving a 20 per cent gain over pre-pregnancy weight, unless the mother was below her ideal body weight at the start of the pregnancy.

2. To attain positive nitrogen balance. This goal has been achieved in all patients studied provided the recommended calorie and nitrogen allowances were given. Positive nitrogen balance is associated with the accrual of nitrogen by the fetal-placental unit in addition to the maintenance of an expanded blood volume of the mother.

3. To provide safe and effective vitamin and mineral therapy. Although precise recommendations for parenteral administration are not known, the adaptation of the requirements for pregnant women from the RDA appears to be satisfactory (see Tables 36–3 and 36–4).

4. To avoid metabolic complications. Metabolic complications are minimized when blood levels are frequently monitored and concentrations of the nutrients in the parenteral solution are adjusted appropriately. It should be remembered, however, that blood volume and plasma concentrations have been

altered by the pregnancy. The goal is to achieve levels appropriate for normal pregnancy, not levels associated with laboratory values observed in nonpregnant women.

5. To avoid sepsis. Meticulous care of the catheter entrance site and standard central vein nutritional protocols will achieve this goal.

Meeting Nutritional Goals

Energy

In order to achieve these goals, central vein nutrition should be instituted. Peripheral venous feedings are possible in some patients, particularly when supplementing enteral feedings. However, in a standard volume of 2.5 L administered per day, only 1700 calories can usually be provided (using two liters of ten per cent dextrose mixed with amino acids and 0.5 L of 20 per cent fat emulsion). In addition to being an inadequate quantity of calories to meet requirements for pregnancy, this intravenous feeding program places undue reliance on fat emulsion as the calorie source. The administration of large quantities of fat emulsion may exacerbate the hyperlipidemia associated with pregnancy, cause premature contractions, and induce labor (see "Complications"). We have, there-

Table 36–4. DAILY MINERAL AND TRACE ELEMENT REQUIREMENTS IN NORMAL PREGNANCY

MINERAL	ENTERAL NUTRITION	PARENTERAL NUTRITION*
Calcium	1200 mg	250 mg
Phosphorus	1200 mg (38 mM)	30–45 mM
Magnesium	450 mg (37.5 mEq)	10–15 mEq
Zinc	20 mg	2.55–3.0 mg[62]
Copper	2.0–3.0 mg†	.5–1.5 mg[64]
Manganese	2.5–5.0 mg†	.15–0.8 mg[64]
Iodine	175 μg	
Selenium	0.05–0.2 mg†	20–40 μg‡
Iron	10 + 30–60 mg supplemental iron	3–6 mg
Chromium	0.05–0.2 mg†	10–15 μg

*Superscript numbers indicate chapter references.
†Estimated safe and adequate daily dietary intakes in nonpregnant adults.[5]
‡Recommended intravenous dose for stable adults.

fore, relied on central vein administration of approximately two liters of hypertonic dextrose solution formulated in the hospital's manufacturing pharmacy by combining 0.5 L of 50 per cent glucose with 0.5 L of 8.5 per cent amino acid solution. Fat emulsion (0.5 L, 10 per cent) is given daily, if tolerated by the patient. This regimen provides approximately 2585 calories and 85 grams of protein per day (Table 36–5).

Amino Acids

Protein requirements for pregnancy can be achieved by using the available commercial amino acid preparations; however, the most appropriate amino acid profile is as yet undetermined.

Normal pregnancy is usually associated with hypoaminoacidemia. The maternal-fetal transfer of amino acids occurs against a concentration gradient from low maternal levels to higher fetal concentrations. Maternal hypoaminoacidemia is probably due to elevations in circulating estrogen and progesterone.[52] Although urinary excretion of amino acids increases during pregnancy, the pattern of excretion has not been related to plasma levels, biochemical structure, or physiologic function.[53] The higher fetal concentrations of amino acids may support the rapid rates of amino acid turnover in fetal tissues.[52]

Schoengold and associates[54] measured plasma amino acid concentrations during normal pregnancies and found that most of the changes occur by the end of the first

Table 36–3. DAILY REQUIREMENTS IN NORMAL PREGNANCY COMPARED WITH A STANDARD INTRAVENOUS VITAMIN PREPARATION

VITAMIN	RDA	MVI-12
A	1000 μg RE	3,300 IU (retinol)*
D	400 IU (10 μg cholecalciferol)	200 IU†
E (di-alpha-tocopheryl acetate)	10 mg α-TE	10 IU*
Ascorbic acid	20 mg	100 mg
Thiamine (B₁)	1.4 mg	3.0 mg
Riboflavin (B₂)	1.5 mg	3.6 mg
Pyridoxine (B₆)	2.6 mg	4.0 mg
Niacin	15 mg	40.0 mg
Pantothenic acid	4–7 mg‡	15.0 mg
Biotin	100–200 μg‡	60 μg
Folic acid	800 μg	400 μg†
B₁₂	4.0 μg	5 μg
K	0.03–1.5 μg/kg (RDA)	—‖

*Equivalent to RDA.
†Requires additional supplementation.
‡Estimated safe and adequate daily dietary intakes in nonpregnant adults (RDA).
‖Must be added to standard vitamin regimens.

Table 36–5. RECOMMENDED PARENTERAL NUTRITION REGIMEN IN NORMAL PREGNANCY*

	CONTENT (GM)	CALORIES	% OF CALORIES
Carbohydrate	500	1700	66
Fat	50	550	21
Nitrogen (85 gm protein)	13.4	335	13
Total		2585	100

*α L daily, each containing 0.5 L of 8.5% amino acid solution and 0.5 L of 50 per cent glucose solution in a hypertonic dextrose solution, plus 0.5 L of a 10% fat emulsion (if tolerated).

trimester and that concentrations return to normal by eight weeks postpartum. "Normal" amino acid concentrations must be interpreted with care, however, because many investigators report large inter- and intra-individual variations.

Amino acids reach the fetus only by active transport across the placental membrane.[52, 55] The fetus depends upon the maternal plasma pool for some nonessential amino acids until the intermediary pathways for their production are developed. This appears to be the case for the amino acids cystine and tyrosine. Fetal enzymes that synthesize the amino acids develop at different stages of gestation, depending upon the species studied.[52]

Rates of placental transport of amino acids may vary, and transport of a specific amino acid may be inhibited by high concentrations of similar amino acids competing for specific transport sites.[55]

Moghissi and colleagues[56] observed that concentrations of some maternal proteins and amino acids in the third trimester correlated significantly with fetal growth and development and that specific amino acids may affect different developmental parameters, such as birth weight, cranial volume, and mental and motor developments. They suggest that dietary deficiencies and excesses of some amino acids may have deleterious effects on the growth of the fetus and on the functional capacity of the brain.

The amino acid formulation used in pregnancy should be selected to avoid excess concentrations and deficiencies. The solution we use in pregnant women is the same as the one we use for the premature infant (Aminosyn). This solution is lower in phenylalanine and glycine than most other formulations, with a suitable ratio of essential to nonessential amino acids. Another product recently introduced to the market, Novamine, may be suitable for use in pregnancy also because it has a nearly complete profile of nonessential amino acids as well as essential amino acids.

Essential Fatty Acids

Essential fatty acids are required by both mother and fetus. They are important for normal fetal lipid development and prostaglandin synthesis.

Within the brain, 50 to 60 per cent of the solid matter is structural lipid (phospholipids and cholesterol) and 20 to 25 per cent of the fatty acids are long-chain derivatives of linoleic and α-linolenic acids. The most active period for the incorporation of the long-chain derivatives of essential fatty acids is during fetal growth and cell division.[57] It has been demonstrated in animal studies that extreme dietary deprivation of essential fatty acids during brain growth may reduce total brain lipid content and impair learning ability.[58, 59]

The second important function of essential fatty acids in fetal development is their role as precursors of prostaglandin synthesis. The most important prostaglandins are those derived from arachidonic acid, which can be obtained directly from the diet or by formation from its precursor, linoleic acid.[60]

The pharmacologic properties of prostaglandins in pregnancy are: (1) placental endocrine function; (2) regulation of uterine and placental blood flow; (3) bronchial dilatation; (4) vasodilatation; (5) lipolysis; (6) prevention of progesterone release by the ovary; and (7) stimulation of contractions of uterine and other smooth muscles.

Prostaglandins may influence fetal development by regulating the supply of substrate to the placenta and fetus through their effects on uterine and placental bloodflow. The local production of prostaglandins in various fetal organs, as determined by changes in synthetic and catabolic activity, may regulate the differentiation and/or development of an organ. Finally, through the effects of prostaglandins on endocrine functions, alterations in the production of those hormones known to influence fetal development may occur.[60]

Prostaglandin synthesis may be inhibited by chronic treatment with indomethacin, which prevents formation of prostaglandins from fatty acid precursors, or by a diet deficient in essential fatty acids. Clinical examples indicate that the inhibition of prostaglandin synthesis may adversely affect human fetal circulation. *In utero* constriction of the ductus arteriosus results in fetal hypertension, which is the most frequently noted clinical symptom in infants exposed *in utero* to inhibitors of prostaglandin synthesis.[60]

The total gain in essential fatty acids by mother and fetus represents approximately 600 to 650 gm, which in terms of energy represents an increase of one per cent of dietary energy over the nonpregnant state. When the low rate of conversion from linoleic acid and α-linolenic acid to their long-chain polyunsaturated fatty acids is accounted for, an additional 0.5 per cent is required.

These increases, added to normal requirements for essential fatty acids (three per cent of dietary energy), equal an intake of 4.5 per cent of dietary energy required from essential fatty acids to maintain essential fatty acid status without depleting maternal stores.[57]

It has been demonstrated that after fat infusions, free fatty acids and triglycerides appear in the fetal blood and are taken up by the fetus. All or part of the increased placental flow of triglycerides and free fatty acids are derived from the emulsion. However, the mechanism by which triglycerides appear in fetal blood is not known. The emulsion may be hydrolyzed by lipase and re-esterified or it may cross the placenta intact.[61]

In general, fat emulsion is provided daily, starting with small aliquots, with gradual increases so that eventually approximately 20 per cent of the calories are provided via fat emulsion. This quantity may be increased to 30 to 40 per cent if tolerated by the patient. Because the role of linolenic acid in parenteral nutrition in pregnancy is not defined, we recommend utilizing fat emulsions that contain both linoleic and linolenic

acid. To avoid complications, the recommended infusion rate is half of the normal maximum rate allowed in nonpregnant adults, i.e., 10 per cent emulsion at 60/ml/hr maximum.

Vitamins, Minerals, and Trace Elements

Vitamin and some mineral requirements in normal pregnancy are well established. Intravenous administration may alter requirements, because the gastrointestinal tract is bypassed. Table 36–3 compares the RDAs in pregnancy with MVI-12, one of several standard intravenous vitamin preparations used in parenteral nutrition.[5] Additional supplements of vitamin D, vitamin K, and folate are necessary when MVI-12 is used.

The requirements for some minerals are less well defined, and the RDAs for calcium, iron, and zinc are subject to the effect of the efficiency of absorption. Tentative recommendations listed in Table 36–4 for calcium, phosphorus, magnesium, zinc, and iron are based on oral requirements for pregnancy, adjusted for the efficiency of gastrointestinal absorption.

The RDA for dietary zinc during pregnancy is 20 mg/day. This recommendation accounts for incomplete absorption of zinc, which is estimated to range from 10 to 40 per cent of intake, depending upon its bioavailability for a given type of diet.[46, 62] Pregnancy *per se* does not appear to influence zinc absorption from the gastrointestinal tract.[48, 63] Parenteral nutrition bypasses the gastrointestinal tract, thus eliminating the influence of the bioavailability of zinc from the diet. Utilizing estimates for total retention and excretion from urine and sweat, one can estimate the zinc requirement in normal pregnancy to be 2.55 to 3.0 mg/day, depending upon gestation (Table 36–6).[46, 62] Zinc requirements will increase with concomitant disease and/or extra losses from the gastrointestinal tract.[46]

Table 36–6. ESTIMATED ZINC REQUIREMENTS IN HEALTHY PREGNANT WOMEN

GESTATION (WEEKS)	PEAK DAILY RETENTION	URINARY EXCRETION	SWEAT EXCRETION	TOTAL EXCRETION REQUIREMENT
0–20	0.55	0.5	1.5	2.55
20–30	0.9	0.5	1.5	2.9
30–40	1.0	0.5	1.5	3.0

(Adapted from Solomons, N. W.: Biological availability of zinc in humans. Am. J. Clin. Nutr., 35:1048–1075, 1982.)

There is little information on pregnancy requirements for other trace minerals. Recommendations for copper, manganese, chromium, and selenium are based on the RDA recommendations for safe and adequate intakes in nonpregnant adults[5] and the AMA recommendations for trace mineral supplementation in stable adults.[64] Trace elements should be administered and monitored carefully.

COMPLICATIONS OF PARENTERAL NUTRITION IN PREGNANCY

Carbohydrate-Related Complications

The complications of central vein nutrition associated with any adult may all occur in the pregnant woman. However, excesses and deficiencies may have profound effects on the fetus and be associated with an untoward outcome. Hence, monitoring schedules and precise provision of nutrient requirements are essential in these patients. Because the nutrient mixture is based on the large glucose load, problems with glucose intolerance may be observed and should be carefully monitored. However, a variety of glucose tolerance tests, both oral and intravenous, have demonstrated adequate insulin responses to glucose loads in nondiabetic pregnant women. For example, Lind[65] examined the insulin response throughout gestation by infusing ten per cent dextrose solutions. Blood glucose rose to between 174 and 213 mg/100 ml, but all patients were capable of a massive insulin response under infusion conditions, with insulin levels reaching 70 to 200 µU/ml. Because of this ability to handle glucose loads, hyperglycemia has not been a major concern in our patients studied to date. It should be noted, however, that changes that occur in renal function may cause glucosuria in the nondiabetic pregnant patient, in spite of near-normal concentrations of blood sugar. Therefore, the administration of insulin based on the presence of glucosuria alone should be avoided. Urine glucose levels should be correlated with blood concentrations before exogenous insulin is administered.

We have not as yet cared for a diabetic pregnant woman who has required intravenous nutrition. We recommend that similar glucose-based nutritional regimens be utilized in such a patient; if glucose control is difficult, we would utilize a servo-control insulin delivery unit (Biostator, Miles Laboratories).

Amino Acid–Related Complications

Hyperaminoacidemia is a concern with the administration of amino acid loads. Amino acid concentrations are generally 20 per cent below normal levels in the serum of pregnant women, and these levels may be markedly elevated with the infusion of amino acid solutions rich in nonessential amino acids such as glycine.

Studies carried out in pregnant rhesus monkeys have examined the question of whether the transplacental gradient for amino acids is maintained in the face of maternal hyperaminoacidemia.[55] Animals were infused with total parenteral nutrient solutions of five per cent mixed synthetic amino acids at a constant rate for eight to ten hours. Simultaneous maternal and fetal plasma samples were taken at hourly intervals and were analyzed for amino acid composition. The gradients for cystine, leucine, and lycine increased, indicating that fetal levels were raised to a proportionally greater degree than maternal levels. The gradients for isoleucine, phenylalanine, and arginine fell only slightly and probably not to a significant degree. The gradients for all other amino acids declined with elevations of the maternal levels, indicating somewhat of a blunting effect on the fetal side of the placenta. Thus, although induced maternal hyperaminoacidemia generally resulted in elevated fetal levels of amino acids, the most common pattern observed was a somewhat disproportionately smaller increase in the fetal compartment than in the maternal compartment. It should be noted, however, that this response was disparate and that marked increases in cystine, leucine, and lysine were observed.[55] The significance of these abnormalities is unknown. Further studies that monitor amino acid concentration in the maternal bloodstream should help improve formulation of amino acids for the pregnant mother.

Fat Emulsion–Related Complications

Although we know essential fatty acids are required for both the mother and fetus, the exact role of the administration of fat emulsion in prostaglandin synthesis and potential induction of labor is unknown.

Arachidonic acid is the precursor of the prostaglandins that predominate uterine tissue. It is generally thought that the availability of free arachidonic acid is rate-limiting in the formation of prostaglandins, because the addition of arachidonic acid to tissue usually results in higher prostaglandin production.[60] In humans, addition of arachidonic acid to the diet will increase overall production of prostaglandins.[66]

An elevation of prostaglandins in uterine tissue could theoretically stimulate contractions. It has been reported that rapid infusions of fat emulsion can cause uterine contractions, presumably because of increased prostaglandin production stimulated by the infusion of linoleic acid in fat emulsion or some component of the lipid emulsion.[67, 68] Elphick and colleagues[61] observed an increase in arachidonic acid production by the placenta in five women infused with the fat emulsion Intralipid just prior to delivery. However, in examining absolute levels of arachidonic acid in maternal and fetal blood and tissues within the pregnant uterus, Filshie and Anstey[69] concluded "there is so much free arachidonic acid in the tissues and in the plasma that it is probable that the substrate level is not the limiting factor in prostaglandin production."[69]

The hyperlipidemia observed in pregnancy is rarely associated with complications. There have been reports of extreme hyperlipidemia in pregnancy associated with abdominal pain; hyperlipidemia has also been associated with abnormalities in placental morphology. Nielsen and associates[70] reported a case of a 25-year-old primigravida who presented just prior to delivery with acute abdominal pain, ketonuria, hypertriglyceridemia, hypercholesterolemia, and a normal serum amylase level. Macroscopic features of the placenta were normal; however, microscopic examination revealed the accumulation of lipid-containing macrophages in the intervillous space. This finding was believed to be a type IV hyperlipidemia exacerbated by the influence of pregnancy.[70] Pregnant women receiving fat emulsion should be carefully monitored for hypertriglyceridemia, because such changes in the placenta may occur.

Complications Related to Vitamins and Minerals

As previously reviewed, addition of a number of nutrients is made to parenteral nutrition mixtures to satisfy the increased requirements for folic acid, calcium, phosphorus, zinc, iron, and magnesium. Maternal deficiencies in these and other nutrients may have deleterious effects on the fetus. However, nutrient excesses or toxicities may be equally harmful.

Compared with the adult, the fetus is at higher risk for nutrient toxicity, because the greatest damage occurs during the developmental process. Also, as with amino acids, the placenta transports nutrients against a concentration gradient, exposing the fetus to higher blood levels of some substances. Finally, fetal exposure to nutrients may increase by recycling through the swallowing of amniotic fluid, resulting in toxic accumulation of the substances.[71]

Excessive intake of vitamin D may lead to fetal hypercalcemia, which may cause fetal growth retardation, aortic stenosis, and deposition of calcium in the brain and other organs. It has been suggested that severe infantile hypercalcemia is due to fetal sensitivity and not to high maternal intakes.[71] Excessive intake of vitamin A has been linked to congenital obstructive lesions of the ureter and malformations of the urinary tract[45, 71, 72] and may be associated with neural tube defects.[73] The transplacental gradient of vitamin C is maintained in the face of elevated maternal levels, thus increasing the exposure of the fetus to the vitamin. Excessive intake may then condition the infant to need high quantities of ascorbic acid, leading to the development of scurvy after birth. Chronically elevated intakes of iodine have been associated with congenital goiter.[71]

The major impact of many of these toxicities is during fetal development in the first trimester, and reported intakes are from dietary or oral supplementation at least ten times the RDA. However, when administering nutrients intravenously without the benefit of the buffering effects of the gastrointestinal tract and liver, one must have adequate knowledge of maternal nutritional history and the potential complications of excessive intake.

CLINICAL EXPERIENCE WITH TPN IN PREGNANCY

Over the past four years, 21 patients have been referred to the Nutrition Support Service from the highly active obstetrical service of Brigham and Women's Hospital. All of the outpatients seen in consultation by our service had previously been counseled both by physicians and nutritionists, and in many cases dietary alterations and food supplements had been provided, but a satisfactory weight gain had not been achieved. In the inpatients, enteral feedings were not possible, and these patients were seen immediately to be evaluated for parenteral nutrition. A summary of these patients' data is given in Table 36–7.

A wide variety of patients have been seen by our service, including those with minimal stress, such as anorexia or hyperemesis, or those with severe medical or surgical problems, such as life-threatening injury and postoperative complications. In patients with minimal degrees of stress, counseling with provision of nutritional supplements allowed normal weight gain. One patient was begun on home tube feedings and was supported for a period of 18 weeks; during this time she gained approximately 20 pounds, increased her strength and appetite, and was able to be weaned from the tube feedings. Throughout that time, ultrasound studies showed normal growth and development of the fetus. She delivered a full-term, 8-lb 4-oz, normal boy.

In the patients with severe stress, such as major trauma and infection, intravenous feedings were initiated. However, the outcome for the fetus was determined by the degree of stress to the mother. In all three cases, cesarean section was performed early in the hospital course, and the mothers continued to be supported by parenteral nutrition during the remainder of their hospitalizations. Other studies have demonstrated that following severe injury, pregnant women will spontaneously abort if early in their pregnancy or will commence labor if a life-threatening complication such as hypoxia, sepsis, or shock occurs.[74]

In the patients with mild to moderate stress who could not eat, long-term intravenous feeding was required. Duration has varied from 2.5 to five weeks and serves as the basis of this more detailed report. One of the patients had prolonged hyperemesis with weight loss requiring hospitalization. A second patient had exacerbation of ulcerative colitis, characterized by bloody diarrhea; she was put on bowel rest and treated with high doses of corticosteroids, at the same time receiving total parenteral nutrition. A third patient had paroxysmal nocturnal hemoglobinuria and was treated throughout her hospitalization; abortion was discussed with the parents but was not considered an acceptable option. Central vein feedings were carried out in all three patients. The average caloric intake ranged from 2000 to 2800, with a nitrogen intake varying from 11 to 12 gm/day. Nitrogen balance results in all patients varied from +10 gm/day in a severely depleted woman to +1.1 gm/day in a woman with more normal body composition. Positive nitrogen balance occurred in the patient with inflammatory bowel disease who was receiv-

Table 36–7. PREGNANT WOMEN REFERRED TO NUTRITION SUPPORT SERVICE, BRIGHAM AND WOMEN'S HOSPITAL, 1980–1983

DEGREE OF STRESS	NO. PATIENTS	DIAGNOSIS*	DISPOSITION*
Minimal	10	Anorexia (2) Hyperemesis gravidarum (8)	Counseling, nutritional supplements (4) Parenteral nutrition (2) Tube feeding (4)
Mild to moderate	9	Crohn's disease (3) Paroxysmal hemoglobinuria (1) Lymphoma (1) Ruptured appendix (2) Bowel obstruction (2)	Dietary counseling (1) See text
Severe	3	40% total body surface burn (1) Head injury (1) Postoperative complications (1)	Short-term IV feedings (<1 wk)

*Numbers in parentheses denote numbers of patients.

ing high doses of corticosteroids, demonstrating the tremendous anabolic effects of pregnancy on protein metabolism. No significant complications occurred in this group of women, and the fetal outcome was satisfactory in two patients with benign disease. A stillbirth occurred during the 26th week of gestation in the patient with paroxysmal nocturnal hemoglobinuria; this patient continued nutritional support but after several months died of the complications of this disease process.

The following case histories typify our experience with parenteral nutrition in pregnancy.

Case Example 1. A 32-year-old female gravida 1, para 0, with a past history of ulcerative colitis, was admitted to the hospital at 32 weeks gestation complaining of bloody diarrhea and weight loss. The diarrhea had commenced approximately one month before and, despite modification of her diet and the administration of exogenous steroids, had continued. She had lost weight, going from a normal pre-pregnancy weight of 84 kg to 70 kg. She was put on bowel rest. A central venous catheter was placed by percutaneous sterile technique, and hypertonic nutrient solutions were started. Caloric requirement was estimated at 2500 kcal/day. Measurement of gas exchange demonstrated a basal energy requirement of 2000 calories; an additional 500 calories were allotted for activity. The estimated nitrogen requirement was 14 gm.

This requirement was satisfied by administering two liters of central vein solution containing 1000 calories and seven grams of nitrogen per liter. Intravenous fat emulsion was given as 0.5 L of a ten per cent emulsion per day; the patient tolerated the infusion without complications. Serial ultrasound studies showed good growth of the fetus during the period of nutritional support (Table 36–8). Amniocentesis showed biochemical evidence of maturation of the fetal lungs, and when the patient commenced labor on the 17th day of intravenous feeding, the child was delivered by a normal, spontaneous vaginal delivery. The child weighed 3,500 grams and was normal. Intravenous feedings were continued while the mother remained in remission for her ulcerative colitis. Requirements were modified somewhat to accommodate breast feeding of the infant. The mother was gradually started on enteral feeding. After parenteral nutrition was discontinued, the patient was discharged, and mother and infant have done well since hospitalization.

Case Example 2. A 29-year-old female, gravida 1, para 0, was admitted to the hospital at 26 weeks gestation with a diagnosis of hyperemesis gravidarum. The hyperemesis began two weeks after her missed period. She was hospitalized several times during the first five months of pregnancy for rehydration and control of vomiting. The disorder was unresponsive to medical treatment and hypnosis. On admission, an abdominal ultrasound showed a normal fetus. A gastrointestinal work-up was negative.

Her height was five feet; pre-pregnancy weight was 61.4 kg, and weight on admission was 55.9 kg. Weight gain at this point should have been five to six kilograms.

Her calorie requirements for normal pregnancy were assessed at 2,200 kcal/day and 70 to 80 gm of protein. She received two liters of central vein solution and 0.5L of 10 per cent fat emulsion per day, as described in Table 36–5. Trace elements and vitamins with extra folate were administered daily. Vitamin K was given as 10 mg IM per week.

She continued on parenteral nutrition for 24 days. Her total mean daily intake was 2,780 kcal, 12.6 gm nitrogen, and 50 gm fat. Protein and fat represented 11 and 20 per cent of calories, respectively. Nitrogen balance was followed daily (Fig. 36–1).

During this period her oral intake began to increase, and vomiting subsided. The central line was removed and discharge was planned.

The patient immediately began vomiting again, taking minimal oral feedings. Peripheral vein infusions were started three days later, consisting of 200 ml of 8.5 per cent amino acids and 800 ml of ten per cent dextrose solution per liter, plus the same vitamin and trace element regimen. During this time, the patient was seen by the psychiatrist, who believed the patient was se-

Table 36–8. CASE EXAMPLE 1: ULTRASOUND FEATURES BEFORE AND AFTER PARENTERAL NUTRITION

FEATURE	GESTATIONAL AGE BY DATE (wk)	
	32	35
Estimated gestational age (wk)	33.5	37–40
Biparietal diameter (mm)	86	94.2
Occipital-frontal diameter (mm)	98	110.9
Abdominal diameter (mm)	87	98.1
Femoral length (mm)	62	70.8
Estimated weight (gm)	2200	3040

Table 36–9. CASE EXAMPLE 2: NEWBORN PROFILE

Weight	3450 gm
Head circumference	34 cm
Length	51 cm
Gestational age	40 wk
Risk factors	None
Abnormalities	None
Observations	Slightly peeling skin, 1/6 systolic murmur

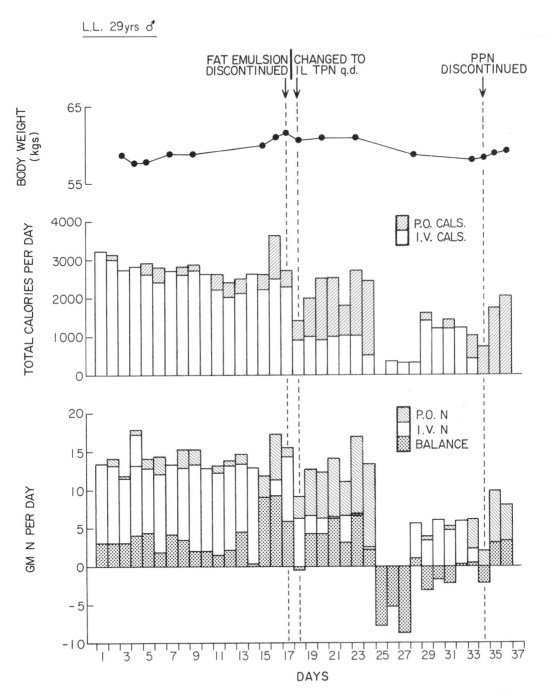

Figure 36–1. Body weight, calorie intake, and nitrogen balance in a 29-year-old female with hyperemesis gravidarum.

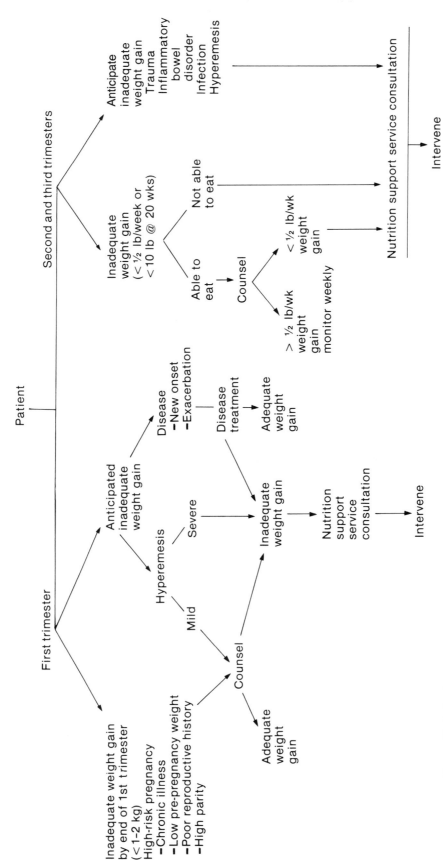

Figure 36–2. Decision process for specialized nutritional care in pregnancy. (This process assumes that a decision has been made to continue the pregnancy.)

verely depressed, because relapses of her hyperemesis occurred every time she was allowed to go home for a visit. Peripheral vein feedings continued for six days, until her vomiting again subsided. The decision was made to keep her in the hospital until delivery. The patient ate and drank well until delivery. A healthy female baby, weighing 7 lb, 9 oz, was delivered by cesarean section. The newborn profile is shown in Table 36–9.

SUMMARY

Increased knowledge of nutritional factors that affect outcome for the fetus allows the application of nutritional support techniques to pregnant women with disease processes precluding enteral feeding. Women who fail to gain weight during pregnancy or in fact demonstrate weight loss may be candidates for such intervention (Fig. 36–2). Our experience and the experience of others demonstrate that intravenous nutrition can be provided safely and effectively to these patients. However, optimal and safe nutritional therapy can be achieved only by central venous infusion of a hypertonic dextrose and amino acid mixture, with supplementation of fat emulsion. Careful monitoring and adjustment of the solutions for the pregnant woman and her fetus are necessary, as fetal growth and development may be altered by an imbalance of nutrients available to the fetus. With careful monitoring of both mother and child, a combination of nutritional support techniques, and modern obstetrical care, a successful outcome for both woman and infant can now be expected when all nutrients are provided by vein.

CASE REPORTS OF PARENTERAL NUTRITION IN PREGNANCY

Cox, K.L., Byrne, W.J., and Ament, M.E.: Home total parenteral nutrition during pregnancy: A case report. J.P.E.N., 5:246–249, 1981.

di Costanzo, J., Martin, J., Cano, N., et al.: Total parenteral nutrition with fat emulsions during pregnancy—nutritional requirements: A case report. J.P.E.N., 6:534–538, 1982.

Hew, L.R., and Deitel, M.: Total parenteral nutrition in gynecology and obstetrics. Obstet. Gynecol., 55:464–468, 1980.

LaKoff, K.M., and Feldman, J.D.: Anorexia nervosa associated with pregnancy. Obstet. Gynecol., 39:699–704, 1972.

Lavin, J.P., Gimmon, Z., and Miodovnik, M.: Total parenteral nutrition in a pregnant insulin requiring diabetic. Obstet. Gynecol., 59:660, 1982.

Main, A.N.H., Shenkin, A., Black, W.P., et al.: Intravenous feeding to sustain pregnancy in patients with Crohn's disease. Br. Med. J., 283:1221–1222, 1981.

Martin, R., and Blackburn, G.: Hyperalimentation during pregnancy. Clin. Con. Nutr. Sup., 2(3): 1982.

Tesadern, J.C., Falconer, G.F., Turnberg, L.A., et al.: Successful completed pregnancy in a patient maintained on home parenteral nutrition. Br. Med. J., 286:602–603, 1983.

Webb, G.A.: The use of hyperalimentation and chemotherapy in pregnancy: A case report. Am. J. Obstet. Gynecol., 137:263–266, 1980.

Weinberg, R.B., Sitrin, M.D., Adkins, G.M., et al.: Treatment of hyperlipidemic pancreatitis in pregnancy with total parenteral nutrition. Gastroenterology, 83:1300–1305, 1982.

REFERENCES

1. van den Berg, B.J.: Maternal variables affecting fetal growth. Am. J. Clin. Nutr., 34:722–726, 1981.
2. Jaffin, H.: Nutrition in pregnancy. In Halpern, S. (ed.): Quick Reference to Clinical Nutrition. Philadelphia, J.B. Lippincott, 1979.
3. Hytten, F.E.: Weight gain in pregnancy. In Hytten, F.E., and Chamberlain, G. (eds.): Clinical Physiology in Obstetrics. Oxford, Blackwell Scientific Publications, 1980, pp. 197–199.
4. Aubrey, R.H., Roberts, A., and Quenca, V.G.: The assessment of maternal nutrition. Clin. Perinatol., 2:207–219, 1975.
5. Food and Nutrition Board: Recommended Dietary Allowances. Washington, D.C., National Academy of Sciences, 1980.
6. Pitkin, R.M.: Nutritional support in obstetrics and gynecology. Clin. Obstet. Gynecol., 19:489–513, 1976.
7. National Research Council: Laboratory Indices of Nutritional Status in Pregnancy. Washington, D.C., National Academy of Sciences, 1978.
8. King, J.C.: Protein metabolism in pregnancy. Clin. Perinatol., 2:243–254, 1975.
9. Frisch, R.E.: Nutrition, fatness, puberty, and fertility. Comprehen. Ther., 7:15–23, 1981.
10. Niswander, K., and Jackson, E.C.: Physical characteristics of the gravida and their association with birth weight and perinatal death. Am. J. Obstet. Gynecol., 119:306–313, 1974.
11. Winick, M.: Nutrition and nerve cell growth. Fed. Proc., 29:1510–1515, 1970.
12. Smithells, R.W., Sheppard, S., Schorah, C.J., et al.: Possible prevention of neural tube defects by periconceptional vitamin supplementation. Lancet, 1:339–340, 1980.
13. Strauss, M.B.: Anemia of infancy from maternal iron deficiency in pregnancy. J. Clin. Invest., 12:345–353, 1933.
14. Gatenby, P.B.B., and Lillie, E.W.: Clinical analysis of 100 cases of severe megaloblastic anemia of pregnancy. Br. Med. J., 2:1111–1114, 1960.
15. Hibbard, E.D., and Smithells, R.W.: Folic acid metabolism and human embryopathy. Lancet, 1:1254, 1965.
16. Jameson, S.: Effects of zinc deficiency in human reproduction. Acta Med. Scand.(Suppl.), 593: 5–89, 1976.

17. Shaw, J.C.L.: Trace elements in the fetus and young infant. Am. J. Dis. Child., 133:1260–1268, 1979.

18. Hambridge, K.M., Krebs, N.F., Jacobs, M.A., et al.: Zinc nutritional status during pregnancy: A longitudinal study. Am. J. Clin. Nutr., 37:429–442, 1983.

19. Watney, P.J.M., Chance, G.W., Scott, P., et al.: Maternal factors in neonatal hypocalcemia. A study in three ethnic groups. Br. Med. J., 2:432–436, 1971.

20. King, E.Q.: Acute cardiac failure in the newborn due to thiamine deficiency. Exp. Med. Surg., 25:173–177, 1967.

21. Winick, M., and Rosso, P.: The effect of severe early malnutrition in cellular growth of human brain. Pediatr. Res., 3:181–184, 1969.

22. Chase, H.P., Welch, N.N., and Dabiere, C.S.: Alterations in human brain biochemistry following intrauterine growth retardation. Pediatrics, 50:403–411, 1972.

23. Fitzhardinge, P.M., and Steven, E.M.: The small for date infant. II. Neurological and intellectual sequelae. Pediatrics, 50:50–57, 1972.

24. Susser, M.: Prenatal nutrition, birth weight, and psychological development: An overview of experiments, quasi-experiments, and natural experiments in the past decade. Am. J. Clin. Nutr., 34:784–803, 1981.

25. Eastman, N.J., and Jackson, E.: Weight relationships in pregnancy. I. The bearing of maternal weight gain and pre-pregnancy weight on birth weight in full term pregnancies. Obstet. Gynecol. Surv., 23:1003–1025, 1968.

26. Peckhans, C.H., and Christianson, R.A.: The relationship between prepregnancy weight and certain obstetric factors. Am. J. Obstet. Gynecol., 111:1–7, 1971.

27. Simpson, J.W., Lawless, R.W., and Mitchell, A.C.: Responsibility of the obstetrician to the fetus. II. Influence of prepregnancy weight and pregnancy weight gain on birthweight. J. Obstet. Gynecol., 45:481–487, 1975.

28. Ten State Nutrition Survey in the United States, 1968–1970. Department of Health, Education and Welfare Publication Number (HSM) 72–8129 through 72–8134. Washington, D.C., U.S.D.H.E.W., 1972.

29. King, J.C.: Assessment of nutrition status in pregnancy—1. Am. J. Clin. Nutr., 34:685–690, 1981.

30. Robertson, E.G., and Cheyne, G.A.: Plasma biochemistry in relation to edema of pregnancy. J. Obstet. Gynaecol. Br. Common 79:769–776, 1972.

31. Jacobi, J.M., Powell, L.W., and Gaffney, T.J.: Immunochemical quantitation of human transferrin in pregnancy and during the administration of oral contraceptives. Br. J. Haematol., 17:503–509, 1969.

32. DeLeeuw, N.K.M., Lowenstein, L., and Hsieh, Y.: Iron deficiency and hydremia in normal pregnancy. Medicine, 45:291–315, 1966.

33. Carr, M.C.: The diagnosis of iron deficiency in pregnancy. Obstet. Gynecol., 43:15–21, 1974.

34. O'Sullivan, J.B., and Mahan, C.M.: Criteria for oral glucose tolerance test in pregnancy. Diabetes, 13:278–285, 1964.

35. Wilkerson, H.L.C., and O'Sullivan, J.B.: A study of glucose tolerance and screening criteria in 752 selected pregnancies. Diabetes, 12:313–318, 1963.

36. Lind, T., Bellewicz, W.Z., and Brown, G.: A serial study of changes occurring in the oral glucose tolerance test in pregnancy. J. Obstet. Gynaecol. Br. Common., 80:1033–1039, 1973.

37. Biezenski, J.J.: Maternal lipid metabolism. Obstet. Gynecol. Ann., 3:203–233, 1974.

38. Wideman, G.L., Baird, G.H., and Bolding, O.T.: Ascorbic acid deficiency and premature rupture of fetal membrane. Am. J. Obstet. Gynecol., 88:592–595, 1964.

39. Clemetson, C.A.B., and Andersen, L.: Ascorbic acid metabolism in pre-eclampsia. Obstet. Gynecol., 24:744–782, 1964.

40. Heller, S., Salkeld, R.M., and Korner, W.F.: Vitamin B_1 status in pregnancy. Am. J. Clin. Nutr., 27:1221–1224, 1974.

41. Pitkin, R.M.: Vitamins and minerals in pregnancy. Clin. Perinatol., 2:221–232, 1975.

42. McGarry, J.M., and Andrews, J.: Smoking in pregnancy and Vitamin B_{12} metabolism. Br. Med. J., 2:74–77, 1972.

43. Chanarin, I.: Megaloblastic anaemia associated with pregnancy. In The Megaloblastic Anaemias. Oxford, Blackwell Scientific Publications, 1969.

44. Wallingford, J.C., Milunsky, A., and Underwood, B.A.: Vitamin A and retinol-binding protein in amniotic fluid. Am. J. Clin. Nutr., 38:377–381, 1983.

45. Committees on Drugs and Nutrition of the American Academy of Pediatrics. Joint Committee Statement: The use and abuse of Vitamin A. Pediatrics, 48:655–656, 1971.

46. Solomons, N.W.: Biological availability of zinc in humans. Am. J. Clin. Nutr., 35:1048–1075, 1982.

47. Hambridge, K.M., and Droegemueller, W.: Changes in plasma and hair concentrations of zinc, copper, chromium, and manganese during pregnancy. Obstet. Gynecol., 44:667–672, 1974.

48. Swanson, C.A., and King, J.C.: Zinc utilization in pregnant and non-pregnant women fed controlled diets providing the zinc RDA. J. Nutr., 112:697–707, 1982.

49. Shaw, J.C.L.: Trace elements in the fetus and young infant. II. Am. J. Dis. Child., 134:74–81, 1980.

50. O'Leary, J.A.: Serum copper levels as a measure of placental function. Am. J. Obstet. Gynecol., 105:636–637, 1969.

51. Hambridge, K.M., and Rodgerson, D.O.: Comparison of hair chromium levels of mulliparous and parous women. Am. J. Obstet. Gynecol., 103:320–321, 1969.

52. Young, M.: Transfer of amino acids. In Chamberlain, G.V.P., and Wilkinson, A.W. (eds.): Placenta Transfer. Tunbridge Wells, Pitman Medical, 1979.

53. Hytten, F.E., and Cheyne, G.A.: The aminoaciduria of pregnancy. J. Obstet. Gynaecol. Br. Common., 79:424–432, 1972.

54. Schoengold, D.M., DeFiore, R.H., and Parlett, R.C.: Free amino acids in plasma throughout pregnancy. Am. J. Obstet. Gynecol., 131:490–499, 1978.

55. Pitkin, R.M.: Amino acid sources for the fetus. In Moghissi, K.S., and Evans, T.N. (eds.): Nutritional Impacts on Women. Hagerstown, Md., Harper & Row, 1977.

56. Moghissi, K.S., Churchill, J.A., and Kurrie, D.: Relationship of maternal amino acids and proteins to fetal growth and mental development. Am. J. Obstet. Gynecol., 123:398–407, 1975.

57. Crawford, C.A.: Estimation of essential fatty acid requirements in pregnancy and lactation. Prog. Food. Nutr. Sci., 4:75–80, 1980.

58. Lamptey, M.S., and Walker, B.L.: Physical and neurological development of the progeny of female rats fed an essential fatty acid deficient diet during pregnancy and/or lactation. J. Nutr., *108*:351, 1978.

59. Lamptey, M.S., and Walker, B.L.: Learning behavior and brain lipid composition in rats subjected to essential fatty acid deficiency during gestation, lactation, and growth. J. Nutr., *108*:358–367, 1978.

60. Heyman, M. (ed.): Prostaglandins in the Perinatal Period: Their Physiologic and Clinical Importance. New York, Grune & Stratton, 1980.

61. Elphick, M.C., Filshie, G.M., and Hull, D.: The passage of fat emulsion across the human placenta. Br. J. Obstet. Gynaecol., *85*:610–618, 1978.

62. World Health Organization: Trace elements in human nutrition. Report of a WHO Expert Committee. (WHO Technical Report, Ser. No. 532.) Geneva, WHO, 1973.

63. Turnlund, J.R., Michel, M.C., Swanson, C.A., et al.: Studies of zinc absorption in human subjects using enriched stable isotopes. Am. J. Clin. Nutr., *34*:650, 1981.

64. American Medical Association, Department of Foods and Nutrition: Guidelines for essential trace element preparations for parenteral use. A statement by an expert panel. J.A.M.A., *241*:2051–2054, 1979.

65. Lind, T.: Carbohydrate metabolism—some aspects of glycosuria. *In* Moghissi, K.S., and Evans, T.N. (eds.): Nutritional Impacts on Women. Hagerstown, Md., Harper & Row, 1977.

66. Seyberth, H., Oelz, O., Kennedy, T., et al.: Increased arachidonate in lipids after administration to man. Effects on prostaglandin biosynthesis. Clin. Pharmacol. Ther., *18*:521–529, 1975.

67. Luukkainen, T.U., and Csapo, A.I.: Induction of premature labor in the rabbit after treatment with phospholipids. Fertil. Steril., *14*:65–72, 1963.

68. Heller, J.: Parenteral Nutrition. Edinburgh, Churchill Livingstone, 1972.

69. Filshie, G.M., and Anstey, M.D.: The distribution of arachidonic acid in plasma and tissue of patients near term undergoing elective or emergency caesarean section. Br. J. Obstet. Gynecol., *85*:119–123, 1978.

70. Nielsen, F.H., Jacobsen, B.B., and Rolschau, J.: Pregnancy complicated by extreme hyperlipidemia and foam cell accumulation in placenta. Acta Obstet. Gynecol. Scand., *52*:83–89, 1973.

71. Pitkin, R.M.: Megadose nutrients during pregnancy. *In* National Research Council, Food and Nutrition Board, Committee on Nutrition of the Mother and Child (eds.): Alternative Dietary Practices and Nutritional Abuses in Pregnancy. Washington, D.C., National Academy Press, 1982.

72. Bernhardt, I.R., and Dorsey, D.J.: Hypervitaminosis A and congenital renal anomalies in a human infant. Obstet. Gynecol., *43*:750–755, 1974.

73. Parkinson, C.E., and Tan, J.C.Y.: Vitamin A concentration in amniotic fluid and maternal serum related to neural-tube defects. Br. J. Obstet. Gynaecol., *89*:935–939, 1982.

74. Taylor, J.: Burns in pregnancy. *In* Artz, C.P., Moncrief, J.A., and Pruitt, B.A. (eds.): Burns: A Team Approach. Philadelphia, W.B. Saunders, 1979, pp. 330–333.

CHAPTER 37

Theoretic and Practical Issues in the Treatment of Obesity

L. JOHN HOFFER
JOHN PALOMBO
BRUCE R. BISTRIAN

The essence of the management (and prevention) of obesity is the appropriate matching, over years, of energy expenditure and nutritional intake. The difficulty lies in the inability of many overweight individuals to bring this state about, even with good will and the assistance of nutrition education programs and hypocaloric diets. For individuals with moderate obesity—130 to 199 per cent of ideal body weight (IBW)—or morbid obesity—200 per cent or more of IBW—a health hazard exists that worsens with increasing obesity. For such individuals seeking professional treatment, two new modalities of therapy have been used in recent years: very-low-calorie diets (fewer than 800 kcal/day) and gastric surgery in selected morbidly obese patients. It is the purpose of this chapter to consider some theoretic and practical aspects of these two recent treatment approaches.

VERY-LOW-CALORIE DIETS FOR MODERATELY OBESE PATIENTS

Numerous diets, some very low in energy, are undoubtedly in common use in the self-treatment of obesity. But it is only relatively recently that physicians have begun to explore very-low-calorie diet therapy systematically and to prescribe it on a wide scale. Although foreshadowed by earlier work,[75, 110, 111] current approaches date from a study by Bolinger and coworkers,[19] in which an attempt was made to ameliorate the body

nitrogen (N) losses accompanying total fasting by providing 40 to 80 gm of albumin daily to already fasting morbidly obese patients. Nitrogen balance improved while rapid weight loss nevertheless continued. Similar findings, and in many cases complete cessation of net nitrogen losses, were subsequently reported with protein-supplemented fasting in obese individuals. Many diets provided only protein, but favorable experiences were also reported with very-low-calorie diets containing both carbohydrate and protein. Patients were found to tolerate the diets well; because of the infrequency or absence of complications known to attend total fasting, coupled with the better nitrogen balance findings, these diets are now commonly prescribed for outpatient use. Their ultimate efficacy is still unknown, and evaluation must await the results of controlled trials comparing traditional methods and long-term follow-up studies.

Because very-low-calorie diets of different composition may bring about different metabolic responses, recent research has been devoted to characterizing different diets, particularly with regard to protein metabolism, and to a determination of the optimal composition in terms of safety, tolerance, and side effects. That severely re-

Part of this chapter is reproduced from Palombo, J. D., and Bistrian, B. R.: Obesity. *In* Hare, J. (ed.): Signs and Symptoms in Endocrine and Metabolism Disorders. Philadelphia, J. B. Lippincott, 1985. Supported in part by grant AM-26349, National Institutes of Health DHHS.

stricted diets are not innocuous was made clear by the diet-related deaths in 1977 and 1978 of a small number of morbidly obese individuals subsisting on hydrolyzed collagen formulas of low biologic value, in which the provision of electrolytes and micronutrients was unreliable.[64, 114]

Physiology of Fasting and Its Modulation by Carbohydrate

When water alone is provided to normal or obese nondiabetic individuals, a coordinated response occurs over the ensuing days to enable endogenous fat to meet the body's energy demands efficiently. A crucial aspect of this response is a diminution of the rate of glucose oxidation in the brain, which after several weeks of total fasting utilizes ketone bodies as a partial fuel replacement. The characteristic patterns of weight and body composition change during the initial days of total fasting and very-low-calorie dieting are now reasonably well understood. This process is excellently described in available reviews,[29-31] but it is useful to recapitulate certain features relating to the conservation of body protein during fasting.

In the first or second day after a fast begins, urinary N excretion fluctuates in a way largely determined by the preceding protein intake and nutritional status. There then occurs a marked increase in the net rate of N lost from the body to approximately 12 gm/day. Body weight decreases rapidly as a result of glycogenolysis, extracellular fluid loss, and the catabolism of body protein. Fat constitutes only a small proportion of this initial weight loss. After two to three weeks, the rate of weight loss decreases, and there is approximate equilibrium of fluid balance or even mild fluid retention. Urinary N excretion diminishes to approximately four to six grams per day, representing a daily lean tissue loss of roughly 100 to 150 gm, and fat oxidation accounts for approximately 95 per cent of energy consumption.[6, 39, 100] The later rate of lean tissue loss is more desirable than the rate in the early days of fasting, but it remains nontrivial and appears to be sustained, although as the lean body mass decreases, the rate of N loss probably slowly diminishes proportionately.[48]

The extensive protein losses in early fasting are attributed to the need for gluconeogenesis to provide for the obligatory glucose needs of the central nervous system. As glycogen is used up, amino acids (and glycerol released when triglycerides are hydrolyzed) must be used in glucose synthesis to meet this requirement. Later in fasting, brain glucose uptake is markedly diminished, and only 50 per cent of this glucose is irreversibly oxidized (the other portion being recirculated as reutilizable lactate). Therefore the need for amino acid catabolism is less, and a physiologic signal, perhaps the rising blood concentration of ketone bodies, then limits the rate of net body protein breakdown.

Even after adaptation to prolonged fasting, body protein losses remain considerable. First, brain glucose oxidation does not diminish to zero; hence there is a continuing need for gluconeogenesis at a moderate level. Second, it is known that N losses of two to three grams per day accompany high-carbohydrate, maintenance-energy, zero-protein diets.[32, 104] This observation indicates that even in the absence of a need for amino acids as glucose precursors, protein turnover in the body is not perfectly efficient. Third, the mild ketoacidosis of fasting stimulates renal ammoniagenesis, resulting in urinary ammonia N losses of approximately two grams per day. A variety of measures, including potassium provision,[101] small amounts (15 gm/day) of glucose, which increases renal ketone reabsorption,[103] and systemic alkalinization with lactate or bicarbonate,[109] diminish ammonia and total N excretion in fasting. These findings indicate that not all the N losses in prolonged fasting are obligatory features of the fasting state.

It has long been known that carbohydrate spares protein during fasting, whereas equivalent calories given as fat have no effect.[81] Presumably the exogenous glucose provides the central nervous system with its obligatory fuel substrate while stimulating insulin secretion, which in turn inhibits amino acid catabolism for gluconeogenesis. The glucose protein-sparing effect is substantial in early fasting, because central nervous system glucose requirements are still high and the need for gluconeogenesis is correspondingly great. However, in prolonged fasting this effect is not necessarily greater than the slower, naturally occurring protein-sparing effect based on the diminution of brain glucose oxidation. When submaintenance energy diets consisting entirely of carbohydrate are given for a prolonged time[24, 83] and when small amounts of glucose (150 gm/day) are administered to individuals well-adapted to prolonged fasting,[3] N losses are reduced only slightly more than the body could bring about by its own adaptation, in the absence of any calories. Thus, although carbohydrate is undeniably protein sparing in short fasts, it is not particularly protein sparing in *prolonged* fasting states such as would be undertaken by obese individuals.

In contrast, protein supplementation during prolonged fasting permits nitrogen losses to approach zero after an adaptation period of one to two weeks. There remain uncertainties about the smallest amount of protein required to bring about effective protein sparing, and whether an additional protein-sparing effect is brought about by supplementing protein diets with carbohydrate.

Very-Low-Calorie Diets and Total Fasting Compared

A variety of very-low-calorie obesity diets described in the literature is shown in Table 37–1. Because these diets are uniformly low in fat and energy, they differ only in the relative proportions of protein and carbohydrate. The diets providing the greatest amounts of protein are carbohydrate-free, whereas those diets that provide carbohydrate do so at the expense of protein. This need not be so, but the consequence of providing generous amounts of both carbohydrate and protein would be to increase the calories so much that weight loss would be slowed. The recommended dietary allowance (RDA) for protein is 0.8 gm/kg/day, or 40 to 50 gm protein per day for many women, 60 to 70 gm/day for many men. Americans customarily consume 100 gm or more protein per day. Therefore, even the "high-protein," very-low-calorie diets cannot be considered extremely high in protein. All very-low-calorie diets in current professional use provide protein with high biological value only and

are carefully supplemented with minerals (particularly potassium) and vitamins.

The metabolic response to very-low-calorie diets is similar qualitatively to that of prolonged fasting, but with important differences in degree. Much of the adaptation to fasting is to carbohydrate exclusion, and, indeed, is similar in many ways to the adaptation by normal subjects to carbohydrate-free diets at normal energy levels.[93] Ketosis occurs with all very-low-calorie diets, although the amount is far less than with fasting. Subjects taking 80 to 100 gm of protein daily as their only food have blood β-hydroxybutyrate concentrations of around 2 mM;[12, 35, 74] these are reduced to approximately 1 mM when the diet provides 40 to 50 gm carbohydrate plus 50 gm protein.[35, 50] These values are subject to considerable daily and interindividual variability, in our experience. In total fasting, blood ketone concentrations are roughly 6 mM.[84, 96, 102] Other substrate changes occurring in total fasting (rises in plasma free fatty acids, decreases in glucose and insulin, and characteristic changes in plasma free amino acids) also occur to a less extreme extent during very-low-calorie dieting.

The early weeks of fasting are associated with a rise of 8 mg/dl or more in serum uric acid in men, followed by a return toward previous levels after a few weeks.[39] Transient hyperuricemia of approximately the same magnitude may accompany very-low-calorie dieting, although, in our experience, rises of this magnitude have not occurred in women. It has been suggested that uric acid rises are greater with carbohydrate-free than carbohydrate-containing very-low-calorie diets,[62] but there is no evidence to support or refute this.

Resting energy expenditure decreases by approximately 25 per cent in total fasting,[42] but by only 10 per cent (or less) with very-low-calorie diets.[4, 43] The failure of resting oxygen consumption to fall to the same extent as in fasting, plus the presumed ther-

Table 37–1. CHARACTERISTICS OF SOME VERY-LOW-CALORIE WEIGHT REDUCTION DIETS

STUDY	PROTEIN SOURCE	KCAL	PROTEIN (GM)	CARBOHYDRATE (GM)	COMMENT
Apfelbaum et al.[4]	Casein	Women 220	55	0	
		Men 300	75	0	
Bistrian[9]	Meat, fish, fowl	400–600	1.5 gm/kg IBW	0	
Genuth et al.[50, 51]	Egg albumin	300	45	30	"Optifast"
Howard[62]	Milk and soy	330	31	15	"Cambridge Diet"

mogenic effect of even low-calorie meals, may explain why adapted rates of weight loss are similar with very-low-calorie diets and total fasting. Weight loss is variable among individuals on similar hypocaloric diets, in part because the rate of weight loss is influenced by existing body weight.[47] As a crude approximation, weight loss after adaptation to prolonged fasting is 0.27 kg per day in women,[100] compared with 0.20 kg per day after adaptation to very-low-calorie diets in our experience. Approximately 0.1 kg per day of weight loss in prolonged fasting is from the lean tissues, a loss that does not occur in low-calorie diets in which nitrogen equilibrium is attained; thus, rates of adipose tissue loss may be almost the same with fasting and very-low-calorie dieting. This is not to deny that *initial* rates of weight loss are usually much greater during total fasting, but as this initial weight loss consists largely of glycogen, extracellular fluid, and protein, it represents no advantage for the patient.

An important effect of carbohydrate on the sympathetic nervous system, which in turn may affect the regulation of energy metabolism, is now recognized.[53, 68, 98] Fasting, calorie restriction, and carbohydrate restriction all are associated with decreased sympathetic nervous system activity or a decrease in catecholamine turnover, and it may be that the provision of even small amounts of carbohydrate during very-low-calorie dieting may be beneficial. De Haven and colleagues[35] observed greater orthostatic decreases in systolic blood pressure in patients following a diet providing 100 gm of protein than one providing 50 gm of protein and 50 gm of carbohydrate. However, the amounts of sodium and potassium provided to the subjects in that study were below those that would normally be provided in a clinical setting, and this difference may have exaggerated an effect that, in our experience, is uncommon with very-low-calorie diets of either type. Orthostatic hypotension in total fasting may be ameliorated (but not entirely prevented) by providing generous amounts of electrolytes and fluids.[55]

Protein Metabolism with Very-Low-Calorie Diets

Very-low-calorie diets were introduced in obesity therapy to retain the desirable features of total fasting (essentially, patient acceptability by restriction of food choices and the reward of rapid weight loss) while preventing lean tissue losses. This aim would appear largely to have been realized, judging from the literature. Table 37–2 summarizes the results of nine nitrogen balance studies in which most or all of the subjects were women. Shown are the average daily nitrogen balances after at least two weeks of adaptation to the diets. We caution that these results represent averages of sample means with large variances, implying that there are subjects with substantially more negative and more positive nitrogen balance than indicated in the table. Men appear to lose more nitrogen than women.[46] Greater existing body weight and greater lean body mass are usually associated with a more negative nitrogen balance,[48] but this fact does not entirely explain the wide variability in N balance observed by workers in this field.[46, 89, 121] Therefore, insofar as protein loss is undesirable, caution is still mandated in the use of very-low-calorie diets because the response of individual patients may not be typical of the arithmetic means indicated in Table 37–2.

It is apparent from Table 37–2 that the mean nitrogen balance obtained with different diets, or even rather similar ones, is quite variable. Some of the variability may be accounted for by differences in the populations studied and the small numbers of subjects, but much of it remains unexplained. One important determining factor is to be found, in our opinion, in the level of protein supplied. In surveying these studies, we have concluded that nitrogen balance tends to be more positive when the protein intake is greater. Such a relation is believed to hold in the maintenance energy range.[82] Moreover, it appears that a submaintenance energy intake results in a higher protein requirement for zero nitrogen balance.[32, 33, 54] As many of the protein intakes shown in Table 37–2 are near or below the Recommended Dietary Allowance (RDA), it might be predicted that nitrogen balance would be suboptimal at these intake levels under conditions of severe energy restriction, and the N balance would be improved by increasing the protein level above the RDA. Testing this hypothesis is difficult in practice because of the meticulous requirements of human balance studies and the long duration of study and large numbers of subjects needed. In one published study in which this was attempted, nitrogen balance after three weeks of adaptation was slightly but not significantly more positive

Table 37–2. AVERAGE DAILY NITROGEN BALANCE AFTER ADAPTATION TO VERY-LOW-CALORIE WEIGHT REDUCTION DIETS

	SUBJECTS			DIET				NITROGEN BALANCE (GM N PER DAY)‡
STUDY	No.	Sex*	Obesity†	kcal	Protein (gm)	Carbo-hydrate (gm)	Duration	
Passmore et al.[89]	7	5F 2M	Severe	400	25	41	6 weeks	−2.5
Apfelbaum et al.[4]	26	F	Moderate	220	55	0	19 days	+1.1
Bistrian et al.[12]	5	F	Moderate	300	75	0	3 weeks	−0.4
Howard et al.[63]	7	F	?	320	31	45	5–6 weeks	−1.4
Marliss et al.[74]	7	6F 1M	Moderate to severe	400	84	3	3 weeks	0.0
Wilson and Lamberts[119]	11	10F 1M	Moderate to severe	320	31	45	4 weeks	−1.8
Contaldo et al.[34]	25	F	Severe	80 180	17 40	0 0	4 weeks 4 weeks	−4 (low protein) −3 (high protein)
De Haven et al.[35]	7	6F 1M	Moderate to severe	400 400	50 100	50 0	3 weeks 3 weeks	−1.6 (low protein) −1.0 (high protein)
Bistrian et al.[13]	5	F	Moderate	440	45	40	3 weeks	−2.0

*F = female; M = male.

†Moderate obesity was defined as 130 to 199 per cent IBW; severe obesity was defined as more than 200 per cent + IBW.

‡Nitrogen balance was defined as the N intake minus measured N losses in urine and stool and estimated N losses from integument and other sources. In those studies in which integumental and other N losses were not estimated, an adjustment of 0.5 gm N was made to account for them.

when 100 gm of protein was provided than when 50 gm of protein plus 50 gm of carbohydrate were provided.[35] A difficulty with this study, however, was that inadequate quantities of potassium and sodium were provided, possibly preventing optimum nitrogen balance from being attained.[92] In a recent trial we have participated in, nitrogen balance was approximately 2 gm/day more positive with a diet providing approximately 85 gm of protein and 500 kcal than with one providing 44 gm of protein, 38 gm of carbohydrate, and 500 kcal.[60]

In addition to nitrogen balance, body protein turnover has been estimated during very-low-calorie dieting and during fasting. It is recognized that nitrogen balance may be acceptable under certain conditions even when protein malnutrition exists.[2] Thus, acceptable nitrogen balance in itself is not proof that body protein metabolism is normal, because undesirable adaptations in protein metabolism may have been necessary in order to conserve body protein.[52] Protein turnover in the hypocaloric state has most frequently been assessed by means of the Picou and Taylor-Roberts technique.[94] In this method, ^{15}N is administered at a steady rate by mouth, and its dilution in urinary N excretion products is used to calculate the rate of turnover in the body nitrogen pool; from that rate, the rates of synthesis and breakdown of body proteins are calculated. In one pediatric study[91] and one adult study,[120] protein kinetic parameters were maintained in the normal range during very-low-calorie dieting using 1.5 gm protein per kg of IBW with zero carbohydrate. Total fasting, in comparison, resulted in marked decreases in protein turnover.[120] The results in two studies using lower protein levels are conflicting. Thus, Garlick and associates[49] found turnover parameters maintained on a diet of 500 kcal and 50 gm of protein, whereas Bistrian and coworkers[13] found substantial decreases with a diet of 440 kcal and 45 gm of protein. Zero-protein diets providing carbohydrate, however, were clearly associated with decreases in body protein turnover.[49] Therefore, it appears that very-low-calorie diets providing at least 50 gm of protein per day are able to maintain protein turnover at normal levels, whereas at some uncertain protein intake below this, protein turnover rates decline. The total energy intake may be important in determining when turnover rates decline. Protein turnover (both synthesis and breakdown) is energetically expensive, and it is conceivable that below a critical energy and protein intake combination, protein turnover may be decreased as occurs in total fasting, as part of an energy-conserving mechanism.[61]

Certain circulating plasma proteins, including albumin, transferrin, retinol-binding protein (RBP), and thyroxin-binding prealbumin (PA), have been used as indexes of nutritional status. In our experience, albumin and transferrin are maintained during very-low-calorie dieting at protein intake levels of 45 or 80 gm, with or without carbohydrate, but RBP and PA decrease by approximately 25 per cent. This finding is similar to the published experience,[67, 105] although in one report of a diet consisting of zero carbohydrate, 70 gm of protein, and 800 kcal, 40 per cent decreases in transferrin, RBP, and PA were observed, but only minor changes resulted when the same diet contained 70 gm of carbohydrate in exchange for fat.[18] The implications of declines in RBP and PA with very-low-calorie diets is not clear, but recent data indicate similar declines in healthy young men maintained on nutritious high-energy carbohydrate-free diets.[66] Thus, in this setting, such declines likely represent a response to carbohydrate deprivation rather than malnutrition. There are no data to compare these results with those obtained in total fasting or with high-energy, zero-protein diets.

Indications for Carbohydrate Provision in Very-Low-Calorie Diets

A number of authors caution against the use of carbohydrate-free, very-low-calorie diets, arguing that hyperuricemia, electrolyte depletion, impaired sympathetic nervous system activity, and symptoms due to ketosis appear or are greater than when small amounts of carbohydrate are included.[35, 62, 74] Our experience with carbohydrate-free and carbohydrate-containing very-low-calorie diets disagrees with this caution. When adequate supplements of potassium, sodium, and fluid have been taken, hypokalemia has not occurred with either type of diet, nor has there been more frequent or more severe postural hypotension to suggest volume depletion or sympathetic nervous system suppression on one type of diet more than the other; they have been rare in both, and almost invariably traceable to inadequate attention to the daily sodium supplement.

It should be recognized that ketosis, even with zero-carbohydrate diets, is not nearly as profound as in total fasting. Dietary protein is readily converted to glucose in the body, so the difference in carbohydrate metabolism between protein-only diets and those containing 40 or 50 gm of carbohydrate is probably slight. We have compared fasting plasma glucose turnover and oxidation in subjects on 350-kcal diets providing roughly either 84 gm of protein or 45 gm of protein plus 30 gm of carbohydrate. After adaptation to the diets, turnover and oxidation decreased approximately 20 and 30 per cent, respectively, with both diets. This finding may be compared with decreases of 40 and 60 per cent, respectively, in the literature on total fasting.[29, 88] These results indicate, as predicted, that dietary protein is readily converted to glucose during very-low-calorie, carbohydrate-free dieting, so that no difference between the diets was observed in fasting glucose kinetics.

Nevertheless, the possibility that there is an important metabolic effect of ingested carbohydrate, even in small amounts, is not excluded. Figure 37–1 shows the immediate effect on serum insulin and whole blood glucose levels of ingesting the breakfast ration of very-low-calorie diets that provide approximately 28 gm of protein three times a day (essentially no change) or 15 gm of protein and 13 gm of carbohydrate three times a day (large rises in glucose and insulin). The four subjects were adapted to their respective diets at the time of the measurements. Similar large rises in circulating insulin and glucose concentrations have previously been reported in response to very-low-calorie meals containing only small amounts (33 gm) of carbohydrate.[14] The implication of these different meal-related metabolic responses to carbohydrate-containing and carbohydrate-free very-low-calorie diets is unknown.

It remains our view that carbohydrate provision in very-low-calorie diets is not essential. Nevertheless, there is no persuasive reason to exclude carbohydrate, provided that it is given in addition to an ample protein ration and not as replacement. Unnecessary carbohydrate will, of course, slow the rate of fat loss by providing exogenous calories.

Clinical Use of Very-Low-Calorie Diets

The practical use of very low calorie diets has been reviewed[9, 10] but may be summarized in light of the foregoing discussion. The diets may be provided as formulas,[50, 63] but our experience is with meat, fish, or fowl purchased and weighed by the patients. Because the total intake is severely restricted,

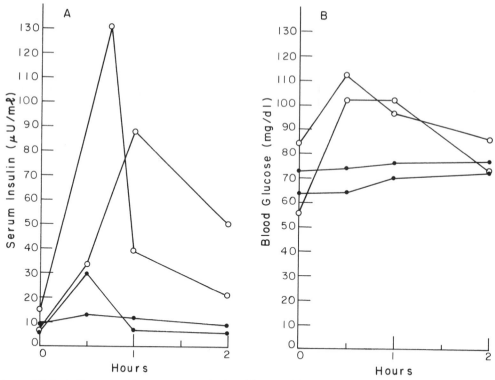

Figure 37-1. *A,* Serum insulin responses to the breakfast meal in moderately obese female subjects during the third week of dieting with very-low-calorie protein diets containing either no carbohydrate *(closed circles)* or 13 gm carbohydrate *(open circles). B,* Whole blood glucose responses to the breakfast meal in the same subjects. The time points are *ante cibum* and 0.5, 1.0, 2.0 hours *post cibum.*

mineral and vitamin supplementation is crucial. The total potassium intake should be at least 50 mEq; in protein-only diets providing 1.5 gm per kg of IBW per day, a daily supplement of K-LYTE 25 mEq has proved sufficient. Additionally, a multivitamin supplement containing folate, 800 gm of calcium, at least 5 gm of sodium chloride, and at least 1.5 L fluids is required daily. The necessity for magnesium supplementation above that found in meat is uncertain.

Outpatients are started on the diets after an initial two to four weeks on balanced weight reduction diets providing 800 to 1200 kcal, during which time a medical evaluation is completed. Contraindications to the diet include only mild overweight, pregnancy, advanced age, cerebrovascular insufficiency, recent myocardial infarction, severe renal or hepatic disease, insulin-dependent diabetes mellitus, and lithium therapy. Adult-onset diabetes and hypertension are not contraindications; indeed, patients with these conditions may expect to derive important benefit from weight reduction. Diuretics are discontinued before beginning the diet, as are oral hypoglycemic agents, because insulin re-

quirements and blood glucose levels invariably decrease. Diabetic patients receiving insulin should be hospitalized for diet initiation in order to discontinue insulin under supervision. If the requirement is 35 units or less, it may be discontinued immediately on starting the diet. Patients in whom it is not possible to discontinue insulin are not candidates for the diet. Patients with gout continue to take their medication. Cases of asymptomatic hyperuricemia are occasionally treated with allopurinol with or without colchicine, starting one to two weeks before the diet is instituted.

Normal concomitants of the diet include moderate decreases in heart rate and mean blood pressure, occasional constipation (which may be treated wth magnesium laxatives or with low-calorie vegetables), mild cold intolerance, temporarily increased rate of hair loss, fatigue, and temporary amenorrhea. Body weight, vital signs, electrolytes, and urine (or breath) ketones are assessed periodically. When the patient is at goal weight, refeeding is accomplished over four to six weeks by the slow introduction of normal foods. The intake of simple sugars is strongly discouraged; this approach minimizes the abrupt gain of fluid that would occur if carbohydrates were reintroduced rapidly. Potassium supplementation is discontinued as the intake increases and ketonuria disappears. Concurrent with the period of rapid weight loss and the reinstitution of a normal intake, an individually tailored program of education, counseling, behavior modification, and exercise continues. Without it, rapid weight regain due to the resumption of prior eating habits is almost certain.

SURGICAL AND MEDICAL THERAPY IN SELECTED MORBIDLY OBESE PATIENTS

Morbid obesity is an abnormal physiologic condition of severe fat deposition, defined as a body weight more than 200 per cent of IBW or 100 pounds overweight according to actuarial standards.[22] The latter definition may not be valid in some instances, however; e.g., a 300-lb male whose IBW is 200 lb is only 150 per cent of IBW.

There is no reliable information on the prevalence of morbid obesity in the United States. The Health and Nutrition Examination Survey (HANES) of 1971 to 1974 indicated that five per cent of the men and seven per cent of the women surveyed were "severely" obese according to skinfold thickness measurements. This "severe" obesity translated into any weight greater than 244 lb for men and 225 lb for women.[39] Another estimate placed the number of morbidly obese in the U.S. at 600,000.[117]

There is no doubt, however, that life expectancy is greatly diminished for morbidly obese individuals. In one survey of 16 severely overweight people, the mean age at the time of death was 35 years, with a range of 22 to 59.[21] In the Study on Build and Blood Pressure by the Society of Actuaries in 1959,[107] insured males weighing more than 250 lb had a mortality rate 168 per cent of that expected. The more recent Study on Build and Blood Pressure of 1979[108] confirms that the severely obese have a significantly reduced life expectancy.

A recent investigation documented the morbidity and mortality of 306 grossly obese men and women over a six-year period.[73] The average age of the 227 females was 41 years and their mean weight was 106 kg. The 79 males averaged 39 years in age with a mean weight of 111 kg. Clinical examination revealed that overt or chemical diabetes occurred in 50 per cent of the subjects, and arterial hypertension was present in 27 per cent of the females and 48 per cent of the males. Cardiorespiratory symptoms were present in 32 per cent of the females and 48 per cent of the males, whereas osteoarthrosis was observed in 75 per cent and 50 per cent, respectively. Cholelithiasis and hyperlipidemias were common. Six deaths had occurred among 142 of these subjects on follow-up two years later.

In a longitudinal study of 200 morbidly obese men (average weight 143.5 kg), the mortality among the 25-to-34-year age group was 12-fold that of normal males and six-fold that of normal males in the 35-to-44-year age group.[40] During an average follow-up period of 7.6 years, 50 of the original 200 subjects had died from a variety of causes, including cardiovascular disease (54 per cent), malignancies (eight per cent), accidents (ten per cent), and diabetes or cirrhosis (eight per cent). The initial clinical screening of the 200 men revealed that diabetes (38 per cent), hypertension (20 per cent), cardiovascular disease (ten per cent), gout (six per cent), arthritis (seven per cent), and Pickwickian syndrome (four per cent) were the most prevalent disorders. In another series of morbidly obese patients (mean weight 135 kg), the prevalence of clinical disorders was as follows: fatty liver, 89 per cent; hypertension, 70 per cent; osteoarthritis, 72 per cent; respiratory distress, 62 per cent; and diabetes, 56 per cent.[36] These and other metabolic disorders have been cited in recent publications.[56, 116]

Aside from the clinical effects of massive obesity, the quality of life for these subjects is often greatly compromised. The morbidly obese frequently have a poor self-image and tend to be physically and socially inactive. Many do not seek employment or are unable to find employment on account of obesity, limiting opportunities for attaining a sense of accomplishment and improving self-esteem. The anguish arising from social isolation and feelings of inferiority may lead to compulsive eating but also may be a motivation to seek relief by extreme measures, including hazardous fad diets and major surgery. Questions about informed consent for such a patient population support the value of patient advocates in many instances.

Medical Treatment for the Morbidly Obese Patient

The use of calorie-restricted regimens in the treatment of morbid obesity has been successful for only a small segment of the obese population.[116] Fasting,[41] semistarvation,[8, 41] and very-low-calorie diets[9, 15] have been tried. Because the morbidly obese have a greater resting energy expenditure and increased energy output associated with standard physical activity on account of their great size, large initial weight losses are commonly observed in compliant patients. At an acceptable weight loss of three to five pounds per week, a morbidly obese patient would have to remain on a calorie-restricted regimen for four to seven months to lose 100 lb. Furthermore, adherence to these diets does not guarantee that body weight will stabilize once the patient stops dieting. Weight regain is often rapid, owing perhaps to the continued presence of a large number of adipose cells and the obligate regain of lean tissue lost during dieting, but most certainly accompanied by the resumption of maladaptive eating habits. Rapid weight regain has been observed both after fasting and very-low-calorie diets.[41, 51] Genuth and colleagues[51] reported that 56 per cent of their patients who had been placed on a supplemented fast regained more than 50 per cent of their weight loss within a two-year period.

Using a very-low-calorie diet providing 1.5 gm of protein per kg of IBW as part of a multidisciplinary weight reduction program, we have observed sizeable weight loss in the morbidly obese.[9, 11] As seen in other studies, however, there is a high rate of recidivism (although 28 per cent of our morbidly obese patients remained more than 40 lb lighter at two- to seven-year follow-up).

Behavior modification techniques have had limited success as unimodal therapy in the treatment of mild to moderate obesity.[112, 118] In virtually all behavioral studies, however, the subjects have weighed less than 200 lb. There are no reports of successful treatment of the morbidly obese by use of behavior modification alone.

Reviews are available regarding the use of pharmacologic agents to control appetite and/or alter fat metabolism in the obese population.[17, 113] As with behavior modification, there is no information about the successful use of these agents in the treatment of morbid obesity. Few clinical studies employing these anorectic drugs last longer than three months, an insufficient period to attain significant weight losses at the slow rates observed with drug therapy. There is valid concern about untoward side effects arising from long-term use of such pharmacologic agents.

Surgical Therapy for the Morbidly Obese

One of the least invasive techniques utilized over the past decade for treatment of morbid obesity is jaw wiring. Weight loss following this procedure is substantial. In one group of 13 patients who had their jaws wired for an average period of eight months, the mean weight loss was 29 kg.[65] On removal of the wires, however, weight regain was steady and rapid in 12 of these patients. The popularity of jaw wiring has declined because of these universal observations.

Many reviews are available regarding the use of jejunoileal bypass operations for treatment of morbid obesity.[7, 25, 36, 44, 99] This operation was originally designed to promote caloric malabsorption by shunting food past the major absorptive areas of the intestine, although in practice a reduction in intake emerged as the principal mechanism of weight loss. Sizable weight losses were commonly observed within one year of surgery.[7, 99] Unfortunately, the metabolic sequelae of vitamin,[7] electrolyte,[36] and mineral[58] inbalances, along with hepatic dysfunction,[80] urolithiasis,[99] and protein malnutrition,[106] have prompted bariatric surgeons to reconsider the value of this procedure.

The use of gastric bypass and gastric partition surgery has increased steadily as the use of jejunoileal bypass operations has declined. Bypass creates a very small stomach pouch (less than 30 ml), which limits total food intake. Since the first report of its use in treatment of the morbidly obese appeared in 1967,[77] numerous clinical studies have described its effectiveness and relatively low complication rate.[59, 78, 87, 97] The rate and amount of weight loss following gastric bypass surgery parallel those reported following jejunoileal bypasses.[1, 99] Weight loss following gastric bypass surgery approaches 45 kg at the end of the first year in the majority of patients.[86, 97] Patients weighing more than 250 per cent of IBW tend to lose more weight than those weighing less than 250 per cent of IBW. Perioperative mortality rates are similar to those in jejunoileal bypass surgery, and complications are fewer and generally less severe.[26, 90]

Because the classic gastric bypass operation is technically difficult,[72, 76] the use of the simpler procedure of gastric partitioning or gastroplasty has developed over the past few years.[70, 76] These surgical variants, however, may not be as effective as gastric bypass techniques in promoting long-term weight loss or weight maintenance.[69, 85] A recent report indicates that vertical banding instead of transverse banding may prove to be the most effective and safest of the gastroplasty procedures.[75]

CURRENT TREATMENT PROGRAM FOR MORBID OBESITY

We have utilized a comprehensive multidisciplinary program in the treatment of morbid obesity prior to surgery.[16, 20] This program provides diet, exercise, and behavior modification therapies as adjuncts to the surgical treatment. The continued use of these concepts appears important for successful long-term weight maintenance following surgically induced weight reduction.[27, 57]

Each patient entering the program is extensively evaluated physically and psychologically to ensure that he or she is a suitable candidate for gastric bypass surgery.[29, 37, 87] The criteria important for patient selection include an adult body weight of more than 200 per cent of IBW or more than 100 lb overweight for three or more successive years, repeated failure of dietary or medical control of body weight, absence of serious psychiatric, hepatic, renal, cardiopulmonary, and gastrointestinal dysfunction, and willingness to forego pregnancy during the one-year period of weight loss. Only subjects between 18 and 55 years of age are accepted.

The presurgical multidisciplinary period lasts for at least one month to allow time for reconsideration, plus a comprehensive medical and psychologic evaluation. Simple aerobic exercises, generally consisting of a walking program, are prescribed along with a conventional moderately restricted weight loss diet. After a few weeks on this diet, the patient may be put on a very-low-calorie diet if there are no contraindications.[15, 16] Even limited weight loss (20 to 40 lb) can markedly improve cardiorespiratory function in certain

patients and mobilize fat from the liver. Absolute cessation of smoking is mandatory for one month prior to surgery, even if it can be accomplished only at the cost of no weight loss. The technical aspects of the preoperative preparation of the patient and the surgical procedures employed have been described.[72, 76, 97]

Our experience with gastric bypass surgery in conjunction with the comprehensive multidisciplinary program has demonstrated that substantial weight loss can be obtained within 12 months and that weight can be maintained for up to 30 months postoperatively.[87] We have currently performed gastric bypass operations on 141 morbidly obese subjects (mean initial weight 134.3 kg) at a female/male ratio of 4:1. The primary surgical technique utilized is a roux-en-Y gastrojejunostomy.[20] Rates and extent of weight loss have been similar to those observed earlier.[87] The mean cumulative weight loss at the end of the first year is 45 kg, reaching a maximum mean of 50 kg by the beginning of the third year. The mean percentage of excess weight above IBW lost by one and two years has been 56 and 61 per cent, respectively. Approximately 34 per cent of the patients reached 130 per cent of IBW by the first year following surgery.

We also examined lean tissue loss subsequent to gastric bypass over time in a subset of morbidly obese patients, using body ^{40}K counting of lean body mass.[87] The fraction of total weight loss represented by lean tissue decreased from 32 per cent at the end of the first post-surgical month to five per cent at the end of the first year. By the beginning of the third year after surgery, lean tissue loss accounted for only three per cent of the total weight loss.[87] We have concluded that gastric bypass surgery produces sizable weight loss which ultimately is of fat; despite initial lean tissue losses, lean tissue is restored after the first postoperative month. Successful maintenance of the reduced weight following surgery is highly dependent on the patient's utilization of the dietary, exercise, and behavior modification techniques as well as total time of participation in the program.

Postoperative Dietary Consideration

Recent studies have focused on dietary intake of subjects several months after gastric bypass surgery. One report revealed that intake of calories, protein, iron, and folate tended to be below RDA levels for most patients studied.[115] Another study evaluated the nutritional status of gastric bypass patients and found significant reductions in the intake of calories, protein, fat, cholesterol, carbohydrate, iron, and vitamin A.[23] Several cases of a peripheral neuropathy responding to thiamine replacement have been described following gastric bypass in patients with particularly poor dietary intake and rapid weight loss.[95] Furthermore, a case of severe neurologic dysfunction culminating in death was described in one patient with severe malnutrition resulting from inadequate intake.[45]

It is imperative that gastric bypass patients undergo periodic dietary biochemical and hematologic assessments. The similarity of a gastric bypass to a Billroth II gastrojejunostomy with bypass of the duodenum suggests that iron, folate, and possibly B_{12} malabsorption could occur. Dietitians should have a major role both in the selection of foods that will provide a balanced diet and in continued support of the use of behavior modification techniques.[28] This dietary counseling is necessary to reduce the risk of development of nutritional deficiencies and to control caloric intake in the prevention of long-term regain of weight.

REFERENCES

1. Alden, J.F.: Gastric and jejunoileal bypass. Arch. Surg., *112*:799, 1977.
2. Allison, B.M., and Baird, J.W.C.: Elimination of nitrogen from the body. *In* Munro, H.N., and Allison, J.B. (eds.): Mammalian Protein Metabolism, Vol 1. New York, Academic Press, 1964, p. 483.
3. Aoki, T.T., Muller, W.A., Brennan, M.F., et al.: Metabolic effects of glucose in brief and prolonged fasted man. Am. J. Clin. Nutr., *28*:507, 1975.
4. Apfelbaum, M., Boudon, P., Dacatis, D., et al.: Effets métaboliques de la diéte protidique chez 41 sujets obèses. Presse Med., *78*:1917, 1970.
5. Apfelbaum, M.: Effects of very restrictive high-protein diets with special reference to the nitrogen balance. Int. J. Obesity, *5*:209, 1981.
6. Ball, M.F., Canary, J.J., and Kyle, L.J.: Comparative effects of caloric restriction and total starvation body composition in obesity. Ann. Int. Med., *67*:60, 1967.
7. Benfield, J.R., Castelnuovo-Teddesco, P., Drenick, E., et al.: Intestinal bypass operation as a treatment for obesity. Ann. Intern. Med. *85*:97, 1976.
8. Bernstein, R.S., and VanItallie, T.B.: An overview of therapy for morbid obesity. Surg. Clin. North Am., *59*:985, 1979.
9. Bistrian, B.R.: Clinical use of a protein-sparing modified fast. J.A.M.A., *240*:2299, 1978.
10. Bistrian, B.R., and Hoffer, L.J.: Obesity. *In* Conn, H.F. (ed.): Current Therapy 1982. Philadelphia, W.B. Saunders, 1982, p. 444.
11. Bistrian, B.R., and Sherman, M.: Results of the treatment of obesity with a protein-sparing modified fast. Int. J. Obesity, *2*:143, 1978.
12. Bistrian, B.R., Winterer, J., Blackburn, G.L., et al.: Effect of a protein-sparing diet and brief fast on nitrogen metabolism in mildly obese subjects. J. Lab. Clin. Med., *89*:1030, 1977.
13. Bistrian, B.R., Sherman, M., and Young, V.R.: The mechanisms of nitrogen sparing in fasting supplemented by protein and carbohydrate. J. Clin. Endocrinol. Metab., *53*:874, 1981.
14. Bistrian, B.R., George, D.T., Blackburn, G.L., and Wannemacher, R.W.: Effect of diet on the metabolic response to infection: Protein-sparing modified fast plus 100 grams glucose and yellow fever immunization. Am. J. Clin. Nutr., *34*:238, 1981.
15. Blackburn, G.L., Bistrian, B.R., Flatt, J.P., et al.: Role of a protein-sparing modified fast in a comprehensive weight reduction program. *In* Howard, A. (ed.): Recent Advances in Obesity Research. London, Newman Publishing, 1975, p. 279.
16. Blackburn, G.L., and Greenberg, I.: Multidisciplinary approach to adult obesity therapy. Int. J. Obesity, *2*:133, 1978.
17. Blundell, J.E.: Pharmacological adjustment of the mechanisms underlying feeding and obesity. *In* Stunkard, A.J. (ed.): Obesity. Philadelphia, W.B. Saunders, 1980, p. 182.
18. Bogardus, C., Lagrange, B.M., Horton, E.S., et al.: Metabolic fuels and the capacity for exercise during hypocaloric diet. Int. J. Obesity, *5*:295, 1981.
19. Bolinger, R.E., Lukert, B.P., Brown, R.W., et al.: Metabolic balance of obese subjects during fasting. Arch. Intern. Med., *118*:3, 1966.
20. Bothe, A., Jr., Bistrian, B.R., Greenberg, I., et al.: Energy regulation in morbid obesity by multidisciplinary therapy. Surg. Clin. North Am., *59*:1017, 1979.
21. Bray, G.A.: The Obese Patient. Philadelphia, W.B. Saunders, 1976.
22. Bray, G.A.: Definition, measurement, and classification of the syndromes of obesity. Int. J. Obesity, *2*:99, 1978.
23. Brown, K.E., Settle, E.A., and Van Rij, A.M.: Food intake patterns of gastric bypass patients. J. Am. Diet. Assoc., *80*:437, 1982.
24. Brozek, J., Grande, R., Taylor, H.L., et al.: Changes in body weight and body dimensions in men performing work on a low calorie carbohydrate diet. J. Appl. Physiol., *10*:412, 1957.
25. Buchwald, H., and Rucker, R.D.: The history of metabolic surgery for morbid obesity and a commentary. World J. Surg., *5*:781, 1981.
26. Buckwalter, J.A., and Herbst, C.A.: Complications of gastric bypass for morbid obesity. Am. J. Surg., *139*:55, 1980.
27. Buckwalter, J.A.: Nonsurgical factors important to the success of surgery for morbid obesity. Surgery, *91*:113, 1982.
28. Bukoff, M., and Carlson, S.: Diet modification and behavioral changes for bariatric gastric surgery. J. Am. Diet. Assoc., *78*:158, 1981.
29. Cahill, G.F., Jr.: Starvation in man. N. Engl. J. Med., *282*:668, 1970.

30. Cahill, G.F., Jr., and Aoki, T.T.: How metabolism affects clinical problems. Med. Times, *98*:106, 1970.

31. Cahill, G.F., Jr.: Starvation in man. Clin. Endocrinol. Metab., *5*:397, 1976.

32. Calloway, D.H., and Margen, S.: Variation in endogenous nitrogen excretion and dietary nitrogen utilization as determinants of human protein requirement. J. Nutr., *101*:205, 1971.

33. Committee on Dietary Allowances, Food and Nutrition Board: Recommended Dietary Allowances. Washington, D.C., National Academy of Sciences, 1980.

34. Contaldo, F., Di Biase, G., Scalfi, L., et al.: Protein-sparing modified fast in the treatment of severe obesity: Weight loss and nitrogen balance data. Int. J. Obesity, *4*:189, 1980.

35. De Haven, J., Sherwin, R., Hendler, R., et al.: Nitrogen and sodium balance and sympathetic-nervous system activity in obese subjects treated with a low-calorie protein or mixed diet. N. Engl. J. Med., *302*:477, 1980.

36. Deitel, M., Bojm, M.A., Atin, M.D., et al.: Intestinal bypass and gastric partitioning for morbid obesity: A comparison. Canad. J. Surg., *25*:283, 1982.

37. Diaz, S.G., and Fernandez, S.G.: Medical and surgical indications for treatment of morbid obesity. World J. Surg., *5*:795, 1981.

38. Drenick, E.J.: Weight reduction by prolonged fasting. *In* Bray, G.A. (ed.): Obesity in Perspective, Vol. 2, Part 2. (Fogarty International Center Series on Preventive Medicine. DHEW Publication No. (NIH) 75–708.) Washington, D.C., U.S. Department of Health, Education and Welfare, 1975, p. 341.

39. Drenick, E.J.: Definition and health consequences of morbid obesity. Surg. Clin. North Am., *59*:963, 1979.

40. Drenick, E.J., Bale, G.S., Seltzer, F., et al.: Excessive mortality and causes of death in morbidly obese men. J.A.M.A., *243*:443, 1980.

41. Drenick, E.J., and Johnson, D.: Weight reduction by fasting and semistarvation in morbid obesity: Long-term follow-up. Int. J. Obesity, *2*:123, 1978.

42. Du Bois, E.F.: Basal Metabolism in Health and Disease. Philadelphia, Lea & Febiger, 1927.

43. Durrant, M.L., Garrow, J.S., Royston, P., et al.: Factors influencing the composition of the weight lost by obese subjects on a reducing diet. Br. J. Nutr., *44*:275, 1980.

44. Faloon, W.W.: Jejunileostomy for obesity. Am. J. Clin. Nutr., *30*:1, 1977.

45. Feit, H., Glasberg, M., Ireton, C., Rosenberg, R.N., and Thau, E.: Peripheral neuropathy and starvation after gastric partitioning for morbid obesity. Ann. Intern. Med., *96*:453, 1982.

46. Fisler, J.S., Drenick, E.J., Blumfeld, D.E., et al.: Nitrogen economy during very low·calorie reducing diets: Quality and quantity of dietary protein. Am. J. Clin. Nutr., *35*:471, 1982.

47. Forbes, G.B.: Weight loss during fasting: Implications for the obese. Am. J. Clin. Nutr., *23*:1212, 1970.

48. Forbes, G.B., and Drenick, E.J.: Loss of body nitrogen on fasting. Am. J. Clin. Nutr., *32*:1570, 1979.

49. Garlick, P.J., Clugston, G.A., and Waterlow, J.C.: Influence of low-energy diets on whole-body protein turnover in obese subjects. Am. J. Physiol., *238*:E235, 1980.

50. Genuth, S.M., Castro, J.H., and Vertes, V.: Weight reduction in obesity by outpatient semistarvation. J.A.M.A., *230*:987, 1974.

51. Genuth, S.M., Vertes, V., and Hazelton, I.: Supplemented fasting in the treatment of obesity. *In* Bray, G.A. (ed.): Recent Advances in Obesity Research: II. London, Newman Publishing, 1978, p. 370.

52. Golden, M.H.N., Waterlow, J.C., and Picou, D.: Protein turnover, synthesis and breakdown before and after recovery from protein-energy malnutrition. Clin. Sci. Mol. Med., *53*:473, 1977.

53. Goodner, C.J., Koerker, D.J., Werrbach, J.H., et al.: Adrenergic regulation of lipolysis and insulin secretion in the fasted baboon. Am. J. Physiol., *224*:534, 1973.

54. Greenberg, G.R., and Jeejeebhoy, K.N.: Intravenous protein-sparing therapy in patients with gastrointestinal disease. J.P.E.N., *3*:427, 1979.

55. Gries, F.A., Berger, M., and Berchtold, P.: Clinical results with starvation and semistarvation. *In* Bray, G.A. (ed.): Recent Advances in Obesity Research: II. London, Newman Publishing, 1978, p. 359.

56. Griffen, W.O., Bivins, B.A., Bell, R.M., et al.: Gastric bypass for morbid obesity. World J. Surg., *5*:817, 1981.

57. Halverson, J.D., and Koehler, R.E.: Gastric bypass: Analysis of weight loss and factors determining success. Surgery, *90*:446, 1981.

58. Halverson, J.D., Scheff, R.J., Gentry, K., et al.: Jejunoileal bypass: Late metabolic sequelae and weight gain. Am. J. Surg., *140*:347, 1980.

59. Halverson, J.D., Zuckerman, G.R., Koehler, R.E., et al.: Gastric bypass for morbid obesity. Ann. Surg., *194*:152, 1981.

60. Hoffer, L.J., Bistrian, B.R., Young, V.R., et al.: Metabolic effects of very low calorie weight reduction diets. J. Clin. Invest., *73*:750, 1984.

61. Hoffer, L.J., Phinney, S.D., Bistrian, B.R., Blackburn, G.L., and Young, V.R.: Whole body protein turnover, studied with ^{15}N-glycine, during weight reduction by moderate energy restriction. *In* Blackburn, G.L., Grant, J.R., Young, V.R., and Wright, J. (eds.): Amino Acids: Metabolism and Medical Applications. Boston, PSG, Inc., 1983, p. 48.

62. Howard, A.N.: The historical development, efficacy and safety of very-low-calorie diets. Int. J. Obesity, *5*:195, 1981.

63. Howard, A.N., Grant, A., and Edwards, O.: The treatment of obesity with a very low calorie liquid-formula diet: An inpatient/outpatient comparison using skim milk protein as the chief protein source. Int. J. Obesity, *2*:321, 1978.

64. Jones, A.O.L., Jacobs, R.M., Fry, B.E., et al.: Elemental content of predigested liquid protein products. Am. J. Clin. Nutr., *33*:2545, 1980.

65. Kark, A.E.: Jaw wiring. Am. J. Clin. Nutr., *33*(Suppl.):420, 1980.

66. Kelleher, P.C., Phinney, S.D., Sims, E.A.H., et al.: Effects of carbohydrate-containing and carbohydrate-restricted hypocaloric and eucaloric diets on serum concentrations of retinol-binding protein, thyroxin-binding prealbumin and transferrin. Metabolism, *32*:95–101, 1983.

67. Krotkiewski, M., Toss, L., Bjorntorp, P., et al.: The effect of a very-low-calorie diet with and without chronic exercise on thyroid and sex hormones, plasma proteins, oxygen uptake, insulin and C

peptide concentrations in obese women. Int. J. Obesity, 5:287, 1981.

68. Landsberg, L., and Young, R.B.: Fasting, feeding and regulation of the sympathetic nervous system. N. Engl. J. Med., 298:1295, 1978.

69. Linner, J.H.: Comparative effectiveness of gastric bypass and gastroplasty. Arch. Surg., 117:701, 1982.

70. MacLean, L.D., Rhode, B.M., and Shizgal, H.M.: Gastroplasty for obesity. Surg. Gynecol. Obstet., 153:200, 1981.

71. Mahmud, K., Ripley, D., and Doscherholmen, A.: Vitamin B$_{12}$ absorption tests: Their unreliability in postgastrectomy states. J.A.M.A., 216:1167, 1971.

72. Maini, B.S., Blackburn, G.L., and McDermott, W.V.: Technical considerations in a gastric bypass operation for morbid obesity. Surg. Gynecol. Obstet., 145:907, 1977.

73. Mancini, M., Contaldo, F., DiBiase, G., et al.: Frequency, relevance, and reversibility of medical complications of obesity. In Mancini, M., Lewis, B., and Contaldo, F. (eds.): Medical Complications of Obesity. New York, Academic Press, 1979, p. 1.

74. Marliss, E.B., Murray, F.T., and Nakhooda, A.F.: The metabolic response to hypocaloric protein diets in obese man. J. Clin. Invest., 62:468, 1978.

75. Mason, E.E.: Vertical banded gastroplasty for obesity. Arch. Surg., 117:701, 1982.

76. Mason, E.E.: Evolution of gastric reduction for obesity. Contemp. Surg., 20:17, 1982.

77. Mason, E.E., and Ito, C.: Gastric bypass in obesity. Surg. Clin. North Am., 47:1345, 1967.

78. Mason, E.E., Printen, K.J., Blommers, T.J., et al.: Gastric bypass in morbid obesity. Am. J. Clin. Nutr., 33(Suppl.):395, 1980.

79. Mason, E.H.: The treatment of obesity. Can. Med. Assoc. J., 14:1052, 1924.

80. Moxley, R.T., Pozefsky, T., and Lockwood, D.H.: Protein nutrition and liver disease after jejunoileal bypass for morbid obesity. N. Engl. J. Med., 290:921, 1974.

81. Munro, H.N.: Carbohydrate and fat as factors in protein utilization and metabolism. Physiol. Rev., 31:449, 1951.

82. Munro, H.N.: General aspects of the regulation of protein metabolism by diet and hormones. In Munro, H.N., Allison, J.B. (eds.): Mammalian Protein Metabolism, Vol. 1. New York, Academic Press, 1964, p. 381.

83. O'Connell, R.C., Morgan, A.P., Aoki, T.T., et al.: Nitrogen conservation in starvation: Graded responses to intravenous glucose. J. Clin. Endocrinol. Metab., 39:555, 1974.

84. Owen, O.E., Felig, P., Morgan, A.P., et al.: Liver and kidney metabolism during prolonged starvation. J. Clin. Invest., 48:574, 1969.

85. Pace, W.G., Martin, E.W., Tetirick, T., et al.: Gastric partitioning for morbid obesity. Ann. Surg., 190:392, 1979.

86. Palombo, J.D., Hayward, E., Reinhold, R.B., et al.: Composition of weight loss after gastric bypass: Long-term analysis. Surg. Forum, 32:114, 1981.

87. Palombo, J.D., Maletskos, C.J., Reinhold, R.B., et al.: Composition of weight loss in morbidly obese patients after gastric bypass. J. Surg. Res., 30:435, 1981.

88. Paul, P., and Bortz, W.M.: Turnover and oxidation of plasma glucose in lean and obese humans. Metabolism, 18:570, 1969.

89. Passmore, R., Strong, R.A., and Richie, F.J.: The chemical composition of the tissue lost by obese patients on a reducing regimen. Br. J. Nutr., 12:113, 1958.

90. Peltier, G., Hermreck, A.S., Moffat, R.E., et al.: Complications following gastric bypass procedures for morbid obesity. Surgery, 86:648, 1979.

91. Pencharz, P.B., Motil, K.J., Parsons, H.G., et al.: The effect of an energy-restricted diet on the protein metabolism of obese adolescents: Nitrogen-balance and whole-body nitrogen turnover. Clin. Sci., 59:13, 1980.

92. Phinney, S.D.: Low calorie protein versus mixed diet. N. Engl. J. Med., 303:158, 1980.

93. Phinney, S.D., Bistrian, B.R., Wolfe, R.R., et al.: The human metabolic response to chronic ketosis without caloric restriction: Physical and biochemical adaptation. Metabolism, 32:757, 1983.

94. Picou, D., and Taylor-Roberts, T.: The measurement of total protein synthesis and catabolism and nitrogen turnover in infants in different nutritional states and receiving different amounts of dietary protein. Clin. Sci., 36:283, 1969.

95. Printen, K.J., and Mason, E.E.: Peripheral neuropathy following gastric bypass for treatment of morbid obesity. Obesity Bariatr. Med., 6:185, 1977.

96. Reichard, G.A., Haff, A.C., Skutches, C.L., et al.: Plasma acetone metabolism in the fasting human. J. Clin. Invest., 63:619, 1979.

97. Reinhold, R.B.: Critical analysis of long-term weight loss following gastric bypass. Surg. Gynecol. Obstet., 155:385, 1982.

98. Rowe, J.W., Young, J.B., Minaker, K.L., et al.: Effect of insulin and glucose infusions on sympathetic nervous system activity in normal man. Diabetes, 30:219, 1981.

99. Rucker, R.D., Horstmann, J., Schneider, P.D., et al.: Comparisons between jejunoileal and gastric bypass operations for morbid obesity. Surgery, 92:241, 1982.

100. Runcie, J., and Hilditch, T.E.: Energy provision, tissue utilization and weight loss in prolonged starvation. Br. Med. J., 2:352, 1974.

101. Sapir, D.G., Chambers, N.E., and Ryan, J.W.: The role of potassium in the control of ammonium excretion during starvation. Metabolism, 25:211, 1976.

102. Sapir, D. G., and Owen, O.E.: Renal conservation of ketone bodies during starvation. Metabolism, 24:23, 1975.

103. Sapir, D.G., Owen, O.E., Cheng, J.T., et al.: The effect of carbohydrates on ammonium and ketoacid excretion during starvation. J. Clin. Invest., 51:2093, 1972.

104. Scrimshaw, N.S., Hussein, M.A., Murray, E., et al.: Protein requirements of man: Variations in obligatory urinary and fecal nitrogen losses in young men. J. Nutr., 102:1595, 1972.

105. Shetty, P.S., Watrasiewicz, K.E., Jung, R.T., et al.: Rapid-turnover transport proteins: An index of subclinical protein-energy malnutrition. Lancet, 2:230, 1979.

106. Shizgal, H.M., Forse, R.A., Spanier, A.H., et al.: Protein malnutrition following intestinal bypass for morbid obesity. Surgery, 86:60, 1979.

107. Society of Actuaries: Build and Blood Pressure Study. Chicago, 1959.

108. Society of Actuaries and Association of Life Insurance Medical Directors: Build Study. 1979.

109. Stinebaugh, B.J., Marliss, E.B., Goldstein, M.B., et

al.: Mechanism for the paradoxical aciduria following alkali administration to prolonged-fasted subjects. Metabolism, *24*:915, 1975.

110. Strang, J.M., McCluggage, HB., and Evans, F.A.: Further studies in the dietary correction of obesity. Am. J. Med. Sci., *179*:687, 1930.

111. Strong, J.A., Passmore, R., and Ritchie, F.: Clinical observations on obese patients during a strict reducing regimen. Br. J. Nutr., *12*:105, 1958.

112. Stunkard, A.J., and Penick, S.B.: Behavior modification in the treatment of obesity. Arch. Gen. Psychiatry, *36*:801, 1979.

113. Sullivan, A.C., and Comai, K.: Pharmacological treatment of obesity. Int. J. Obesity, *2*:167, 1978.

114. Talbot, J.: Research needs in management of obesity by severe caloric restriction. (Bureau of Goods, Food and Drug Administration, Department of Health, Education and Welfare.) Bethesda, Life Sciences Research Office, Federation of American Societies for Experimental Biology, 1979.

115. Updegraff, T.A., and Neufeld, N.J.: Protein, iron and folate status of patients prior to and following surgery for morbid obesity. J. Am. Diet. Assoc., *80*:437, 1982.

116. Van Itallie, T.B.: "Morbid obesity": A hazardous disorder that resists conservative treatment. Am. J. Clin. Nutr., *33*(Suppl.):358, 1980.

117. Van Itallie, T.B., and Kral, J.G.: The dilemma of morbid obesity. J.A.M.A., *246*:999, 1981.

118. Wilson, G.T.: Behavior modification and the treatment of obesity. *In* Stunkard, A.J. (ed.): Obesity. Philadelphia, W.B. Saunders, 1980, p. 325.

119. Wilson, J.H.P., and Lamberts, S.W.J.: Nitrogen balance in obese patients receiving a very-low-calorie liquid formula diet. Am. J. Clin. Nutr., *32*:1612, 1979.

120. Winterer, J., Bistrian, B.R., Bilmazes, C., et al.: Whole body protein turnover studies with ^{15}N-glycine and muscle protein breakdown in mildly obese subjects during a protein-sparing diet and a brief total fast. Metabolism, *29*:575, 1980.

121. Yang, M-U, Barbos-Saldivar, J.L., Pi-Sunyer, F.X., et al.: Metabolic effects of substituting carbohydrate for protein in a low-calorie diet: A prolonged study in obese patients. Int. J. Obesity, *5*:231, 1981.

CHAPTER 38

Total Parenteral Nutrition: Considerations in the Elderly

RONNI CHERNOFF
DAVID A. LIPSCHITZ

Many hospitalized patients who are maintained on parenteral nutrition are greater than 65 years of age. However, consideration of the special and unique requirements of individuals in this age group are rarely addressed. The nutritional requirements of elderly patients must be adjusted for the physiologic and metabolic changes that occur as a natural part of the aging process, and they must be modified for chronic illness and those special needs caused by episodes of critical illness, such as those requiring parenteral nutrition. In spite of the frequency with which elderly patients are noted as part of patient populations that are defined by diagnosis or treatment, they have not been identified in the parenteral nutrition literature as a group with special nutritional requirements.

Protein-calorie malnutrition in hospitalized aged patients may be secondary to the primary disease or it may be a contributing factor to that primary disease. Decreased cell-mediated immunity, diminished muscle strength and coordination, weakness, anemia, malabsorption, and depressed tissue synthesis may all be related to prolonged protein-calorie malnutrition in this patient population.[1] Although it is accepted that parenteral nutrition may be used successfully to reverse the sequelae of protein-calorie malnutrition, the unique requirements imposed by the aging process must be addressed to best meet the needs of the elderly hospitalized patient. The first step in this process is to evaluate nutritional status in this age group. The nutritional assessment of elderly persons presents some limitations and special considerations because of the lack of appropriate norms for comparison.[2]

NUTRITIONAL ASSESSMENT OF THE ELDERLY PATIENT

The physical measures that are routinely used to assess nutritional status may not be suitable for an elderly population. Height and weight tables do not usually include subjects past the age of 65 years because the most commonly used references (e.g., Metropolitan Life Insurance Tables) are derived from actual studies developed for insurance policy purposes. The standard tables for the height and weight of Americans 65 to 94 years of age developed by Master and associates may be more appropriate. Unfortunately, the study was limited to whites of relatively high socioeconomic group and therefore does not provide a broad-based sample that is applicable to the entire population. It is also known that height decreases with age because of a shortening of the spinal column. Losses may be as great as 4.2 cm every 20 years.[2] In both cross sectional and longitudinal studies, it has been shown that this phenomenon exists in many populations.[3]

Weight is not a stable measure throughout adulthood either. Weight changes occur during the adult years, with a pattern of decreasing body weight after the age of 54 years.[3] However, weight change is also accompanied by changes in body composition.

With age, lean body mass decreases, and adipose tissue—both subcutaneous and that surrounding the internal organs—increases. This results in an altered subcutaneous fat/total body weight ratio, a change in lean body mass/weight ratio, and a change in weight to height proportion.

Changes in body composition that occur with aging have been demonstrated through the use of total body potassium, total body water, or radiographic techniques.[2] These sophisticated techniques have indicated that water, fat, lean body mass, visceral protein, and mineral changes occur.[3] Estimating body composition by crude measures, such as skinfold thickness, presents several problems. First, skinfolds thicken with increasing age, muscle mass decreases, distribution of subcutaneous fat changes, and bone density diminishes. Second, there are no reasonable standards against which to compare a sample of elderly subjects.[3] Lean body mass has also been estimated by measuring urinary creatinine excretion, which is related either to height or to total arm length. Recent evidence indicates that this parameter is of little value in assessing reductions in lean body mass in older subjects. The estimate may be important, however, in assessing the response to nutritional intervention.

The biochemical indices commonly used for assessing nutritional status have been shown to be affected by age. Estimates of visceral protein using serum albumin or transferrin as indicators[4] may be less accurate in elderly persons; their organs are smaller and the liver production of circulating proteins is reduced.[3] In addition, hepatic and renal disease, cancer, and congestive heart failure are also known to reduce levels of circulating albumin. Serum transferrin levels also vary with tissue iron stores. Thus, in older subjects transferrin levels are reduced, not because of altered nutritional status but because of an increase in iron stores. Hydration status in the aged patient is another factor that may affect the results of biochemical measurements. Dehydration or excess fluid may concentrate or dilute serum values of albumin, transferrin, enzymes, or other proteins.

Cell-mediated immunity, which is frequently used to assess nutritional status, is also altered as a result of the aging process.[5] The incidence of anergy is increased in older persons, and lymphocytopenia is more common. Absolute T-cell number is reduced with a relative increase in T-helper cells. B-cell number and function are largely unaffected.

These age-related declines in normal immune function are thought to be important to the increased incidence of infection, autoimmune diseases, and cancer in older persons. The alterations in cell-mediated immunity that occur with aging are very similar to those described in protein-calorie malnutrition. As a result, interpretation of host-defense abnormalities in elderly persons is difficult.

Clinical judgment is very important in the diagnosis of protein-calorie malnutrition in the geriatric patient. It should always be suspected when a disorder associated with malnutrition (cancer, chronic infections, hepatic and renal disease) is present. Dehydration and confusion are common, and hypoalbuminemia (less than 3 gm/dl) that is not due to hepatic disease or renal losses is invariably present. Anemia, hypotransferrinemia, anergy, and lymphocytopenia are the most useful supporting measurements.

CALORIC REQUIREMENTS

The caloric requirement is usually the first nutritional parameter identified in a patient receiving nutritional support. This is usually determined using a standard formula, nomogram, or reference table. Basal heat production and basal energy expenditure diminish with age. On the average, basal metabolism falls from about 38 Kcal/m²/hour at age 30 years to about 30 Kcal/m²/hour at age 80 years (Fig. 38–1).[6] This fall in basal metabolism is simply a reflection of a loss of metabolizing tissue or an increase in body fat, or both, with advancing age. In addition to basal heat production, the production of energy related to activity is lowered. Reduced and slowed physical activity among elderly persons leads to a lower total daily requirement of calories. In addition, the total heat elimination required in elderly subjects is less than in young subjects (Fig. 38–2). These facts must be considered when calculating daily caloric requirements of patients receiving parenteral support. Tables employing basal energy requirements for young adults may provide an inappropriate excess of calories for aged persons.

PROTEIN REQUIREMENTS

Although there is little information available on protein requirements in aging, it is known that the rate of protein synthesis and turnover is modestly reduced in older per-

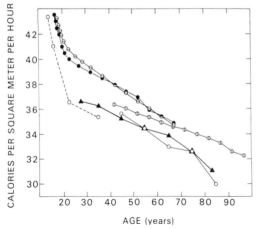

Figure 38–1. Age differences in basal metabolism of males aged 15 to 95 years. ◯––––◯, data from Shock, 1955; ●——●, data from Boothby, Berkson, and Dunn, 1936; ⊖——⊖, data from Dubois, 1936; ◯——◯, data from Shock and Yiengst, 1955; ▲——▲, data from GRC Longitudinal Study–Shock, Andres and Norris, unpublished. (*From* Shock, N. W.: Systems integration. *In* Finch, C. E., and Hayflick, L. (eds.): Handbook of the Biology of Aging. New York, Van Nostrand Reinhold Company, 1977, with permission.)

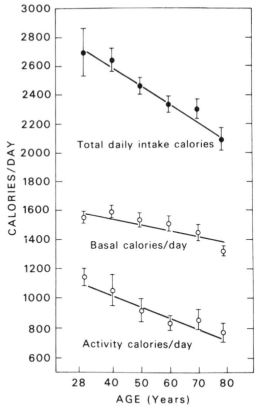

Figure 38–2. Daily caloric intake and expenditure in normal males. ●——●, total daily caloric intake; ◯——◯ *(upper curve)*, basal caloric expenditure per day; ◯——◯ *(lower curve)*, daily caloric expenditure for activity. Vertical lines represent ± 1 standard curve of the mean. (*From* Shock, N. W.: Energy metabolism, caloric intake and physical activity of the aging. *In* L. A. Carlson (ed.): Nutrition in Old Age. (X Symposium of the Swedish Nutrition Foundation), Uppsala: Almquist and Wilkbell, 1972, pp. 12–23.)

sons.[7] There is also mounting evidence that the 30 per cent reduction in caloric intake is not paralleled by or equal to the decrease in requirements of other nutrients, particularly protein. Since the intake of food and nutrients is primarily regulated by energy needs, it is very likely that protein nutriture in the elderly person is severely compromised. It is conceivable that this alteration in protein nutriture may play an important role in the reduction of lean body mass that occurs with aging.

In the elderly patient requiring parenteral feeding, these facts are complicated by the presence of other primary disease processes that may affect protein nutriture. In general, in older individuals a protein intake of 1 gm/kg body weight seems appropriate,

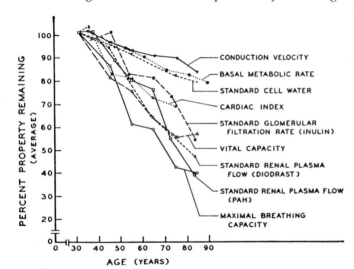

Figure 38–3. Data compiled by Shock and colleagues clearly document the loss of organ functional capacity that occurs with advancing age. (*From* Shock, N. W.: Physiologic aspects of aging. *J. Am. Diet. Assoc.,* 56:491, 1970, with permission.)

with adequate adjustments made to accommodate for losses that are illness-related. Acute febrile illnesses and trauma lead to immediate and often large losses of body protein, which must be replaced. However, high-protein diets are contraindicated under several circumstances. Patients who have severely compromised renal function require restrictions on the type and amount of protein provided. Parenteral protein solutions specifically developed for renal failure are appropriate to use in this situation (see Chapter 34).

The amount and type of protein must also be very carefully monitored in patients with severely impaired liver function. Products with moderate amounts of protein, high levels of branched-chain amino acids, and low levels of aromatic amino acids have been tested for use with these patients.

It has also been theorized that high-protein diets may cause increased bone resorption in patients who have osteoporosis.[7] This is a factor not often considered when supporting elderly patients with parenteral nutrition. A careful balance must be established among meeting physiologic needs for protein, replacing protein losses from trauma and illness, and not overloading the system with extraneous supplies of protein. One important factor is the provision of adequate calories from nonprotein sources.

CARBOHYDRATE METABOLISM

The usual nonprotein calorie source in parenteral nutrition is glucose. Hypertonic glucose solutions can effectively meet the caloric needs of the parenterally supported patient. However, glucose tolerance deteriorates progressively with age.[8] This phenomenon is supported by a variety of diagnostic tests, such as the oral glucose tolerance test, the intravenous glucose tolerance test, the intravenous tolbutamide tolerance test, and so on. The mechanism for decreased glucose tolerance is controversial. One theory is that impaired tissue sensitivity to insulin is the primary factor, the possible mechanism being a decrease in hormone receptor levels that may occur with aging. Studies assessing the effect of age on the serum insulin response to glucose have failed to confirm this possibility.[8] A second theory suggests that the biologic feedback mechanisms do not work as efficiently in older subjects as in younger subjects. In studies performed by Andres and

associates,[9] insulin release relative to investigator-controlled hyperglycemia was identical in all age subjects, leading to the conclusion that pancreatic beta-cell sensitivity to glucose does not change with age. Regardless of the reasons for decreased glucose tolerance in older subjects, infusing insulin with the parenteral solution is common practice in patients with impaired glucose tolerance.

FAT REQUIREMENTS

There has been an increase in the use of intravenous fat emulsions in parenteral hyperalimentation. The major indication is to provide more calories in a smaller volume. Intravenous fat emulsions are contraindicated in patients who have an impaired ability to clear lipids from the blood. Since all serum lipids increase in concentration with age,[10] it is a wise precaution to monitor lipid clearance at regular intervals in older patients.

VITAMIN REQUIREMENTS

Although there are no reliable data available on vitamin requirements in the elderly population,[11, 12] the dosages prescribed for younger adults are probably adequate. At present, the American Medical Association Nutritional Advisory Group guidelines for parenteral vitamins are generally used to calculate water-soluble- and fat-soluble-vitamin needs.[13]

It has been shown that when low plasma levels of vitamins occur in older persons, administration of the deficient nutrient corrects the abnormality. There is no evidence that absorption of vitamins is impaired with aging. It must be emphasized that absorption may be affected by a variety of diseases that are common in elderly patients. Interference with vitamin utilization by various drugs, medications, and chemotherapeutic agents must also be considered. Drug metabolism and clearance is slower in older persons than in younger persons. The problem may be compounded by the presence of associated diseases and malnutrition that interfere with drug metabolism.

An attempt to reverse nutritional deficiencies by giving therapeutic doses of some vitamins may cause deleterious effects. Fat-soluble-vitamin toxicity is a danger, especially in elderly patients who have smaller livers. Some water-soluble vitamins, such as vitamin C and niacin, occasionally cause cardiac arrhythmias and gastrointestinal problems even at therapeutic doses.[12]

MINERAL REQUIREMENTS

Minerals in solutions are added as individual salts. Because of the insoluble precipitate that occurs when they are in the same solution, calcium and phosphorus are added separately. Requirements for calcium in elderly persons are only estimates. It has been suggested that the amount required to maintain equilibrium ranges from 840 to 1020 mg;[14] however, there is a large variability in reported studies and in the ability of subjects to achieve equilibrium at various levels of intake. In establishing levels of calcium in parenteral solutions for the geriatric patient, attention must be paid to renal status, state of bone mineralization, and soft-tissue calcification.

Phosphorus and calcium are generally given in approximately equivalent amounts. Phosphate is also an important consideration when infusing hypertonic glucose solutions so as to avoid hypophosphatemia. Therefore, phosphorus should be infused in amounts that are sufficient to meet the needs of bone maintenance, intermediary metabolism, and nucleic acid formation.

Magnesium is essential for the normal metabolism of calcium and as a coenzyme in tissue-protein synthesis. Although dietary deficiencies are rare, magnesium must be added to parenteral solutions in adequate amounts—2 mEq/gm of nitrogen in the solution has been suggested.[15]

Potassium must be included in parenteral solutions for elderly patients in amounts adequate to maintain normal serum concentrations. The same precautions must be taken for patients receiving diuretic or steroid therapy and for patients suffering large fistulous losses, diarrhea, or chronic renal disease. Hyperkalemia in aged persons may be related to acute dehydration, acute or chronic renal failure, adrenal insufficiency, or severe metabolic or respiratory acidosis. Potassium balance in the elderly patient can be managed easily in parenteral nutrition if it is carefully monitored.

Sodium requirements for parenteral solutions in the geriatric patient must be adequate to meet individual needs. Considera-tion of chronic medical problems must be addressed even through a phase of acute illness. Many older persons are on sodium-restricted diets because of congestive heart failure, hypertension, cirrhosis, or compromised renal function. Maintenance of normal serum sodium levels and compensation for sodium-containing medication should be the goal of parenteral nutrition in this population. Other minerals—chloride, iron, iodine, zinc, copper, chromium, and manganese—should be provided in parenteral solutions in adequate amounts to meet individual needs.

FLUID BALANCE

Water balance in elderly patients may be affected by a diminished efficiency of the kidney resulting from a decrease in the number of functioning nephrons. Fever, polyuria, diarrhea, excessive losses from vomiting, or fistulous losses will increase fluid requirements. Meeting the fluid requirements of aged patients via parenteral feeding would not seem to be a problem; however, this mode of feeding, which provides several liters of fluid a day by the circulatory system, may cause stresses of its own.

Cardiac output decreases with age, as does stroke volume and stroke index.[16] The large arteries stiffen with age; increased vessel stiffness will cause increased systolic blood and pulse pressure. There is a functional decrease in the ability of the heart to contract and an increase in peripheral resistance.[17] These changes must be accounted for when perfusing the large volume of fluid required for total parenteral nutrition (TPN). When the decline in renal blood flow and glomerular filtration rate are accounted for, it must be recognized that fluid balance in elderly patients must be monitored very carefully.[18]

ACID-BASE BALANCE

Another consideration in parenteral nutritional support for older persons is acid-base balance. Respiratory rate and volume changes that control the elimination from or retention of carbon dioxide in the blood compose the first of two mechanisms that control acid-base balance. Although there are significant age changes in pulmonary characteristics—such as vital capacity, residual volume, and maximum breathing capacity—these factors have only minor effects on the elimination of carbon dioxide from the blood via the lungs. However, the permeability of the lung cells that separate capillary blood from the air spaces in the lungs does play a significant role in carbon dioxide elimination. There is a significant age decrement of about eight per cent/decade in the diffusion capacity of the lung, indicating a less-efficient acid-base control mechanism.[6]

The second mechanism for the control of acid-base balance is the kidney, which eliminates fixed acids. An adequate blood supply to the kidney is essential for the proper functioning of this mechanism. However, the kidney's response to a normal physiologic stimulus is less effective in older subjects when compared to young subjects. This deficit in the elderly population is due primarily to the age-related decrease in the glomerular filtration rate. Older persons require more time than do young persons to achieve the same results to a stimulus because fewer glomeruli are available to contribute to the formation of urine.[6]

SUMMARY AND CONCLUSIONS

There is a great deal that is not yet known about the use of parenteral nutrition in geriatric patients. Areas for future research are parenteral nutrient requirements in geriatric patients—including protein, vitamins, minerals, and trace elements. The clearance rates of fat emulsions may well be an important concern. Additional important variables are changes in the cardiac output and stroke index of patients receiving large-volume parenteral infusions, the effect of multiple-drug therapies on nutrient utilization, the effects of parenteral support on subsequent gastrointestinal function, the renal response to large-volume parenteral infusions, and the response rates to parenteral-solution electrolyte composition changes.

Aging *per se* is not a contraindication to parenteral hyperalimentation. Patients must be treated with caution and monitored regularly and frequently. Consideration of the physiologic alterations that occur as part of normal aging, the effects of chronic disease, and the stresses of critical illness must all be addressed when providing parenteral nutritional support in the aged patient.

REFERENCES

1. Lipschitz, D.A.: Protein calorie malnutrition in the hospitalized elderly. Primary Care. 9(3):531–543, 1982.
2. Mitchell, C.O., and Lipschitz, D.A.: The effect of age and sex on the routinely used measurements to assess the nutritional status of hospitalized patients. Am. J. Clin. Nutr., 36:340–349, 1982.
3. Rossman, I.: Anatomic and body composition changes with aging. In Finch, C.E., and Hayflick, L. (eds.): Handbook of the Biology of Aging. New York, Van Nostrand Reinhold Co., 1977.
4. Bistrian, B.R., Blackburn, G.L., Scrimshaw, N.S., and Flatt, J.P.: Cellular immunity in semi-starved states in hospitalized adults. Am. J. Clin. Nutr., 28:1148, 1975.
5. Makinodan, T.: Immunity and aging. In Finch, C.E., and Hayflick, L. (eds.): Handbook of the Biology of Aging. New York, Van Nostrand Reinhold Co., 1977.
6. Shock, N.W.: System integration. In Finch, C.E., and Hayflick, L. (eds.): Handbook of the Biology of Aging. New York, Van Nostrand Reinhold Co., 1977.
7. Kao, K.T., and Lakshmanan, E.L.: Protein nutrition and aging. In Hsu, J.M., and Davis, R.L. (eds.): Handbook of Geriatric Nutrition. Park Ridge, New Jersey, Noyes Publications, 1981.
8. Reiser, S., and Hallfrisch, J.: Carbohydrate nutrition and aging. In Hse, J.M., and Davis, R.L. (eds.): Handbook of Geriatric Nutrition. Park Ridge, New Jersey, Noyes Publications, 1981.
9. Andres, R., Pozefsky, T., Swerdloff, R.S., and Tobin, J.D.: Effect of aging on carbohydrate metabolism. In Camerini-Davalos, R.N., and Cole, H.S. (eds.): Early Diabetes. New York, Academic Press, 1970.
10. Sanadi, D. R.: Metabolic changes and their significance in aging. In Finch, C.E., and Hayflick, L. (eds.): Handbook of the Biology of Aging. New York, Van Nostrand Reinhold Co., 1977.
11. Watkin, D.M., and Lipschitz, D.A.: Enteral nutrition for older persons. In Rombeau, J., and Caldwell, M.: Clinical Nutrition. Vol. 1. Enteral Nutrition and Tube Feeding. Philadelphia, W.B. Saunders, 1984.
12. Roe, D.A.: Geriatric Nutrition. Englewood Cliffs, New Jersey, Prentice-Hall, 1983.
13. American Medical Association: Multivitamin preparations for parenteral use: a statement by the Nutrition Advisory Group. J.P.E.N., 3(4):258–262, 1979.
14. Barrows, C.H., and Roeder, L.M.: Nutrition. In Finch, C.E., and Hayflick, L. (eds.): Handbook of the Biology of Aging. New York, Van Nostrand Reinhold Co., 1977.
15. Silberman, H., and Eisenberg, D.: Parenteral and Enteral Nutrition for the Hospitalized Patient. Appleton-Century-Crofts, East Norwalk, Connecticut, 1982.
16. Steffee, W.P.: Nutrition intervention in hospitalized geriatric patients, Bull. N.Y. Acad. Med., 56(6):564–574, 1980.
17. Kohn, R.R., Heart and cardiovascular system. In Finch, C.E., and Hayflick, L. (eds.): Handbook of the Biology of Aging. New York, Van Nostrand Reinhold Co., 1977.
18. Ausman, R.K.: A standardized approach to parenteral nutrition for the geriatric patient. J. Am. Geriatr. Soc., 29(4):172–176, 1981.

CHAPTER 39

Home Parenteral Nutrition

EZRA STEIGER
FAITH SRP
MICHELENA I. HELBLEY
PATRICE M. MISNEY
CATHY MARIEN
JOHN SHARP
A. DALE GULLEDGE
RIYAD TARAZI

Total parenteral nutrition (TPN), which was introduced by Dudrick, Wilmore, Vars, and Rhoades[1] at the University of Pennsylvania in 1968, demonstrated that patients without adequate gastrointestinal tract function could achieve a normal nutritional status with intravenous feeding. Since its introduction, TPN has become a widely used and accepted means of achieving weight gain, positive nitrogen balance, wound healing, and spontaneous closure of enterocutaneous fistulas in hospitalized patients with inadequate gastrointestinal tract function. A small group of patients may require a prolonged course of TPN or TPN for the rest of their lives to achieve or maintain an adequate nutritional status. This group includes patients with extensive Crohn's disease involving multiple bowel resections or severe disease of the remaining intestinal tract, or both;[2] patients with radiation enteritis;[3] patients with superior mesenteric artery or vein thrombosis, resulting in extensive resection of the small bowel;[4, 5] patients with multiple enterocutaneous fistulas;[6, 7] patients with volvulus of the small bowel, with resultant gangrene and massive resection;[6] and patients with pseudo-obstruction of the intestine.[8] The remaining intestinal tract in these patients is unable to absorb enough nutrients, because of either residual disease or massive resection, or both. The alternative methods of treatment for these patients include (1) permanent hospitalization for TPN, (2) intermittent prolonged hospitalizations for TPN, or (3) home parenteral nutrition (HPN).

In the United States, in 1970, Shils and then Scribner[4] pioneered the use of parenteral nutrition at home for a patient with severe Crohn's disease. Also in the early 1970s, Solassol and Joyeaux[9] in France and Jeejeebhoy and coworkers[10] in Canada investigated the use of intravenous nutrient solutions for patients at home. Since then, HPN has gained acceptance as a means of promoting optimal nutritional status in patients with inadequate gastrointestinal tract function. The person who has been on an HPN program for the longest period of time (since 1969) is one of Dr. Bozian's patients at the University of Cincinnati. Many medical centers in the United States, Europe, and Canada have established HPN programs to train patients in the principles and procedures of HPN. The Home Parenteral Nutrition Registry, maintained by Dr. Maurice Shils of the New York Academy of Medicine, shows that 552 patients were discharged on HPN in the United States prior to 1980.[12] As of November 1982, 66 patients had been discharged on a full program of HPN at the Cleveland Clinic Foundation (CCF) since the program began in 1976.

CANDIDATES FOR HPN

Most patients who are started on HPN have anatomic short-bowel syndrome, including those who have had multiple resections over many years for Crohn's disease, patients with radiation enteritis, or patients who have had a mesenteric infarction with resultant gangrene and massive small-bowel resection. Survival from massive small-bowel resection is felt to be impossible if less than 300 cm of small bowel remains. However, a patient with only 18 cm of small bowel, along with the ileocecal valve and the entire colon, has survived without HPN.[13] Long-term followup of a patient with only 45 cm of proximal jejunum anastomosed to the transverse colon was also presented by Meyer.[14] Patients with radiation enteritis or intestinal malabsorption syndromes may have larger segments of intestine remaining, but they have active disease that interferes with normal digestion and absorption of nutrients.

The medical management of the short-bowel syndrome includes frequent small feedings, decreasing total fat from the feeding, increasing caloric intake, and using medium-chain triglycerides, food supplements, and antidiarrheal agents such as opium tincture, diphenoxylate hydrochloride and atropine (Lomotil), or codeine. The use of continuous overnight or 24-hour-a-day enteral feeding can be tried to maintain adequate nutrition. It is only after the preceding methods and techniques have failed to control stool and stoma output and to allow for enhanced absorption, or when there is extreme anatomic short-bowel syndrome, that the more expensive HPN should be considered.[15] Various types of absorption, motility, and x-ray studies are difficult to use to objectively identify the patients in need of HPN. The most consistent guidelines seem to be the patient's requirements for intravenous fluid in order to achieve normal fluid balance, despite all dietary manipulations or medications, or both. Intake and output records, along with daily weights, blood urea nitrogen (BUN), and creatinine determinations, will indicate if adequate fluid balance can be maintained with all these maneuvers, whereas repeated nutritional assessment parameters will indicate the adequacy of calorie and protein absorption. Some patients may just need fluid and electrolyte replacement at home to maintain adequate kidney function, whereas most patients will also require the added nutrients to maintain normal protein nutriture.

There are other groups of patients who have catastrophic intra-abdominal conditions that can be best treated by a diverting-loop jejunostomy to allow for drainage and excision of diseased intestinal parts, along with staged re-establishment of the gastrointestinal tract continuity over a period of months or years.[6] Patients with concrete impenetrable abdominal cavities who have distal diseased or inflammatory processes for which dissection is impossible because of the intense inflammatory response that is secondary to radiation ulcers, intestinal fistulas, or severe inflammatory bowel disease can be managed by diverting the fecal stream proximally with the jejunostomy and placing the patient on a program of HPN for three to six months or longer. This allows for resolution of the inflammatory process. Further surgery can then be done to excise diseased segments and re-establish gastrointestinal tract continuity. Management would otherwise be a very complicated or surgically impossible process requiring prolonged hospitalization. Instead, the patient can return to the home setting, allowing the bypassed inflammatory processes to subside, and eventually staged resection and reconstruction of the intestine can be undertaken. HPN is stopped after the return of adequate gastrointestinal tract function.

DISEASE STATES REQUIRING HPN

The 1980 survey from the Registry of Patients on Home Parenteral Nutrition, which was initiated by Shils, showed that 812 patients were discharged on HPN, with 260 of these patient discharged in 1980 alone. These data are said to represent a moderate underestimate of the total number of HPN patients in the United States and Canada, since not all institutions known to have HPN patients responded to the questionnaire. The data collected represent 63 institutions in the United States and Canada that have discharged patients on HPN. The following disease processes required the initiation of HPN in the 260 patients discharged in 1980, as reported by Shils and coworkers.[12]

1. Malignancy or its treatment, involving obstruction, fistulas, radiation enteritis, massive bowel resection due to tumors, and

various other problems (85 patients; 32.6 per cent of total).

2. Inflammatory bowel disease with or without resection or fistulas (83 patients; 31.9 per cent of total).

3. Ischemic bowel infarction with resection (38 patients; 14.6 per cent of total).

4. Motility disorders—pseudo-obstruction, scleroderma (17 patients; 6.5 per cent of total).

5. Cystic fibrosis, pathologic conditions of head and neck, chronic pancreatitis, sclerosing cholangitis, chronic diarrhea of unknown cause, cystinosis with growth failure, chronic obstructive pulmonary disease, and celiac disease (14 patients; 5.4 per cent of total).

6. Persistent bowel fistulas or short-bowel syndrome unrelated to the preceding disease entities (13 patients; five per cent of total).

7. Congenital malformation (nine patients; 3.5 per cent of total).

8. Trauma (one patient; 0.1 per cent of total).

In our review of CCF patients started on HPN from January 1976 to September 1981, the following clinical conditions requiring HPN were noted:

1. Inflammatory bowel disease—Crohn's disease (19 patients; 38 per cent of total) (Fig. 39–1).

2. Radiation enteritis (13 patients; 26 per cent of total).

3. Ischemic bowel infarction (seven patients; 14 per cent of total).

4. Short-bowel syndrome—Gardner's syndrome–volvulus (three patients; six per cent of total).

5. Multiple small-bowel fistulas unrelated to the preceding diseases (two patients; four per cent of total).

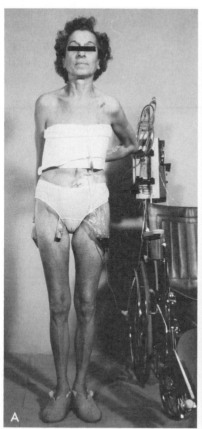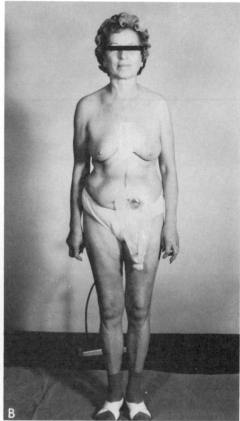

Figure 39–1. *A,* This patient with inflammatory bowel disease involving the large and small intestines had undergone multiple resections over a number of years. She had a persistent enterocutaneous fistula and had lost a great deal of weight. She was hospitalized approximately one out of every three days during the year before home parenteral nutrition was started. *B,* The patient is shown one year after having started home parenteral nutrition and having regained 35 pounds, back to her normal weight. She was able to remain at home without need for hospitalization for that one-year period, since home hyperalimentation was started.

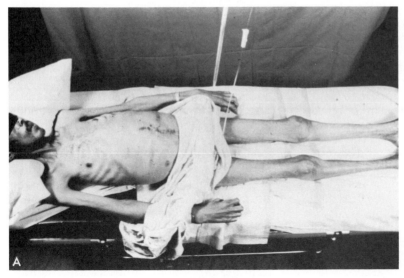

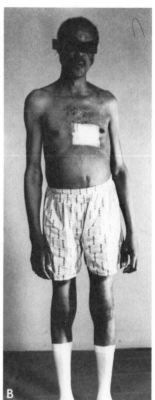

Figure 39–2. *A,* This patient with pseudo-obstruction had lost 35 per cent of his body weight and required multiple hospitalizations in the year preceding the institution of home parenteral nutrition. *B,* The patient regained his weight after one year of home parenteral nutrition and was able to avoid rehospitalization. (*From* Steiger, E.: Total Parenteral Nutrition, Part II. New York, Med Com, Inc., 1982, with permission.)

6. Malabsorption syndrome unrelated to the preceding diseases (two patients; four per cent of total).

7. Intra-abdominal malignancy (two patients; four per cent of total).

8. Motility disorders—pseudo-obstruction, scleroderma (two patients; four per cent of total) (Fig. 39–2).

The three major disease categories of patients requiring HPN in the Shils Registry and the CCF patient data are the same; however, the primary diagnosis of patients requiring HPN at CCF is Crohn's disease. Shils reports that the range of age of patients discharged on HPN in 1980 varied from less than 1 year to more than 65 years of age, with the largest group of patients being between 31 and 40 years of age. In the CCF patients, the ages ranged between 15 and 69 years of age, with a mean patient age of 35 years. The patients discharged on HPN are young and have many years of potentially productive life ahead.

DETERMINING ELIGIBILITY FOR HPN

To be eligible for HPN a patient must have short-bowel syndrome or malabsorp-

tion to such an extent that it has not responded to intensive dietary and medical management. Consultation with gastroenterology, general surgery, colon and rectal surgery, and dietary departments may be required. In addition, the patient should be trainable and able to carry out the program in the home setting. A trainable patient is required to have a basic minimal intelligence level in order to understand the program. In our experience, this requirement can be met by almost any patient who is capable of carrying out the independent activities of daily living. However, those patients who are addicted to narcotics will have great difficulty learning, and a drug withdrawal program should be carried out before starting HPN training. Very old patients will have difficulty with the training process, and caution should be exercised before instituting a program of HPN in them. The patient and his or her spouse should be able to carry out the program independent of family members or health-care professionals who live outside of the patient's primary residence. Patients whose quality of life will not be improved by HPN should not be started on the program. Thus, the patient who is dying with metastatic cancer and has resisted conventional treatment should not have the suffering pro- longed by parenteral nutrition. The indica- tions for parenteral nutrition in these patients are very limited.[16] Also, the very aged or infirm whose quality of life will not be im- proved should not be started on a program of intensive nutritional support. Financial and insurance considerations must be care- fully evaluated so that the financial implica- tions of HPN are well understood by the patient, the family, and the health-care pro- viders. Requirements for disability and its effect on the other family members must be appreciated. Assistance from a variety of so- cial service agencies might be necessary. The patient should have sufficient manual dex- terity to perform the various tasks associated with catheter care, solution preparation, and delivery. The help of a spouse at certain times during the day might be essential. The pa- tient should be healthy and strong enough to carry out these tasks independently, or with minimal help, prior to discharge. All members of the team involved in training and following the patient should meet with the patient. The attending physician, training nurse, pharmacist, social worker, psychia- trist, and dietitian should confer from their professional vantage points prior to deciding whether or not HPN is appropriate for a particular patient.

SOCIAL AND ECONOMIC CONSIDERATIONS

Family, vocational, and economic issues play a major role in the candidate's adjust- ment to HPN. Family patterns need assess- ment to screen for dysfunctional family sys- tems as well as for adaptive role changes. Role changes fall into three groups: (1) pa- tients with chronic bowel disease who are entrenched in a dependent sick role in the family, (2) those with chronic bowel disease who maximize independent functioning, and (3) those with acute onset of bowel dysfunc- tion. With acute onset and "because of pro- longed hospitalization, the family often had been forced to assume all the patient's tra- ditional duties . . . the sharing of responsi- bilities was in a state of flux. Family members were reluctant to relinquish their new roles for two reasons: (1) they do not want to overtax the patient physically and emotion- ally; (2) they were not willing to risk another reshuffle should the patient resume his du- ties and it be only temporary."[17]

Even with the patient with chronic bowel disease who functioned independently prior to admission, hospitalization results in this role shift. Some authors observe that patients with chronic disease and their families seem to cope more effectively with HPN ini- tially.[17, 18] We observe satisfactory adjustment during the training process in many chronic- bowel-disease patients. They are well accli- mated to the hospital environment and ex- press gratitude for relief of past symptoms. However, the chronic-bowel-disease patient proceeds into one of two types of long-term adjustment that affect the family as well as the HPN team. The patient who has a history of dependent, sick-role behavior in the family is more likely to balk during training. These patients find it difficult to make the transition from the dependent stance fostered by mul- tiple hospitalizations to the independence of self-care expected of most HPN candidates. Because of recurrent hospitalizations and personality factors, the role shifts described previously are permanent and resistant to the emphasis of home training. Substance- abuse problems, sometimes supported by the family system, complicate this situation. The patient or family, or both, may experience secondary gain from the hospitalization (un- conscious motivation to prolong it) and stall the training process and future adjustment.

The patient with a satisfactory life ad- justment to chronic disease may have the fewest problems in HPN training and long- term adjustment. They characteristically demonstrated independence in self-care pre- vious to HPN and utilized relationships for emotional support rather than physical care. The patient with an acute bowel catastrophe goes through an initial period of mourning[17] but seems motivated to return to normal functioning once the acute phase of the ill- ness and grief is past.

The amount of stress on the family caused by HPN is directly related to who is responsible for daily care in the home. If the patient assumes total responsibility for self- care, the burden on the family is minimized. However, this creates the need for the family to be well informed of the treatment regimen outside of the instruction session. When the family is unable to visit and is at a distance from the HPN center, their ignorance about HPN can give way to irrational fears of the treatment modality. If the family is well in- formed, they are able to prepare themselves cognitively and prepare the physical environ- ment of the home for the return of the patient, thus alleviating some anxiety.

At times a parent or spouse may take primary responsibility because of the patient's debility or inability to learn. This family member is particularly stressed when he or she is the primary wage earner in addition to the HPN caregiver. A more common and less stressful situation is sharing the caregiver role. Often the patient will care for the catheter and the spouse will mix the solutions. In some cases, the vendor will assume major responsibility in mixing, initiating, and monitoring infusions in the home. Typically, if the patient does not take full responsibility for care at the time of discharge, it is unlikely that he or she ever will. Therefore, assessing the patient's willingness and ability to assume responsibility for care is necessary before initiating HPN training.

Two pre-existing family circumstances can influence future compliance. First, the presence of small children in the home may lead to poor compliance because the needs for child care assume primary responsibility. Second, pre-existing family problems can be exacerbated by the institution of HPN.[19]

Another concern besides family issues is the home environment. Three aspects of the home deserve consideration. First, a clean location for mixing the solution is necessary. This includes a formica table top that can be cleaned with alcohol. Some husbands of our female patients have built their own tables specifically for this purpose. Second, storage of the solution is a major concern. Most vendors deliver a month's supply at one time, which can be more than 90 1-L bottles plus catheter-care materials. Storage is rarely a problem if the patient and family anticipate this need. Some insurers now cover the cost of a rental refrigerator for storage of premixed solutions. Third, there is the location of the infusion pump in relation to the floor plan of the home. Easy access to a bathroom is essential during infusion because of nocturia and high stoma output. This is rarely a problem and is often anticipated by the patient and family. Vendors typically assist the family in solving storage problems on the first delivery. Some vendors do an assessment for the HPN center by sending a social worker or a public health nurse for a home visit prior to discharge from the hospital.

In the assessment of the HPN candidate, vocation is a minor but consequential factor. The patient's career may enhance the ability to learn HPN, for example, an accounting student became particularly interested in keeping his input and output records. Obsessive personality traits expressed through a vocation usually enhance learning of HPN, as in the preceding example.

A financial assessment is essential. Insurance coverage of HPN has improved greatly since its inception. Private insurance companies now typically cover HPN under major medical provisions of the contract. Public programs—Medicaid and Medicare—now cover many patients. Effective August 1981, the Medicare Intermediary Manual allows coverage under Part B for a list of seven diagnoses.[20] Medical justification is required in the form of a statement of medical necessity. Fortunately, most vendors now accept assignment for HPN and have reimbursement services, which simplifies the insurance claims process for the physician and the patient.

Prior medical bills often plague the patient and family considering HPN. Although not a contraindication for HPN, the extent of these debts and the family's concern about medical bills need assessment.

The employment status of the patient and the family also needs careful assessment. Initial data on HPN patients show a significant return to previous employment or activities, either full- or part-time.[18, 19] Loss of income is always a great fear of the HPN patient who is the family wage earner. Often the lengthy hospitalization that is required to stabilize and train the patient exhausts sick-time benefits. The motivation to return to work may be indicative of the patient's sense of self-worth. Some who consider themselves disabled because of the need for HPN also lack motivation for self-care. Those returning to full-time employment appear to have the highest motivational levels. A "catch-22" situation exists in the relationship between Medicare and Medicaid and employment for these patients. For those younger than 65 years of age who are in either program, gainful employment threatens their continued coverage under these programs. Program reform is needed to enable the HPN patient to maintain public insurance while pursuing gainful employment.[18]

In summary, assessment of the HPN patient should include family, home environment, and vocational and economic factors. Family history and insurance coverage are essential prior to training; other social and economic factors need assessment to plan for the complete rehabilitation of the HPN patient in his home, work, and family setting.

PSYCHOLOGIC ISSUES

Common psychiatric variables that are frequently seen with HPN include depression, delirium, drug use, grief, anxiety, and, on occasion, impaired cognition from prior central nervous system problems.[21] Each of these problems can impede the acquisition of needed information about home care, and they require careful evaluation to determine their significance because they might affect what information can be learned and subsequently utilized as the patient proceeds with an HPN program.[17] It has been clearly recognized, for example, that if a patient has acquired a short-bowel problem from a series of operative procedures for Crohn's disease, the risks of narcotic addiction and chronic-illness behavior need to be considered and treated as one helps the patient adjust to HPN—the former often requiring detoxification and a formal chemical dependency program if subsequent narcotic abuse problems are to be avoided during HPN.[21, 22]

The *sudden* loss of one's gut without prior chronic gut problems, and the inability to eat like others with all of the associated social pleasures, usually brings normal grief reactions from both patient and family, and time, not antidepressants, is required to work through the grief.[23] Moreover, the usual doses and routes of psychiatric medications often cannot be utilized because of an inadequate amount of gut function. Excessive intramuscular fibrosis from prior injections often makes the use of anxiolytic narcotics and antidepressants more difficult when one needs to treat pathologic anxiety or depression, and considerable time is often required to find the effective doses for treating the symptoms of inertia, diminished concentration, decreased attention span, and reduced self-esteem. Psychotic states are most frequently associated with encephalopathic processes and are uncommon as "psychologic reactions" to medical or surgical issues. If psychosis is present with a delirium, judicious use of antipsychotic medication through injection is usually efficacious while reversing the causes of the delirium.

Often, anxiety represents an encephalopathic process secondary to electrolyte imbalance, hypo- or hypervolemia, central anticholinergic syndromes, and "central clouding" from anxiolytic, hypnotic, or analgesic medications. For example, hyperosmolar states, vitamin deficiencies, infections from impaired immunocompetence, a variety of anemias, and trace element problems can present with anxiety symptoms and signs, yet frequently are manifestations of an encephalopathy.[24, 25] Etiologic pursuits are necessary while providing a supportive milieu, structured reality, and consistency of input by staff until *the cause* of the anxiety is rectified; the key approach is to recognize the delirium early by doing a very careful mental status examination that establishes cognitive dysfunction as the cause of the anxiety rather than psychologic reactions to a very stressful medical-surgical situation.[21]

In contrast, anxiety can be a "primary" reaction because of the fear of loss of control over one's physical or psychologic functions, the fear of being placed in a strange or overwhelming environment, or the fears of having to deal with strangers, being confronted with chronic pain, or trying to adjust to an altered body image.[21] Sleep changes associated with night infusions often seem to influence circadian rhythms, with day-night reversals being a problem that, if prolonged, can lead to "out-of-phase" living with one's environment or family, which, in turn, can induce anxiety or depression.

Certainly, as one studies the patient's adjustment and the family's reactions, there is a need for evaluation that is not only in the context of current medical issues but also takes into account the prior attitudes of these persons, so as to better understand them as they plan for the future.[26]

Briefly, just as there are growth and development cycles for each person, each family passes through certain milestones as it acquires its own unique identity and functions.[27] Hence, before one can identify strain or dysfunction in the family as they deal with HPN, the HPN team needs to know what "was normal" for this family unit and how illness and treatment affected the family *prior* to the institution of HPN. HPN means different things to each family member, since the needs of each are significantly influenced and altered, depending on whether the member is a child, adolescent, spouse, parent, or grandparent. Depending on beliefs, attitudes, social support surrounding the family, and the sensitivity of the HPN team, psychologic reactions need to be recognized and dealt with in type and extent to prevent maladaptive behavior and responses as the family passes through its own cycle while dealing with the many issues of HPN.

Frequently, it is at this nodal point in a family's life that community resources, friends, religion, and ethnic and social surroundings become critical in easing the patient and family entry into HPN. If family struggles have been excessive in the past, HPN does not suddenly make family members a new, close-knit unit. Thus, awareness of the processes that result from the integration of HPN into the course of the illness with the stage of the family's development becomes critical to facilitating patient and family entry into HPN.

Thus, when beginning HPN, inquiries should be made into the following:

1. Has the family's style been one that has "openly" dealt with issues? If not, communication with the HPN team will usually be more difficult to achieve, trust will be harder to establish, and the HPN team members will need to "model" how "openness" improves situations. More time and energy will be required for this kind of family.

2. Has the family pattern been one of closeness and stability? Are family members showing strain because the ill member has been the primary force in establishing family cohesion and stability? Particular attention should be directed toward the HPN effects on young children and adolescents to be sure basic emotional needs are being met and the "well parent" is getting help in adapting to new roles.

3. Where and who are the nonfamily resources? Has prior illness made health-care providers the primary support resources, or is there evidence that reliable other persons and the community can be of aid in an HPN program and that the family shows a willingness to allow outside support. If the willingness is not there, more dependence on the HPN team probably will ensue, and this may lead to the problems associated with chronic-illness behavior, which require more intensive psychologic treatment. If these problems are not dealt with, the independence and the opportunity for a more active life offered by HPN may not be realized.

The HPN process embraces fully the "biopsychosocial" approach, and without such an approach, successful evaluation and treatment of patient and family are fraught with potential difficulties. Careful psychosocial evaluation of patient and family, coupled with detailed mental status determinations, is the keystone to the successful identification of problems when they can be appropriately treated. Focusing only on physiologic problems, ignoring family, and being unaware of the common normal "reactions" to losses will lead to such problems as compliance difficulties, poor adjustment to HPN, and often repeated hospitalization for catheter problems, narcotic abuse, and unresolved depressions.[17, 22, 23, 26]

LONG-TERM VENOUS ACCESS

Once the decision has been made to proceed with HPN, safe long-term venous access is achieved to permit infusions. Solutions containing carbohydrates, amino acids, vitamins, and electrolytes are infused through a catheter that can remain in place for extended periods of time. The infusion system should not restrict joint mobility or otherwise interfere with physical activity. The high osmolality of the solution requires administration into a large vein with a high blood flow to avoid pain, phlebitis, and thrombosis. These requirements limit the site of catheter tip location to the superior vena cava, right atrium, inferior vena cava, or a surgically created arteriovenous (AV) shunt.

The concept of an "artificial gut" system for patients without functional gastrointestinal tracts was first introduced by Scribner and associates in 1970[4] using a standard AV shunt as was used for hemodialysis, thus allowing long-term access to the circulation. The basic principle of this system was that by introducing an irritating, sclerosing, hypertonic nutrient solution such as HPN into the shunt itself, local phlebitis and pain would be eliminated and the rapid dilution by blood flow through the shunt would prevent phlebitis and thrombosis of the vein distal to the shunt. Infection and clotting of the shunt, however, did occur,[28] and its use for HPN was abandoned. Also, the debilitated and malnourished patients needing the shunt were relatively hypovolemic and lacked veins suitable for the construction of a well-functioning shunt. The standard AV shunts clotted frequently when placed in these hypovolemic patients.[28]

In 1973, Broviac and colleagues[29] modified the Tenckhoff peritoneal dialysis catheter for use in the right atrium after determining that long-term venous access with the AV shunt was unsuccessful. They incorporated the Tenckhoff catheter's Dacron cuff and the subcutaneous tunnel beyond the cuff in the new right atrial catheter. The cuffed portion of the catheter was placed in the subcutaneous tunnel to allow for the ingrowth of fibrous tissue to anchor the catheter and to serve as a barrier against infection by skin microorganisms.[30] The main complication found in a patient with this type of catheter was superior vena cava thrombosis thought to be caused by mechanical trauma to the vein from the Teflon catheter itself. Soft silicone rubber was then substituted for the Teflon, making this catheter and a wider-bore modification, the Hickman catheter, a very safe and widely used means of achieving long-term venous access.[31–33]

A manual explaining the entire home program[34] is given to the patient to read prior to catheter insertion. He or she is shown the catheter, and the procedures that will be experienced during venography and catheter insertion are explained. Prior to catheter insertion, bilateral subclavian venography is performed to determine the optimal site for catheterization. Collateralization at the subclavian vein indicates the presence of thrombosis. Subclinical thrombosis, which renders the subclavian vein unsatisfactory for permanent catheter placement, is often seen in

patients whose subclavian veins have been used for temporary in-hospital TPN. In most instances of subclavian vein thrombosis, the internal jugular vein on the same side can often be used because it usually empties into the subclavian or innominate vein central to the thrombosed area. If the subclavian vein is patent, the catheter may be inserted into the external jugular vein, the cephalic vein, or the muscular branches of the subclavian vein under the pectoralis major muscle (Fig. 39–3).

In the operating room with the patient under local anesthesia, a cutdown is made, usually over the cephalic vein in the delto-pectoral groove. The extravascular portion of the catheter is tunneled subcutaneously from the cutdown site to the exit site on the anterior chest wall. The exit site is marked preoperatively by the nutrition support team (NST) nurse to ensure that it can be easily seen by the patient so that he or she can properly care for it, to avoid its interfering with wearing clothing or undergarments, and to make sure it is not too close to stoma or fistula sites. When the saphenous vein is used for venous access, the catheter can be tunneled through the subcutaneous tissue on the anterior thigh. The Dacron cuff is positioned to lie midway between the cutdown site and the exit site.

The intravascular portion of the catheter is trimmed so that its tip will lie in the

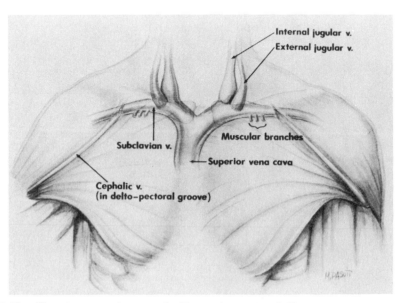

Figure 39–3. The different access veins on each side are demonstrated. There are at least three to five different access routes that can be used on each side to gain entry into the superior vena cava. Preoperative venograms are important to delineate the patency of the subclavian vein on the anticipated side of venous access. (*From* Steiger, E.: Total Parenteral Nutrition, Part II. New York, Med Com, Inc., 1982, with permission.)

superior vena cava. Under fluoroscopic control it is threaded into the access vein, down the subclavian vein, and into the superior vena cava. A suture is placed at the exit site to anchor the catheter in place until tissue growth into the Dacron cuff occurs. This exit-site suture is removed after one month. After a chest x-ray film is taken to verify placement, the catheter can be used immediately for fluid infusion. All solutions infused through the catheter should contain at least 1 U heparin/ml. Percutaneous catheter placement techniques have been described, but they are more appropriately used for patients needing the catheter for relatively short periods of time.[35]

After the catheter has been inserted, the patient is taught to care for it. The principles of aseptic technique are explained and employed as the patient is instructed on how to change the dressing over the catheter exit site and to heparinize the catheter. Both procedures are performed daily, and the dressing is changed more frequently if it falls off or becomes soiled. The procedure for the catheter dressing change is designed to minimize the possibility of catheter infection.[34]

Between infusions, the catheter is kept patent by filling it with a heparin solution. HPN patients are taught to heparinize their catheter once daily, usually at the completion of their hyperalimentation infusion.

EMERGENCY PROCEDURES

In the event that air should enter the catheter, the patient is instructed to clamp the catheter immediately and lie on the left side for 20 minutes. This will help prevent passage of air into the pulmonary artery and will allow the air embolus to gradually break up and disperse.[36] Care must be taken to avoid pulling, bending, or kinking the catheter to prevent cracking or splitting. If the catheter does become cracked or torn, a temporary repair can be made with an emergency repair kit having a blunted 15-gauge needle for the Hickman catheter and a blunted 18-gauge needle for the Broviac catheter. A new catheter cap is fitted onto the end of this needle. A permanent repair, which is made by the physician by splicing a new catheter end onto the original catheter, should be done within one or two weeks. There has been no increased incidence of catheter infection observed with the use of this type of temporary catheter repair.[37]

CATHETER COMPLICATIONS

The most common catheter complication is infection. Whether the infection is intravascular or at the catheter exit site, it usually necessitates hospitalization of the patient. A catheter exit-site infection is evidenced by inflammation, redness, and induration at the exit site and may involve the tissues along the length of the subcutaneous tract. If purulent exudate can be expressed from the site, it is sent for culture, as is blood drawn from the catheter. Antibiotics appropriate for a *Staphylococcus* infection are started. Repeat blood cultures are drawn daily. If the blood culture results are negative, the catheter does not have to be removed unless the infection is resistant to antibiotic therapy.

Intravascular infection, most often caused by *Staphylococcus* and *Candida*, is evidenced by positive blood cultures and fever, and the catheter should be removed. Antibiotic treatment is usually not required. The fever usually resolves within 24 hours, and a new catheter can be placed in five to seven days if blood culture results remain negative. The use of a combination of antibiotics and urokinase to lyse and sterilize the infected catheter thrombus in an attempt to save the catheter from removal has been described by Glynn and coworkers.[38]

To further prevent catheter infection, antibiotic coverage should be initiated whenever the patient undergoes a procedure that might be associated with transient bacteremia, such as dental work, drainage of superficial skin infections, uterine dilatation and curettage, prostatectomy, instrumentation of the urinary tract, and similar procedures.[34] The risk of infection can also be reduced by avoiding catheter use for multiple purposes. Blood and blood products should neither be infused nor withdrawn through the catheter used for hyperalimentation except in extreme circumstances in which the patient has no other route of venous access.[39] In Riella and Scribner's work with indwelling catheters, they have avoided the use of local antibiotic preparations, feeling these applications may predispose the catheter to fungal infection.[33]

Thrombosis of the catheter is another potential complication and is more likely to occur in the smaller-lumen Broviac catheter than in the larger-lumen Hickman catheter. The thrombus can almost always be lysed by instilling streptokinase or urokinase into the catheter. A volume of streptokinase equal to the internal volume of the catheter should be instilled in a concentration of 2500 U/ml. After being left in place for one-half hour, repeated aspirations every five minutes will usually dislodge the dissolved clot.[40] If patency is not restored after several attempts, the streptokinase can be left in the catheter overnight or for 24 to 48 hours.[40]

Catheter-induced subclavian vein or superior vena cava thrombosis can also occur, causing obstruction to the venous flow and, occasionally, venous occlusion. In the event of a subclavian vein thrombosis, the patient may experience fever and arm swelling, distention of veins in the shoulder and anterior chest wall, and shoulder pain in the side of the body on which the catheter is inserted. A superior vena cava thrombosis is suspected when the patient presents with symptoms of arm swelling, neck or throat pain, puffiness of the face, excessive tearing or rhinorrhea, distended shoulder and chest wall veins, and fever. A venogram is obtained to confirm the diagnosis. If there is thrombosis, obstruction to the flow of contrast material and collateralization will be noted. (If the venogram shows apparent obstruction but no collateralization, this is a flow phenomenon and not a true obstruction.) Rubenstein and Creger,[41] in their work with iatrogenic central vein thrombosis, have found that heparin is an ineffective treatment modality but have achieved successful thrombolysis with the use of streptokinase. Although streptokinase can be infused locally in an attempt to dissolve the thrombus, in most cases the thrombus renders the catheter useless, necessitating its removal. Blood drawn from the catheter and the catheter tip are then sent for culture.

VENOUS ACCESS SITES FOR DIFFICULT RIGHT ATRIAL CATHETER INSERTION

Superior vena cava catheter placement has been achieved predominantly through venous entry routes in the upper thoracic and jugular venous network. The usual entry sites are the cephalic, jugular, or muscular branches of the subclavian veins. Of more than 130 CCF HPN catheters inserted since January 1976, only four CCF patients have required alternate routes of venous entry. The predominant reason for using alternate venous access routes was thrombosed upper or lower anatomic venous entry sites resulting from the use of multiple jugular or subclavian catheters for central venous pressure (CVP) monitoring and in-hospital TPN or from previous Hickman-Broviac catheter placements. Two patients had no upper thoracic or jugular venous access sites and were able to have catheters inserted via cutdowns over and insertion into the saphenous vein.[42] The catheters were successfully directed up the inferior vena cava area just below the right atrium, and the distal end of the catheter was tunneled to exit on the anterior thigh in one patient and to the anterior chest wall in an infant patient. Two patients who lacked patency of both the upper and lower venous system had catheters inserted directly into the right atrium.[43] One of these patients expired prior to discharge on HPN, unrelated to the direct right atrial catheter placement. The remaining three patients continue to have successful use of their catheters for HPN use. No complications have yet been observed in using the saphenous or direct right atrial catheterization route for placement of Hickman-Broviac catheters for HPN. The technique of catheter-care management for these catheters remains the same as for those catheters inserted via the upper thoracic venous entry sites. The catheters inserted via the saphenous vein and tunneled to the anterior thigh require special care in protecting the catheter and exit site from intestinal stoma drainage.

HPN SOLUTION PREPARATION

Given adequate time and with the proper instruction, the majority of HPN candidates can learn to safely mix their own TPN solutions. An average of 10 to 14 days of hospitalization is required to complete the pharmacy training. The exact time required varies, depending on each patient's learning capabilities; therefore, the instruction is paced according to the patient's actual abilities.

Patients can also be sent home to use premixed solutions. Several supply companies now offer the service of providing premixed, patient-specific TPN solutions. The use of premixed solutions greatly decreases the amount of time required for training, since there are usually only two to three substances that must be added to the premixed solution by the patient just prior to administration. This training can usually be accomplished in just two to three days. However, because using premixed solutions is more expensive than having patients prepare solutions themselves, using these solutions is usually reserved only for those patients who are unable to mix solutions or for those patients who will require TPN for only a short period of time (i.e., less than six months). For these short-term TPN patients, it becomes more cost-effective to provide them with premixed solutions in order to avoid the cost of their spending an extra 10 to 14 days in the hospital for training.

Prior to discharge, a stable HPN formula is decided upon. Each patient's HPN solution is individualized according to the computed fluid, electrolyte, caloric, and protein requirements. The patient's intake and output records, daily weights, and BUN and creatinine concentrations are checked frequently to ensure that the fluid provision is adequate. Nitrogen balance and nutritional assessment parameters are also checked periodically to ensure the adequacy of calorie and protein provisions.[44] Appropriate quantities of calcium, magnesium, sodium, potassium, phosphate, chloride, and acetate are also included in the formula and are based upon the patient's serum electrolyte concentrations.

Requirements for calcium and phosphorus in TPN have recently been reviewed.[45] It has been suggested that at least 15 mEq of calcium be given daily, along with 15 mm of phosphorus, to patients receiving TPN in hospitals. Hypercalciuria is commonly noted in hospitalized as well as HPN patients. It is important to perform calcium balance studies in HPN patients to be certain that calcium is being given in adequate amounts. Klein and coworkers[46] and Shike and coworkers[47] have reported a syndrome of bone pain that in some patients is accompanied by hypercalcemia or hypercalciuria. Other authors have coined the term *paradoxic vitamin D–dependent metabolic bone disease*. These patients develop demineralization of bone, with biopsy evidence of osteomalacia, normal or increased serum calcium levels, normal parathormone levels, and compression fractures. Shike and associates[48] reported that correction of this disorder followed discontinuation of vitamin D. Low levels of some vitamin D metabolites have been noted by others.[49] More clinical studies are needed to correlate the bone disease in HPN with vitamin D and calcium balance studies. Heparin is usually added in

dosages of 1 U/ml to prevent fibrin deposition within the catheter. Insulin is added as required to maintain blood glucose control. Vitamins are included in the TPN solution in accordance with the recommendations of the AMA Nutrition Advisory Group regarding parenteral vitamin supplementation for adults.[50] Ten milliliters of MVI-12 is usually added to the patient's TPN solution daily to provide recommended adult dosages of all the water- and fat-soluble vitamins except for vitamin K (Table 39–1). Since vitamin K is not routinely given intravenously,[51] patients are instructed to give themselves intramuscular injections of phytonadione (vitamin K_1), 10 mg twice monthly.

Trace elements are also added to the TPN solution in accordance with the Guidelines for Essential Trace Element Preparations for Parenteral Use, developed by the AMA Nutrition Advisory Group (Table 39–2).[52] Usually, 4 mg zinc, 1 mg copper, 10 μg chromium, and 0.5 mg manganese are given daily to provide doses within the AMA's recommended dosage range. In addition, 120 μg selenium are also given daily because of preliminary evidence that it is essential for humans.[53, 54] Iron dextran is not added routinely to TPN solutions, but it is given separately in bolus doses if needed to maintain normal hematologic variables.[55] Until just a few years ago, trace-element supplementation could be achieved only with the use of special pharmacy-compounded solutions. However, commercial single-component injections of zinc, copper, chromium, manganese, and selenium are now available. In addition, several companies also produce multiple-component injections of zinc, copper, chromium, and manganese that offer the advantage of providing usual recommended adult dosages of all four trace metals in one small-volume injection, thereby permitting easier dose delivery (Tables 39–3 and 39–4). The AMA Nutrition Advisory Group discourages the use of multiple-component injections because of the risk of overdosage when the requirement for one trace metal is more than the requirement of the others.[52] However, a multiple-component injection increases patient convenience in solution preparation. Trace element levels are monitored and if normal levels cannot be achieved by supplementation with a multicomponent injection, each mineral is titrated individually using single-component injections. The intravenous infusions are started on a continuous

Table 39–1. INTRAVENOUS VITAMIN RECOMMENDATIONS

| | | | AMA GUIDELINES* | |
| | | MVI-12 (USV LABORATORIES) PROVIDES/10 ML | ADULT REQUIREMENT | PEDIATRIC REQUIREMENT (<11 YR OF AGE) |
VITAMIN	UNITS			
C	mg	100.0	100.0	80.0
Thiamin	mg	3.0	3.0	1.2
Riboflavin	mg	3.6	3.6	1.4
Niacin	mg	40.0	40.0	17.0
B_6 (pyridoxine)	mg	4.0	4.0	1.0
Pantothenic acid	mg	15.0	15.0	5.0
Folacin	mg	0.4	0.4	0.14
B_{12}	μg	5.0	5.0	1.0
Biotin	μg	60.0	60.0	20.0
A	IU	3300.0	3300.0	2300.0
D	IU	200.0	200.0	400.0
E	IU	10.0	10.0	7.0
K	IU	—	—	0.2

*Adapted from Dudrick, S. J., Wilmore, D. W., Vars, H. M., and Rhodes, J. M.: Long-term parenteral nutrition with growth and development and positive nitrogen balance. Surgery, *64*:134–142, 1968.

Table 39–2. SUGGESTED DAILY INTRAVENOUS INTAKE OF ESSENTIAL TRACE ELEMENTS

	ADULT	STABLE ADULT WITH INTESTINAL LOSS	CHILD
Zinc	2.5–4.0 mg (additional 2 mg if catabolic)	Add 12.2 mg/L small bowel fluid lost; 17.1 mg/kg of stool or ileostomy output	Premature infants (weighing <1500 gm up to 3 kg): 300 μg/kg Full-term infants up to 5 years: 100 μg/kg; More than 5 years: same as adults (max. 4 mg/day)
Copper	0.5–1.5 mg	—	20 μg/kg
Chromium	10–15 μg	20 μg	0.14–0.2 μg/kg
Manganese	0.15–0.8 mg	—	2–10 μg/kg

(Adapted from Fleming, C. R., McGill, D. B., and Berkner, S.: Home parenteral nutrition as primary therapy in patients with extensive Crohn's disease of the small bowel and malnutrition. Gastroenterology, *73*:1077–1081, 1977.)

Table 39–3. EXAMPLES OF COMMERCIAL SINGLE-ENTITY TRACE ELEMENTS

TRACE ELEMENT	COMPOUND	MANUFACTURER	CONCENTRATION	SIZE
Zinc	Zinc chloride	USV	1 mg/ml	10 ml
	Zinc chloride	Abbott	1 mg/ml	10 ml, 50 ml
	Zinc sulfate	Travenol	1 mg/ml	10 ml
	Zinc sulfate	IMS	4 mg/ml	20 ml
	Zinc sulfate	Lypho-Med	5 mg/ml	5 ml
			1 mg/ml	10 ml, 30 ml
	Zinc sulfate	American Quinine	1 mg/ml	10 ml, 30 ml
Copper	Cupric chloride	USV	0.4 mg/ml	10 ml
	Cupric chloride	Abbott	0.4 mg/ml	10 ml, 30 ml
	Cupric sulfate	Travenol	0.4 mg/ml	10 ml
	Cupric sulfate	IMS	1 mg/ml	20 ml
	Cupric sulfate	Lypho-Med	2 mg/ml	5 ml
			0.4 mg/ml	10 ml, 30 ml
	Cupric sulfate	American Quinine	0.4 mg/ml	10 ml, 30 ml
Manganese	Manganese chloride	USV	0.1 mg/ml	10 ml
	Manganese chloride	Abbott	0.1 mg/ml	10 ml, 50 ml
	Manganese sulfate	Travenol	0.1 mg/ml	10 ml
	Manganese sulfate	IMS	0.5 mg/ml	10 ml, 20 ml
	Manganese sulfate	Lypho-Med	0.5 mg/ml	5 ml
			0.1 mg/ml	10 ml, 30 ml
	Manganese sulfate	American Quinine	0.1 mg/ml	10 ml, 30 ml
Chromium	Chromic chloride	USV	4 μg/ml	10 ml
	Chromic chloride	Abbott	4 μg/ml	10 ml, 30 ml
	Chromic chloride	Travenol	4 μg/ml	10 ml
	Chromic chloride	IMS	10 μg/ml	10 ml, 20 ml
	Chromic chloride	Lypho-Med	20 μg/ml	5 ml
			4 μg/ml	10 ml, 30 ml
	Chromic chloride	American Quinine	4 μg/ml	10 ml, 30 ml
Selenium	Selenous acid	Lypho-Med	40 μg/ml	10 ml

Table 39–4. TRACE ELEMENT FORMULATIONS

EXAMPLES OF COMMERCIAL MULTIPLE-ENTITY TRACE ELEMENTS

Product Name	Multiple Trace Metals Additive	MTE-4	MTE (conc.)	Trace Metals Additive	Multiple Trace Element Injection
Manufacturer	IMS	Lypho-Med Travenol	Lypho-Med	Abbott	American Quinine
Concentration/ml					
Zinc	4 mg/ml	1 mg/ml	5 mg/ml	4 mg/5 ml	1 mg/ml
Copper	1 mg/ml	0.4 mg/ml	1 mg/ml	1 mg/5 ml	0.4 mg/ml
Manganese	0.5 mg/ml	0.1 mg/ml	0.5 mg/ml	0.8 mg/5 ml	1.0 mg/ml
Chromiun	10 μg/ml	4 μg/ml	10 μg/ml	10 μg/5 ml	4 μg/ml
Size	1 ml, 5 ml, 10 ml	3 ml, 10 ml, 30 ml	1 ml, 10 ml	5 ml, 50 ml	10 ml

EXAMPLES OF CLEVELAND CLINIC FORMULATIONS OF TRACE ELEMENTS

Trace Elements (CCF formulation)—Each ml provides:

Copper	1.5 mg (as the chloride)
Manganese	0.8 mg (as the chloride)
Chromium	15 μg (as the nitrate)
Selenium	120 μg (as the acid)

Zinc sulfate (CCF formulation)—Each ml provides:

Zinc (Zn^{++})	3 mg (as the sulfate)

Selenium injection (special CCF formulation)—Each ml provides:

Selenium	120 μg (as selenous acid)

basis, 24 hours a day, and as the patient learns to take care of the infusion catheter and to heparinize the catheter when it is not being used, the infusions are gradually tapered and the fluid is administered over a shorter and shorter period of time during the night.

Clinical anabolism and weight gain are readily achieved with either a continuous or an overnight infusion regimen. Continuous infusions with a vest system[56] might be particularly useful in patients with severe heart or lung disease who cannot tolerate overnight infusions of their daily fluid requirements. The continuous system of infusion is also preferred by an occasional patient who wants to sleep unattached to any intravenous infusion system. Most patients, however, prefer to be unencumbered and free of the intravenous infusion during the day. The average patient being given 2 to 3 L of TPN fluid/day will have the infusion tapered from 24 hours to 20 hours, then 16 hours, and then 12 hours. Those patients receiving 2 L of TPN fluid can usually receive their fluids over eight hours. The patient's ability to tolerate the infused glucose and fluid volume determines how rapidly one can infuse the prescribed fluid. Patients with congestive heart failure should be given their fluids over longer time intervals. Infusion blood glucose should usually be 250 mg/dl or less during the infusion itself, and two-hour postinfusion blood values should be back to normal. If blood glucose exceeds 200 to 250 mg/dl during the infusion, insulin is added to the solutions to control them.

Prior to pharmacy instruction, the required TPN solution contents are reviewed by the HPN team pharmacist to determine the feasibility of adjusting the specific electrolyte salts and base solutions to develop the easiest equivalent solution for the patient to mix. The final TPN solution formula is then typed onto a special TPN solution worksheet prior to working with the patient (Fig. 39–4). The sheet is set up similar to a "recipe" so that the patient can add the ingredients in the amounts specified in the volume column, in the exact order listed on the sheet, to avoid physical incompatibilities. The sheet is enclosed in an acetate protector page so that the patient can check off the ingredients with a wax pencil as they are added, in order to avoid confusion.

The ingredients listed on the TPN solution worksheet and the purposes of each ingredient are explained to the patient on the first day of pharmacy instruction. While in the hospital, this instruction takes place in the pharmacy so that the patients can mix their solutions under laminar air flow sterile conditions. To ensure safe mixing conditions at home, patients are instructed on selecting a properly disinfected home admixture area (Fig. 39–5). In addition, a 0.22-μ filter will be used as part of the infusion delivery system in order to filter out any bacteria and particulate matter that might be introduced during the admixture process. As training commences, the patient is given a thorough explanation of aseptic techniques, and the proper use of sterile equipment is reviewed. The admixture process is then demonstrated to the patient, and the patient practices the admixture procedures daily until they are mastered.

The solutions themselves can be prepared in either bottles or bags. If bottles are used, 2 L of fluid can be infused at once with the use of a Y-type administration set. Since many patients require more than 2 L of TPN fluid/day, the use of 2-L and 3-L bags often decreases the time necessary for solution preparation because 2 or 3 L of fluid can be prepared at once, allowing the use of larger syringes to combine electrolyte additives of all solutions together, thereby decreasing the total number of syringe transfers. The use of a 3-L bag for a patient who requires more than 2 L of fluid also permits the patient to have uninterrupted sleep and avoid the need to get up in the middle of the night to remove empty bottles and hang up new bottles.

Fat emulsions are also given as part of the infusion. These solutions are given either immediately before or immediately after the infusion, since the emulsified fat particles cannot pass through the 0.22-μ filter. Usually 500 ml of a 20 per cent fat emulsion or two 500-ml units of a 10 per cent emulsion are given each week to provide the amount of linoleic acid required to prevent essential fatty acid deficiency.[57]

As the patient nears the completion of training, discharge plans are made. A final review of admixture techniques is conducted, and the patient is instructed about the storage and ordering of supplies. A list is supplied as a reminder about items that must be refrigerated. The contents of the TPN solutions and a list of necessary supplies will be communicated to a nutritional products supply company that will deliver the necessary

THE CLEVELAND CLINIC HOSPITAL PHARMACY DEPARTMENT

HOME TPN WORKSHEET

TPN SOLUTION NO. 1

for

Mr. John Doe
(1-234-567-8)

VOLUME	SOLUTION OR ADDITIVE	PRESCRIBED DOSE
500 ml	Dextrose 50% Injection	500 ml
500 ml	Freamine III 8.5% Injection	500 ml
20 ml	Calcium Gluconate 10% Injection (0.46 mEq/ml)	9.2 mEq
2 ml	Magnesium Sulfate 50% Injection (4.06 mEq/ml)	8.1 mEq
10 ml	Potassium Chloride Injection (2 mEq/ml)	20 mEq
2.3 ml	Potassium Phosphate Injection (4.4 mEq K^+/ml)	10 mEq K^+
6.25 ml	Sodium Chloride 23.4% Injection (4 mEq/ml)	25 mEq
12.5 ml	Sodium Acetate 16.4% Injection (2 mEq/ml)	25 mEq
1 ml	Heparin Sodium Injection (1,000 units/ml)	1,000 units
1 ml	Trace Elements Injection	1 ml
1 ml	Zinc Sulfate Injection (3 mg Zn^{++}/ml)	3 mg
5 ml	MVI-12 Injection (Vial #1)	Total of
5 ml	MVI-12 Injection (Vial #2)	10 ml

Note: Add the calcium gluconate and magnesium sulfate to the dextrose bottle.
Add all other additives to the Freamine bottle. Then transfer the contents
of the Freamine bottle into the dextrose bottle. Mix the solutions
thoroughly after each addition and transfer.

INFUSION INSTRUCTIONS AND SCHEDULE OF VITAMIN K INJECTIONS AND I.V. FAT EMULSIONS

1.   Infuse Solution #1 together with Solution #2 via a Y-type administration set
over an 8-hour period.

2.   Inject 1 ml (10 mg) of Vitamin K (aquamephyton 10 mg/ml) I.M. twice a month.

3.   Infuse 500 ml of 20% IV fat emulsion (Intralipid) once a week.

Figure 39–4. Special TPN worksheet showing typical formula for one liter of home PN fluid.

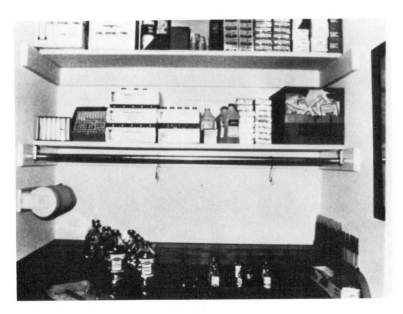

Figure 39–5. The patient's closet area has been changed into an admixture area. There is room for storage of supplies as well as for mixing of the intravenous solutions. (*From* Steiger, E.: Total Parenteral Nutrition, Part II. New York, Med Com, Inc., 1982, with permission.)

supplies directly to the patient's home upon discharge and will continue to deliver supplies monthly. In addition to delivering supplies, several companies also offer other valuable services, such as maintaining patient inventories, billing insurance companies directly, and helping to monitor patient compliance to therapy. Several also offer other nursing and pharmacy services and in many ways serve as a liaison between the patient and the physician.

Occasionally, adjustments are made to the patient's HPN solution as part of the outpatient monitoring process. These changes are communicated by the NST physician to the patient as well as to the NST pharmacist and the nutritional supply company. The NST pharmacist then provides all parties with a revised TPN solution worksheet reflecting these changes, and the supply company makes adjustments in the supplies delivered to reflect the patient's current needs.

ANCILLARY MEDICATION

Patients with mesenteric vascular infarction are often placed on anticoagulants for long-term management. Although vitamin K is often required to maintain normal prothrombin values in patients on HPN with extreme short-bowel syndrome, some of these patients may instead require sodium warfarin (Coumadin) to maintain therapeutic prothrombin time values to prevent thrombosis. The sodium warfarin is given orally, and the prothrombin time is monitored to ensure that adequate absorption can be achieved with an oral dosage. For those patients who require digitalis preparations for congestive heart failure, oral medications may also be given as long as blood levels are monitored to be sure that therapeutic levels are achieved. Most drug absorption occurs proximally in the duodenum and proximal small bowel, and if the medications are given in liquid form adequate absorption occurs. If there are questions about adequate absorption, therapeutic efficacy can be monitored by serum levels or appropriate clinical response. If appropriate blood levels are not achieved or therapeutic efficacy cannot be measured clinically, intramuscular or intravenous administration of the medication becomes necessary. Examples of medication that can be tried orally with blood values monitored include digoxin, phenobarbital, phenytoin, and certain antibiotics. A list of the patient's usual medications and their routes of administration should be kept as a separate sheet in the patient's HPN notebook.

USE OF FILTERS

The National Coordinating Committee on Large Volume Parenterals (NCCLVP) recommended that inline particulate-matter filters be considered for use in the intravenous administration of electrolytes, medications, and nutrients. The use of such filters can reduce the amount of particulate matter and the possibility of bacterial contamination and provide protection from the infusion of air.[58]

Special considerations must be made for patients receiving HPN. Patients who mix their own HPN fluids without laminar-flow air filtration and filtration needles are at the greatest risk. Final inline filtration is an absolute necessity. Patients who receive a premixed HPN fluid supply from a hospital pharmacy or commercial facility must also be assured of proper filtration, even though the techniques of mixing HPN solutions in these areas are very sophisticated.

Filters are commercially available with a wide range of micron pore size, from 0.22 μ, to 0.45 μ, to 1 μ, through 10 μ. The 0.22-μ inline filter is the smallest filter-pore size available and is the only pore-size filtration device that will assure the sterilization of fluids passing through it.[59] The NCCLVP recommends that patients receiving hyperalimentation solutions use an inline filter that is particulate- and microbe-retentive.[60] Inline filters can be used effectively when administering fluids through an infusion pump as long as instructions from the filter manufacturer are carefully followed.[61] The ideal features recommended for the filtration of parenteral nutrition fluids include (1) a 0.22-μ pore size, (2) an air-venting system within the filter to prevent the occurrence of an air lock, (3) ability of the filter to remain structurally sound with pressure produced by concomitant use of an infusion pump, and (4) adequate surface filtration area to maintain accurate flow rates.

All of our HPN patients use a 0.22-μ inline filter at the final intravenous connection closest to the Hickman-Broviac catheter. The entire intravenous tubing–filter system is discarded daily after it is used.

The use of inline filtration for the administration of parenteral nutrition fluids in the home should reduce the infusion of solution–intravenous tubing system contaminants that can lead to sepsis.

FLUID INFUSION PUMPS

Hyperalimentation fluid administration in the home setting must be done with the assurance of accuracy and safety. The majority of HPN programs administer parenteral nutrition fluids intermittently on an overnight or cyclic HPN infusion schedule.[7, 62–65] The method of 24-hour continuous adminis-

tration of HPN fluids is generally called ambulatory HPN.[56] Parenteral nutrition fluids are more safely infused with the use of mechanical-electronic intravenous infusion devices.[66–68] Gravity drip administration of parenteral nutrition fluids is not accurate or reliable and can lead to significant complications. Therefore, HPN programs use one of the many types of infusion devices to assure proper controlled administration of parenteral nutrition fluids.

Pipp[69] described how selection of an infusion device can be done carefully with special consideration given to the following:

1. Physical characteristics—weight, size, balance, sound level of pump operation, ease in setting controls, and ability to attach device to intravenous fluid pole.

2. Electrical characteristics—automatic power switch from AC to DC, low-current leakage, safety plug, length of battery operation, and explosion hazard control.

3. Control characteristics—accuracy of volume and rate, and wide range of flow rate and volume settings.

4. Alarm characteristics—visual and audible alarm signals for air inline, infusion completion, occlusion, and low battery level, plus ability to change volume of audible alarm.

5. Miscellaneous characteristics—ability to infuse various viscosities of parenteral nutrition fluids, cost of administration set, ability for pump operation to be taught and easily managed by the HPN patient, minimal requirements for maintenance, availability of manufacturer to properly service unit, and cost of unit.

The selection process for an infusion device for hospital-home use must be done with scrutiny by knowledgeable members of the health-care team.

A review and current update of infusion pumps and controllers was presented by Turco.[66] He described the methods of intravenous administration by gravity flow, infusion controllers (volumetric and nonvolumetric), and infusion pumps (syringe, peristaltic, cassette), along with each of their characteristics. There are many products available for optimal safety and accuracy of parenteral nutrition fluid administration.

Our program has successfully used a volumetric, cassette-type infusion pump for the last four years. Programs designed for 24-hour infusion of parenteral nutrition fluids, or ambulatory HPN, have utilized a vest system to deliver the fluids. This vest system enables the patient to wear bags of parenteral nutrition fluids and a peristaltic infusion pump and tubing and to be mobile throughout the 24-hour infusion period.

The type of infusion device chosen for HPN use must be continually evaluated for efficiency and ease of use by the patient. Awareness and comparison of the new infusion devices available should be an ongoing process.

METABOLIC MONITORING

The metabolic monitoring of HPN patients is divided into two areas—laboratory monitoring and home self-monitoring. Laboratory monitoring is ordered by the HPN team physician at routine followup clinic visits or at the patient's local hospital. The reports are phoned to the HPN team physician, and the patient is then examined by his or her local physician. The patient receives a copy of the laboratory studies and enters the values on a flow sheet that is kept in the HPN notebook. The notebook also includes records of daily intake and output, weight, urinary dextrose levels, medications taken, and an HPN teaching manual that serves as a reference source. The HPN team physician evaluates the patient's blood tests plus intake and output records to determine the efficacy of the HPN formula the patient is infusing.

The requirements for electrolytes vary widely in individual patients, depending on volume and type of fluid loss, renal status, and amount of nutrients given. Initially, electrolyte levels, along with glucose, BUN, creatinine, calcium, phosphorus, and magnesium values, are determined weekly after the patient is discharged from the hospital. They are then determined once every two weeks and then monthly as the patient stabilizes. Also included with the monthly blood studies are a complete blood count, liver function tests, cholesterol and uric acid levels, and prothrombin time. Changes in the amounts of amino acids infused are dependent on the evaluation of BUN, nitrogen balance, albumin, and transferrin measurements. Changes in the amounts of sodium added are dependent on serum values and the clinical detection of peripheral edema. Potassium, chloride, acetate, phosphorus, and magnesium additives are dictated by serum levels. Trace element, fatty acid, and vitamin levels are measured every six months, and these meas-urements dictate the amounts of these nutrients required. Calcium requirements are determined by doing balance studies.

In the patient who has been on HPN for one year or more without a wide variation of blood value changes, the frequency of the laboratory studies is reduced to every two months. Every 6 to 12 months, trace element and serum vitamin levels are drawn. Essential fatty acid levels and serum transferrin levels are also measured every 6 to 12 months. The intravenous fluid formulation that a patient is infusing when discharged home usually does not require changing more than once or twice a year. The most common single change in formulation usually decreases the amount of dextrose infused because of excessive weight gain. All blood studies have to be carefully monitored, compared to previous studies, and correlated with the various additives in the intravenous solution and with the patient's clinical course.

Self-monitoring of daily weight, urinary glucose measurement, intravenous fluid intake, oral fluid intake, and urine, stoma, and fistula output is part of the patient's daily routine (Fig. 34–6). The adequacy of the infused fluid volume is assessed by noting urine output, daily weights, and BUN and creatinine determinations. If the daily urine output is 1000 to 1500 ml/day, and the BUN, creatinine, and weight measurements are stable, the fluid volume administered is adequate. Ideally, total intake should be about 500 ml greater than total output. If the patient develops new or increased peripheral edema or experiences a urine output of less than 600 ml for two consecutive days, he or she is advised to contact the physician. A urine output this low, especially if associated with increased BUN and decreased weight measurements, usually calls for the administration of more fluids. The increased fluid volume required to maintain normal hydration in a patient who had otherwise been stable may be due to increased stomal output or diarrhea caused by an exacerbation of the inflammatory bowel disease, dietary indiscretions, or cessation of the use of antidiarrheal agents. Increased amounts of fluid may also be required in the hot summer months.

A volume of urine output greater than 1700 ml/day in the average adult usually means that the patient is getting too much fluid. The volume of intravenous fluid infused is reduced by 500 ml/day, which can be expected to decrease urine output by 500

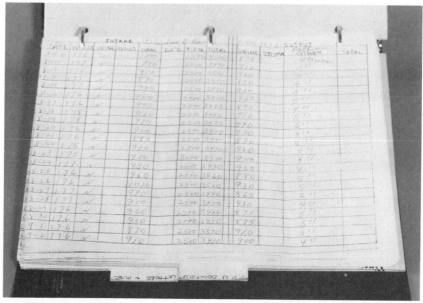

Figure 39–6. The patient's home parenteral nutrition notebook is demonstrated. Daily weights, urinary dextrose measurements, oral and intravenous intake, as well as urine output and frequency of bowel movements are charted. These records are reviewed monthly by the physician managing the patient.

ml/day. Thereafter, the remaining nutrients are more concentrated, or they might be reduced along with the fluid volume reduction. In the absence of glycosuria, a gradually increasing urine output in a patient whose urine output has been adequate and stable usually signifies enhanced absorption from the remaining intestinal tract, especially if the patient is also gaining weight. In this instance, fluid volume and nutrients should be reduced.

Weight should be measured at the same time daily, with the patient wearing similar articles of clothing. Expected weight gain or loss will of course vary with each patient, but a loss or gain greater than 10 lb should be reported to the physician so that it can be determined if the loss or gain is due to fluid overload or dehydration. If there is too much weight gain in the absence of fluid retention, that is, the urine output is adequate and stable, and there is no peripheral edema, the kilocalorie content of the solution can be reduced by decreasing the concentration of dextrose. Usually, significant reductions of 20 per cent or more of infused calories are needed to stabilize weight gain.

To ensure that the HPN patient is tolerating the high-dextrose concentration in the solution, he or she checks the urine with Testape shortly after completing the infusion and six to eight hours later. The physician is notified if the urine reduction is persistently 2+ or greater over a 24-hour period. Insulin

can be added to the infusion to control blood glucose as needed. The sudden onset of glycosuria in an otherwise stable HPN patient may signify impending sepsis, hypokalemia, or a chromium deficiency.

In addition to the reasons just outlined for physician notification, the HPN patient is also instructed to notify the physician if elevated temperature, chills, or sweats are experienced, since these things may signify infection, or if any signs of metabolic complications such as nausea, vomiting, weakness, muscle tingling, double vision, convulsions, or muscle twitching occur.

Prior to leaving the hospital the patient is provided with a three-ring notebook, in which daily records of self-monitoring, laboratory results, and the hyperalimentation formula sheet are kept. It is brought when the patient visits the NST physician and is used by the physician to evaluate the patient's response to the current HPN formula. A similar notebook is kept in the physician's office for recording laboratory values, the patient's formula, along with any changes needed in the formula, and patient-related information.

REHOSPITALIZATION AND MORTALITY RATES

The goal of HPN is to nutritionally support patients with minimal risks of compli-

Table 39–5. CCF HPN PATIENT DATA—JANUARY 1976 TO SEPTEMBER 1981

NO. OF ADMISSIONS	PRIMARY CAUSE OF ADMISSION	PER CENT OF ADMISSIONS	PER CENT OF REHOSPITALIZATION TIME
73	Related to primary disease	43	54
40	Suspected sepsis	24	17
39	Not related to HPN or primary disease	23	22
11	Catheter-related	7	1
2	Fluid-electrolyte imbalance	1	1
2	Psychologic problems	1	1
2	HPN retraining	1	4

cations related to this method of nutritional support in the home setting.

The CCF HPN program investigated the causes for rehospitalization in 50 consecutive patients discharged on HPN up to September 1981. The total HPN patient experience was 32,353 days. Rehospitalization of 41 patients (82 per cent of the total) accounted for 4228 days spent in the hospital after discharge on HPN. Nine patients (18 per cent of the total) had no hospital admissions after the initial HPN discharge. The average length of hospital stay for the 169 admissions was 25 days, ranging from 1 to 206 days. The primary causes for readmission are noted in Table 39–5. The largest number of rehospitalizations (73 patients) were related to the HPN patient's primary disease (Table 39–6). Thirty-nine rehospitalizations were nonrelated to HPN or to the patient's primary disease. Suspected sepsis was the primary HPN-related cause for the admission of 43 patients; however, sepsis was ruled out in 33 per cent of those cases. Further information on the admissions related to suspected sepsis is noted in Table 39–7. Sixty-six per cent of the admissions and 76 per cent of the rehospitalization time were due to causes unrelated to HPN; 53 per cent of the admissions and 58 per cent of the rehospitalization time were attributed to 8 of the 41 patients, 6 of whom had Crohn's disease and 2 of whom had radiation enteritis. HPN was not the major cause for rehospitalization of the CCF HPN patient population.

Shils[12] reports in the 1980 survey of the Registry of Patients on Home Total Parenteral Nutrition that 59.3 per cent of all patients on HPN in 1980 had no hospital admission related to HPN (Table 39–8). The average length of hospital stay for the HPN-related problems was 12.5 days per admission; 15.4 per cent of all patients on HPN in 1980 were responsible for 62.4 per cent of the HPN-related admissions.

The mortality rate of 39 of the 50 CCF HPN patients comprising the three major clinical conditions that required HPN therapy was reported by Steiger.[70] The rehospitalization and mortality rates were considered low in this group of patients with extensive and advanced disease processes and were largely due to the primary disease process and not to HPN.

The CCF HPN patient experience for five and one-half years has resulted in the following observations: (1) 54 per cent of all patients started on HPN continue to be managed on HPN successfully; (2) 12 per cent of all patients started on HPN no longer required HPN support, which has been discontinued; and (3) the total mortality rate of 50 patients started on HPN is 34 per cent. More information on these patients is tabulated in Table 39–9.

The Shils study reports that 385 of the 812 patients started on HPN since 1970 remain on HPN. Respondents to the Shils study state that 89 per cent of their patients

Table 39–6. CCF HPN PATIENT DATA—JANUARY 1976 TO SEPTEMBER 1981. REHOSPITALIZATIONS RELATED TO PRIMARY DISEASE

ADMISSIONS (73)	PATIENT DIAGNOSIS
67%	Crohn's disease
18%	Radiation enteritis
15%	Other

Table 39–7. CCF HPN PATIENT DATA—JANUARY 1976 TO SEPTEMBER 1981. REHOSPITALIZATION RELATED TO SUSPECTED SEPSIS

DETERMINATION	% OF PATIENTS
Sepsis ruled out	33
Sepsis determined	67
Infected catheter	(55)
Infected catheter exit site	(12)

Table 39–8. HPN-RELATED HOSPITAL ADMISSIONS FROM THE REGISTRY OF PATIENTS ON HOME TOTAL PARENTERAL NUTRITION

CAUSE OF ADMISSION	% OF PATIENTS
Sepsis: known or suspected at time of admission (sepsis confirmed by culture—33.3%)	51.4
Catheter-related problems	25.2
Fluid or electrolyte problems	11.4
Bone disease workup or treatment	3.3
Retraining of HPN techniques	1.4
Hypoglycemia or hyperglycemia, or both	1.0
Organ failure or dysfunction (e.g., liver, kidney)	0.5
Psychologic problems	0.5
Other, including abdominal pain of unknown cause, zinc deficiency, clotted shunt, gallstones, others not specified	5.2

would expire or be institutionalized without the use of HPN.

HPN is a modality of therapy that must be monitored and managed carefully in patients who are appropriate candidates and who cannot be managed with any other form of nutritional support. There must be a continued awareness and effort made to maintain low rehospitalization and mortality rates in HPN patients.

SOCIAL ASPECTS

In evaluating the results of HPN, one must review the patient's quality of life in relation to the family and other interpersonal relationships. Role changes can occur. The motivated patient often returns to work once physical rehabilitation has taken place. The additional family task of the HPN regimen is typically assumed by the patient. If another family member (spouse or parent) assumes some of this responsibility at the time of discharge, this role is usually maintained. The exception is the motivated patient who needs extensive physical rehabilitation who then assumes his or her premorbid family roles. This usually takes place three to six months after HPN is initiated and may coincide with the achievement of ideal body weight.

When family dysfunction occurs during HPN, one must distinguish the causal elements. Is the stress on the family due to the underlying illness or HPN, or both, and is there a history of family problems? In relation to married HPN patients, most authors report that when there was a previously stable relationship, couples continued to exhibit sharing and empathy when one partner began HPN. When the relationship was already dysfunctional, HPN added significantly to the discord.[19]

If the HPN patient is an adolescent or young adult living with parents, the psychologic issues of separation and autonomy may be exacerbated. Usually this resolves through a supportive relationship. In other cases the child fails to mature into adulthood or regresses into a dependent sick role in the family.

For some patients there are changes that occur at mealtimes, in social life, and in relationships with children. For most families, mealtime is the basic forum for family interaction; when an HPN patient has signif-

Table 39–9. CCF HPN PATIENT DATA—JANUARY 1976 TO SEPTEMBER 1981

CLINICAL CONDITION	NO. OF PATIENTS	NO. REMAINING ON HPN	NO. OFF HPN	NO. EXPIRED	MORTALITY RATE
Crohn's disease	19	12	2	5	26%
Radiation enteritis	13	7	1	5	38%
Mesenteric vascular infarction	7	4	0	3	43%
Short-bowel syndrome (Gardner's syndrome–volvulus)	3	2	1	0	0
Multiple small-bowel fistulas	2	0	2	0	0
Malabsorption syndrome	2	1	0	1	50%
Malignancy	2	0	0	2	100%
Scleroderma	1	0	0	1	100%
Pseudo-obstruction	1	1	0	0	0
TOTALS	50	27	6	17	34%

icant dietary or fluid restrictions, this family time may be disrupted by the patient's absence or limited participation. These food restrictions also limit social life. One HPN patient found that family visits to his mother's home, which were once amiable and always associated with pastry and other food, had now become stilted and quiet with his mother withholding food for fear of offending him. Perl[19] notes that parent-child relationships are altered through the HPN parent feeling inhibited or the children expressing disgust or fear of the catheter and pump.

Vacations and traveling logistics are complicated for the HPN patient. The physician can facilitate transporting the infusion pump on airlines with an appropriate letter of explanation. Travel by auto is facilitated by the use of specially designed wheeled carts for the pump and fluids.[71] One author reports an incident of a patient who was refused intravenous fluids as an outpatient at a rural hospital that was unfamiliar with HPN.[19] To prevent difficulties in emergencies for the HPN patient, especially while traveling, we recommend the use of a Medic-Alert bracelet.[71] One of our patients, a woman in her 20s, reported a feeling of loss if she could not go camping—an enjoyable hobby for her and her husband prior to HPN. Fortunately, the major vendors now provide assistance in travel, including a rental pump and solutions that are delivered to the site of the vacation. Travel and vacation anywhere in the United States and most countries abroad are now almost unlimited.

Sexual functioning on HPN relates to the broader psychologic issue of self-image in relationship to others. Although no detailed study of HPN and sexual function is available to date, descriptive data indicate patterns similar to those of hemodialysis patients.[72] Organic causation is suspicious in males, particularly in the case of zinc deficiency. Perl did not find any such cases in his survey.[19] In contrast to hemodialysis patients, a rehabilitated HPN patient may have more energy and vigor to actively participate in sexual relations. The first months on HPN are the most difficult, since many patients are gradually returning to normal physical activities and adjusting psychologically to a new body image.[1] Johnston found that "many of these patients have adjusted sexually to ileostomies and colostomies and are not unduly distraught over sexual concerns

with catheter placement." Most patients disconnect their TPN line from their monitor or pump during sexual relations.[18]

As with hemodialysis, reactive depression in the first months can reduce sexual desire; depression seems less chronic with HPN patients as time passes, and so Perl noted improvement in functioning with time. The partner's fear of harming the patient may also inhibit sexual relations, but this seems to be a transient problem with an understanding partner. Although there are no data on the incidence of sexual dysfunction, the most likely cause is psychogenic, relating to body image, the ostomy, the interference of the catheter and pump, and general weakness from protein depletion.

With the growth of HPN, patients have developed alternative social supports. The Lifeline Foundation is a well-established national group with a regular newsletter; it is encouraging the establishment of local chapters near the major HPN medical centers (Lifeline Foundation, 2 Osprey Road, Sharon, Massachusetts 02067). Some centers established newsletters and pen pals for their patients.[73] Others suggest support groups for local patients led by a social worker to assist in adjustment to HPN, but there are no reports of successful groups to date.[18] Public exposure in the press and at medical conferences appears to have a beneficial effect on these patients.[71] The social consequences for the patient on long-term HPN reach every area of the patient's interactions with others. Yet there is the potential for a good quality of life after an initial period of adjustment.

The use of HPN in patients having active malignancy and in the terminal phase of illness affects the gamut of social relationships, but in a drastically different manner. Here the main issue is maintaining a quality of life in the face of impending death. Weiss's work illustrates criteria for this special category of HPN candidates with followup data demonstrating that limited and select patients who meet strict criteria can enjoy their last months at home.[16]

FINANCIAL AND VOCATIONAL CONCERNS

Any chronic or catastrophic illness requiring serial hospitalizations and operations takes a toll on the patient's financial resources. Chronic bowel disease and massive bowel resection are no exceptions. The typical HPN candidate experiences extended hospital stays and at least one operation. Even the most comprehensively insured person faces the loss of income, the fear of large hospital bills, the cost of home supplies, the fear of long periods of unemployment and disability, and the hidden costs of travel and medical followup.

Initial data indicate that the ability of the HPN patient to return to premorbid activities is higher than that for hemodialysis patients. Johnston's sample of 18 cases found two thirds of these patients active—one third were gainfully employed and the remainder were retired or housewives. The remaining third were "disabled by narcotic dependency, depression, or primary disease."[18] Perl[19] cites that of five patients previously employed, three continued their occupations. Price and Levine[17] report that of 10 patients who had been the primary income source for their families, five returned to work. These authors note that "the self-employed patients had greater potential to return to work because of the flexibility they could build into their working hours."[17] Psychosocial factors—for example, chemical dependence and depression—are as significant as causes of disability as is underlying disease in these patients. The HPN regimen is not in itself an obstacle to employment and full activity. In a few cases, the combination of the bowel disease and HPN precipitate the patient's decision to take early retirement.

Funding for long-term HPN patients continues to be a complicated issue. Third-party reimbursement, whether government or private, considers these patients on an individual basis. Our experience is that once the insurer agrees to cover the HPN claims, it will continue to do so. With an average annual cost in excess of $40,000, even a substantial private major medical contract can be exhausted as these patients survive beyond five years. Vendors with efficient reimbursement services have a reassuring policy of not refusing supplies to those who exhaust insurance resources. An impasse is reached when patients younger than 65 years of age who are on Medicaid or Medicare wish to return to work; by doing so they become ineligible. A similar problem is encountered by those patients applying for government benefits who are employed or are full-time students. They are not disabled but they also are not insurable, yet they require HPN to prevent hospitalization and death. The trend toward work incentives for disabled persons on Medicaid and Medicare will go a long way toward enhancing the financial and psychologic independence of HPN patients who rely on these programs.

In spite of reassurance from vendors and the availability of insurance from public sources for HPN, these patients continue to have concerns about the cost. At times this concern is greater than the medical threats to the patient.[74] Unlike some other disease groups, patients with chronic bowel disease have no private foundations that provide financial assistance or other concrete patient services. Finally, there are hidden costs for the HPN patient. Most centers attempt to limit the need for return office appointments to minimize unnecessary travel and loss of income. The need for assistance from a spouse in the HPN regimen may limit or interrupt that spouse's employment and curtail much needed income.

The financial repercussions of HPN are substantial. The HPN team's emphasis on independent self-care and maximum rehabilitation enhances the patient's ability to return to a high level of functioning, including employment. Future changes in public insurance for these patients will enable them to realize this potential for independence rather than encourage dependence. Further studies on a national level are needed to examine the incidence of family, sexual, and financial problems and to demonstrate the degree of independence that can be achieved by most HPN patients.

CONCLUSION

HPN is an effective life-sustaining method of caring for patients who have severe gastrointestinal tract disability that would otherwise lead to significant malnutrition. The only alternatives to a program of HPN are permanent or repeated hospitalizations for nutritional rehabilitation or the death of the patient from malnutrition. There are many specialized health-care personnel whose expertise is needed for the complete and adequate teaching of the patient requiring HPN. A formal program of followup and monitoring is carried out by a team of knowledgeable and concerned health-care professionals to allow for the success of the program. Careful attention must be paid to meeting all nutrient requirements and to monitoring the patient to be certain that this is indeed accomplished. Further refinements in the solutions administered and in defining precise requirements, methods, techniques, and apparatus for delivering these nutrients will be made over the ensuing years to allow the system to be used with greater safety. Social issues and insurance reimbursement policies have to keep pace with medical and technical advances to allow for optimal rehabilitation of patients with gastrointestinal tract failure requiring HPN.

REFERENCES

1. Dudrick, S.J., Wilmore, D.W., Vars, H.M., and Rhoades, J.M.: Long-term parenteral nutrition with growth and development and positive nitrogen balance. Surgery, 64:134–142, 1968.
2. Fleming, C.R., McGill, D.B., and Berkner, S.: Home parenteral nutrition as primary therapy in patients with extensive Crohn's disease of the small bowel and malnutrition. Gastroenterology, 73:1077–1081, 1977.
3. Lavery, I.C., Steiger, E., and Fazio, V.W.: Home parenteral nutrition in the management of patients with severe radiation enteritis. Dis. Colon Rectum, 23:91–93, 1980.
4. Scribner, B.H., Cole, J.J., and Christopher, T.C.: Long-term total parenteral nutrition: the concept of an artificial gut. J.A.M.A., 212:457–463, 1979.
5. Langer, B., McHattie, J.D., Zohrab, W.J., and Jeejeebhoy, K.N.: Prolonged survival after complete small bowel resection using intravenous alimentation at home. J. Surg. Res., 15:226–233, 1973.
6. Oakley, J.R., Steiger, E., Lavery, I.C., et al.: Catastrophic enterocutaneous fistulae: the role of home hyperalimentation. Cleve. Clin. O., 46:133–136, 1979.
7. Byrne, M.D., Burke, M., Fonkalsrud, E.W., and Ament, M.E.: Home parenteral nutrition: an alternative approach to the management of complicated gastrointestinal fistulas not responding to conventional medical or surgical therapy. J.P.E.N., 3:355–359, 1979.
8. Faulk, D.L., Anuras, S., and Freeman, J.B.: Idiopathic chronic intestinal pseudo-obstruction: use of central venous nutrition. J.A.M.A., 240: 2075–2076, 1978.
9. Solassol, C., Joyeaux, H., Etco, L., et al.: New techniques for long-term intravenous feeding and artificial gut in 75 patients. Ann. Surg., 179:519–522, 1974.
10. Jeejeebhoy, K.N., Sohrab, W.J., Langer, B., et al.: Total parenteral nutrition at home for 23 months without complication and with good rehabilitation: a study of technical and metabolic features. Gastroenterology, 65:811, 1973.
11. Bozian, R.C.: Personal communication, 1982.
12. Shils, M.E., Ament, M.E., Blackburn, G.L., and Jeejeebhoy, K.N.: Registry of patients on home total parenteral nutrition. N.Y. Acad. Med., Questionnaire 5, 1981.
13. Winawer, S.J., Broitman, S.A., Wolochow, M., et al.: Successful management of massive small

bowel resection based on assessment of absorption defects and nutritional needs. N. Engl. J. Med., 274:72–78, 1966.
14. Meyer, H.W.: Extensive resection of small and large intestine: a further twenty-two year follow-up report. Ann. Surg., 168:287–289, 1968.
15. Wateska, L.P., Sattler, L.L., and Steiger, E.: Cost experiences with a home parenteral nutrition program. J.A.M.A., 244:2303–2304, 1980.
16. Weiss, S.M., Worthington, P.H., Prioleau, M., and Rosato, F.E.: Home total parenteral nutrition in cancer patients. Cancer, 50:1210–1213, 1982.
17. Price, B.S., and Levine, E.L.: Permanent total parenteral nutrition: psychology and social responses of the early stages. J.P.E.N., 3(2):48–52, 1979.
18. Johnston, J.E.: Home parenteral nutrition: the "cost" of patient and family participation. Soc. Work Health Care, 7(2):49–66, 1981.
19. Perl, M., Hall, R.C.W., Dudrick, S.J., et al.: Psychological aspects of long-term home hyperalimentation. J.P.E.N., 4(6):554–560, 1980.
20. Medicare Intermediary Manual: Part III—Claims Process, Transmittal No. 923, Section 65–10, 1981.
21. Gulledge, A.D., Gipson, W.T., Steiger, E., Hooley, R.D., and Srp, F.: Home parenteral nutrition for the short bowel syndrome. Psychol. Issues, 2:271–281, 1980.
22. Gulledge, A.D., Juguilon, B.C., and Ahluwalia, S.: Psychological issues in evaluating patients for HPN. J.P.E.N., 3:32, 1979.
23. Gulledge, A.D., and Gipson, W.T.: Short bowel syndrome and psychological issues for home parenteral nutrition. Presented at the McGaw Home TPN Team Concept Seminar, Las Vegas, Nevada, December 1979.
24. Malcolm, R., Bovson, J.R.K., Vanderveen, T.W., and O'Neal, P.M.: Total parenteral nutrition: psychosocial aspects. Psychosomatics, 21(2):115–125, 1980.
25. Malcolm, R.: The psychosocial aspects of total parenteral nutrition. Presented at the annual meeting of the Academy of Psychosomatic Medicine, San Francisco, October 28–31, 1979.
26. Gulledge, A.D.: Home parenteral nutrition and the family. Nutr. Supp. Serv., 2(5):44–46, 1982.
27. Barnhill, L.R., and Longo, D.: Fixation and regression in the family life cycle. In Howells, J.G. (ed.): Advances in Family Psychiatry. New York, International Universities Press, 1981, pages 51–56.
28. Scribner, B.H., and Cole, J.J.: Evolution of the technique of home parenteral nutrition. J.P.E.N., 3:58–61, 1979.
29. Broviac, J.W., Cole, J.J., and Scribner, B.H.: A silicone rubber right atrial catheter for prolonged parenteral alimentation. Surg. Gynecol. Obstet., 136:602–606, 1973.
30. Grundfest, S., and Steiger, E.: Experience with the Broviac catheter for prolonged parenteral alimentation. J.P.E.N., 3:45–47, 1979.
31. Grundfest, S., and Steiger, E.: Home parenteral nutrition. J.A.M.A., 244:1701–1703, 1980.
32. Jeejeebhoy, K.N., Langer, B., Tsallas, G., Chu, R.C., et al.: Total parenteral nutrition at home: studies in patients surviving 4 months to 5 years. Gastroenterology, 71:943–953, 1976.
33. Riella, M.C., and Scribner, B.H.: Five years' experience with a right atrial catheter for prolonged parenteral nutrition at home. Surg. Gynecol. Obstet., 143:205–208, 1976.
34. Sattler, L., Wateska, L.P., Siska, B., et al.: Cleveland Clinic Home TPN Manual. Irvine, California, McGaw Laboratories, 1978.

35. Hawkins, J., and Nelson, E.W.: Percutaneous placement of Hickman catheter for prolonged venous access. Am. J. Surg., 144:624–626, 1982.

36. Ostrow, L.S.: Air embolism and central venous lines. Am. J. Nurs., 81:274–276, 1981.

37. Montague, N., Srp, F., and Steiger, E.: Emergency catheter repairs in the home parenteral nutrition patient (Abstract). J.P.E.N., 4:597, 1980.

38. Glynn, M.F.X., Langer, B., and Jeejeebhoy, K.N.: Therapy for thrombotic occlusion of long-term intravenous alimentation catheters. J.P.E.N., 4:387–390, 1980.

39. Copeland, E.M., III: Catheter care and intravenous hyperalimentation. J.P.E.N., 6:93–94, 1982.

40. Hurtubise, M.R., Bottino, J.C., Lawson, M., and McCredie, K.B.: Restoring patency of occluded central venous catheters. Arch. Surg., 115:212–213, 1980.

41. Rubenstein, M., and Creger, W.P.: Successful streptokinase therapy for catheter-induced subclavian vein thrombosis. Arch. Intern. Med., 140:1370–1371, 1980.

42. Wilson, S.E., and Owens, M.L. (eds.): Vascular Access Surgery. Chicago, Year Book Medical Publishers, Inc., 1980, page 24.

43. Oram-Smith, J.C., Mullen, J.L., Harken, A.H., and Fitts, W.T., Jr.: Direct right atrial catheterization for total parenteral nutrition. Surgery, 83:274–276, 1978.

44. Hooley, R.A.: Nutritional assessment: a clinical perspective. J. Am. Diet. Assoc., 77:861–866, 1980.

45. Sloan, G.M., White, D.E., and Brennan, M.F.: Calcium and phosphorous metabolism during total parenteral nutrition. Ann. Surg., 197:1–6, 1983.

46. Klein, G.L., Ament, M.E., Bluestone, R., et al.: Bone disease associated with total parenteral nutrition. Lancet, 2:1041–1045, 1980.

47. Shike, M., Harrison, J.E., Sturtridge, W.C., Tam, C.S., Bobechko, P.E., Jones, G., Murray, T.M., and Jeejeebhoy, K.N.: Metabolic bone disease in patients receiving long-term total parenteral nutrition. Ann. Intern. Med., 92:343, 1980.

48. Shike, M., Sturtbridge, W.C., Tam, C.S., et al.: A possible role of vitamin D in the genesis of parenteral nutrition induced metabolic bone disease. Ann. Intern. Med., 95:560–568, 1981.

49. Klein, G.L., Horst, R.L., Norman, A.W., Ament, M.E., Slatopolsky, E., and Coburn, J.W.: Reduced serum levels of 12,25-dihydrosy vitamin D during long-term total parenteral nutrition. Ann. Intern. Med., 94:638–643, 1981.

50. American Medical Association Department of Foods and Nutrition: Multivitamin Preparations for Parenteral Use. A statement by the Nutrition Advisory Group. J.P.E.N., 3:258–262, 1978.

51. Butler, V.E., and O'Donnel, J.: Vitamin K preparations: guidelines and cautions for intravenous use. Infusion, 5:154–155, 1982.

52. American Medical Association: Guidelines for Essential Trace Element Preparations for Parenteral Use. A statement by the Nutrition Advisory Group. J.P.E.N., 3:263–267, 1979.

53. Van Rij, A.M., McKenzie, J.M., Robinson, M.F., et al.: Selenium and total parenteral nutrition. J.P.E.N., 3:235–239, 1979.

54. Van Rij, A.M., Thompson, C.D., McKenzie, J.M., and Robinson, M.F.: Selenium deficiency in total parenteral nutrition. Am. J. Clin. Nutr., 32:2076–2085, 1979.

55. Trissel, L.: Handbook on Injectable Drugs. Edition 2. Washington, D.C., American Society of Hospital Pharmacy, Inc., pages 281–282.

56. Englert, D.M., and Dudrick, S.J.: Principles of ambulatory home hyperalimentation. Am. J. Intravenous Ther., 5:11–28, 1978.

57. Barr, L.H., Dunn, G.D., and Brennan, F.M.: Essential fatty acid deficiency during total parenteral nutrition. Ann. Surg., 193:304–311, 1981.

58. Schneider, P.J.: Should inline filters be used when administering TPN solutions? Infusion, 6:66–67, 1982.

59. Boomus, M.: Intravenous filtration: why and how. N.I.T.A., 4:187–192, 1981.

60. National Coordinating Committee on Large Volume Parenterals: Problems and Benefits of Inline Filtration. Am. J. Intravenous Therapy, Clin. Nutr. 7:45–44, 1980.

61. Lorenzen, B.A.: Final filtration. N.I.T.A., 4:322–327, 1981.

62. Ivey, M., Riella, M., Mueller, W., and Scribner, B.H.: Long-term parenteral nutrition in the home. Am. J. Hosp. Pharm., 32:1032–1036, 1975.

63. Langer, B., McHattie, J.D., Zohrab, W.J., and Jeejeebhoy, K.N.: Prolonged survival after complete small bowel resection using intravenous alimentation at home. J. Surg. Res., 15:226–233, 1973.

64. Srp, F., Steiger, E., Montague, N., et al.: Patient preparation for cyclic home parenteral nutrition: a team approach. Nutr. Supp. Serv., 1:30–34, 1981.

65. Shils, M.: A program for total parenteral nutrition at home. Am. J. Clin. Nutr., 28:1429–1435, 1975.

66. Turco, S.J.: Mechanical and electronic equipment for parenteral and enteral use: an update. Am. J. Intravenous Ther. Clin. Nutr., 9:9–43, 1982.

67. Goldfarb, I.W., and Slater, H.: Techniques of administration. Am. J. Intravenous Ther. Clin. Nutr., 8:25–34, 1981.

68. Labry, J.: Infusion monitoring devices. N.I.T.A., 4:366–367, 1981.

69. Pipp, T.L.: Intravenous infusion pumps: justification and selection and utilization. Infusion, 2:45–58, 1978.

70. Steiger, E., and Srp, F.: Morbidity and mortality related to home parenteral nutrition in patients with gut failure. Am. J. Surg., 145(1):102–105, 1983.

71. Lifeline Letter: Vol. IV, No. 4, Autumn 1982.

72. Levy, N.B.: Sexual adjustment to maintenance hemodialysis and renal transplantation. National Survey by Questionnaire: Preliminary Report. Trans. Am. Soc. Artif. Organs, 19:138–143, 1973.

73. HPN Newsletter: Seattle, Washington 98195, University of Washington.

74. Grover, M., Gulledge, A.D., and Steiger, E.: Long-term psychological issues of the HPN patient. Abstract for the 1982 Congress of the American Society for Parenteral and Enteral Nutrition, San Francisco, February 1982.

CHAPTER 40

Developmental Considerations in Neonatal TPN

CHRISTINE KENNEDY-CALDWELL
MICHAEL D. CALDWELL

Advances in neonatal care and parenteral nutrition have made it possible to support almost indefinitely many infants who less than 15 years ago would have died early in life from starvation. Improved survival, rather than a change in the percentage of high-risk infants born, is cited as the primary reason for the decline in infant mortality since 1961—from 50 to 20 per cent for the 1- to 1.5-kg infant and 50 per cent for those infants less than 1 kg.[1] There are now 7500 newborn intensive care unit (NICU) beds in approximately 600 hospitals. It is estimated that six per cent of all live births enter an NICU, with an average length of stay ranging from 8 to 18 days.[2]

Assessment of the nutritional status of the hospitalized pediatric population in United States' medical centers revealed that a 20 to 50 per cent incidence of nutritional deficits existed in these patients.[6-9] Thus, the problem of pediatric malnutrition is not limited to Third World countries or the impoverished. Its occurrence in hospitalized patients reflects the secondary effect of illness or disease as opposed to only a primary lack of nutrient intake.

Feeding problems are paramount in the clinical management of this population.[3] It has been calculated that an infant without food will die on the 4th to 11th postnatal day, depending on birth weight.[4] The premature infant is particularly at risk because not only is the gastrointestinal tract unable to efficiently process and absorb ingested nutrients but also these infants are frequently too immature to maintain the sucking and swallowing reflexes necessary for oral feedings.[5] Often, feeding via the gastrointestinal tract is contraindicated because of complica-

tions such as aspiration or necrotizing enterocolitis. Parenteral feedings have thus been used not only to nourish postoperative infants and children but also to serve as the sole source of nutrients for the growth and development of low-birth-weight and premature infants.

Most of the studies to date regarding neonatal and pediatric parenteral nutrition have dealt exclusively with the biochemical and technologic aspects of this form of therapy. The science of nutrient function and the requirements for somatic maintenance, restoration and growth, and metabolism regulation have been illuminated elsewhere in this volume (see Chapters 41 and 42). It is necessary to consider that food is something more than metabolic substrates, and feeding is something more than the ingestion of nutrients. Thus, this chapter seeks to delineate those neurophysiologic factors that have implications for parenterally fed infants and children. The nutrient milieu required for optimal development and functioning of the brain and central nervous system (CNS) has not been defined. It is nevertheless clear that these processes depend upon an adequate nutrient supply. Eating is one of the earliest exposures involving human interaction in the child's world. Because of the immediate and long-range implications alternative feeding modalities may hold, this chapter will also seek to clarify normative developmental findings in regard to the care of children requiring specialized nutrition.

The growth and development of the human brain is the result of several factors. Metabolic, genetic, and environmental components are so closely intertwined that the isolation of nutrition as an independent factor in the development of intelligence or as a causal agent in behavior is difficult. This chapter will explore those studies that have demonstrated a role for nutrition in the neurophysiologic and developmental aspects of infant growth.

METABOLIC FACTORS

Parenteral feeding of premature infants causes the clinician to act as the "fetal placenta." However, fetal nutrition is an arena that is still filled with many unanswered questions. In utero, the fetus requires a continuous influx of glucose, essential fatty acids, amino acids, vitamins, minerals, water, and oxygen for combustion and somatic construction.[10] The primary thesis of this discussion will be that to adequately nourish children, we must address those issues that go beyond the past criterion of successful nourishment—somatic growth.

Glucose Metabolism in the Developing Brain

The mature human brain is composed of approximately 100 billion neurons and an equivalent number of glial cells. By the age of two years, the brain approaches its adult size, weight, and number of cells. It composes only 2 per cent of the adult body weight, yet it receives 15 per cent of the cardiac output and accounts for 20 to 30 per cent of the resting metabolic rate.[11] In contrast to other tissues and organs and despite its high energy requirements, the brain lacks the storage capability to meet these energy requirements. Human fetal glucose is derived from maternal glucose.[12] The concentration of D-glucose is higher in maternal plasma than in fetal plasma;[13–37] even when an intravenous glucose infusion creates maternal and fetal hyperglycemia, the fetal plasma concentration remains below that of the maternal concentration.[17, 18] Glucose serves as an obligatory energy source for the developing brain, with the respiratory quotient (RQ) being close to 1. There are two sources of glucose available to the brain—blood glucose and brain glycogen. The concentration of brain glycogen is relatively small and is therefore rapidly exhausted. During the early growth and development of the brain, 50 per cent of glucose oxidation is via the hexose

monophosphate (HMP) shunt[20] (see Fig. 40–1). In the adult brain, 90 per cent of glucose undergoes glycolysis via the Embden-Meyerhof pathway. Thus, the significant use of the HMP shunt affords the developing brain direct oxidation of glucose, generating the reduced form of nicotinamide-adenine dinucleotide phosphate (NADPH), for rapid lipid synthesis for the myelination process, and ribose molecules for nucleic acid metabolism.[20]

Glycolysis in the brain is normally limited by hexokinase. The normal brain glucose level is 2 to 3 μmol·gm^{-1} or 3 to 4 mM, which greatly exceeds the Km of hexokinase. In fact, the usual brain/plasma ratio for glucose exceeds the extracellular volume of distribution. In this regard, the brain differs from other peripheral tissues in that its glycolysis is not limited by substrate under normal circumstances.[21]

Alpha-ketoglutarate and oxaloacetate produced from the entrance of pyruvate into the tricarboxylic acid (TCA; Krebs) cycle are converted into glutamate and aspartate; thus, glucose also serves as carbon sources for amino acid synthesis.[22]

In the CNS, the uptake of fructose is considerably less than that of glucose; indeed, it appears that the brain can utilize large amounts of fructose only after its conversion to glucose. Because fructose cannot be rapidly taken up by the brain, it cannot as such sustain the normal metabolic activity of the brain. Therefore, its attributes for use in parenteral feeding are limited to its being less irritating to the veins than glucose and more readily taken up by tissues other than the brain.

Necropsy evidence of neurologic damage has been observed in both humans and experimental animals following severe hypoglycemia.[23, 24] Neurologic damage has been found in the cerebral cortex and hippocampus in rats and monkeys.[24, 25] Hypoglycemia, uncomplicated by undernutrition, results in reduced incorporation of ^{35}S into brain sulfatides, thus adversely affecting myelination.[26]

Protein Metabolism in the Developing Brain

Parenteral protein is necessary to provide amino acids for the synthesis of body proteins. Since there is no storage pool, a continuous supply is necessary for the growing child. Beyond the essential amino acids leucine, isoleucine, valine, lysine, threonine, methionine, phenylalanine, and tryptophan, there is evidence that cystine, histidine, tyrosine, and taurine may need to be exogenously supplied to infants.[27–37]

Amino acids play key roles in brain function as substrates for protein and neurotransmitter synthesis. The transport of amino acids is carrier-mediated from the circulating blood into the brain; however, carrier properties are not identical for many of the amino acids.[38] Protein synthesis in the developing brain occurs at a similar overall rate to its synthesis in muscle. Therefore, as in muscle, protein accumulation is thought to be linear from the sixth month of gestation until the second postnatal year.

Studies of protein malnutrition, or kwashiorkor, in either the mother during pregnancy or in the infant, or both, have yielded abundant proof that malnutrition can adversely affect the somatic development of animals and humans.[39–52] More recently, studies have demonstrated that alterations in behavior, brain electrophysiologic properties, and neurotransmitter metabolism are induced in the fetus or newborn animal by protein deprivation during pregnancy and lactation.[53–59]

Inadequate nutrition has been documented as adversely affecting the total number of brain cells, the size of the cells, the number of synaptic connections, the rate of protein synthesis, the activity of enzymes, and the amount of neurotransmitters.[60–93]

Of particular importance is the role of protein nutriture on neurotransmitters. About two dozen different neurotransmitters are known (Table 40–1). Neurotransmitters

Table 40–1. KNOWN AND POTENTIAL NEUROTRANSMITTER SUBSTANCES

Acetylcholine
Catecholamines
  Dopamine
  Norepinephrine
Other Monoamines
  Serotonin
Amino acids
  Glycine
  Alpha-aminobutyric acid
  Glutamic acid
  Aspartic acid
  Histamine

(Adapted from Dhopeshwarkar, G. A.: Nutrition and Brain Development. Chapter 9, Figure 29, page 131.)

Table 40–2. AMINO ACID PRECURSORS FOR BRAIN NEUROTRANSMITTER SYNTHESIS

AMINO ACID	REGULATORY ENZYME	NEURO-TRANSMITTER
Tryptophan	Hydroxylase	Serotonin
Tyrosine	Hydroxylase	Dopamine or noradrenaline
Histidine	Decarboxylase	Histamine
Threonine	Serine hydroxymethyl-transferase	Glycine

(Adapted from Anderson, G. H.: Diet neurotransmitters and brain function. Br. Med. Bull., 37(1):95, 1981.)

act as chemical signals between the nerve fiber ending and a postsynaptic nerve cell. The ability to synthesize several neurotransmitters depends directly on the composition of the blood. Cohen and Wurtman[85] have reviewed four mechanisms in which changes in brain neurotransmitter concentrations may be affected by nutritional variations: (1) "chronic malnutrition in the developing animals affects absolute and relative numbers of particular groups of neurons . . . thereby decreasing the number of cellular units capable of synthesizing and storing particular neurotransmitters, (2) suppressed arborization of growing neurons and the impaired formation of boutons and terminals (the loci of most neurotransmitter molecules) as well as synapses, (3) effect (on) the brain's levels of cofactors necessary for the optimal activity of enzymes involved in neurotransmitter synthesis or catabolism and (4) variations in the availability to neurons of circulating compounds that are the precursors of the neurotransmitters."[85]

Table 40–2 lists the four neurotransmitters that are known to be influenced by the availability of their precursors from a dietary protein source. Extensive research in the last decade has pointed toward a relationship among diet, brain neurotransmission, and brain function.[93–114] It is for this reason that the role of amino acids in parenteral feedings should not be viewed solely for their tissue-synthetic properties.

As an example of this, one can review current discussions surrounding the provision of cystine and taurine to infants.[115–140] Figure 40–1 portrays the trans-sulfuration pathway, which is a series of metabolic reactions involving the four sulfur-containing amino acids—methionine, cystine, cysteine, and taurine. Methionine is an essential amino acid for human metabolism. Cystine and cys-

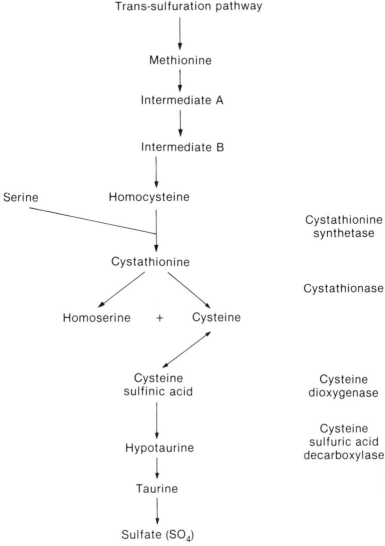

Figure 40–1. Trans-sulfuration pathway.

teine or cyst(e)ine (which is the mixture in any proportion of the sulfhydryl cysteine and the disulfide cystine) are considered nonessential in adults, as is taurine. In adults, 90 per cent of ingested methionine is converted to cyst(e)ine, and cystathionine is normally present in high concentrations in the adult brain, though it is barely detectable in the liver.[141–143]

Questions arose concerning the essentiality of sulfur-containing amino acids in infants and children because of an early report citing depressed growth rates and reduced nitrogen retention in a premature infant fed cystine-free formula[32, 35] and a series demonstrating negligible hepatic cystathionase levels in young infants.[29] At the same time, other studies[118, 121] found decreased plasma cystine in infants receiving cystine-free parenteral solutions. Subsequent studies demonstrated that (1) cystathionase activity was absent from the human placenta and the fetal liver and brain in the presence of considerable methionine-activating enzyme and cystathionine synthase activity;[119] (2) the fetal liver is not able to synthesize more than trace amounts of cystathionase;[120] (3) approximately 75 per cent of maximal cystathionase enzyme activity is present in the human fetal kidney by the second trimester of pregnancy;[123] and (4) unlike other free amino acids, the concentration of cyst(e)ine in fetal plasma was equal to or lower than maternal concentrations.[122] One study suggested, however, that the hepatic cystathionase activity in premature and full-term infants matured rapidly after birth to achieve 70 per cent of adult values by the ninth and third postnatal intake days, respectively.[123] These data were interpreted to mean that if given adequate methionine intake, even premature infants could produce sufficient cysteine to meet protein synthesis requirements.[130] Yet, despite the elevation of plasma methionine from the intake of methionine-rich mixtures, Pohlandt found low plasma cystine concentrations in premature infants, suggesting that cystine biosynthesis in the newborn is independent of substrate concentration.[124] Complicating interpretation of the earlier studies, data from a recent report[133] show that measurement of plasma and urinary 1/2 cystine by an amino acid analyzer does not accurately reflect the effect of administered cysteine and therefore measurement of both sulfhydryl and disulfide cyst(e)ine is necessary to interpret the fate of parenterally administered cysteine hydrochloride.

Thus, the role of cyst(e)ine in infant metabolism is still unanswered. The metabolic function of this amino acid is of particular concern because of its role in the production of taurine. Several studies have suggested that taurine is involved in a number of physiologic functions, especially in the CNS. This area has been extensively reviewed by Baskin[117, 127, 145–154] (Table 40–3). In the neonate taurine conjugates with bile salts, preferentially in a ratio of 3:1, until three months of age, when development of the glycine–bile acid conjugate reverses the ratio to that found in the adult.[144] The essen-

Table 40–3. POSSIBLE ROLE OF TAURINE IN THE CNS HUMAN AND ANIMAL MODELS

Inhibitory neurotransmitter
Antiarrhythmic agent
Control of body temperature
Control of water regulation
Involvement in psoriasis
Endogenous antiepileptic agents
Neurotransmitter in retina
Involvement in retinitis pigmentosa
Regulation of melatonin in pineal gland
Central depressant
Involvement in schizophrenia
Control of osmolarity
Regulation of pain threshold
Regulation of glucose metabolism
Regulation of oxygen utilization
Involvement in stress reaction
Regulation of tissue excitability

(Adapted from Baskin, S. I., Leibman, A. J., and Cohn, E. M.: Possible functions of taurine in the central nervous system. Adv. Biochem. Psychopharm., 15:153, 1976.)

tiality of taurine in infant feeding, as measured by its effect on bile salt metabolism, has resulted in conflicting reports. In a series of five studies the following was found: (1) taurine supplementation did not affect growth,[134] though it maintained plasma and urinary taurine concentrations similar to those in infants fed human milk;[135, 155–156] (2) it had little effect on bile salt metabolism;[136, 138] and (3) it had no effect on intestinal fat absorption.[137] However, age and health status may be an important variable in regard to these studies. Okamoto and colleagues[139] found significantly lower stores of taurine at birth and a difference in plasma and urinary taurine concentration in term low-birth-weight appropriate for gestational age (mean birth weight 1476 gm and 31.7-week gestational age) than did Rassin and coworkers,[135] who studied slightly larger, more mature, and healthier infants (mean birth-weight 1700 gm and 33-week gestational age).

Caution must be urged in discounting a role for cyst(e)ine and taurine because of a lack of changes in growth or nitrogen retention,[130, 139] since these studies do not address the possibility of taurine's function in the brain as a modulator or a neurotransmitter. The very large concentrations of taurine that are reported in the human fetal brain as compared to the adult brain are striking, and the slow postnatal decrease in taurine concentration has led to the suggestion that taurine may be associated in some way with brain development, *per se*, in addition to its functional role in more mature brains.[126] Because propriety cows' milk–based formulas contain negligible amounts of taurine, some products are now fortified with taurine at levels comparable to term breast milk (45 mg/L). Soy-based formulas contain no taurine. It has been shown, and is of particular significance regarding the parenteral provision of taurine, that the high brain concentrations of this amino acid are probably not the result of its increased synthesis, since the enzyme activity of cysteine sulfinic acid decarboxylase has been shown to be low in the newborn rat brain,[117] and as its activity increases with age the concentration of taurine decreases.[147] Sturman speculates that the brain responds during metabolic stress states with changes in taurine turnover rather than changes in taurine concentration.[126] Therefore, the human infant, who cannot synthesize adequate taurine from cyst(e)ine and methionine precursors,[29, 123, 155] may be dependent on a dietary taurine source.[128]

Lipid Metabolism in the Developing Brain

There is evidence that less than 10 per cent of fetal calorie needs are supplied by ketones. Much of this use of lipid-derived substrate is reserved for the CNS, since large amounts of β-hydroxybutyrate are oxidized by the fetal brain (Fig. 40–2).[159] The fetal whole-body lipid content increases markedly during the last trimester of pregnancy. From a content of 0.5 per cent of body weight at 12 weeks, and only 3.5 per cent of body weight at 7 months of gestation, fat content rises rapidly to 16 per cent by term.[157–159] Fetal fat is thought to be derived from free fatty acids via placental transfer as well as from fetal fatty acid synthesis from carbohydrate and acetate.

Total lipid content and concentration are also increased in the fetal brain during development. The major increase occurs in the white matter in which myelination is occurring. The white matter attains 90 per cent of its total lipid content in 2 years, and the remainder is attained by 10 years of age. Lipid accrual proceeds rapidly in gray matter following glial proliferation, and the adult composition is reached by the third month of postnatal age.[90] The absolute and relative increase in cerebral lipids with maturation is most closely linked to the development of myelin. Analysis of mature myelin shows that on a dry weight basis it accounts for 50 per cent of the total lipid in the brain and more than 25 per cent of the brain's total weight.[160–161] In most species, myelin is the major membrane to be formed quantitatively in postnatal life, and therefore it is one of the most susceptible to nutritional insult. In the human, the peak rate of myelin formation is during the perinatal period, with the majority of myelination completed by 18 months. Once formed, myelin is thought to be a relatively stable membrane, so malnutrition has less of an adverse effect on it once synthesis is completed.[162]

The importance of the role myelin plays in neuronal function cannot be underestimated. It is thought to have evolved as a means of conserving the neuron's metabolic energy and has enabled animals to greatly increase the number of their fastest signaling channels without making extra demands on anatomic space. Along the axon, the membrane is specialized to propagate an electric impulse so that, in general, myelinated nerve fibers conduct nerve impulses faster than unmyelinated fibers. This is why vertebrates have been able to retain thin fibers and yet vastly increase the speed of impulse to approximately 100 m/second (225 miles/hour). In addition, the membrane appears to be one factor in mediating the recognition of other cells in embryonic development so that each cell finds its proper place in the network of the total 1×10^{11} cells.

Myelin composition is characterized by small amounts of water and 15 to 30 per cent protein, with the balance of dry weight being lipid (Table 40–4). The chemical composition of the sheath represents a cholesterol/

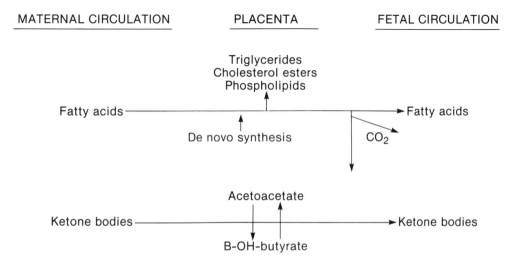

Figure 40–2. Placental transport and metabolism of fatty acids and ketone bodies. (From Robertson, A. F., and Karp, W. B.: Placental transport of nutrients. South. Med. J., *69*:1358–1362, 1976, with permission.)

Table 40–4. CHARACTERISTICS OF BRAIN LIPID COMPOSITION (DRY WEIGHT BASIS)

Total lipids (mg/gm)	Newborn 27–30
	1–15 days 55–60
	Adult 100–110
Triglycerides	Found only in trace amounts
Free cholesterol	Adult (20–22 mg/gm)
Esterified cholesterol	Small amounts up to 3 weeks
Desmosterol	Only trace-adult
Total phospholipids (mg/gm)	12 days 28
	Adult 47
Phosphatidylcholine	Major component approximately 48–50 mole %
Phosphatidylserine	Approximately 11–12% mole
Phosphatidylinositol	Contains mono-, di-, and triphosphate inositides
Phosphatidylethanolamine	Diacyl type major component before myelination; alkeneyl-acyl type major after myelination (70%)
Sphingolipids	Sphingomyelin, cerebrosides, sulfatides. Very rapid increase during myelination (myelin lipids)

Fatty Acids
  Hydroxy fatty acids
  Odd-number carbon-chain fatty acids
  Long-chain fatty acids (>24)
  Polyunsaturated fatty acids
    Very small amounts of 18:2w6 or 18:3w3
    High amounts of longer-chain 20:4w6 and 22:6w3

(Adapted from Dhopeshwarkar, G. A.: Nutrition and Brain Development. New York, Plenum Press, 1983, pages 61–62 [Tables 3 and 4].)

phospholipid/galactolipid molar ratio of approximately 4:3:2. The phospholipid and glycolipid fractions are particularly vulnerable to essential fatty acid deficiency (EFAD).[163–164] To date, most of the work related to cerebral lipid development centers around the effect EFAD has on the developing brain. However, changes in brain lipid composition are also found when the diet is lacking other nutritional substrates such as protein. Conversely, lack of essential fatty acids can cause alterations in nonlipid components of the brain as well. Several studies have documented that fat deprivation induced marked changes in brain weight and the fatty acid composition of brain phospholipids.[165–177] In addition, studies using titrated glucosamines have demonstrated that the myelin of under-nourished animals was unstable, with a shorter than normal half-life.[160]

Clinicians in the past have mainly been concerned with the role lipids played in providing calories and preventing gross somatic evidence of deficiency. Additional concerns now center around the role essential fatty acids play as precursors of prostaglandin biosynthesis and the further elucidation of the essentiality of linolenic acid.[178, 179]

The relative effectiveness of linolenic acid (18:3w3) in curing EFAD symptoms is only one-tenth that of linoleic acid (18:2w6).[180] Also, it has to be converted to eicosapentaenoic acid (20:5w3) to be an effective precursor of prostaglandins of the PGF_3 series, and this conversion is not a major process; thus, doubt is cast on its essentiality for human metabolism. The competitive and inhibitory effects of W3 fatty acids on the metabolism of W6 fatty acids (e.g., linoleic acid) was cited as a possible deleterious side effect of the administration of linolenic acid. Given as 0.1 per cent of the total energy intake, linolenic acid induces a 50 per cent inhibition of linoleic acid conversion to 22:5w6.[181, 182] For these reasons, second-generation commercial intravenous fat emulsions formulated from safflower (0.1 per cent linolenic acid) rather than soybean oil (9 per cent linolenic acid) were made clinically available.

However, the CNS—along with the human retina, testes, and sperm—contains large amounts of W3 (primarily 22:6w3) fatty acids whose half-life is rather short at 15 days.[183–187] The low content of 22:6w3 induced in brains of rats by low linolenic–acid diets has been reported to result in abnormal physical activity and ability to learn. Only one case of human linolenic acid–deficiency has been reported and it did involve neurologic abnormalities.[188] The authors concluded that the symptomatology resulted not only from a deficit of linolenic acid but also from the altered ratio of 18:2w6/18:3w3 in the parenteral fat emulsions.

Carnitine is a carrier molecule that is necessary for the transport of long-chain fatty acids into the cell mitochondria. It also serves to transport the end product of fatty acid oxidation, acetylcoenzyme A (acetyl-CoA), into the cytoplasm. Carnitine is of particular concern in premature infants who are born with a relative fat deficit and who are also in need of fat the most for brain growth. Postnatal changes in the activity of carnitine palmitoyl transferase parallel the development of fatty acid oxidation in a number of organs, suggesting that it may have a central role in regulating the development of fatty acid oxidation.[189]

In both human and rat neonates, plasma and tissue carnitine stores are lower than in the adult.[190–191] In human neonatal livers, the γ-butyrobetaine hydrolase activity (the last enzyme in the carnitine pathway) is only 12 per cent of the adult level. By two and one-half years of age, it has reached only 30 per cent of this level, and does not obtain 100 per cent of the adult value until 15 years of age.[192, 193] Neonates who are receiving parenteral feedings only must rely entirely on their meager endogenous carnitine synthesis and tissue stores to fully utilize fatty acids, since parenteral products do not currently contain carnitine. Plasma and muscle carnitine concentrations in premature infants drop after 5 to 15 days of total parenteral nutrition (TPN) if carnitine is not enterally supplemented.[194–196]

Vitamins

By definition, all vitamins are essential for the growing infant. However, some of them are particularly important for the sick infant because a deficiency state can occur more rapidly in these infants than in healthy infants (Table 40–5). Fat-soluble vitamins are provided in the placenta via simple and facilitated diffusion that is dependent upon a maternal-fetal concentration gradient, and therefore energy expenditure is not required.[197] With the exception of vitamin E, circulating fetal concentrations correspond to maternal levels.[198] Accumulation takes place primarily in the third trimester of pregnancy. Transfer of water-soluble vitamins is relatively independent of concentrations in the maternal circulation and occurs via active transport or pinocytosis (Table 40–6).[199] However, Hurley and others feel the evidence is

Table 40–5. PREDISPOSING FACTORS FOR VITAMIN DEFICIENCY

Decreased body stores
Decreased availability or intake
Decreased absorption
Increased need or utilization
Special conditions of low birth-weight infants

(From Orzalesi, M., and Colarizi, P.: Critical vitamins for low birthweight infants. Acta Paediatr. Scand. (Suppl.) 296:105, 1982, with permission.)

Table 40–6. FETAL/MATERNAL VITAMIN BLOOD LEVEL RATIO

Vitamin A	1/1
Vitamin D	0.8/1
Vitamin E	0.3/1
Vitamin K	0.9/1
Vitamin B_1	2/1
Vitamin B_2	4/1
Vitamin B_6	3/1
Vitamin B_{12}	4/1
Folate	2/1
Vitamin C	2/1

(Adapted from Orzalesi, M., and Coralizi, P.: Critical vitamins for low birthweight infants. Acta Paediatr. Scand. (Suppl.), 296:105, 1982.)

inconclusive for active transport, since placental metabolism may affect the concentrations measured.[159, 200]

Neither the mechanism of uptake nor the factors affecting vitamin content of the brain has been fully described.[201] Inadequacy of the vitamin supply is of concern because of the role they play as cofactors in key metabolic pathways within the brain. Adequate parenteral provision of vitamins is uncertain because of (1) the questionable practice of using the recommended daily allowance (RDA) for orally fed term infants as a standard for the hospitalized parenterally fed premature infant[202, 203] and (2) the large variability in the stability of the vitamins in TPN solutions.[204–213]

Vitamins that are known to be light-labile are vitamins A, D, E, K, B_2, B_6, B_{12}, C, and folic acid. Only biotin and niacin have been documented as being light-stable. The fate of pantothenic acid is unknown.

Under regular lighting conditions in a hospital nursery, Ostrea and associates determined that riboflavin in parenteral solution decreased 33 per cent ($p < 0.001$) at concentrations of 20 and 40 µg/ml when compared to control groups of solutions that were wrapped in aluminum foil to protect them from light.[204] Simulating clinical conditions, Bhatia and colleagues studied riboflavin and amino acid mixtures while they were exposed to phototherapy over a 24-hour period.[205] The riboflavin decreased more than 50 per cent, from 1.09 to 0.57 mg/L ($p < 0.001$). Chen and associates observed that the concentration of riboflavin-5-phosphate in solutions that were exposed to direct sunlight for four hours dropped by 98 per cent, when measured by microbiologic assay, and by 59 per cent by absorbance measurements. Under fluorescent lighting, changes were undetectable during an eight-hour exposure time by both microbiologic and absorbance measurements. Indirect sun exposure resulted in a 47 and 18 per cent decrease, respectively, within eight hours.[206]

To date, no specific effects of riboflavin deficiency can be related to brain biochemistry. Although the liver loses 60 per cent of its riboflavin in moderate deficiency, the loss in brain tissue is marginal.[214] It has been postulated that because of riboflavin's cofactor role for monoamine oxidase activity, a deficiency would lead to a disturbance in neurotransmitter metabolism; however, no such data have been established.[20] In riboflavin-deficient monkeys, neurologic symptoms such as partial paralysis of hindlimbs has been produced, the mechanism possibly being due to degeneration of myelin in the peripheral nerves.[215]

Pyridoxine (B_6) is involved in more than 50 enzymatic reactions as the coenzyme pyridoxal phosphate. The conversion of pyridoxine to pyridoxamine 5-phosphate occurs in the brain *in situ*.[216] Vitamin B_6 plays a major role in brain metabolism specifically within the metabolic pathway of γ-aminobutyric acid (GABA).[217, 218] γ-Aminobutyric acid is metabolized to form succinic acid, an important component of the Krebs (TCA) cycle. Decarboxylation of serine requires pyridoxine. This reaction effects the synthesis of sphingosine, a component of sphingoglycolipids. Pyridoxine deficiency leads to a decreased synthesis of cerebroside and sulfatides, two important myelin lipids.[219] Several animal studies have confirmed the effect of vitamin B_6 deficiency on neurologic impairment.[220–228]

Neurologic involvement secondary to pyridoxine metabolism in infants was demonstrated by Synderman and colleagues in the early 1950s.[228] In addition, a tragic demonstration of its necessity for infant metabolism occurred when, because of a manufacturing problem, the vitamin was destroyed in a commercial infant formula, resulting in a vitamin B_6-deficiency epidemic of seizures.[229–231]

Using a microbiologic assay in the only study to date on the stability of parenteral pyridoxine hydrochloride, Chen and associates demonstrated a decrease of 86 per cent over an eight-hour exposure to direct sun. In fluorescent and indirect light, the concentration remained relatively stable at 15 μ/ml.[206]

In general, the other water-soluble vitamins function in nerve cells as they do in other cells; thus, dietary deficiency might be expected to alter brain metabolism. However, "the point at which neurochemical transmission is affected and whether this aspect of nerve cell metabolism is more or less susceptible than other aspects of metabolism is undefined." Thus, evidence for neurotransmitter involvement is still limited but promises to be a new frontier.[201]

Ascorbic acid is the only other water-soluble vitamin that has been studied for stability during parenteral provision. There was no significant change in the TPN-effluent vitamin C concentration when measurements were taken every 6 hours over a 24-hour experimental period.[207]

"The fat-soluble vitamins A and E are directly involved in neuronal metabolism, whereas the involvement of vitamin D is likely to be indirect, because of its effect on calcium metabolism."[201] Because of limited transplacental acquisition of fat-soluble vitamins (a largely third-trimester phenomenon), premature infants are at a higher risk for deficiency.

Shenai and coworkers studied 39 premature infants who were born at less than 36 weeks' gestation and found that 82 per cent had lower plasma vitamin A ($p < 0.001$), plasma retinol-binding protein (RBP) ($p < 0.001$), and a lower molar ratio of plasma vitamin A/RBP ($p < 0.02$) than 32 term control infants.[232] These data confirmed earlier studies by Brandt.[233] They postulated four explanations for their findings: (1) maternal deficiency of vitamin A, (2) inadequate transplacental transfer of vitamin A, (3) inadequate storage and release of vitamin A from the neonatal liver, or (4) inadequate tissue utilization of vitamin A.

There is controversy as to the extent of vitamin A involvement in the metabolism of the developing brain. Manifestations of vitamin A toxicity have been well documented and range from gross anomalies of the skull and brain to possible interference with DNA synthesis in neuroepithelial cells.[234–237] Cases of mild hypervitaminosis in rats cause functional deficits, without producing visible malformations of the CNS.[238, 239]

Keating and Feigin observed increased intracranial pressure associated with vitamin A deficiency of short duration in an infant with cystic fibrosis.[240]

Based on dog studies, Mellanby concluded that vitamin A deficiency resulted in obstructive hydrocephalus by producing an interruption of cerebrospinal fluid (CSF) flow.[241] Periosteal bone formation was found to be obstructing CSF circulation in chicks with vitamin A deficiency.[242] Different mechanisms have been proposed for these developments,[243, 244] and there is still disagreement as to the reliability of these findings.[245]

Six studies examining vitamin A delivered parenterally have been published since 1976.[208–213] Results documented a decrease in effluent delivery of vitamin A from 30 to 75 per cent of that expected. The clinician is in the precarious position of dealing with babies of various gestational ages who thus have different stores and requirements of vitamin A, and he or she faces a varying reliability of parenteral delivery of the vitamin while trying to avoid toxicity and deficiency!

Five postulates have been forwarded to account for low levels of vitamin E in premature infants: (1) inadequate dietary intake, (2) impaired absorption of fat and fat-soluble vitamins via the gastrointestinal tract, (3) inadequate concentration of transport lipoproteins, (4) increased requirements produced by rapid growth, and (5) increased requirements by high–polyunsaturated fatty acid (PUFA) diets.

Bell has documented a dramatic linear increase in the total body tocopherol content of infants with an increase in gestational age and body weight.[246] From five months to term, vitamin E increases from 1 mg to 20 mg.

Several animal studies have substantiated that vitamin E deficiency results in CNS-related alterations.[247–250] No reports have documented a similar role in humans. It has been suggested that the role of vitamin E in brain metabolism relies on its powerful antioxidant properties to prevent peroxidation of brain lipids.[256–258] Recent findings reported axonal lesions in children with cholestatic liver disease and concomitant low vitamin E levels.[259] Neuroaxonal dystrophy was also described in children with congenital biliary atresia[260] and cystic fibrosis,[261] though others have concluded that there is no relationship between infantile neuroaxonal dystrophy and vitamin E deficiency.[262]

There are several recent studies that indicate a role for vitamin E, especially its possible pharmacologic effect on retrolental fibroplasia (RLF).[251–255]

The parenteral provision of vitamin E is also a difficult issue. In the two studies to date on the parenteral provision of vitamin E, Shenai and associates[207] estimated a net delivery of 88 per cent over a 24-hour period from the effluent. The concentration in the TPN bottle remained stable over time. They suggested that the absorptive loss of 12 per cent took place via the progressive saturation of the delivery tubing and was characterized by initial low levels that increased over 8 hours, and then plateaued for the next 16 hours. Gillis and coworkers[213] published similar results, with minimal concentrations in the effluent over the first 1 to 1½ hours, reaching a plateau at 6 hours, with a total delivery every 24 hours of approximately 64 per cent of the initial concentration.

DEVELOPMENTAL FACTORS

The critical interrelationship of nutrition with physical and psychosocial development is never more apparent than in the premature sick infant requiring parenteral nourishment. Alternative feeding modalities have an impact on the child's biologic function, personality development, social skills, and general well-being.

The majority of infants and children who require parenteral nutrition receive it for a relatively short duration, a few days to a few weeks. However, there is a growing population that is receiving TPN as the sole source of feeding for an extensive period, consisting of a few months to indefinitely. The interface of this technologic mode with normal developmental achievements is unexplored.

Eating is one of the earliest repetitive activities of an infant. The following questions arise. If the psychomotor skills involved in oral feeding progression are not utilized, does the child experience developmental imbalance? If the missing experience is short-lived, is there compensation for the effect? If the situation is long-term, is normalcy irretrievable? There are no studies to date that address these issues. A significant complicating factor in assessing the role of early feeding difficulties in development is the target population. Infants requiring TPN are always sick children. The sequelae to prematurity alone makes teasing out a singular factor for study in followup very difficult. Currently available animal models lack the depth and complexity needed to study the issue. For these reasons many of the rationales for care plans have been derived from observational data and work in related areas.

What does oral feeding with its progression over the first few years of life provide the child other than nutrients for somatic use? Although by no means comprehensive, Table 40–7 attempts to delineate some aspects that need to be addressed if an infant is alternatively nourished.

The foundation of the feeding behavior pattern of infants lies within the neuromotor complexes of the brain and CNS. Although the fetus demonstrates oral reflexes as early as seven weeks of gestation, the utilization of these reflexes and the physiopsychologic readiness for feeding are not well established until late gestation (35 to 36 weeks). Therefore, the integrity of neuromuscular function sets the stage for resultant psychosocial interactions.

Freud, Erikson, and Piaget all viewed feeding during infancy as more than the obtainment of nutritional substance. Erikson and Freud emphasized the importance of the experience in the infant's development of a sense of trust. If the infant's physical and emotional needs are met through sensitive care, a state of trust is created. Through this consistent associated sense of well-being, the infant acquires experiences with satisfaction and nonsatisfaction of his basic needs. Feeding leads to the emergence of interpersonal interactions. O'Grady[263] analyzed the reciprocity of feeding behavior and suggested five stages:

1. Prefeeding behavior. The level of arousal demonstrated by the infant, indicating hunger to others.

2. Approach behavior. The predominant physical mode of reaching out to food or showing readiness to eat.

3. Attachment behavior. Activities enacted during nipple engagement and nursing.

4. Consummatory behavior. Sucking and swallowing.

5. Satiety behavior. Acts that indicate saturation-completion. Successful completion and interpretation of these actions provide cues to the feeder. Failure to enact the feeding behaviors and, conversely or jointly, the failure of the reciprocal feeder-parent to react to the infant's behavior leads to inappropriate action and confusion on the part of the participants. This early recognition and re-enforcement of hunger, food, and social interaction is thus lacking in the environment of the TPN-fed child. It is possible to accept that the alteration of this competency might interfere with the development of other competencies.

Therefore, the social setting that is eliminated by providing nutrients with parenteral nutrition needs to be recreated. It is important that instead of focusing on the technologic equipment or other needs of the infant, the parent or nursing staff, or both, should set aside regular intervals when the infant enjoys an opportunity to (1) experience adult verbal and emotional attention; (2) discover colors, shapes, textures, smells, and if not contraindicated, tastes; (3) exercise with the fine- and gross-motor skills that are usually enacted in feeding (fingering and grasping of bottles, utensils, plates, and cups; and (4) recreate tongue action beyond that provided by non-nutritive sucking (pacifier).

The parents' roles need to be addressed and their contribution incorporated into actions that will provide positive interaction with the infant. Food is highly symbolic and frequently equated with love and caring in our culture. Moore describes eating as human and feeding as maternal; the mother's self-esteem is deeply involved.[264] Failure to accomplish the task of feeding the child brings into question the mother's basic competency in our society. Exclusive focus on mother-infant interaction is, however, too narrow. One must also address the mother-father-child family system,[265–268] the role of a formal and informal support system,[269–272] and finally, the role of the cultural-ethnic system.[273, 274] In addition to the disequilibrium initiated by the infant who is alternatively nourished (e.g., additional tasks associated with caregiving, modifications of schedules and activities, readjustment of the marital relationship), the infant is often at risk because of the sequelae of prematurity, which further increase familial stress in a number of ways.[275–278]

Table 40–7. ASPECTS OF ORAL FEEDING IN THE INFANT

FUNCTION	EFFECT
Psychosocial	Comfort and sense of satiety
	Primary behavioral re-enforcement
	Orientation to time
	Establishment of trust
	Social interaction skills
Oral stimulation	Progression of babbling to speech and language
Visual	Perceptual stimulation
Neuromuscular coordination	Gross and fine motor skills

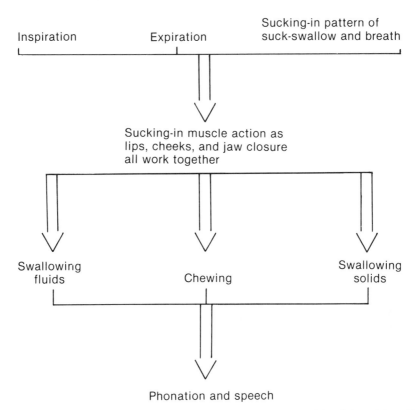

Figure 40–3. Interrelationship of oral motor activities to feeding and speech skills. (Adapted from Heiniger, M. C., and Randolph, S. L.: Muscle spindle and Golgi tendon organ: Stability against gravity. *In*: Neurophysiological Concepts in Human Behavior. St. Louis, C. V. Mosby Co., 1981.)

The development of speech is a complex process related to the maturation of cognitive and motor skills and can be substantially delayed by dysfunction in the oral motor area. Several components of the feeding process interrelate with the development of early speech attempts (Fig. 40–3). Before an infant can learn to speak, he or she must be capable of chewing, sucking, blowing, and swallowing. Babbling (prespeech) occurs around the same time as the development of self-feeding skills during late infancy.

"Neurophysiological studies indicate that the vestibular system is intimately connected with the propioceptive, visual and motor systems in the acquisition of developmental reflexes and postural control" (Table 40–8).[279, 280] Gross motor deficits reported in children on TPN may reflect the lack of sufficient experiences in these areas resulting from prolonged hospitalization and attachment to heavy equipment and its attendant limitation of mobility.[281] The social and emotional consequences of limited mobility should not be ignored. The emergence of self-produced locomotion has a role in the infant's sense of exploration and self-control.[283–284] It has been speculated that the onset of self-produced locomotion may facilitate the shift from the use of egocentric to allocentric frames of reference, especially between six and nine months of age.[284] Abercrombie argues that limitations of an individual's capacity to exhibit active movement may retard perceptual development because of a conflict in attentiveness to different stimuli.[285] Motor impediment thus can "increase dependency and decrease mastery motivation, resulting in a more passive individual and a greater difficulty in establishing independence from the caregiver."[286, 287]

A study of eight children who had received 75 per cent or more of their nutrition parenterally at home since infancy (average length five years), revealed perceptual-motor coordination problems, with a mean delay of 9.8 months. Deficits were also demonstrated in visual-spatial planning ability. Seven of the eight children showed delay in fine-motor coordination ranging from mild to severe. The same children demonstrated strength in verbal-conceptual skills, six of eight of the

Table 40–8. THE VESTIBULAR SYSTEM IN ASSOCIATION WITH DEVELOPMENTAL REFLEXES AND POSTURAL CONTROL

| NORMAL ORAL REFLEX | RETENTION BEYOND USUAL EXTINCTION | |
	Produces	*Interferes with*
Moro reflex	Total body responses to stimuli	Sitting balance, hand-to-mouth activities
Asymmetrical tonic neck reflex	Asymmetric postures	Sitting balance, hand-to-mouth activities
Hand grasp	Fisted hands; difficulty in opening hands	Holding utensils
Suckle-swallow	Sucking response to any oral stimuli	Taking food from spoon with lips, drinking from cup, chewing
Rooting	Asymmetric oral response to stimuli; head turning to oral stimuli	Maintaining head position for appropriate feeding
Gag	Increased oral sensitivity	*Hyperactive*—food pushed forward and out of mouth *Hypoactive*—food passively enters esophagus or trachea
Bite	Biting all objects placed in the mouth	Mouthing activities, ingesting food, more mature biting, chewing

(Adapted from Howard, R. B., and Herbold, N.: Nutrition in Clinical Care. New York, McGraw-Hill Co., 1978.)

children scored in the average range of intellectual functioning, and the other two children were considered "borderline." Thus, the delays were not necessarily linked with cognitive dysfunction. However, primary diagnoses, length, and number of hospitalization visits were not reported, making interpretation limited.[288]

The early formation of a child's body schema (the internal unconscious postural model of the body), may affect proper development of their body image (what an individual feels about one's body) and body concept (knowledge of body parts and their function).[289] This model is based on the tactile and proprioceptive input arising from the body as it interacts with the environment. Input also is acquired from social interactions with family and other people, thus affecting attitude, affect, and social perceptions. The totality is labeled body awareness. For example, in one report[290] children and adolescents who had been on ventilators for long periods of time (undefined) tended to incorporate their respirators into their body images, often having trouble accepting their actual bodies when they were disconnected from the equipment. Relatively few systematic studies have been done of the body-image problems of chronically ill or technology-dependent children.

Conflicting information has so far been garnered from studies in regard to body awareness.[291–295] However, one study offers some insight for the TPN-dependent child.[296] In that study, three groups of children were asked to make figures of people from soft plastic. One group was composed of children at home with spina bifida, the second group consisted of children living in an institution also with spina bifida, and the third group was composed of normal, nonhandicapped children living at home. The two groups living at home made similar figures. The institutionalized children made consistently smaller figures with many of them lacking one or more limbs. These findings are consistent with the perceptions by these children of themselves as "deformed" and insignificant persons. These observations are supportive of Garrard and Richmond's[297] findings that how the child's family handles and accepts the child's chronic illness or handicap is the most important determinant of his or her adaptation and social adjustment.

Parenterally-fed children also suffer from a deprivation of sensory stimuli. Through its organoleptic characteristics, food provides the child with a variety of stimuli, such as texture, color, aroma, flavor, and temperature. Odors that promote parasympathetic responses and suck-swallow motions are useful in an alternative feeding program. Steiner[298] found that term infants less than a day old relax their facial muscles, smile, and perform sucking and licking movements when presented with sweet smells (bananas and vanilla extract). Aversive disgustlike responses were seen in the presence of unpleasant odors-tastes (rotten eggs). He concluded that these were instinctive responses mediated through the limbic system to assist the individual in determining the ingestibility of substances. Evaluation of facial responses, muscle tone, spontaneous behavior, and verbal behavior should be documented in the therapeutic use of odors because of the variability in normal individual responses.[299]

Closely aligned with the sense of smell is the sense of taste, which includes sensations of sweet, sour, bitter, and salty. It is mediated over one of three cranial nerves, depending on the area of the tongue involved.[300] However, the experience of tasting food includes smell, taste, sight, temperature, touch, memory, and social milieu. The therapeutic use of sense intervention for this population offers promise as a preventative measure in early development.

Experimental studies are needed to enhance our understanding of the mechanisms influencing the senses and normal development. Growth in our knowledge should result in the development of tools that determine which intervention techniques are most effective in fostering the development of the alternatively-nourished infant or child.

EVALUATION

Psychometric tests as evaluation tools pose particularly serious problems for children lacking normal early experiences because of dependency on medical technology. Many problems with conventional tests result from assumptions of sensorimotor intelligence and cephalocaudal development.[301–304] The basic assumption is that intelligence among infants and toddlers is reflected through gross- and fine-motor actions. CNS maturation is believed to follow a cephalocaudal pattern, thus dictating the sequence of items on tests of neuromotor skills.[302, 303] Because these tests are standardized on normal children with intact capabilities, the results often yield lower estimates of intellectual functioning from children whose fine and gross motor skills and senses are delayed (Table 40–9). Alternatives have been designed that may be more appropriate for technology-dependent children.[305]

Utilization of evaluation results as predictors should be used reluctantly to avoid the possibility of a self-fulfilling prophecy.[306] Lindsley has stated: "Children are not retarded. Only their behavior in average environments is sometimes retarded. In fact, it is modern science's ability to design suitable environments for these children that is retarded."[307] Alternatively-nourished children should be challenged to actualize their fullest capability. The practices of parents and caretakers need to be directed to accommodate the infants' behaviors without establishing learned incompetence.[308]

Table 40–9. EXAMPLE OF CONVENTIONAL TEST WITH LIMITING VARIABLE

BAYLEY SCALE OF INFANT DEVELOPMENT (1969)	LIMITOR
Gross-and fine-motor items measured directly on motor skill—predictor for intellectual ability	Basis is that neuromotor normalcy is equivalent to normal intellectual function, thus poor neuromotor skills would indicate impaired intellectual ability
Mental scale—imitation items (emphasis 2 years old)	Requires motor facility of upper extremities
Mental scale—language comprehension items (2nd year)	Requires facility of upper extremities for unambiguous pointing
Language production as measure of intelligence	Used as dominant role in measurement from 3rd year forward, ability to talk (motor component required)
Requires compliance with examiner's verbal request	Does not take into account responses that indicate cognition without compliance

(Adapted from Zelazo, P.: Alternative assessment procedures for handicapped infants and toddlers: Theoretical and practical issues. *In* Bricker, D. D. (ed.): Intervention with At-Risk and Handicapped Infants. Baltimore, University Park Press, 1982.

REFERENCES

1. Lee, K. S.: Neonatal mortality: An analysis of the recent improvement in the United States. Am. J. Public Health, *70:*15, 1980.
2. The Costs and Effectiveness of Neonatal Intensive Care. Washington, D.C., U.S. Government Printing Office, 1981.
3. Klaus, M. H., and Fanaroff, A. A.: Care of the High Risk Neonate. Philadelphia, W. B. Saunders Co., 1979.
4. Heird, W. C.: Intravenous alimentation in pediatric patients. J. Pediatr., *80:*351, 1972.
5. Kennedy-Caldwell, C., and Caldwell, M. D.: Pediatric enteral nutrition. *In* J. Rombeau and M. Caldwell (eds.): Clinical Nutrition: Enteral and Tube Feeding. Philadelphia, W. B. Saunders Co., 1984.
6. Merritt, R. J., and Suskind, R. M.: Nutritional survey of hospitalized pediatric patients. Am. J. Clin. Nutr., *32:*1320, 1971.

7. Parson, H. G. et al.: The nutritional status of hospitalized children. Am. J. Clin. Nutr., 33:1140, 1980.
8. Cooper, A.: Nutritional assessment—An integral part of the pre-operative surgical evaluation. J. Pediatr. Surg., 16:554, 1981.
9. Mize, C.: Undernutrition of pediatric inpatients: Repeated nutrition status evaluation. Nutr. Support Serv., 4:27, 1984.
10. Faber, J. J., and Thornburg, K. L.: Placental Physiology. New York, Raven Press, 1983.
11. Sokoloff, L., Fitzgerald, G. G., and Kaufman, E. E.: Determinants of the availability of nutrients to the brain. In Wurtman, R. J., and Wurtman, J. J. (eds.): Nutrition and the Brain. New York, Raven Press, 1977.
12. Setchell, B. P., Bassett, J. M. et al.: The importance of glucose in the oxidative metabolism of the pregnant uterus and its contents in conscious sheep with some preliminary observation on the oxidation of fructose and glucose by fetal sheep. Q. J. Exp. Physiol., 57:257, 1972.
13. Simmons, M. A., Battaglia, F. C., and Meschia, G.: Placental transfer of glucose. J. Dev. Physiol., 1:243, 1979.
14. Tsoulos, N. G., Colwill, J. R. et al.: Comparison of glucose, fructose and oxygen uptakes by the fetuses of fed and starved ewes. Am. J. Physiol., 221:234, 1971.
15. Kalhan, S. C., D'Angelo, L. J. et al.: Glucose production in pregnant women at term gestation. J. Clin. Invest., 63:388, 1979.
16. Oakley, N. W., Beard, R. W., and Turner, R. C.: Effect of sustained maternal hyperglycemia on the fetus in normal and diabetic pregnancies. Br. Med. J., 1:466, 1972.
17. Morriss, F. H., Makowski, E. L. et al.: The glucose/oxygen quotient of the term human fetus. Biol. Neonate, 25:44, 1975.
18. Cordero, L., Yeh, S. Y. et al.: Hypertonic glucose infusion in labor. Am. J. Obstet. Gynecol., 107:295, 1970.
19. Oldendorf, W. H.: Brain uptake of radiolabeled amino acids, amines, hexoses after intercranial injection. Am. J. Physiol., 221:1629, 1971.
20. Dhopeshwarkar, G. A.: Nutrition and Brain Development. New York, Plenum Press, 1983.
21. Pardridge, W. M.: Brain metabolism: A perspective from the blood-brain barrier. Physiol. Rev., 63:1481, 1983.
22. Patel, A. J., and Balazs, R.: Effect of x-ray irradiation of the biochemical maturation of rat cerebellum: Metabolism of [14C] glucose and [14C] acetate. Radiat Res., 62:456, 1975.
23. Anderson, J. M., Milner, R. D. G., and Strich, S. J.: Effects of neonatal hypoglycemia on the nervous system: A pathological study. J. Neurol. Neurosurg. Psychiatry, 30:295, 1967.
24. Jones, E. L., and Smith, W. T.: Hypoglycemic brain damage in neonatal rat. Clin. Dev. Med., 39/40:231, 1971.
25. Brierley, J. B., Brown, A. W., and Mendrum, B. S.: The nature and time course of the neurological alterations resulting from oligamenia and hypoglycemia in the brain of Macacca mulata. Brain Res., 25:483, 1971.
26. Chase, P. H., Marlow, R. A. et al.: Hypoglycemia and brain development. Pediatrics, 52:513, 1973.
27. Gaull, G. E., Rassin, D. K. et al.: Milk protein quantity and quality in low-birth-weight infants.

III. Effects on sulfur amino acids in plasma and urine. J. Pediatr., 90:348, 1977.
28. Gaull, G. E., Sturman, J. A., and Raiha, N. C. R.: Development of mammalian sulfur metabolism. Absence of cystathionase in human fetal tissues. Pediatr. Res., 6:538, 1972.
29. Sturman, J. A., Gaull, G. E., and Raiha, N. C. R.: Absence of cystathionase in human fetal liver: Is cystine essential? Science, 169:74, 1970.
30. Pascal, T. A., Gillam, B. M., and Gaull, G. E.: Cystathionase: Immunochemical evidence for absence from human fetal liver. Pediatr. Res., 6:773, 1972.
31. Synderman, S. E., Boyer, A. et al.: The histidine requirement of the infant. Pediatrics, 31:786, 1963.
32. Synderman, S. E.: The protein and amino acid requirement of the premature infant. In Visser, M. K. A., and Travoelstra, J. A. (eds.): Metabolic Processes in the Fetus and Newborn Infant. Leiden, H. E. Stenfert Kroese, 1971.
33. Jacobsen, J. G., and Smith, L. M.: Biochemistry and physiology of taurine and taurine derivatives. Physiol. Rev., 48:425, 1968.
34. Sturman, J. A., Russin, K. D., and Gaull, G. E.: Taurine in development. Life Sci., 21:1, 1977.
35. Synderman, S. E.: Amino acid requirements. In Winter, R. W., and Hasselmeyer, E. G., (eds.): Intravenous Nutrition in the High Risk Neonate. New York, John Wiley & Sons, 1975.
36. Rose, W. C.: The amino acid requirements of man. XIII. The sparing effect of cystine on the methionine requirements. J. Biol. Chem., 216:763, 1955.
37. Pohlandt, E.: Cysteine: A semi-essential amino acid in the newborn infant. Acta Paediatr. Scand., 63:801, 1974.
38. Padridge, W. M.: In Wurtman, R. J., and Wurtman, J. J. (eds.): Nutrition and the Brain, Volume 1: Determinants of the Availability of Nutrients to the Brain. New York, Raven Press, 1977.
39. Proctor, R. A. W.: Paper on the first clinical description of kwashiorkor presented to the BMA International Conference. Kenya Med. J., 3:284, 1927.
40. Williams, C. D.: A nutritional disease of childhood associated with a maize diet. Arch. Dis. Child., 28:423, 1933.
41. Spies, T. D.: Influence of pregnancy, lactation, growth and aging on nutritional processes. J.A.M.A., 153:185 ,1953.
42. Gomez, F., Ramos Galvan, R., and Cranoto, J.: Nutritional recovery syndrome: Preliminary report. Pediatrics, 10:513, 1952.
43. Gomez, F., Ramos Galvan, R. et al.: Malnutrition in infancy and childhood with specific reference to kwashiorkor. Adv. Pediatr., 7:131, 1955.
44. Holt, L. E., Synderman, S. E. et al.: The plasma aminogram in kwashiorkor. Lancet, 2:1343, 1963.
45. Hadden, D. R.: Glucose, free fatty acid and insulin interrelations in kwashiorkor and Marasmus. Lancet, 2:589, 1967.
46. Smith, R.: Total body water in malnourished infants. Clin. Sci., 19:275, 1960.
47. Hadden, D. R., and Rutishauser, H. E.: Effect of human growth hormone in kwashiorkor and marasmus. Arch. Dis. Child., 42:9, 1967.
48. Tandon, B. N., Magotra, M. L. et al.: Small intestine in protein malnutrition. Am. J. Clin. Nutr., 21:813, 1968.
49. Dodge, P. R., Prensky, A. L., and Feigin, P. P.

(eds.): Protein-calorie malnutrition and somatic growth. *In* Nutrition and the Developing Nervous System. St. Louis, The C. V. Mosby Co., 1975.

50. Barry, L. W.: The effects of inanition in the pregnant albino rat, with special reference to the changes in the relative weights of the various parts, systems and organs of the offspring. Carnegie Inst. Contr. Embryol., *11*:91, 1920.

51. Widdowson, E. M.: Effects of premature and dysmaturity in animals. *In* Jonxis, J. H. P., Visser, H. K. A., and Troelstra, J. A. (eds.): Nutrica Symposium: Aspects of Praematurity and Dysmaturity. Springfield, Illinois, Charles C Thomas, 1968.

52. Zeman, F. J., and Stanbrough, E. C.: Effects of maternal protein deficiency on cellular development in the fetal rat. J. Nutr., *99*:274, 1969.

53. Chanez-Bel, C., Priam, M., Hamon, A. et al.: Neurotransmitters in early life and in intrauterine growth retardation. *In* Intensive Care in the Newborn. III. New York, Masson Publishing, 1981.

54. Morgane, P. J., Miller, M., Kemper, T. et al.: The effects of protein malnutrition on the developing central nervous system in the rat. Neurosci. Biobehav. Rev., 2:137, 1978.

55. Zamenhof, S., von Marthens, E., and Margolis, F. L.: DNA (cell number) and protein in neonatal brain: Alterations by maternal dietary protein restriction. Science, *160*:322, 1968.

56. Zamenhof, S., van Marthens, E., and Grauel, L.: DNA cell number and protein in rat brain: Second generation (F_2) alterations by maternal (F_0) dietary protein restriction. Nutr. Metab., *14*:262, 1972.

57. Zamenhof, S., Hall, S. M., Grauel, L. et al.: Deprivation of amino acids and prenatal brain development in rats. J. Nutr., *104*:1002, 1974.

58. Zeman, F. J., and Stanbrough, E. L.: Effects of maternal protein deficiency on cellular development of fetal rat. J. Nutr., *99*:274, 1969.

59. Zeman, F. J.: Effect of protein deficiency during gestation on postnatal cellular development in young rat. J. Nutr., *100*:530, 1970.

60. Dobbing, J., and Sands, J.: Vulnerability of developing brain not explained by cell number/cell size hypothesis. Early Hum. Dev., 5:227, 1981.

61. Bedi, K. S., Hall, R. et al.: A stereological analysis of the cerebellar granule and Purkinje cells of 30-day old and adult rats undernourished during early postnatal life. J. Comp. Neurol., *193*:863, 1980.

62. Sands, J., Dobbing, J., and Gratrix, C. A.: Cell number and cell size: Organ growth and development and the control of catch-up growth in rats. Lancet, 2:309, 1979.

63. Smart, J. L., and Dobbing, J.: Increased thirst and hunger in adult rats undernourished as infants: An alternative explanation. Br. J. Nutr., 37:421, 1977.

64. Smart, J. L., Tricklebank, M. D. et al.: Nutritionally small-for-dates rats: Their subsequent growth, regional brain 5-hydroxytryptamine turnover and behavior. Pediatr. Res., 10:807, 1976.

65. Adlard, B. P., and Dobbing, J.: Maze learning by adult rats after inhibition of neuronal multiplication in utero. Pediatr. Res., 9:139, 1975.

66. Smart, J. L., Adlard, B. P., and Dobbing, J.: Further studies of body growth and brain development in "small-for-date" rats. Biol. Neonate, 3:135, 1974.

67. Lynch, A., Smart, J. L., and Dobbing, J.: Motor coordination and cerebellar size in adult rats undernourished in early life. Brain Res., 83:249, 1975.

68. Dobbing, J.: The later development of the brain and its vulnerability. *In* Davis, J. A., and Dobbing, J. (eds.): Scientific Foundations of Paediatrics. London, Heinemann, 1981.

69. Smart, J. L., Dobbing, J. et al.: Vulnerability of developing brain: Relative effects of growth restriction during the fetal and suckling periods on behavior and brain composition of adult rats. J. Nutr., *103*:1327, 1973.

70. Dobbing, J.: Vulnerable periods of brain development. Lipids, Malnutrition and the Developing Brain. Amsterdam, Ciba Foundation Symposium, 1971, page 9.

71. Dobbing, J.: Nutrition and the developing brain. Lancet, *1*(793):48, 1973.

72. Adlard, B. P., and Dobbing, J.: Vulnerability of developing brain. V. Effects of fetal and postnatal undernutrition on regional brain enzyme activities in three-week-old rats. Pediatr. Res., *6*(1):38, 1972.

73. Adlard, B. P., and Dobbing, J.: Vulnerability of developing brain. VIII. Regional acetylcholinesterase activity in the brains of adult rats undernourished in early life. Br. J. Nutr., *28*(1):139, 1972.

74. Dobbing, J., and Sands, J.: Vulnerability of developing brain. IX. The effect of nutritional growth retardation on the timing of brain growth-spurt. Biol. Neonate, *19*(4):363, 1971.

75. Smart, J. L., and Dobbing, J.: Vulnerability of developing brain. VI. Relative effects of foetal and early postnatal undernutrition on reflux ontogeny and development of behaviour in the rat. Brain Res., *33*(2):303, 1971.

76. Dobbing, J., and Hopewell, J. W.: Permanent deficit of neurons in cerebral and cerebellar cortex following early mild nutrition. Arch. Dis. Child., *46*(249):736, 1971.

77. Dobbing, J., Hopewell, J. W., and Lynch, A.: Vulnerability of developing brain. VII. Permanent deficit of neurons in cerebral and cerebellar cortex following early mild nutrition. Exp. Neurol., *32*(3), 1971.

78. Adlard, B. P., and Dobbing, J.: Vulnerability of developing brain. III. Development of four enzymes in the brains of normal and undernourished rats. Brain Res., *28*(1):97, 1971.

79. Smart, J. L., and Dobbing, J.: Vulnerability of developing brain. II. Effects of early nutritional deprivation on reflex ontogeny and development of behaviour in the rat. Brain Res., *28*(1):85, 1971.

80. Dobbing, J., and Widdowson, E. M.: The effect of undernutrition and subsequent rehabilitation on myelination of rat brain as measured by its composition. Brain, *88*(2):357, 1965.

81. Dobbing, J., and Sands, J.: Vulnerability of developing brain not explained by cell number/cell size hypothesis. Early Hum. Dev., 5:227, 1981.

82. Katz, H. B., and Davis, C. A.: The effects of early life undernutrition and subsequent environment on morphological parameters of the rat brain. Behav. Brain Res., 5:53, 1982.

83. Katz, H. B., Davis, C. A., and Dobbing, J.: Effects of undernutrition at different ages early in life

and later environmental complexity on parameters of the cerebrum and hippocampus in rats. J. Nutr., 112:1362, 1982.

84. Cohen, E. L., and Wurtman, R. J.: Brain acetylcholine: Control by dietary choline. Science, 191:561, 1976.

85. Cohen, E. L., and Wurtman, R. J.: Nutrition and brain neurotransmitters. In Winick, M. (ed.): Pre- and Post-natal Development. New York, Plenum Press, 1979.

86. Winick, M.: Nutrition and nerve cell growth. Fed. Proc., 29:1510, 1970.

87. Winick, M.: Malnutrition and Brain Development. London, Oxford Press, 1976.

88. Winick, M., and Noble, A.: Cellular responses in the rat during malnutrition at various ages. J. Nutr., 89:300, 1966.

89. Winick, M., and Rosso, P.: Effects of severe early malnutrition on cellular growth of human brain. Pediatr. Res., 3:181, 1969.

90. Winick, M., and Biasel, J. A., Rosso, P.: Nutrition and cell growth. In Nutrition and Development. Vol. 1. Current Concepts in Nutrition. New York, John Wiley & Sons, 1972.

91. Winick, M., Rosso, P., Brasel, J. A.: Malnutrition and cellular growth in the brain; Existence of critical periods. In Elliot, K., and Knight, J. (eds.): Lipids, Malnutrition and the Developing Brain. Amsterdam, Elsevier, 1972.

92. Duckett, S., and Winick, M.: Malnutrition and brain dysfunction. In Black, P. (ed.): Brain Dysfunction in Children: Etiology, Diagnosis and Management. New York, Raven Press, 1981.

93. Anderson, G. H.: Diet, Neurotransmitters and brain function. Br. Med. Bull., 37(1):95, 1981.

94. Wurtman, R. J., and Fernstrom, J. D.: Control of brain monoamine synthesis by diet and plasma amino acids. Am. J. Clin. Nutr., 28:638, 1975.

95. Wurtman, R. J.: In Garattini, S., and Saminin, R. (eds.): Central Mechanisms of Anorectic Drugs. New York, Raven Press, 1978.

96. Hess, S. M., and Doepfner, W.: Behavioral effects and brain amine content in rats. Arch. Int. Pharmacodyn. Ther., 134:89, 1961.

97. Ashcroft, G. W., Eccelston, P., and Crawford, T. B.: 5-Hydroxyindole metbolism in rat brain. A study of intermediate metabolism using the technique of tryptophan loading. I. Methods. J. Neurochem., 12:483, 1965.

98. Fernstrom, J. D., and Wurtman, R. J.: Effect of chronic corn consumption on serotonin content of rat brain. Nature (New. Biol.), 234:62, 1971.

99. Fernstrom, J. D., and Wurtman, R. J.: Brain serotonin content: Physiological dependence on plasma tryptophan levels. Science, 173:149, 1971.

100. Fernstrom, J. D., and Wurtman, R. J.: Brain serotonin content: Increase following ingestion of carbohydrate diet. Science, 174:1023, 1971.

101. Wurtman, R. J., Larin, F., Mostafapour, S. et al.: Brain catechol synthesis: Control by brain tyrosine concentration. Science, 185:183, 1974.

102. Gibson, C. J., and Wurtman, R. J.: Physiological control of brain norepinephrine synthesis by brain tyrosine concentration. Life Sic., 22:1399, 1978.

103. Fernstrom, J. D., Larin, F., and Wurtman, R. J.: Correlations between brain tryptophan and plasma neutral amino acid levels following food consumption in the rat. Life Sci., 13:517, 1973.

104. McMenamy, R. H., and Oncley, J. L.: Specific binding of tryptothan to serum albumin. J. Biol. Chem., 223:1436, 1958.

105. Fernstrom, J. D., and Faller, D. V.: J. Neurochem., 30:1531, 1978.

106. Schwartz, J. C., Lampart, C., and Rose, C.: Properties and regional distribution of histidine decarboxylase in rat brain. J. Neurochem., 17:1527, 1970.

107. Schwartz, J. C., Lampart, C., and Rose, C.: Histamine formation in rat brain in vivo: Effects of histidine loads. J. Neurochem., 19:801, 1972.

108. Enwonwu, C. O., and Worthington, B. S.: Concentrations of histamine in brain of guinea pig and rat during dietary protein malnutrition. Biochem. J., 144:601, 1974.

109. Maher, T. J., and Wurtman, R. J.: L-Threonine administration increases glycine concentrations in the rat central nervous system. Life Sci., 26:1283, 1980.

110. Blundell, J. E.: Is there a role for serotonin (5-hydroxytryptamine) in feeding? Int. J. Obes., 1:15, 1977.

111. Anderson, G. H.: Control of protein and energy intake: Role of plasma amino acids and brain neurotransmitters. Can. J. Physiol. Pharmacol., 57:1043, 1979.

112. Southwell, P. R., Evans, C. R., and Hunt, J. N.: Effect of a hot milk drink on movements during sleep. Br. Med. J., 2:429, 1972.

113. Hartmann, E.: L-Tryptophan: A rational hypnotic with clinical potential. Am. J. Psychiatr., 134:366, 1977.

114. Brezinova, V., and Oswald, I.: Sleep after a bedtime beverage. Br. Med. J., 2:431, 1972.

115. Hope, D. B.: Studies of taurine and cystathionine in brain. Proc. Int. Congr. Biochem. 13:63, 1958.

116. Jacobsen, J. G., and Smith, L. H.: Biochemistry and physiology of taurine and taurine derivatives. Physiol. Rev. 48:424, 1968.

117. Agrawal, H. C., Davison, A. N., and Kaczmarek, L. K.: Subcellular distribution of taurine and cysteine sulphinate decarboxylase in developing rat brain. Biochem. J., 122:759, 1971.

118. Stegink, L. D., and Baker, G. L.: Infusion of protein hydrolysates in the newborn infant: Plasma amino acid concentrations. J. Pediatr., 78:595, 1971.

119. Gaull, G., Sturman, J. A., and Raiha, N. C. R.: Development of mammalian sulfur metabolism: Absence of cystathionase in human fetal tissues. Pediatr. Res., 6:538, 1972.

120. Pascal, T. A., Gillam, B. M., and Gaull, G. E.: Cystathionase: Immunochemical evidence for absence from human fetal liver. Pediatr. Res., 6:773, 1972.

121. Wei, P., Hamilton, J. R., and LeBlanc, A. E.: A clinical and metabolic study of intravenous feeding technique using peripheral veins as the initial infusion site. Can. Med. Assoc. J., 106:969, 1972.

122. Gaull, G. E., Raiha, N. C. R. et al.: Transfer of cyst(e)ine and methionine across the human placenta. Pediatr. Res., 7:908, 1973.

123. Gaull, G. E., VonBerg, W. et al.: Development of methyltransferase activities of human fetal tissue. Pediatr. Res., 7:527, 1978.

124. Pohlandt, F.: Cystine: A semi-essential amino acid in the newborn infant. Acta Paediatr. Scand., 63:801, 1974.

125. Hayes, K. C., Carey, R. C., and Schmidt, S. Y.: Retinol degeneration associated with taurine deficiency in the cat. Science, *188*:949, 1975.

126. Sturman, J. A., and Gaull, G. E.: Taurine in the brain and liver of the developing human and monkey. J. Neurochem., *25*:831, 1975.

127. Baskin, S. I., Leibman, A. J., and Cohn, E. M.: Possible functions of taurine in the central nervous system. Adv. Biochem. Psychopharm., *15*:153, 1976.

128. Sturman, J. A., Rassin, D. K., and Gaull, G. E.: Taurine in developing rat brain: Transfer of [³⁵S] taurine to pups via the milk. Pediatr. Res., *11*:28, 1977.

129. Sturman, J. A., Rassin, D. K., Hayes, K. C., et al.: Taurine deficiency in the kitten: Exchange and turnover of [³⁵S] taurine in brain, retina and other tissues. J. Nutr., *108*:1462, 1978.

130. Zlotkin, S. H., Bryan, M. H., and Anderson, G. H.: Cysteine supplementation to cysteine-free intravenous feeding regimens in newborn infants. Am. J. Clin. Nutr., *34*:914, 1981.

131. Batta, A. K., Salen, G., Shefer, S. et al.: The effect of taurous odeoxycholic acid and taurine supplementation on biliary bile acid composition. Hepatology, *2*:811, 1982.

132. Geggel, H. S., Ament, M. E. et al.: Evidence that taurine is an essential amino acid in children receiving total parenteral nutrition. Clin. Res., *30*:486A, 1982.

133. Malloy, M. H., Rassin, D. K. et al.: Cyst(e)ine measurements during total parenteral nutrition. Am. J. Clin. Nutr., *37*:188, 1983.

134. Jarvenpaa, A. L., Raiha, N. C. R. et al.: Feeding the low birth weight infant. I. Taurine and cholesterol supplementation formula does not affect growth and metabolism. Pediatrics, *71*:171, 1983.

135. Rassin, D. K., Gaull, G. E. et al.: Feeding the low birth weight infant. II. Effect of taurine and cholesterol supplementation on amino acids and cholesterol. Pediatrics *71*:179, 1983.

136. Jarvenpaa, A. L., Rassin, D. K. et al.: Feeding the low birth weight infant. III. Diet influences bile acid metabolism. Pediatrics, *72*:677, 1983.

137. Jarvenpaa, A. L.: Feeding the low birth weight infant. IV. Fat absorption as a function of diet and duodenal bile acids. Pediatrics, *72*:684, 1983.

138. Watkins, J. B., Jarvenpaa, A. L., Van Leevrren, P. S. et al.: Feeding the low birth weight infant. V. Effects of taurine, cholesterol and human milk on bile acid kinetics. Gastroenterology, *85*:793, 1983.

139. Okamoto, E., Rassin, D. K. et al.: Role of taurine in feeding the low birth weight infant. J. Pediatr., *104*:936, 1984.

140. Sturman, J. A., Wen, G. Y. et al.: Retinal degeneration in primates raised on a synthetic human formula. Int. J. Dev. Sci., in press.

141. Rose, W. C., and Wixom, R. L.: Amino acid requirements of man; sparing effect of tyrosine on phenylalanine requirement. J. Biol. Chem., *216*:95, 1955.

142. Tallan, H. H., Moore, S., and Stein, W. H.: L-Cystathionine in human brain. J. Biol. Chem., *230*:707, 1958.

143. Brenton, D. P., Cusworth, D. C., and Gaull, G. E.: Homocystinuria—biochemical studies of tissues including a comparison with cystathioninuria. Pediatrics, *35*:50, 1965.

144. Poley, J. R., Dower, J. C. et al.: Bile acids in infants and children. J. Lab. Clin. Med., *25*:831, 1975.

145. Sieghart, W., and Karobath, M.: Evidence for specific synaptosomal localization of exogenous accumulated taurine. J. Neurochem., *23*:911, 1974.

146. Jasper, H. H., and Koyama, I.: Rate of release of amino acids from the cerebral cortex in the cat as affected by brain stem and thalamic stimulation. J. Physiol. (London), *47*:889, 1969.

147. Oja, S. S., and Lahdesmaki, P.: Is taurine an inhibitory neurotransmitter? Med. Biol., *52*:138, 1974.

148. Crawford, J. M.: The effect upon mice of intraventricular injection of excitant and depressant amino acids. Biochem. Pharmacol., *12*:1443, 1963.

149. Purpura, D. P., Girado, M. et al.: Structure activity determinants of pharmacological effects of amino acids and related compounds on central synapses. J. Neurochem., *5*:238, 1959.

150. Holsi, L., Holsi, E. et al.: Amino acid transmitters—action and uptake in neurons and glial cells of humans and rat CNS tissue culture. Golgi Cent. Symp. Proc. 473, 1975.

151. Kaczmarek, L. K., and Adey, W. R.: Factors affecting the release of [¹⁴C] taurine from cat brain: The electrical effects of taurine on normal and seizure prone cortex. Brain Res., *76*:83, 1974.

152. Hayashi, T.: Comments on the excitine-inhibitine hypothesis. *In* Florey, E. (ed.): Proceedings of the Second Frie Harbor Symposium, pages 378–385.

153. Read, W. O., and Welty, J. D.: Effect of taurine on epinephrine and digoxin induced irregularities of the dog heart. J. Pharmacol. Exp. Ther., *139*:283, 1963.

154. Robert, J., and Modell, W.: Phamacologic evidence for the importance of catecholamines in cardiac rhythmicity. Circ. Res., *9*:171, 1961.

155. Gaull, G. E., Rassin, D. K. et al.: Milk protein quantity and quality in low birth weight infants. III. Effects on sulfur amino acids in plasma and urine. J. Pediatr., *90*:348, 1977.

156. Jarvenpaa, A. L., Rassin, D. K. et al.: Milk protein quantity and quality in the term infant. II. Effects of acidic and neutral amino acids. Pediatrics, *70*:221, 1982.

157. Widdowson, E. M.: Growth and composition of the fetus and newborn. *In* Assali, N. S. (ed.): Biology of Gestation. Vol. 2. New York, Academic Press, 1968.

158. Avery, G. B.: Neonatology. Philadelphia, J. B. Lippincott Co., 1979.

159. Hurley, L. S.: Developmental Nutrition. Englewood Cliffs, Prentice-Hall, 1980.

160. Dickerson, J. W. T.: Nutrition, brain growth and development. *In* Clinics in Developmental Medicine. Maturation and Development: Biological and Psychological Perspectives. Philadelphia, J. B. Lippincott Co., 1981.

161. Chase, H. P.: Undernutrition and growth and development of the human brain. *In* Lloyd-Grill, J. (ed.): Malnutrition and Intellectual Development. Lancaster, M.T.P., 1976.

162. Davison, A. N., and Dobbing, J.: Myelination as a vulnerable period in brain development. Br. Med. Bull., *22*:40, 1966.

163. McKenna, M. C., and Capagnoni, A. T.: Effect of pre- and post-natal essential fatty acid deficiency on brain development and myelination. J. Nutr., *109*:1195, 1979.

164. Galli, G.: Effects of essential fatty acid deficiency and various subcellular structures in rat brain. J. Neurochem., *19*:1863, 1972.

165. Biran, L. A.: Studies on essential fatty acid deficiency. Effect of the deficiency on the lipids in various rat tissues and the influence of dietary supplementation with essential fatty acids on deficient rats. Biochem. J., 93:492, 1964.

166. Rathbone, L.: The effect of diet as the fatty acid compositions of serum, brain, brain mitochondria and myelin in the rat. Biochem. J., 97:620, 1965.

167. Caldwell, D. F., and Churchill, J. A.: Learning impairment in rats administered a lipid free diet during pregnancy. Psychol. Rep., 19:99, 1966.

168. Walker, B.: Recovery of rat tissue lipids from essential fatty acid deficiency: Brain, heart and testes. J. Nutr., 94:469, 1968.

169. Peifer, J. S.: Effects of minimal intakes of specific polyenoic acids on brain lipids, development and behavior of rats. Fed. Proc., 19:495, A(1410), 1970.

170. Galli, C., White, H. B., and Paoletti, R.: Lipid alterations and their reversion in the central nervous system of growing rats deficient in essential fatty acids. Lipids, 6:378, 1971.

171. White, H. B., Galli, C., and Paoletti, R.: Brain recovery from essential fatty acid deficiency in developing rats. J. Neurochem., 18:869, 1971.

172. Galli, C., Trzeciak, H. I., and Paoletti, R.: Effects of essential fatty acid deficiency on myelin and various subcellular structures in rat brain. J. Neurochem., 19:1863, 1972.

173. Sun, G. Y.: Effects of a fatty acid deficiency on lipids of whole brain microsomes and myelin in the rat. J. Lipid Res., 13:56, 1972.

174. Svennerbol, M. L.: Effects on offspring of maternal malnutrition in the rat. In Lipids, Malnutrition and the Developing Nervous System. Ciba Foundation, Amsterdam, Elsevier, 1972.

175. Seifter, E., and Rettura, G.: Enhanced brain maturation due to cholesterol feeding. J. Nutr., 103:A14, 1973.

176. Sinclair, A. J., and Crawford, M. A.: The effect of a low fat diet on neonatal rats. Br. J. Nutr., 29:127, 1973.

177. Sun, G. Y., Go, J., and Sun, A. Y.: Induction of essential fatty acid deficiency in mouse brain: Effects of fat deficient diet upon acyl group composition of myelin and synaptosome-rich fractions during development and maturation. Lipids, 9:450, 1974.

178. Hornstra, G., Haddenman, E., and Ten Hoor, F.: Fish oils, prostaglandins, and arterial thrombosis. Lancet, 2:1080, 1979.

179. Needleman, P.: Triene prostaglandins: Prostacyclin and thromboxane biosynthesis and unique biological properties. Proc. Natl. Acad. Sci., 76:944, 1979.

180. Mead, J. F., and Fulco, J. F.: The Unsaturated and Polyunsaturated Fatty Acids in Health and Disease. Springfield, Illinois, Charles C Thomas, 1976.

181. Holman, R. T.: Nutritional and metabolic interrelationships between fatty acids. Proc. Fed. Am. Soc. Exp. Biol., 23:1062, 1964.

182. Hwang, D. H., and Carroll, A. E.: Decreased formation of prostaglandins derived from arachidonic acid by dietary linolenate in rats. Am. J. Clin. Nutr., 33:590, 1980.

183. Dhopeshwarkar, G. A., and Mead, J. F.: Age and lipids of the CNS: Lipid metabolism in the developing brain. In Brody, H. et al. (eds.): Aging,

Vol. 1. Clinical, Morphologic and Neurochemical Aspects in the Aging CNS. New York, Raven Press, 1975.

184. Svennerhold, L.: Distribution and fatty acid composition of phosphoglycerides in normal human brain. J. Lipid Res., 9:570, 1968.

185. Anderson, R. E.: Lipids of ocular tissues. IV. Comparison of the phospholipids from the retina of six mammalian species. Exp. Eye Res., 10:339, 1970.

186. Cotman, C.: Lipid composition of synaptic plasma membranes isolated from rat brain by zonal centriguation. Biochemistry, 8:4606, 1969.

187. Anderson, R. E. et al.: Polyunsaturated fatty acids of photoreceptor membranes. Exp. Eye Res., 18:205, 1974.

188. Holman, R. T., Johnson, S. B., and Hutch, T. F.: A case of human linolenic acid deficiency including neurological abnormalities. Am. J. Clin. Nutr., 35:617, 1982.

189. Warshaw, J. B., and Maniscalco, W. M.: Perinatal adaptations in carbohydrate and lipid metabolism. In Stern, L., Oh, W., and Friss-Hansen, B. (eds.): Intensive Care of the Newborn. II. New York, Masson Publishing Inc., 1978.

190. Borum, P. R.: Variation in tissue carnitine concentration with age and sex in the rat. Biochem. J., 176:677, 1978.

191. Battistella, P. A.: Tissue levels of carnitine in human growth. In Berra, B. and DiDonato, S. (eds.): Perspectives in Inherited Metabolic Diseases. Milan, Italy, Edi. Ermes, 1980.

192. Borum, P. R.: Role of carnitine in fat metabolism of the neonate. In Filer, L. J., and Leathem, W. D. (eds.): Parenteral Nutrition in the Infant Patient. Chicago, Abbott Laboratories, 1983.

193. Rebouche, J., and Engel, A. G.: Tissue distribution of carnitine biosynthesis enzymes in man. Biochem. Biophys. Acta, 630:22, 1980.

194. Schiff, D.: Plasma carnitine levels during intravenous feeding of the neonate. J. Pediatr., 95:1043, 1979.

195. Penn, D.: Carnitine deficiency in premature infants receiving total parenteral nutrition. Early Hum. Dev., 4:23, 1980.

196. Penn, D.: Decreased carnitine concentrations in newborn infants receiving total parenteral nutrition. J. Pediatr., 98:976, 1981.

197. Malone, J. L.: Vitamin passage across the placenta. Clin. Perinatol., 2:295, 1975.

198. Mino, M., and Nishmo, H.: Fetal and maternal relationship in serum vitamin E level. J. Nutr. Sci. Vitaminol., 19:475, 1973.

199. Orzalezi, M., and Colansi, P.: Critical vitamins for low birth weight infants. Acta Paediatr. Scand. [Suppl.], 296:105, 1982.

200. Foundation for Child Development: Villee, C. A. (ed.): The Placenta and Fetal Membranes. New York, Williams & Wilkins, 1960.

201. Anderson, G. H.: Diet, neurotransmitters and brain function. Br. Med. Bull., 37(1):95, 1981.

202. American Medical Association: Guidelines for Multivitamin Preparation for Parenteral Use. Nutrition Advisory Group. Department of Foods and Nutrition, American Medical Association, Chicago, 1975.

203. Zenk, K. E., Huxtable, R. F., and Dunaway, D.: Advisable daily vitamin intake for preterm infants [letter]. J.P.E.N., 5(5):447, 1981.

204. Ostrea, E. M., Greene, C. D., and Bahen, J. E.:

Decomposition of TPN solutions exposed to phototherapy. J. Pediatr., *100*:670, 1982.

205. Bhatia, J., Steglink, L. D., and Ziegler, E. S.: Riboflavin enhances photo-oxidation of amino acids under simulated clinical condition. J.P.E.N., 7(3):277, 1983.

206. Chen, M. F., Boyce, H. W., and Triplett, L.: Stability of the B vitamins in mixed parenteral solution. J.P.E.N., 7(5):462, 1983.

207. Shenai, J. P., Borum, P. R., and Duke, E. A.: Delivery of vitamins E and C from parenteral alimentation solution. J. Pediatr. Gastroenterol., *1*:537, 1982.

208. Hartline, J. V., and Zachman, R. D.: Vitamin A delivery in total parenteral nutrition solutions. Pediatrics, *58*(3):448, 1976.

209. McKenna, M. C., and Bieri, J. G.: Loss of vitamin A from TPN solutions. Fed. Proc., *39*:561, 1980.

210. Howard, L., Chu, R. et al.: Vitamin A deficiency from long-term parenteral nutrition. Ann. Intern. Med., *93*(4):576, 1980.

211. Shenai, J. P., Stahlman, M. T., and Chytil, F.: Vitamin A delivery from parenteral alimentation solutions. J. Pediatr., *99*:661, 1981.

212. Riggle, M. A., Brandt, R. B., and Mueller, D. G.: Letter to the editor. J. Pediatr., *100*:670, 1982.

213. Gillis, J., Jones, G. et al.: Delivery of vitamins A, D, and E in total parenteral solutions. J.P.E.N., 7:11, 1983.

214. Burch, H. S., Lowry, O. H. et al.: Effect of riboflavin deficiency and realimentation of flavin enzymes of tissues. J. Biol. Chem., *223*:29, 1956.

215. Mann, G. V., Watson, P. L. et al.: Primate nutrition. II. Riboflavin deficiency in cerbus monkey and its diagnosis. J. Nutr., *47*:225, 1952.

216. Tiselius, H. G.: Metabolism of tritum labeled pyridoxe and pyridoxine-5¹-phosphate in the central nervous system. J. Neurochem., *20*:937, 1973.

217. Awapara, J., Landua, A. J. et al.: Free γ-aminobutyric acid in brain. J. Biol. Chem., *187*:35, 1950.

218. Roberts, E., and Frankel, S.: γ-Aminobutyric acid in brain: Its formation from glutamic acid. J. Biol. Chem., *187*:55, 1950.

219. Kutz, D. J., Lery, H., and Kanfer, J. N.: Cerebral lipids and amino acids in vitamin B_6 deficient suckling rats. J. Nutr., *102*:291, 1972.

220. Tews, J. K.: Pyridoxine deficiency and brain amino acids. *In* Kelsall, M. A. (ed.): Vitamin B_6 in Metabolism of the Nervous System. Ann. N.Y. Acad. Sci., *166*:74, 1969.

221. Higgins, E. S.: The effects of ethanol on GABA content of rat brain. Biochem. Pharmacol., *11*:394, 1962.

222. McKhann, G. M., Mickelson, O., and Tower, D. B.: Oxidative metabolism of incubated cerebral slices from pyridoxine-deficient kittens. Am. J. Physiol., *200*:34, 1961.

223. Massieu, G. H., Ortega, B. G. et al.: Free amino acids in brain and liver of deoxypyridoxine-treated mice subject to insulin shock. J. Neurochem., *9*:143, 1962.

224. Perez De La Mora, M., Feira-Velasco, A., and Tupia, R.: Pyridoxal phosphate and glutamate decarboxylase in subcellular particles of mouse brain and their relationship to convulsions. J. Neurochem., *20*:1575, 1973.

225. Alton-Mackey, M. G., and Walker, B. L.: Graded levels of pyridoxine in the rat diet during gestation and the physical and neuromotor development of offspring. Am. J. Clin. Nutr., *26*:420, 1973.

226. Bayoumi, R. A., and Smith, W. R. D.: Some effects of dietary B_6 deficiency on γ-aminobutyric acid metabolism in developing rat brain. J. Neurochem., *19*:1883, 1972.

227. Baxter, C. F., and Roberts, E.: The γ-aminobutyric acid-alpha-ketoglutaric acid transaminase of beef brain. J. Biochem., *233*:1135, 1958.

228. Synderman, S. E., Holdt, L. E. et al.: Pyridoxine deficiency in the human infant. J. Clin. Nutr., *1*:200, 1953.

229. Tomarrelli, R. M., Linden, E., and Bernhart, F. W.: Nutritional quality of milk thermally modified to reduce allergic reaction. Pediatrics, *9*:89, 1952.

230. Coursin, D. B.: Convulsive seizures in infants with pyridoxine-deficient diet. J.A.M.A., *154*:406, 1954.

231. Moloney, C. J., and Parmalee, A. H.: Convulsions in young infants as a result of pyridoxine (vitamin B_6) deficiency. J.A.M.A., *154*:405, 1954.

232. Shenai, J. P., Chytil, F. et al.: Plasma vitamin A and retinol-binding protein in premature and term neonates. J. Pediatr., *99*:302, 1981.

233. Brandt, R. B., Mueller, D. G. et al.: Serum vitamin A in premature and term neonates. J. Pediatr., *92*:101, 1978.

234. Bernhardt, I. B., and Dorsey, D. J.: Hypervitaminosis A and congenital renal anomalies in a human infant. Obstet. Gynecol., *43*:750, 1974.

235. Cohlan, S. Q.: Excessive intake of vitamin A as a cause of congenital anomalies in the rat. Science, *117*:535, 1953.

236. Morriss, G. M.: Morphogenesis of the malformation induced in rat embryos by maternal hypervitaminosis Am. J. Anat., *113*:241, 1972.

237. Wilson, J. G., Roth, C. B., and Warkany, J.: An analysis in the syndrome of malformations induced by maternal vitamin A deficiency. Effects of restoration of vitamin A at various times during gestation. Am. J. Anat., *92*:189, 1953.

238. Butcher, R. E., Brunne, R. L. et al.: A learning impairment associated with maternal hypervitaminosis A in rats. Life Sci., *11*:141, 1972.

239. Hutchings, D. E., Gibbon, J., and Kaufman, M. A.: Maternal vitamin A excess during the early fetal period: Effects on learning and development in the offspring. Dev. Psychobiol., *6*:445, 1973.

240. Keating, J. P., and Feigin, R. D.: Increased intracranial pressure associated with probable vitamin A deficiency in cystic fibrosis. Pediatrics, *46*:41, 1970.

241. Mellanby, E.: Skeletal changes affecting the nervous system produced in young dogs by diets deficient in vitamin A. J. Physiol., *99*:467, 1941.

242. Howell, J. M., and Thompson, J. N.: Lesions associated with the development of ataxia in chicks. Br. J. Nutr., *21*:741, 1967.

243. Wolbach, S. B., and Hegstead, D. M.: Vitamin A deficiency in the chick. Arch. Pathol., *54*:13, 1952.

244. Millen, J. W., Woollam, O. H. M., and Lamming, G. E.: Congenital hydrocephalus due to experimental hypovitaminosis A. Lancet, *2*:679, 1954.

245. Dodge, P. R., Prensky, A. L., and Feigin, R. D.: Nutrition and the Developing Nervous System. St. Louis, The C. V. Mosby Co., 1975.

246. Bell, E. F.: Vitamin E in the premature infant. *In* Feeding the Neonate Weighing < 1,500 Grams: Nutrition and Beyond. 79th Ross Conference on Pediatric Research. Columbus, Ross Publications, 1979.

247. Einarson, L., and Ringstead, A.: Effect of chronic vitamin E deficiency on the nervous system and

the skeletal musculature in adult rats. Copenhagen, Levin and Munksgaard, 1938.

248. De Gutierrez-Mahoney, W.: Neural myotrophy and vitamin E. South. Med. J., *34*:389, 1941.

249. Einarson, L., and Telford, R.: Effects of vitamin E deficiency on the CNS in various laboratory animals. Biol. Dan. Vid. Selsk., *11*:1, 1960.

250. Verman, K., and Wei King, D.: Disorders of the developing nervous system of vitamin E deficient rats. Acta Anat., *67*:623, 1967.

251. Owen, W. C., and Owen, E. U.: Retrolental fibroplasia in premature infants. II. Studies on the prophylaxis of the disease. The use of alphatocopherol acetate. Am. J. Ophthalmol., *32*:1631, 1949.

252. Johnson, L. H., Schaffer, P. et al.: The role of vitamin E in retrolental fibroplasia (Abstract). Pediatr. Res., *10*:425, 1976.

253. Curran, J. S., and Contollino, S. J.: Vitamin E (injectable) administration in the prevention of retinopathy of prematurity (Abstract). Pediatr. Res., *12*:404, 1978.

254. Hittner, H. M., Godio, L. B. et al.: Retrolental fibroplasia: Efficacy of vitamin E in a double-blind clinical study of pre-term infants. N. Engl. J. Med., *305*:1365, 1981.

255. Finer, N. N., Grant, G. et al.: Effect of intramuscular vitamin E on frequency and severity of retrolental fibroplasia. Lancet, *1(8281)*:1087, 1982.

256. Horwitt, M. K.: Vitamin E in human nutrition—An interpretive review. Borden Rev. Nutr. Res., *22*:1, 1961.

257. Witting, L. A.: The effect of antioxidant deficiency on tissue lipid composition in the rat. IV. Peroxidation and interconversion of polyunsaturated fatty acids in muscle phospholipids. Lipids, *2*:109, 1967.

258. Draper, H. H.: The tocopherols. *In* Fat Soluble Vitamin. International Encyclopedia of Food and Nutrition. Vol. 19. New York, Pergamon Press, 1976.

259. Perlmutta, G. H., Gross, P. T. et al.: Neurophysiology of vitamin E deficiency in childhood cholestatic liver disease (Abstract). Pediatr. Res., *31*:198a, 1983.

260. Sung, J. H., and Stadlan, E. M.: Neuroaxonal dystrophy in congenital biliary atresia. J. Neuropathol. Exp. Neurol., *25*:341, 1966.

261. Sung, J. H.: Neuroaxonal dystrophy in mucoviscidosis. J. Neuropathol. Exp. Neurol., *23*:567, 1964.

262. Huttenlocher, P. R., and Gilles, F. H.: Clinical, pathologic and histochemical findings in a family with three affected siblings. Neurology, *17*:1174, 1967.

263. O'Grady, R.: Feeding behavior in infants. Am. J. Nurs., *71*(4):736, 1967.

264. Moore, H. B.: The meaning of food. Am. J. Clin. Nutr., *5*(1):79, 1957.

265. Belsky, J.: Early human experience: A family perspective. Dev. Psychol., *17*:3, 1981.

266. Lewis, M., and Feiring, C.: Direct and indirect interactions in social relationships. *In* Lipsitt, L. (ed.): Advances in Infancy Research. Vol. 1. New York, Albex Publishing Corp., 1981.

267. Parke, R. D., Power, T. G., and Gottman, J. M.: Conceptualizing and quantifying influence patterns in the family with three affected siblings. *In* Lamb, W. E. (ed.): Social Interaction Analysis: Methodological Issues. Madison, The University of Wisconsin Press, 1979.

268. Pedersen, F. A. (ed.): The Father-Infant Relationship: Observational Studies in the Family Setting. New York, Praeger Special Studies, 1980.

269. Bronfenbrenner, U.: The Ecology of Human Development. Cambridge, Harvard University Press, 1979.

270. Cochran, M. D., and Brassard, J. A.: Child development and personal social networks. Child Dev., *50*:601, 1979.

271. Garbaniro, J., and Gilliam, G.: Understanding Abusive Families. Lexington, Massachusetts, Health, 1980.

272. Parke, R. D.: Socialization into child abuse: A social interactional perspective. *In* Tapp, J. L., and Levine, P. J. (eds.): Law, Justice and the Individual in Society: Psychological and Legal Issues. New York, Holt, Rinehart and Winston, 1977.

273. LeVine, R. A.: Child rearing as cultural adaptation. *In* Leiderman, P. H. et al. (eds.): Culture and Infancy: Variations in the Human Experience. New York, Academic Press, 1977.

274. Parke, R. D., Grossman, K., and Tinsley, B. R.: Father-mother-infant interaction in the newborn period: A German-American comparison. *In* Field, T. (ed.): Culture and Early Interactions. Hillsdale, New Jersey, Lawrence Erlbaum Assoc., 1981.

275. Lynch, M. A.: Risk factors in the child: A study of abused children and their siblings. *In* Martin, H. P. (ed.): The Abused Child: A Multi-Disciplinary Approach to Developmental Issues and Treatment. Cambridge, Ballinger, 1976.

276. Goldberg, S.: Premature birth: Consequence for the parent-infant relationship. Am. Sci., *67*:214, 1979.

277. Field, T. M., Sostek, A. M., Goldberg, S., and Shuman, H. H. (eds.): Infants Born at Risk: Behavior and Development. New York, S. P. Medical and Scientific Books, 1979.

278. Engeland, B., and Brunnquell, D.: An at-risk approach to the study of child abuse: Some preliminary findings. J. Am. Acad. Psychoanal., *18*:219, 1979.

279. Heiniger, M. C., and Randolph, S. L.: Muscle spindle and golgi tendon organ: Stability against gravity. *In* Neurophysiological Concepts in Human Behavior. St. Louis, The C. V. Mosby Co., 1981.

280. Eviatar, L., Eviatar, A., and Navay, I.: Maturation of neurovestibular responses in infants. Dev. Med. Child. Neurol., *16*:435, 1974.

281. Allen, S. S., and Harper, K. L.: Developmental delays in infants on long-term total parenteral nutrition. Nutr. Supp. Serv., *3*:4, 1983.

282. Decarie, T. A.: The study of mental and emotional development of the thalidomide child. *In* Foss, B. (ed.): Determinants of Infant Behavior. Vol. 4. London, Methuen and Co., Ltd., 1969.

283. Dearie, T., and O'Neill, M.: Quelques aspects du developpement cognitif d'enfants souffrant de malformations du a la thalidomide. Bull. Psychologie, *24*:286, 1973–1974.

284. Bremer, J., and Bryant, P.: Place versus response as the basis of spatial errors made by young infants. J. Exp. Child Psychol. *23*:162, 1977.

285. Abercrombie, M.: Some notes on spatial disability: Movement, intelligence quotient, and attentiveness. Dev. Med. Child Neurol., *10*:206, 1968.

286. Campos, J. J., Svejda, M. J. et al.: The emergence of self-produced locomotion: Its importance for psychological development in infancy. *In* Bricker,

D. D. (ed.): Intervention with At-Risk and Handicapped Infants. Baltimore, University Park Press, 1982.

287. Mahler, M., Pine, F., and Bergman, A.: The Psychological Birth of the Human Infant. New York, Basic Books, 1975.

288. Ament, M. E., and O'Connor, M. J.: Long-term cognitive development of children raised on home total parenteral nutrition for 42–96 months. Clin. Res., 32:96A, 1984.

289. Frostig, M., and Horne, D.: Teacher's Guide: The Frostig Program for the Development of Visual Perception. Chicago, Follett Educational Corp., 1974.

290. Prugh, D. B., and Tagiuri, C. K.: Emotional aspects of the respirator care of patients with poliomyelitis. Psychosom. Med., 16:104, 1954.

291. Silverstein, A. B., and Robinson, H. A.: The representation of physique in children's figure drawings. J. Consult. Clin. Psychol., 25:146, 1961.

292. Green, M., and Levill, E. E.: Constriction of body image in children with congenital heart disease. Pediatrics, 29:438, 1962.

293. Cassell, W. A.: Body perception and symptom localization. Psychosom. Med., 27:71, 1965.

294. Schwab, J. J., and Harmeling, J. D.: Body image and medical illness. Psychosom. Med., 30:51, 1968.

295. Johnson, F. A.: Figure drawings in subjects recovering from poliomyelitis. Psychosom. Med., 34:19, 1972.

296. Fischer, S.: Body image and psychopathology. Arch. Gen. Psychiatry, 10:519, 1964.

297. Garrard, S. D., and Richmond, J. B.: Psychological aspects of the management of chronic diseases and handicapping conditions of childhood. In Lief, H. I. et al. (eds.): The Psychologic Basis of Medical Practice. New York, Harper & Row, 1963.

298. Steiner, J. E.: Innate discriminative human facial expressions to taste and smell stimulation. Ann. N.Y. Acad. Sci., 237:229, 1974.

299. Farber, S. P.: Olfaction in health and disease. Am. J. Occup. Ther., 32:155, 1978.

300. Haagen-Smit, A. J.: Smell and taste. Sci. Am., 186:28, 1952.

301. Zelazo, P.: Comments on genetic determinants of infant development: An overstated case. In Lipsitt, L. (ed.): Developmental Psychobiology: The Significance of Infancy. Hillsdale, New Jersey, Lawrence Erlbaum Assoc., 1976.

302. Zelazo, P.: From reflexive to instrumental behavior. In Lipsitt, L. (ed.): Developmental Psychobiology: The Significance of Infancy. Hillsdale, New Jersey, Lawrence Erlbaum Assoc., 1976.

303. Zelazo, P.: Reactivity to perceptual-cognitive events: Application for infant assessment. In Kearsley, R., and Sigels, I. (eds.): Infants at Risk: Assessment of Cognitive Functioning. Hillsdale, New Jersey, Lawrence Erlbaum Assoc., 1976.

304. Zelazo, P.: An information processing approach to infant cognitive assessment. In Lewis, M. and Taft, L. (eds.): Developmental Disabilities: Theory, Assessment, and Intervention. Jamaica, New York, S. P. Medical and Scientific Books, 1981.

305. Zelazo, P.: Alternative assessment procedures for handicapped infants and toddlers: Theoretical and practical issues. In Bricker, D. D. (ed.): Intervention with At-Risk and Handicapped Infants. Baltimore, University Park Press, 1982.

306. Rosenthal, R., and Jacobson, L.: Pygmalion in the Classroom: Teachers' Expectation and Pupils' Intellectual Development. New York, Holt, Reinhart and Winston, 1968.

307. Lindsley, O. R.: Direct measurement and prosthesis of retarded behavior. J. Educ., 147:62, 1964.

308. Kearsley, R.: Iatrogenic retardation: A syndrome of learned incompetence. In Infants at Risk. Assessment of Cognitive Functioning. Hillsdale, New Jersey, Lawrence Erlbaum Assoc., 1979.

CHAPTER 41

Parenteral Nutrition in the Neonate

GILBERTO R. PEREIRA
MARK GLASSMAN

DEVELOPMENT OF PARENTERAL NUTRITION

In many ways the development of parenteral nutrition has been an essential adjunct to the advancement of modern neonatology. The emergence and refinement of this pediatric subspecialty has led to an increase in the quality and length of survival for premature and intrauterine growth–retarded infants. The immaturity of the gastrointestinal tract and the frequent occurrence of intestinal disease in these infants commonly require the use of either intravenous nutritional supplementation to enteral feedings or total parenteral nutrition (TPN).

As the experience with parenteral nutrition evolves, we are more able to refine our understanding of the nutritional uniqueness of the term infant, the premature infant, and infants who are malnourished during their gestation. As we have become more sensitive to these issues, the use of the parenteral route of feeding has increased. This, in turn, has resulted in an appreciation of the frequency and severity of the associated complications and the methods that may minimize them.

It is our hope that this chapter will serve as a reference for those who care for neonates and as a basis for the development of a rational approach to their nutritional management.

History

The first use of intravenous "nutrition" is credited to Claude Bernard, who in 1843 successfully infused sugar solutions into animals.[1] Seventy years later, Henriques and Andersen[2] used a hydrolysate of goat-muscle protein, carbohydrate, and salt as the sole nutritional support for goats over a two-week period. In 1939, parenteral nutrition was first used in humans by Elman and Weiner,[3] who were able to maintain a positive nitrogen balance in postoperative patients and in patients with unresectable carcinoma.

Despite these advances, nutritional support by intravenous infusion could not meet the increased requirements of the hypermetabolic trauma patient. The search for an infusate of high-caloric density culminated in the development of fat emulsions that were suitable for intravenous use. Although they were first marketed in the 1950s, the unacceptable frequency of significant toxic side effects (thrombosis, embolism, fever, vomiting, rash, and eosinophilia) led to their recall in 1964. Seven years later, a soybean oil and egg emulsion (known as Intralipid) was released for general use. Concomitantly, the development of a technique for catheterization of the superior vena cava[4] permitted the use of hypertonic carbohydrate solutions. With such an approach, it was possible to maintain growth and development as well as a positive nitrogen balance in Beagle pups and postoperative surgical patients. As more experience with intravenous feeding was acquired, its use in the neonate became possible. The last major advance in the field occurred in the mid-1970s with the replacement of the fibrin hydrolysate for crystalline amino acid solutions. The decreased ammonia and fixed-acid content successfully reduced the degree of observed complications, allowing for its use in premature infants. Finally, appreciation of the vitamin and trace element requirements necessitated the development of infusible solutions designed to meet these needs.

Additional knowledge of the physiology and metabolism of newborn infants will allow further refinement of our methods for matching their nutritional demands. In addition, as the impact of nutritional support on the survival and long-term outcome of the neonate is realized, the use of parenteral nutrition will become more integrated into the subspecialty of neonatology.

Clinical Use and Implications

In 1975, Heird and Winters[5] used the data of Friis-Hansen[6] and Widdowson[7] to define the body composition of premature and term infants. Based upon these calculations, it was determined that the small premature infant had energy stores that were sufficient to withstand only four days of starvation. In addition, neonatal malnutrition has been shown to result in long-term deficits in brain growth and development.[8] These data support the use of intravenous feedings as either a supplement or as the sole source of nutrition soon after delivery in all neonates who are unable to be adequately fed via the gastrointestinal tract.[9] Hughes and Ducker[10] list the principal indications for parenteral nutrition in neonates as follows: (1) congenital malformation of the gastrointestinal tract, (2) gastroschisis, (3) meconium ileus, (4) short-bowel syndrome, (5) necrotizing enterocolitis, (6) substrate transport defects, and (7) paralytic ileus. To this list, we would add (8) acute renal failure, (9) respiratory distress syndrome, (10) malabsorption syndromes, (11) chylothorax and lymphangiectasia, and (12) extreme prematurity.

It should be emphasized that if tolerated the enteral route is preferable to intravenous parenteral nutrition. In addition to a decrease in the frequency of complications, enteral feeding stimulates the development of gastrointestinal function. The prolonged omission of oral feedings results in pancreatic and small-intestine hypoplasia and decreased efficiency of intestinal absorption, and it may be a risk factor for the development of cholestatic liver disease. These are, however, only relative contraindications for parenteral nutrition and should not dissuade the physician from using this therapeutic modality when necessary.

FETAL GROWTH PATTERNS

The understanding of fetal growth patterns provides the basis upon which nutritional recommendations are determined for its continuum—the neonate. This knowledge is particularly important for the premature infant, whose growth standards and nutritional requirements are derived from those of the intrauterine period.

From the time of conception to birth, fetal weight increases 6 billion times. As shown in Figure 41–1, *in utero* growth in weight is not uniform but increases progressively during gestation, with birth taking place at the steepest point of the curve (3 kg). Figure 41–1 also shows a change in the slope of the fetal growth curve after 36 weeks of gestation, beyond which time growth rates

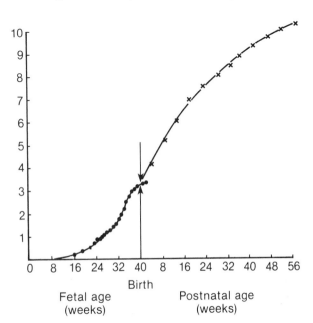

Figure 41–1. Growth of the human fetus and newborn. (*From* Widdowson, E. M.: Growth and composition of the fetus and newborn. *In* Assalin, N. S. (ed.). Biology of Gestation. New York, Academic Press, 1972, pp. 1–44.)

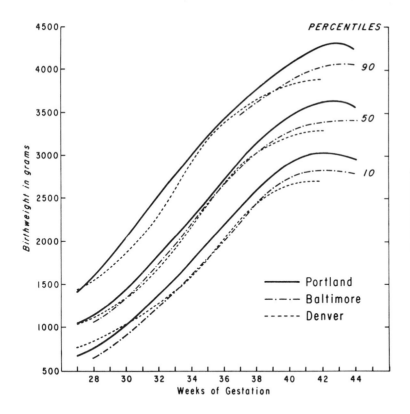

Figure 41–2. Comparisons of fetal weight curves for different populations in the United States. (*From* Babson, S. G., Behrman, R. E., and Lessel, R.: Fetal growth. Liveborn birth weights for gestational age of white middle class infants. Pediatrics, *45*:937–944, 1970.)

begin to fall, probably secondary to the inadequacy of the placental food supply.

A variety of growth charts are available for the assessment of intra- and extrauterine growth in clinical settings.[11–13] Comparing these charts (Fig. 41–2) discloses significant differences among growth parameters (weight, head circumference, and length) at the same gestational ages. These differences are attributed to demographics of the various populations used for compiling the data. Another major criticism of these charts is that the fetal growth curves were constructed using measurements of live-born infants delivered prematurely at different gestational ages. Therefore, these data have an inherent bias because the conditions that result in premature labor are also known to affect fetal size. Nevertheless, until noninvasive methods for estimating fetal size *in utero* become available, postnatal data, by necessity, continue to be used.

Body Composition of the Fetus

The amounts of various body constituents of the developing fetus at different body sizes are presented in Table 41–1. These data, extrapolated from the work of several investigators,[15–18] are regarded as approximate values representing a given body weight rather than a particular gestational age. A more detailed discussion on the fetal deposition rates of fat, carbohydrate, protein, water, and minerals during intrauterine life follows.

Fats. In the early stages of gestation, the fetus lays down no fat apart from essential lipids in the nervous system and phospholipids in the cell membranes. Despite the fact that stored fat represents a major caloric reserve, fat in the human fetus consists of only 0.5 per cent of body weight until midgestation. After that time, the percentage of body weight as fat progressively increases from 3.5 per cent at 28 weeks to 7.5 per cent at 34 weeks to 16 per cent at 40 weeks gestation (term).[19] Infants born to diabetic mothers are known to accumulate body fat at higher rates, so their body fat content may approach 20.8 per cent.[20]

Carbohydrates. Mucopolysaccharides and glycogen are the main carbohydrates deposited in different fetal organs. Mucopolysaccharides are laid down in skeletal muscle, skin, and other fetal organs early in gestation in concentrations that decrease with gestational age. Comparatively, large concentrations of mucopolysaccharides in the body are characteristic of the immature fetus.

Table 41–1. TOTAL AMOUNTS OF WATER, FAT, NITROGEN, AND MINERALS IN THE BODY OF THE DEVELOPING FETUS

APPROXIMATE WEIGHT (gm)	FETAL AGE (wk)	WATER (gm)	FAT (gm)	N (gm)	Ca (gm)	P (gm)	Mg (gm)	Na (mEq)	K (mEq)	Cl (mEq)	Fe (mg)	Cu (mg)	Zn (mg)
30	13	27	0.2	0.4	0.09	0.09	0.003	3.6	1.4	2.4	—	—	—
100	15	89	0.05	1.0	0.3	0.2	0.01	9	2.6	7	5.1	—	—
200	17	177	1.0	2.8	0.7	0.6	0.03	20	7.9	14	10	0.7	2.6
500	23	440	3.0	7.0	2.2	1.5	0.10	49	22	33	28	2.4	9.4
1000	26	860	10	14	6.0	3.4	0.22	90	41	66	64	3.5	16
1500	31	1270	35	25	10	5.6	0.35	125	60	96	100	5.6	25
2000	33	1620	100	37	15	8.2	0.46	160	84	120	160	8.0	35
2500	35	1940	185	49	20	11	0.58	200	110	130	220	10	43
3000	38	2180	360	55	25	14	0.70	240	130	150	260	12	50
3500	40	2400	560	62	30	17	0.78	280	150	160	280	14	53

(Adapted from Camerer, W. J. R.: Z. Biol., 39:173, 1900, Camerer, W. J. R.: Z. Biol., 43:1, 1902, Iob, V., and Swanson, W. W.: Am. J. Dis. Child., 47:302, 1934, Widdowson, E. M., and Spray, C. M.: Arch. Dis. Child., 26:205, 1951, and Widdowson, E. M., and Dickson, J. W. T.: *In* Cornar, C. L., and Bronner, F. (eds.): Mineral Metabolism. Vol. 2. The Elements. New York, Academic Press, Part 2A, pages 1–247.)

Most mucopolysaccharides in fetal skin are in the form of hyaluronic acid.[21] Glucose is the main carbohydrate utilized by the fetus and neonate as an energy source. Glucose is deposited as glycogen in the fetal liver, the skeleton, and the heart muscles during the last two months of pregnancy. Because carbohydrates reach the fetus as glucose, the synthesis of glycogen is dependent upon the appearance of the enzyme necessary for its synthesis. In the liver, a significant rise in glycogen synthesis occurs at about 36 weeks of gestation. Soon after birth, these stores are rapidly consumed and are replenished only after adequate feedings are being taken by the newly born infant.[22] Liver glycogen stores alone provide sufficient energy to the neonate for a period of four to six hours postnatally. Infants who are either small for gestational age or are born prematurely have decreased liver glycogen stores and are, therefore, less equipped to withstand long fasting periods. The size of the glycogen stores is smaller than that of the fat stores at all periods of gestation. In infants born at term, fat stores exceed glycogen stores by 16 times.

Water. Both the volume and the distribution of body fluids change considerably during fetal life, and these trends persist during postnatal life. The smallest fetus analyzed (0.5 gm) was shown to contain 93 to 95 per cent water. The total amount of body water decreases progressively during fetal life to values of 88 per cent at 20 weeks of gestation to 70 to 75 per cent at term. Concomitant with these changes is a progressive reversal in the ratio of extracellular/intracellular water as the fetus matures. As such, the extracellular/intracellular water ratios during gestation vary from 4:1 at 10 weeks to 2.5:1 at 20 weeks to 1.8:1 at 30 weeks to 1:1 at term.[23]

Protein. The protein content of the body weight of the fetus has been determined from measurements of total body nitrogen and is derived by using the protein/nitrogen ratio of 6.5:1. Nitrogen content as a percentage of body weight increases during pregnancy from values of 0.8 per cent at 8 weeks' gestation to 2.4 per cent at 40 weeks' gestation. Most nitrogen reaches the fetus through the placenta in the form of amino acids. The consistently higher concentration of amino acids in the fetal circulation, as compared to the maternal circulation, suggests the presence of active amino acid transport across the placenta. Fetal swallowing of amniotic fluid is known to progressively increase during the pregnancy, and at term the fetus swallows nearly one half of the total volume of amniotic fluid daily. This supplies the fetus at term with approximately 0.6 gm/kg/day of protein.

Minerals (Calcium, Phosphorus, Magnesium). Although body deposition of calcium, phosphorus, and magnesium increases during fetal life, their relative accretion rates vary. As such, the total concentration of calcium, phosphorus, and magnesium in the fetal body from 12 to 40 weeks of gestation increases five, two and one-half, and two times, respectively. Calcium is deposited predominantly in the skeleton, whereas phosphorus and magnesium are distributed between bone and soft tissues. These minerals cross the placental barrier against a concentration gradient, suggesting that their transfer also occurs by active transport.

Sodium and Potassium. Sodium is present in the fetal body in two main pools, the extracellular fluid (ECF) and the skeleton. Early in gestation, most sodium is present in the ECF. As the ECF decreases with maturation, the total sodium body concentration also decreases. Later in gestation, the fall in the total body sodium concentration levels off because of increased sodium deposition in the mineralizing skeleton.[24] Unlike sodium, the fetal body concentration of potassium increases during the pregnancy; however, the total concentration of sodium is higher than that of potassium at all gestational ages. In the fetus, a significant amount of potassium is present outside the cells.

Iron, Copper, and Zinc. Iron and copper are deposited in several fetal organs at progressively higher concentrations during the last trimester of pregnancy.[24] However, a similar trend is not seen with zinc. Although body zinc increases during fetal life, the body concentration of this trace element does not change significantly from 16 weeks to 40 weeks of gestation.[24]

NEONATAL GROWTH PATTERNS

Fetal growth is dependent upon the supply of nutrients that reach the fetus through the umbilical vessels from the maternal circulation. After birth, growth of the newly born infant is dependent on his or her own ability to utilize nutrients provided orally, via the gastrointestinal tract, or intravenously, via parenteral nutrition solutions. Because the full-term, the premature, and the growth-retarded infant differ considerably in their biochemical development and nutritional requirements, their growth characteristics will be presented separately.

Full-Term Infants

A postnatal weight loss of five to eight per cent is seen in term neonates during the first few days of life. This "physiologic" weight loss has been attributed mainly to the loss of edema fluid and to a lesser extent to losses from other body components, such as meconium, urine, the remnant of the umbilical cord, vernix, and energy stores (glycogen, fat). The magnitude of the physiologic weight loss is known to be affected by feeding practices, by conditions associated with increased energy expenditure (respiratory distress, hypothermia), and by increased fluid losses through the skin (radiant warmers) and the gastrointestinal tract (diarrheal stools). In healthy neonates, the upturn of the weight curve takes place between the fourth and sixth days of life at a time when the nutritional intake is adequate for the resumption of growth. With adequate nutrition, most healthy full-term infants regain birth weight by the tenth day of life and continue to grow in weight, head circumference, and length at the same percentiles of the growth chart exhibited at birth.

Although full-term infants are born with the energy reserves (glycogen and fat) necessary for adaptation to extrauterine life, they do not tolerate fasting periods in excess of four to six hours without developing hypoglycemia, increased protein catabolism, and more severe weight loss. Therefore, neonates should be fed within the first six hours after birth. Under circumstances in which enteral feedings cannot be provided (e.g., gastrointestinal anomalies, severe respiratory distress), the intravenous administration of fluids and nutrients is recommended.

Premature Infants

Premature infants exhibit postnatal weight losses of a higher degree than do full-term infants (10 to 12 per cent), and they do not regain birth weight until the end of the second week of life. The weight-loss curve of these infants is magnified by the degree of prematurity, intercurrent illnesses, and delay in initiating nutritional support. Weight curves of premature infants weighing 750 to 2000 gm have been reported by Dancis and O'Connell (Fig. 41–3).[25] This grid displays mean physiologic weight losses of 5 per cent in babies born weighing 2000 gm and significantly higher weight losses of 25 per cent in babies born weighing 750 gm. These data, however, reflect feeding practices from a time prior to the routine administration of early feeding to neonates and the advent of parenteral nutrition. A recent study by Cashore and associates[26] demonstrates that premature infants could resume post-

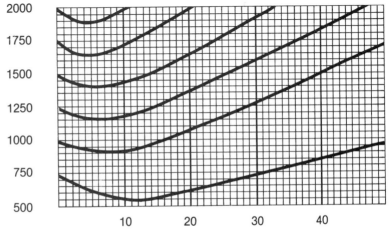

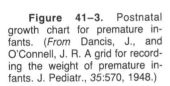

Figure 41–3. Postnatal growth chart for premature infants. (*From* Dancis, J., and O'Connell, J. R. A grid for recording the weight of premature infants. J. Pediatr., *35*:570, 1948.)

2000
1750
1500
1250
1000
750
500

10   20   30   40

AGE IN DAYS

natal growth at intrauterine rates if their enteral feedings were supplemented with intravenous protein, dextrose, and fat emulsions to maintain a total caloric intake between 100 and 120 kcal/kg/day.

Under conditions of suboptimal caloric intake (60 to 85 kcal/kg/day), the growth of premature infants is not uniform. As such, the head circumference increases at a faster rate than the body weight and length, demonstrating the phenomenon of head sparing.[27] Also, during nutritional recovery, premature infants exhibit catchup growth, which is characterized by growth rates exceeding those of the intrauterine period and by crossing percentiles in the growth charts.[28]

Small-for-Gestational-Age Infants

Postnatal growth patterns of infants who are small for gestational age differ from those of full-term and premature infants. They vary according to the time of onset and the degree of intrauterine growth retardation (IUGR) during the pregnancy. Growth impairment during the last trimester of pregnancy often results in mild IUGR and in "asymmetric" small-for-gestational-age infants. These infants usually have normal head circumferences but a low ponderal index (weight/length ratio). Postnatal nutritional recovery promotes continuation of normal head growth and a slow return of the other growth parameters to the appropriate percentiles on the growth chart. Infants who are born with severe growth retardation are affected early in gestation, and all growth parameters are more "symmetrically" impaired. Long-term followup of these babies throughout infancy demonstrates a continuum of their reduced fetal growth pattern.[29]

NUTRITIONAL REQUIREMENTS OF THE NEONATE

This section reviews the nutritional requirements of the neonate, taking into account gestational age, age after birth, and the route for the administration of nutrients.

The estimation of nutritional requirements of babies born prematurely takes into account the biochemical immaturity that affects most of their organ systems.

A rapid metabolic maturation occurs during the first few days of life in full-term and premature neonates as part of their adaptation to extrauterine life. These metabolic changes allow progressive increases in the oral and intravenous intake of nutrients necessary for the resumption of postnatal growth.

The estimation of oral nutritional requirements also varies, depending upon the route of nutrient administration—oral versus intravenous. The calculation of oral requirements is based on the efficiency of nutrient absorption by the gastrointestinal tract, which is often assessed by measurements of nutrient losses in stools. The estimation of intravenous requirements takes into account urinary losses of nutrients. As such, amino acids, vitamins, and trace elements infused to neonates can be lost in the urine in significant amounts. These losses result from renal clearance of the nutrients preceding their hepatic uptake. Differences between oral and intravenous requirements have not been established for all nutrients in the neonate. In fact, oral and intravenous requirements are often used interchangeably. For the purpose of this chapter, intravenous requirements of nutrients will be presented preferentially over oral requirements depending on data availability.

This section outlines the requirements for water, calories, amino acids, protein, fat, carbohydrates, minerals, and vitamins that should be provided to neonates during parenteral nutrition.

Water

The principles used for the intravenous administration of fluids to neonates are different from those used for older children and reflect the unique body water composition of the neonate (70 to 75 per cent of total body weight).

The recommended rates for the initiation and maintenance of intravenous-fluid intake in full-term and premature babies are presented in Table 41–2. The higher fluid rates required by low-birth-weight infants result from their large body surface/weight ratio and their limited ability to concentrate urine. Additionally, premature infants have high rates of insensible water losses through their skin, which is thin and has a rich blood supply, a high water content, and increased permeability. Adjustments in fluid rates are commonly needed under the clinical conditions described in Table 41–3.

Table 41–2. RECOMMENDATIONS FOR STARTING PARENTERAL FLUID MAINTENANCE IN LOW-BIRTH-WEIGHT NEWBORN INFANTS

TYPE OF BED	WEIGHT (gm)			
	600–800	*801–1000*	*1001–1500*	*1501–2000*
Radiant warmer				
Volume, ml/kg/day*	120	90	75	65
Dextrose, %	5	10	10	12.5
Saline, %†	0.1	0.2	0.2	0.2
Incubator				
Volume, ml/kg/day*	90	75	65	55
Dextrose, %	7.5	10	10	12.5
Saline, %†	0.1	0.2	0.2	0.2
Either, with shield				
Volume, ml/kg/day*	70	55	50	45
Dextrose, %	7.5	10	12.5	12.5
Saline, %†	0.1	0.2	0.2	0.2

*Plus 30% with phototherapy.
†After first day of life.
(Adapted from Baumgart S., et al.: Clin. Pediatr., *21*(4):199, 1982.)

All infants receiving intravenous fluids should be carefully monitored for fluid intake and output. Measurements of fluid output should include the volume of urine as well as the volume of fluids lost to nasogastric, ileostomy, colostomy, and chest tube drainages. Abnormal fluid losses should be added in equal volume and mineral composition to daily maintenance fluids. Urine volume greater than 2 ml/hour and urine specific gravity less than 1010 suggest an adequate state of hydration in the neonate who is free of renal disease.

The treatment of a variety of cardiorespiratory diseases in the newborn period requires fluid restriction, which unfortunately limits fluid intake and consequently caloric intake during parenteral nutrition. Under these circumstances, attempts should be made to provide parenteral nutrition solutions of a high-caloric density in order to prevent caloric deprivation.

Table 41–3. FLUID INTAKE OF THE NEONATE IN VARIOUS ENVIRONMENTAL AND CLINICAL CONDITIONS

INCREASE FLUID INTAKE	DECREASE FLUID INTAKE
Gastrointestinal fluid losses	Congestive heart failure
Renal failure (diuretic phase)	Respiratory distress
Low ambient humidity	Inappropriate ADH syndrome
Phototherapy	Renal failure (oliguric phase)
Radiant warmer bed	Plastic shield over body

Energy

In the absence of external work, energy intake equals the sum of energy expenditure, energy excreted, and energy deposited. Therefore, the calories provided during parenteral nutrition should be sufficient to compensate for the metabolic expenditure, energy losses, and growth requirements of the neonate. The recommended levels of energy intake and the partition of energy utilized by full-term and premature infants after the first week of life are presented in Figure 41–4. The high energy requirements of the premature infant reflect the increased energy losses (urine, stools) and faster growth rates. Adjustments in caloric intake are necessary under a variety of clinical conditions. Caloric requirements are increased in infants with respiratory distress, congenital heart disease, cold stress, and IUGR, and in infants recovering from malnutrition. Caloric requirements are reduced in conditions associated with reduced physical activity.

Amino Acids

Approximately 10 per cent of the total caloric intake during parenteral nutrition should be provided as amino acids. Ideally, the amino acids infused should be spared for protein synthesis rather than utilized as an energy source. Nitrogen-sparing in the neonate can be achieved when the nitrogen (gram)/nonprotein calorie (kcal) ratio is maintained above 1:150.

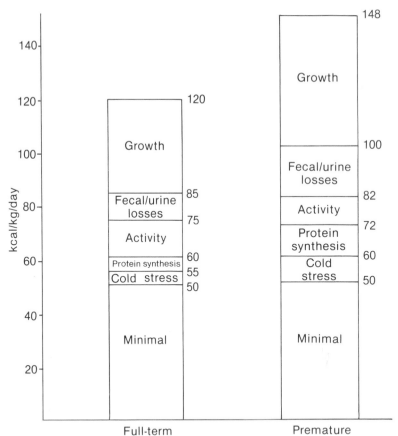

Figure 41–4. Partition of energy requirements in full-term and premature infants. (*Data from* Sinclair, J. C., Driscoll, J. M., Jr., Heird, W. C., et al.: Supportive management of the sick neonate. Parenteral calories, water, and electrolytes. Pediatr. Clin. North Am., *17*:863–893, 1970; Winters, R. W.: The body fluids in pediatrics. *In*: Maintenance Fluid Therapy. Boston, Little, Brown and Company, 1973, p. 267; and Reichman, B. L., Chessex, P., Putet, G., et al.: Partition of energy metabolism and energy cost of growth in the very low-birth-weight infant. Pediatrics, *69*:446–451, 1982.)

The daily intravenous requirement of amino acids for neonates varies from 1.5 to 3 gm/kg, with the small infant requiring the higher values of intake. A recent study using N_{15} glycine to measure its incorporation into the protein pool of premature infants demonstrates a progressive increase in net tissue-protein gain as protein intake increases from 1 to 3 gm/kg. Additionally, the study shows that intakes in excess of 3 gm/kg were not accompanied by increased tissue-protein gain, suggesting that optimal protein intake was achieved at this level. The requirements for protein or amino acids, or both, are increased in conditions associated with excessive protein losses in either urine or stools.

Inadequate provision of amino acids to neonates is associated with failure to thrive, hypoalbuminemia, and edema. Excessive amino acid intake can be detrimental and may be associated with the following metabolic complications: hyperammonemia,[30] serum amino acid imbalance,[31] metabolic acidosis,[32] and possibly cholestatic jaundice.[33]

During parenteral nutrition, the amino acid requirement depends upon the concentration as well as the composition of the amino acids provided (essential and nonessential). There is a need at present to reformulate the composition of amino acid preparations for the neonate, especially for those who are premature. Such solutions should contain tyrosine, cystine, and taurine, three amino acids that are considered essential for the immature infant and that are either absent or present in insufficient amounts in today's amino acid preparations.

Carbohydrates

Carbohydrates represent a major metabolic source during parenteral nutrition and should provide a minimum of 35 to 55 per cent of the total caloric intake. Dextrose, so called because of the dextrorotatory position of the glucose molecule, is the most commonly used carbohydrate for parenteral nutrition in infants. Dextrose infusions are well tolerated if the initial rate of administration does not exceed the hepatic rate of glucose production (6 to 8 mg/kg/minute). The premature infant, however, may develop hyperglycemia at lower levels of glucose infusion. The tolerance to glucose loads increases steadily with postnatal age. High dextrose concentrations (20 to 30 per cent) can be infused continuously to neonates and even to premature babies provided that the increments in concentration are made progressively and slowly. Each gram of dextrose metabolized provides 3.4 kcal of energy.

Other carbohydrates such as fructose, sorbitol, and ethanol have been evaluated in the neonate. Tolerance to the intravenous administration of fructose also increases postnatally but not with the same magnitude noted for glucose.[34] The use of fructose in infants has been associated with increased urinary losses of this carbohydrate and with the production of lactic acid, resulting in metabolic acidosis.[35] The intravenous administration of sorbitol is followed by its rapid conversion to fructose and the occurrence of similar complications.[36] Despite its use in adults, ethanol is not indicated for parenteral nutrition in infants. In the newborn, the activity of alcohol dehydrogenase (the liver enzyme that metabolizes ethanol) is reduced to 15 to 27 per cent of adult levels,[37] which places the newborn infant at high risk for ethanol toxicity.

In summary, the intravenous use of fructose, sorbitol, and ethanol offers no clinical advantage over the use of dextrose for parenteral nutrition in the neonate.

Fats

Along with amino acids and dextrose, fats are an essential component of a parenteral nutrition regimen. There are at least three major advantages for using fats intravenously. They are a source of essential fatty acids, their caloric density is high (1 gm = 11 kcal), and they have a low osmolality that makes them suitable for peripheral vein use. Although fat emulsions represent a major source of energy during parenteral nutrition, their intake should not exceed 50 per cent of the total daily calories.

There are currently two fat emulsions available for clinical use: soybean and safflower oil emulsions. Both products are manufactured at concentrations of 10 and 20 per cent and are comparably effective in preventing essential fatty acid deficiency and sparing of nitrogen in neonates.[38]

The fatty acid compositions of soybean and safflower oils are compared in Table 41–4. In both emulsions, there is sufficient linoleic acid to supply the minimal requirements of this essential fatty acid in infants at minimal fat intakes of three to four per cent of the total daily calories. The essentiality of another fatty acid, linolenic acid, has recently been suggested for parenteral nutrition in children.[39] The concentration of linolenic acid is lower in the safflower oil emulsion compared with the soybean oil emulsion, but the clinical significance of this difference is not known at present and deserves to be studied.

The metabolic process that follows the intravenous infusion of fat emulsions is summarized in Figure 41–5. The infused triglycerides are initially hydrolyzed by capillary lipoprotein lipase, an enzyme that is known to be activated by heparin. The resultant free fatty acids circulate bound to albumin and follow two metabolic pathways: they are either oxidized in the liver to form ketone bodies or are re-esterified to triglycerides and deposited in the adipose tissue for energy storage.

The premature and the small-for-gestational-age infant have a decreased ability to clear both free fatty acids and triglycerides from their serum. Shennan and colleagues[40] suggested that this impaired clearance of triglycerides was secondary to a decreased activity of lipoprotein lipase resulting from reduced adipose tissue mass or hepatic immaturity. Dhainreddy and associates[41] attempted to increase lipoprotein lipase activity with a heparin infusion, which had only a transient effect. More recently, the same investigators documented improved triglyceride clearance in low-birth-weight infants receiving parenteral nutrition with "in-line" heparin, which was accomplished by increased circulating levels of hepatic lipase.[42] Evidence that the acquisition of lipoprotein

Table 41–4. FATTY ACID COMPOSITION OF FAT EMULSIONS

FATTY ACIDS	SOYBEAN OIL	SAFFLOWER OIL
Linoleic acid (%)	50	75
Linolenic acid (%)	9	0.5
Oleic acid (%)	26	12.9
Palmitic acid (%)	10	6.7
Stearic acid (%)	2.5	2.7
Others (%)	2.5	2.2
Total (%)	100	100

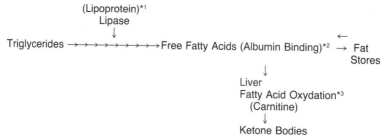

Figure 41–5. Metabolism of intravenous fats. (*) indicates a metabolic step that is impaired in small premature infants.

lipase activity is a developmental phenomenon was provided by Sigmura[43] and Filer,[44] who noted that the activity of this enzyme increases with gestational age. Shennan and coworkers[40] studied the clearance rates of intravenous fat infusions in premature infants. They discovered that premature neonates less than 33 weeks' gestational age cleared fat at a rate of 0.16 gm/kg/hour and that infants greater than 33 weeks' gestation cleared fat at a rate of 0.3 gm/kg/hour. We believe that these values should serve as guidelines for the institution of lipid therapy in premature infants.

In all infants there is an improvement in fat tolerance with an increase in postnatal age. Under most clinical conditions, fat calories can be advanced in amounts parallel to carbohydrate calories in order to provide comparable amounts of metabolizable energy from each source. This approach should be routinely taken during parenteral nutrition in small infants. Further studies are currently needed to identify specific clinical conditions in which either carbohydrate or fat calories are preferably utilized.

Minerals

Suggested daily intakes of minerals for premature and full-term infants are presented in Table 41–5. Higher levels of some minerals are recommended for the premature baby. Serial monitoring of serum mineral levels is necessary during parenteral nutrition of neonates even when the intake provided is within the indicated ranges.

Vitamins

Specific vitamin requirements for neonates have not been precisely defined. Estimated requirements of vitamins during in-

fancy and the composition of multivitamin preparations available for clinical use are presented in Table 41–6. The table points out the vitamins that premature infants require at higher levels as well as some of the vitamins not included in commercial preparations that need to be added separately to parenteral nutrition solutions.

COMPLICATIONS AND MANAGEMENT

The complications associated with the use of TPN are legion, but they are primarily associated with the use of central hyperalimentation. Cashore and associates[9] used peripheral nutritional supplementation in 23 premature infants without significant complications. This has been the experience in many other nurseries. The occurrence of skin sloughs following accidental infiltration of the infusate represents the major complication of peripheral hyperalimentation. To prevent or minimize this complication, the dex-

Table 41–5. DAILY INTRAVENOUS INTAKE OF MINERALS FOR NEONATES

MINERAL	FULL TERM	PREMATURE
Sodium (mEq)	2–3	3–5*
Potassium (mEq)	1–2	1–2
Magnesium (mEq)	0.3–0.5	0.3–0.5
Calcium (mg)	20–40	40–60†
Phosphorus (mg)	20–40	20–40†
Iron (mg)	1	1
Zinc (μg)	100–200	400–600*
Copper (μg)	10–20	20
Chromium (μg)	0.14–0.2	0.14–0.2
Manganese (μg)	2–10	2–10
Fluoride (μg)	1	1‡
Iodine (μg)	3–5	3–5‡

*Upper ranges suggested during rapid growth.
†Higher intake needed for premature infants weighing less than 1500 gm.
‡Requirements not well defined.

Table 41–6. VITAMINS FOR INFANTS
RECEIVING PARENTERAL NUTRITION

	RDA FOR NEONATES* (units/kg body wt)	MVI PEDIATRIC (per 5 ml solution)
Vitamin A (IU)	233	2300
Vitamin D (IU)	66	400
Vitamin E (IU)	0.66	7
Vitamin K1 (mg)	—	0.2
Vitamin C (mg)	6	80
Folacin (mg)	8	140
Niacin (mg)	0.9	17
Riboflavin (mg)	0.07	1.4
Thiamin (mg)	0.055	1.2
Vitamin B_6 (μg)	0.05	1.0
Vitamin B_{12} (μg)	0.04	1.0
Pantothenic acid (mg)	0.3*	5.0
Biotin (μg)	30*	20

*Adapted from American Medical Association Department of Foods and Nutrition, 1975. Multivitamin preparations for parenteral use. A statement by the Nutrition Advisory Group. J. Parent. Ent. Nutr. 3:258, 1979; American Academy of Pediatrics Committee on Nutrition: Profound changes in food and drug administration regulations concerning formula products and vitamin-mineral dietary supplements for infants. Pediatrics, 40:916, 1967; and Shenkin, A., and Wretlind, A.: Parenteral nutrition. World Rev. Nutr. Diet., 28:1, 1978.

trose concentration of peripheral solutions should not exceed 10 gm/dl.

The hazards of central hyperalimentation can be divided into three categories: those related to infection, those related to the catheter, and those related to metabolic derangements.

Infectious Complications

Four large series surveying the relative complication rates of central hyperalimentation in pediatric and neonatal patients have reported rates of infection that vary from 21 to 45 per cent.[45–47] This wide variation in the incidence of infection is explained in part by the varying percentage of neonates and premature infants in the different samples. In addition, infants requiring parenteral nutrition often have other risk factors for sepsis. As such, the effect of malnutrition upon immune function contributes to this relative risk. Support for this hypothesis comes from the data of Filston and Geant[46] and Eichelberger and colleagues,[47] who noted that the catheter tip was the only source of infection in 25 and 68 per cent of their respective patients with sepsis. Thus, it appears that sepsis in patients on TPN has a multifactorial

etiology. The most commonly encountered organisms are coagulase-positive and -negative *Staphylococcus, Streptococcus viridans, Escherichia coli, Pseudomonas* sp., *Klebsiella* sp., and *Candida albicans*.

The mechanisms by which pathogens can contaminate central hyperalimentation lines include (1) catheter contamination at the insertion site either during initial placement or during maintenance of the line; (2) catheter contamination secondary to the use of the central line for the administration of blood products and medications, blood sampling, and monitoring of central venous pressure; and (3) catheter contamination secondary to another source of infection.

Contamination of the hyperalimentation fluid is a theoretic source of infection. Felts and coworkers[48] reported an outbreak of sepsis following the nonaseptic preparation of intravenous fluids. Since then, other authors have shown that both lipid emulsions and glucose-dextrose solutions support the growth of staphylococcal and candidal species as well as several gram-negative organisms responsible for confirmed cases of sepsis. Aseptic preparation of infusates by trained pharmacists working under laminar-flow hoods is known to minimize the risk of contamination of hyperalimentation solutions.

The newborn infant is particularly vulnerable to infection. Abnormalities in chemotaxis, phagocytosis, bactericidal functioning, and splenic immaturity prevent the neonate from adequately clearing organisms that enter the circulation. Fat emulsions have been noted to further compromise the chemotactic and bactericidal activity of the leukocyte;[49, 50] however, these *in vitro* studies utilized fat emulsions at concentrations much higher than those utilized clinically. Friedman and coworkers[51] found that following the intravenous infusion of fat, lipid droplets were found in the alveolar macrophages. These authors hypothesized that "reticuloendothelial blockade" could enhance the susceptibility of the newborn to sepsis because the reticuloendothelial system plays a major role in immunocompetence. It is important to note that the immunologic effect of the lipid emulsion on immune function seems to occur in a dose-response pattern.[52] This may be of particular relevance for premature and small-for-gestational-age infants who are less able to clear the infused triglycerides from the blood stream.[52] Finally, the particle size of the lipid infusate precludes the use of filtration systems, which act as a barrier against the transmission of bacteria.

Suggested guidelines to reduce the incidence of central hyperalimentation–related sepsis include (1) aseptic preparation of the infusate, (2) aseptic technique for catheter insertion and for dressing changes, (3) use of less thrombogenic silastic/silicone catheters, (4) use of the central line for parenteral nutrition solution exclusively, and (5) routine use of in-line bacterial filters.

Catheter Complications

The incidence of technical complications related to central line placement varies from 4 to 9.2 per cent and among the most common are pneumothorax, pneumomediastinum, arterial puncture, and hemorrhage. When radiologic confirmation was routinely done, Mitchell and Clark[53] noted that 29 per cent of the venous catheters were malpositioned. The importance of determining tip placement has been emphasized by Brady and Weinberg[54] and Franciosi and associates,[55] who reported serious cardiac arrhythmias and sudden death as a result of myocardial necrosis in infants and children whose catheter tips had slipped into the right atrium or ventricle. Based on these reports, we recommend that line placement be confirmed on a regular basis.

Thrombosis of the vein adjacent to the catheter tip is the most common thrombotic complication of TPN[56] and may result in a "superior vena cava syndrome," with edema of the face, eyes, and neck. This syndrome resolves spontaneously as collateral circulation is established. A more serious complication of catheter thrombosis is pulmonary embolism, which may result in sudden death. To date, there have been reports of 16 patients on TPN with such a complication.[57–59]

Extravasation of the infusate resulting from malpositioned catheters may result in fluid collection in the pleural cavity with associated chylothorax,[60, 61] pericardial space with resultant tamponade,[62, 63] and mediastinum associated with tracheal compression.[64] Lam and associates[65] reported that paralysis of a hemidiaphragm resulted from the inflammatory reaction to hyperalimentation solution in the hemithorax.

Metabolic Complications

This section reviews the common metabolic complications that are related to either toxicity or the inadequate composition of parenteral nutrition solutions used in the neonate. Guidelines for the prevention and the management of these complications are also discussed.

Amino Acids. Protein hydrolysates, the original source of amino acids for intravenous use, were first made available three decades ago. Both casein and fibrin hydrolysates suffered from deficiencies that were particularly relevant to the neonate. First, there was a large variability in the composition of the same products from different batches.[66] Second, approximately 50 per cent of the amino acids in these solutions were peptides, which have an uncertain metabolic fate in the small infant. Third, these solutions caused mild hyperammonemia in premature babies.[30]

Hyperammonemia was first reported by Ghadimi and associates[67] and was later found to be proportional to the amount of the protein hydrolysate infused.[30] Initially thought to result from the high-ammonia and fixed-acid loads of the hydrolysates, hyperammonemia was shown to occur at equal frequencies with either the fibrin or the casein preparations, and it occurred at infusion rates below those necessary to maintain positive nitrogen balance. Later, it was suggested that the delay in the maturation of the metabolic pathways for nitrogen excretion contributed to the hyperammonemia. In support of this theory, Heird and coworkers[68] found that administration of arginine would correct the hyperammonemia. Thus, it appeared that a combination of substrate deficiency and metabolic immaturity was responsible for the abnormalities in ammonia metabolism in premature babies.

In the 1970s, crystalline amino acid solutions replaced the protein hydrolysates, and they had the main advantage of a more precise and reproducible amino acid composition. However, even the revised formulations of these solutions are still inadequate for the immature neonate, and complications associated with their use include (1) prerenal azotemia, which correlates with the amount of amino acid infused and reflects decreased glomerular filtration rates by the immature kidney; (2) hyperchloremic metabolic acidosis resulting from excessive infusion of chloride salts of the crystalline amino acids; (3) serum amino acid imbalances characterized by excessive levels of glycine and methionine and low levels of cystine, tyrosine, and taurine; and (4) possibly cholestatic liver disease.

There is a need at present to more precisely define the amino acid requirements of neonates and formulate solutions that are more adequate for these infants.

Dextrose. The metabolic hazards of carbohydrate infusions include both hypoglycemia and hyperglycemia. Abrupt discontinuation of a hypertonic glucose solution can result in a precipitous fall in serum glucose concentrations. In view of the insulin-glucose imbalance that occurs, it is recommended that hypertonic dextrose solutions be decreased gradually over 24 to 48 hours in order to avoid this complication. Hyperglycemia is seen in very low-birth-weight infants and is often secondary to the administration of the glucose infusion at rates that exceed those of hepatic glucose production (6 to 8 mg/kg/minute).[69, 70] Additionally, stressed premature neonates have increased catecholamines in the umbilical cord blood,[71] which may contribute to peripheral insulin resistance and result in hyperglycemia.[72] This phenomenon, also noted in small-for-gestational-age infants, has led some investigators to support the use of supplemental insulin in low-birth-weight infants receiving parenteral nutrition. Hyperglycemia has also been described in association with neonatal sepsis[73] and the use of intravenous fat emulsions as a dose-dependent complication.[74]

Hyperglycemia can lead to hyperosmolality and osmotic diuresis, resulting in dehydration. Neonates are particularly vulnerable to these complications as a result of their immature renal function and their decreased glomerular threshold for glucose. The glycosuria seen in these infants occurs at lower absolute glucose concentrations than in older infants. The immature kidney's decreased ability to conserve salt also prevents the neonate from compensating for increased urinary water loss.

The effect of carbohydrate load on pulmonary function has recently been studied in adult patients. Respiratory quotient (RQ) elevations above 1 were noted when glucose was used to support lipogenesis. Therefore, as glucose utilization increases, the rate of carbon dioxide production and the RQ also increase. Askanazi and associates[75] reported that excessive infusion of carbohydrates precipitated respiratory distress in an adult with borderline pulmonary function. Similarly, Covelli and colleagues[76] noted the development of respiratory distress, acidosis, hypercapnea, and increased alveolar and minute ventilation in three patients given a high carbohydrate load. Although these observations have not been reproduced in neonates, we hypothesize that intravenous carbohydrate loads may have an adverse effect in infants with compromised pulmonary function.

Fat Emulsions. The major complications of fat emulsions in the neonate are related to the elevated levels of serum triglycerides and serum free fatty acids that follow the infusion of fat. Hypertriglyceridemia, often associated with "cloudy serum," may cause impairments in both the immune response and the pulmonary function of neonates.

The effect of lipid infusions upon pulmonary function was first reported by Greene and coworkers[77] who described the association between hyperlipemia and decreased pulmonary diffusion capacity in healthy adults. This complication, noted to be prevented by the administration of heparin, was shown to resolve spontaneously as the infused lipid was cleared from the serum. Decreased oxygen transport secondary to either lipid coating of the red cell or to alterations in the red cell membrane have been well documented.[78] Pereira and associates[79] noted decreased oxygenation in premature infants receiving intravenous fats, which correlated with serum triglyceride concentrations but was unrelated to changes in pulmonary dynamics.

Carnitine is the protein necessary for transporting medium-chain fatty acids from the cytosol to the mitochondria in which they undergo oxidation. Deficiency of carnitine has been documented in infants as early as five days after receiving fat-free parenteral nutrition.[80, 81] Schmidt-Sommerfield[82] studied the accumulation of carnitine in the newborn infant and found that its oral absorption plays an essential role in its postnatal increase. Although the neonate has adequate concentrations of the precursors lysine and methionine, the premature infant may not have the synthetic capability to produce carnitine. This may contribute to decreased oxidation and delayed clearance of serum free fatty acids.

Free fatty acids resulting from the hydrolysis of triglycerides may compete with bilirubin for albumin sites and cause displacement in bilirubin, increasing its free fraction in the serum. This complication is of particular significance in premature babies suffering from concomitant hyperbilirubinemia and hypoalbuminemia. *In vitro* displacement of bilirubin was shown to occur at serum free fatty acid/albumin molar ratios greater than 6:1.[83] Under these circumstances, fat infusions should be temporarily decreased or discontinued.

False elevations in the estimation of serum bilirubin have been reported in neonates during the infusion of fat emulsions.[84] This complication may result in an unnecessary exchange transfusion and can be easily prevented by further centrifugation of blood samples prior to bilirubin determinations.

Deficiencies of the essential fatty acids have occurred in many patients receiving fat-free parenteral nutrition. Friedman and co-workers reported biochemical evidence of essential fatty acid deficiency after ten days of fat-free TPN in full-term neonates and as early as two days of fat-free TPN in one premature infant.[85] Essential fatty acid deficiency is associated with decreased platelet aggregation, supposedly secondary to thromboxane A_2 deficiency,[86] poor weight gain, scaly eczematoid rash, sparse hair growth, and thrombocytopenia. Prevention of the deficiency state can be achieved by supplying two to four per cent of the total caloric intake as essential fatty acids or by applying sunflower seed oil to the skin of deficient patients.[87, 88] Biweekly plasma and blood transfusions at doses of 10 ml/kg body weight are impractical and unreliable therapies for the prevention of essential fatty acid deficiency in neonates.[74]

Minerals. Mineral deficiencies are common during parenteral nutrition in neonates. Because most minerals are transferred to the fetus during the last trimester of pregnancy, the premature neonate has decreased mineral reserves and is therefore at high risk for developing mineral deficiencies.

Osteopenia, rickets, and pathologic fractures have been extensively reported in association with parenteral nutrition in premature and full-term neonates. Etiologic factors related to these complications include (1) inadequate intake of vitamin D (less than 400 IU/day), (2) inability of premature infants to convert vitamin D_3 to its active metabolites 25 OH and 1,25 $(OH)_2$ vitamin D, (3) inadequate intake of calcium and phosphorus, and (4) excessive urinary losses of these two minerals. The adverse effect of decreased physical activity on bone mineralization as described in older patients has not been reported in neonates. It has recently been shown that the average recovery of vitamin D in hyperalimentation solutions infused over a 24-hour period is reduced to 68 per cent of its original concentration, possibly because of the adherence of this vitamin to the bag and tube. Therefore, concentrations of this vitamin in parenteral nutrition solutions need to be adjusted to guarantee adequate intake. Calcium and phosphorus should be provided to premature neonates at concentrations approximating intrauterine accretion rates. However, when these two minerals are present in the same solution, calcium-phosphate precipitation may occur. To prevent this phenomenon, which is concentration-dependent, the product of the calcium and phosphorus concentration in solution should not exceed 75 mM^2.[89] A calcium/phosphorus ratio of 3:1 in hyperalimentation solutions minimizes the urinary losses of these two minerals by the premature kidney.[89]

A progressive decline in zinc levels occurs in premature neonates after four weeks of parenteral nutrition if zinc is not supplemented. Zinc is required for RNA-DNA metabolism, skin regeneration, and lymphocyte transformation. Zinc deficiency results in poor growth, diarrhea, alopecia, susceptibility to infection, and skin desquamation surrounding the mouth and anus (acrodermatitis enteropathica). Zinc requirements are increased during active growth and in all infants with short-bowel syndrome. The latter results from malabsorption and increased enteric losses of zinc from either ileostomy or colostomy drainage.[90] The presence of aminoaciduria, stress, and catabolism also increases zinc requirements because of the chelation of zinc and its renal wasting.[91]

Copper deficiency in the neonate is characterized by osteoporosis, hemolytic anemia, neutropenia, and depigmentation of the skin. Rickets is also noted in copper-deficient patients,[92] though it becomes manifest only in growing infants. Because there is no hepatic accumulation of manganese, chromium, or cobalt prior to birth,[93] deficiencies of these minerals may also occur in infants maintained on parenteral nutrition without trace element supplementation. Deficiencies of chromium or selenium, which are accompanied by glucose intolerance[94] and cardiomyopathy,[95] respectively, have not been reported in neonates.

Hepatic Dysfunction. The incidence of hepatic dysfunction associated with parenteral nutrition ranges from 8.6 to 42 per cent. In 1971, Johnson and colleagues[30] first described abnormal liver function in patients receiving fibrin hydrolysates. Since then, several attempts to determine the pathogenesis of this significant and often reversible hepatocellular dysfunction have revealed a multifactorial etiology. Amino acid toxicity,[33] the use of hypertonic dextrose solutions,[96] the lack of oral alimentation or the prolonged use of hyperalimentation,[97] and associated bacterial sepsis[98] have been described as possible etiologic factors. The high incidence of hyperalimentation-induced cholestasis in premature infants was described by Pereira[99] and suggests that the liver immaturity and the tendency to cholestasis observed in premature infants predispose them to this complication. More recently, impaired bile flow from amino acid solutions[100] and abnormal metabolism of bile acids, interfering with the bile salt independent flow,[101] have been suggested as contributing to the development of cholestasis.

The course of the intrahepatic cholestasis has recently been outlined.[99] Clinical improvement beginning two weeks after discontinuation of parenteral nutrition often becomes complete by five months. However, serial liver biopsies revealed that histopathologic changes may not resolve completely by ten months.[102] Attempts to initiate oral feedings and progressively discontinue parenteral nutrition are recommended as the early signs of liver dysfunction are observed.

SUMMARY

Although different nutrients have been administered intravenously to patients for many decades, it has only been during the past 15 years that the concept of TPN was developed and rapidly incorporated into many areas of medicine.

Intravenous supplementation of enteral feedings and TPN are currently used on a routine basis for neonates who are unable to receive milk feedings in the amounts necessary to promote growth.

The nutrient intake and the growth velocity of the fetus are two parameters that are used as standards for providing nutritional recommendations to premature infants. These infants have higher requirements of calories and almost all other nutrients than their full-term counterparts.

Caloric deprivation in the neonate has unique adverse effects on their growth patterns. As such, growth in weight and length are more significantly affected than growth of the head, which is relatively spared. Also, prolonged caloric deprivation has long-term consequences on brain growth, brain function, and somatic growth in neonates.

Major complications of parenteral nutrition in the neonate are related to (1) bacterial infection, (2) arterial catheters, and (3) metabolic derangements. The toxicity, intolerance, and deficiency of almost every component of the hyperalimentation infusate have caused metabolic complications in the neonate.

Overall, the complications of parenteral nutrition can be minimized by following standard recommendations for preparing solutions, caring for the central catheter, and biochemically monitoring the patient.

Despite the wide clinical use of parenteral nutrition and its effectiveness in improving nutritional status, further research is needed to improve the composition of TPN infusates and to better meet the nutritional demands of the neonate.

REFERENCES

1. Bernard, C.: Cited by Dudrick, S. J., and Rhoads, J. E.: New horizons for intravenous feeding. J.A.M.A., 215:939, 1971.
2. Henriques, V., and Andersen, A. C.: Cited by Greenstein, I. P., and Winitz, M.: Chemistry of the amino acid. Vol. 1. New York, John Wiley & Sons, 1961, page 332.
3. Elman, R., and Weiner, D. O.: Intravenous alimentation: With special reference to protein (amino acid) metabolism. J.A.M.A., 112:796, 1939.
4. Dudrick, S. J., Wilmore, D. W., Vars, H. M., et al.: Long-term total parenteral nutrition with growth, development and positive nitrogen balance. Surgery, 64:134, 1968.
5. Heird, W. C., and Winters, R. W.: Total parenteral nutrition. The state of the art. J. Pediatr., 86:2, 1975.
6. Friis-Hansen, B.: Body composition during growth: In vivo measurements and biochemical data correlated to differential anatomical growth. Pediatrics, 47:264, 1971.
7. Widdowson, I. E.: Changes in body proportions and composition during growth. In Davis, I. A., and Dobbing, J. (eds.): Scientific Foundations of Paediatrics. London, William Heinemann Medical Books Ltd., 1974, Chapter 12, page 153.

8. Dobbing, J.: Later growth of the brain. Its vulnerability. Pediatrics, 53:2, 1974.
9. Cashore, W. J., Sedaghatian, M. R., and Usher, R. N.: Nutritional supplements with intravenously administered lipid, protein hydrolysate and glucose in small premature infants. Pediatrics, 56:8, 1975.
10. Hughes, C. A., and Ducker, D. A.: Indications for total parenteral nutrition in preterm infants. Acta Chir. Scand. (Suppl.), 507:282, 1980.
11. Lubchenco, O., Hansman, C., and Boyd, E.: Intrauterine growth in length and head circumference as estimated from liveborn birthweight data at 24 to 42 weeks gestation. Pediatrics, 37:403, 1966.
12. Babson, S. G., and Benda, G. I.: Growth graphs for clinical assessment of infants of varying gestational age. J. Pediatr., 89:814, 1976.
13. Gruenwald, P.: Growth of the human fetus. I. Normal growth and its variation. Am. J. Obstet. Gynecol., 94:1112, 1966.
14. Camerer, W. J. R.: Die chemische Zusammensetzung des Neugeborenen. Z. Biol., 39:173, 1900.
15. Camerer, W. J. R.: Die chemische Zusammensetzung des Neugeborenen Menschen. Z. Biol., 43:1, 1902.
16. Iob, V., and Swanson, W. W.: Mineral growth of the human fetus. Am. J. Dis. Child., 47:302, 1934.
17. Widdowson, E. M., and Spray, C. M.: Chemical development in utero. Arch. Dis. Child., 26:205, 1951.
18. Widdowson, E. M., and Dickerson, J. W. T.: In Cornar, C. L., and Bronner, F. (eds.): Mineral Metabolism. Vol. 2. The Elements. New York, Academic Press, 1964, Part 2A, pages 1–247.
19. Widdowson, E. M.: Chemical composition of newly born mammals. Nature, 166:626, 1950.
20. Fee, B., and Weil, W. M.: Body composition of a diabetic offspring by direct analysis. Am. J. Dis. Child., 100:718, 1960.
21. Loewi, G.: The acid mucopolysaccharides of human skin. Biochem. Biophys. Acta, 52:435, 1961.
22. Shelley, H. J., and Neligan, G. A.: Neonatal hypoglycemia. Br. Med. Bull., 22:34, 1966.
23. Widdowson, E. M., and Spray, C. H.: Chemical development in utero. Arch. Dis. Child., 26:205, 1951.
24. Widdowson, E. M.: Growth and composition of the fetus and newborn. In Assali, N. S. (ed.): Biology of Gestation. New York, Academic Press, 1972, pages 1–44.
25. Dancis, J., and O'Connell, J. R.: A grid for recording the weight of premature infants. J. Pediatr., 33:570, 1948.
26. Cashore, W. J., Sedaghatian, M. R., and Usher, R. N.: Nutritional supplements with intravenously administered lipids, protein hydrolysate and glucose in small premature infants. Pediatrics, 56:8, 1975.
27. Georgieff, M. K., Hoffman, J., and Pereira, G. R.: Minimal nutritional requirements for ideal head growth and weight gain in premature infants. Pediatr. Res., 17(4):313a, 1983.
28. Sher, P. K., and Brown, S. B.: A longitudinal study of head growth in the preterm infant. I. Differentiation between "catchup" head growth and infantile hydrocephalus. Dev. Med. Child. Neurol., 17:711, 1975.
29. Holmes, G. E., Miller, H. C., Hassanein, K., et al.: Postnatal somatic growth in infants with atypical growth patterns. Am. J. Dis. Child., 131:1978, 1977.
30. Johnson, J. D., Albritton, W. C., and Sunshine, P.: Hyperammonemia accompanying parenteral nutrition in newborn infants. J. Pediatr., 81:154, 1972.
31. Winters, R. W., Heird, W. C., Dell, R. B., and Nicholson, J. E.: Plasma amino acids in infants receiving parenteral nutrition. In Green, H. L., Holliday, M. A., and Munro, H. N. (eds.): Clinical Nutrition Update. Chicago, American Medical Association Publishing Co., 1977, pages 147–157.
32. Heird, W. C., Dell, R. B., Driscoll, J. N., Jr., et al.: Metabolic acidosis resulting from intravenous alimentation mixtures containing synthetic amino acids. N. Engl. J. Med., 287:943, 1972.
33. Veleisis, R. A., Inwood, R., and Hunt, C. R.: Prospective controlled study of parenteral nutrition associated cholestatic jaundice: Effect of protein uptake. Pediatrics, 96:893, 1980.
34. Cornblath, M., Wybright, S. H., and Baens, G. S.: Studies on carbohydrate metabolism in the newborn infant. VII. Tests on carbohydrate tolerance in premature infants. Pediatrics, 32:1007, 1963.
35. Kaye, R., Williams, M. L., and Barbero, G.: A comparative study of the metabolism of glucose and fructose in infants. Am. J. Dis. Child., 93:85, 1957.
36. Van den Berghe, G., and Hers, H. G.: Dangers of intravenous fructose and sorbitol. Acta Pediatr. Belg., 31:115, 1978.
37. Pikkarainen, P. H., and Raiha, N. C. R.: Development of alcohol dehydrogenase activity in the human liver. Pediatr. Res., 1:165, 1967.
38. Pereira, G. R., Yudkoff, M., and Moskowitz, S.: Effect of Intralipid therapy on nitrogen retention in premature infants. J.P.E.N., 4:112, 1981.
39. Holman, R. T., Johnson, S. B., and Hatch, T. F.: A case of human linolenic acid deficiency involving neurological abnormalities. Am. J. Clin. Nutr., 35:617, 1982.
40. Shennan, A. T., Bryan, M. H., and Angel, A.: The effect of gestational age on Intralipid tolerance in newborn infants. J. Pediatr., 91:134, 1977.
41. Dhainreddy, R., Hamosh, M., Sivasubramanian, K. N., et al.: Post-heparin lipolytic activity and Intralipid clearance in very low birthweight infants. J. Pediatr., 98:617, 1981.
42. Zaidan, H., Dhainreddy, R., Hamosh, M. et al.: Lipid clearance in premature infants: Role of hepatic lipase. Pediatr. Res., 17(4):297A, 1983.
43. Sigmura, F. C., Brynn, H., and Angel, A.: Post-heparin lipase activity in newborn infants. In Hahn, P., Segal, S., and Israels, S. (eds.): The Role of Fat in Intravenous Feeding of the Newborn. Dorval, Quebec, Pharmacia (Canada) Ltd., 1974, page 129.
44. Filer, R. M., Takada, Y., Carreras, T., and Heim, T.: Serum Intralipid levels in neonates during parenteral nutrition: The relation to gestational age. J. Pediatr. Surg., 15:1405, 1980.
45. Johnson, D. G.: Total intravenous nutrition in newborn surgical patients: A 34 year perspective. J. Pediatr. Surg., 5:601, 1970.
46. Filston, H. C., and Geant, J. P.: A safer system for percutaneous subclavian venous catheterization in newborn infants. Pediatr. Surg., 14:564, 1980.
47. Eichelberger, M. R., Rous, P. G., Hoelzer, D., et al.: Percutaneous subclavian venous catheters in

neonates and children. Pediatr. Surg., 16(1):547, 1981.

48. Felts, S. K., Schaffner, W., Melly, M. A., et al.: Sepsis caused by contaminated intravenous fluids. Epidemiologic, clinical, and laboratory investigation of an outbreak in one hospital. Ann. Intern. Med., 77:881, 1972.

49. Nordenstrom, J., Jarsteand, C., and Wiernik, A.: Decreased chemotactic and random migration of leukocytes during Intralipid infusion. Am. Clin. Nutr., 32:2416, 1979.

50. Fischer, G. W., Wilson, S. R., Hunter, K. W., and Mease, A. D.: Diminished bacterial defenses with Intralipid. Lancet, 2:819, 1980.

51. Friedman, Z., Marks, K. H., Maisels, M. E., et al.: Effect of parenteral fat emulsion on the pulmonary RES in the newborn infant. Pediatrics, 61:694, 1978.

52. Andrew, G., Chan, G., and Schiff, D.: Lipid metabolism in the neonate. I. The effects of Intralipid infusion on plasma triglyceride and free fatty acid concentrations in the neonate. Pediatrics, 88:273, 1976.

53. Mitchell, S. E., and Clark, R. A.: Complications of central venous catheterization. Am. J. Roentgenol., 133:467, 1979.

54. Brady, R. E., and Weinberg, P. M.: Arterioventricular conduction disturbance during total parenteral nutrition. J. Pediatr., 88:113, 1976.

55. Franciosi, R. A., Ellefson, R. D., Uden, D., and Drake, R. M.: Sudden unexpected death during central hyperalimentation. Pediatrics, 69:305, 1982.

56. Pliam, M. B., McGough, E. C., Nixon, G. W., and Rutenberg, H. D.: Right atrial ball valve thrombosis: A complication of central venous alimentation in an infant. J. Thorac. Cardiovasc. Surg., 78:579, 1981.

57. Nichols, M. M., and Tyson, K. R.: Saddle embolus occluding pulmonary arteries. Am. J. Dis. Child., 132:926, 1978.

58. Ryan, J. A., Abel, R. M., Abbott, W. M., et al.: Catheter complications in total parenteral nutrition: A prospective study in 200 consecutive patients. N. Engl. J. Med., 290:757, 1974.

59. Mahoney, L., Snider, A. H., and Silverman, N. H.: Echocardiographic diagnosis of intracardiac thrombi complicating total parenteral nutrition. J. Pediatr., 98:469, 1981.

60. Vain, N. B., Swarney, O. W., and Cha, C. C.: Neonatal chylothorax: A report and discussion of nine consecutive cases. J. Pediatr. Surg., 15:261, 1980.

61. Curei, M., and Dobbins, A. W.: Bilateral chylothorax in a newborn. J. Pediatr. Surg., 15:663, 1980.

62. Kulicarni, P. B., Dorand, R. D., and Simmons, E. M., Jr.: Pericardial tamponade, a complication of total parenteral nutrition. J. Pediatr. Surg., 16:735, 1981.

63. Grebnall, M. J., Blewitt, R. W., and McMahon, M. T.: Cardiac tamponade and central venous catheters. Br. Med. J., 2:595, 1980.

64. Ayalon, A., Borlatzicy, Y., Annev, H., and Schiller, M.: A life-threatening complication of the infusion pump. Lancet, 8:858, 1978.

65. Lam, D. S., Ramus, A. D., and Ratzker, A. C. G., et al.: Paralysis of diaphragm complicating central venous alimentation. Am. J. Dis. Child., 135:382, 1981.

66. Winters, R. W., Heird, W. C., and Dell, R. B.: Parenteral amino acid nutrition in infants. In Grant, J. P., and Young, V. R. (eds.): Amino Acids, Metabolism and Medical Applications. Boston, John Wright–PSG Inc., 1983, page 327.

67. Ghadimi, H., Abaci, F., Kumar, S., et al.: Biochemical aspects of intravenous alimentation. Pediatrics, 48:955, 1971.

68. Heird, W. C., Nicholson, J. F., Driscoll, J. M., et al.: Hyperammonemia resulting from intravenous alimentation using a mixture of synthetic L-amino acids: A preliminary report. J. Pediatr., 81:162, 1972.

69. Dweck, H. S., and Cassady, G.: Glucose intolerance in infants of very low birthweight. I. Incidence of hyperglycemia in infants of birthweight 1,000 grams or less. Pediatrics, 53:189, 1974.

70. Bier, D. M., Leake, R. D., Gruenke, L. D., and Sperling, M. A.: Measurement of deuterium-labelled glucose flux in newborn infants by the continuous isotopic infusion technique. In Klein, P. (ed.): Second International Conference on Stable Isotopes. Argonne, Illinois, Argonne National Laboratory, 1975, pages A–Y.

71. Lagercrantz, H., and Bistoletti, P.: Catecholamine release in the newborn infant at birth. Pediatr. Res., 11:889, 1977.

72. Goldman, S. L., and Hirata, T.: Attenuated response to insulin in very low birthweight infants. Pediatr. Res., 14:50, 1980.

73. James, T., III., Blesa, M., and Boggs, T. R., Jr.: Recurrent hyperglycemia associated with sepsis in a neonate. Am. J. Dis. Child., 133:645, 1979.

74. Vileisis, R. A., Cowett, R. M., and Oh, W.: Glycemia response to lipid infusion in the premature neonate. J. Pediatr., 100:108, 1982.

75. Askanazi, J., Elwyn, D. H., Silverberg, P. A., et al.: Respiratory distress secondary to a high carbohydrate load: A case report. Surgery, 87:596, 1980.

76. Covelli, H. D., Black, J. W., Olsen, M. S., and Beekman, J. F.: Respiratory failure precipitated by high carbohydrate loads. Ann. Intern. Med., 95:579, 1981.

77. Greene, H. L., Hazlett, D., and DeMaree, R.: Relationship between Intralipid-induced hyperlipemia and pulmonary function. Am. J. Clin. Nutr., 29:127, 1976.

78. Greene, H. L.: Effects of Intralipid in the lung. In Winters, R. N., and Hasselmeyer, E. G. (eds.): Intravenous Nutrition in the High Risk Infant. New York, John Wiley & Sons, 1975, pages 369–375.

79. Pereira, G. R., Fox, W. W., Stanley, S. A., et al.: Decreased oxygenation and hyperlipemia during intravenous fat infusions in premature infants. Pediatrics, 66:26, 1980.

80. Schiff, D., Chan, G., Seccombe, D., et al.: Plasma carnitine levels during intravenous feeding of the neonate. J. Pediatr., 95:1043, 1979.

81. Penn, D., Schmidt-Sommerfield, N. D., and Wolf, H.: Carnitine deficiency in premature infants receiving total parenteral nutrition. Early Hum. Dev., 4:23, 1980.

82. Schmidt-Sommerfield, E., Novak, M., Penn, D., et al.: Carnitine and development of newborn adipose tissue. Pediatr. Res., 12:660, 1978.

83. Andrew, G., Chan, G., and Schiff, D.: Lipid metabolism in the neonate. II. The effect of Intralipid on bilirubin binding in vitro and in vivo. J. Pediatr., 88:279, 1976.

84. Shennan, A. R., Cherian, A. G., Angel, A., and

Brynn, M. H.: The effect of Intralipid on the estimation of serum bilirubin in the newborn infant. J. Pediatr., 88:285, 1976.

85. Friedman, S., Danon, A., Stahlman, M. T., et al.: Rapid onset of essential fatty acid deficiency in the newborn. Pediatrics, 58:640, 1976.

86. Friedman, Z., Lamberth, E. L., Stahlman, M. T., and Oates, J. A.: Platelet dysfunction in the neonate with essential fatty acid deficiency. J. Pediatr., 90:439, 1977.

87. Press, M., Hartop, P. J., and Prottey, C.: Correction of essential fatty acid deficiency in man by the cutaneous application of sunflower seed oil. Lancet, 1:597, 1974.

88. Friedman, Z., Shochat, S. J., Maisels, M. J., et al.: Correction of essential fatty acid deficiency in newborn infants by cutaneous application of sunflower seed oil. Pediatrics, 58:650, 1976.

89. Knight, P., Heer, D., and Abdenour, G: Ca × P and Ca/P in parenteral feedings of preterm infants. J.P.E.N., 7:110, 1983.

90. Palma, P. A., Conley, S. B., Crandell, S. S., and Denson, S. E.: Zinc deficiency following surgery in zinc supplemented infants. Pediatrics, 69:800, 1982.

91. Van Rij, A. M., Godfrey, P. T., and McKenzie, J. M.: Amino acid infusions and urinary zinc excretion. J. Surg. Res., 26:293, 1973.

92. Allen, T. M., Maroli, A., II, and Lamont, R. L.: Skeletal changes associated with copper deficiency. Clin. Orthop., 168:206, 1981.

93. Widdowson, E. M., Chan, H., Hawison, G. E., and Milner, R. D. G.: Accumulation of Co, Zn, Mn, Cr, and Cb in the human liver before birth. Biol. Neonate, 20:360, 1972.

94. Jeejeebhoy, K. N., Chu, R. C., Marliss, E. D., et al.: Chromium deficiency, glucose intolerance and neuropathy reversed by chromium supplementation in a patient receiving long-term total parenteral nutrition. Am. J. Clin. Nutr., 30:531, 1977.

95. Johnson, R. A., Baker, S. S., Fallon, J. T., et al.: An accidental case of cardiomyopathy and selenium deficiency. N. Engl. J. Med., 304:1210, 1981.

96. Vileisis, R. A., Inwood, R., and Hunt, C. R.: Prospective controlled study of parenteral nutrition–associated cholestatic jaundice: Effect of protein intake. J. Pediatr., 96:893, 1980.

97. Roger, R., and Finegold, M. J.: Cholestasis in immature newborn infants. Is parenteral alimentation responsible? J. Pediatr., 86:264, 1975.

98. Manginello, F. P., and Javitt, N.: Parenteral nutrition and cholestasis. J. Pediatr., 94:296, 1979.

99. Pereira, G. R., Sherman, M. S., DiGiacomo, J., et al.: Hyperalimentation induced cholestasis: Increased incidence and severity in premature infants. Am. J. Dis. Child., 135:842, 1981.

100. Fouin-Fortunet, H., LeQuernec, L., Erlinger, S., et al.: Hepatic alterations during total parenteral nutrition in patients with inflammatory bowel disease: A possible consequence of lithocholate toxicity. Gastroenterology, 82:932, 1982.

101. Black, D. D., Suttle, E. A., Whitington, P. F., et al.: The effect of short-term total parenteral nutrition on hepatic function. A prospective randomized study demonstrating alteration of hepatic canalicular function. J. Pediatr., 99:445, 1981.

102. Dahms, B. B., and Halpin, T. C., Jr.: Serial liver biopsies in parenteral nutrition–associated cholestasis of early infancy. Gastroenterology, 81:136, 1981.

CHAPTER 42

Parenteral Nutrition in the Pediatric Patient

RAJ N. VARMA
ROBERT M. SUSKIND

Total parenteral nutrition (TPN) has been extensively used in the pediatric patient in whom enteral feeding is impossible, inadequate, or hazardous. TPN has additional significance in the malnourished child, for it provides a means of achieving rapid repletion of lean body mass and resumption of normal body growth, thereby allowing the child to return rapidly to an optimal metabolic state while recovering from illness or injury. Hence, TPN is also becoming increasingly valuable in the long-term management of the pediatric patient.

Despite its proven feasibility and efficacy, one must be concerned about potential metabolic and catheter-related complications. TPN should, therefore, be reserved for those children who cannot be nourished by bolus or continuous tube feeding. It should not be regarded as an alternative to nutrient delivery by the enteral route. In addition, TPN should never be considered a substitute for adequate surgical or medical therapy.

Prior to initiation of TPN, it is important to evaluate the child's underlying nutritional and metabolic state. Conditions of stress, infection, and starvation are known to affect the hormonal and/or metabolic response. The child should be evaluated for such conditions periodically and nutritional support therapy should be modified accordingly. Several important questions should be addressed during implementation of the TPN program: Will TPN be used as the sole nutritional support or as an adjunct to enteral feeding? Will the route of administration be central or peripheral? What will be the composition of the formula with regard to carbohydrate, fat, protein, vitamins, and minerals? What will be the volume of the formulation to be administered over 24 hours and the rate at which it will be administered?

CLINICAL INDICATIONS

The decision as to when and how TPN should be administered to a child ultimately depends on the clinical judgment of the physician responsible for the patient. Pediatric conditions that usually require the administration of TPN are listed in Table 42–1.

TPN has been of particular value in treating patients with congenital anomalies of the gastrointestinal tract[1] and intractable diarrheal syndrome.[2, 3] Since the advent of TPN, mortality from these conditions has decreased from 75 per cent to less than 10 per cent.[4]

Promising results have been obtained using TPN for the treatment of children with Crohn's disease, either alone or as a supplement to oral intake.[5] Marked increase in caloric intake, total body weight, and lean body mass, sustained accelerated growth velocity, and improvement in nitrogen balance have been achieved with TPN.[6] The value of TPN in increasing the weight of patients with ulcerative colitis has also been demonstrated.[7, 8] In patients with inflammatory bowel disease, TPN provides bowel rest, thus facilitating control of symptoms such as abdominal pain, anorexia, weight loss, and diarrhea.[5] TPN therapy also improves healing of fistulas in patients with either surgical complications or inflammatory bowel disease, resulting in closure of fistulas without surgical intervention.[5, 9]

For over a decade, TPN has been a major contributing factor to the improved survival and growth of low-birth-weight (LBW) infants, particularly those weighing less than 1000 gm.[10, 11] It is now feasible to sustain adequate weight gain in LBW infants with TPN as the sole source of nutritional support. However, several questions remain unan-

Table 42–1. PEDIATRIC CONDITIONS THAT USUALLY REQUIRE APPLICATION OF TPN

Congenital anomalies of the gastrointestinal tract (chronic intestinal obstruction due to adhesion or peritoneal sepsis, bowel fistulas, inadequate intestinal length)
Intractable diarrhea (chronic, severe diarrhea)
Inborn errors of metabolism
Chronic diseases in children and adolescents (malignancy, various cardiorespiratory disorders, gastrointestinal diseases, hepatic dysfunction, renal failure, trauma, and/or infection)
Abdominal tumors treated by surgery, irradiation, and chemotherapy
Inflammatory bowel disease
Severe thermal injury
Low birth weight

swered. For example, what is "normal" growth for the LBW infant? What is the composition of the weight gain? How does the IQ of children who received TPN during the neonatal period compare with that of normal children? A detailed discussion of the application of TPN in perinatology appears in Chapter 41.

TPN has been used effectively to treat starvation and cachexia associated with childhood malignancies.[12] Although it is difficult to delineate the role of improved nutrition on the cure rate, there are short-term beneficial effects associated with improved nutrition. The principal reasons for recommending TPN in children with malignancy are anorexia, vomiting, diarrhea, intestinal complications or surgery, and preoperative correction of malnutrition.

Nutritional support for children and adolescents with various chronic disease states such as cardiorespiratory disorders,[4] pancreatic insufficiency,[13] hepatic dysfunction,[14, 15] and renal failure[16] as well as those with trauma and/or infection and severe thermal injury[17] may be successfully accomplished by the intravenous route.

ADMINISTRATION OF TPN

Composition of the Nutrient Infusate

Nonprotein Calories

Glucose is the sole or major source of calories used in TPN infusates. In central parenteral nutrition, glucose solutions are well tolerated up to a concentration of 20 per cent and an infusion rate of 135 ml/kg/day by pediatric patients.[19] In the absence of glucose intolerance, 150 ml/kg/day of the infusate containing 20 per cent glucose may be safely used.[20] To reduce glucose intolerance, glucose may be provided at a concentration of 10 per cent on the first day, 15 per cent the second day, and 20 per cent the third day and thereafter. Fructose, galactose, sorbitol, glycerol, and ethanol all have been used as a source of calories in infants. They offer no advantage over glucose and can produce serious complications in premature infants.

To enhance the caloric value of the infusate and to prevent essential fatty acid deficiency, iso-osmolar fat emulsions (Intralipid 10% or 20%) may be delivered with the glucose–amino acid mixture (containing vitamins, minerals, and trace elements) as tolerated by the child. In peripheral hyperalimentation, glucose solutions exceeding a concentration of 10 per cent cannot easily be infused, and supplemental calories in the form of Intralipid may be provided to meet the energy needs of the infants. Even so, with a fluid and fat intake of 150 ml/kg/day and 4 gm/kg/day, respectively, the maximum caloric delivery that can be achieved is approximately 90 kcal/kg/day. The essential fatty acid requirement of the pediatric patient can be easily met by infusing 0.5 to 1 gm/kg/day of intravenous lipid.

Protein

The source of nitrogen may be fibrin or casein hydrolysate, or one of the synthetic mixtures of amino acids. Commercial preparations of amino acids are available as 3.5 to 10 per cent mixtures that can be diluted to meet the nutritional needs of infants at different ages.[2] These preparations do not contain cysteine, an amino acid considered essential in premature infants because of the decreased activity of hepatic cystathionase, which is involved in the biosynthesis of cysteine.[22] Cysteine is available as a separate preparation that can be added to TPN formulations. Taurine, another amino acid considered important for the premature infant, is also absent from commercial solutions. None of the available solutions contains carnitine, which is required for the optimal oxidation of fatty acids.[23]

Vitamins, Minerals, and Trace Elements

Guidelines for the parenteral use of multivitamin and essential trace element preparations have been established.[24, 25] Current

Table 42–2. RECOMMENDED DIETARY ALLOWANCES AND ESTIMATED SAFE AND ADEQUATE INTAKES OF NUTRIENTS

NUTRIENT	INFANTS (0–1.0 years)	CHILDREN AND ADOLESCENTS		
		1–10 Years	11–18 years	
			MALES	FEMALES
Fat-Soluble Vitamins				
Vitamin A (μg RE)*	400–420	400–700	1000	800
Vitamin D (μg)	10	10	10	10
Vitamin E (mg α-TE)†	3–4	5–7	8–10	8
Vitamin K (μg)‡	12–20	16–60	50–100	50–100
Water-Soluble Vitamins				
Vitamin C (mg)	35	45	50–60	50–60
Thiamin (mg)	0.3–0.5	0.7–1.2	1.4	1.1
Riboflavin (mg)	0.4–0.6	0.8–1.4	1.6–1.7	1.3
Niacin (mg NE)§	6–8	9–16	18	14–15
Vitamin B_6 (mg)	0.3–0.6	0.9–1.6	1.8–2.0	1.8–2.0
Folacin (μg)	30–45	100–300	400	400
Vitamin B_{12} (μg)	0.5–1.5	2.0–3.0	3.0	3.0
Biotin (μg)‡	35–50	65–120	100–300	100–200
Pantothenic acid (mg)‡	2–3	3–5	4–7	4–7
Electrolytes				
Sodium (mg)‡	115–750	325–1800	900–2700	900–2700
Potassium (mg)‡	350–1275	550–3000	1525–4575	1525–4575
Chloride (mg)‡	275–1200	500–2775	1400–4200	1400–4200
Minerals				
Calcium (mg)	360–540	800	1200	1200
Phosphorus (mg)	240–360	800	1200	1200
Magnesium (mg)	50–70	150–250	350–400	300
Iron (mg)	10–15	15–10	18	18
Zinc (mg)	3–5	10	15	15
Iodine (μg)	40–50	70–120	150	150
Trace Elements				
Copper (mg)‡	0.5–1.0	1.0–2.5	2.0–3.0	2.0–3.0
Manganese (mg)‡	0.5–1.0	1.0–3.0	2.5–5.0	2.5–5.0
Fluoride (mg)‡	0.1–1.0	0.5–2.5	1.5–2.5	1.5–2.5
Chromium (mg)‡	0.01–0.06	0.02–0.2	0.05–0.2	0.05–0.2
Selenium (mg)‡	0.01–0.06	0.02–0.2	0.05–0.2	0.05–0.2
Molybdenum (mg)‡	0.03–0.08	0.03–0.3	0.15–0.5	0.15–0.5

*1 μg RE = 1 μg retinol equivalent = 1 μg retinol or 6 μg β-carotene.
†1 mg α-TE = 1 mg α-tocophenol equivalent = 1 mg D-α-tocophenol.
‡Estimated safe and adequate intake. See reference 26 for details.
§1 mg NE = 1 mg niacin equivalent = 1 mg niacin or 60 mg of dietary tryptophan.
(Adapted from National Research Council, Food and Nutrition Board: Recommended Dietary Allowances. Washington, D.C., National Academy of Sciences, 1980.)

recommendations are derived from Recommended Dietary Allowances, which are the best estimates of oral nutritional requirements of healthy people (Table 42–2).[26] Parenteral requirements are estimated after allowing for the efficiency of enteric absorption. No currently available formulation meets all recommendations. Metabolic complications have been derived from deficiencies as well as excesses of some of these nutrients in patients receiving TPN.[27]

Compositions of suitable solutions for central and peripheral vein infusion of infants and children are given in Table 42–3. The suggested amount of calcium is inadequate for optimal bone mineralization in growing children. However, additional calcium may cause precipitation of calcium phosphate. Iron may be added to the intravenous mixture or may be given as a biweekly intramuscular injection of iron dextran. Reduced renal function of the patient may necessitate readjustment of the electrolyte concentration of the infusate.

Catheter Placement and Care

In infants and small children, catheters for central vein TPN are usually inserted through the internal or external jugular vein by cutdown and threaded into the superior vena cava. The subclavian vein may be used in the older children and adolescents. To

Table 42–3. COMPOSITION OF SUITABLE SOLUTIONS FOR TPN IN CHILDREN

NUTRIENT	DAILY AMOUNT (per kg)
Glucose	
For central vein infusate	20–30 gm
For peripheral vein infusate	10–15 gm
Lipid	0.5–3.0 gm
Amino acids (protein hydrolysate or crystalline)	2.5–3.0 gm
Sodium (as chloride)	3–4 mEq
Potassium (as phosphate and chloride)*	2–4 mEq
Calcium (as gluconate)	1–4 mEq
Magnesium (as sulfate)	0.25 mEq
Phosphorus (as potassium phosphate)	1.36 mM
Zinc (as sulfate)	150–300 μg
Copper (as sulfate)	20–40 μg
Multivitamin preparation†	1–3 ml
Volume	
For central vein infusion	120 ml
For peripheral vein infusion	150 ml

*To prevent hyperphosphatemia, potassium, as phosphate, should be limited to 2 mEq/kg/day; additional potassium may be provided as the chloride salt.

†MVI (U.S.V. Pharmaceutical Corp., Tuckahoe, N.Y.) plus folic acid, 1 to 2 mg IM every 2 weeks; vitamin B_{12}, 50 μg IM monthly; vitamin K_1, 1 mg IM every 2 weeks.

(Adapted from Heird, W. C.: Total parenteral nutrition. In Lebenthal, E. (ed.): Textbook of Gastroenterology and Nutrition. New York, Raven Press, 1981, p. 659.)

minimize bloodstream contamination from the skin, the proximal end of the catheter is tunnelled subcutaneously to exit in the parieto-occipital area of the scalp. The catheter should be inserted under strict aseptic conditions, preferably in an operating room or cardiac catheterization laboratory. Specific steps for catheter insertion via the jugular vein are available.[18] A silicon rubber (Silastic) catheter should be used, and the entry of the catheter tip into the vena cava should be verified radiologically by the use of a radiopaque catheter or one filled with contrast material. An antibacterial ointment and sterile dressing are applied to the skin exit site. For peripheral feeding, any vein that can be cannulated may be used.

Meticulous care of the catheter is essential for prolonged complication-free use. The catheter exit site should be dressed at least three times weekly with both a defattening agent and an antiseptic agent (Betadine). The antiseptic ointment should then be reapplied and a fresh occlusive dressing applied. With proper care, a single catheter may be used for up to 90 days.

The nutrient infusate may be delivered from a plastic bag through a calibrated burette. To assume an even flow rate, a constant-flow propulsion pump may be used. A Millipore filter (0.22 m) in the circuit will remove any particulate matter and/or microorganisms that may have contaminated the system. When a fat emulsion is employed, it must be delivered by means of a second pump and mixed with the infusate proximal to the site where the tubing joins the needle. The catheter should never be used for purposes other than infusion of the nutrient solution.

Central versus Peripheral Feeding

Central vein TPN involves the use of hypertonic formulas and is a more logical choice for supporting normal growth and maintaining existing body composition (e.g., in a LBW infant), especially when the clinical course necessitates prolonged (more than two weeks) intravenous infusion. In general, peripheral parenteral nutrition is indicated in patients for whom TPN is required but in whom central vein catheterization is not possible or in whom the catheter has been removed because of sepsis. Peripheral parenteral nutrition may also be useful to meet the nutritional needs of patients being started on total enteral nutrition. In this case, peripheral parenteral nutrition is decreased simultaneously with increasing enteral alimentation.

In most patients (e.g., those with postoperative complications, necrotizing enterocolitis, intractable diarrhea, or surgically correctable lesions), parenteral nutrition may be required for a period of ten to 18 days. Thus, the choice between central and peripheral feeding in these patients is determined by such factors as the extent of nutritional depletion, the duration of illness, and the clinical course prior to initiation of parenteral nutrition.

COMPLICATIONS

Potential complications with the use of TPN fall into two categories—catheter-related and metabolic (Table 42–4).

Catheter-Related Complications

One of the major problems associated with parenteral nutrition therapy is catheter

Table 42–4. COMPLICATIONS OF TPN IN CHILDREN

COMPLICATION	POSSIBLE CAUSE
Catheter-Related	
Malposition	
Pneumothorax	Failure to confirm site of catheter tip
Hemothorax	
Sepsis	Inadequate care of catheter and catheter exit site
Thrombosis	Unknown pump dysfunction
Catheter dislodgement	Unknown
Metabolic	
Hyperglycemia	Excessive glucose concentration
	Increased infusion rate
	Change in metabolic state (e.g., sepsis, surgical stress)
Hypoglycemia	Sudden cessation of infusion
Metabolic acidosis	High acid load of the infusate
Hyperammonemia	Hepatic immaturity
	Subclinical liver disease
	Ammonia in the infusate
	Amino acid imbalance
	Arginine deficiency
Azotemia	Excessive nitrogen intake
Vitamin and mineral disorders	Excessive or inadequate intake
Electrolyte disorders	Excessive or inadequate intake
Essential fatty acid deficiency	Inadequate intake
Abnormal plasma aminogram	Amino acid pattern of intake
Hepatic disorders; cholelithiasis; cholecystitis	Unknown

(Adapted from Heird, W. C.: Total parenteral nutrition. *In* Lebenthal, E. (ed.): Textbook of Gastroenterology and Nutrition. New York, Raven Press, 1981, p. 659).

related sepsis. Bloodstream infection due to bacteria and fungi carried along the catheter or through the infusate may cause infection in the patient. The major cause of infection is improper care of the catheter, especially too-infrequent dressing changes. High incidences of fungal septicemia and death have been reported by some institutions.[28] The likelihood of sepsis appears to be related to the duration of therapy. The early indications of infection are fever, leukocytosis, and/or unexplained glycosuria. Infection is confirmed when microorganisms are cultured from blood obtained through the central ve-nous line. The infection may be treated with antibiotics, usually after removal of the central venous line.

Other catheter-related complications include malposition of the central venous catheter outside the vein, with infusion of hypertonic solutions into the pleural or pericardiac space, catheter dislodgement, thrombophlebitis (due to pump malfunctioning and blood flowing back into the catheter), pneumothorax and brachial plexus injuries, air embolus, and catheter emboli.

Metabolic Complications

Some of the metabolic complications relate to the procedure itself whereas others result from the patient's limited capacity to metabolize various components of the infusate and/or from an inappropriate composition of the infusate. The latter may be easily controlled with appropriate monitoring (Table 42–5).

Hyperglycemia and Hypoglycemia

Glucose intolerance and hyperglycemia have been seen in low-birth-weight, premature infants and in children with renal and central nervous system abnormalities. The acute consequences of glucose intolerance include serum hyperosmolarity and osmotic diuresis. Both of these conditions may be avoided through careful monitoring of the patient. In premature infants, gradually increasing the glucose infusion rate from 5 mg/kg/min to 15 mg/kg/min over a two-day period may reduce the intolerance seen when large amounts of glucose are infused initially. Insulin added to the infusate may lead to unpredictable responses. Therefore, when acute hyperglycemic episodes are managed by this method, close monitoring of the patient's serum glucose level is required. Hypoglycemia may occur when TPN is abruptly stopped. To avoid this complication, the child should be gradually changed from parenteral to enteral alimentation.

Metabolic Acidosis

In low-birth-weight, premature infants and children with renal or hepatic failure, the increased acid load of the TPN solution may lead to metabolic acidosis.[3] The acid-base regulatory mechanisms of the average infant or child are adequate to compensate for the acid load. Frequent monitoring of the blood pH is necessary to avoid acidosis.

Hyperammonemia

Hyperammonemia is another complication that has been reported in infants less than six months of age.[29, 30] Hepatic immaturity or subclinical liver disease may be only one of the reasons for this abnormality. Other factors contributing to this complication may be large quantities of ammonia present in the protein hydrolysate used in the infusate, imbalance of amino acids, and arginine deficiency.[19]

Nutritional Disorders

Hypocalcemia, hypercalcemia, hypophosphatemia, and hyperphosphatemia have all occurred in patients on TPN.[31, 32] Hypomagnesemia causing seizures has been described in several patients. In each case, the patient had prolonged diarrhea prior to the institution of TPN.[19] Seizures were largely eliminated as the magnesium content of the standard infusate was increased.

Pediatric patients maintained on TPN for long periods have been known to develop zinc[33] and copper[34, 35] deficiencies. The clinical features of an acquired zinc deficiency state include skin lesions, diarrhea, and alopecia, and those of copper deficiency include anemia, neutropenia, and fractures. The development of spontaneous biotin deficiency during parenteral alimentation has been reported in a one-year-old girl with short-gut syndrome.[36] The symptoms of biotin deficiency include erythematous rash in the facial areas, loss of body hair, waxy pallor, irritability, lethargy, and mild hypotonia. Chromium deficiency, with glucose intolerance and subjective ataxic and peripheral neuropathy,[37] and carnitine deficiency, with persistently elevated plasma bilirubin levels, reactive hypoglycemia, and generalized skeletal muscle weakness,[38] have been described in adult patients maintained on TPN. These complications could also occur in pediatric patients fed intravenously. Decreased carnitine levels have been reported in neonates and infants receiving TPN.[39, 40] Essential fatty acid deficiency routinely occurs with fat-free parenteral nutrition.[41, 42] However, with the administration of lipid emulsions rich in linoleic acid, essential fatty acid deficiency has been easily avoided.[43]

Hepatic Complications

The single most important gastrointestinal complication of TPN in the pediatric patient is the development of liver disease, presenting clinically as hepatomegaly and jaundice and histologically as cholestasis, hepatocellular necrosis, and, in far advanced cases, cirrhosis or hepatic failure.[44] The etiology remains obscure.[45] The serum transaminase, bilirubin, and alkaline phosphatase levels become elevated, usually two weeks after the initiation of TPN. The longer the infusions are administered, the greater the risk of cholestasis. The liver abnormalities are seen with or without Intralipid and are reversed in most nonadvanced cases after the intravenous feeding is stopped.

Recent evidence suggests that prolonged administration of TPN may induce cholelithiasis and cholecystitis in children.[46] Fasting and aberrant eating patterns may remove the physiologic, neural, and hormonal stimuli that regulate emptying of the gallbladder, resulting in biliary stasis and sequestration of bile salts within the gallbladder. This situation, in addition to an early expansion of the bile salt pool, may result in biliary sludge and development of calcium bilirubinate stones.

Other Gastrointestinal Complications

Much less is known about the long-term effects of TPN on gastric, pancreatic, and small bowel structure and function. Animal studies show pancreatic hyposecretion and intestinal mucosal atrophy, which are reversible on the resumption of enteric feeding.[47] Similar observations have been made in human subjects.[48]

Enteral feeding should be initiated as soon as the gastrointestinal tract is functional. Initially, enteral feeding may act as a supplement to TPN, which should be continued until the patient is able to tolerate enteral feedings well enough to meet nutritional requirements.

Potential Hazards of Intravenous Fat Emulsions

For several reasons, fat emulsions have found widespread use in the parenteral support of pediatric patients. Fat has the highest caloric density of any nutrient. Intravenously infused fat emulsions exert negligible osmotic effects and make it possible to deliver adequate calories solely by peripheral vein, thus avoiding the use of the central vein catheter in many patients. Fat emulsions also provide essential fatty acids.

Several potential hazards associated with the use of intravenous fat emulsions need to be more fully evaluated. Less mature infants are unable to dispose of the infused lipid as rapidly as mature infants.[49, 50] The malnourished child tolerates these products less well than the normal child. Failure to "clear" the infused emulsion may have an adverse effect on pulmonary diffusion capacity.[51] In addition, hyperlipemia may partially block reticuloendothelial function,[52, 53] alter erythrocyte membrane composition, and enhance red cell platelet clumping.[54-56] Thus, infants with either infection or pulmonary disease should receive intravenous fat emulsions only under conditions that guarantee normolipemia.[57, 58]

Even with adequate metabolism of the infused fat, the released free fatty acids may displace albumin-bound bilirubin.[59-61] Infants with plasma bilirubin concentrations greater than 8 to 10 mg/100 ml (assuming an albumin concentration of 2.5 to 3 gm/100 ml) should not receive more parenteral fat emulsion than is required to meet the essential fatty acid requirement, i.e., 0.5 to 1.0 gm/kg/day.

The accumulation of "intravenous fat pigment" in the reticuloendothelial cells of the liver, spleen, bone marrow, and lymph nodes has been known for several years in human subjects given fat emulsions intravenously.[62] No gross abnormalities of either hepatic or reticuloendothelial function have been observed in such patients, and the deposition of the pigment in the tissue apparently imposes no serious complications.[63]

Serum concentrations of triglycerides, phospholipid, and cholesterol all increase with the chronic administration of intravenous fat emulsions.[64-67] These changes appear to be transient and *per se* do not usually pose any serious threat to the health of the recipient of these products.

The high content of linoleic acid in the intravenous fat emulsions results in elevated levels of this fatty acid in both plasma and tissue lipids. Despite the high linoleic acid levels, plasma arachidonic acid levels and tissue lipid levels are similar to those observed in essential fatty acid deficiency.[43] In addition, the urinary excretion of prostaglandin E metabolites by infants receiving soybean oil emulsion is similar to that of infants with EFA deficiency and lower than that of control infants.

MONITORING

Careful monitoring is essential if the full potential of TPN is to be realized. A suggested schedule of monitoring of patients on TPN is presented in Table 42–5. Such a schedule obviously requires that the patient initially be housed in a unit where continuous nursing care is available.

Routine monitoring of blood glucose is not included in the schedule. If the urine is free of glucose, it may be safe to assume that the blood glucose concentration is not sufficiently high to cause problems. Routine plasma aminograms are not recommended, because (1) this determination is expensive and difficult to obtain and (2) some derangement of the plasma aminogram is seen with all available mixtures of amino acids. Visual inspection or nephelometry should be performed for the presence of lipemia. Serum triglyceride and free fatty acid concentrations may be determined, providing that microtechniques for these assays are available.

CONCLUSIONS

TPN, when properly used, is an extremely valuable technique in pediatric patients in whom gastrointestinal function is compromised or absent. Attention must be directed toward patient selection and management so as to assure that patients are not unnecessarily exposed to this potentially hazardous procedure. To fully understand the benefits and limitations of TPN in pediatric patients, further research is needed in several areas. These areas include the effects of nutritional support on the growth and development of individual organs, composition of "growth" tissue gained during TPN therapy, the effects of long-term TPN on IQ, development of noninvasive methods for the assessment of nutritional status, and the determination of the contribution of malnutrition to the morbidity associated with various acute and chronic disease states such as cancer, heart disease, and respiratory, hepatic, and renal disorders. It is essential to establish clearly the beneficial effects of nutritional support in reducing mortality and morbidity in such patients, to determine the nutrient

Table 42–5. SUGGESTED SCHEDULE OF MONITORING DURING TPN OF PEDIATRIC PATIENTS

| | SUGGESTED FREQUENCY (TIMES PER WEEK) | |
VARIABLE MONITORED	*Initial Period**	*Later Period*†
Weight	7	7
Height (length)	1	1
Head circumference (for infants)	1	1
Serum glucose	‡	‡
Serum sodium, potassium, and chloride	3–4	1
Serum calcium, magnesium, and phosphorus	2	1
Serum acid-base status	3–4	1
Serum ammonia	2	1
Serum area nitrogen	2	1
Serum protein (electrophoresis or albumin/globulin)	1	1
Liver function studies	1	1
Hemoglobin	2	2
Urine glucose	2–6/day	2/day
Clinical observations (activity, temperature, etc.)	Daily	Daily
WBC count and differential count	As indicated	As indicated
Cultures	As indicated	As indicated
Serum triglyceride	As indicated	As indicated

*Initial period is time before full glucose intake is achieved or any period of metabolic instability.
†Later period is time during which patient is in a metabolic steady state.
‡Blood glucose should be monitored closely during period of glucosuria (to determine degree of hyperglycemia) and for 2 to 3 days after cessation of parenteral nutrition (to detect hypoglycemia). Dextrostix determinations are useful for monitoring for hypoglycemia.
(Adapted from Heird, W. C.: Total parenteral nutrition. *In* Lebenthal, E. (ed.): Textbook of Gastroenterology and Nutrition. New York, Raven Press, 1981, p. 659.)

requirements in various diseases, and to evaluate the safety and efficacy of intravenously administered fat in reference to the pathophysiology of hepatic dysfunction frequently found in very young patients who received parenteral nutrition.

REFERENCES

1. Filler, R. M., Eraklis, A. J., Rubin, V. G., et al.: Long term parenteral nutrition in infants. N. Engl. J. Med., *281*:589, 1969.
2. Keating, J. P., and Ternberg, J. L.: Amino acid-hypertonic glucose treatment for intractable diarrhea in infants. Am. J. Dis. Child., *122*:123, 1971.
3. Heird, W. C., and Winters, R. W.: Total parenteral nutrition. The state of the art. J. Pediatr., *86*:2, 1975.
4. Heird, W. C.: Panel report on nutritional support of pediatric patients. Am. J. Clin. Nutr., *34*:1223, 1981.
5. Grand, R. J.: Model for the treatment of growth failure in children with inflammatory bowel disease. *In* Suskind, R. M. (ed.): Textbook of Pediatric Nutrition. New York, Raven Press, 1981, p. 483.
6. Grand, R. J., Shew, G., Werlin, S. L., et al.: Reversal of growth arrest in Crohn's disease: A new approach. Pediatr. Res., *11*:444, 1977.
7. Franklin, F. A., and Grand, R. J.: The use of parenteral nutrition for the management of inflammatory bowel disease in childhood and adolescence. *In* Romieu, C., Solassol, C., Joyeaux, H., et al. (eds.): Proceedings, International Congress

on Parenteral Nutrition. Montpelier, France, University of Montpelier Press, 1976, p. 583.
8. Werlin, S. L., and Grand, R. J.: Severe colitis in children and adolescents: Diagnosis, course and treatment. Gastroenterology, *73*:828, 1977.
9. Byrne, W. J., and Ament, M. E.: Home parenteral nutrition: Results of its use in the management of enterocutaneous and hectovaginal fistulas. J.P.E.N., *3*:25, 1979.
10. Peden, V. H., and Karpel, J. T.: Total parenteral nutrition in premature infants. J. Pediatr., *81*:137, 1972.
11. Driscoll, J. M., Jr., Heird, W. C., Schullinger, J. N., et al.: Total intravenous alimentation in low-birthweight infants. A preliminary report. J. Pediatr., *81*:145, 1972.
12. Filler, R. M., Jaffe, N., Cassady, J. E., et al.: Parenteral nutritional support in children with cancer. Cancer, *39*:2665, 1977.
13. Schwachman, H.: Nutritional considerations in the treatment of children with cystic fibrosis. *In* Suskind, R. M. (ed.): Textbook of Pediatric Nutrition. New York, Raven Press, 1981, p. 511.
14. Cohen, M. I., Boley, S. J., Daum, F., et al.: The role and effect of parenteral nutrition on the liver and its use in chronic inflammatory bowel disease in childhood. *In* Bode, H. H., and Washaw, J. B. (eds.): Parenteral Nutrition in Infancy and Childhood. New York, Plenum Press, 1974, p. 214.
15. Watkins, J. B.: Nutritional considerations in treatment of liver diseases in children. *In* Suskind, R. M. (ed.): Textbook of Pediatric Nutrition. New York, Raven Press, 1981, p. 493.
16. Fischer, J. E.: Parenteral nutrition of renal disease. *In* Bode, H. H., and Warshaw, J. B. (eds.): Par-

enteral Nutrition in Infancy and Childhood. New York, Plenum Press, 1974, p. 225.

17. Postuma, R.: Nutrition in pediatric surgical patients. *In* Pediatric Nutrition Handbook. American Academy of Pediatrics, 1979, p. 335.

18. Dudrick, S. J., and Copeland, E.: Parenteral hyperalimentation. *In* Nyhus, L. M. (ed.): Surgery Annual. New York, Appleton-Century-Crofts, 1973, p. 69.

19. Filler, R. M.: Parenteral support of the surgically ill child. *In* Suskind, R. M. (ed.): Textbook of Pediatric Nutrition. New York, Raven Press, 1981, p. 341.

20. Pediatric Parenteral Nutrition Manual. Boston, Children's Service, Massachusetts General Hospital, 1983.

21. Ghadim, H.: Newly devised amino acid solutions for intravenous administration. *In* Ghadim, H. (ed.): Total Parenteral Nutrition, Premises and Promises. New York, John Wiley & Sons, 1975, P. 393.

22. Sturman, J. A., Gaull, G., and Raiha, N. C. R.: Absence of cystathionase in human fetal liver: Is cystine essential? Science, *169*:74, 1970.

23. Schiff, D., Chan, G., Secombe, D., et al.: Plasma carnitine levels during intravenous feeding of the neonate. J. Pediatr., *95*:1043, 1979.

24. American Medical Association, Department of Food and Nutrition: Multivitamin preparations for parenteral use: A statement by the Nutrition Advisory Group. J.P.E.N., *3*:258, 1979.

25. American Medical Association, Nutrition Advisory Group: Guidelines for essential trace element preparations for parenteral use. J.P.E.N., *3*:263, 1979.

26. National Research Council, Food and Nutrition Board: Recommended Dietary Allowance, 9th ed. Washington, D.C., National Academy of Sciences, 1980.

27. Shils, M. E.: Parenteral nutrition. *In* Goodhart, R. S., and Shils, M. E. (eds.): Modern Nutrition in Health and Disease, 6th ed. Philadelphia, Lea & Febiger, 1980, p. 1125.

28. Curry, C. R., and Quie, P. G.: Fungal septicemia in patients receiving parenteral hyperalimentation. N. Engl. J. Med., *285*:1221, 1971.

29. Ghadimi, G. H., Abaci, F., Kumar, S., et al.: Biochemical aspects of intravenous alimentation. Pediatrics, *48*:955, 1971.

30. Johnson, J. C., Albritton, W. L., and Sunshine, P.: Hyperammonemia accompanying parenteral nutrition in newborn infants. J. Pediatr., *81*:154, 1972.

31. Shils, M. E.: Guidelines for total parenteral nutrition. J.A.M.A., *220*:1721, 1972.

32. Special Communications: Guidelines for essential trace element preparations for parenteral use. A Statement by an Expert Panel. J.A.M.A., *241*:2051, 1979.

33. Hambidge, M.: Trace element deficiencies in childood. *In* Suskind, R. M. (ed.): Textbook of Pediatric Nutrition. New York, Raven Press, 1981, p. 163.

34. Ashkenazi, A., Levin, S., Djaldetti, M., et al.: The syndrome of neonatal copper deficiency. Pediatrics, *52*:525, 1973.

35. Karpel, J. T., and Peden, V. H.: Copper deficiency in long-term parenteral nutrition. J. Pediatr., *80*:32, 1972.

36. Mock, D. M., deLorimer, A. A., Liebman, W. M., et al.: Biotin deficiency: An unusual complication of parenteral alimentation. N. Engl. J. Med., *304*:820, 1981.

37. Jeejeebhoy, K. N., Chu, R. C., Marliss, E. B., et al.: Chromium deficiency, glucose intolerance and neuropathy reversed by chromium supplementation in a patient receiving long-term total parenteral nutrition. Am. J. Clin. Nutr., *30*:531, 1977.

38. Worthley, L. I. G., Fishlock, R. C., and Snoswell, A. M.: Carnitine deficiency with hyperbilirubinemia, generalized skeletal muscle weakness and reactive hypoglycemia in a patient on long-term total parenteral nutrition. Treatment with intravenous L-carnitine. J.P.E.N., *7*:176, 1983.

39. Schiff, D., Chang, G., Seccombe, D., et al.: Plasma carnitine levels during intravenous feeding of the neonate. J. Pediatr., *95*:1043, 1979.

40. Penn, D., Sommerfeld, E. S., Pascu, F.: Decreased tissue carnitine concentrations in newborn infants receiving total parenteral nutrition. J. Pediatr., *98*:976, 1981.

41. Paulsrud, J. R., Pensler, L., Whitten, C. F., et al.: Essential fatty acid deficiency in infants induced by fat-free intravenous feedings. Am. J. Clin. Nutr., *25*:897, 1972.

42. Friedman, Z., Danon, A., Stahlman, M. T., et al.: Rapid onset of essential fatty acid deficiency in the newborn. Pediatrics, *58*:640, 1976.

43. Friedman, A., and Frolich, J. C.: Essential fatty acids and major urinary metabolites of the E prostaglandins in thriving neonates and infants receiving parenteral fat emulsions. Pediatr. Res., *13*:932, 1979.

44. Cohen, M. I.: changes in hepatic function in intravenous nutrition. *In* Winters, R. W., and Hasselmeyer, E. (eds.): Intravenous nutrition in the high risk infant. New York, John Wiley & Sons, 1975, p. 295.

45. Sondheimer, J. M., Bryan, H., Andrews, W., et al.: Cholestatic tendencies in premature infants on and off parenteral nutrition. Pediatrics, *62*:984, 1978.

46. Roslyn, J. J., Berquist, W. E., Pitt, H. A., et al.: Increased risk of gallstones in children receiving total parenteral nutrition. Pediatrics, *71*:784, 1983.

47. Feldman, E. J., Dowling, R. H., McNaughton, J., et al.: Effects of oral versus intravenous nutrition on intestinal adaptation after small bowel resection in the dog. Gastroenterology, *70*:712, 1976.

48. Kolter, D. P., and Levine, G. M.: Reversible gastric and pancreatic hyposecretion after long-term total parenteral nutrition. N. Engl. J. Med., *300*:271, 1979.

49. Gustafson, A., Kjellman, I., Olegård, R., et al.: Nutrition in low-birth-weight infants. I: Intravenous injection of fat emulsions. Acta Pediatr. Scand., *61*:149, 1972.

50. Shennan, A. T., Bryan, M. H., and Angel, A.: The effect of gestational age on Intralipid tolerance in newborn infants. J. Pediatr., *91*:134, 1977.

51. Greene, H. L., Hazlett, D., and Demarec, R.: Relationship between Intralipid-induced hyperlipidemia and pulmonary function. Am. J. Clin. Nutr., *29*:127, 1976.

52. DeLuzio, N. R., and Wooles, W. R.: Depression of phagocytic activity and immune response by methyl palmitate. Am. J. Physiol., *296*:939, 1964.

53. Nordenstrom, J., Jarstrand, C., and Wiernik, A.:

Decreased chemotactic and random migration of leukocytes during Intralipid infusion. Am. J. Clin. Nutr., 32:2416, 1979.

54. Bagdade, J. D., and Ways, P. O.: Erythrocyte membrane lipid composition in exogenous and endogenous hypertriglyceridemia. J. Lab. Clin. Med., 75:53, 1970.

55. Cullen, C. F., and Swank, R. L.: Intravascular aggregation and adhesiveness of the blood elements associated with alimentary lipemia and injections of large molecular substances: Effect on blood-brain barrier. Circulation, 9:335, 1954.

56. Branemark, P. I., and Lindstrom, J.: Microcirculatory effects of emulsified fat infusions. Circ. Res., 15:124, 1964.

57. McKee, K. T., Melly, M. A., Greene, H. L., et al.: Gram-negative bacillary sepsis associated with use of lipid emulsion in parenteral nutrition. Am. J. Dis. Child., 133:649, 1979.

58. Fischer, G. W., Hunter, K. W., and Wilson, S. R.: diminished bacterial defences with 'Intralipid'. Lancet, 2:819, 1980.

59. Thiessen, H., Jacobsen, J., and Brodersen, R.: Displacement of albumin-bound bilirubin by fatty acids. Acta Pediatr. Scand., 61:285, 1972.

60. Jacobsen, J.: Binding of bilirubin to human serum albumin. F.E.B.S. Lett., 5:112, 1969.

61. Starinsky, R., and Shafrir, E.: Displacement of albumin-bound bilirubin by free fatty acids: Implications for neonatal hyperbilirubinemia. Clin. Chim. Acta, 29:311, 1970.

62. Thompson, S. L.: Histologic and ultrastructural changes following intravenous administration of fat emulsions. In Meng, H. C., and Law, D. H. (eds.): Parenteral Nutrition. Springfield, Charles C Thomas Publisher, 1970, p. 408.

63. Levene, M. I., Wigglesworth, J. S., and Desai, R.: Pulmonary fat accumulation after 'Intralipid' infusion in the preterm infant. Lancet, 2:815, 1980.

64. Thompson, G. R., Segura, R., Hoff, H., et al.: contrasting effects of plasma lipoproteins of intravenous versus oral administration of a triglyceride-phospholipid emulsion. Eur. J. Clin. Invest., 5:373, 1975.

65. Broviac, J. W., Riella, M. C., and Scribner, B. H.: The role of Intralipid in prolonged parenteral nutrition. I: As a calorie substitute for glucose. Am. J. Clin. Nutr., 29:255, 1976.

66. Franklin, F. A., Jr., Watkins, J. B., Heafitz, L., et al.: Serum lipids during total parenteral nutrition with Intralipid (abstracted). Pediatr. Res., 10:354, 1976.

67. Press, M., Kikuchi, H., Shimoyama, T., et al.: Diagnosis and treatment of essential fatty acid deficiency in man. Br. Med. J., 2:247, 1974.

68. Heird, W. C.: Total parenteral nutrition. In Lebenthal, E. (ed.): Textbook of Gastroenterology and Nutrition. New York, Raven Press, 1981, p. 659.

CHAPTER 43

Home Parenteral Nutrition in Infants and Children

MARVIN E. AMENT

HISTORY OF HOME PARENTERAL NUTRITION

Home parenteral nutrition is a technique that was first described by Dr. Belding Scribner at the University of Washington in 1970.[1] Dr. Scribner referred to home parenteral nutrition by the name of "the artificial gut." The initial patients he put on the system had Crohn's disease with short-bowel syndrome or diffuse small-bowel disease, or both. This was followed by the description of a technique by others, including Dr. Jeejeebhoy in Toronto, Dr. Salassol in France, and ourselves in Los Angeles.[2-9]

In all instances, the techniques for intravenous nutritional support at home were developed because patients were being kept hospitalized solely to receive intravenous fluids and nutrition.

Two of the original patients studied by Dr. Scribner were children. One patient was a nine-year-old girl with diffuse mast cell disease in whom the intestinal lining was replaced by flat mucosa, and the other was a boy with end-stage acrodermatitis enteropathica.

Silastic Catheters

Initially, Dr. Scribner tried to use arterial venous shunts to administer the solutions. However, the shunts became easily thrombosed by the hypertonic dextrose and protein solutions that were used. This problem led to the development of a semipermanent Silastic catheter that made it possible to deliver the solutions to the central venous circulation.

The use of Silastic catheters had many advantages, for example, greater flexibility in the catheter, reduced risk of catheter brittleness, and decreased thrombogenicity. Dr. Scribner, in conjunction with Dr. John Broviac, developed a special Silastic catheter that had a Dacron cuff at its midpoint, which allowed the catheter to become adherent to the chest or the abdominal wall once it was implanted in the central venous circulation. The Dacron cuff precipitated a fibrous reaction around it, which resulted in its becoming securely fixed in place. The catheter's other advantage was its Luer lock adaptor, which had only to be closed off when not being used for the administration of parenteral nutrition. The catheter was filled with a heparin and saline solution when it was not in use to prevent clotting. The catheter's other advantage was its ability to be spliced if it cracked or was cut.

Until 1975, there were no catheters specifically developed for infants who required home parenteral nutrition. The miniaturized Broviac catheter became available in 1976. Once this happened, it was feasible to find out if infants could be managed on a home total parenteral nutrition (TPN) program.[10]

Prior to the development of the infant Broviac catheter, older children had standard Broviac catheters placed for home care.

INDICATIONS FOR HOME PARENTERAL NUTRITION IN INFANTS AND CHILDREN

Short-bowel syndrome is the most frequent condition associated with the need for home TPN. It occurs because of either congenital intestinal atresias or malrotation and volvulus with strangulation, or it can develop secondary to resections performed because of necrotizing enterocolitis. Rare youngsters may have congenital short intestine.

Crohn's disease in the pediatric age group rarely leads to multiple and massive intestinal resection; however, there is an occasional patient in whom this occurs as well as those patients who have diffuse small-bowel disease that is refractory to medical management.

Chronic idiopathic intestinal pseudo-obstruction syndrome is another condition in which home TPN has made the difference between life and death. This is a chronic motility disorder that can present in the neonatal period, during infancy, or later in childhood. These youngsters have either a defect in the intramural plexuses of nerves or a degenerative process of the smooth muscle. Children with the congenital form of the disease are often misdiagnosed as having total aganglionosis because they develop bilious vomiting and microcolon. Many of these youngsters are operated on two or three times before the condition is recognized. Typically, they are operated on for obstruction and are given an ileostomy to relieve it, but the intestinal contents fail to be delivered through the ostomy. They often undergo a second operative procedure to explore for adhesions before the physicians become aware of the lack of intestinal motility. Some children with this condition who require home TPN do not become symptomatic until later.

Rare infants develop obstruction secondary to prior intra-abdominal surgeries that lead to intestinal resection.

Some youngsters are born without functional intestinal villi. These cases are rare. Some are familial. These patients usually do not improve with the passage of time. Typically, they have diarrhea from birth and have difficulty with even the simplest of nutrients. If a physician recognizes this type of condition shortly after birth, the youngster should have an upper gastrointestinal and small-bowel series as well as intestinal biopsies performed in an attempt to confirm the le-

sion. This is one reason why youngsters who develop diarrhea even with feeding of dextrose and electrolytes should have these studies done. Children with intra-abdominal malignancies occasionally require home parenteral nutrition, because of damage resulting to the intestine from radiation therapy and intra-abdominal operative procedures. In some, the need for parenteral nutrition is temporary; in others it is life-long. Some patients have obstruction to the gastrointestinal tract from intra-abdominal and intraintestinal malignancy. Some of these patients may benefit from chemotherapy. In such youngsters, parenteral support at home may allow them to survive while these therapies are attempted.

Patients with immunodeficiency disorders of the combined type or those with selective IgA deficiency may require prolonged parenteral support because of intractable diarrhea. In some of these youngsters, a severe mucosal lesion develops for which no specific cause can be found. Patients such as these should be carefully evaluated for giardiasis, strongyloidiasis, cryptosporidium, cytomegalovirus, and chronic rotovirus excretion. Some of these conditions are treatable and result in improved digestion and absorption, whereas there is no specific treatment available for other conditions.

Cystic fibrosis is another condition in which the placement of a Broviac catheter may be used both to support the nutrition of the patient and as a means for providing home antibiotics.

Intestinal lymphangiectasia is typically thought of as a condition that can be managed by dietary means. However, a substantial number of these patients do not benefit from low-fat diets with medium-chain triglycerides. Their ascites persists as does their diarrhea and malabsorption. These patients may benefit from parenteral support on a long-term basis at home.

Communication with Parents

The physician who decides to place the patient on a home TPN program should discuss with the parents what it is hoped will be accomplished by such a program. The benefits as well as the risks to the patient should be discussed. Complications and the possibility of death must be mentioned.

When patients have had intestinal resection, the physician may indicate that the youngster may achieve intestinal adaptation if supported for a sufficient length of time. However, it is an established fact that a youngster who has an infarct or an atresia of the entire jejunum and ileum is never going to adapt and will be on a home TPN program for the rest of his or her life.

Ninety per cent of children who have at least 40 cm of small intestine and an intact ileocecal valve will eventually be able to discontinue parenteral support. Those children who have an intact ileocecal valve and 15 to 20 cm of small intestine may ultimately adapt completely, but they will definitely have partial adaptation.

ESTABLISHING A PATIENT ON A HOME TPN PROGRAM

Once a decision is made to place a patient on such a program, the surgeon places a central venous catheter in the femoral saphenous, subclavian, or external jugular vein. In female infants and children, the femoral saphenous vein placement is more commonly used because of the cosmetic effect. Catheters placed in this region do not have a greater risk of becoming infected, nor is this placement better than in other areas.

The size of the Broviac catheter used depends in part on the size of the child and the major vein as well as the purposes for which the central catheter will be used. A Hickman catheter is a larger version of the Broviac catheter. It has a greater internal as well as external diameter and is typically used for four purposes: (1) TPN, (2) administration of drug products, (3) obtaining blood samples, and (4) giving chemotherapy. The Broviac catheter is smaller than the Hickman catheter and is designed specifically for infants and younger children, as already discussed. Physicians should be aware that there is an infant Broviac catheter as well as a standard Broviac catheter. Both of these catheters have screw caps and Luer locks. These caps can be reused if sterilized each day in 1.5 per cent formalin, or disposable ones may be substituted each day. The catheter is filled with heparin and saline each day after being used.

Planning the Solutions for Home Use

The determination of the patient's nutritional requirements is based on the expected weight and height of the patient according to age. Fluid requirements are determined by the patient's clinical condition as well as by anthropometric measurements. We try to provide 25 per cent of the energy calories in the form of a fat emulsion to decrease the risk of liver dysfunction. The remainder of the energy calories are derived from glucose. The determination of electrolytes, trace metals, and vitamins to be added are based on the patient's weight and height. Additional electrolytes and minerals may be necessary, depending on the losses. A vial of a multiple-vitamin infusion for children is used because it contains all the necessary vitamins, including vitamin K.

Infusion Time

Initially, the patient is established on a 24-hour infusion in the hospital. Once the maximal concentration of dextrose solution and the maximal amount of fat to be used is reached, we begin to decrease the number of hours of support by one hour/day, but the rate of administration is increased to keep the volume administered constant. Over a period of 12 to 13 days, the duration of the infusion is decreased to 10 to 12 hours. We attempt to infuse all solutions during the night-time. This allows the patient a maximal amount of time to be free from being attached to an infusion system.

At the end of the infusion, the rate of administration is reduced twice by 50 per cent over a period of 30 minutes. Occasional patients require the infusion rate to be reduced over an hour's time. Some school-aged children are able to participate in and perform a portion of their care. Occasionally, youngsters 10 years old have been taught to perform all their care except for the hanging of the plastic bags containing the solution. Certainly most teenagers, unless they are critically ill, can perform all of the care required for their support.

In the case of the infant, it is the parent or parents who are required to learn the techniques for home TPN. The parent or parents are given a booklet to read on the techniques. They are shown a video tape of how the techniques are performed and are given a demonstration by our nurses. They work on a mannequin under the supervision of our nurses until their techniques are perfected, after which they are allowed to work with their own child under supervision.

Once they have demonstrated successfully to the nurses that the techniques have been mastered for both stopping and starting parenteral nutrition, they are put in a room alone with their child. They stay overnight in the hospital for a period of three days to practice both starting and stopping parenteral support. If they have need for a nurse, they can always call for one. In this way, the infant or child is prepared for going home. The parents are taught the problems they may encounter as well as emergency situations and how to act if they occur.

Planning Discharge

The family must decide whether to mix their own solutions or use premixed ones. Solutions mixed in the home have only two advantages: (1) they require no extra refrigeration and (2) they may be potentially less expensive. In contrast, it takes 30 to 45 minutes to mix the solution; therefore it reduces the amount of time available for other activities. Premixed solutions must be kept refrigerated but are typically good for 60 days in storage.

Our social worker goes to the home of the patient to assess it for cleanliness and to determine the amount of storage space available for supplies. The typical family takes home 30 days worth of supplies. A family may choose to pick up supplies and solutions or have them delivered. In our institution, we provide such a service. Other commercial home parenteral nutritional services provide similar services. The family may have to purchase additional refrigeration space because of the needs of the patient who requires home parenteral nutrition.

Before the patient is discharged, the family is given a group of telephone numbers to call in case of emergency. They are given the 24-hour phone number of the physicians and are also provided with the phone number of the hospital paging service if they should fail to get a response from the physicians. Physicians who care for such patients must work out an arrangement with another physician or nurse or both, to be available for such patients 24 hours a day 7 days a week.

The families must be instructed that if no one is reachable by telephone and their youngster is febrile, they should bring the patient to the hospital to be examined.

Ongoing Care

Following discharge from the hospital, the patient is usually seen within one week. At that and subsequent visits, anthropometric measurements are taken, and the nutritional support received is recalculated to determine if there is a need to change any of the nutrients.

Pediatric patients differ from adults in that their weight and height is constantly changing. This is the reason for the continuous attention given to anthropometric determinations and for following the patient along growth channels. Subsequent visits during the first month after discharge are on an alternate-week basis. If the patient is stable, subsequent visits will be on a monthly basis through the first year of life, and every two to three months thereafter. Laboratory tests performed at each visit should consist of a complete blood count (CBC), and electrolyte, calcium, and magnesium determinations. Serum protein and albumin determinations should also be done. A CBC should always be performed. Trace metal determinations should be done twice a year. Liver function tests should be done quarterly. These determinations are all necessary for the optimal management of the patient.

In home parenteral nutrition patients who have some functioning of the intestine, an attempt should always be made to feed him or her the proportion of calories that can be readily digested and absorbed. At times, this means that there is a risk that the patient will not get all the calories and nutrients necessary. However, it is necessary to do this in order to ensure maximal stimulation of the gastrointestinal tract for growth. We believe that any infant started on parenteral nutrition from the time of birth should have enteral nutrition provided as early as possible and in amounts compatible with their digestion and absorption capabilities.

COMPLICATIONS OF HOME TPN

Sepsis

Sepsis is the most serious and frequent complication of home TPN.[11, 13, 14] In all instances, complications are usually due to some known or unsuspected break in the technique for which the patients or parents were instructed.[12] In infants and preschool children, fever can occur not only from breaks in the technique of administering the parenteral nutrition but also from usual childhood illnesses. This is why physicians who care for children must carefully examine them each time a fever develops in order to try and identify its source. If there is no recognizable source, the most likely possibility is either a catheter infection or a viremia. Each time a patient develops a fever, we take a careful history to determine if there are any simple explanations. Parents are always asked to bring the child in for an examination, which must be done carefully. The parents must be questioned carefully concerning the routine they have used for catheter care in administering the solution. They should be asked if they are aware of any lapse in technique that may have occurred.

If there is no obvious source of infection, the patient should have blood cultures drawn from both the catheter and the peripheral veins if possible. A CBC with a differential count should be done as should a urinalysis.

Other tests would depend on the clinical findings and suspicions of the examining physician.

If a specific source of infection is identified, the patient should be treated appropriately. If an infant or child on home TPN develops otitis media or streptococcal pharyngitis, antibiotic therapy should be started.

In those patients who have insufficient intestine to absorb antibiotics and other oral medications, the home parenteral nutrition nurses should teach the parents how to administer antibiotics intravenously. Frequently, we attempt to use antibiotics that can be given three times/day in order to minimize the number of times the line must be entered.

Typically, we admit the patient to the hospital for the first two days of antibiotic therapy and until we can educate the parents in the means of giving the antibiotics. Once this has been mastered and the patient is afebrile, the family is sent home to complete the course of antibiotic therapy. Once the parents have learned these techniques, they can be applied in the future if similar problems occur.

If no focus of infection is found, a white blood cell count is taken. If it is elevated or has a shift to the left with increased numbers of band forms, antibiotic coverage may be started to treat the suspected infection in the catheter.

Since the most common organisms belong to either *Staphylococcus aureus* or *Staphylococcus epidermidis*, amoxicillin or vancomycin should be started.

If sensitivity to these agents becomes apparent, different, more appropriate antibiotics can be given at that time.

Patients who have catheters infected with the *Staphylococcus* organism usually can be effectively treated by a four- to six-week course of antibiotics. Fungal and gram-negative infections cannot be treated by leaving the catheter in place; it must be removed in this case. A new central venous catheter may be replaced after the patient has been afebrile for 72 hours and the blood cultures do not grow the offending organism.

Catheter Occlusion

Occlusion of the central venous catheter is another problem that has potentially serious consequences.[10, 11, 13, 14] Occlusion usually happens because of inadequate flushing of the catheter with heparin and saline or because of increased thrombogenicity of the patient's blood, or both. Catheter occlusion is uncommon if the catheters are properly cared for and are flushed on a daily basis. If the patient observes that the catheter is becoming increasingly difficult to infuse, we usually check this personally by flushing the catheter or injecting it with a radiopaque dye to determine if clots have formed at its end. If this is verified and the catheter is not completely occluded, we fill it with a solution of urokinase, typically using a solution that contains 2500 units/ml and diluting it to 2 ml or the volume of the catheter with saline. The catheter is flushed and capped and is allowed to remain closed for a period of one hour. At the end of that time the urokinase solution is aspirated back and then the catheter is flushed with a heparin and saline solution and is tested for its patency.

If it again proves difficult to infuse or injection studies continue to show persistence of the clot, we repeat the procedure a second time. As a rule, if the clots fail to break up after the second one-hour period of filling with urokinase, we allow the catheter to remain filled with the urokinase solution for 24 hours. If this fails to clear the catheter it must be removed. Once a catheter becomes totally occluded and cannot be filled, it is unlikely that declotting can be accomplished.

Other Problems

Electrolyte imbalances are uncommon in patients on parenteral nutrition, because the electrolyte needs of the patients are determined prior to discharge from the hospital. Unless there is some major clinical change in the patient to alter the electrolyte losses, patients seldom have any alteration in this nutritional need. We monitor these patients as indicated earlier in this chapter in order to ensure that changes and losses have not occurred.

Hypoglycemia is one of the more common problems that develop in patients on long-term parenteral nutrition. Carnitine deficiency is likely to develop in infants and children, especially in those who have very short small intestines and are virtually dependent on parenteral support for almost all their nutrition. Carnitine is an amino acid by-product that is necessary intracellularly for the transport of fatty acids to the mitochondria for the generation of energy bonds. If patients become deficient in carnitine, difficulties with glucose instability often develop and they become hypoglycemic. This deficit can only be corrected by giving the patients intravenous or oral carnitine.

Any patient with unexplained hypoglycemia during or following infusion of a TPN solution should be tested. If one does not find evidence of carnitine deficiency, it is possible that the patient may be releasing more insulin than is required. Hypoglycemia may be avoided in these patients by lengthening the tapering infusion time of the parenteral nutrition solutions.

Hyperglycemia is uncommon. It is particularly unusual in the pediatric age group. Sepsis or some other major change in the patient's condition should be suspected when patients on long-term TPN who are glucose-tolerant suddenly develop hyperglycemia and glycosuria. We have rarely added insulin to the parenteral nutrition solutions of pediatric patients. On the rare occasions when this has been necessary, we typically provide one unit of insulin for every 10 gm of dextrose. Half of this adheres to the plastic container in which the solutions are administered or in the tubing. Additional insulin or glucose, or both, can be provided when necessary.

Gastroesophageal reflux is a common problem in patients who have extremely short small intestines and are on home par-enteral nutrition. It typically develops because of a delay in gastric emptying that results from the administration of the TPN solution. Patients secrete gastric acid in response to the amino acid load administered. The intravenous fat emulsion also contributes to the problem by its effect in delaying gastric emptying. If a patient has a problem with vomiting or night-time awakening with irritability, we typically add cimetidine to the TPN solution. We provide a dose of 10 to 15 mg/kg to be administered with the parenteral nutrition solution.

Cholelithiasis is an uncommon occurrence in pediatric patients. It has been reported in as few as 1 case in 16,000 infants and children who have come to autopsy.[15, 16] In patients on home parenteral nutrition who have received parenteral support for three months or more, the incidence is more than 40 per cent. We believe cholelithiasis develops for a variety of reasons, for example, (1) lack of stimulation of the bile flow from the liver and the gallbladder, (2) decreased availability of bile salts for solubilization of cholesterol, and (3) lack of gallbladder contractility. Any pediatric patient on home parenteral nutrition who has unexplained upper abdominal pain, with or without vomiting and fever, should be suspected of having cholecystitis or acalculous cholecystitis.

These patients typically have white blood cell counts that are elevated or have a shift to the left with a normal count, or both. The liver function tests typically become acutely altered and the patient may become jaundiced if the stone is passed down the common duct and obstructs the ampulla.

Acalculous cholecystitis is another complication that can occur and that we believe is secondary to stasis itself.

CHRONIC LIVER DISEASE

Chronic liver disease in patients on long-term TPN appears to correlate with the early onset of parenteral nutrition administration in immature or premature infants who have minimal enteral feeding.

In the earlier years of our home parenteral nutrition program, we saw the problem only in infants who were started on parenteral nutrition from the time of birth.[17] None of the children we started on parenteral support after six months of age have developed chronic liver disease. Some of the infants who have developed this condition might have problems secondary to aluminum toxicity. Aluminum was a contaminant of the casein hydrolysate solutions that at one time were used for home parenteral nutrition. In recent years, liver disease has been much less frequent in patients receiving long-term parenteral support.

Trace Metal Deficiency

Trace metal deficiencies in patients on home parenteral nutrition should not occur commonly provided that patients are supplemented with appropriate amounts of copper, zinc, chromium, selenium, and possibly molybdenum.

We saw zinc deficiency in only one pediatric patient early in the history of our home parenteral nutrition program.[9] In that patient, losses from the gastrointestinal tract were not taken into consideration when the individual's home parenteral nutrition solutions were formulated. Physicians must be aware that extra zinc must be provided in patients who have a large volume of diarrhea or ostomy output.

Copper deficiency is highly uncommon and we have never recognized it in any patient.

Patients with selenium deficiency have primarily been described as having cardiac arrhythmias and heart failure. We have seen patients with selenium deficiency who presented with pure cerebellar ataxia, having loss of motor strength and decreased mental capacity. Findings such as this have not been described before. This patient had no recognizable heart lesion. Other patients we have seen with documented low levels of selenium and chromium have not shown any evidence of heart disease or obvious neurologic disease.

Vitamin deficiency has never been apparent in any of our patients on home parenteral nutrition. It is exceedingly uncommon and should not occur provided that full and appropriate supplementation is given. It is important that when the patient adds the vitamins to the TPN solution it is done just before administration to minimize losses while the solution hangs and sufficient volume of vitamins is given to provide appropriate dosage.

DEVELOPMENTAL DELAY AND SOCIAL PROBLEMS

Most patients on home TPN programs that start in early infancy may develop more slowly because of their prolonged hospitalization prior to discharge. However, if patients are promptly discharged from the hospital and are successfully managed at home without rehospitalization, the best chance for developing in a completely normal fashion is provided. The more that patients are rehospitalized for complications, the greater the risk that their development will be slowed by being taken out of the home environment.

In general, when our patients have been tested by standard developmental tests for infants and children, they have shown normal or near-normal intelligence and motor function.[18] We have had only two patients with severe brain damage on our home parenteral nutrition program. One was an infant with a midline facial cleft defect and a dysmorphic brain. The second was a patient born to a diabetic mother who suffered severe hypoglycemic insult in the neonatal period.

DIAGNOSES OF 85 PEDIATRIC PATIENTS ON THE HOME TPN PROGRAM

Of all the patients aged 18 years and younger in our home TPN program, those with short-bowel syndrome, Crohn's disease, and pseudo-obstruction syndrome make up the largest group. Nearly 27 per cent of our patients fit into the category of short-bowel syndrome. They have varied from those who had only a duodenum connected to the transverse colon to those who have had limited small-intestine resections.

Of the 18 patients with Crohn's disease, one third were placed on home parenteral nutrition because of growth failure.[14] Others in this group were referred because of intractable disease, enterocutaneous fistula, perianal fistula and ulcers, and diffuse disease that was unresponsive to medical therapy and was unresectable.

One third of this group of patients gained a remission for more than one year following four months of parenteral nutrition therapy. All those who had not entered puberty or had a delayed bone age of two or more years had an acceleration of height and catchup growth. All gained weight at normal or accelerated levels. This occurred in some despite the persistence of active disease. All patients were provided with 60 to 80 calories/kg/day. The bowel rest provided by the parenteral nutrition did not result in the reversal of any chronic obstruction from the disease.

Eight patients have had intestinal pseudo-obstruction syndrome. All but one had onset of disease early in infancy, during the first week of life. All but two have had improvement in digestion and absorption with the passage of time. Two youngsters who had no ileostomy output from birth to six months of age spontaneously began to flow. These patients and several others have ultimately been able to gain the majority or near-majority of their nutrition enterally and they need parenteral support only as a supplement. None of the patients with pseudo-obstruction syndrome, however, have been able to discontinue the parenteral support. We have learned from this group of patients that if the protein and amino acids are withdrawn for more than 48 hours, ileus develops.

Intractable diarrhea of infancy, probably secondary to protein intolerance, was treated in four patients. All these patients ultimately had healing of the intestinal mucosa and were returned to elemental enteral formulas.

Surprisingly, we have had three patients with intestinal lymphangiectasia who were unresponsive to dietary management. At one time we thought that patients with intestinal lymphangiectasia could be managed by a low-fat diet that was high in medium-chain triglycerides. We have subsequently learned that some patients with this condition are not manageable by dietary measures. Although TPN did allow such patients to gain weight and grow, it did not result in a major reduction in their ascites. Although TPN allows alternative care in this type of patient, it is still not the optimal one.

Patients with cystic fibrosis receive parenteral support as well as antibiotics at home through their central venous catheters. They pose special problems in management. Patients with cystic fibrosis require more concentrated solutions of dextrose and protein because they typically do not tolerate the standard volumes administered to such patients. Because of cor pulmonale, they would go into congestive failure if administered normal volumes of fluid. It might benefit patients with cystic fibrosis to start parenteral support earlier, but there is a reluctance to do this on the part of many physicians. The longevity of these patients might be improved if TPN is started sooner.

Some patients with carcinoma of the stomach were managed with home parenteral nutrition because there was obstruction of the intestinal tract by tumors. Attempts were made to provide these patients with experimental chemotherapy, but these attempts were unsuccessful and the patients died. Patients with immune-deficiency disorders seem to be managed without an increased incidence of infections from contamination of the catheter. Patients with immune-deficiency disease typically require a more sterile technique in order to ensure that the risk of infection is not increased.

One of our patients with selective IgA deficiency and intractable diarrhea with severe mucosal damage had complete reversal of his lesion within six months. Of the patients with familial and nonfamilial congenital failure of the villi, there was no improvement in absorptive function over time. This was despite attempts to stimulate development of the villi with feeding or drugs, or both.

A limited number of patients with dysautonomia were started on home TPN. Because of malnutrition, we could not see any long-term benefit in these particular patients. One patient with congenital stenosis of the superior mesenteric artery benefitted from long-term parenteral support by developing bowel adaptation following a period of intestinal ischemia. He was on parenteral support for nearly two years before adaptation took place.

Typically, we do not recommend the use of home parenteral nutrition for patients with anorexia nervosa unless they are carefully supervised. Patients who are sufficiently debilitated from this disease and cannot feed themselves may require tube feeding or hospitalization.

We supported one unique patient who had a hyper-IgE syndrome with more than 7000 IU of IgE/ml of blood. This particular patient had total rejection and sloughing of his intestinal tract following challenges with whole proteins. He never had sufficient healing of his intestinal tract to discontinue parenteral nutrition.

Duration of Time on TPN and Survival

Of the 85 pediatric patients who received TPN in our program during the past decade, 35 have received it for more than two years, 11 have received it for more than five years, and 2 have received it for more than eight years.

During the past decade, 15 of our patients have died from infection. Eleven of these infections have been either bacterial or fungal, and four infections have been viral. *Staphylococcus aureus* or *S. epidermidis* have been the most common organisms. Gram-negative infections have not been common. *Candida* was the cause of death in one patient. Cytomegalovirus was the presumed cause of death in four patients who were either immunocompetent or severely compromised secondary to radiation and drug therapy. Aspiration pneumonia and occlusion of the trachea occurred in one patient with a tracheoesophageal fistula who developed a stenosis of the esophagus and aspirated secretions into her lungs. This patient had severe brain damage. Fluid overload occurred in one patient whose mother used four times the solutions recommended in a matter of four hours. Cancer was the cause of death in two patients and one patient succumbed to leukemia. One patient died an accidental death when his spleen ruptured after playing. One patient died of a pneumococcal pneumonia. He had had a splenectomy but had also received Pneumovax (a pneumococcal vaccine). Nursing error in the hospital was the cause of death in one patient when her parenteral fluids were administered intrajejunally rather than intravenously. This patient developed severe dehydration. Liver failure was a contributing factor to death in eight patients. Of those patients who died, eight had short-bowel syndrome, three had adenocarcinoma of the stomach, two had combined immune deficiency, two had intestinal lymphangiectasia, two had congenital failure of the development of villi, one had pseudo-obstruction syndrome, and another had mucocutaneous candidiasis. One patient with cystic fibrosis died from chronic pulmonary insufficiency. A patient with hyper-IgE syndrome and severely damaged intestinal mucosa died from chronic lung disease. One patient with ulcerative colitis and short-bowel syndrome died secondary to a gram-negative infection.

The average patient on parenteral nutrition had one occlusion, breakage, or cutting of the catheter/550 days. Infections occurred at a rate of 1/1800 days of home TPN.

We believe home parenteral nutrition can be a life-saving technique in infants and children who require it. The technique can be carried out safely. This is shown by two of our patients on TPN for longer than six years who never became infected and never had serious catheter complications.

All school-aged children on our program attend school full time, and preschoolers attend school after the age of four years.

There have been no divorces among our parents, but there was one separation. Several mothers have become pregnant one or more times despite having a child on a home TPN program.

It is too early to say whether this group of infants and children will have special problems at school, though we have had youngsters who do superior work as well as children who have failed in school. Two youngsters who started home TPN as teenagers have completed high school and college and have overcome the problems of coping with the need to do nightly home TPN.

REFERENCES

1. Scribner, B. H., Cole, J. J., and Christopher, T. G.: Long-term total parenteral nutrition. J.A.M.A., *212*:457, 1970.
2. Jeejeebhoy, K. N., Zohrab, W. J., Langer, B. et al.: Total parenteral nutrition at home for 23 months without complications and with good rehabilitation. A study of technical and metabolic features. Gastroenterology, *65*:811, 1973.
3. Solassol, C., Joyeux, H., Etco, L., et al.: New techniques for long-term intravenous feeding and artificial gut in 75 patients. Ann. Surg., *179*:519, 1974.
4. Steiger, E.: Home parenteral nutrition. ASPEN Update, *3*(4):1, 1981.
5. Fleming, C. R.: Home parenteral nutrition. Mayo Clin. Proc., *56*:132, 1981.
6. Steiger, E. (ed.): Home Parenteral Nutrition. New York, Pro Clinica, 1981.
7. Byrne, W. J., Ament, M. E., Burke, M. et al.: Home parenteral nutrition. Surg. Gynecol. Obstet., *149*:593, 1979.
8. Goldberger, J. H., DeLuca, F. G., Wesselhoeft, C. W., et al.: A home program of long-term total parenteral nutrition in children. J. Pediatr., *94*:325, 1979.
9. Strobel, C. T., Byrne, W. J., Fonkalsrud, E. W., et al.: Home parenteral nutrition: Results in 34 pediatric patients. Ann. Surg., *188*:394, 1978.
10. Maksimak, M., Ament, M. E., and Fonkalsrud, E. W.: Comparison of the pediatric Silastic catheter

with a standard No. 3. French silastic catheter from central venous alimentation. J. Pediatr. Gastroenterol. Nutr., *1*(2):227, 1982.

11. Byrne, W. J., Burke, M., Fonkalsrud, E. W., et al.: Home parenteral nutrition: An alternative approach to the management of complicated gastrointestinal fistulas not responding to conventional medical or surgical therapy. J.P.E.N., *3*:355, 1979.

12. Ament, M. E.: Home parenteral nutrition in infants and children. Course in Intravenous Nutrition in the Pediatric Patient. San Francisco, Letterman Army Medical Center, February 13, 1981, p. 326.

13. Cannon, R. A., Byrne, W. J., Ament, M. E., et al.: Home parenteral nutrition in infants. J. Pediatr., *96*:1098, 1980.

14. Strobel, C. T., Byrne, W. J., and Ament, M. E.: Home parenteral nutrition in children with Crohn's disease: An effective management alternative. Gastroenterology, *77*:272, 1979.

15. Pitt, H. A., King, W., Mann, L. L., Roslyn, J. J., Berquist, W. E., and Ament, M. E.: Prolonged parenteral nutrition increases the risk of cholelithiasis. Am. J. Surg., *145*:106, 1983.

16. Roslyn, J. J., Berquist, W. E., Pitt, H. A., Mann, L. L., Kangaloo, H., Denbesten, L., and Ament, M. E.: Increasing risk of gallstones in children receiving total parenteral nutrition. Pediatrics, *71*:784, 1983.

17. Kibort, P. M., Ulich, T. R., Berquist, W. E., et al.: Hepatic fibrosis and cirrhosis in children on long-term parenteral nutrition. Clin. Res., *30*:115A, 1982.

18. Ament, M. E., and O'Connor, M. J.: Long-term cognitive development of children on home total parenteral nutrition. Pediatr. Res., *18*(4):100A, 1984.

Index

Note: Page numbers in *italics* refer to illustrations; page numbers followed by t refer to tables.